VOLUME
TWO

Diagnostic
Cytology
and Its Histopathologic Bases

VOLUME
TWO

Diagnostic Cytology
and Its Histopathologic Bases

LEOPOLD G. KOSS, M.D.

Professor and Chairman, Department of Pathology,
Albert Einstein College of Medicine at Montefiore Hospital;
Chairman, Department of Pathology,
Montefiore Hospital and Medical Center
New York, New York

FOURTH EDITION

J.B. Lippincott Company   Philadelphia

Acquisitions Editor: Richard Winters
Sponsoring Editor: Elizabeth Orem
Project Editor: Tom Gibbons
Design Coordinator: Kathy Kelley-Luedtke
Cover Designer: Patti Maddaloni
Production Manager: Helen Ewan
Production Coordinator: Nannette Winski
Compositor: Digitype
Printer/Binder: Arcata Graphics/Halliday
Color Insert Printer: Princeton Polychrome

Fourth Edition

Library of Congress Cataloging in Publications Data

Koss, Leopold G.
    Koss's diagnostic cytology and its histopathologic bases /
Leopold G. Koss.—4th ed.
        p. cm.
    Rev. ed. of: Diagnostic cytology and its histopathologic
bases.
    3rd ed. c1979.
    Includes bibliographical references and index.
    ISBN 0-397-51049-7 (set).—ISBN 0-397-51223-6 (v. 1).
—ISBN 0-397-51222-8 (v. 2)
    1. Diagnosis, Cytologic.   2. Histology, Pathological.   I.
Koss, Leopold G. Diagnostic cytology and its histopathologic
bases.
    II. Title. III. Title: Diagnostic cytology and its histopathologic
bases.
    [DNLM: 1. Cytodiagnosis.   2. Neoplasms—
diagnosis.   QY 95 K86d]
    RB43.K67 1992
    616.07′582—dc20
    DNLM/DLC
    for Library of Congress   91–31224
                                                                                CIP

The authors and publishers have exerted every effort to ensure
that drug selection and dosage set forth in this text are in
accord with current recommendations and practice at a time
of publication. However, in view of ongoing research, changes
in government regulations, and the constant flow of
information relating to drug therapy and drug reactions, the
reader is urged to check the package insert for each drug for
any change in indications and dosage and for added warnings
and precautions. This is particularly important when the
recommended agent is a new or infrequently employed drug.

To my teachers in science and to my teachers in humanities, and most of all to the memory of my parents and sister, Stephanie, who perished during the Holocaust.

L.G.K.

Contributors

Gunter F. Bahr, M.D.
Chapter 35, *Image Analysis*
Chairman Emeritus,
Department of Cellular Pathology,
Armed Forces Institute of Pathology;
Clinical Professor of Pathology Emeritus,
Georgetown University,
Washington, D.C.,
Research Professor of Anatomy and Clinical
Professor of Pathology, Emeritus,
Uniformed Services University of the Health
Sciences,
Bethesda, Maryland

Carol E. Bales, CT(ASCP), CT(IAC), CFIAC
Chapter 33, *Cytologic Techniques*
Former Teaching Supervisor, Cytology Division,
Department of Pathology,
Montefiore Medical Center,
Albert Einstein College of Medicine,
Bronx, New York

Peter H. Bartels, Ph.D.
Chapter 35, *Image Analysis*
Professor, Optical Science Center
University of Arizona,
Tucson, Arizona

Harvey Dytch, S.B.
Chapter 35, *Image Analysis*
Head, Image Analysis Laboratory,
Departments of Obstetrics and Gynecology and
Pathology,
Pritzker School of Medicine, University of
Chicago,
Chicago, Illinois

Grace R. Durfee, B.S., CT(ASCP)
Chapter 33, *Cytologic Techniques*
Former Chief Cytotechnologist,
Memorial Sloan-Kettering Cancer Center,
New York, New York

Cecilia M. Fenoglio-Preiser, M.D.
Chapter 34, *Immunocytochemistry*
MacKenzie Professor and Director,
Department of Pathology and Laboratory
Medicine,
University of Cincinnati Medical School,
Cincinnati, Ohio

Xiao Man Liang, M.D.
Appendix II to Chapter 34, *In Situ Hybridization*
Visiting Research Fellow,
Department of Pathology,
Montefiore Medical Center,
Bronx, New York

Margaret B. Listrom, M.D.
Chapter 34, *Immunocytochemistry*
Former Chief, Cytopathology,
Veterans Administration Medical Center,
Associate Professor of Pathology,
University of New Mexico School of Medicine,
Albuquerque, New Mexico
Currently Associate Pathologist
Clinical Pathology Laboratories, Inc.,
Austin, Texas

Myron R. Melamed, M.D.
Chapter 30, *Circulating Cancer Cells*
Professor and Chairman,
Department of Pathology,
New York Medical College,
Valhalla, New York

Avery Sandberg, M.D., D.Sc. (Hon.)
Chapter 6, *The Chromosomes and the
Cell Cycle*; Chapter 7, *Cytogenetics of
Human Neoplasia*
Director,
The Cancer Center of the Southwest Biomedical
   Research Institute,
Scottsdale, Arizona

Rosemary Wieczorek, M.D.
Appendix II to Chapter 34, *In Situ Hybridization*
Former Assistant Professor of Pathology,
Montefiore Medical Center,
Albert Einstein College of Medicine;
Currently Assistant Professor of Pathology,
New York University Medical School,
New York, New York

George L. Wied, M.D.
Chapter 31, *Automated Cytology*
Professor Emeritus of Pathology and
   Blum-Riese Professor of Obstetrics
   and Gynecology,
Pritzker School of Medicine,
University of Chicago,
Chicago, Illinois

Josef Zajicek, M.D.
Chapter 29, *Aspiration Biopsy*
The late Chief, Cytology Division,
Department of Pathology,
Radiumhemmet, Karolinska Institute,
Stockholm, Sweden

Preface to the Fourth Edition

Nearly 12 years have elapsed since the publication of the third edition of this book. During this time period many changes have occurred; diagnostic cytology has been recognized as an important component of pathology. Since 1989 the American Board of Pathology has offered a speciality examination in this discipline and, I am happy to say, several hundred American pathologists have availed themselves of the opportunity to document their expertise in this field.

Although the status of diagnostic cytology in countries other than the United States and Canada has, as yet, not been crystallized, the trend is clear: increasingly, the regulatory agencies insist on a thorough education in this field before allowing practice privileges to the interested physicians.

Therefore the purpose of this book has remained unchanged since its first publication in 1961 — to assist the interested reader in gaining an understanding of the cellular manifestations of diseases, compared with their histologic patterns.

The decade of the 1980s brought a great many other changes. From the scientific point of view, there has been an increasing interest in measuring cell components, not only those visible under the light microscope in conventionally stained preparations, but also those that can be revealed by molecular biologic and immunologic techniques. It is for this reason that new chapters on principles of molecular biology, immunocytochemistry, image analysis, and flow cytometry have been written. Progress in cytogenetics of human tumors is re-flected in the completely rewritten chapters on this topic.

In reference to diagnostic cytology, major textual changes have been introduced throughout this edition. The observations on the role of human papillomaviruses in neoplastic events in the female genital tract have been newly summarized. Consequently, a major reorgnization of this part of the book was required. In reference to other organs and organ systems, every attempt has been made to update this book through 1991. In view of the increasing importance of aspiration biopsy as a diagnostic technique, the chapter on this subject has been totally restructured and nearly tripled in size.

As a consequence of these changes, some 3,000 new references have been added and integrated into the bibliographies at the end of each chapter.

This book has grown to a substantial size. The choices were few — either to omit information of possible value and reduce this book to the size of a handy laboratory manual, or to make every effort for this book to remain an authoritative source of references and information for some years to come. The author, with the help of several colleagues listed as contributors, elected the second path.

The task was quite significant, and it can only be hoped that the product of this labor will meet with the needs and approval of its readers.

LEOPOLD G. KOSS, M.D.
New York, December 1991

Contents

Part Two   Diagnostic Cytology of Organs

Diagnostic Cytology

and Its Histopathologic Bases

22

The Urinary Tract in the Absence of Cancer

ANATOMY

The urinary tract is composed of the kidneys, the ureters, the urinary bladder, and the urethra. The structure of the kidney is extremely complex and, since it has but little bearing on the cytology of the urinary tract, it will not be described here. However, tumors of renal origin that may exfoliate into the urinary tract will be dealt with briefly in Chapter 23. Aspiration biopsy of renal tumors is described in Chapter 29. The urine excreted by the kidneys is channeled through the renal pelvis into the ureters. In their course toward the bladder, the ureters cross the pelvic brim and enter the pelvis (Fig. 22–1).

In the female the ureters pass near the lowest segment of the uterus to reach the bladder. This relationship is especially important, because cancers of the cervix extending into the pelvis may readily surround and damage the ureters. The bladder is a balloon-shaped organ provided with an extremely elastic muscular wall that allows expansion while accumulating urine and collapse with voiding. A vestigial organ, the urachus, connects the bladder with the umbilicus. The embryologic derivation of the bladder is from the anterior portion of the cloaca, hence, the terminal portion of the embryonal intestinal tract. This origin accounts for the variety of epithelial types that may occur in the bladder (see below).

The basal portion of the urinary bladder contains the trigone, a triangular area with the apex directed forward. The two ureters enter the bladder at the two posterior angles of the trigone. The urethra leaves the bladder at the apex of the trigone. In the female the trigone overlies the vesicovaginal septum and the vagina. In the male the immediately underlying organ is the prostate.

The female urethra has only a very short course and opens into the upper portion of the vestibule, somewhat behind and below the clitoris. In the male the urethra runs across the prostate and enters the penis. The anatomy of the prostate will be discussed in Chapter 23.

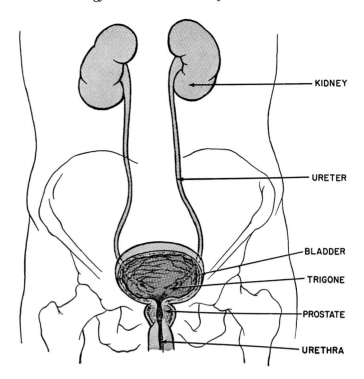

FIGURE 22–1. Diagram of the urinary tract in the male: frontal view. Compare with the diagram of the female genital tract in Fig. 8–1, which outlines the anatomic relationship of the lower urinary tract in the female.

HISTOLOGY AND ULTRASTRUCTURE OF THE UROTHELIUM (TRANSITIONAL EPITHELIUM)

The renal pelves, the ureters, the bladder, and the urethra are lined by a highly specialized type of epithelium that, because of its unique structure, should be referred to as the *urothelium*, but is often called by the traditional term—transitional epithelium.

The microscopic appearance of human urothelium is extremely characteristic. Normal urothelium is composed of no more than seven layers of cells, although the number of cell layers may appear smaller in dilated bladders. The deeper cell layers are made up of cuboidal cells with a single nucleus. The superficial cells of the urothelium are very large and often have multiple nuclei of variable sizes (Fig. 22–2). The superficial cells in the ureters often have a larger number of nuclei than similar cells in the bladder. Because each superfi-

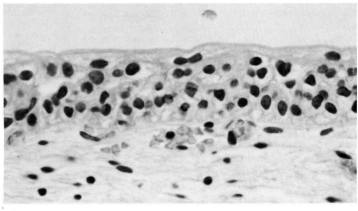

FIGURE 22–2. Normal human urothelium (transitional epithelium), moderately distended bladder. Note four to five layers of epithelial cells resting on a lamina propria provided with capillary vessels. The superficial cells (umbrella cells) are very large, sometimes multinucleated, and each stretches over several of the deeper epithelial layer. (×560)

cial cell covers several smaller cells of the underlying deeper layer, the term *umbrella cells* has been used to describe them. The umbrella cells in histologic sections vary in shape, according to the state of dilatation of the bladder. In the dilated bladder, they appear flat; in the contracted bladder they are more cuboidal. The schematic representation of the dilated and contracted mammalian urothelium is shown in Fig. 22–3.

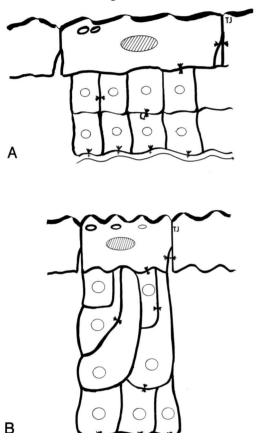

FIGURE 22–3. Diagrammatic representation of a dilated (*A*) and contracted (*B*) bladder urothelium to show the changes in cell configuration and the mechanism of cell movement. The superficial cells (umbrella cells) are shown lined by thick plaques of the asymmetric unit membrane, with intercalated segments of thin, symmetric membrane. The structure of the membrane can be compared with medieval armor in which flexible links between metal plates provided mobility for the bearer. Near the surface, the umbrella cells are linked by tight junctions (TJ). Abundant desmosomes bind the epithelial cells. Hemidesmosomes bind the epithelium to the lamina densa (LD). Note the difference in the configuration of the superficial cells in the dilated and contracted bladder. (Modified from Koss, L.G.: Some ultrastructural aspects of experimental and human carcinoma of the bladder. Cancer Res. *37*:2824–2835, 1977)

Cordon-Cardo et al. (1984) and Fradet et al. (1987) documented immunologic differences between deeper and superficial cells of the urothelium by means of monoclonal antibodies.

The lower urinary tract contains urine, which is a highly toxic excretion product of the kidney. Hence, there must be a barrier that prevents the penetration of the urine into the bloodstream. To some extent the superficial cells may constitute the first such barrier. Ultrastructural observations disclosed that the superficial cells of the urothelium in all mammals yet examined, including humans, are lined on their surface facing the bladder lumen by a unique membrane.

The membrane has two components: rigid, thick plaques and intervening segments of ordinary thin plasma membrane. The plaques, measuring about 13 nm in thickness, are composed of three layers: the two outer layers are electron opaque and of unequal thickness, the central layer is electron lucent. Because of the difference in thickness of the electron-opaque components, the membrane has been named *asymmetric unit membrane* (AUM). It is assumed that the plaques may play a role in the urine–blood barrier, whereas the intervening segments of ordinary plasma membrane act like hinges, providing flexibility to the plaques, thereby assuring that the umbrella cells can adapt to changing urinary volume requirements (see Fig. 22–3). There is some experimental evidence that the destruction of the superficial cells increases the permeability of the bladder to lithium ions (Hicks, 1966). Still, the urine–blood barrier remains in place, even in the absence of umbrella cells or if the asymmetric plaques are absent, as is common in older persons (Jacob et al., 1978). Hence, this function of the bladder must be also vested in other components of the epithelium, most likely the basement lamina.

The AUM is produced in the Golgi complex of the superficial cells and travels to the surface packaged into oblong vesicles (Fig. 22–4), as was documented several years ago (Hicks, 1966; Koss, 1969, 1977). The urothelium continues to receive much attention from molecular biologists because of its unique structure and properties. Most recently (1990), Yu et al. described a specific protein, named uroplakin, as a characteristic component of AUM.

Detailed description and discussions of urothelial ultrastructure and function may be found in the accounts by Hicks (1975) and Koss (1969, 1977).

Urothelial cells can be successfully cultured from the sediment of voided urine (Herz et al.,

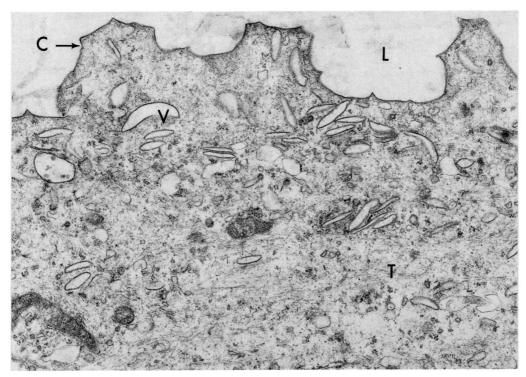

FIGURE 22–4.   Electron micrograph of a superficial cell of moderately dilated rat bladder. Note the characteristic oblong vesicles (V) lined by a rigid, asymmetric unit membrane, morphologically identical with segments of the cell membrane (C). L = lumen of bladder. Fine tonofilaments (T) are evident as well as a few round vesicles and mitochondria. (×20,400)

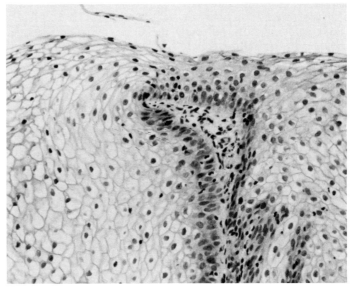

FIGURE 22–5.   Squamous epithelium of vaginal type in the trigone of an asymptomatic adult woman. (×250)

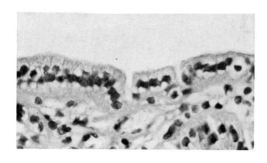

FIGURE 22–6.   Mucus-producing columnar epithelium lining the bladder. (×350)

1979). The AUM may persist in several generations of these cells (Shokri-Tabibzadeh et al., 1982).

Epithelial Variants in the Lower Urinary Tract

Squamous Epithelium of the Vaginal Type

The lower urinary tract may contain a significant admixture of epithelia of histologic types other than the urothelium. The trigone of the bladder in approximately 50% of normal adult women and in a small proportion of men contains areas of squamous epithelium of the vaginal type (Fig. 22–5). Although this is merely an anatomic variant of bladder epithelium, this condition has been recorded clinically as "urethrotrigonitis," "epidermidization" or "membranous trigonitis," although evidence of inflammation is usually absent. In women, this epithelium appears to be under hormonal control and is the most likely source of cells in urocytograms, described on p. 299.

Intestinal Type Epithelium

Areas of mucus-producing epithelium may also be noted, undoubtedly reflecting the origin of the bladder in the embryonal cloaca (Fig. 22–6).

Brunn's Nests and Cystitis Cystica

The urothelium of the bladder may form small, usually round, buds that extend into the lamina propria, occasionally to the level of the muscularis. These are the nests of von Brunn (Brunn's nests) that occur in approximately 80% of normal bladders. Within the center of Brunn's nests, formation of cysts, often lined by mucus-producing columnar epithelium, may be noted (Fig. 22–7). The cysts may become quite large and distended, with mucus giving rise to the so-called cystitis cystica or glandularis (Fig. 22–8). Glandlike cystic structures may also arise directly from the urothelium, without going through the stage of Brunn's nests. It is interesting that some foci in these structures may express the prostate-specific antigen (Nowels et al.). It is customary to consider Brunn's nests and cystitis cystica as an expression of abnormal urothelial proliferation, either caused by an inflammatory process or as an expression of a neoplastic potential. This most emphatically is not true. The studies by Morse (1928) and more recent studies by Wiener and Koss (1979) disclosed that such findings are common in normal bladders. Brunn's nests and cystitis cystica must be considered as mere anatomic variants of the urothelium. The frequency of these epithelial variants is summarized in Table 22–1.

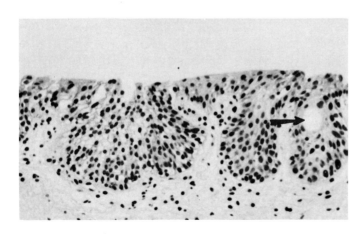

FIGURE 22–7.   Brunn's nests with an incipient cyst formation (*arrow*). (×250)

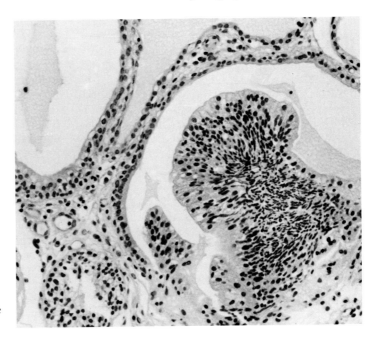

FIGURE 22–8. Cystitis glandularis (see text). (×250)

CYTOLOGY OF NORMAL URINE

Urine is an acellular liquid product of renal excretory function. As the liquid passes through the excretory renal tubules, renal pelvis, urether, bladder, and urethra, it picks up desquamating cells, derived from the epithelia of these organs. Thus, the main cellular components of normal voided urine are the renal tubular cells and the cells derived from the urothelium and its variants. The urine usually has a low acid pH and a high content of urea and other organic components; therefore, it is not isotonic. Consequently, the urine is not a hospitable medium for desquamated cells, which are often poorly preserved and sometimes difficult to assess on microscopic examination. Still, the

Table 22–1
Frequency of Epithelial Variants in 100 Consecutive Normal Bladders (61 Male, 39 Female; 8 Children and 92 Adults)

Total bladders with one or more lesions: 93

	Male	*Female*
Brunn's nests	53	36
Cystitis cystica	32	28
Vaginal metaplasia	3	19
None	6*	1*

*Two newborns: 1 male, 1 female. 5 males: 4 adults, 1, age 13.

voided urine is a very valuable diagnostic medium for the study of renal function (which is discussed in this book only when it produces cytologic abnormalities) and in the diagnosis of tumors of the lower urinary tract and, sometimes, the kidneys, as discussed in Chapter 23.

A number of direct sampling techniques have been developed to study the status of the urothelium. These are bladder washings or barbotage, cell collection by retrograde catheterization of the ureters and renal pelves, and direct brushings. All of these techniques result in major modifications in the normal population of urothelial cells and their variants, described below. The understanding of the complexities of the normal cell population under various clinical circumstances is an important first step for proper diagnostic utilization of cytology of the urinary tract. Knowledge of clinical circumstances and clinical procedures and their consequences may prevent major errors of interpretation, particularly in low-grade urothelial tumors.

Voided Urine

Processing

Voided urine is usually submitted for cytologic examination for the diagnosis of tumors or for monitoring patients with past histories of tumors. The sediment can be processed in a variety of ways: a *di-*

rect smear can be made on albumin-coated slides; the urine can be filtered using one of the commercially available filtering devices, either for direct viewing or for preparation of smears by placing the filtered cells on a glass slide (reverse filtration); or by cytocentrifugation, preferably using the method developed by Bales (1981) in our laboratory. For further details on processing, see Chapter 33. Unless the urine is processed without delay, the addition of a fixative is recommended. In our hands, the best fixative is 2% polyethylene glycol (Carbowax) solution in 70% ethanol.

Specimen Collection

Morning urine specimens have the advantage of highest cellularity, but also the disadvantage of marked cell degeneration. A specimen from the morning's second voiding is usually best. Three samples obtained on 3 consecutive days are diagnostically optimal (Koss et al., 1985). Hydration of patients has been recommended by some investigators as increasing the yield of desquamated urothelial cells.

Normal Urothelial Cells

Normal urothelial cells have several features that set them apart from other epithelial cells. The cells vary greatly in size: the superficial cells may be very large and multinucleated, but such cells are rarely seen in the absence of prior instrumentation (see below). The average superficial cell seen in voided urine is about the size of a large superficial squamous cell, as seen in the sputum or the vaginal smear. They are usually flat and polygonal and often show one flat or convex smooth surface, corresponding to the lumen of the bladder. It is not uncommon for such cells to have relatively large nuclei (Fig. 22–9A), probably the expression of increased amount of DNA (polyploidy). Smaller polygonal or round urothelial cells originating in the deeper layers of the urothelium, when fresh and well preserved, have finely granular nuclei (see Fig. 22–9B). Similar small cells in voided urine usually have pale nuclei (Fig. 22–10). On close inspection (Fig. 22–11) the fine granularity of the nuclear chromatin pattern is better demonstrated, as is the presence of single, round nucleoli. The latter are *normal*, even in superficial cells. Occasionally mitotic figures (see Fig. 22–11D) and columnar cells may be noted, but these are more common after instrumentation (see below).

A very important property of normal urothelium is its propensity to desquamate in fragments or clusters. Although this feature is markedly enhanced in urines obtained by bladder catheterization, lavage, or any type of instrumentation, urothelial cell clusters may also occur in spontaneously voided urine. Abdominal palpation, the slightest trauma, or inflammatory injury to the bladder may enhance the shedding of clusters. The clusters may be small and flat, composed of only a few clearly benign cells (see Figs. 22–10 and 22–11A), but they also may be substantial and composed of several hundred superimposed cells. The clusters may round up and appear to be of spherical, oval, or "papillary" configuration, but occasionally, they are distorted and may be thought to be derived from a low-grade papillary tumor (Fig. 22–12A). The distortion may be increased if frosted slides are used for preparation. On close inspection of the transparent segments of the cluster, the edge of the cluster is sharply demarcated, and the component cells of normal urothelium may be readily observed (see Fig. 22–12B). In our experience, at least 20% of normal voided

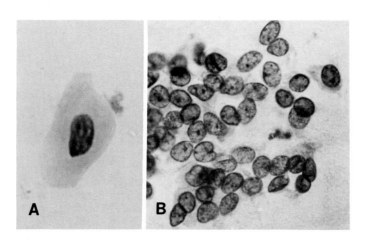

FIGURE 22–9. Urothelial cells from a normal urinary sediment. (*A*) Voided urine: large superficial urothelial cell. Note one smooth surface corresponding to the lumen of the bladder, and a large, granular nucleus. (*B*) Bladder washing: cluster of deeper epithelial cells with finely granular nuclei and tiny chromatin granules. The nucleus of the superficial cell shown in (*A*) is much larger than the nuclei shown in (*B*). This may reflect polyploidy of the large cell. (*A, B* ×560)

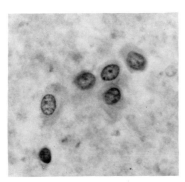

FIGURE 22–10. Poorly preserved urothelial cells in normal, spontaneously voided urine. (×560. Melamed, M.R., et al.: Cytohistological observations on developing carcinoma of the urinary bladder in man. Cancer, *13*:67–74, 1960)

urine sediments, especially if processed by filtration or cytocentrifuge, will display at least one, and often more, clusters of benign urothelial cells. *It is paramount in urinary cytology to avoid making the diagnosis of a papillary tumor based on this type of evidence.* For further discussion of cytology of bladder tumors, see Chapter 23.

In normal urine, the background is clean, free of leukocytes, and with only an occasional erythrocyte.

Normal, spontaneously voided urine from a

male patient contains very few urothelial cells. All but freshly desquamated cells may display a measure of degeneration. The occasional squamous cells of superficial type are of urethral origin. Sometimes, for reasons unknown, the squamous cells may be numerous. Schmid et al. observed periodic exfoliation of squamous and urothelial cells in the male, with cyclic variations ranging from 18 to 22 days, depending on age. The origin of the cells was probably in the male urethra. The dependence of the rhythmic exfoliation on gonadal function could not be documented.

In the *female* patient there may be considerable admixture of squamous cells of all types, which represent vaginal contamination and cells derived from the vaginal-type epithelium in the area of the trigone commonly observed in normal women (Fig. 22–13). The value of urinary sediment in estimating the hormonal status of the woman is discussed (urocytograms) in Chapter 9.

In the *newborn*, both boys and girls, the urinary sediment may contain a fairly large proportion of mature squamous cells, reflecting the effect of maternal hormones. It is likely that areas of vaginal-type epithelium may occur in the bladders of newborns of both sexes.

The use of other microscopic techniques, such as phase microscopy (de Voogt et al.), and the use of supravital stains (Sternheimer) in the assessment of urine cytology has been suggested.

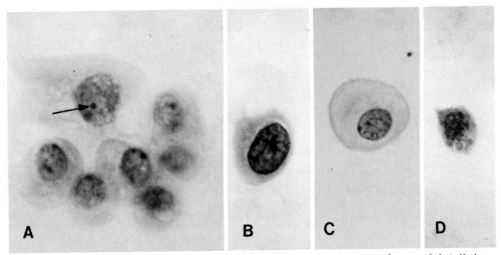

FIGURE 22–11. Benign urothelial cells in urinary sediment—higher magnification. (*A*) Cell cluster containing one large umbrella cell and several smaller cells from deeper epithelial layers. Note fine granularity of the nuclear chromatin and nucleoli (*arrow*). The nucleoli of this size are normal. (*B, C*) Variations in nuclear sizes and finely granular nuclear chromatin. In cell (*C*) note a sex chromatin body. Cell (*D*) shows a mitotic figure. (*A–D* ×1,000)

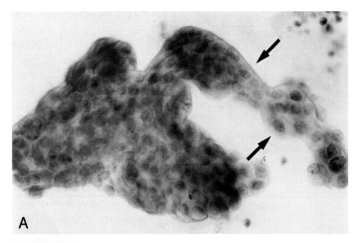

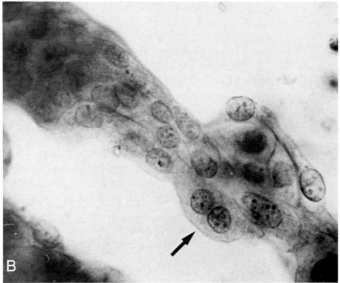

FIGURE 22–12. Voided urine, possibly after iatrogenic trauma to the bladder. There was no evidence of tumor. (*A*) A large thick cluster of urothelial cells of unusual shape, mimicking a frond of a papillary tumor. Note that the cluster has sharp edges (*arrows*), suggestive of origin in surface epithelium. (*B*) Higher-powered view of the transparent part of the large cluster again shows a sharp edge. A binucleated umbrella cell is evident (*arrow*). The nuclei of the component cells show the normal fine granulation of chromatin and one or two chromocenters or nucleoli. (*A* ×350; *B* ×1,000)

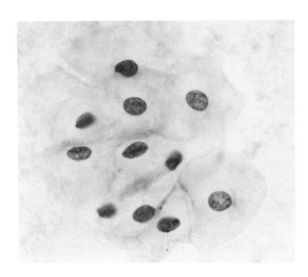

FIGURE 22–13. Urinary sediment, normal female. Cluster of intermediate squamous cells. (×1,000)

Urine Obtained by Catheterization, Bladder Washings (Barbotage), and Instrumentation

Catheterized Urine

Catheterized bladder urine is often rich in desquamated cells, which may appear singly or in clusters. Single cells may vary enormously in size and configuration (Fig. 22–14). Next to large polyhedral superficial urothelial cells, which may be bi- or multinucleated, smaller elongated cells may be noted. The latter may be columnar with a single cytoplasmic process at the end, reminiscent of origin in columnar epithelium (see Fig. 22–14A). Harris et al. noted ciliated columnar cells in bladder washings. Urothelial cells in clusters may display cell-to-cell attachments (see Fig. 22–14B,C), and there may be some, however slight, superposition of cells.

Urine obtained by retrograde catheterization, hence, of ureteral and renal pelvic origin, is charac-

terized by a large number of exfoliated urothelial cells occurring singly and in large clusters and by a marked variety of cell types. The single cells may be round, oval, spindly, columnar, or polyhedral. (Fig. 22–15 and see Fig. 22–18B). The cytoplasm of such cells is clear and may contain fat (Masin and Masin, 1976). The nuclei are of normal size, round or oval, sometimes double, with a finely granular chromatin pattern. Nucleoli are very uncommon. Occasionally, ciliated cells may be noted.

The clusters may be numerous and sometimes several dozen of them may be observed in a single specimen. The origin of the clusters has been traced to areas of ureteral epithelium scraped by the tip of the catheter, leaving large segments of the ureter completely denuded (see Plate 22–1). On closer analysis of such clusters the component cells of normal urothelium are readily observed (Fig. 22–16). The superficial urothelial cells in clusters are characterized by sharply demarcated surfaces, large and variable sizes, clear cytoplasm, and con-

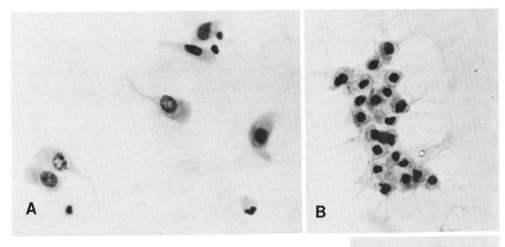
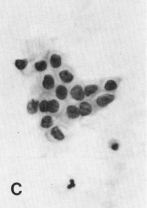

FIGURE 22–14. Urothelial cells in catheterized bladder urine. (*A*) Single cells of bladder origin may often display columnar configuration with long processes. (*B, C*) Clusters show cytoplasmic processes, remnants of cell-to-cell attachments. (*A, B, C* ×560. *B*: Melamed, M.R., et al.: Cytohistological observations on developing carcinoma of the urinary bladder in man. Cancer, *13*:67–74, 1960)

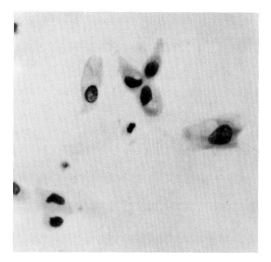

FIGURE 22–15.   Catheterized ureteral specimen. Note the variations in cell shape and slight nuclear hyperchromasia. A columnar cell (*top, left*) is shown. (×560)

siderable variability in nuclear sizes. A slight nuclear hyperchromasia may be observed (see Fig. 22–16*A*). Cells from the deeper layers of the urothelium are smaller and show less variability in nuclear sizes and generally less hyperchromasia (see Fig. 22–16*B,C*). Perhaps the most striking cell component is the multinucleated umbrella cell (Figs. 22–17, 22–18*A*). These cells may vary in size from 10 to 40 μm or more and may contain from 2 to 50 or more nuclei of variable sizes. The nuclei may appear unduly large and may contain specks of chromatin or prominent chromocenters readily visible against the pale background. The nuclear membrane is often prominent. Occasionally, the nuclei in the large superficial cells are clumped and degenerated, and they may impress one as malignant, were it not for the general configuration of the cell (Fig. 22–19).

The large multinucleated cells are normal superficial umbrella cells of the urothelium, described above. Such cells may be derived from the urothelium of the bladder. However, they appear to be particularly large and may contain a very large number of nuclei when derived from the urothelium of the ureters. The reason for this is not definitely known, but this finding may reflect a relatively low epithelial turnover in the ureters, resulting in formation of larger and perhaps older superficial epithelial cells, with more numerous nuclei.

The presence of the large nuclei reflects the tendency of the urothelium to form tetraploid or even octaploid nuclei (Levi et al., Farsund). This tendency to polyploidy appears to be part and parcel of the pattern of normal urothelial differentiation. The nuclear enlargement resulting therefrom is more evident in specimens obtained by means of catheterization or after instrumentation and is not nearly as noticeable in spontaneously voided specimens. Although the nuclei may appear large and may vary in size, they usually have the "salt-and-pepper" speckled appearance of granules of chromatin distributed against a clear background that affords their easy identification as benign (see Fig. 22–18).

Bladder Washings (Barbotage)

The procedure has been introduced on a large scale for purposes of DNA analysis by flow cytometry in bladder cancer (see p. 989). It consists of instilling 50 to 100 ml of saline or Ringer's solution and aspirating and reinjecting it several times. The procedure is performed during cytoscopy or through a catheter.

In the absence of cancer, the specimens offer an excellent panorama of the component cells of the urothelium (Fig. 22–20). A broad variety of superficial umbrella cells and deeper urothelial cells may be seen. Cell clusters are common and may be numerous.

Brushings of Ureters and Renal Pelves

The brushing procedure is occasionally used in the investigation of space-occupying lesions in the ureters or renal pelves. Most common application of the procedure is in the differential diagnosis between a stone and tumor. The samples, usually prepared as smears by the urologist, are rarely of any value. If the brush is placed in a fixative and forwarded for processing to the cytology laboratory, better samples can be obtained. In the absence of cancer, the cytologic findings are very similar to those described for retrograde catheterization. The principal pitfall is the diagnosis of a tumor based on the presence of numerous clusters of benign urothelial cells of various sizes with prominent chromocenters (see Plate 22–1).

It is a safe rule in diagnostic cytology of the urinary tract that in the absence of a markedly altered nucleocytoplasmic ratio and changed nuclear texture (see p. 948), one should not attempt to establish the diagnosis of a malignant tumor. This is particularly important with specimens obtained by brushing, retrograde catheterization or immediately thereafter, after instrumentation such as cystoscopy, or in bladder washings obtained under

Color Plate 22 – 1

Plate 22–1. Benign urothelial cells. (*A*, and *B*) Bladder washings or barbotage: (*A*) Note the two populations of cells: the large umbrella cells and clusters of small cells from the deeper layers of the urothelium. (*B*) Cluster of small urothelial cells. Note the presence of prominent chromocenters. (*C*, *D*, *E*, *F*) Urethral and renal pelvic brushings in the absence of disease. (*C*, *D*, *E*) Various aspects of the smears, showing a mixture of umbrella cells and of deeper, small urothelial cells arranged in papillary clusters. Note the presence of prominent chromocenters, particularly in (*C*) and (*E*). A false diagnosis of papillary urothelial carcinoma was made on this preparation. (*F*) The appearance of the ureter stripped of its epithelial lining, with early regeneration in a crypt. This was interpreted as "dysplasia." (*H*) Other benign papillary clusters of urothelium obtained by retrograde brushings. There was no evidence of tumor in either patient. Both clusters reflect perfectly benign urothelium. (*G*) Slightly overstained and shows uniform, darker nuclei; (*H*) shows prominent chromocenters mimicking enlarged nucleoli. (Original magnification *A–E, G, H* ×160; *F* ×40; enlarged × 2)

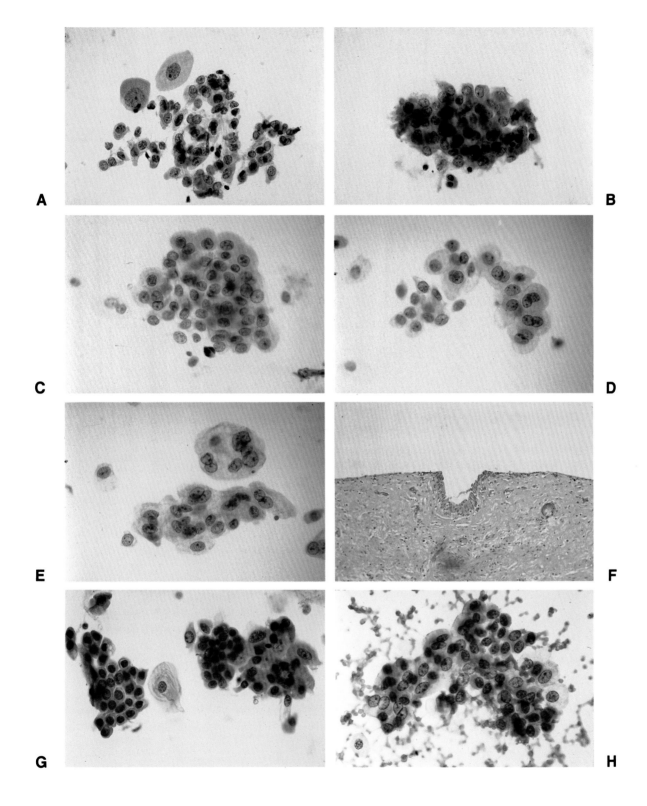

A

B

C

D

E

F

G

H

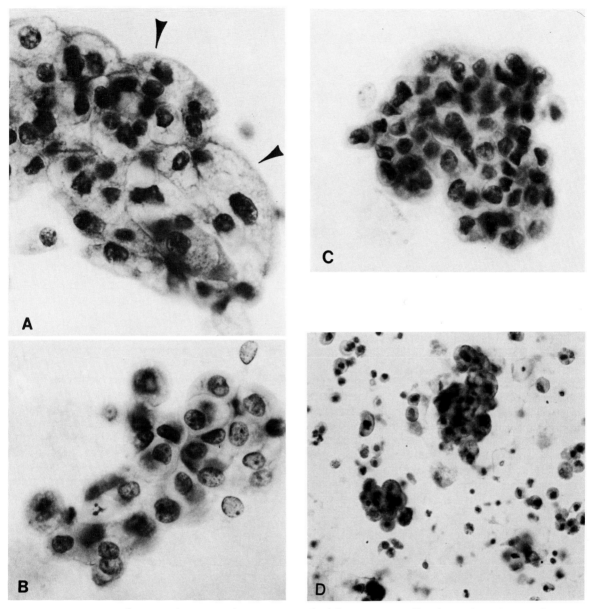

FIGURE 22–16. Normal urinary sediment: retrograde catheterization and brushing. Three clusters of urothelial cells found side-by-side on the same smear. Cluster (*A*) shows a smooth surface (*arrowheads*) suggestive of origin from the epithelial surface. Note the characteristic clear cytoplasm, the variability of nuclear sizes, and some hyperchromasia. (*B*) Cluster of smaller urothelial cells. Note transparent nuclei and small nucleoli. (*C*) Cluster of still smaller urothelial cells. The nuclear sizes in clusters (*B*) and (*C*) are approximately the same. (*D*) Renal brushing: there was no evidence of disease. Note the numerous thick clusters and single urothelial cells. (*A, B, C* ×560; *D* ×350)

cystoscopic control. The enormous morphologic variability of the normal cellular components of urothelial derivation and the presence of prominent chromocenters mimicking large nucleoli must be recognized and mastered before any attempt at diagnosis of cancer is made.

Cytologic Expressions of Epithelial Variants

It has been pointed out on p. 893 that several epithelial variants may occur in bladder epithelium. There are no specific cytologic findings corre-

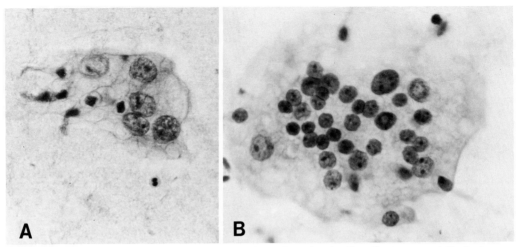

FIGURE 22–17. Catheterized ureteral urine: multinucleated umbrella cell. Note especially the large nuclei and prominent chromocenters in (*A*). Also note the variability of the nuclear sizes (*B*). (*A*, *B* ×560)

sponding to Brunn's nests and cystitis cystica. Intestinal type epithelium may be reflected in the columnar, sometimes mucus-producing cells that are frequently observed in bladder washings and catheterized specimens (see Fig. 22–15). Squamous epithelium sheds squamous cells of various degrees of maturity. The finding is exceedingly common and normal in adult women, but less frequent in men. In both sexes the harmless squamous epithelium, may become fully keratinized (leukoplakia), presumably as a consequence of chronic irritation. The cytologic findings and significance of leukoplakia of the bladder are discussed on p. 916.

Other Cells and Acellular Components in Normal Urinary Sediment

Normal urinary sediment may contain benign, mature squamous cells derived from the external genitalia in the female and from the distal part of the urethra in the male. A few leukocytes may occasionally be observed in the absence of inflammation. It is generally assumed that normal urinary sediment does not contain any red blood cells. Yet, Freni (1977), using a careful collection technique, documented that a few erythrocytes may be ob-

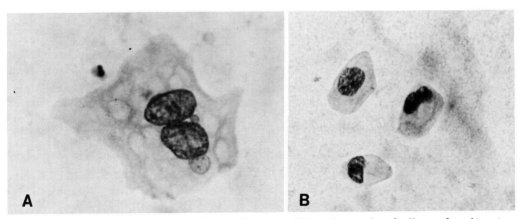

FIGURE 22–18. Catheterized ureteral urine. These are additional examples of cell types found in urinary sediment following retrograde catheterization. Note the giant umbrella cell with cytoplasmic vacuoles in (*A*) and the variation in cell shape and nuclear appearance in cells shown in (*B*). Such cells are often mistaken for cancer cells, and yet thy reflect no abnormalities whatever. The "salt-and-pepper" nuclear configuration of nuclear chromatin is well shown. (*A*, *B* ×560)

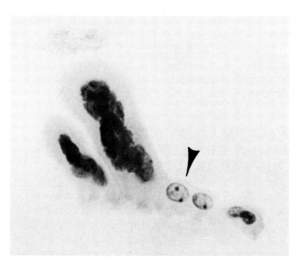

FIGURE 22-19. Retrograde catheterization: no evidence of disease. Huge multinucleated superficial urothelial cells, identified by a smooth cell border, with nuclear degeneration. Note two normal nuclei in adjacent cells (*arrowhead*). (×560)

served in virtually all healthy adults. In 8.8% of this healthy population, there were 10 erythrocytes per single, high-power field.

These observations were important because the presence of microscopic blood in urine has been suggested as a means of detecting bladder tumors.

Microhematuria in asymptomatic persons has been the subject of several other studies. Unfortunately, the populations studied were different and, therefore, no simple conclusion can be drawn. In an earlier study by Greene et al. (1956), 500 Mayo Clinic *patients* with microhematuria were investigated and 11 of them were found to have cancer (7 of bladder and 2 of kidney). Most other patients had trivial and incidental disorders. In a study by Carson et al. (1979), of 200 Mayo Clinic patients referred for a urologic workup, 22 (11%) had a tumor of the bladder and 2 had carcinoma of the prostate. It is of note that synchronous cytologic examination of urine was positive in 9 patients with occult carcinoma in situ and negative in 5 patients with low-grade papillary tumors (see also p. 951). Similar results were observed by Golin and Howard (1980). On the other hand, in a study of 1,000 asymptomatic male Air Force personnel, Froom et al. (1984) found microhematuria in 38.7%. In 1 subject, a "transitional cell carcinoma," not further specified, was observed. In a randomized 1986 study, Mohr et al. observed microhematuria in 13% of asymptomatic adult men and women, with neoplasms of the bladder in 0.1% and of the kidney in 0.4% of the population studied. Bard (1988) observed no significant disease in 177 women with microhematuria, followed for over 10 years.

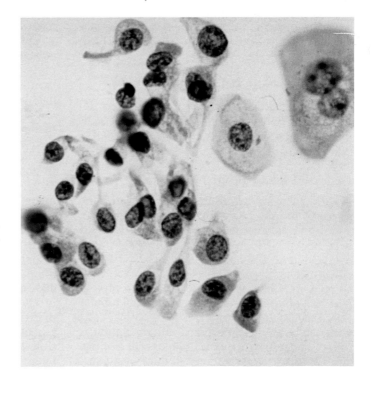

FIGURE 22-20. Normal urinary sediment in bladder washings. The field shows two large umbrella cells (one of them binucleated and not fully in focus) and a large cluster of smaller epithelial cells from deeper layers of the urothelium. The smaller cells are often oddly shaped, with elongated cytoplasmic processes that result mainly from stretching of the cytoplasm during smear preparation. Note the finely granular "salt-and-pepper" nuclei, each containing two or more chromocenters. In the large umbrella cell, one nucleus has four chromocenters. There was no evidence of tumor in this patient. (×560)

The initial views on the significance of microhematuria suggested an aggressive investigation of all patients with this disorder. More recent opinions, notably by Mohr et al., Messing et al., and Bard, suggest that a conservative follow-up of most asymptomatic patients is appropriate, with cystoscopic workup reserved for the patients with persisting significant hematuria or other evidence or suspicion of an important urologic disorder.

As Messing et al. (1987) noted, microhematuria is a sporadic event that may occur intermittently and may not occur at all in patients with significant disease. Therefore, it seems quite unlikely that microhematuria may be used as a screening test for bladder tumors. Of note, however, is the Carson study which suggested that a synchronous cytologic evaluation of the urinary sediment may lead to diagnosis of a carcinoma in situ of the bladder, a highly dangerous lesion (see p. 954 for further discussion).

The presence of *eosinophils* in urine (eosinophiluria) may be an indication of a drug-induced acute interstitial cystitis. Nolan et al. (1986) suggested the use of Hansel's stain (methylene blue and eosin-Y in methanol) to facilitate the recognition of eosinophils.

In a rare form of amaurotic familial idiocy, known as ceroid lipofuscinosis, Dolman et al. (1980) documented the presence of the characteristic cytoplasmic inclusions by electron microscopy of a spun-down urinary sediment. This may be used as a screening test for the disease, but is inferior to a suspension of lymphocytes isolated from blood.

Cells of Prostatic Origin

Cells of prostatic or testicular origin and seminal vesicle cells may be observed in the urinary sediment of moles, particularly after a prostatic palpation or massage (see p. 1001).

Casts and Renal Tubular Cells

By preserving voided urine in a 2% polyethylene glycol (Carbowax) solution (Bales, 1981; see p. 1465), the presence of renal casts was observed with unexpected frequency in patients without overt evidence of renal pathology. The casts were either hyaline or granular. The hyaline casts were composed of homogeneous eosinophilic protein material, often with a few peripheral renal tubular cells attached at the periphery. The granular casts were composed of debris mixed with renal tubular cells or of degenerating renal tubular cells (see Fig. 22–52). Such casts are very common in renal transplant patients during episodes of rejection (see p. 927).

An increase in the number of casts and renal tubular cells may also occur after urography during the period of elimination of the dye used for this purpose (Fischer et al., 1982).

INFLAMMATORY PROCESSES WITHIN THE LOWER URINARY TRACT

Inflammatory processes involving the lower urinary tract may be either primary or secondary. Of the primary ones, bacterial infection is by far the most common. Cornish et al. (1988) pointed out that the loss of mucus layer facilitates bacterial invasion. A variety of pyogenic bacteria, especially cocci but also *Escherichia coli* and *Pseudomonas aeruginosa* (*Bacillus pyocyaneus*), may be the predominant organisms. Obstructive processes, such as strictures, compression, calculi, diverticula or prostatic enlargement, which may interfere with the free flow of urine, either in a portion of or in the entire lower urinary tract, are the backbone of infection. Cancers, intrinsic or extrinsic to the lower urinary tract, may also create a favorable terrain for infection or may produce obstruction with the same effect. Some of the long-standing infectious processes are of a secondary nature. For instance, tuberculosis of the bladder is usually secondary to renal tuberculosis.

The result of the inflammatory processes is the appearance of red blood cells and, subsequently, purulent material in the urine. The presence of numerous red blood cells in the urine should be thoroughly investigated as to cause and origin, since it may reflect serious renal disease or a benign or a malignant neoplasm within the urinary tract (see comments on microhematuria, above).

The epithelial cellular constituents often appear in increased numbers in the urine. The cells are sometimes concealed by a heavy inflammatory exudate. Degeneration and necrosis are the characteristic cellular changes (Fig. 22–21). The degenerated cells are of variable size and configuration and are often large because of a markedly vacuolated cytoplasm that may be infiltrated with polymorphonuclear leukocytes (see Fig. 22–21B). Of special diagnostic interest are the nuclei of the atypical urothelial cells. They may be of variable sizes and of irregular outline, but usually show a clear, transparent center surrounded by a rim of chromatin (Fig. 22–22). This is a very important point of differential diagnosis between inflammatory atypias

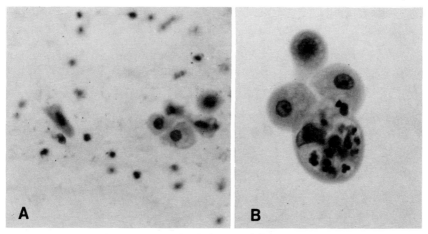

FIGURE 22-21. Chronic cystitis: voided urine. (*A*) Note the background of inflammatory cells and debris. (*B*) Vacuolization and infiltration of the cytoplasm of an epithelial cell by polymorphonuclear leukocytes. (*A, B* ×560. *B*: Melamed, M.R., et al.: Cytohistological observations on developing carcinoma of the urinary bladder in man. Cancer, 13:67–74, 1960)

and urothelial cancer. In the latter, the nuclear texture is quite different (see p. 948).

In severe inflammatory processes because of extensive epithelial damage, the urothelial cells may sometimes appear in sheets or clusters of variable sizes, usually showing the changes described above (Fig. 22–23).

Essentially similar inflammatory changes may be observed in urinary sediment following transurethral resection of the prostate or other surgical procedures. Electrocautery causes nuclear enlargement and pyknosis associated with cell distortion, occasionally closely simulating bladder cancer (Fig. 22–24). These changes may persist for several days following the procedure. Epithelial regeneration that follows the surgical procedure may also result in some atypia of urothelial cells and mitotic activity that may be observed in urinary sediment. As a rule, these changes do not last more than 6 weeks after the procedure. If significant cell abnormalities persist beyond that period, the possibility of a malignant event cannot be ruled out. For further comments on changes induced by therapeutic agents see p. 918.

Other Cells Seen in Inflammation

Macrophages may make their appearance in the urine, accompanying in varying numbers the more chronic inflammatory processes. Mononucleated or multinucleated varieties, with the characteristic faintly vacuolated basophilic cytoplasm and faintly stippled nuclei, may occur. They may be confused with vacuolated urothelial cells. Occasionally, plasma cells may be noted. In eosinophilic cystitis (see below), eosinophils may appear in the urinary sediment.

Specific Forms of Inflammation

Bacterial Infections

There are few if any specific cytologic findings in common bacterial infections. Occasionally the offending organism may be observed in the urinary sediment, but its exact identification must depend on bacteriologic data. Examination of the urinary sediment by phase microscopy may give a general idea as to whether the bacteria are cocci or rods.

Granulomatous Inflammation

Tuberculosis. Kapila and Verma (1984) described the presence of comma-shaped epithelioid cells in the urinary sediment of a patient with tuberculosis of the bladder. For description of epithelioid cells, see pp. 340 and 727. Piscioli et al. (1985) described the cytologic findings in the urinary sediment of 11 patients with tuberculosis. In 5 of them epithelioid cells were observed, although the illustration provided was not convincing. In all 11 patients, multinucleated cells of Langhans' type were observed. In my experience, this type of giant

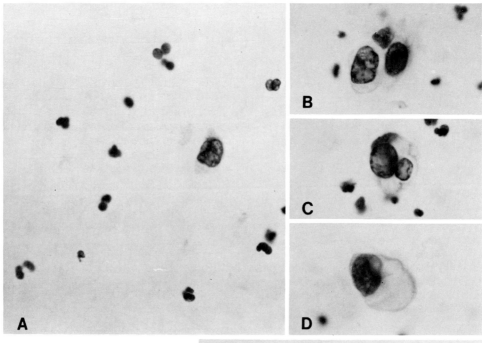

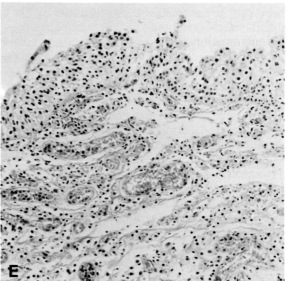

FIGURE 22–22. Cystitis with formation of inflammatory pseudopolyp. Urinary sediment and tissue. (*A, B, C, D*) Urothelial cells with inflammatory changes. The cells are enlarged, mainly because of cytoplasmic swelling and vacuolization. The nuclei, of variable sizes and configuration, consistently show a central clear, translucent area, surrounded by a thin rim of chromatin. Note in (*A*) smear background with numerous leukocytes. (*E*) Bladder biopsy of a polypoid lesion caused by inflammation. Note the frayed epithelium. (*A, B, C, D* ×560; *E* ×150)

cell is extremely rare in urinary sediment, and their presence may well prove to be of diagnostic value. Piscioli et al. also described in 2 patients the presence of markedly atypical urothelial cells resembling cancer cells, which they traced to the atypical hyperplastic urothelium, some of which appeared similar to flat carcinoma in situ.

Effects of Treatment with Bacillus Calmette-Guérin.   As will be discussed in Chapter 23, this form of immunotherapy is now extensively used for treatment of flat carcinoma in situ. The monitoring of these patients by cytologic examinations of urinary sediment is mandatory and the findings are described on p. 987. Granulomas, mimicking

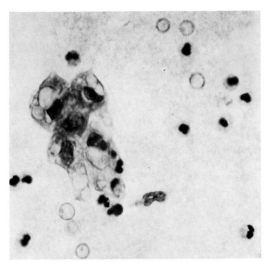

FIGURE 22 – 23. Acute cystitis: urinary sediment. Cluster of degenerated epithelial cells. Note cytoplasmic vacuolization. The background contains erythrocytes and polymorphonuclear leukocytes. (×560)

tuberculosis, may occasionally be observed and may shed giant cells of Langhans' type in the background of inflammation.

Granulomas After Bladder Surgery. Spagnolo et al. (1986) described the presence of granulomas in bladder walls of patients with two or more surgical procedures for bladder tumors. There were two types of granulomas: one type with necrosis and palisading of peripheral cells resembled rheumatoid nodules; the other type was composed of foreign body giant cells. There is no known cytologic presentation of these granulomas, and the entity is cited as a potential source of confusion with tuberculosis.

Fungal Infections

The most common fungus observed in the urinary sediment is *Candida albicans*. In the urine, the organism is observed mainly as fungal spores, but pseudohyphae may occasionally be observed (Fig. 22 – 25). This infection is particularly serious in renal transplant recipients and other immunosuppressed patients. It may lead to generalized fungal infection or, in a rare case, to obstruction of the ureters by a fungal ball.

Other fungi are uncommon. Eickenberg et al. pointed out that the urinary tract may be affected in patients with systemic North American blastomycosis, and that the organism can be identified in urine.

Viral Infections

Cytomegalic Inclusion Disease. The identification of cytomegalovirus in the urinary sediment of infants and children has been a recognized diagnostic procedure for many years. More recently, the spread of the acquired immunodeficiency syndrome (AIDS), the manipulation of the immune status of many patients, notably, recipients of renal transplants, and patients with leukemia or other forms of cancer, has increased significantly the frequency of this infection. Urinary sediment remains one of the methods of diagnosis of this serious disorder.

This disease is due to a virus of the herpesvirus group and is often fatal to infants, small children, and patients with AIDS. It causes a variety of vague clinical symptoms, fever, petechiae, jaundice, and

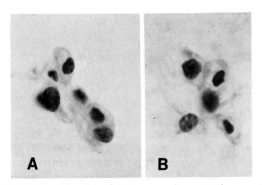

FIGURE 22 – 24. (*A, B*) Urinary sediment. Changes in urothelial cells following the use of intravesical cautery. Note nuclear pyknosis and variability in nuclear sizes. (*A, B* ×560)

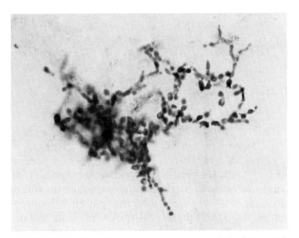

FIGURE 22 – 25. Urinary sediment. *Candida (Monilia) albicans* in yeast form (conidia) and pseudohyphae. (×560)

may affect a great many organs, particularly in patients with AIDS. The conclusive diagnosis intra vitam is made by cytologic examination of gastric washings, sputum, or of the urinary sediment. Virologic methods of diagnosis are now available as well. The virus can also be demonstrated by in situ hybridization techniques.

In the early stages of cellular transformation, the multiple, small, basophilic viral inclusions are distributed throughout the nucleus and the cytoplasm and are surrounded by individual halos (Fig. 22–26*A*). In more advanced, classic forms of the disease, the epithelial cells are markedly enlarged and carry within their nuclei very large, basophilic inclusions, surrounded by a conspicuous clear halo. The residual chromatin is condensed at the nuclear periphery (see Fig. 22–26*B*). In the advanced stage of the cellular disease, cytoplasmic inclusions are less frequent. Cellular inclusions of cytomegalovirus have been observed in the urinary sediment of renal transplant recipients (Johnston et al.; Bossen et al., 1969), in patients with leukemia (Chang), in those with other forms of cancer, and in AIDS. It is of particular interest that the identification of the virus in otherwise healthy adults does not carry with it the ominous prognosis of this disease in infancy and early childhood. Apparently, many of

the patients are carriers of the virus without suffering any direct ill effect. This virus has been identified in patients with some forms of infectious mononucleosis. The survival of the virus in the semen of a young asymptomatic man who recovered from infectious mononucleosis has been reported by Lang et al. (1974). The virus was found in seminal fluid, but presumably also within the spermatozoa. Sexual transmission of the virus to a young woman has been recorded in this case. The differential diagnosis of cytomegalovirus from the human polyomavirus is discussed below. Cytomegalovirus infection is now treatable with antiviral agents.

Herpes Simplex.   Herpetic infection of the urinary tract was a rarity 20 years ago. The recognition of the typical multinucleated epithelial cells with molded, ground-glass nuclei and, on rare occasions, of typical eosinophilic intranuclear inclusions has not posed any diagnostic dilemmas (see pp. 351 and 733 and Figs. 10–49 and 19–62). This virus has now been recognized in recipients of renal allografts (Bossen and Johnston, 1975) and in a patient with squamous cancer of the urinary bladder (Murphy, 1976). Several such cases were

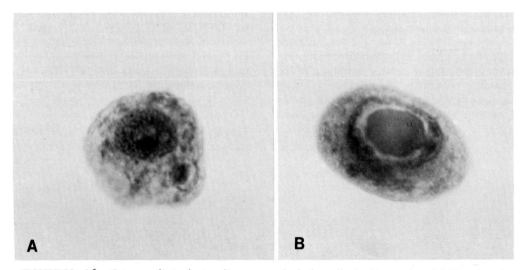

FIGURE 22–26.   Cytomegalic inclusion disease: renal tubular cells shed into urine. (*A*) Note heavily textured cytoplasm containing numerous particles; three cytoplasmic inclusion bodies along the right show well-defined peri-inclusion halos. The nucleus retains a moderately well-preserved chromatin net pattern, while a few noncoalescent inclusion bodies are forming. (*B*) A more advanced change, still demonstrating the coarsely textured cytoplasm, but without cytoplasmic inclusions. The nuclear chromatin net pattern has been lost, whereas the intranuclear inclusions have coalesced, increased in size, and become hyperchromatic to occupy nearly the entire nucleus. Around the inclusion there is the characteristic clear halo with the distinctly thick, irregular membrane sharply demarcating it from the surrounding cytoplasm. (*A, B* ×1,600. Courtesy Dr. John K. Frost, Baltimore, Maryland)

personally observed in patients with and without cancer.

Human Polyomavirus (Decoy Cells). In the 1950s, the late Mr. Andrew Ricci, senior cytotechnologist at Memorial Hospital for Cancer in New York, recognized, in the urinary sediment, cells with large, homogeneous, hyperchromatic nuclei, mimicking cancer cells, but not associated with bladder cancer (Fig. 22–27). Mr. Ricci named these cells *decoy cells*. The nature of the decoy cells remained unknown for many years. In the 1968 edition of this book it was speculated that the change was due to an unidentified virus. This virus has been identified as human polyomavirus by Gardner et al. (1971) and has been extensively studied by Coleman and her coworkers (1973, 1975, 1980, 1984). The virus belongs to the Papovaviridae family and is related to the human papillomavirus implicated in genital cancer (see p. 374). Two strains of the human polyomavirus have been identified: the JC strain, isolated from a patient with a rare disease, progressive multifocal leukoencephalopathy (Pagett et al., 1971), and the BK strain, isolated from a patient with renal transplant (Gardner et al., 1971). The two strains differ from each other by the size of virus particles and by serologic characteristics. The polyoma group of DNA viruses has been previously identified in the animal kingdom and extensively studied in experimental systems because of their oncologic properties.

It has been documented by serologic studies that the human infection with polyomavirus is acquired in childhood and is nearly universal (Padgett and Walker, 1976). Thus, the cytologic manifestations of this infection reflect an activation of, or a superinfection with, the virus, a sequence of events also proposed for the human papillomavirus (Koss, 1989; see also p. 381). There is, however, a major difference between these two viruses.

Although the human papillomavirus is implicated in neoplastic events in the skin, female genital tract, larynx, and perhaps even the bronchus and the esophagus, there is no evidence that the polyomavirus plays a similar role in humans, although it appears to play some role in tumor formation in experimental animals.

The activation of polyomaviruses occurs in immunosuppressed individuals who are receiving chemotherapy, in diabetics, in bone marrow transplant recipients (O'Reilly et al., 1981; Apperly et al., 1987), and in patients with AIDS. *Most importantly, however, virus activation may occur without any obvious cause* (Kahan et al., 1980) and last for a few weeks or even months, without any ill effects (Table 22–2).

The virus appears to play an important role in the previously very rare progressive multifocal encephalopathy currently on the rise in AIDS patients, and, possibly, in interstitial nephritis (Rosen et al., 1983). Houff et al. (1988) documented that the JC type polyomavirus may proliferate in bone marrow cells and in mononuclear cells. They proposed that the lesions in progressive multifocal leukoencephalopathy may be due to viruses carried to the brain by mononuclear cells.

A case of uretheral obstruction in viral presence was reported by Coleman, and the possibility that the virus contributed to the obstruction of the cystic duct in a liver transplant recipient has been raised. It may be questioned, however, whether these events were actually due to human polyomavirus infection. A suggestion by Arthur et al. (1986) that the virus is the cause of hemorrhagic cystitis in bone marrow transplant recipients has been disproved (Cottler-Fox et al., 1989).

The effects of human polyomavirus activation may be observed occasionally in endocervical cells

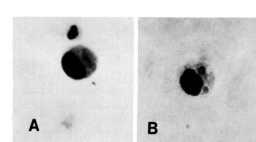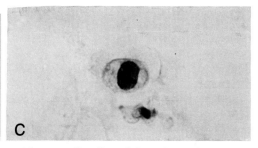

FIGURE 22–27. "Decoy cells" in urinary sediment. These small cells with large hyperchromatic, smooth nuclei closely imitate cancer cells, except for total lack of nuclear structure. The cell in (*B*) shows two incidental small eosinophilic inclusion bodies in the cytoplasm. The nuclear abnormalities are diagnostic of an infection with human polyomavirus (cf. Fig.22–28). (*A, B, C* ×560)

Table 22–2
*Human Polyoma Virus in Urinary Sediment**

	No. of Patients Studied	Virus-Infected Cells Identified†
Recent renal transplant recipients	7	1
Past renal transplant recipients	21	0
Diabetic outpatients	84	2
Disseminated lupus erythematosus patients on therapy	23	0
Cancer patients on chemotherapy	37	5

*Survey carried out by Allayne Kahan, MD
†Millipore filter technique was used.

in cervical smears of pregnant women and in bronchial cells, but, for reasons unknown, the most important and common manifestations are observed in urothelial cells in urinary sediment.

In a person shedding the virus, the number of affected urothelial cells in a urinary specimen varies from an occasional cell (see Fig. 22–27) to a massive manifestation of infection, affecting nearly all cells (Fig. 22–28). Two stages of the infection may be recognized and both are diagnostic of the disorder.

Inclusion Stage. The infected cells vary in size, and many are markedly enlarged. The virus forms single, dense basophilic homogeneous, or less basophilic, opaque intranuclear inclusions that fills completely, or nearly so, the enlarged nucleus. A narrow, clear halo may be seen between the edge of the inclusion and the marginal rim of nuclear chromatin (see Fig. 22–28). Similar inclusions may be observed in a fortuitous tissue biopsy from an infected person (see Fig. 22–28*C*) and in cytologic preparations from progressive multifocal encephalopathy (Suhrland et al., 1987).

Electron microscopy of polyomavirus inclusions shows many similarities to the human papillomavirus (HPV) infection (Fig. 22–29, cf. Fig. 11–5). Both viruses form crystalline arrays of viral particles. The polyomavirus particles are somewhat smaller than the papillomavirus particles.

Although the similarities between the polyomavirus inclusions and cytomegalovirus (CMV) inclusions are slight (cf. Fig. 22–26 with 22–28 and 22–29), inasmuch as the polyomavirus inclusions have no large halo and are not accompanied by satellite inclusions, nonetheless sometimes the differentiation cannot be securely made. In these cases, virologic or serologic methods may be used. In situ

hybridization techniques with specific viral probes are also available. Electron microscopy may prove decisive because the CMV particles are very large (about 150 nm in diameter), encapsulated, as are all the particles of the herpesvirus family (see Fig. 10–51), and do not form crystalline arrays.

Postinclusion Stage. Presumably because of the leaching-out of the virus particles, the nuclei of the infected cells that lost their viral content acquire a new appearance that, in my judgment, is just as characteristic of this infection as the inclusions. The enlarged nuclei of the cells that lost the inclusion have an "empty" appearance, with a distinct network of chromatin filaments wherein scattered chromocenters may be observed. Transition forms between the inclusion-bearing cells and the "empty" cells may be observed (Fig. 22–30). The scanty cytoplasm and the large size of the "empty" nuclei must also be noted for comparison with normal urothelial cells (cf. Fig. 22–11).

The host organism appears to be unaffected by the virus in most cases: virus-infected cells have been observed in the urinary sediment in many patients or normal individuals over a period of many months or even years. The shedding of the affected epithelial cells may be intermittent.

The principal significance of the urothelial cell changes caused by polyomavirus activation is in an erroneous diagnosis of urothelial cancer. The so aptly named *decoy cells* have been mistaken for cancer cells on many occasions and frequently resulted in a very extensive and unnecessary clinical workup, which included biopsies of the bladder, and cost vast sums of money. An example of the cells causing such an error many years ago in our own institution is shown in Fig. 22–31.

Unfortunately, polyomavirus infection may also occur in patients with urothelial cancer, par-

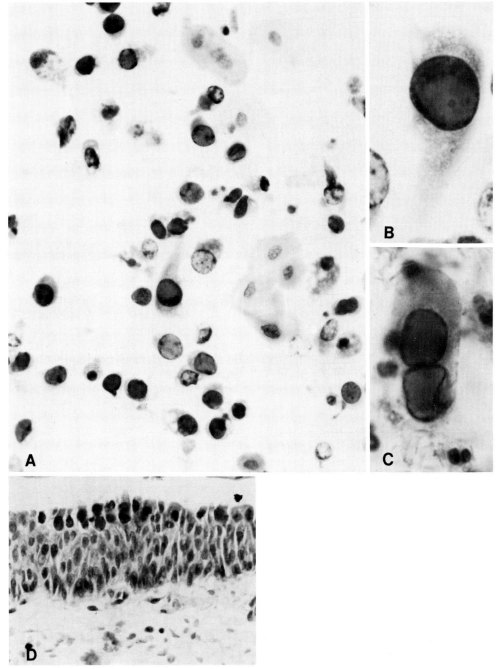

FIGURE 22–28. Human polyomavirus, urinary sediment: Millipore filter preparation. (*A*) Low-power view to show numerous, large virus-infected cells with very large, dark nuclei (*B, C*) Detailed view of virus-infected cells. The cell nuclei are markedly enlarged and filled with homogeneous, sometimes opaque basophilic inclusions. In some cells a very narrow clear rim separates the inclusion from the peripheral band of nuclear chromatin. (*D*) Epithelium of ureter showing numerous virus-infected cells in the luminal layers of the urothelium. (*A* ×500; *B, C* ×1,500; *D* ×350. *A, B, C:* Case courtesy of Drs. D.V. Coleman and E.F.D. MacKenzie, photographs courtesy Dr. J. Bate, London, England. *D:* Tissue courtesy of Dr. D.V. Coleman)

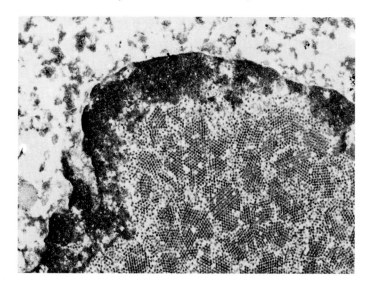

FIGURE 22–29. Electron micrograph of a cell in the human urinary sediment infected with human polyomavirus. The crystalline arrays of virus particles, measuring about 45 nm in diameter, are clearly shown. (×32,000. Courtesy Dr. D.V. Coleman, London, England)

ticularly if treated with cytotoxic drugs. In these fairly rare cases the inclusion-bearing and the "empty" cells may appear side by side with cancer cells. As is discussed in Chapter 23, the characteristic features of urothelial cells *do not* include smooth, homogeneous appearance of the nucleus or the characteristic filamentous chromatin pattern of empty cells.

Human Papillomavirus (HPV). Infection of the lower urinary tract with HPV occurs with a fair frequency. Because the infection is related to condylomata acuminata and possibly cancer of the urethra and bladder, the topic is discussed in Chapter 23. However, it may be noted that koilocytes in the urinary sediment in women may occur as a consequence of a "pick-up" of cells from the genital tract. In such cases further investigation of the genital organs is suggested before the much more complex investigation of the urinary tract is undertaken.

Other Viruses. Other viruses, such as herpes zoster, have been observed in recipients of renal allograft transplants (Spencer and Anderson).

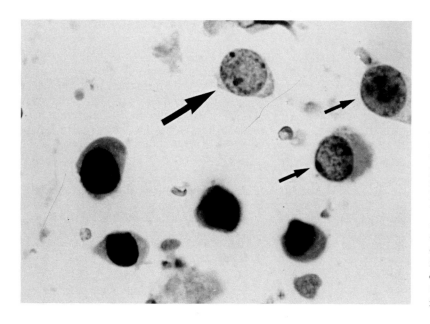

FIGURE 22–30. Severe polyomavirus infection in a young bone marrow transplant recipient. Several very large urothelial cells show the typical homogeneous nuclear inclusions. The nuclei of two cells (*small arrows*) show partial loss of the inclusion material and begin to show the underlying chromatin network. One "empty" large nucleus (*large arrow*) shows merely a peculiar chromatin network with scattered chromocenters. This appearance is also very characteristic of polyomavirus activation (see text). (×700). Case courtesy of Dr. Denise Hidvegi, Chicago, Illinois)

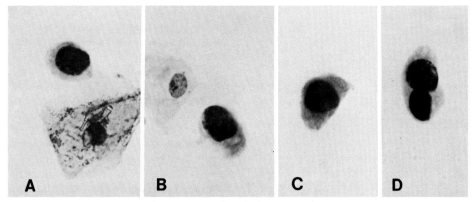

FIGURE 22–31. Human polyomavirus-induced changes in the urinary sediment of a 54-year-old woman with diabetes, hypertension, and symptoms of cystitis. The large infected cells with nuclear inclusions were interpreted in 1970 as cancer cells. There was no evidence of cancer in 1977. (×560)

Cellular Inclusions in Urinary Sediment Not Caused by Viral Infection

Several types of cell inclusions that may be observed in the urinary sediment must be differentiated from viral inclusions.

Intracytoplasmic Eosinophilic Inclusions. On frequent occasions, red, eosinophilic, opaque cytoplasmic inclusions, single or multiple, may be noted within the epithelial cells in the urinary sediment. Most of the inclusions appear in cells with a degenerated or absent nucleus. However, in some instances the nucleus may still be well preserved (Fig. 22–32). Similar inclusions are frequently observed in cells derived from ileal bladders (see p. 918). Dorfman and Monis established that the inclusions contained mucopolysaccharides. Kobayastin et al. (1984) reported a case of the rare Kawasaki disease with identical inclusions.

Melamed and Wolinska (1961) studied these inclusions in a large number of cases. In this study there was no evidence of a specific association of the cytoplasmic inclusions with any known disease state. Bolande's suggestion that these inclusions correlate with specific viral diseases of childhood was surely in error. Naib (personal communication) failed to identify any viral organisms in these inclusions and considers them as products of cell degeneration, possibly the result of prior viral infection. Similar inclusions may be observed in degenerating cells of the respiratory tract (ciliocytophthoria, see p. 709) and occasionally in other organs. Most patients with intracytoplasmic eosinophilic inclusions have some form of urinary tract disease or injury.

Eosinophilic *nuclear* inclusions in urinary sediment of women were described by Rouse et al. (1986). Extensive investigations failed to uncover the nature of these inclusions. Electron microscopy was not performed.

Inclusions Caused by Lead Poisoning. Lead poisoning is not uncommonly observed in children and results in the formation of intranuclear acid-fast inclusion bodies in renal tubular cells (Fig. 22–33). It was proposed that examination of the urinary sediment may lead to the correct diagnosis of the disease (Landing and Nakai).

FIGURE 22–32. Intracytoplasmic eosinophilic inclusions in urothelial cells. (*A*) The cell is undergoing the common degenerative change. (*B*) The inclusion (*arrow*) is present next to a relatively well-preserved nucleus. (*A, B* ×560. *B*: Melamed, M.R., et al.: Cytohistological observations on developing carcinoma of the bladder in man. Cancer, *13*:67–74, 1960)

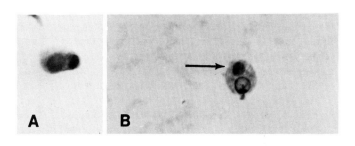

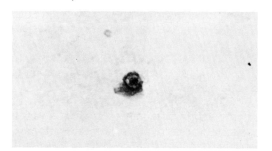

FIGURE 22–33. Lead poisoning. An intranuclear inclusion in an epithelial cell in urinary sediment (Hematoxylin–eosin; ×560. Courtesy of Dr. Benjamin Landing, Cincinnati, Ohio.)

Parasites

The presence of *Trichomonas vaginalis* in the male may be established on urinary sediment, particularly after prostatic massage (for description of the parasite see p. 346). In female patients the parasites are usually of vaginal origin.

***Schistosoma Hematobium* Infestation.** Infestation with the trematode worm *S. hematobium* is extremely widespread in certain parts of Africa, particularly along the Nile. The disease is transmitted from man to man through an intermediate host, a sweet-water snail. The adult worms travel to the veins of the pelvis, particularly the veins of the bladder, where they copulate. The ova, provided with a terminal spine (Fig. 10–44*B*), are deposited mainly in the submucosa of the distal ureter and the urinary bladder, although the rectum may also be involved. The major importance of this infestation is its frequent association with carcinoma of the bladder (see p. 964). The reasons for this association are unclear; it may somehow be related to the severe inflammatory reaction and fibrosis of the bladder wall caused by the ova. Squamous metaplasia of the epithelium is frequently observed. The urinary sediment reflects such changes very closely: marked inflammatory epithelial changes, often associated with purulent exudate, are the rule in advanced schistosomiasis. Numerous squamous cells corresponding to squamous metaplasia were observed in 18 of 51 urine sediments from patients from Zimbabwe with schistosomiasis (Houston et al.), a much higher ratio than that in material from patients in New York City. Ova were not seen in this material. Somewhat similar observations were reported by Dimmette et al.

Because of air travel and movement of infected people, the finding of *Schistosoma* is no longer confined to endemic areas. Clements and Oko (1983) reported such a case from New York City, and more such cases may be expected to occur in the Western world.

Filariasis. For similar reasons, filariasis, previously confined to endemic areas, may now be observed in other geographic settings. Webber and Eveland (1982) observed *Wuchereria bancrofti* filariae in urinary sediment of a patient in New York City.

Other Specific Forms of Inflammation

Interstitial Cystitis (Hunner's Ulcer). This is a rare form of ulcerative chronic cystitis of unknown causes, first described by Hunner and, more recently, discussed by Smith and Denner. There is no known specific cytologic presentation of this disease. However, Utz and Zincke pointed out that nonpapillary carcinoma in situ may masquerade clinically as interstitial cystitis. The cytologic presentation of carcinoma in situ is discussed on p. 954.

Eosinophilic Cystitis. Infiltration of the bladder wall with numerous eosinophils is most commonly observed after cautery treatment, although spontaneous forms of this disease may also occur (Hellstrom et al., 1979). Occasionally, however, dense eosinophilic infiltrates may be observed in patients with asthma or other allergic disorders. A true eosinophilic granuloma, with simultaneous proliferation of eosinophils and macrophages, may also occur (Koss, 1974). In such cases the urinary sediment may contain numerous eosinophils.

URINARY CALCULI (LITHIASIS)

Urinary calculi (stones) cause two types of important abnormalities of the urothelial cells: the abrasive effect and atypias of urothelial cells.

Abrasive Effect

A stone or stones, particularly when lodged in the renal pelvis or ureter, or when being actively expelled through the narrow lumen of the ureter, may act like an abrasive instrument. Significant and sometimes massive exfoliation of urothelial cells, singly and in clusters, may occur and may be observed in the urinary sediment. Among the single cells, numerous large multinucleated umbrella cells are sometimes quite striking. Because of the customary variation in the sizes of the nuclei (see Fig. 22–17) such cells have been mistaken for cancer cells by inexperienced observers. Cell clusters, as is customary with urothelial cells, may form compact balls or "papillary" clusters (see Figs. 22–16, 22–20, and Plate 22–1) that may be mistaken for cells from a low-grade papillary tumor.

The most common situation leading to these errors is the presence of a space-occupying lesion in a renal pelvis in a patient with hematuria. The differential diagnosis in such cases includes a stone, a blood clot, and a tumor. The urologist, believing that a cytologic examination will clarify the issues, proceeds to obtain a sample by retrograde catheterization or by direct brushing. Under these circumstances, the large number of clusters of normal or somewhat atypical urothelial cells generated by the procedures (see p. 900) are mistaken for a papillary tumor, and the kidney and ureter are surgically removed. Because the damaged urothelium may show evidence of regeneration within 3 or 4 days after the retrograde procedure, the mitotic activity and slight atypia of the regenerating epithelium are interpreted as showing an early neoplastic process, and the term *dysplasia* is sometimes used to describe it; (see Plate 22–1) and the error is compounded still further.

It must be clearly stated that the cytologic diagnosis of low-grade papillary tumors (papillomas, grade I papillary carcinomas), particularly when located in the renal pelvis or ureter, cannot be reliably established on cell clusters. Retrograde cell samples are not helpful in these situations and tend to confuse the picture still further. The differentiation of lithiasis from low-grade tumors cannot be accomplished by cytology and must be based on clinical and radiologic data. For example, past or present history or renal pain (colic), strongly supports the diagnosis of lithiasis. On the other hand, high-grade tumors can usually be recognized cytologically in voided urine sediment (for further discussion, see Chap. 23, pp. 951 and 954).

Calculus-Induced Atypias of Urothelial Cells

Highman and Wilson (1982) observed papillary clusters of urothelial cells in slightly over 40% of 154 patients with calculi. They proposed that such clusters are predictive of calculi. They tested this hypothesis on over 6,000 routine urine specimens and found similar clusters in 48 patients, of whom 30 were subsequently shown to harbor calculi.

In my experience, however, the presence of papillary clusters in voided urine, especially after palpation of the bladder, occurs in about 10% to 15% of all specimens from patients in whom no stones can be found. The Highman and Wilson observation still should be tested.

Urinary calculi, perhaps more than any other benign disorder, are likely to produce a variety of unusual and occasionally striking alterations in the shapes and sizes of urothelial cells. Moreover, there may be a degree of nuclear hyperchromasia that, in the absence of any other nuclear changes, should be interpreted with caution (Fig. 22–34). Crystalline deposits may be observed in the cytoplasm.

The Dutch investigator, Beyer-Boon, has recorded 11 cases of lithiasis that resulted in sufficiently abnormal cytologic patterns to warrant the diagnosis of bladder cancer, occasionally of high grade. She supported her findings with a careful review of the literature, strongly suggesting that next to effects of treatment and certain drugs (see p. 920) lithiasis may be the most important source of diagnostic error in cytology of the urinary tract.

Highman and Wilson (1982) observed markedly atypical urothelial cells in 10 of 154 patients with calculi. In one of the patients a major abnormality of the urothelium was observed on biopsy. None of the patients developed bladder cancer after a follow-up of 1 to 3 years.

Personal experience does not completely support these views. In the past 15 years there were only two patients seen in my laboratories wherein a presumably erroneous diagnosis of urothelial cancer was made in the presence of lithiasis (Fig. 22–35). One must keep in mind that cancer of the urothelium and lithiasis may coexist and, in most instances of highly abnormal urothelial cells, some form of cancer is present (see p. 942). In fact, Wynder, in his epidemiologic studies, considered

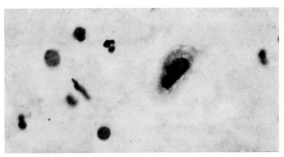

FIGURE 22–34. Cells found in urinary sediment in case of nephrolithiasis. Note marked nuclear hyperchromasia and irregularity of nuclear shape. The cytoplasm contains minute spicules of crystals seen as clear areas. (×560)

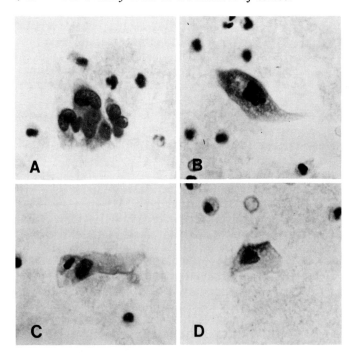

FIGURE 22–35.   (*A, B, C, D*) Urinary sediment in bladder lithiasis. Significant abnormalities of urothelial cells, mainly abnormalities in nuclear shape and significant hyperchromasia resulted in the diagnosis of urothelial carcinoma. This diagnosis could not be confirmed during the ensuing 3 years of follow-up. (*A–D* ×560)

lithiasis as an important factor associated with bladder cancer. It must also be pointed out that cytologic evidence of bladder cancer, particularly nonpapillary carcinoma in situ, may precede by many months or even years clinical evidence of disease (see p. 946). Hence, in the presence of cytologic findings suggestive of cancer, further investigation of patients is necessary, whether or not there is associated lithiasis.

sediment. Some of these cells may be fully keratinized to the point of nuclear loss. These nucleated or anucleated squames have a yellow cytoplasm in Papanicolaou stain (cf. Fig. 10–54). The diagnostic significance of such findings varies. In a voided urine specimen from female patient, the presence of squamous cells is of no diagnostic value. In the

LEUKOPLAKIA OF BLADDER EPITHELIUM

The presence of the vaginal-type squamous epithelium in the area of bladder trigone in women was described above (see p. 893). This must be considered a common anatomic variant of no diagnostic or prognostic significance.

Chronic inflammatory processes in the urinary bladder, often associated with lithiasis or, in Africa, with schistosomiasis, may result in the formation of a fully differentiated squamous epithelium or squamous metaplasia, which may occur anywhere in the bladder or the renal pelvis. The process may progress to stages of excessive keratinization with the resulting formation of white plaques or leukoplakia (Fig. 22–36). Keratinizing squamous cancer of the bladder may follow this disorder (see Chap. 23). Leukoplakia of the bladder contributes numerous mature squamous cells to the urinary

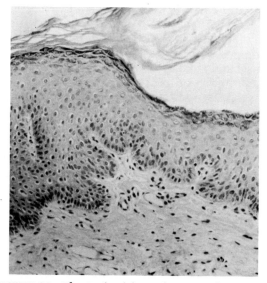

FIGURE 22–36.   Leukoplakia or keratinized squamous metaplasia of bladder epithelium. Note keratin formation on the surface. (×150)

male patient it may indicate the remote possibility of squamous metaplasia. In a catheterized specimen, there is again a sex difference that must be considered. In the female the squamous cells may indicate the harmless vaginal squamous epithelium, previously discussed, although this rarely results in complete keratinization. In the male the possibility of leukoplakia becomes higher. In both sexes, *if the catheterized specimen contains anucleated squamae, the presence of leukoplakia in the urinary tract becomes a virtual certainty.* Contrary to the benign vaginal-type epithelium, leukoplakia must be considered as a potentially dangerous lesion that may lead to squamous carcinoma with which it may share similar cytologic presentation (see p. 964).

MALACOPLAKIA OF BLADDER

Malacoplakia is a rare disorder characterized grossly by formation of yellow plaques within the bladder wall. Histologically, the lesions are com-

posed of sheets of mononucleated macrophages, somewhat similar to the epithelioid cells. The cytoplasm of these cells contains spheroid, laminated, sometimes calcified concretions (Michaelis–Gutmann bodies). In a case reported by Melamed (1962) from my laboratory, and in other cases subsequently observed by me and others, numerous cells in the urinary sediment of patients with malacoplakia contained one or more Michaelis–Gutmann bodies. Concentric laminations were readily identifiable in some of the bodies, although some took a uniform eosin or hematoxylin stain (Fig. 22–37). It must be noted that such cells very rarely appear in the urinary sediment prior to biopsies because malacoplakia is separated from the lumen by normal bladder epithelium.

Malacoplakia has now been described in several other organs besides the urinary bladder (see pp. 357 and 747). It has been shown that malacoplakia represents an enzymatic deficiency of macrophages which are unable to digest bacterial agents, mainly coliform bacteria. The Michaelis–Gutmann bodies represent cytoplasmic lysosomes that

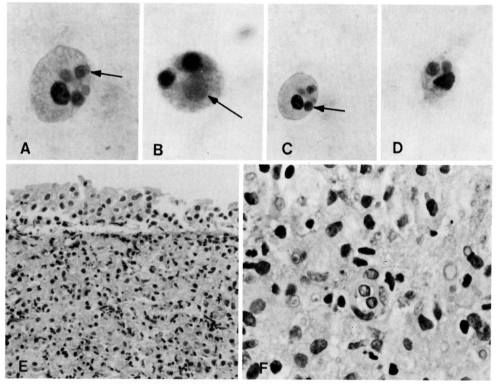

FIGURE 22–37. Malacoplakia of bladder. Urinary sediment and biopsies. (*A, B, C, D*) Cells in the urinary sediment containing single or multiple Michaelis–Gutmann bodies (*arrows*). The latter vary in size; some are calcified and resemble small psammoma bodies (*A*); others are not calcified. (*E, F*) Biopsies of bladder. Low-power view (*E*) shows the characteristic lesion made up of sheets of epithelioid cells beneath normal urothelium. The high-power view (*F*) shows numerous calcified and noncalcified Michaelis–Gumann bodies or inclusions. (*A–D* ×1,000; *E* ×250; *F* ×560)

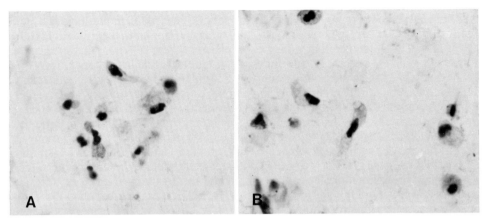

FIGURE 22–38.   (*A, B*) Urinary sediment: ileal bladder. Some of the cells of small-bowel origin have still preserved their columnar appearance. Others, however, have become smaller, of oval or irregular shape. Nuclear pyknosis and karyorrhexis are frequent in this type of material. Many cells have a vacuolated cytoplasm and resemble small macrophages. (*A, B* ×560)

phagocytose the bacteria and later become calcified in a concentric fashion. Although epithelial cells may occasionally contain specks of calcium in the presence of lithiasis (see Fig. 22–34), the Michaelis–Gutmann bodies have a sufficiently unique appearance to be considered diagnostic of malacoplakia.

URINE OBTAINED THROUGH AN ILEAL BLADDER

An ileal bladder or ileal conduit is constructed surgically to bypass the natural urinary bladder, most often at the time of cystectomy for cancer. For reasons that are discussed in detail on p. 977, cytologic follow-up of such patients is of considerable importance and familiarity with the makeup of the urinary sediment is important.

Urinary sediments obtained from an ileal bladder are always rich in epithelial cells of intestinal origin, which occur singly and in large clusters. Rarely, the original columnar configuration of such cells is well preserved (Fig. 22–38). More often these cells are round, oval, or somewhat irregular (Fig. 22–39). Their cytoplasm may show vacuolization, and the nuclei, although of monotonous size, may appear somewhat hyperchromatic. A characteristic change frequently observed in the cells derived from the epithelium of the ileum is cellular degeneration in the form of nuclear pyknosis and karyorrhexis and the presence of numerous pink or red cytoplasmic inclusions of the type discussed on p. 913 (Fig. 22–40). There is no

known clinical significance to this finding, which is present in most patients with an ileal bladder.

CYTOLOGIC CHANGES IN BLADDER EPITHELIUM CAUSED BY THERAPY

Changes Caused by Radiation Therapy

Irradiation of the pelvic organs produces marked changes in the urinary bladder. Edema of the bladder wall is usually marked (Fig. 22–41*A*). The epithelial cells share the fate of irradiated cells elsewhere (cf. p. 666) and become enlarged. Their nuclei are blown up, occasionally showing pyknosis and karyorrhexis; the cytoplasm becomes vacuolated and at times eosinophilic (see Fig. 22–41*B*). The value of cytologic assessment of radiotherapy for primary carcinoma of the bladder is discussed on page 991.

Radiation changes in the bladder following treatment of carcinoma of the cervix by irradiation have resulted in serious diagnostic problems. Evaluating the presence or absence of metastatic carcinoma of the cervix within the bladder on the basis of the urinary sediment is at times difficult and, on at least one occasion, it was erroneous because irradiated urothelial cells were mistaken for cells of epidermoid carcinoma. As elsewhere in similar situations, it appears wise to withhold diagnostic judgment in the presence of radiation changes until clear-cut evidence of cancer has been obtained.

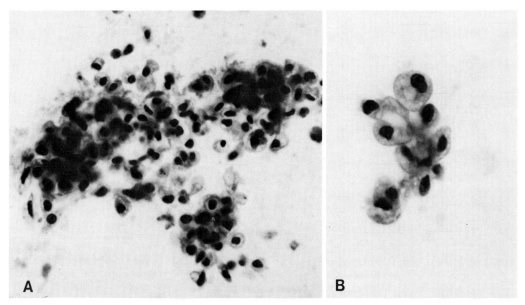

FIGURE 22–39. Ileal bladder urine. The sediment contains large clusters of cells or cells of intestinal derivation, although the columnar shape of such cells is only occasionally noted (*A*). Most cells are round, oval, or irregular and have cytoplasmic vacuoles and somewhat hyperchromatic nuclei of even sizes (*B*). (*A* ×350; *B* ×560)

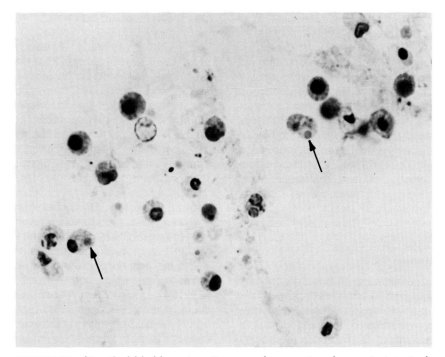

FIGURE 22–40. Ileal bladder urine. Common degenerative changes in intestinal cells. There is nuclear pyknosis and karyorrhexis. Numerous eosinophilic cytoplasmic inclusions may be observed (*arrows*). (×560)

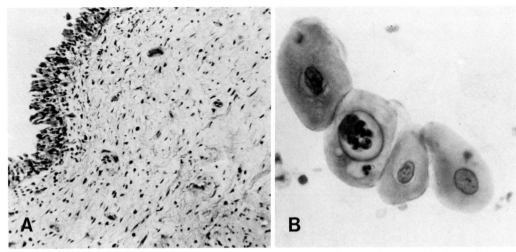

FIGURE 22–41. (*A*) Wall of irradiated bladder. Note the characteristic subepithelial edema. (*B*) Radiated benign cells of bladder epithelium. Proportionate nuclear and cellular enlargement, cytoplasmic and nuclear vacuolization, and karyorrhexis are characteristic of the change. (*A* ×150; *B* ×560)

Changes Caused by Chemotherapy

Certain alkylating drugs, particularly cyclophosphamide, administered for the treatment of cancer, exercise a marked effect on the epithelium of the urinary bladder.

Cyclophosphamide (Cytoxan, Endoxan) is related to nitrogen mustard, but is per se inactive until metabolized in the liver. The products of metabolism of the drug exercise a marked cytotoxic effect and are rapidly excreted in the urine. The characteristic clinical change is hemorrhagic cystitis, which may lead to an intractable hemorrhage necessitating surgical treatment. The concentration of the drug in the urine accounts for these changes. By deviating the urinary stream in the experimental animal (Bellin and Koss), the bladder was protected from the effect of the cytotoxic effects of the drug. The cytologic changes in patients receiving cyclophosphamide for a variety of malignant diseases have been described in detail by Forni et al. from my laboratory.

The Effects of Cyclophosphamide on Bladder Epithelial Cells

The changes observed were somewhat similar to those following radiation treatment to the urinary bladder, although more pronounced. The most striking feature was marked but variable cell enlargement, usually pertaining to both the nucleus and the cytoplasm (Fig. 22–42). The study of patients from the very beginning of treatment suggested that the nuclear enlargement preceded cytoplasmic abnormalities. The enlarged nucleus was often eccentric, slightly irregular in outline, and nearly always markedly hyperchromatic. The chromatin granules were at times coarse, but their distribution was usually fairly even, giving the nucleus a "salt-and-pepper" appearance (Figs. 22–42 and 22–43). A chromocenter or a nucleolus or two were often well in evidence and sometimes very large. The large nucleoli were frequently distorted, with irregular and sharp edges. In female patients the sex chromatin body was often visibly enlarged (Fig. 22–43*D*). Occasionally, multinucleated cells with some variability in the sizes of the component nuclei were noted. Nuclear pyknosis and karyorrhexis were common late effects, resulting in large and hyperchromatic nuclei; in some cells the chromatin texture was lost, and the nucleus appeared "glassy." The cytoplasm commonly showed marked vacuolization. At times it contained particles of foreign material or was infiltrated by polymorphonuclear leukocytes. In numerous cells, elongation and vacuolization of cytoplasmic material were seen, probably as a result of mechanical trauma during the preparation of smears (see Fig. 22–42). In cases showing such marked cell changes as those just described, the smear background often contained numerous erythrocytes, cellular debris, and leukocytes. In some instances, the cytologic changes due to cyclophosphamide therapy may be extremely severe and imitate urothelial carcinoma to perfection (see Fig. 22–43).

An example of the relationship of the cytologic abnormalities to treatment with cyclophosphamide is illustrated in Fig. 22–44. It must be noted

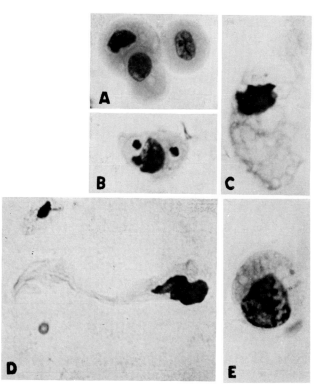

FIGURE 22–42. Urinary sediment. Epithelial cell changes caused by cyclophosphamide therapy. (*A*) Nonspecific slight nuclear enlargement. (*B–E*) Marked cellular enlargement, combined with pyknosis and cytoplasmic vacuolization and smudging in (*C*) and (*D*). Nucleolar enlargement in a coarsely granular, abnormally shaped large nucleus is noted in (*E*). (*A–E* ×560. Forni, A.M., et al.: Cytological study of the effect of cyclophosphamide on the epithelium of the urinary bladder in man. Cancer, *17*:1348–1355, 1964.)

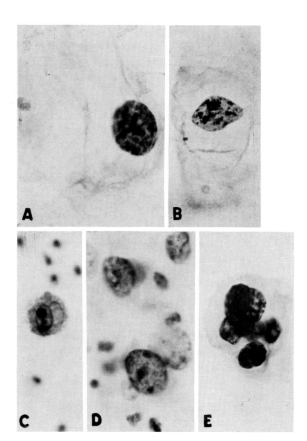

FIGURE 22–43. Urinary sediment. Epithelial cell changes caused by cyclophosphamide therapy. (*A, B*) "Salt-and-pepper" distribution of coarse chromatin granule in enlarged nuclei. (*C*) A markedly enlarged nucleolus. (*D*) A large sex chromatin body in an enlarged nucleus. (*E*) Atypical multinucleated cell. (*A–E* ×560. Forni, A.M., et al.: Cytological study of the effect of cyclophosphamide on the epithelium of the urinary bladder in man. Cancer, *17*:1348–1355, 1964)

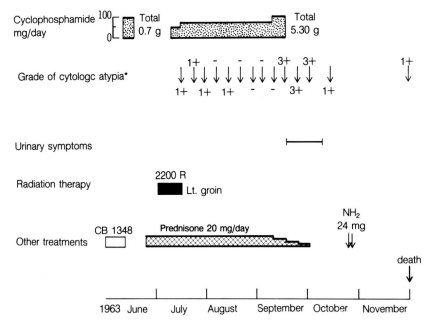

FIGURE 22-44. Diagram illustrating the case history of a 69-year-old woman treated with cyclophosphamide and also by other mans for a large-cell lymphoma. It may be noted that treatment with prednisone does not affect urinary tract cytology. Cytologic changes in the urinary sediment are designated as 1+, 2+, or 3+. (Forni, A. M., et al.: Cytological study of the effect of cyclophosphamide on the epithelium of the urinary bladder in man. Cancer, *17*: 1348–1355, 1964)

that there was no direct correlation between the degree of cytologic atypia and the dosage of the drug, as shown in Table 22-3. Histologic changes in biopsies of the bladder show very marked epithelial abnormalities, which, at the height of the cyclophosphamide effect, are akin to carcinoma in situ (Fig. 22-45), but can regress after cessation of therapy. It has been shown by Jayalakshmamma and Pinkel that simultaneous radiotherapy enhances the effects of cyclophosphamide on the bladder.

The cytologic changes caused by cyclophosphamide should not be confused with synchronous urothelial cell abnormalities due to human polyomavirus infection (Fig. 22-46). The drug has an immunosuppressive effect, and thus, it may contribute to reactivation of the virus. The polyomavirus-induced changes are quite common in these patients. As discussed on p. 909, there is no evidence whatever that the polyomavirus activation has any bearing whatever on the occurrence of hemorrhagic cystitis in patients with bone marrow transplants (Cottler-Fox et al., 1989).

Experimental evidence (Koss, 1967) supports the view that metabolites of cyclophosphamide exercise a direct and marked effect on the epithelium of the bladder: in the rat, a single intraperitoneal injection of the drug in the dose of 200 or 400 mg/kg produced a rapid necrosis of the bladder epithelium, followed by a marked atypical hyperpla-

Table 22-3
The Effect of Cyclophosphamide on the Epithelium of the Urinary Bladder

Dose/Day (mg)	Administration	Total Dose (g)	Effect
150	Oral	3.6	Marked
50–100	Oral	6.0	Marked
100–300	Oral	226.0	Marked
300–350	Oral	25.0	Marked
15 Patients		5–25	Slight to moderate
3 Patients		5.0	Slight

(Modified from Forni, A.M., et al.: Cytological study of the effect of cyclophosphamide on the epithelium of the urinary bladder in man. Cancer, *17*:1348–1355, 1964)

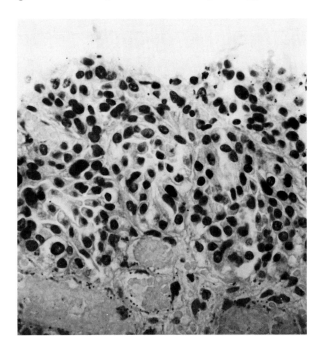

FIGURE 22-45. Effects of cyclophosphamide: bladder biopsy. Marked hyperplasia and atypia observed at the height of hemorrhagic cystitis in a patient with a malignant lymphoma. Note hemorrhage in the lamina propria beneath the epithelium. (×250)

sia. Cells from the hyperplastic epithelium showed a marked atypia, comparable with that observed in human material (Fig. 22–47).

Cyclophosphamide-induced abnormalities are not confined to the epithelium. There is experimental evidence that subepithelial blood vessels and smooth muscle of the bladder may be severely damaged. It has also been recorded that, in children, fibrosis of the bladder wall may occur after exposure to this potent drug.

In most patients, the effects of cyclophosphamide are transient and may be prevented by proper administration of the drug. However, the most significant complication of cyclophosphamide therapy has been the occurrence of bladder cancer recorded in several patients after long-term administration of large doses of the drug for unrelated malignant disease, usually a lymphoma (Worth; Dale and Smith; Wall and Clausen). A case of carcinoma of the renal pelvis was also recorded under

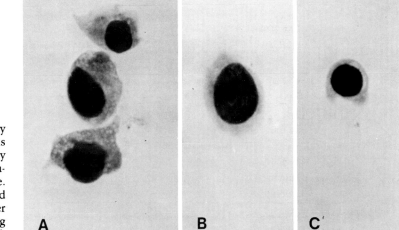

FIGURE 22-46. (*A, B, C*) Urinary sediment. Enlarged urothelial cells with nuclear inclusions caused by human polyomavirus infection in a patient treated with cyclophosphamide. Patient with malignant lymphoma and hemorrhagic cystitis, observed after the administration of 15 g of the drug in large daily doses. (*A, B, C* ×1,000)

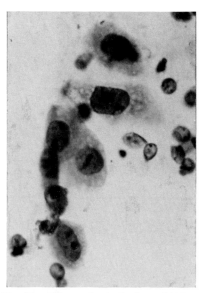

FIGURE 22–47. Effects of a single dose of 200 mg/kg of cyclophosphamide on the epithelium of the urinary bladder in the rat. Note striking abnormalities of epithelial cells, particularly large nucleoli, occurring 72 hours after the administration of the drug. (×560)

similar circumstances (Fuchs et al.). An excess of bladder cancer was observed in patients treated with cyclophosphamide for Hodgkin's disease (Pedersen-Bjergaard, 1988) and non-Hodgkin's lymphomas (Travis et al., 1989). Although in some of the older patients, the bladder cancer may have been an incidental new primary tumor, some of the observed patients were sufficiently young to suggest that the drug acted as a carcinogenic agent. This possibility is not unique to cyclophospha-

mide, and it has also been suggested for other alkylating agents (see p. 679). Recently, a squamous carcinoma of the bladder was personally observed in a 19-year-old girl with a history of 24 months of cyclophosphamide therapy (Fig. 22–48). A case of leiomyosarcoma of the bladder has also been observed, (Fig. 22–49). These still-sporadic observations strongly suggest that cytologic follow-up of patients receiving cyclophosphamide therapy is prudent. In patients in whom cell abnormalities develop and persist after cessation of therapy, a clinical investigation of the bladder is warranted.

The Effect of Other Akylating Agents on Urinary Tract Epithelia

Busulfan, the marked effects of which on the epithelia of the cervix and the lung were described on pages 675 and 753, also exercises such an effect on the urinary tract. Large cells with atypical large nuclei may be observed in renal tubules (Fig. 22–50*A*). The epithelium of the renal pelvis and of the urinary bladder may show striking changes closely resembling those of carcinoma in situ (Fig. 22–50*B*; cf. Fig. 23–26). Therefore, it is not surprising that the urinary sediment of patients receiving busulfan may contain abnormal epithelial cells, difficult to differentiate from cancer cells (see Fig. 22–50*C*). The role of busulfan as a possible carcinogenic agent was discussed in extenso in Chapter 19, to which the reader is referred for further information.

Effects of Intravesical Therapy

A number of drugs such as triethylenethiophosphoramide (thiotepa), doxorubicin hydrochloride

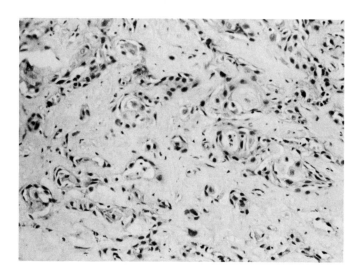

FIGURE 22–48. Infiltrating squamous carcinoma of bladder observed in a 19-year-old woman with a history of 24 months of cyclophosphamide therapy. (×150)

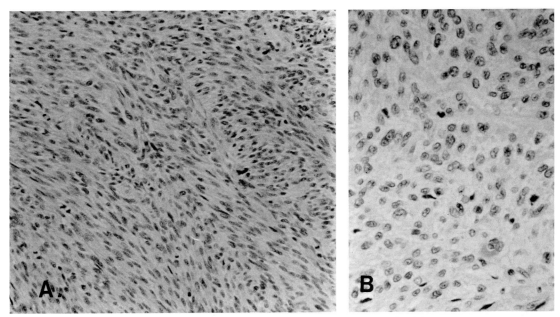

FIGURE 22-49. (*A, B*) A huge low-grade leiomyosarcoma of the urinary bladder, necessitating cystectomy, observed in a 17-year-old man after several hundred grams of cyclophosphamide therapy for a malignant lymphoma (*A* ×150; *B* ×350. Case courtesy of Dr. Lawrence Roth, Indianapolis, Indiana)

(Adriamycin), mitomycin, and immunotherapy with the attenuated *Mycobacterium bovis* strain, bacillus Calmette-Guérin (BCG), are being used intravesically for treatment of some bladder cancers, mainly carcinoma in situ and for prevention of recurrences of papillary tumors. In my experience, urothelial cell changes observed with these drugs are relatively trivial and consists of a radiomimetic effect (cell and nuclear enlargement) and multinucleation. I have not seen any drug-induced nuclear abnormalities that mimic carcinoma (except for an occasional polyomavirus activation; see above). Thus, the presence of identifiable cancer cells in the urinary sediment during the monitoring of such patients usually indicates a lack of tumor response to treatment. (For further discussion, see Chap. 23, p. 990.)

In experimental dogs treated with intravesical doxorubicin and thiotepa similar observations were recorded: cell and nuclear enlargement, multinucleation, and karyorrhexis were the principal transient abnormalities noted (Rasmussen et al., 1980).

As discussed on p. 906, tubercles, indistinguishable from other forms of tuberculosis, may occur in bladder wall during treatment with BCG. Epithelial cells and Langhans' -type giant cells may be observed in the urinary sediment.

Aspirin and Phenacetin

Prescott pointed out that the nephrotoxic effect of these drugs may be assessed in urinary sediment by performing counts of renal tubular cells. This is best accomplished by staining the sediment by the method described by Prescott and Brodie (see p. 933), which stains leukocytes deep blue, renal tubular cells pink, and erythrocytes red. This method was used by Prescott to demonstrate a marked increase in the desquamation of renal tubular cells in patients receiving aspirin, phenacetin, and related drugs. The significance of these drugs in the causation of carcinoma of the renal pelvis is discussed on p. 972.

URINARY SEDIMENT IN ORGAN TRANSPLANTATION

One of the greatest medical advances of our era has been the ability to substitute a diseased organ of a patient with a transplanted organ (allograft) obtained either from a living or deceased donor. Although the knowledge of human immunology has made great strides and much more is known about the mechanisms of tissue matching and prevention of tissue rejection than a few years ago, neverthe-

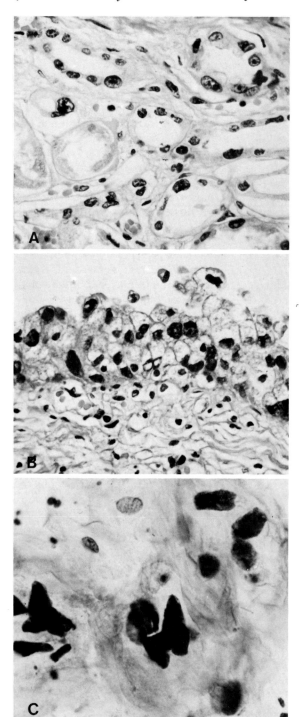

FIGURE 22–50.   Effects of busulfan on the urinary tract epithelial. (*A*) Renal tubules, showing variable numbers of cells with substantially enlarged nuclei. (*B*) Epithelium of urinary bladder, showing changes closely similar to those of spontaneously occurring carcinoma in situ. (*A*, *B*) are from the same patient, who received busulfan for nearly 10 years for chronic myelogenous leukemia. (*C*) Urinary sediment from a patient receiving busulfan for 30 months. Striking cell abnormalities are evident. (*A*, *B* ×350; *C* ×560. *C*: Koss, L.G., et al.: The effect of busulfan on human epithelia. Am. J. Clin. Pathol., *44*:385–397, 1965)

less, the rejection of the transplanted organ by the recipient remains a serious risk in every case. It is beyond the scope of this work to discuss all the manifestations of organ rejection phenomena. Only some of the effects on the urinary sediment will be discussed here in reference to bone marrow and renal transplantation.

Bone Marrow Transplantation

The procedure is used in patients with treatment-resistant leukemias and lymphomas and in the treatment of some solid tumors. More recently, attempts have been made to treat in this fashion patients with nonmalignant blood disorders (summary in Stella et al., 1987). The preparation of the patients for a bone marrow transplant involves total body irradiation and large doses of drugs, such as cyclophosphamide and busulfan (summary in Cottler-Fox et al., 1989). Both radiation and drugs may affect the urothelial cells when applied singly, as discussed above. The combination of these procedures may be very difficult to interpret.

Perhaps the most common event is the activation of polyomavirus infection, with resulting nuclear inclusions, described and illustrated on p. 909. Changes caused by radiotherapy and by cyclophosphamide may also occur simultaneously. Cell changes mimicking (or perhaps representing) cancer may be observed. Thanks to Dr. Denise Hidvegi of Chicago, tissue evidence supporting the cytologic findings could be recorded in Fig. 22–51. Because the patient died, the long-term clinical significance of the epithelial abnormalities illustrated in Fig. 22–51 *C, D* is unknown. On the other hand, it is known that organ transplant patients are prone to develop various forms of cancer, including carcinomas and malignant lymphomas (see discussion of this topic in Chap. 18). Hence, it remains a possibility that carcinomas in situ of the urinary bladder may occur in transplant patients.

Renal Transplantation

The monitoring of renal rejection by urinary sediment analysis was proposed in the late 1960s. Bossen et al. (1970) studied a profile of urinary sediment that was composed of seven features observed before and during episodes of renal allograft rejection. These features were nuclear degeneration, tubular casts, erythrocytes, necrotic material forming background of smears ("dirty background"), mixed cell clusters (epithelial and leukocytes), lymphocytes, and tubular cells. At least five of these features were observed in every patient prior to episodes of rejection. The two most constant features were the presence of lymphocytes and of tubular cells. The mere cellularity of the smears was a hint of impending rejection. In the absence of rejection, the urinary sediment had low cellularity and a clean background. Prior to and during rejection episodes the sediment was cellular and the background contained necrotic material. If the rejection episode was controlled by therapy, there was an improvement in the profile of features discussed above. Bossen et al. recommend an evaluation of the urinary sediment profile for monitoring renal transplants as more reliable than any single feature, such as the presence of lymphocytes or tubular cells, as previously advocated by Kauffman et al., and by Taft and Flax. Schumann et al. advocated the use of the cytocentrifuge for the study of urinary sediment and confirmed that the presence of tubular cells, singly or in casts, was of great prognostic value of impending rejection (Fig. 22–52).

In a subsequent communication, Schumann et al. (1981) discussed at length the criteria for recognition of renal fragments and tubular cells in the urinary sediment. These authors stressed the close relationship of tubular cells with casts and the cylindric fragments corresponding to tubular cells. With the use of Bales' method of urine fixation and processing, the recognition of casts in the sediment is significantly enhanced (see Fig. 22–52).

Cyclosporine Effect

Cyclosporine is an immunomodulatory drug extensively used in organ transplant recipients to prevent rejection. The drug affects renal function in about 30% of the patients. Winkelmann et al. (1985) and Stella et al. (1987) described necrosis of epithelial cells derived from renal tubular epithelium and the presence of "tissue fragments" in the urine of bone marrow transplant patients as evidence of cyclosporine toxicity. So far as one could judge from the photographs, the changes were not specific. Similar conclusions were reached by Stilmont et al. (1987). Most unfortunately, many people knowledgeable about organ transplants who write about the cytologic findings in the urinary sediment are not familiar with the scope of urinary cytology. A number of published articles confuse common findings with transplant-specific findings. The reader should be skeptical reading much

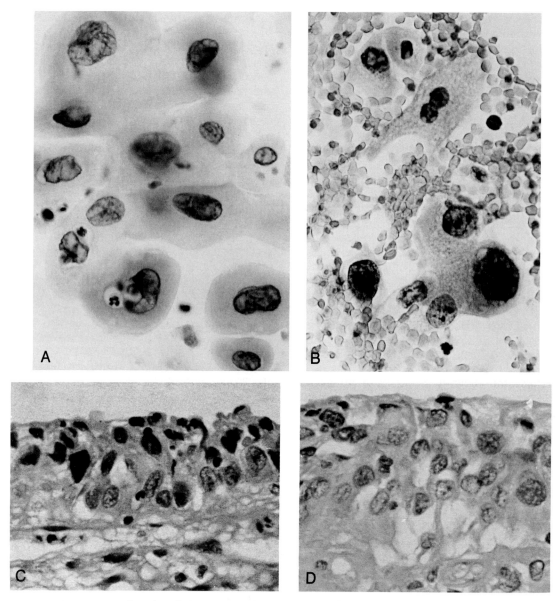

FIGURE 22–51. (*A–D*) Cell abnormalities in voided urine and bladder tissue in a 43-year-old man, who was a recipient of a bone marrow transplant. (*A*) Urothelial cells with radiomimetic effect. Note the symmetric enlargement of the cells and their nuclei and the presence, in some cells, of intranuclear and intracytoplasmic vacuoles. (*B*) Urothelial cells with distortion of shape, huge hyperchromatic, densely granular nuclei and altered nucleocytoplasmic ratio. For all intents and purposes, these are cancer cells. (*C*) Bladder biopsy showing epithelial changes consistent with a flat carcinoma in situ (cf. Figs. 23–21, 23–25). (*D*) Bladder epithelium obtained at autopsy 6 weeks later. There is a persistent major epithelial abnormality, similar to that shown in (*C*). (*A, B* ×560; *C, D* ×430. Courtesy Dr. Denise Hidvegi, Chicago, Illinois)

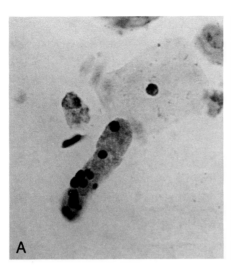
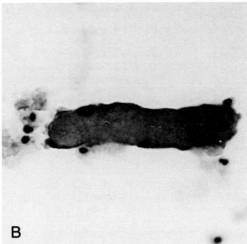

FIGURE 22–52. (*A, B*) Renal casts in voided urine specimens prepared by the method of Bales (see p. 1465). (*A*) Cellular cast composed of renal tubular cells. (*B*) Hyaline cast. (*A, B* ×560)

of the published work on this subject by people with limited experience.

Because the allograft recipients routinely receive immunosuppressive drugs, they are subject to infections by agents that are uncommonly observed in nonsuppressed patients. These are mainly viral agents which have been discussed in detail on p. 907. Such patients also run a substantial risk of developing malignant tumors, such as malignant lymphomas or other cancers, as discussed in Chapter 18.

OTHER RENAL DISORDERS

Eggensperger et al. (1989) described the use of "cytodiagnostic urinalysis" as a "new laboratory test," applicable to the diagnosis of renal disorders. The authors used fairly conventional cytologic techniques for routine urinalysis to identify renal tubular cells and casts as an expression of renal parenchymal disease (see also comment on Holmquist's work on p. 986).

BIBLIOGRAPHY

Urothelium: Structure and Function

Alm, P., and Colleen, S.: A histochemical and ultrastructural study of human urethral uroepithelium. Acta Pathol. Microbiol. Immunol. Scand., *90*:103–111, 1982.

Alroy, J., Pauli, B.U., Weinstein, R.S., and Merk, F.B.: Association of asymmetric unit membrane plaque formation in the urinary bladder of adult humans with therapeutic radiation. Experientia, *33*:1645–1647, 1977.

Foot, N.C.: Glandular metaplasia of the epithelium of the urinary tract. South. Med. J., *37*:137–142, 1944.

Herz, F., Gazivoda, P., Papenhausen, P.R., Katsuyama, J., and Koss, L.G.: Normal human urothelial cells in culture. Subculture procedure, flow cytometric and chromosomal analyses. Lab. Invest., *53*:571–574, 1985.

Herz, F., Schermer, H.F., and Koss, L.G.: Short term culture of epithelial cells from urine of adults. Proc. Soc. Exp. Biol. Med., *161*:153–157, 1979.

Hicks, R.M.: The function of the Golgi complex in transitional epithelium. Synthesis of the thick cell membrane. J. Cell Biol., *30*:623–643, 1966.

Hicks, R.M.: The mammalian urinary bladder: An accommodating organ. Biol. Rev., *50*:215–246, 1975.

Hicks, R.M.: The permeability of rat transitional epithelium. Keratinization and the barrier to water. J. Cell Biol., *28*:21–31, 1966.

Hicks, R.M., and Newman, J.: Scanning electron microscopy of urinary sediment. *In* Koss, L.G., and Coleman, D.V. (eds): Advances in Clinical Cytology, vol. 2, pp. 135–161. Masson Publishing, New York, 1984.

Hicks, R.M., Wakefield, J.S.J., and Chowaniec, J.: Evaluation of a new model to detect bladder carcinogens or co-carcinogens: Results obtained with saccharin, cyclamate and cyclophosphamide. Chem. Biol. Interact., *11*:225–233, 1975.

Ito, N., Hirose, M., Shirai, T., Tsuda, H., Nakanishi, K., and Fukushima, S.: Lesions of the urinary bladder epithelium in 125 autopsy cases. Acta Pathol. Jpn., *31*:545–557, 1981.

Jacob, J., Ludgate, C.M., Forde, J., and Tulloch, W.S.: Recent observations on the ultrastructure of human urothelium.

1. Normal bladder of elderly subjects. Cell Tissue Res., *543*:543–560, 1978.

Kittredge, W.E., and Brannan, W.: Cystitis glandularis. J. Urol., *81*:419–430, 1959.

Koss, L.G.: The asymmetric unit membrane of the epithelium of the urinary bladder of the rat. An electron microscopic study of a mechanism of epithelium maturation and function. Lab. Invest., *21*:154–168, 1969.

Koss, L.G.: Some ultrastructural aspects of experimental and human carcinoma of the bladder. Cancer Res., *37*:2824–2835, 1977.

Levi, P.E., Cooper, E.H., Anderson, C.K., and Williams, R.E.: Analysis of DNA content, nuclear size and cell proliferation of transitional cell carcinoma in man. Cancer, *23*:1074–1085, 1969.

Martin, B.F.: Cell replacement and differentiation in transitional epithelium; a histological and autoradiographic study of the guinea-pig bladder and ureter. J. Anat., *112*:433–455, 1972.

Morse, H.D.: The etiology and pathology of pyelitis cystica, ureteritis cystica, and cystitis cystica. Am. J. Pathol., *4*:33–50, 1928.

Newman, J., and Hicks, R.M.: Surface ultrastructure of the epithelia lining the normal human lower urinary tract. Br. J. Exp. Pathol., *62*:232–251, 1981.

Pund, E.R., Yount, H.A., and Blumberg, J.M.: Variations in morphology of urinary bladder epithelium. Special reference to cystitis glandularis and carcinomas. J. Urol., *68*:242–251, 1952.

Shokri-Tabibzadeh, S., Herz, F., and Koss, L.G.: Fine structure of cultured epithelial cells derived from voided urine of normal adults. Virchows Arch. [B], *39*:41–48, 1982.

Streitz, J.M.: Squamous epithelium in the female trigone. J. Urol., *90*:62–66, 1963.

Tyler, D.E.: Stratified squamous epithelium in the vesical trigone and urethra: Findings correlated with the menstrual cycle and age. Am. J. Anat., *111*:319–325, 1962.

Wiener, D.P., Koss, L.G., Sablay, B., and Freed, S.Z.: The prevalence and significance of Brunn's nests, cystitis cystica and squamous metaplasia in normal bladders. J. Urol., *122*:317–321, 1979.

Yu, J., Manabe, M., Wu, X.R., Xu, C., Surya, B., and Sun, T.T.: Uroplakin I: A 27-kD protein associated with the asymmetric unit membrane of mammalian urothelium. J. Cell Biol. *111*:1207–1216, 1990.

Benign Disorders and Effects of Treatment in Urinary Sediment

Apperley, J.F., Rice, S.J., Bishop, J.A., et al.: Late-onset hemorrhagic cystis associated with urinary excretion of polyomaviruses after bone marrow transplantation. Transplantation, *43*:108–112, 1987.

Arthur, R.R., Shah, K.V., Baust, S.T., Santos, G.W., and Saral, R.: Association of BK viruria with hemorrhagic cystis in recipients of bone marrow transplants. N. Engl. J. Med., *315*:230–234, 1986.

Ashton, P.R., and Lambird, P.A.: Cytodiagnosis of malakoplakia. Report of a case. Acta Cytol., *14*:92–94, 1970.

Bales, C.E.: A semi-automated method for preparation of urine sediment for cytologic evaluation. Acta Cytol., *25*:323–326, 1981.

Bancroft, J., Seybolt, J.F., and Windhager, H.A.: Cytologic diagnosis of cytomegalic inclusion disease. Acta Cytol., *5*:182–186, 1961.

Bard, R.H.: The significance of asymptomatic hematuria in women and its economic implications—a ten year study. Arch. Intern. Med., *148*:2629–2632, 1988.

Bellin, H.J., Cherry, J.M., and Koss, L.G.: Effects of a single dose of cyclophosphamide. V. Protective effect of diversion of the urinary stream on dog bladder. Lab. Invest., *30*:43–47, 1974.

Berger, J.R., Kaszovitz, B., Post, M.J., and Dickinson, G.: Progressive multifocal leukoencephalopathy associated with human immunodeficiency virus infection: A review of the literature with a report of sixteen cases. Ann. Intern. Med., *107*:78–87, 1987.

Berkson, B.M., Lome, L.G., and Shapiro, I.: Severe cystitis induced by cyclophosphamide. Role of surgical management. JAMA, *225*:605–606, 1973.

Blanc, W.A.: Cytologic diagnosis of cytomegalic inclusion disease in gastric washings. Am. J. Clin. Pathol., *28*:46–49, 1957.

Bolande, R.P.: Inclusion-bearing cells in urine in certain viral infections. Pediatrics, *24*:7–12, 1959.

Bonikos, D.S., and Koss, L.G.: Acute effects of cyclophosphamide on rat urinary bladder muscle. Arch. Pathol., *97*:242–245, 1974.

Bossen, E.H., and Johnston, W.W.: Exfoliative cytopathologic studies in organ transplantation. IV. The cytologic diagnosis of herpesvirus in the urine of renal allograft recipients. Acta Cytol., *19*:415–419, 1975.

Bossen, E.H., and Johnston, W.W.: Exfoliative cytopathologic studies in organ transplantation. V. The diagnosis of rejection in the immediate postoperative period. Acta Cytol., *21*:502–507, 1977.

Bossen, E.H., Johnston, W.W., Amatulli, J., and Rowlands, D.T.: Exfoliative cytopathologic studies in organ transplantation I. The cytologic diagnosis of cytomegalic inclusions disease in the urine of renal allograft recipients. Am. J. Clin. Pathol., *52*:340–344, 1969.

Bossen, E.H., Johnston, W.W., Amatulli, J., and Rowlands, D.T.: Exfoliative cytopathologic studies in organ transplantation. III. The cytologic profile of urine during acute renal allograft rejection. Acta Cytol., *14*:176–181, 1970.

Buckner, C.D., Rudolph, R.H., Fefer, A., Clift, R.A., and Epstein, R.B.: High dose cyclophosphamide therapy for malignant disease. Toxicity, tumor response, and the effects of stored autologous marrow. Cancer, *29*:357–365, 1972.

Carson, I.C.C., Segura, J.W., and Greene, L.F.: Clinical importance of microhematuria. JAMA, *241*:149–50, 1979.

Chang, S.C.: Urinary cytologic diagnosis of cytomegalic inclusion disease in childhood leukemia. Acta Cytol., *14*:338–343, 1970.

Chappell, L.H., and Lundin, L.: A pitfall in urine cytology. A case report. Acta Cytol., *20*:162–163, 1976.

Clark, B.G., and Gherardi, G.J.: Urethrotrigonitis or epidermidization of the trigone of the bladder. J. Urol., *87*:545–548, 1962.

Clements, M.S., and Oko, T.: Cytologic diagnosis of schistosomiasis in routine urinary sediment. Acta Cytol., *27*:277–280, 1983.

Coleman, D.V.: The cytodiagnosis of human polyomavirus infection. Acta Cytol., *19*:93–96, 1975.

Coleman, D.V.: The cytological diagnosis of human polyomavirus infection and its value in clinical practice. *In* Koss, L.G., and Coleman, D.V. (eds): Advances in Clinical

Cytology, vol. 1, pp. 136–159. London, Butterworths, 1981.

Coleman, D.V., Wolfendale, M.R., Daniel, R.A., et al.: A prospective study of human polyomavirus infection in pregnancy. J. Infect. Dis., *142*:1–8, 1980.

Coleman, D.V., Field, A.M., Gardner, S.D., Porter, K.A., and Starzi, T.E.: Virus-induced obstruction of the ureteric and cystic duct in allograft recipients. Transplant. Proc., *5*:95–98, 1973.

Coleman, D.V., Gardner, S.D., and Field, A.M.: Human polyomavirus infection in renal allograft recipients. Br. Med. J., *3*:371–375, 1973.

Colin, A.L., and Howard, R.S.: Asymptomatic microscopic hematuria. J. Urol., *124*:389–91, 1980.

Connery, D.B.: Leukoplakia of the urinary bladder and its association with carcinoma. J. Urol., *69*:121–127, 1953.

Cordon-Cardo, C., Bander, N.H., Fradet, Y., Finstad, C.L., Whitmore, W.F., Lloyd, K.O., Oettgen, H.F., Melamed, M.R., and Old, L.J.: Immunoanatomic dissection of the human urinary tract by monoclonal antibodies. J. Histochem. Cytochem., *32*:1035–1040, 1984.

Cornish, J., Lecamwasam, J.P., Harrison, G., Vanderwee, M.A., and Miller, T.E.: Host defense mechanisms in the bladder. II. Disruption of the layer of mucus. Br. J. Exp. Pathol., *69*:759–770, 1988.

Cottler-Fox, M., Lynch, M., Deeg, H.J., and Koss, L.G.: Human polyomavirus: Lack of relationship of viruria to prolonged or severe hemorrhagic cystitis after bone marrow transplant. Bone Marrow Transpl., *4*:279–282, 1989.

Cowen, P.N.: False cytodiagnosis of bladder malignancy due to previous radiotherapy. Br. J. Urol., *47*:405–412, 1975.

Crabbe, J.G.S.: "Comet" or "decoy" cells found in urinary sediment smears. Acta Cytol., *15*:303–305, 1971.

Crabtree, W.N., and Murphy, W.M.: The value of ethanol as a fixative in urinary cytology. Acta Cytol., *24*:452–455, 1980.

Csapo, Z., Kuthy, E., Lantos, J., and Ormos, J.: Experimentally induced malakoplakia. Am. J. Pathol., *79*:453–462, 1975.

Dale, G.A., and Smith, R.B.: Transitional cell carcinoma of the bladder associated with cyclophosphamide. J. Urol., *112*:603–604, 1974.

deVoogt, H.J., Beyer-Boon, M.E., and Brussee, J.A.M.: The value of phase contrast microscopy for urinary cytology. Reliability and pitfalls. Acta Cytol., *19*:542–546, 1975.

deVoogt, H.J., Rathert, P., and Beyer-Boon, M.E.: Urinary Cytology. New York, Springer-Verlag, 1977.

Dolman, C.L., McLeod, P.M., and Chang, E.C.: Lymphocytes and urine in ceroid lipofuscinosis. Arch. Pathol. Lab. Med., *104*:487–490, 1980.

Dorfman, H.D., and Monis, B.: Mucin-containing inclusions in multinucleated giant cells and transitional epithelial cells of urine: Cytochemical observations on exfoliated cells. Acta Cytol., *8*:293–301, 1964.

Eggensperger, D.L., King, C., Gaudette, L.E., Robinson, W.M., and O'Dowd, G.J.: Cytodiagnostic urinalysis. Three years experience with a new laboratory test. Am. J. Clin. Pathol., *91*:202–206, 1989.

Eickenberg, H.-U., Amin, M., and Lich, R.J.: Blastomycosis of the genitourinary tract. J. Urol., *113*:650–652, 1975.

Failde, M., Eckert, W.G., and Patterson, J.N.: A comparison of a simple centrifuge method and the Millipore filter technic in urinary cytology. Acta Cytol., *7*:199–206, 1963.

Fetterman, G.H.: New laboratory aid in clinical diagnosis of inclusion disease of infancy. Am. J. Clin. Pathol., *22*:424–425, 1952.

Fisher, E.R., and Davis, E.: Cytomegalic-inclusion disease in adult. N. Engl. J. Med., *258*:1036–1040, 1958.

Forni, A.M., Koss, L.G., and Geller, W.: Cytological study of the effect of cyclophosphamide on the epithelium of the urinary bladder in man. Cancer, *17*:1348–1355, 1964.

Fradet, Y., Islam, N., Boucher, L., Parent-Vaugeois, C., and Tardif, M.: Polymorphic expression of a human superficial bladder tumor antigen defined by mouse monoclonal antibodies. Proc. Natl. Acad. Sci. USA, *84*:7227–7231, 1987.

Freni, S.C., and Freni-Titulaer, L.W.J.: Microhematuria found by mass screening of apparently healthy males. Acta Cytol., *21*:421–423, 1977.

Froom, P., Ribak, J., and Benbassat, J.: Significance of microhaematuria in young adults. Br. Med. J., *288*:20–22, 1984.

Fuchs, E.F., Kay, R., Poole, R., Barry, J.M., and Pearse, H.D.: Uroepithelial carcinoma in association with cyclophosphamide ingestion. J. Urol., *126*:544–545, 1981.

Gardner, S.D., Field, A.M., Coleman, D.V., and Hulme, B.: New human papovavirus (B.K.) isolated from urine after renal transplantation. Lancet, *1*:1253–1257, 1971.

Gardner, S.D., MacKenzie, E.F.D., Smith, C., and Porter, A.A.: Prospective study of the human polyomaviruses BK and JC and cytomegalovirus in renal transplant recipients. J. Clin. Pathol., *37*:578–86, 1984.

Glucksman, M.D.: Bladder cancer after cyclophosphamide therapy. Urology, *16*:553, 1980.

Goudsmit, J., Wertheim-van Dillen, P., van Strein, A., and van der Noordaa, J.: The role of BK virus in acute respiratory tract disease and the presence of BKV DNA in tonsils. J. Med. Virol., *10*:91–99, 1982.

Greene, L.F., O'Shaughnessy, E.J., Jr., and Hendricks, E.D.: Study of five hundred patients with asymptomatic microhematuria. JAMA, *161*:610–613, 1956.

Gupta, R.J., Schuster, R.A., and Christian, W.D.: Autopsy findings in a unique case of malakoplakia. Arch. Pathol., *93*:42–48, 1972.

Harris, M.J., Schwinn, C.P., Morrow, J.W., Gray, R.L., and Brownell, B.M.: Exfoliative cytology of the urinary bladder irrigation specimen. Acta Cytol., *15*:385–399, 1971.

Hellstrom, H.R., Davis, B.K., and Shonnard, J.W.: Eosinophilic cystitis. A study of 16 cases. Am. J. Clin. Pathol., *72*:777–784, 1979.

Henry, L., and Fox, M.: Histological findings in pseudomembranous trigonitis. J. Clin. Pathol., *24*:605–608, 1971.

Heritage, J., Chesters, P.M., and McCance, D.J.: The persistence of papovavirus BK DNA sequences in normal human renal tissue. J. Med. Virol., *81*:143–150, 1981.

Hicks, R.M., and Newman, J.: Scanning electron microscopy of urinary sediment. *In* Koss, L.G., and Coleman, D.V. (eds.): Advances in Clinical Cytology, vol. 2, pp. 135–1961. New York, Masson Publishing, 1984.

Highman, W., and Wilson, E.: Urine cytology in patients with calculi. J. Clin. Pathol., *35*:350–356, 1982.

Hogan, T.F., Borden, E.C., McBain, J.A., Padgett, B.L., and Walker, D.L.: Human polyomavirus infection with JC and BK virus in renal transplant patients. Ann. Intern. Med., *82*:373–378, 1985.

Houff, S.A., Major, E.O., Katz, D.A., Kufta, C.V., Sever, J.L., Pittaluga, S., Roberts, J.R., Gitt, J., Saini, N., and Lux, W.: Involvement of JC virus-infected mononuclear cells from the bone marrow and spleen in the pathogenesis of progressive multifocal leukoencephalopathy. N. Engl. J. Med., *318*:301–305, 1988.

Hunner, G.L.: A rare type of bladder ulcer in women: Report of cases. Boston Med. Surg., *172*:660–664, 1915.

Jayalakshmamma, B., and Pinkel, D.: Urinary-bladder toxicity following pelvic irradiation and simultaneous cyclophosphamide therapy. Cancer, *38*:701–707, 1976.

Johnson, W.W., and Meadows, D.C.: Urinary bladder fibrosis

and telangiectasia associated with long term cyclophosphamide therapy. N. Engl. J. Med., *284*:290–294, 1971.

Johnston, W.W., Bossen, E.H., Amatulli, J., and Rowlands, D.T.: Exfoliative cytopathologic studies in organ transplantation. II. Factors in the diagnosis of cytomegalic inclusion disease in urine of renal allograft recipients. Acta Cytol., *13*:605–610, 1969.

Kahan, A.V., Coleman, D.V., and Koss, L.G.: Activation of human polyomavirus infection—detection by cytologic technics. Am. J. Clin. Pathol., *74*:326–332, 1980.

Kapila, K., and Verma, K.: Cytologic detection of tuberculosis of the urinary bladder. Acta Cytol., *28*:90–91, 1984.

Kauffman, H.M., Clark, R.F., Magee, J.H., Ritenbury, M.S., Goldsmith, C.M., Prout, G.R., and Hume, D.M.: Lymphocytes in urine as an aid in the early detection of renal homograft rejection. Surg. Gynecol. Obstet., *119*:25–36, 1964.

Kaye, W.A., Adri, M.N.S., Soeldner, J.S., Rabinowe, S.L., Kaldany, A., Kahn, C.R., Bistrian, B., Srikanta, S., Ganda, O.P., and Eisenbarth, G.S.: Acquired effect in interleukin-2 production in patients with type I diabetes mellitus. N. Engl. J. Med., *315*:920–924, 1986.

Koss, L.G.: A light and electron microscopic study of the effects of a single dose of cyclophosphamide on various organs in the rat. I. The urinary bladder. Lab. Invest., *16*:44–65, 1967.

Koss, L.G.: Formal discussion of "clinical observations on 69 cases of in situ carcinoma of the urinary bladder." Cancer Res., *37*:2799, 1977.

Koss, L.G.: Urinary tract cytology. *In* Connolly, J.C. (ed.): Carcinoma of the Bladder, pp. 159–163. New York, Raven Press, 1981.

Koss, L.G.: Tumors of the Urinary Bladder. Atlas of Tumor Pathology, and series, Fascicle 11. Armed Forces Institute of Pathology, 1975 (Supplement), 1985.

Koss, L.G.: From koilocytosis to molecular biology: The impact of cytology on concepts of early human cancer. Mod. Pathol., *2*:526–535, 1989.

Koss, L.G., Bartels, P.H., Sychra, J.J., and Wied, G.L.: Computer analysis of atypical urothelial cells. II. Classification by unsuperivsed learning algorithms. Acta Cytol., *21*:261–265, 1977.

Koss, L.G., Melamed, M.R., and Mayer, K.: The effect of busulfan on human epithelia. Am. J. Clin. Pathol., *44*:385–397, 1965.

Koss, L.G., and Sherman, A.B.: Image analysis of cells in the sediment of voided urine. *In* Greenberg, S.D. (ed.): Computer Assisted Image Analysis Cytology. pp. 148–162. Basel, Karger, 1984.

Koss, L.G., Sherman, A.B., and Eppich, E.: Image analysis and DNA content of urothelial cells infected with human polyomavirus. Anal. Quant. Cytol., *6*:89–94, 1984.

Landing, B.H., and Nakai, H.: Histochemical properties of renal lead-inclusions and demonstration in urinary sediment. Am. J. Clin. Pathol., *31*:499–503, 1959.

Lang, D.J., Kummer, J.F., and Hartley, D.P.: Cytomegalovirus in semen. persistence and demonstration in extracellular fluids. N. Engl. J. Med., *291*:121–123, 1974.

Lawrence, H.J., Simone, J., and Aur, R.J.A.: Cyclophosphamide-induced hemorrhagic cystitis in children with leukemia. Cancer, *36*:1572–1576, 1975.

Lewin, K.J., Harell, G.S., Lee, A.S., and Crowley, L.G.: Malacoplakia. An electron-microscopic study: Demonstration of bacilliform organisms in malacoplakic macrophages. Gastroenterology, *66*:28–45, 1974.

Limas, C., and Lange, P.: T-antigen in normal and neoplastic urothelium. Cancer, *58*:1236–1245, 1986.

Loveless, K.J.: The effects of radiation upon the cytology of benign and malignant bladder epithelia. Acta Cytol., *17*:355–360, 1973.

Madersbacher, H., and Bartsch, G.: Eosinophile Infiltrate der Harnblase. Urol. Int., *27*:149–159, 1972.

Masukawa, T., Garancis, J.C., Rytel, M.W., and Mattingly, R.F.: Herpes genitalis virus isolation from human bladder urine. Acta Cytol., *16*:416–428, 1972.

Melamed, M.R.: The urinary sediment cytology in a case of malakoplakia. Acta Cytol., *6*:471–474, 1962.

Melamed, M.R., Koss, L.G., Ricci, A., and Whitmore, W.F.: Cytohistological observations on developing carcinoma of the urinary bladder. Cancer, *13*:67–74, 1960.

Melamed, M.R., and Wolinska, W.H.: On the significance of intracytoplasmic inclusions in the urinary sediment. Am. J. Pathol., *38*:711–718, 1961.

Messing, E.M., Young, T.B., Hunt, V.B., Emoto, S.E., and Wehbie, J.M.: The significance of asymptomatic microhematuria in men 50 or more years old: Findings of a home screening study using urinary dipsticks. J. Urol., *137*:919–922, 1987.

Mohr, D.N., Offord, K.P., Owen, R.A., and Melton, I.L.J.: Asymptomatic microhematuria and urologic disease. JAMA, *256*:224–229, 1986.

Murphy, W.M.: Herpesvirus in bladder cancer. Acta Cytol., *20*:207–210, 1976.

Myerson, D., Hackman, R.C., Nelson, J.A., Ward, D.C., and McDougall, J.K.: Widespread presence of histologically occult cytomegalovirus. Hum. Pathol., *15*:430–439, 1984.

Nolan, I.C.R., Anger, M.S., and Kelleher, S.P.: Eosinophiluria —a new method of detection and definition of the clinical spectrum. N. Engl. J. Med., *315*:1516–1519, 1986.

Norkin, L.C.: Papovaviral persistent infections. Microbiol. Rev., *46*:384–425, 1982.

Nowels, K., Kent, E., Rinsho, K., and Oyasu, R.: Prostate specific antigen and acid phosphatase-reactive cells in cystitis cystica and glandularis. Arch. Pathol. Lab. Med., *112*:734–737, 1988.

O'Conor, V.J., and Greenhill, J.P.: Endometriosis of the bladder and ureter. Surg. Gynecol. Obstet., *80*:113–119, 1945.

O'Flynn, J.D., and Mullaney, J.: Leukoplakia of the bladder. Br. J. Urol., *39*:461–471, 1967.

O'Morchoe, P.J., Riad, W., Cowles, L.T., Dorsch, R.F., and Frost, J.K.: Urinary cytological changes after radiotherapy of renal transplants. Acta Cytol., *20*:132–136, 1976.

O'Reilly, R.J., Lee, F.K., Grossbard, E., et. al.: Papovavirus excretion following marrow transplantation: Incidence and association with hepatic dysfunction. Transplant. Proc., *13*:262–266, 1981.

Oravisto, K.J.: Epidemiology of interstitial cystitis. Ann. Chir. Gynaecol. Fenn., *64*:75–77, 1975.

Padgett, B.L., Walker, D.L., Zu Rhein, G.M., Eckroade, R.J., and Dessel, B.H.: Cultivation of papova-like virus from human brain with progressive multifocal encephalopathy. Lancet, *1*:1257–1260, 1971.

Padgett, B.L., and Walker, D.L.: New human papillomaviruses. Prog. Med. Virol., *21*:1–135, 1976.

Pedersen-Bjergaard, J., Ersboli, J., Hansen, V.L., Sorensen, B. L., Christoffersen, K., Hou-Jensen, K., Nissen, N.I., Knudsen, J.B., and Hansen, M.M.: Carcinoma of the urinary bladder after treatment with cyclophosphamide for non-Hodgkin's lymphoma. N. Engl. J. Med., *318*:1028–1032, 1988.

Piscioli, F., Pusiol, T., Polla, E., Failoni, G., and Luciani, L.: Urinary cytology of tuberculosis of the bladder. Acta Cytol., *29*, 125–131, 1985.

Prescott, L.F.: Effects of acetylsalicylic acid, phenacetin, paracetamol, and caffeine on renal tubular epithelium. Lancet, *1*:91–96, 1965.

Prescott, L.F., and Brodie, D.E.: A simple differential stain for urinary sediment. Lancet, *2*:940, 1964.

Rasmussen, K., Petersen, B.L., Jacobo, E., Penick, G.D., and Sall, J.: Cytologic effects of thiotepa and adriamycin on normal canine urothelium. Acta Cytol., *24*:237–243, 1980.

Reeves, D.S., Thomas, A.L., Wise, R., Blacklock, N.J., and Soul, J.O.: Lack of homogeneity of bladder urine. Lancet, *1*:1258–1259, 1974.

Rosen, S.H., Harmon, W., Krensky, A.M., et al.: Tubulointerstitial nephritis associated with polyomavirus (BK type) infection. N. Engl. J. Med., *308*:1192–1196, 1983.

Rouse, B.A., Donaldson, L.D., and Goellner, J.R.: Intranuclear inclusions in urinary cytology. Acta Cytol., *30*:105–109, 1986.

Schmid, G.H., Hornstein, O.P., Munstermann, M., and Potyka, J.: Periodical epithelial exfoliation of the urinary ducts in the male. Acta Cytol., *16*:352–362, 1972.

Schneider, V., Smith, M.J.V., and Frable, W.J.: Urinary cytology in endometriosis of the bladder. Acta Cytol., *24*:30–33, 1980.

Schumann, G.B., Berring, S., and Hill, R.B.: Use of the cytocentrifuge for the detection of cytomegalovirus inclusions in the urine of renal allograft patients. A case report. Acta Cytol., *21*:167–172, 1977.

Schumann, G.B., Burleson, R.L., Henry, J.B., and Jones, D.B.: Urinary cytodiagnosis of acute renal allograft rejection using the cytocentrifuge. Am. J. Clin. Pathol., *67*:134–140, 1977.

Schumann, G.B., Johnston, J.L., and Weiss, M.A.: Renal epithelial fragments in urine sediment. Acta Cytol., *25*:147–153, 1981.

Schumann, G.B., Lerner, S.I., Weiss, M.A., Gawronski, L., and Lohia, G.K.: Inclusion bearing cells in industrial workers exposed to lead. Am. J. Clin. Pathol., *74*:192–196, 1980.

Sinclair-Smith, C., Kahn, L.B., and Cywes, S.: Malacoplakia in childhood. Case report with ultrastructural observations and review of the literature. Arch Pathol., *99*:198–203, 1975.

Slavin, R.E., Millan, J.C., and Mullins, G.M.: Pathology of high dose intermittent cyclophosphamide therapy. Hum. Pathol., *6*:693–709, 1975.

Smith, B.H., and Dehner, L.P.: Chronic ulcerating interstitial cystitis (Hunner's ulcer). A study of 28 cases. Arch. Pathol., *93*:76–81, 1972.

Smith, M.G., and Vellios, F.: Inclusion disease or generalized salivary gland virus infection. Arch. Pathol., *50*:862–884, 1950.

Spagnolo, D.V., and Waring, P.M.: Bladder granulomata after bladder surgery. Am. J. Clin. Pathol., *86*:430–437, 1986.

Stella, F., Troccoli, R., Stella, C., Battistelli, S., Biagione, S., Giardini, C., Baroncoani, D., and Manenti, F.: Urinary cytologic abnormalities in bone marrow transplant recipients of cyclosporin. Acta Cytol., *31*:615–619, 1987.

Sternheimer, R.: A supravital cytodiagnostic stain for urinary sediments. JAMA, *231*:826–832, 1975.

Stilmant, M.M., Freelund, M.C., and Schmitt, G.W.: Cytologic evaluation of urine after kidney transplantation. Acta Cytol., *31*:625–630, 1987.

Suhrland, M.J., Koslow, M., Perchick, A., Weiner, S., Alba Greco, M., Colquhoun, F., Muller, W.D., and Burstein, D.: Cytologic findings in progressive multifocal leukoencephalopathy. Report of two cases. Acta Cytol., *31*:505–511, 1987.

Taft, P.D., and Flax, M.H.: Urinary cytology in renal transplantation; association of renal tubular cells and graft rejection. Transplantation, *4*:194–204, 1966.

Travis, L.B., Curtis, R.E., Boice, J.D., Jr., and Fraumeni, J.F., Jr.: Bladder cancer after chemotherapy for non-Hodgkin's lymphoma. N. Engl. J. Med., *321*:544–545, 1989.

Valente, P.T., Atkinson, B.F., and Guerry, D.: Melanuria. Acta Cytol., *29*:1026–1028, 1985.

Wall, R.L., and Clausen, K.P.: Carcinoma of the urinary bladder in patients receiving cyclophosphamide. N. Engl. J. Med., *293*:271–273, 1975.

Webber, C.A., and Eveland, L.K.: Cytologic detection of *Wuchereria bancrofti* microfilariae in urine collected during a routine workup for hematuria. Acta Cytol., *26*:837–840, 1982.

Wenzel, J.E., Greene, L.F., and Harris, L.E.: Eosinophilic cystitis. J. Pediatr., *64*:746–749, 1964.

Winkelman, M., Burrig, K.F., Koldovsky, U., Witkowski, M., Grabensee, B., and Pfitzer, P.: Cyclosporin A altered renal tubular cells in urinary cytology. Lancet, *2*:667, 1985.

Worth, P.H.L.: Cyclophosphamide and the bladder. Br. Med. J., *3*:182, 1971.

23

Tumors of the Urinary Tract and Prostate in Urinary Sediment

TUMORS OF THE UROTHELIUM (TRANSITIONAL EPITHELIUM) OF THE BLADDER

Within recent years, a statistically significant increase in the rate of urothelial tumors, mainly tumors of the urinary bladder, has been observed in most industrialized countries (Clemmesen et al., Cole et al., Wynder et al.). It has been known since the publications of Rehn (1895 and 1896) that workers in certain chemical industries are at a high risk for developing bladder tumors and that this risk knows no national frontiers because it is observed in the West and in the East (Hueper; Temkin). However, the increase is not confined to industrial workers. Whether it is general industrial pollution, cigarette smoking, or a combination of these and other, yet unknown, factors, cancer of the lower urinary tract is on the increase. The chemicals 2-naphthylamine, 4-aminodiphenyl (xenylamin), and 4-4'-diaminobiphenyl (benzidine) are known as bladder carcinogens, as is the drug chlornaphazine (Laursen; Videbaek). The compound MBOCA, [4,4' methylenobis (2-chloroaniline)], an analogue of benzidine, has been shown to be tumorigenic (Ward et al., 1988). Women, heavy users of phenacetin, a common analgesic, are also at increased risk for bladder tumors (Piper et al., 1985). There is also evidence that workers in rubber and cable, leather, and shoe repair industries are at a high risk for bladder cancer, although the specific carcinogenic substances have not always been clearly identified. The association of bladder cancer with prostatic enlargement is discussed on p. 1005.

Urothelial tumors of the bladder, ureters, or the renal pelves, regardless of mechanism of origin, share certain common characteristics: most of them are, initially at least, papillary in configuration. It is not uncommon to see patients in whom all three areas are involved by synchronous or metachronous tumors.

There is excellent evidence that the prognosis of papillary tumors depends not only on the grade of tumor abnormality, but also on the level of histologic abnormality of the urothelium peripheral to the visible lesion. The nonpapillary tumors of the urothelium have a natural history different from the papillary tumors.

Classification and Natural History

Within the last 35 years, a major conceptual evolution pertaining to tumors derived form the urothelium has taken place. Cytologic examination of the urinary sediment played a very important role in this regard. At the time of this writing (1991), the urothelial tumors may be classified into two fundamental, although, to some extent, overlapping groups, with different behavioral patterns and prognosis: the low-grade papillary tumors, rarely capable of invasive growth; and the high-grade tumors, papillary or nonpapillary, usually capable of invasive growth, hence, metastases. The separation of these two groups of tumors is based primarily on their morphologic characteristics, but is supported by a number of biologic features, listed in Table 23–1.

Papillary Tumors

Papillary urothelial tumors are by far the most common form of urothelial tumors seen in the practice of urology. The fundamental structure of all papillary tumors is the same. The tumors form a cauliflower, or sea anemone-like protrusion into the lumen of the organ, be it urinary bladder, renal pelvis, or the ureter (Fig. 23–1). On histologic examination, the tumors are composed of a branching central core of connective tissue and vessels, supporting epithelial folds of varying degrees of thickness and abnormality. The thin and delicate branches of the papillary tumor break off easily, leading to the principal symptom of papillary tumors, hematuria. The bleeding is often intermittent, with episodes of hematuria occurring sporadically at the time of voiding. Hematuria may be significant, resulting in grossly bloody urine, or it may be relatively minor, resulting in microhematuria (for discussion of the significance of microhematuria, see p. 903). Hematuria may be associated with other symptoms, such as dysuria and frequency of urination.

The papillary tumors may have a single, thin stalk of connective tissue, commonly observed in tumors of low grade, or may be sessile, i.e., have a broad base, derived from a larger segment of the urothelium.

Grading of Papillary Tumors. In the 1920s Broders, of the Mayo Clinic, observed that the behavior of papillary tumors of the bladder depended significantly on their morphologic make up, hence, grading. The system of histologic grading in current use (Koss, 1975) is summarized in Table 23–2. The grading is based on the degree of epithelial abnormality. Papillomas and papillary tumors grade I share in common urothelial lining that

Table 23–1
Characteristics of Two Groups of Urothelial Tumors

Feature	Low-Grade Papillary Tumors	High-Grade Papillary Tumors and Invasive Carcinomas
Epithelial abnormality of origin	hyperplasia	Flat carcinoma in situ and related abnormalities: atypical hyperplasia (or dysplasia)
Invasive potential	Low	High
Urine cytology	Negative or atypical	Positive
DNA ploidy pattern (see p. 988)	Predominantly diploid	Predominantly aneuploid
Density of nuclear pores (see p. 990)	Normal	Increased
Expression of Ca antigen (epitectin) (see p. 990)	As in normal urothelium	Increased
Blood group isoantigen expression (see p. 988)	Usually present	Usually absent

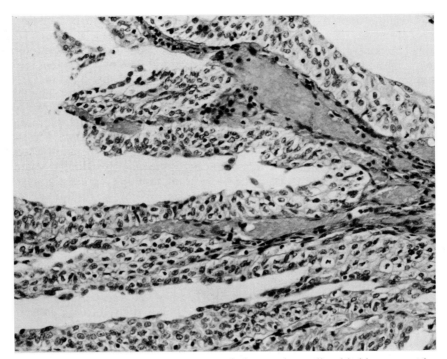

FIGURE 23–1.   Basic histologic structure of a low-grade papillary bladder tumor. The core of the slender papillae is made up of connective tissue carrying capillary blood vessels. The epithelial lining is made up of slightly atypical urothelium (papillary tumor, grade I). (×250)

shows either no deviation or only minor deviation from normal urothelium (see Fig. 23–1). In reference to grade I tumors the term "carcinoma" should not be used. Papillary tumors of higher grades, which are often broad-based or sessile, are usually referred to as *papillary carcinomas*. Papil-lary carcinomas grade III are characterized by a lining composed of highly abnormal cells with major nuclear abnormalities, readily recognized as cancer cells (Fig. 23–2). The common papillary carcinomas grade II are intermediate between the two groups: while retaining the fundamental struc-

Table 23–2
Grading of Papillary Tumors of the Bladder*

	Number of Epithelial Cell Layers	*Superficial Cells*	*Nuclear Abnormalities*	
			Enlargement	*Hyperchromasia*
Papilloma	No more than 7	Present albeit small	Not significant	Absent
Papillary tumors grade I	More than 7	Usually present albeit small	Slight to moderate	Slight in occasional cell
Papillary carcinoma grade II	More than 7 usually marked increase	Variable	Moderate to marked	Slight to moderate in 25–50% of cells
Papillary carcinoma grade III	More than 7 often marked increase	Usually absent	Marked; extreme variability of sizes	Marked in 50% or more of cells

*Note: In practice it may prove difficult to fit any given case into this classification. Intermediate classifications such as I-II or II-III have been used. For all intents and purposes, a separation of tumors grade III from tumors grade IV is not warranted biologically and both groups can be considered as one.
(Modified from Koss, L.G.: Tumors of the Urinary Bladder. Atlas of Tumor Pathology, 2nd series, fascicle 11. Washington, D.C., Armed Forces Institute of Pathology, 1975)

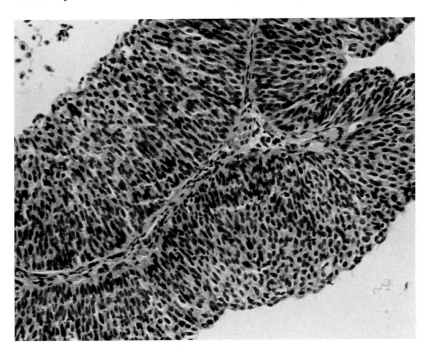

FIGURE 23–2. High-grade papillary tumor, (papillary carcinoma, grade II to III), lined by densely packed small cancer cells. (cf. Fig. 23–1). Such tumors are capable of invasive growth and are often accompanied on their periphery by flat carcinoma in situ and related lesions. (×150)

ture of the urothelium, they show varying degrees of nuclear abnormality and may be difficult to classify precisely. In practice, it is not unusual to observe tumors with a mixture of patterns side by side. Thus, intermediate grades of classification may have to be used, such as grade I–II, II–III, etc. The problems of precise grading, and accordingly, behavior and prognosis of papillary tumors, particularly of the intermediate grade II, have led to several methods of objective analysis, summarized on p. 988. There is good evidence that the grade II tumors may be separated into two prognostic groups, according to their DNA content and perhaps by morphometry. The DNA content of these tumors may be either within normal range (diploid range), or abnormal (aneuploid), a feature that appears to play a major role in clinical behavior (see p. 989).

Behavior Pattern. Papillary tumors, when first seen by a urologist, are either single or multiple and are usually superficial (i.e., they are confined to the urothelium or, at most, extending to the lamina propria). After surgical removal and with the passage of time, new tumors may be observed, usually in other areas of the urothelium, not necessarily within the same organ. Thus patients with initial tumors in the bladder may develop new such tumors in the ureters or the renal pelvis and vice versa. The new tumors may be single or multiple

(Fig. 23–3). The term *recurrence,* which is in common use to describe these events, is inaccurate, inasmuch as the original tumors, if carefully removed, do not recur. Newly formed tumors may be similar to the original papillary tumor or may show different degree of abnormality. The probability of "recurrence" varies with the grade of the tumor: low-grade tumors, such as papillomas or grade I tumors, are less likely to be followed by new tumors than are tumors of grade II or III.

These initial events are shared by all papillary tumors. Subsequent events, however, may vary significantly according to tumor grade. *Low-grade tumors (papillomas, tumors grade I, and some carcinomas grade II, mainly those with a diploid DNA content) very rarely progress to invasive cancer, whereas high-grade tumors [some carcinomas grade II, mainly those with abnormal (aneuploid) DNA content, and all carcinomas grade III] often lead to invasive and metastatic carcinoma.* Invasive carcinoma may develop directly from sessile higher-grade papillary tumors, but it more commonly occurs from adjacent areas of invisible urothelial abnormality, such as carcinoma in situ and related lesions (see below).

Nonpapillary Tumors

Nonpapillary tumors occur in two forms: invasive carcinoma and its precursor lesion, flat carcinoma in situ and related abnormalities.

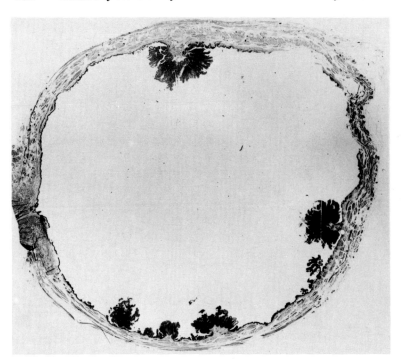

FIGURE 23-3. Cross section of a whole mount of a urinary bladder to show multiple coexisting "recurrent" papillary tumors simultaneously present in several areas. (Courtesy of Dr. R.O.K. Schade, Newcastle-upon-Tyne, U.K. From Koss, L.G.: Tumors of the Urinary Bladder. Washington, D.C., Armed Forces Institute of Pathology, 1975)

Invasive Carcinomas. It has now been documented that, in about 80% of the cases, primary invasive carcinomas of the bladder are *not* preceded by papillary tumors (Brawn, 1982; Kay and Lange, 1982); hence, the conclusion that most of these tumors are derived from invisible and asymptomatic flat lesions, namely, carcinoma in situ (see below).

Invasive carcinomas of the bladder can be graded, usually as grade II or III, and they may show a broad variety of histologic patterns, ranging from urothelial carcinomas, mimicking papillary tumors, to highly anaplastic small-cell cancers, akin to oat cell carcinoma. Other variants, such as squamous carcinoma, adenocarcinoma, or a mixture of types are frequently observed (Fig. 23-4). These variants are reflected in cytologic material (see below).

In the approximately 20% of cases of invasive carcinoma, preceded by papillary tumors, it has been documented by mapping the urinary bladders that invasive cancer is usually derived not from the papillary tumors, but from adjacent epithelial segments showing abnormalities consistent with carcinoma in situ or related lesions (Koss et al., 1974, 1077; Koss, 1979) (Fig. 23-5).

PRECURSOR LESIONS OF INVASIVE UROTHELIAL CARCINOMA

Flat Carcinoma In Situ. Carcinoma in situ of the bladder was first described as "Bowen's dis-

ease" of bladder epithelium by Melicow and Hollowell (1952), a microscopic abnormality of bladder epithelium, accompanying visible papillary tumors (Fig. 23-6). For several years the significance of the lesion was not recognized until a major follow-up study of workers exposed to a potent carcinogen, *p*-aminodiphenyl (Melamed et al., 1960; Koss et al., 1965; Koss et al., 1969). As narrated in some detail below, this study documented that clinically invisible primary carcinoma in situ, identified in the sediment of voided urine by the presence of cancer cells, is a precursor lesion of invasive cancer. Subsequent studies of the origins of primary invasive cancer, cited above, confirmed that carcinoma in situ is the principal precursor lesion of invasive carcinoma.

Thus, two forms of carcinoma in situ can be identified: a primary form, occurring as the initial lesion, and a secondary form, accompanying papillary lesions of the bladder (see Figs. 23-5 and 23-6).

Carcinoma in situ of the urinary bladder cannot be recognized as a tumor on cystoscopic examination. The most common visible alteration is redness of the epithelial surface, sometimes described as "velvety redness," caused by inflammatory changes and vascular dilatation in the underlying stroma. Other changes may mimic inflammation, cobblestone mucosa, interstitial cystitis, etc. However, *many carcinomas in situ do not form any visible abnormalities at all.* The diag-

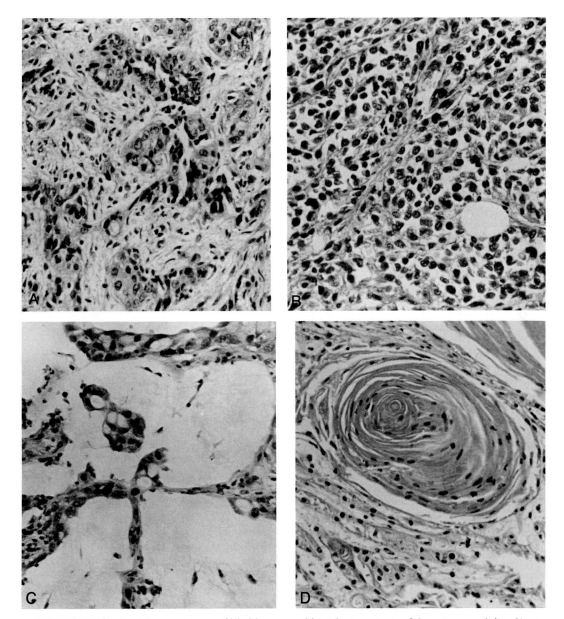

FIGURE 23-4. Invasive carcinoma of bladder: several histologic variants of these tumors. (*A*) Infiltrating urothelial carcinoma; (*B*) solidly growing urothelial carcinoma; (*C*) mucus-producing colloid carcinoma; (*D*) well-differentiated squamous carcinoma. (×150)

nosis of the lesion depends, therefore, either on recognition of cancer cells in the urinary sediment or on a fortuitous biopsy of the epithelium.

Flat carcinoma in situ is recognized histologically as an abnormality of the urothelium composed of cancer cells throughout its thickness (Fig. 23-7D). The epithelium may occasionally show some surface flattening or differentiation. The thickness of the cancerous epithelium and the size of the component cells may vary from one case to

another and is reflected in the size of the cancer cells in the urinary sediment (see Figs. 23-21 to 23-26). Another rare form of carcinoma in situ may mimic Paget's disease and is characterized by the presence of large, clear cancer cells (Koss, 1974; Yamada et al., 1984). Carcinoma in situ may be multicentric and involve several areas of the urothelium. Extension of carcinoma in situ to the nests of von Brunn should not be considered as evidence of invasion. Carcinoma in situ may extend

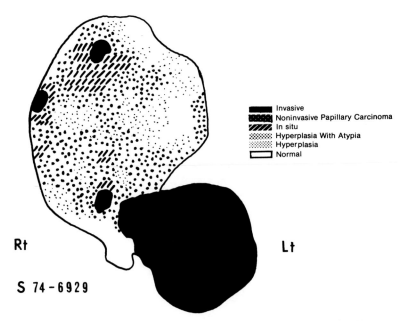

FIGURE 23–5. Map of bladder showing one large, bulky superficially invasive tumor on *right* and three foci of occult invasive carcinoma originating from areas of carcinoma in situ and atypical hyperplasia (Koss, L.G., et al.: Nonpapillary carcinoma in situ and atypical hyperplasias in cancerous bladders. Further studies of surgically removed bladders by mapping. Urology, *9*:422, 1977)

to the ureters. In male patients carcinoma in situ may also extend into the penile urethra and the prostatic ducts.

The most important property of flat carcinoma in situ is its ability to progress to invasive carcinoma. Because the invasion occurs from the deeper portions of the cancerous epithelium, it may completely escape the attention of the urologist, even in patients under close surveillance (Fig. 23–8). Before any major progress in therapy of this disease was made, the rate of progression of untreated carcinoma in situ to invasive cancer was about 60% in 5 years (summary in Koss, 1974). Similar observations were reported by Utz et al. (1970), Schade and Swinney (1973), and Farrow et al. (1977).

There appears to be some difference in behavior of primary carcinoma in situ when compared with the secondary lesions, preceded by or accompanying papillary disease. Prout et al., (1983, 1987) claimed that the progression of the "secondary" carcinoma in situ is less likely to occur. However, in our experience, the difference, if any, is not significant, as documented in Fig. 23–9.

For many years the only form of effective ther-

apy for carcinoma in situ was a cystectomy. At the time of this writing (1991), several alternative forms of therapy are available, such as intravesical immunotherapy or chemotherapy. There is evidence that immunotherapy with bacillus Calmette-Guérin (BCG) has significantly modified the natural history of carcinoma in situ, although it may fail in a substantial proportion of patients. Regardless of mode of therapy, monitoring the patients with flat carcinoma in situ by cytologic techniques is mandatory, as is described on p. 990. The principal features of carcinoma in situ of the urinary bladder are summarized in Table 23–3.

OTHER PRECURSOR LESIONS OF UROTHELIAL TUMORS: THE CONCEPT OF INTRAUROTHELIAL NEOPLASIA

As shown in Fig. 23–7*A–C*, there are other abnormalities of urothelium that can be construed as precursor lesions of urothelial tumors, although not necessarily of invasive cancer. It was proposed (Koss et al, 1985), that all these lesions may be conveniently included under the term *intraurothelial neoplasia* (IUN), and subject to grading in a manner similar to precancerous epithelial abnormali-

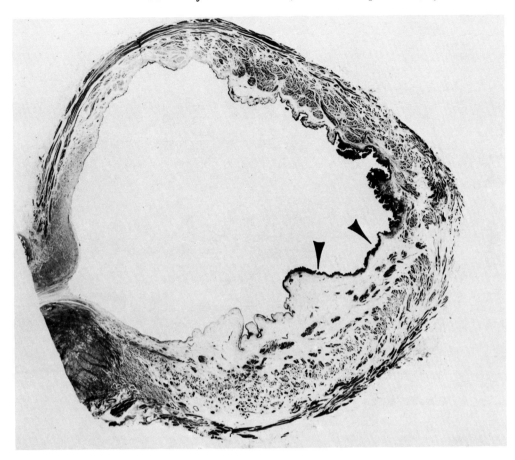

FIGURE 23–6. Whole mount of the urinary bladder to show the association of nonpapillary carcinoma in situ (*arrowheads*) with a papillary carcinoma. (Courtesy of Dr. R.O.K. Schade, Newcastle-upon-Tyne, U.K. From Koss, L.G.: Tumors of the Urinary Bladder. Washington, D.C., Armed Forces Institute of Pathology, 1975)

Table 23–3
Characteristics of Nonpapillary Carcinoma in Situ of the Bladder

- The lesion cannot be recognized cystoscopically as a tumor.
- Cystoscopic abnormalities may mimic inflammation; "velvety redness," "cobblestone epithelium," or "interstitial cystitis" were recorded. In other cases there are no cystoscopic abnormalities whatever.
- The lesion may extend into the ureters.
- In males, the lesion often extends into the prostatic ducts and the penile urethra.
- Because the lesion produces only nonspecific symptoms or may be asymptomatic, its diagnosis is based either on cytology of voided urine or on incidental biopsies of bladder epithelium.
- If untreated, carcinoma in situ will progress to invasive carcinoma in at least 60% of all patients within 5 years.

ties of the uterine cervix (CIN) (see p. 390). Three grades of abnormality of the urothelium may be distinguished: simple hyperplasia (UIN-I), atypical urothelium or atypical urothelial hyperplasia (UIN-II), and markedly atypical hyperplasia ("dysplasia"), which together with carcinoma in situ forms the group of UIN-III.

Simple Urothelial Hyperplasia (UIN-I). As shown in Fig. 23–7*A*, this lesion is represented by a mere increase in the number of epithelial cell layers without any nuclear abnormalities. Two types of hyperplasia may be distinguished: reactive hyperplasia and neoplastic hyperplasia. Reactive hyperplasia may occur in inflammatory processes or as a consequence of an underlying tumor. Neoplastic hyperplasia is the source of well-differentiated low-grade papillary tumors, as shown in experimental

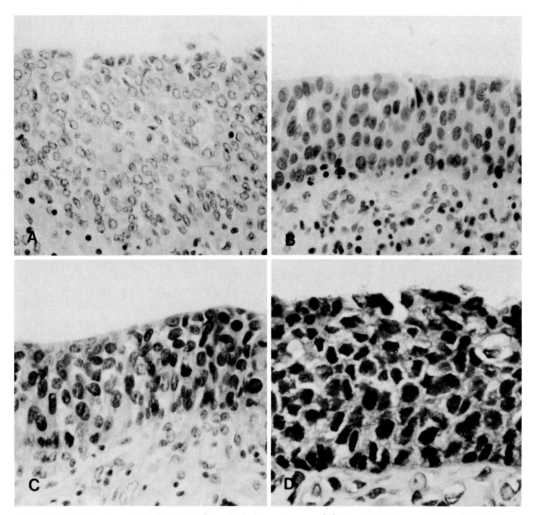

FIGURE 23–7. Precursor lesions of urothelial carcinoma. (*A*) Urothelial hyperplasia (IUN I) — simple increase in the number of cell layers without cytologic abnormalities. (*B*) Atypical urothelial hyperplasia (IUN II). The nuclei of the constituent cells of the epithelium are markedly enlarged when compared with simple hyperplasia. (*C*) Markedly atypical urothelial hyperplasia (IUN III). The makeup of the epithelium is similar to that shown in (*B*) except for marked variation in nuclear sizes and a few hyperchromatic nuclei. (*D*) Nonpapillary carcinoma in situ. The epithelium is made up of cancer cells. (*A–D* ×350)

systems by Koss and Lavin (1971) and Koss (1977). Morphologically, the two types of hyperplasia are identical, and the diagnosis depends on the environment in which this change occurs. The lesion cannot be identified cytologically.

Urothelial Atypia or Atypical Urothelial Hyperplasia (UIN-II). As shown in Fig. 23–7*B*, the urothelial cells show moderate nuclear enlargement, but no significant hyperchromasia. This epithelial abnormality may be a precursor lesion of papillary carcinomas grade II, but its exact signifi-

cance is not fully known. I have not seen an invasive cancer derived from this level of urothelial abnormality, but this possibility can not be excluded. Cytologic atypia may be observed in the presence of this lesion.

Markedly Atypical Urothelial Hyperplasia (UIN-III). As shown in Fig. 23–7*C*, The urothelium shows markedly abnormal enlarged and hyperchromatic nuclei. Although the degree of abnormality is somewhat less than in classic carcinoma in situ (see Fig. 23–7*D*), the differentiation between the two lesions is highly subjective. This

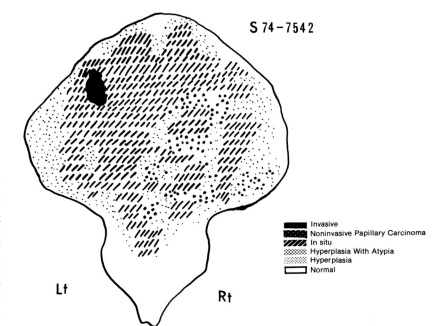

S 74-7542

Lt   Rt

Invasive
Noninvasive Papillary Carcinoma
In situ
Hyperplasia With Atypia
Hyperplasia
Normal

FIGURE 23–8. Map of a bladder with a very extensive secondary carcinoma in situ. An unexpected focus of occult invasive carcinoma was observed (*top left*). (Koss, L.G., et al.: Nonpapillary carcinoma in situ and atypical hyperplasias in cancerous bladders. Further studies of surgically removed bladders by mapping. Urology, *9*:442, 1977)

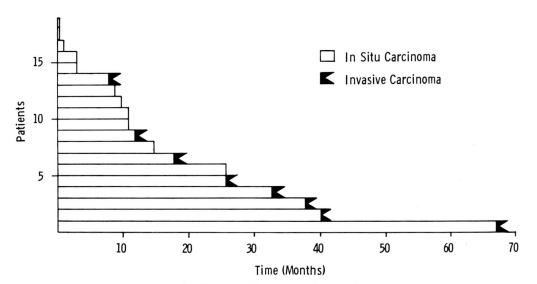

☐ In Situ Carcinoma

◄ Invasive Carcinoma

Patients

15

10

5

10   20   30   40   50   60   70

Time (Months)

FIGURE 23–9. Follow-up study of a group of patients with secondary sessile carcinoma in situ, conservatively treated. There was no history of carcinogen exposure in any of these patients. The black arrows indicate the time of diagnosis of invasive carcinoma. (Melamed, M.R., et al.: Natural history and clinical behavior of in situ carcinoma of the human urinary bladder. Cancer, *17*:1533–1545, 1964)

type of lesion has been designated as "dysplasia" (Murphy and Soloway, 1982), or "carcinoma in situ grade II" (Mostofi, 1979), but all available evidence suggests that the lesion is equivalent in its biologic behavior to carcinoma in situ, described above, and that it has a high potential for progression to invasive cancer (Wolf and Hjgaard, 1983; Harving et al., 1988; Rosenkilde Olsen et al., 1988). The lesion cannot be differentiated cytologically from a carcinoma in situ.

Clinical Significance of Urothelial Abnormalities

In 1960, it was noted by Eisenberg et al. that the prognosis of papillary tumors of the bladder was related to abnormalities in peripheral urothelium adjacent to tumors. In patients with atypical peripheral epithelium, the probability of recurrent tumor or invasive cancer was significantly greater than in patients with normal urothelium. This casual observation was repeatedly confirmed in retrospective studies of bladder tumors by mapping (Koss et al., 1974, 1977; Koss, 1979) and in prospective studies, shown in Table 23–4. It may be noted that the probability of occurrence of invasive cancer in patients with urothelial abnormalities increases with the level of atypia and is very high for patients with peripheral carcinoma in situ. Cytologic monitoring of patients with papillary tumors of whatever grade has for its purpose the detection of such peripheral abnormalities of major prognostic significance.

Table 23–4
Development of Invasive Bladder Cancer in Patients with Grade I or II Papillary Tumors Within 5 Years, According to Status of Peripheral Epithelium

Status of Peripheral Epithelium	No. Patients	Development of Invasive Cancer No. Patients	(%)
Normal	41	3	7
Atypia	25	9	36
Carcinoma in situ	12	10	83
TOTAL	78	22	

(Althausen, A.F., et al.: Non-invasive papillary carcinoma of the bladder associated with carcinoma in situ. J. Urol. *116*:575–580, 1976, with permission)

Staging of Bladder Tumors

The diagram in Fig. 23–10 shows the currently accepted principles of staging of bladder tumors. The staging is also applicable to tumors of the renal pelvis and ureters, although in these organs the therapeutic options are very limited (see p. 975). It may be noted that the staging, hence, prognosis, depends on the depth of invasion and the presence or absence of metastases. In practice, deeply invasive tumors (stages C and D) have a very poor prognosis and do not respond well to radiotherapy or chemotherapy, although there are some rare exceptions to this rule.

The most important concept shown in the left side of Fig. 23–10 pertains to noninvasive tumors. Many years were required for the staging system to recognize the major behavioral and prognostic differences between noninvasive papillary tumors—now designated as Ta—and flat carcinoma in situ—now designated as Tis. Still, even today, it is not uncommon for urologists to speak of noninvasive tumors of both categories as "superficial carcinomas," without recognizing the major differences between the two entities. The difference is particularly significant from the cytologic point of view, as will be set forth below.

The Role of Cytology in the Diagnosis of Urothelial Tumors

Papillary urothelial tumors may be lined either by morphologically normal urothelium or by a urothelium with only slight cellular or nuclear abnormalities. *For obvious reasons, such tumors cannot be identified in cytologic material with any degree of certainty.* Thus, the general concept that all malignant or potentially malignant tumors can be identified in cytologic material because they are made up of abnormal cells does not apply here. *Cytology of the urinary tract is useful only in the identification of tumors or conditions that are associated with perceptible morphologic abnormalities of cells.* This pertains mainly to papillary and nonpapillary carcinomas of high grade and to nonpapillary carcinoma in situ and related atypical hyperplasia (IUN-III). Swedish investigators have used cytologic techniques to assess the grade of urothelial tumors of the bladder. This technique, however, has found little following in the United States.

Thus the primary areas of application of cytologic techniques to the urinary tract are (1) detection and diagnosis of tumors and precancerous

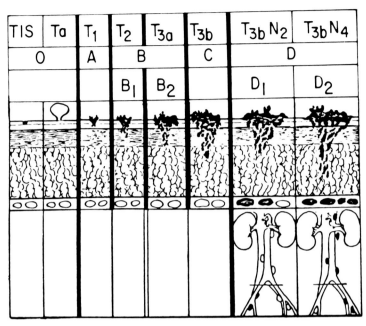

AJC : TNM	TIS	Ta	T_1	T_2	T_{3a}	T_{3b}	$T_{3b} N_2$	$T_{3b} N_4$
JEWETT, STRONG & MARSHALL	O		A	B		C	D	
				B_1	B_2		D_1	D_2

FIGURE 23–10. Modified clinical staging of bladder cancer according to the TNM system. It was recognized that there are two types of noninvasive tumors: flat carcinoma in situ (TIS) and papillary tumors (Ta). The two entities have unequal prognosis inasmuch as most invasive cancers (T_2 and T_3) are derived from TIS (see text). N indicates lymph node metastases to pelvic nodes (N_2) and aortic nodes (N_4). The prognosis of invasive tumors depends on stage.

states of the urinary tract, other than well-differentiated papillary lesions; (2) monitoring of patients treated for neoplastic lesions of the lower urinary tract; and (3) follow-up of high-risk, asymptomatic industrial workers exposed to known carcinogens.

Methods

The simplest way to investigate neoplastic lesions of the lower urinary tract is by cytologic study of voided urine (see p. 895). Bladder barbotage or washings may serve a special purpose, such as DNA measurements by flow cytometry, but, in my experience, they add little to the cytologic diagnosis. Special procedures such as retrograde catheterization and brushings of renal pelvis are discussed on pp. 899 and 900.

Sequential Cytologic Abnormalities in Industrial Workers

An opportunity to observe a group of workers exposed to a potent bladder carcinogen (*p*-aminodiphenyl) over a 12-year period permitted us to es-

tablish cytologic changes in the development of invasive carcinoma of the bladder. The study was based on analysis of cytologic findings in the sediment of voided urine.

Although the sequence of events to be described has been observed primarily in this quasi-experimental industrial situation, there is satisfactory evidence that the natural history of spontaneously occurring carcinoma of the urinary bladder is similar, if not identical. The main difference lies in the nature of the carcinogenic stimulus that, in spontaneous cancer of the bladder, is unknown and, therefore, cannot be accurately timed.

Exposure to *p*-aminodiphenyl results in a high proportion of bladder carcinomas, the disease occurring in no fewer than 10% of the exposed population. The accurate figure may not be available for many years to come.

p-Aminodiphenyl is inhaled, and the products of its metabolism are excreted in the urine within a very short time—no later than 48 to 72 hours after exposure. The initial exposure is usually accompanied by an episode of transient hematuria, with a prompt return to normalcy. There is no evidence that either *p*-aminodiphenyl or its metabolites are stored in the body. Hence it has to be assumed that the genetic damage to the cells of the bladder epithelium, whatever its nature, occurs during the few hours following exposure, even though it may not manifest itself clinically for many years. There appears to be no direct correlation between the amount and length of exposure and the development of cancer of the bladder (Table 23–5). Persons with a casual contact with the carcinogen may develop carcinoma of the bladder, whereas numerous others with prolonged contact may remain free of disease for many years. Thus, a process of natural selection of an unknown nature protects some people from cancer of the bladder, even under most unfavorable conditions.

The Earliest Cytologic Changes

The period of clinical normalcy, accompanied by normal cytologic findings in the urinary sediment, may last for an unpredictably long period, often as long as 10 to 15 or more years. Low-grade papillary tumors may occur during this time.

There follows a period of increasing and identifiable cytologic abnormalities. The earliest changes are slight and affect the nuclei of the epithelial cells; they are akin to dyskaryosis occurring in early precancerous changes of the epithelium of the uterine cervix. Thus, variation of nuclear size, nuclear enlargement, and slight hyperchromasia may be observed. The latter is due to fairly coarse clumping of chromatin and should not be confused with the bland nuclei of "decoy" cells (cf. p. 909). Such dyskaryotic cells appear in the urine intermittently and call for a close follow-up, often lasting several years. These are precursor changes of a high-grade carcinoma. The cystoscopic findings in patients during this stage of the disease may disclose a papillary lesion of low grade or are often essentially neg-

ative. Occasionally, an area of redness or "cystitis" may be observed. A biopsy may yield an area of epithelial hyperplasia with slight nuclear abnormalities (Fig. 23–11).

The Stage of Positive Cytology

Following an unpredictably long period of slight, nonspecific cytologic abnormalities, there follows a period of clearly positive cytologic findings. This may be associated with papillary or nonpapillary clinically obvious high-grade bladder cancer or with nonpapillary (sessile) carcinoma in situ. In the latter situation, the clinical identification of the lesion is difficult. Patients with carcinoma in situ have no specific symptoms. Gross hematuria as the initial symptom is rare. *It is of particular importance that about one-quarter of the patients with carcinoma in situ of the bladder are completely asymptomatic.* Routine urine analysis often shows slight microscopic hematuria and occasional leukocytes. Proteinuria is infrequent in the absence of concomitant renal disease and rarely exceeds a trace. Cystoscopic findings in nonpapillary carcinoma in situ are variable and nonspecific, as discussed on p. 938.

The most commonly affected area, as documented by biopsies, is the floor of the bladder, including the periureteral areas, and the bladder neck. The posterior and lateral walls are next in frequency of involvement. The anterior wall or the dome is rarely affected.

Transition of Carcinoma in Situ to Invasive, Clinically Obvious Carcinoma

The follow-up studies on workers exposed to *p*-aminodiphenyl permitted the accumulation of data pertaining to the duration of the stage of carci-

Table 23–5
Approximate Duration and Amount of Exposure to p-*Aminodiphenyl of 20 Workers With Bladder Cancer*

Relative Intensity of Exposure	Number of Workers	Duration of Exposure Range (yr)	Duration of Exposure Average (Yr)
Maximum exposure, full time	7	2–13	5.3
Maximum exposure, intermittent	4*	2–10	7.0
Moderate exposure	7	4–20	9.6
Slight exposure	2	2–15	

*Two consecutive cancers in one patient.
(Koss, L.G., et al.: Carcinogenesis in the human urinary bladder. Observations after exposure to para-aminodiphenyl. N. Eng. J. Med., *272*:767–770, 1965)

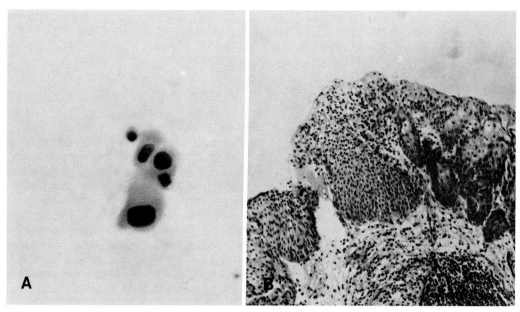

FIGURE 23–11. Borderline lesion of bladder mucosa. (*A*) Very well-differentiated abnormal ("dys-karyotic") cells from the urinary sediment of a 34-year-old woman. There was no known carcinogen exposure in this case.(*B*) The tissue (same case) disclosed hyperplastic epithelium with nuclear atypia (IUN II). Cystoscopically, there was an area of redness. (*A* ×500; *B* ×350)

noma in situ, as diagnosed cytologically. In this group of patients, treatment was usually not instituted before the appearance of a clinically identifiable tumor. This experience is summarized in Table 23–6. At the conclusion of this study in 1970, there were 13 histologically documented instances of primary nonpapillary carcinoma in situ. In 7 of these patients invasive carcinoma developed within 1 or 2 years after the initial diagnosis. The follow-up was inadequate in 3 patients, and in 3 remaining workers cytology remained positive for 1 to 3 years. Unfortunately, no information is yet available on the ultimate fate of these last 6 patients. These data are in general similar to those summarized by Melamed et al. (1964), which pertained to patients seen at the Memorial and James

Table 23–6
Duration of Suspicious or Positive Cytology Until Histologic Proof of Carcinoma — Comparison of Data From 1969 and 1965

	1969		1965	
Duration	Prior carcinoma	No prior carcinoma	Prior carcinoma	No prior carcinoma
<1 yr	1	6	0	0
12–20 mo	0	2	2*	1
21–32 mo	1	2	1	2
33–38 mo	1	1	2	1
50 mo	0	0	1	0
60 mo	0	1	0	0
77 mo	0	0	0	1
Total (26 patients)	3	12	6	5

(Koss, L.G., et al.: Further cytologic and histologic studies of bladder lesions in workers exposed to para-aminodiphenyl: progress report. JNCI, *43*:233–243, 1969)
*One patient with papilloma only.

Ewing Hospitals (see Fig. 23–9). Additional data on several personally observed patients with sessile carcinoma in situ of the bladder occurring ab initio support the view that from 2 to 7 years elapse from the time of initial cytologic observation until the development of invasive carcinoma. This is also in keeping with data from other sources (see p. 940).

Schulte et al. (1986), Crosby, Allsbrook et al. (1991) made fundamentally similar observations on a cohort of workers exposed to β-naphthylamine and benzidine.

The genesis of human bladder cancer may be compared with the processes within the human cervix, the only organ that has had the benefit of similar sustained investigative attention. The cell changes observed in precancerous lesions of the uterine cervix are comparable with the changes observed in developing in situ carcinomas of the urinary bladder. Also, in both organs, the stage of carcinoma in situ appears to precede the appearance of invasive cancer, but it has not yet been proved that every in situ cancer will necessarily proceed to invasive carcinoma within the life span of the patient. However, regression of untreated carcinoma in situ of the bladder appears to be extremely rare. Another major difference between the cervix and the bladder is the time lapse between the occurrence of carcinoma in situ and its progression to invasive carcinoma: this appears to be considerably shorter for the urinary bladder.

Benefits of Cytologic Screening for Industrial Bladder Cancer

The ultimate measure of success in a cancer detection endeavor is the extension of life of good quality for the patients. Unfortunately, the survival rate of workers developing bladder cancer after exposure to *p*-aminodiphenyl was unsatisfactory. The majority of patients died with or of bladder cancer after a survival period of from 5 to 8 years. The usual final events were either metastatic cancer or major complications related to the obstruction of the lower urinary tract.

While the follow-up of high-risk industrial workers has been scientifically a highly rewarding exercise that clarified many points of natural history of bladder cancer, the direct benefit of these studies to the workers in terms of protection from disease and survival remains unclear. Similar doubts were expressed in the United Kingdom (Fox and White). Yet the actual benefits to the society may be more substantial than the survival data may suggest: better medical care for the high-risk patients in general and, in the future, prevention of

exposure to industrial carcinogens, and preventive treatment of nonpapillary carcinoma in situ, may ultimately prove to be of considerable advantage to all patients with bladder cancer.

Cytology of Urothelial Carcinoma

The cytologic diagnosis of neoplastic urothelial lesions is, at times, difficult. The reasons for this difficulty, on one hand, lie in the great morphologic variability of normal urothelial cells and their natural tendency to cluster formation and to polyploidy, resulting in nuclear enlargement (see p. 900). On the other hand, the papillary neoplastic lesions of low-grade (papilloma and papillary carcinoma, grade I) shed cells and cell clusters that usually differ very little from the normal. Consequently, this group of neoplastic urothelial lesions cannot be identified cytologically with any degree of reliability, as will be set forth below.

There is good evidence, discussed in detail on p. 985, that the DNA content of the tumor nuclei goes hand-in-hand with the level of cytologic abnormalities (Koss et al., 1985). Thus, low-grade papillary and other tumors with near diploid DNA content do not form cells that can be morphologically recognized as malignant. Tumors with abnormal (aneuploid) DNA content usually produce recognizable abnormalities.

Urothelial Cancer Cells

The urothelial cancer cells vary in size and may be either smaller or larger than normal urothelial cells. The configuration of cancer cells is variable and may be very bizarre, but the cell shape alone is not a sufficient criterion of identification. The cytoplasm is usually cyanophilic. The nuclei of cancer cells are, as a rule, large for cell size, and a conspicuous change in the nucleocytoplasmic ratio may be noted. The nucleus may be of abnormal shape, although most are spherical or oval, sometimes with small peripheral protrusions. The most important nuclear abnormality in urothelial cancer is hyperchromasia caused by abnormal *nuclear texture:* the chromatin is arranged in large, coarse, tightly packed or superimposed granules, rendering the nucleus dark and nontransparent (Fig. 23–12). This is in marked contrast with benign cells, which have a "salt-and-pepper" appearance due to small chromatin granules, separated from each other by areas of translucent nucleoplasms (cf. Figs. 22–9 and 22–11). Practically speaking, one can "see through" a normal nucleus, but not through the nucleus of a cancer cell. Multi-

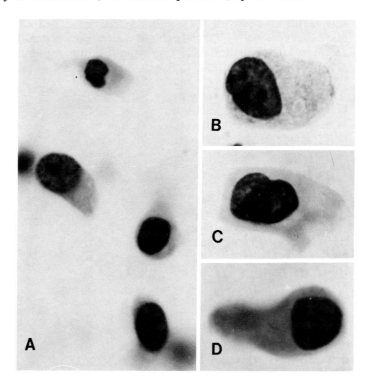

FIGURE 23-12. (*A, B, C, D*) Urothelial cancer cells, voided urine. Urothelial carcinoma, grade III. Note the variability in sizes and shapes of the malignant cells. Note also the altered nucleocytoplasmic ratio. The nuclear features of these cells are well shown and comprise marked hyperchromasia and very coarse nuclear texture, rendering the nuclei nontransparent. Note large nucleoli in some cells. (*A–D* ×1,000)

ple and large nucleoli may occasionally be present particularly in flat carcinoma in situ and in invasive cancer, although they may be difficult to observe because of the marked nuclear hyperchromasia.

Atypical Urothelial Cells

Atypia of urothelial cells is a common finding, particularly in voided urine. Such cells show changes intermediate between normal cells and cancer cells: slight change in the nucleocytoplasmic ratio and an increase in nuclear density, although often below the level associated with obvious cancer (Fig. 23–13). Most of the atypical cells are poorly preserved. Atypical urothelial cells are a common finding in inflammatory conditions (p. 904), lithiasis (p. 914), as a consequence of effects of alkylating drugs (p. 920), and may also occur in the presence of urothelial tumors. In a computerized image-analysis study of atypical cells, an effort has been made to determine whether, by sophisticated objective criteria, atypical cells originating in benign conditions could be separated from those associated with urothelial tumors. Initial statistical analysis disclosed that urothelial cells form a group intermediate between normal and malignant cells. However, the group was made up of two clusters, one sharing cell features with benign cells and the other with malignant cells (Koss et al., 1977). As a consequence of this study, a careful morphologic review of atypical urothelial cells was undertaken on the basis of cell features, with resulting subdivision of atypical cells into two groups. Urothelial cells with nuclei of round or oval configuration and only slight to moderate increase in hyperchromasia were classed as atypical I (ATY-I) and cells with irregular configuration of cytoplasm and of nuclei and greater nuclear hyperchromasia were classed as atypical II (ATY-II) (Fig. 23–14). Subsequent application of this classification rule to the study of 12 patients disclosed that the presence of a high proportion of ATY-II cells was commonly associated with bladder cancer (Koss et al., 1978). It may be assumed from this study that, in spite of the frequent poor preservation of atypical cells, their careful assessment may be of diagnostic benefit. *Although the atypical cells per se do not allow any diagnostic conclusions, the presence of markedly abnormal cells should trigger further search for identifiable cancer cells.*

Scanning Electron Microscopy in the Identification of Urothelial Cancer Cells

Jacobs et al. reported in 1976 the results of scanning electron microscopy of cell surfaces in experimental bladder cancer. The presence of irregular

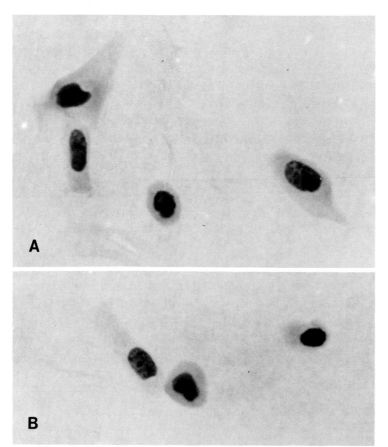

FIGURE 23–13. (*A, B*) Markedly atypical (suspicious) urothelial cells: voided urine. There is considerable variability in cell sizes and shapes. However, the nuclear enlargement is not conspicuous and the degree of nuclear hyperchromasia is only moderate (cf. Fig. 23–12). (*A, B* ×1,000)

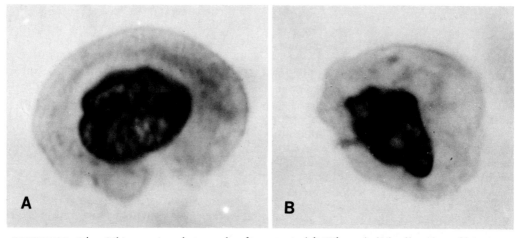

FIGURE 23–14. Oil immersion photographs of two atypical (ATY) urothelial cells, selected by computer as representative of the two groups: ATY I and ATY II. The ATY I cells (*A*) have a cell configuration akin to benign superficial urothelial cells, with a generally smooth cell border. The nucleus, although enlarged and hyperchromatic, approximately follows the configuration of the cytoplasm. The ATY II cells (*B*) have an irregular outline. The irregularly shaped nucleus is dense, but its texture is not quite as coarse as that of frank cancer cells. Although not conclusively diagnostic, ATY II cells suggest the possibility of urothelial cancer (see text).

surface microvilli may be observed during the early stages of carcinogenesis. The applicability of this method to the human sediment was tested in our laboratories (Domagala et al., 1979). The studies disclosed poor preservation of many urothelial cancer cells in the urinary sediment, with loss of surface structure. Some of the better-preserved cancer cells had numerous surface microvilli of uneven length and configuration, similar to those observed in cancer cells in effusion (see p. 1134). The surfaces of benign urothelial and some squamous cells also disclosed the presence of sparse microvilli, albeit of fairly regular configuration. It is of interest that some of the most typical cancer cells in light microscopy failed to disclose surface markers of note. These observations suggest that scanning electron microscopy will not contribute in a major way to the diagnosis of human urothelial cancer in the urinary sediment.

Application of Cytology to the Diagnosis of Urothelial Tumors

Papillary Tumors

Papillary Tumors of Low Grade (Papillomas and Papillary Tumors, Grade I). By definition, papillary tumors of low grade (papillomas and papillary carcinomas, grade I) are lined by normal or only slightly abnormal urothelium (see p. 936). Hence, cells derived therefrom cannot be identified as malignant. Small papillary clusters of cells may sometimes be observed in preparations of spontaneously voided urine. Occasionally, the cells in such clusters are elongated and show either side-by-side arrangement (palisading) or a rosette-like arrangement, with tips of cells converging upon a central point (Fig. 23–15). If this is observed *prior to catheterization or any instrumentation* the possibility of a papillary tumor of low grade may be raised. One must keep in mind, however, that similar findings may also be observed in lithiasis, in marked inflammation, and occasionally without an obvious cause. Perhaps the only exception to this rule is the finding of a papillary cluster of urothelial cells with a central capillary. This very rare finding strongly suggests that the cell cluster represents a broken fragment of a papillary tumor. In filter preparations whereby the urinary sediment is collected and examined directly on the filter membrane, papillary clusters of urothelial cells may be observed in the presence of large or multiple papillary tumors of low grade (Fig. 23–16). Morphologically the cells in such clusters are benign, although the evaluation of the cell detail is often difficult. Again the reservations expressed above must be considered before a cytologic diagnosis of low-grade papillary tumor is rendered with any degree of reliability. Similar conclusions have been reached by the Swedish investigators Esposti and Zajicek (1972).

Wolinska et al. (1985) systematically compared the findings in the voided urine sediment from 51 patients known to have low-grade papillary tumors and 30 controls. The material was obtained from patients without prior cystoscopy. Except for somewhat increased cellularity, an occasional

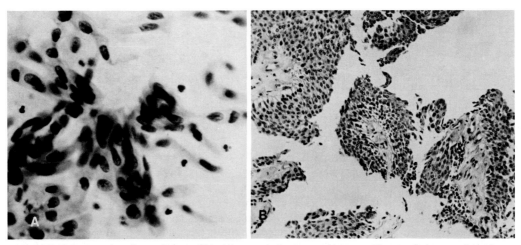

FIGURE 23–15. *(A, B)* Papilloma of bladder: voided urine and biopsy. Cluster of elongated urothelial cells that is sometimes seen in these tumors. The finding is not of diagnostic value, especially if observed after cystoscopy. *(A ×560; B ×150)*

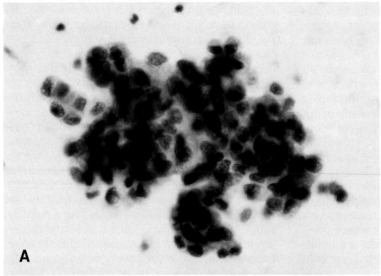

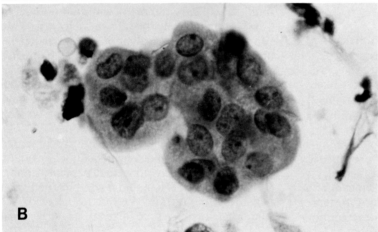

FIGURE 23–16. (*A, B*) Papillary tumors, grade I: voided urine, millipore filter preparations. Large clusters of essentially benign urothelial cells are seen. Although the general configuration of such clusters is suggestive of a papillary tumor, the finding is of diagnostic value only in the absence of any prior manipulation or instrumentation, lithiasis, or inflammation. Note conspicuous chromocenters in (*B*). This finding has no diagnostic value. (*A* ×560; *B* ×1,000)

presence of atypical cell shapes, such as elongated cells, there were no diagnostic findings of note, confirming that the cytologic diagnosis of low-grade papillary tumors cannot be reliably established. These observations and our experience strongly contradict Murphy et al. (1984) who claimed that low-grade papillary tumors could be identified in 62% of patients.

Direct washings or brushings of the urinary bladder contribute little to the diagnosis of low-grade papillary tumors. Harris et al. were able to diagnose such lesions only in cell blocks wherein biopsy-sized fragments of such tumors were observed. Such fragments may also occur in spontaneously voided urine in the absence of a tumor (Fig. 23–17). Kern, using planimetric studies, confirmed the essentially normal configuration of cells derived from such tumors.

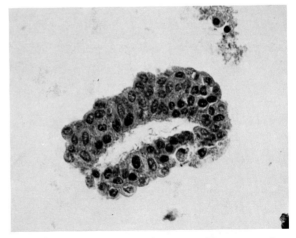

FIGURE 23–17. Papillary fragment of benign urothelium in a cell block preparation of urinary sediment. There was no evidence of tumor. (×350)

Cytology of the urinary sediment does not lend itself to the diagnosis of papillary tumors of low grade. On the other hand, *if the urinary sediment shows obvious cancer cells and the biopsy discloses only a low-grade papillary lesion, the finding is of great clinical importance:* it strongly suggests that a high-grade malignant lesion is present in the urinary tract. This may be another papillary lesion of high grade or, more often, nonpapillary carcinoma, in situ or invasive, located in the bladder, ureters, renal pelvis, or even within the prostatic ducts and the urethra. Every effort must be made to localize and evaluate this lesion or lesions, because of their ominous prognosis.

Papillary Tumors of High Grade (Papillary Carcinomas, Grades II and III).

Most of these lesions are characterized by the presence of urothelial cancer cells, singly and in clusters. Generally the number of single cancer cells increases with the tumor grade. Not all grade II tumors can be recognized cytologically. In 20 of 68 such tumors studied by Koss et al. (1985), only benign or atypical urothelial cells were observed, and the diagnosis could not be established. These were most likely grade II tumors with a DNA content in the diploid range. In aneuploid papillary tumors, grade II, small clusters of cancer cells are fairly common (Fig. 23–18), but cancer cells occurring singly are also invariably present.

Nearly all papillary tumors grade III can be identified by cytology. These tumors shed cancer cells that are often smaller and of variable configuration (Fig. 23–19). The papillary tumors, even highly anaplastic, may shed cancer cells in large clusters, sometimes reminiscent of papillary arrangement of cells. However, single cancer cells are always present. The background usually shows evidence of inflammation and necrosis. Under these circumstances it is impossible to determine whether or not a tumor is invasive. The variability in size and configuration of cancer cells does not offer a helpful clue here (Fig. 23–20). It must be remembered that in the presence of papillary tumors, particularly of high grades, peripheral epithelium of the bladder may be abnormal and show atypical hyperplasia or nonpapillary carcinoma in situ whence occult invasion may take place (see Fig. 23–5). Therefore, a careful investigation of the peripheral bladder by multiple biopsies is always advisable in the presence of positive cytology.

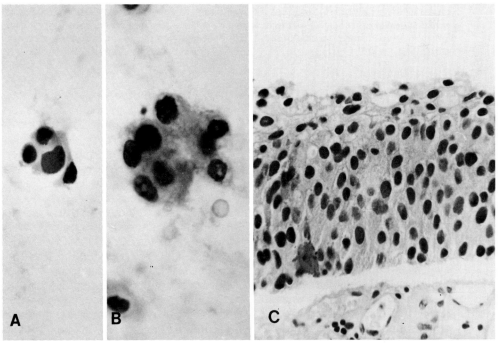

FIGURE 23–18. Papillary carcinoma, grade II. (*A, B*) Clusters of malignant urothelial cells with altered nucleocytoplasmic ratio and the characteristic nuclear changes: hyperchromasia and coarse texture. (*B*) Area of the epithelial surface of the tumor showing nuclear variability and hyperchromasia. (*A, B* ×560; *C* ×350)

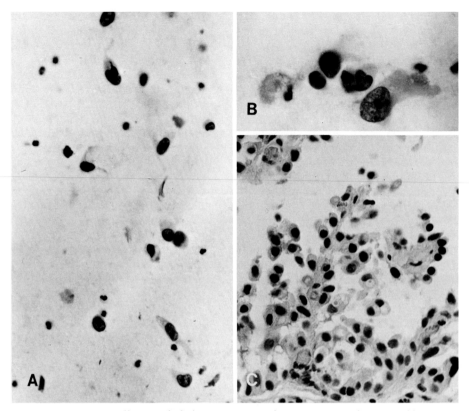

FIGURE 23-19. Papillary urothelial carcinoma, grade III: urinary sediment and biopsies, (*A*) Low-power view of a smear of the urinary sediment to show the great variability in size and configuration of cancer cells. (*B*) Higher-power view of a cluster of cancer cells. The characteristic nuclear features may be noted. (*C*) Biopsy showing the makeup of the tumor. (*A*, *C* ×350; *B* ×560)

Nonpapillary Urothelial Carcinoma

Virtually all nonpapillary urothelial cancers are made up of clearly identifiable cancer cells; hence, the problems encountered with low-grade papillary tumors do not play a role in the cytologic diagnosis. These lesions, particularly the nonpapillary carcinoma in situ, are the principal target of cytologic studies of the urinary tract.

Nonpapillary Carcinoma in Situ. Voided urine sediment is the ideal diagnostic medium for the primary diagnosis of nonpapillary carcinoma in situ, whether located in the bladder, the renal pelvis, the ureters, or the urethra. The processing of urinary sediment by the method of Bales (see p. 1465) usually yields abundant evidence of cancer (see Fig. 23-25). Although the shedding of cancer cells is sometimes intermittent, three specimens of urine obtained on consecutive days are a secure means of diagnosis.

A rather monotonous population of cancer cells of the urothelial type characterizes most, but not all, carcinomas in situ of the bladder. The nuclei are hyperchromatic, dark, and irregular and, unless there is considerable pyknosis, abnormal chromatin texture may be discerned. A coarse filamentous arrangement of the chromatin is especially frequent. Enlarged nucleoli may occasionally be noted. Most carcinomas in situ of the bladder shed small malignant cells and only occasional larger cancer cells (Figs. 23-21 to 23-26). The cancer cells usually appear singly, but occasionally, cells in clusters display similar features. In about one-third of the patients, the population of cancer cells is pleomorphic and cannot be separated from patterns of invasive carcinoma, except by smear background. In the presence of carcinoma in situ, the urine rarely contains more than a few inflammatory cells, and there is usually little evidence of necrosis—contrary to invasive cancer. Rarely, the cellular aberrations in carcinoma in situ may be so

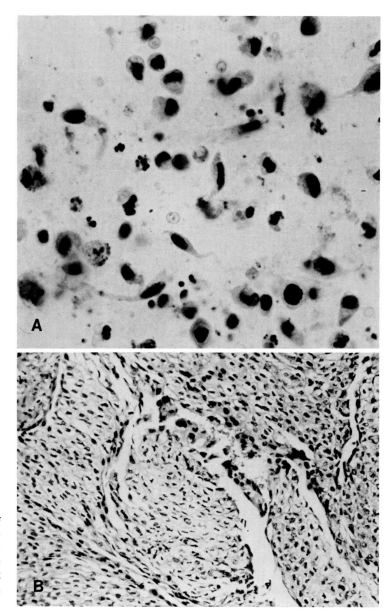

FIGURE 23–20. Invasive urothelial carcinoma, grade III of the urinary bladder. (*A*) Urinary sediment, showing tremendous variability in the shapes and sizes of cancer cells. (*B*) Histologic section of the same tumor. It is evident that the cytologic preparation reflects better than the histologic section the highly malignant nature of this invasive tumor. (*A* ×560; *B* ×150)

inconspicuous that an inexperienced eye may confuse them with inflammatory changes, unless very close attention is paid to the nuclear abnormalities (see Fig. 23–22). However, in most patients the diagnosis is obvious.

Voutsa and Melamed reported from my laboratory a systematic cytologic study of 20 patients with urothelial carcinoma in situ of the bladder. This study generally confirmed the observations reported above. The cell pattern did not differ in patients with a past history of treated papilloma or

carcinoma of the bladder. Voutsa pointed out that, following a biopsy or a fulguration, there is marked alteration of the smear pattern, usually appearing within 24 hours after the procedure and lasting up to 4 weeks. A general increase in the number of both benign and malignant cells and occasionally bizarre changes mimicking radiation changes were observed following such procedures (see Fig. 23–23). When this occurs, the cytologic pattern becomes indistinguishable from that of invasive carcinoma (see below).

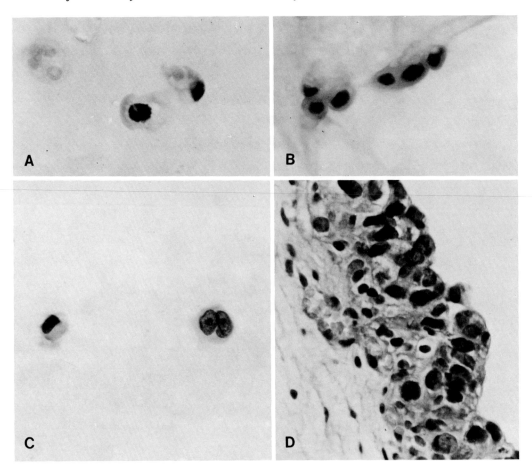

FIGURE 23-21.   A case of carcinoma in situ of the bladder. Primary diagnosis by smear of voided urine. (*A, B*) Typical "dyskaryotic" cells. Note the relatively abundant and well-differentiated cytoplasm surrounding the hyperchromatic nuclei. (*C*) Frank cancer cells. (*D*) Carcinoma in situ as seen in tissue section of the bladder biopsy. Note the nuclear abnormalities and the loose arrangement of the epithelium. (*A–D* ×500. *C:* Melamed, M.R., et al: Cytohistological observations on developing carcinoma of the urinary bladder in man. Cancer, *13*:67–74, 1960)

It must be noted that Beyer-Boon, who studied 13 patients with primary carcinoma in situ and 10 patients with secondary carcinoma in situ of the bladder, did not fully agree with the observations recorded above. She found preponderantly pleomorphic cancer cells in 21 and clusters of cancer cells in 19 of the 23 patients. The differences may be due to a different technical approach to the study of the urinary sediment.

Complete mapping of bladders with carcinoma in situ (see Fig. 23–24*E*) is required to appreciate the full extent of the lesion and to determine the presence or the absence of occult invasion (see Fig. 23–8) or of extension into prostatic ducts.

As has been discussed in reference to natural history of carcinoma of the bladder in industrial workers (p. 947), the cytologic diagnosis of carcinoma in situ may remain unconfirmed for many years in the absence of an aggressive approach to bladder biopsies. A case in point with a diagnostic delay of 5 years is illustrated in Fig. 23–26. This has been repeatedly observed in patients whose primary clinical problem is due to prostatic disease and whose bladders did not receive the necessary attention (see also p. 1005).

Clinical Handling and Confirmatory Biopsy of Carcinoma in Situ.   The unequivocal cytologic diagnosis of urothelial carcinoma in the absence of

(text continues on page 959)

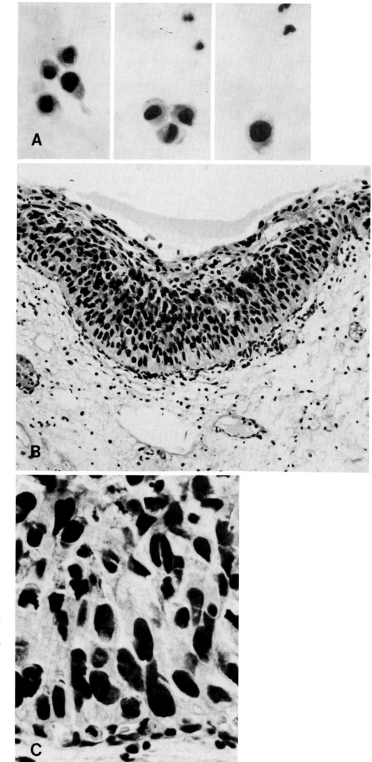

FIGURE 23–22. A case of carcinoma in situ of the urinary bladder. Primary diagnosis by cytologic examination of urinary sediment. (*A*) Composite picture of cell abnormalities, characteristic of this lesion. Note the uniform appearance of small cancer cells with moderate nuclear atypia. (*A, C*) Low- and high-power views of epithelial abnormalities. (*A, C* ×560; *B* ×150. Voutsa, N.G., and Melamed, M.R.: Cytology of in situ carcinoma of the human urinary bladder. Cancer. *16*:1307–1316, 1963)

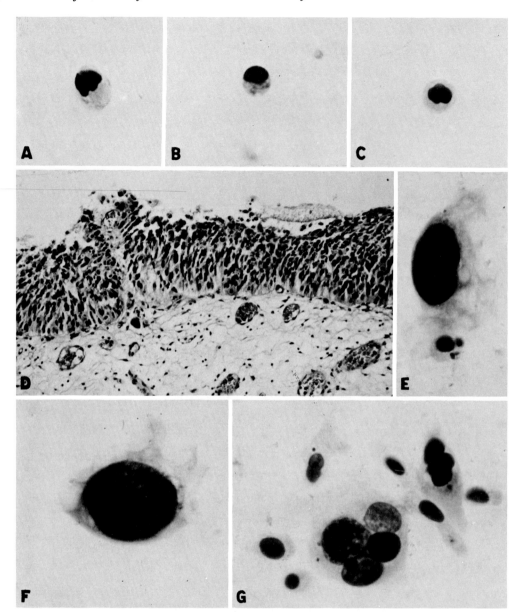

FIGURE 23–23.   A case of carcinoma in situ of the urinary bladder. (*A, B, C*) Classic cell abnormalities of carcinoma in situ. (*D*) Biopsy of the lesion. (*E, F, G*) Cell changes observed following the biopsy. Cell gigantism and multinucleation are evident. (*A, B, C, E, F, G* ×560; *D* ×150. Voutsa, N.G., and Melamed, M.R.: Cytology of in situ carcinoma of the human urinary bladder. Cancer, *16*:1307–1316, 1963)

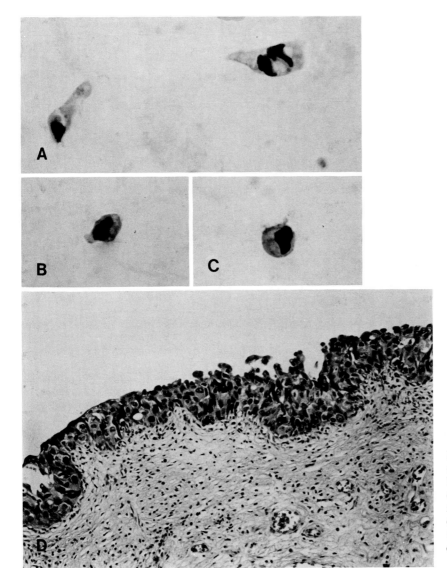

FIGURE 23-24. A case of carcinoma in situ of the urinary bladder. Primary diagnosis by cytologic examination of urinary sediment. (*A, B, C*) Cancer cells in the urinary sediment. (*D*) The histologic appearance of the lesion.

(continued)

clinical evidence of primary or residual tumor is usually diagnostic of a flat carcinoma in situ. This diagnosis is virtually always perplexing to the urologist who is often quite sure that the diagnosis is a laboratory error. On the rare occasion, carcinoma in situ may be primary in the renal pelvis or ureter and requires special handling described on p. 977. In most cases, however, the disease is present in the urinary bladder. The urologist must often be convinced that multiple biopsies of the bladder epithelium should be obtained to localize the disease and define its size. Besides biopsies of any visible, however trivial, abnormalities, multiple areas of the bladder must be sampled, at least the trigone, the four lateral walls, and the dome. In male patients biopsies of the prostatic bed should also be obtained to rule out extension into the prostatic ducts. (For further comments on evaluation of patients with tumors of the bladder, see p. 986).

Because the tissue composing carcinoma in situ is often quite fragile and is readily detached from the underlying stroma, one must always search for detached fragments of cancerous urothelium. De-Bellis and Schumann (1986) proposed that the fixative in which such biopsies are placed should be processed by filtration (or cytocentrifuge), as it may often contain small fragments of cancerous epithelium or detached cancer cells. Boon et al. (1986) also observed frequent failure of denuded

(text continues on page 963)

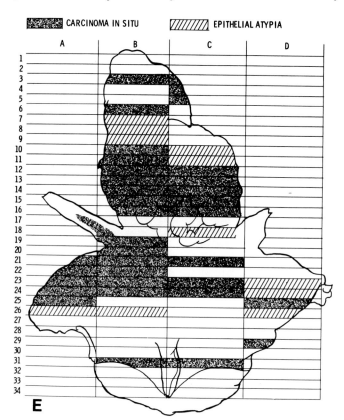

FIGURE 23–24 *(Continued).*
(*E*) Distribution of carcinoma in situ and lesser degrees of epithelial atypia in the operative specimen. Note extension of carcinoma in situ into the ureter. (*A, B, C* ×560; *D* ×150. Melamed, M.R., et al.: Carcinoma in situ of bladder: clinico-pathologic study of case with a suggested approach to detection. J. Urol., *96*:466–471, 1966)

FIGURE 23–25.   Flat carcinoma in situ of bladder—a classic presentation in voided urine sediment processed by the method of Bales (see p. 1465). (*A*) A low-power view of the sediment. Numerous dispersed and clustered cancer cells may be recognized, next to scattered benign squamous cells. (*B, C, D*) Higher-power view of the small cancer cells that were, on the whole, fairly monotonous in size, but demonstrated various configurations, ranging from approximately spherical (*C*), to polygonal (*B*), to columnar (*D*). Regardless of configuration, the cells had a significant enlargement of the hyperchromatic and coarsely granular nuclei, particularly well shown in (*C*). The size of the enlarged nuclei can be compared with those of benign squamous cells in the same fields. (*E*) Flat carcinoma in situ. Note the transformed malignant epithelium and the presence of an inflammatory infiltrate in the lamina propria. (*A, E* ×150; *B, C, D* ×560)

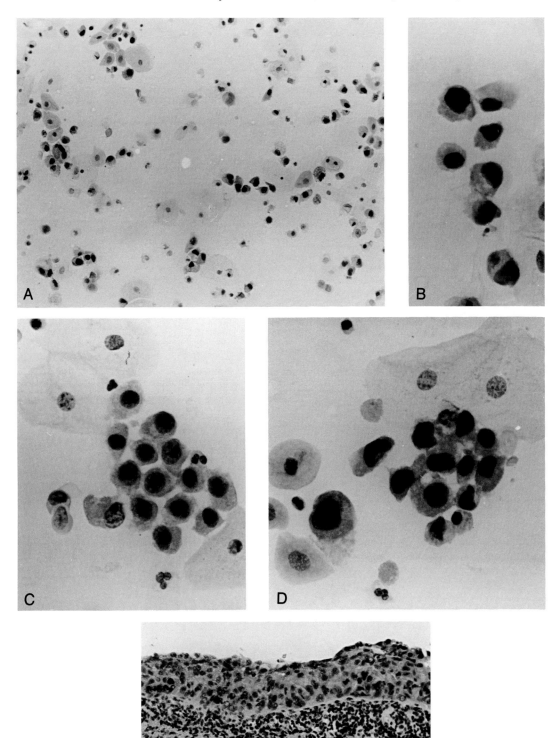

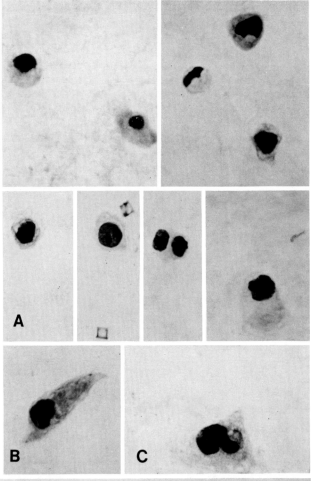

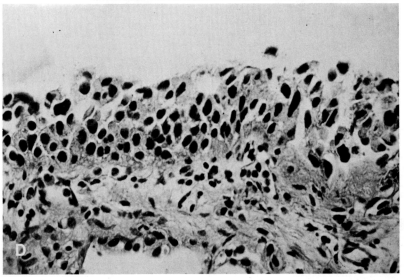

FIGURE 23–26. (*A*) Composite picture of cells observed in the urinary sediment of a 73-year-old man. The diagnosis of carcinoma in situ was established 5 years later. The small size and considerable uniformity of cell appearance are evident. There was no clinical evidence of disease, except for the enlarged prostate. In resecting this, an early prostatic carcinoma was removed. The patient continued to shed cancer cell in his urine, and with the passage of time they became more abnormal. (*B, C*). Five years after the initial cytologic diagnosis, a carcinoma in situ of the bladder was found in the area of the trigone (*D*). (*A, B, C* ×560; *D* ×350)

bladder biopsies to confirm a cytologic diagnosis of carcinoma in situ of the bladder. In such rare instances the biopsies must be repeated with an appropriate instrument.

Invasive Nonpapillary Urothelial Carcinoma. Invasive carcinoma may shed cells identical with a carcinoma in situ. However, this is exceptional in fully developed cancer and, as a rule, the predominant cancer cells are of variable sizes, of irregular configuration, with scanty cytoplasm and promi-

nent, obviously abnormal, hyperchromatic nuclei (Figs. 23–20 and 23–27). The degree of cellular abnormality and often tremendous variation in the appearance of the cells is suggestive of invasive cancer. Although most cancer cells have a basophilic cytoplasm, the presence of single keratinized cancer cells with eosinophilic cytoplasm is not rare (see Fig. 23–29A). This is a common component of invasive urothelial carcinoma. There is usually evidence of marked inflammation and necrosis.

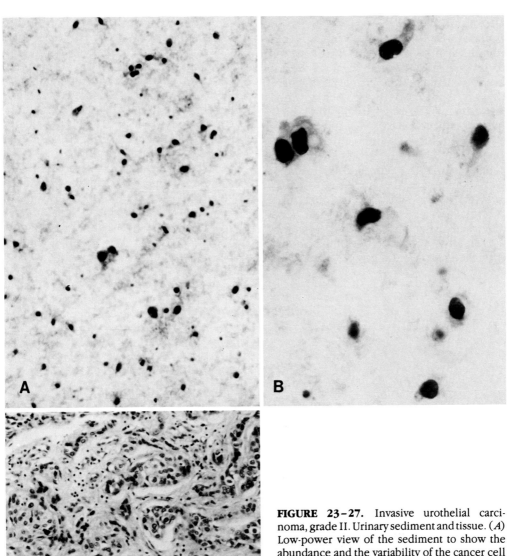

FIGURE 23–27. Invasive urothelial carcinoma, grade II. Urinary sediment and tissue. (*A*) Low-power view of the sediment to show the abundance and the variability of the cancer cell population. (*B*) High-power view of some of the cancer cells. Note the generally small size, poorly preserved cytoplasm, and nuclear hyperchromasia. (*C*) Area of the invasive urothelial carcinoma, grade II. (*A, C* ×150; *B* ×560)

Histologic Variants of Urothelial Carcinoma

Squamous (Keratinizing) Carcinoma

Histology and Natural History. The presence of a focal squamous component in urothelial carcinoma is a common finding. Squamous pearls may occasionally occur, even in papillary urothelial tumors, grade I, and may appear in urinary sediment (Fig. 23–28). Bladder cancers made up predominantly or exclusively of squamous (keratinizing) cell types are less frequent in the Western world than urothelial carcinomas, although they are common among patients with *Schistosoma hematobium* infestation (see p. 914). It is generally assumed that such tumors originate from areas of squamous metaplasia or leukoplakia, although this cannot always be conclusively documented. Squamous carcinomas, like urothelial carcinomas, may be graded according to the degree of differentiation (Koss, 1975). The very well-differentiated grade I variety is notorious for local growth and late metastases. Patients with this type of bladder disease, particularly common in the presence of *Schistosoma*, may die of uremia rather than metastases because of bladder obstruction by tumor. Squamous cancers of higher grades are fully capable of metastases and may occur not only in the bladder, but also in the ureters and the renal pelvis.

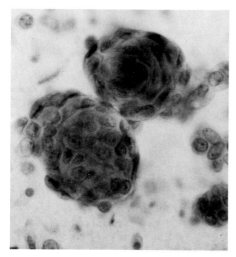

FIGURE 23–28. Papillary tumor, grade I, with squamous component. Urinary sediment, filter preparation. Concentrically arranged structures of urothelial derivation, resembling squamous pearls. This rare finding is diagnostic of this tumor type. (×1,000)

Cytology. Cytologic presentation of squamous carcinoma of the urothelium closely resembles similar lesions of the uterine cervix and bronchus (see pp. 469, 774). The tumors shed squamous cancer cells with eosinophilic, often markedly keratinized cytoplasm. The nuclei are pyknotic and, occasionally, may be totally submerged by keratin formation, with resulting formation of "ghost" cells, not unlike those observed in squamous carcinoma of the lung (see p. 775) (Fig. 23–29). Similar cells may be observed in cell block preparations of urinary sediment (Fig. 23–30). Condylomata acuminata of the bladder may mimic to a substantial degree the cytologic findings in squamous carcinoma (see p. 969). Flat condylomata acuminata may be mistaken for squamous carcinoma in situ (see p. 970 and Fig. 23–37).

In cytologic material from patients with *S. hematobium* infestation, fragments of keratinized epithelium were frequently observed in the urinary sediment next to exceedingly well-differentiated squamous cancer cells. The presence of blood, pus, and necrotic debris rendered the diagnosis of bladder cancer very difficult in some of these patients. As a result, only 15 diagnoses of cancer were rendered in 29 patients with schistosomiasis and proved cancer of the bladder (Houston et al.) There is little doubt that the results could be substantially improved, since, in this particular study, the urinary sediment was mailed in plastic bags from Bulawayo to New York, where the processing of the material took place. El-Bolkainy and Chu (1981) discussed at length the cytologic and histologic findings in bladder cancer in Egypt.

In women, the presence of squamous cancer cells in the sediment of voided urine may indicate the presence of a lesion in the female genital tract. The uterine cervix, vagina, or vulva may be the source of such cells.

Adenocarcinoma

Histology and Natural History. Occasional foci of glandular differentiation in urothelial carcinoma are common. Primary adenocarcinomas of the urothelium are predominantly of the enteric type (Fig. 23–31), although occasionally a tumor of clear cell type, resembling vaginal or endometrial carcinoma, may be observed (Fig. 23–32). Adenocarcinomas may occur anywhere in the lower urinary tract, most commonly in the bladder, but occasionally in the renal pelvis or the ureter. The tumors usually closely resemble carcinomas of the colon and may be made up of columnar, mucus-producing cells or signet-ring

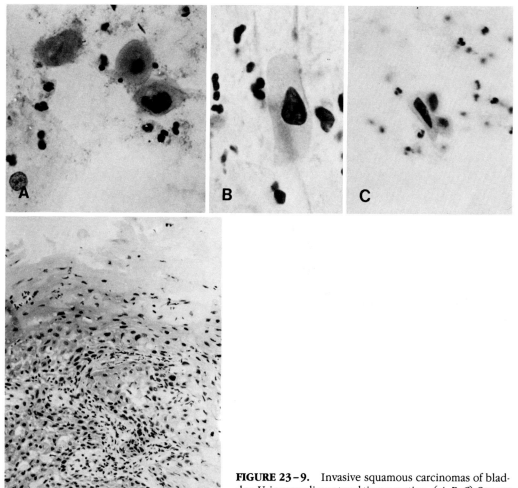

FIGURE 23–9. Invasive squamous carcinomas of bladder. Urinary sediment and tissue section. (*A, B, C*) Cancer cells with varying degrees of cytoplasmic keratinization. "Ghost cells" and cytoplasmic refactility are shown in (*A*). (*D*) Invasive squamous carcinoma of bladder corresponding to cells shown in (*A*). (*A, B, C* ×560; *D* ×150)

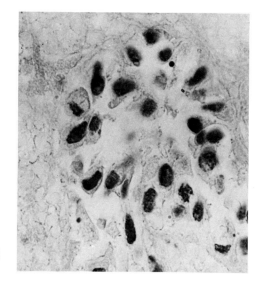

FIGURE 23–30. Squamous carcinoma of bladder. Cell block of urinary sediment. (×560)

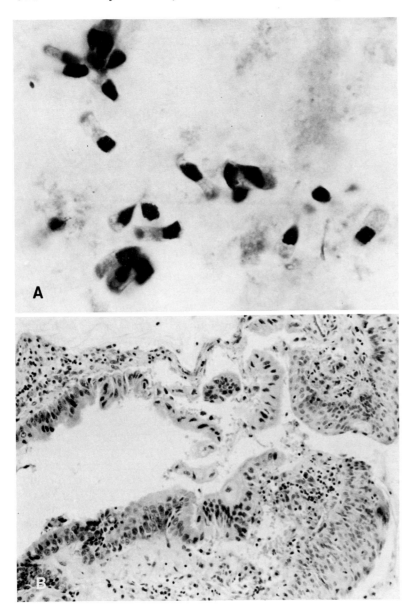

FIGURE 23–31. Adenocarcinoma of bladder: urinary sediment and tissue section. (*A*) Cancer cells in the urinary sediment have a columnar configuration, akin to colonic carcinoma (cf. Fig. 23–56). (*B*) Adenocarcinoma of bladder. The tumor originated from an invagination of glandular epithelium, with normal urothelium still lining the lumen of the bladder (*right*). (*A* ×1,000; *B* ×250)

type cancer cells. Similar tumors may occur in extrophic bladders. Although most such tumors are derived from areas of intestinal metaplasia on the epithelial surface, derivation of such tumors from cystitis glandularis (see p. 893) has also been documented. The prognosis of urothelial adenocarcinoma is generally poor, and metastases occur early.

Adenocarcinomas derived from rests of the embryonal omphaloenteric duct (the urachus) may also occur in the dome of the bladder and along the course of the duct, which terminates at the umbilicus. The urachal carcinomas have no specific histologic features that would permit their separation from other adenocarcinomas of the lower urinary tract.

Adenocarcinoma in situ of the bladder has also been observed.

Cytology. Most adenocarcinomas shed cells resembling those of colonic carcinoma. These are often columnar in configuration and have large, hyperchromatic nuclei and vacuolated cytoplasm (see Fig. 23–31*A*). Occasionally, smaller cancer cells, resembling the signet-ring type, may be observed. Neither cell type can be differentiated from

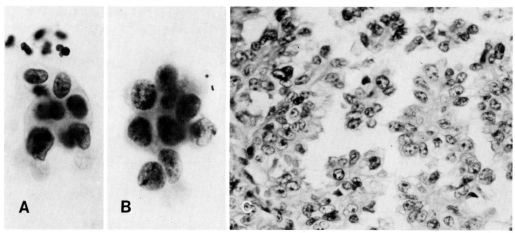

FIGURE 23–32. Papillary adenocarcinoma of urinary bladder, clear cell type in a 54-year-old woman: urinary sediment and biopsy. (*A, B*) Papillary clusters of malignant cells with markedly granular nuclei, occasional nucleoli, and clear cytoplasm. (*C*) The tumor has many similarities to adenocarcinomas of vaginal and endocervical origin, observed in daughters of DES-exposed women. (*A, B* ×560; *C* ×350)

the cells of metastatic colonic carcinoma (see Figs. 23–55 and 23–56). In the rare cases of clear-cell-type adenocarcinoma, papillary clusters of malignant cells with large nuclei, nucleoli, and clear cytoplasm may be observed (see Fig. 23–32). Single case reports of adenocarcinomas by Frillo et al. (1981) and DeMay and Grathwohl (1985) added no new information.

In a case of adenocarcinoma in situ, numerous columnar cancer cells have been observed in the urinary sediment. The cells were very similar to those shown in Fig. 23–31.

Diagnosis of Urothelial Tumors in Special Situations

Lithiasis

It was mentioned on p. 915 that lithiasis may give rise to significant atypia of urothelial cells. Wynder considers lithiasis as a major factor in epidemiology of carcinoma of the bladder. Lithiasis may conceal the presence of carcinoma. In the presence of lithiasis, the urinary sediment must be very carefully evaluated. In the presence of significant cellular abnormalities the presence of a coexisting carcinoma must be ruled out.

Carcinoma of the Bladder and Prostatic Disease

Carcinoma of the bladder may occur, occasionally as an occult lesion, in the presence of prostatic carcinoma of prostatic hypertrophy (see Fig. 23–26). There is persuasive evidence, discussed on p. 1005,

that the association of bladder cancer with prostatic enlargement is a fairly common event.

Diverticula of the Bladder

Several cases of carcinoma originating in diverticula of the bladder have been observed in this laboratory (Fig. 23–33), and several cases have been reported by Crabbe. The cytologic presentation of these lesions did not in any way differ from other such lesions in other locations. However, the clinical localization of the lesions to a diverticulum proved at times very difficult. It must be kept in mind that diverticula may have a very inconspicuous opening into the bladder, readily overlooked on cystoscopy.

RARE TUMORS OF THE BLADDER

Benign Tumors

Condylomata Acuminata. Condylomata acuminata may occasionally be observed in the urinary bladder (Koss, 1975). Petterson et al. (1976) observed two such tumors in immunosuppressed patients following a renal transplant. With the passage of time, additional tumors of this type have been observed (summary in Del Mistro et al., 1988).

The recognition of the relationship of condylomata acuminata with human papillomavirus, particularly types 6 and 11 (see p. 377), has led to further analysis of these tumors. In a report from this laboratory (Del Mistro et al., 1988), three patients were studied in depth. Several important features

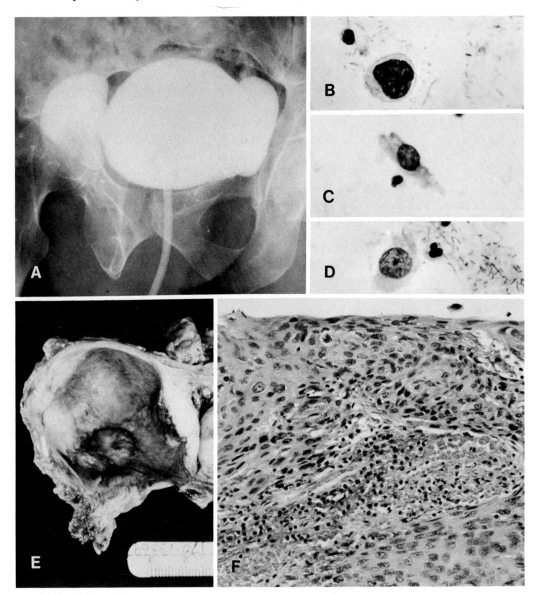

FIGURE 23–33.   Carcinoma in a diverticulum of the bladder. (*A*) Cystogram of the bladder showing a large diverticulum on patient's right and a smaller one on the left. (*B, C, D*) Cancer cells in the urinary sediment. (*E*) Flat tumor was present in the bisected right diverticulum. (*F*) Histologic appearance of invasive urothelial carcinoma with squamous differentiation. (*B, C, D* ×1,000; *F* ×250)

of these tumors became apparent. Condylomas of the bladder are often associated with condylomas of external genitalia, but may also occur as discrete tumors. By in situ hybridization, the presence of HPV types 6 and 11 could be documented. The tumors are very difficult to treat and have a marked tendency to recur. The possibility of progression to verrucous carcinoma, or for that matter, difficulties in precise classification of these tumors as either benign or malignant must be noted. In fact, in one of the patients studied by Del Mistro et al., fol-low-up information strongly suggested that the lesion progressed to an invasive and metastatic squamous carcinoma of the bladder. The proof of this event could not be obtained, however.

Histologically, the tumors resemble genital condylomata acuminata, characterized by the presence of koilocytes in the superficial epithelial layers. In some tumors, marked nuclear abnormalities may be observed in epithelial cells (Fig. 23–34). It is of note that the DNA content of the bladder condylomas is aneuploid.

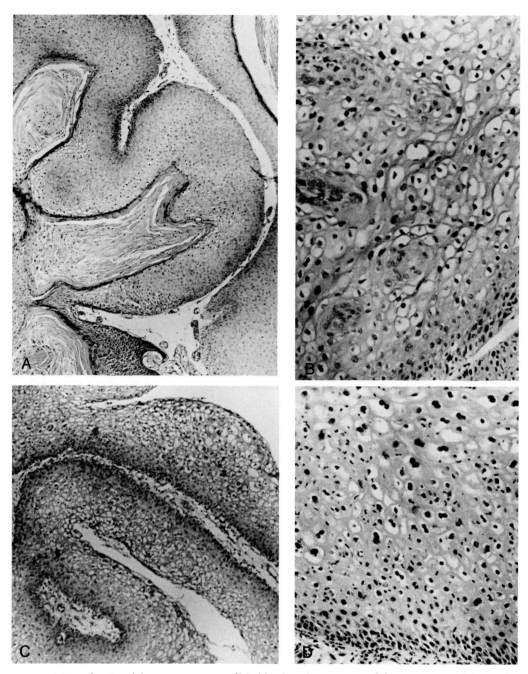

FIGURE 23–34. Condylomata acuminata of bladder: histologic aspects. (*A*) Recurrent condyloma of bladder neck in a 48-year-old woman. Note the epithelial folds and keratin formation on the surface. (*B*) Same patient as (*A*) — first lesion: higher-power view of the epithelium to document koilocytosis. (*C*) Lesion of trigone in a 28-year-old woman. (*D*) Same patient as (*C*): higher-power view of the epithelium to show koilocytosis with marked nuclear atypia. (*A, C* ×22; *B* ×150; *D* ×140)

In voided urine koilocytes can be observed (Fig. 23–35). In a female patient, the possibility of origin of these cells in the uterine cervix must be ruled out. In male patients such cells may also originate in penile urethra (see p. 977). More importantly, perhaps, in two of our patients, the urinary sediment contained large, highly abnormal squamous cells with keratinized cytoplasm and large, hyperchromatic and pyknotic nuclei (Fig. 23–36). "Cell-in-cell" arrangement was observed. Al-

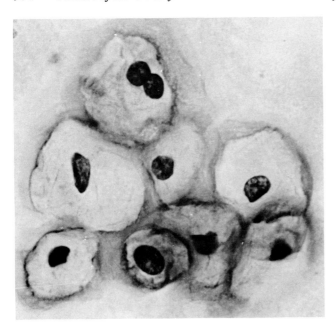

FIGURE 23-35. Koilocytosis in urinary sediment. In a female patient the origin from the female genital tract cannot be ruled out. (×1,000)

though, in some of the cells, perinuclear halos suggested a similarity to koilocytes, such cells were very difficult to distinguish from cells of squamous carcinoma (cf. Fig. 23-29). In the previous edition of this book, a lesion of the bladder with similar cytologic presentation was classified as "squamous carcinoma in situ" (Fig. 23-37). The question of whether this lesion represented a flat condyloma of the bladder or, in fact, a squamous carcinoma cannot be resolved in the absence of follow-up information. Clearly, condylomata acuminata of the urinary bladder are not easily eradicated, truly benign lesions, but straddle the border between benign and malignant tumors, not unlike similar precancerous lesions of the uterine cervix (see Chaps. 11 and 12 for further discussion of cervical lesions).

Inverted Papilloma. An uncommon tumor of the urinary bladder, first described by Potts and Hirst in 1963, it is made up of anastomosing strands of urothelium (Koss, 1975). The tumor is benign and there are no known cytologic abnormalities associated with it.

Endometriosis. Schneider et al. (1980) observed clusters of endometrial cells in voided urine in a case of endometriosis of the bladder.

Eosinophilic Granuloma. The rare eosinophilic granuloma may occur in the bladder or ureter. There are no known specific cytologic findings.

Nephrogenic Adenoma (Adenosis of Bladder). In this rare entity; the lesion is composed of ducts and tubules, probably of enteric origin (Koss, 1985). There are two reports suggesting that nephrogenic adenomas may be recognized in urinary sediment. Stilman et al. (1986) reported the presence of markedly abnormal cells in four patients. Three of the patients, however, had documented bladder cancer with carcinoma in situ. The cells shown in the illustrations could have well originated from the malignant epithelium. Troster et al. (1986) observed papillary urothelial clusters in the urine of one patient. To this observer the cluster had no specific features. It is doubtful that nephrogenic adenoma can be recognized in urinary sediment. However, adenocarcinomas may develop in such lesions and may shed cancer cells (see p. 964).

Villous Adenoma. Villous adenoma is a rare tumor of bladder of enteric origin that resembles similar tumors of the colon and rectum. There are no known cell abnormalities associated with this disorder.

Malignant Tumors

Rare primary tumors may occasionally shed cells in the urinary sediment. Spindle- and giant-cell carcinomas, small-cell (oat cell) carcinomas, carcinomas with pseudosarcomatous stroma, and primary melanomas have been observed (Koss,

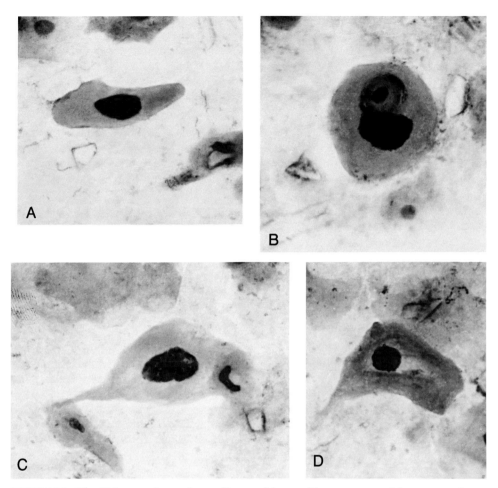

FIGURE 23–36. Urinary sediment from a 42-year-old man with recurrent condylomata acuminata of the urinary bladder. (*A, B*) Markedly keratinized cells very similar to cells of a squamous carcinoma. In (*B*) a "cell-in-cell" structure is shown. (*C, D*) Abnormal squamous cells with a perinuclear halo, hence, resembling koilocytes. (*A–D* ×1,000)

1975). The exact cytologic identification of such exceedingly rare tumors usually cannot be made.

Mesodermal mixed tumors (heterologous carcinosarcomas), which closely resemble similar tumors observed in the female genital tract (see Chap. 17), may shed a mixture of cells, some of which have features of carcinoma cells, and others, which may be traced to a differentiated sarcoma, such as a chondrosarcoma (Fig. 23–38). Such tumors are extremely uncommon.

Sarcomas of the bladder, chiefly rhabdo- and leiomyosarcomas (Koss, 1975) occasionally shed cancer cells in urine. Krumerman and Katatikaru described a case of rhabdomyosarcoma with epithelial involvement. Generally, cells of sarcoma in the urine look malignant, but cannot be accurately identified in the absence of prior histologic diagnosis or clinical history (Figs. 23–39 and 23–40).

Cells of the very rare primary malignant lymphoma of the urinary bladder cannot be differentiated from the cells of systemic tumors of the same type (see p. 993).

A case of primary choriocarcinoma of the bladder was observed in this laboratory (Obe et al., 1983). The urinary sediment contained numerous malignant cells, most of which resembled cells of urothelial carcinoma (Fig. 23–41*A,B*) and some that were multinucleated (see Fig. 23–41*C*). The tumor, which gave a strongly positive reaction for human chorionic gonadotropin (see Fig. 23–41*D*), was accompanied by a flat urothelial carcinoma

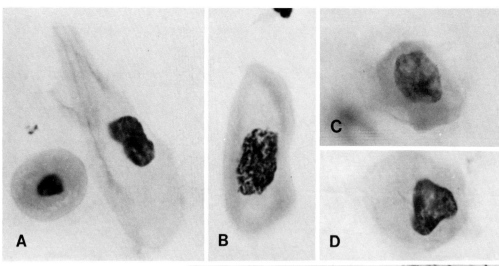

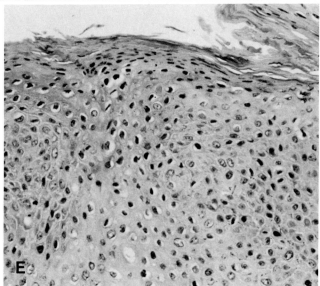

FIGURE 23–37. Flat condyloma or a squamous carcinoma in situ of the bladder. Urinary sediment and biopsy. (*A, B, C, D*) Well-differentiated large squamous cells with abnormal nuclei, resembling dyskaryotic squamous cells of the uterine cervix. In (*A*) and (*B*) a perinuclear halo suggests a marked similarity to koilocytes. Cell (*C*) is almost completely ketatinized and has a pale nucleus. (*E*) Histologic appearance of lesion, resembling a well-differentiated squamous carcinoma in situ of cervix or vagina. (*A–D* ×1,000; *E* ×250)

in situ, hence, probably represented an unusual transformation of a carcinoma.

CARCINOMAS OF THE RENAL PELVIS AND THE URETER

Carcinoma of the Renal Pelvis

Histology and Natural History

Primary tumors of the renal pelvis encompass the full scale of urothelial tumors described in the bladder. The majority of the tumors are urothelial, papillary and nonpapillary in type, but keratinizing carcinomas and adenocarcinomas of intestinal type may also be observed. The most frequent clinical symptom is hematuria, sometimes associated with evidence of renal failure.

Primary carcinomas of the renal pelvis have been observed in association with use and abuse of analgesic drugs containing a common ingredient, phenacetin. Although most of such cases reported originated in Scandinavian countries, sporadic observations on this association have been recorded in other countries as well (review in Johansson et

(text continues on page 975)

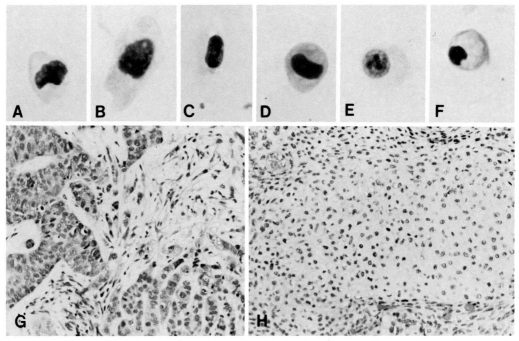

FIGURE 23-38.   Mesodermal mixed tumor of the bladder in a 63-year-old man: urinary sediment and surgical specimen. (*A–F*) Cells in urinary sediment. Cells (*A*) through (*D*) resemble cells of urothelial carcinoma. Cells (*E*) and (*F*) may have originated from the chondrosarcoma. (*G*) Field of tumor showing carcinoma and spindle cell sarcoma. (*H*) Another field of the same tumor with small-cell sarcoma and chondrosarcoma. (*A–E* ×560; *G, H* ×150)

FIGURE   23-39. Embryonal rhabdomyosarcoma of bladder in a 9-year-old child: urinary sediment and tissue. (*A, B*) Small cancer cells in the urinary sediment. Cell (*B*) is somewhat elongated and has a prominent nucleolus. (*C*) Tissue section with a large "strap cell" with eosinophilic cytoplasm. (*A, B, C* ×560)

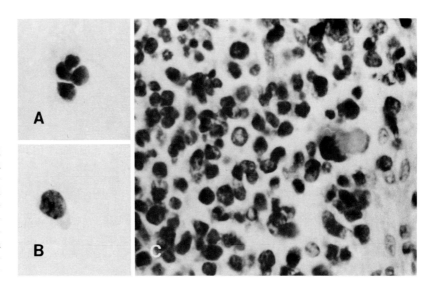

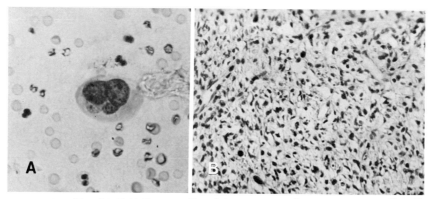

FIGURE 23–40.   (*A, B*) Malignant cell and tissue sections from a primary spindle cell sarcoma (not further classified) in the bladder of an adult male. (*A* ×560; *B* ×150)

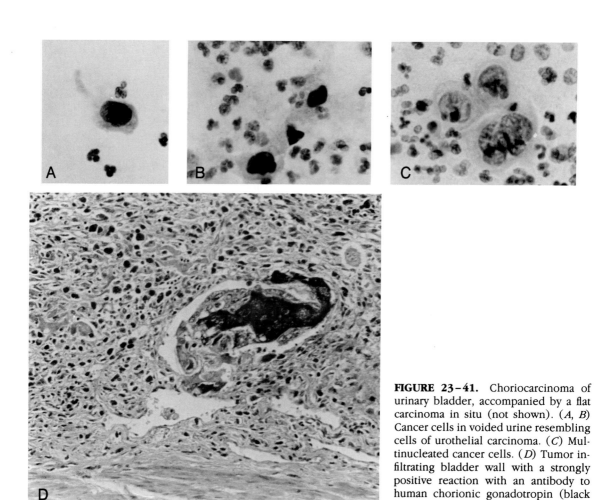

FIGURE 23–41. Choriocarcinoma of urinary bladder, accompanied by a flat carcinoma in situ (not shown). (*A, B*) Cancer cells in voided urine resembling cells of urothelial carcinoma. (*C*) Multinucleated cancer cells. (*D*) Tumor infiltrating bladder wall with a strongly positive reaction with an antibody to human chorionic gonadotropin (black precipitate). (*A, B, C* ×560; *D* ×150)

al., 1974). An important corollary of phenacetin toxicity is papillary necrosis, which occurs in more than half of the patients. A case of carcinoma of the renal pelvis in a patient receiving cyclophosphamide therapy has been recorded (see Chap. 22).

In a significant proportion of patients, carcinomas of the renal pelvis are synchronous or metachronous with urothelial tumors of other organs. Carcinomas of the ureters and of the bladder may either precede or follow renal pelvic cancer. In a series of 41 patients with carcinoma of the renal pelvis and ureters, 50% of the patients developed bladder tumors (Kakizoe et al., 1980). The sequence of events cannot be anticipated, and the presence of carcinoma in one of these locations must automatically trigger the search for other tumors and long-term follow-up in which cytology of urinary sediment plays a major role (Smart; Sherwood; Koss, 1977). Renal pelvic tumors are frequently bilateral. These may occur simultaneously or in sequence and create a major diagnostic and therapeutic dilemma. Between 1974 and 1976 I observed four such patients.

Mahadevia et al. (1983) mapped seven carcinomas of the renal pelvis and two of the ureters and observed peripheral atypical urothelium in five tumors and flat carcinoma in situ in four tumors. Hence, it may be assumed that the sequence of events in renal pelvic and ureteral tumors is exactly the same as in the bladder. The findings were similar to the observations by Chasko et al. Extensive in situ carcinoma and related abnormalities were also observed in analgesic users, who are prone to develop renal pelvic urothelial carcinomas (Lomax-Smith and Seymour, 1980).

The presence of carcinoma in situ in Mahadevia's study was of prognostic significance, inasmuch as two of four such patients developed metachronous carcinoma of the bladder, and one died of disseminated cancer. One of five patients with peripheral atypical urothelium also developed a tumor of the bladder.

A few cases of primary nonpapillary carcinoma in situ of the renal pelvis were recorded: the first was reported by Papanicolaou and Foote; another by Murphy et al. I have also observed one such case by courtesy of Dr. Harold Block of El Paso, Texas (see below and Fig. 23–44). It must be pointed out that the drug busulfan is capable of inducing major changes in renal pelvic epithelium that may mimic a carcinoma in situ (see p. 924, and Burry, 1974).

The prognosis of renal pelvic tumors depends on tumor size and grade, the degree of invasion of surrounding tissue, and the presence or absence of metastases. The grading is identical with that of urothelial cancers of the bladder (see p. 935). Large tumors of high grade have a poor prognosis. Although renal pelvic carcinomas are theoretically fully curable by surgery if diagnosed early, the mortality in the Johansson's series of 62 patients was in excess of 50%. The results were not significantly improved in a more recent series of cases (Huber et al., 1988).

Carcinoma of the Ureter

Histology and Natural History

Primary carcinomas of the ureters share the histologic types and prognosis with similar tumors of the bladder and the renal pelves. Fromowitz et al. (1981) reported from this laboratory on two cases of inverted papillomas of the ureter. The report must be considered of questionable value because one of the tumors recurred with features of urothelial carcinoma, grade II. The second patient developed an adenocarcinoma of bladder. As was recorded in a subsequent publication (*Supplement to Atlas on Tumors of the Urinary Bladder*, Koss, 1985), urothelial carcinomas of the ureter may develop a flat surface, probably for anatomic reasons, and mimic an inverted papilloma. Such tumors may be the source of the occasional reports of positive cytologic findings in the benign inverted papilloma.

It is of special interest that in the presence of carcinoma of the bladder, carcinoma in situ of adjacent distal ureters is a very common finding (summary in Koss, 1975; Koss et al., 1977; Richie and Skinner, 1978).

Cytology of Carcinomas of Renal Pelves and Ureters

Voided Urine

Cytologic presentation of primary renal pelvic and ureteral carcinomas closely resembles that described for bladder tumors (see pp. 948–967). In general, well-differentiated papillary urothelial tumors cannot be diagnosed. In urothelial carcinomas, grade II or higher, the population of malignant cells is sometimes surprisingly abundant and readily identified (Figs. 23–42 and 23–43). The presence of malignant cells of squamous type is common in urothelial tumors. Such cells predominate in keratinizing carcinomas. Cytologic findings in a case of adenocarcinoma of the renal pelvis were reported by Kobayashi et al. (1985).

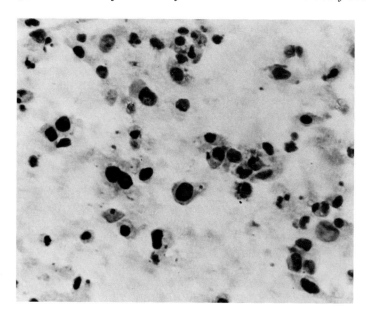

FIGURE 23-42. Urinary sediment: urothelial carcinoma of renal pelvis (voided urine). Note numerous cancer cells. (×560)

In Mahadevia's study (1983), cited above, the urinary sediment disclosed cancer cells in four of nine patients, all with grade II or higher cancers. The appearance of the sediment was suspicious in three additional patients, atypical in one, and not examined in one.

Retrograde Catheterization

The most common reason for retrograde catheterization is a space-occupying lesion of renal pelvis associated with gross or microscopic hematuria. The urologist expects that the problem of differen-

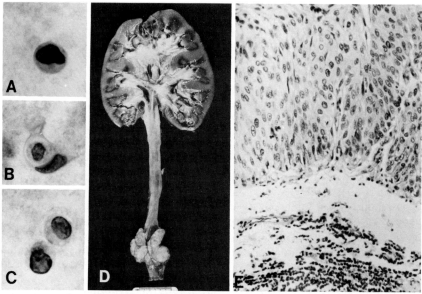

FIGURE 23-43. Papillary urothelial carcinoma, grade II, of ureter: urinary sediment and surgical specimen. (*A, B, C*) Urothelial cancer cells observed in voided urine. They cannot be identified as to site of origin. (*D*) Gross appearance of the tumor located at the lower (distal) end of the ureter. (*E*) Histologic presentation of the tumor. (*A, B, C* ×560; *E* ×150)

tial diagnosis among lithiasis, blood clot, and a tumor will be resolved by cytologic examination. As was discussed at length on p. 900 this expectation is usually frustrated because the cytologic techniques are not suitable for the identification of low-grade tumors. *Cytologic examination of urine obtained by retrograde catheterization is appropriate only under well-defined circumstances, namely for localization of a high-grade tumor to either urether or renal pelvis.* Such events are rare and occur under the following conditions: the patient's voided urinary sediment contains unequivocal cancer cells, but there is no evidence of a bladder lesion; and the roentgenologic examination of the urinary tract is either negative or inconclusive. In such instances the cytologic investigation of renal pelves by retrograde catheterization is appropriate. The urine specimens must be collected separately for each side, and great care must be exercised to avoid cross-contamination of the samples. The cytologic findings are usually very complex because of the population of benign urothelial cells, which may be difficult to interpret and may obscure the presence of malignant cells (see p. 900). Under these circumstances, great diagnostic caution is advised: the diagnosis of carcinoma should not be made unless the cytologic evidence is unequivocal.

This procedure was applied to the diagnosis of an occult carcinoma in situ of the renal pelvis in an 80-year-old woman with hematuria and voided urine showing abundant evidence of a high-grade carcinoma. The lesion was localized to the right kidney on urine obtained by retrograde catheterization (Fig. 23–44). The method is of no value in the diagnosis of low-grade tumors.

Retrograde Brushing

Retrograde brushing as a method of direct sampling of the ureters, renal pelves, and renal calices offers, in skilled hands, the option of obtaining direct cytologic and histologic material for diagnosis (Gill et al.). Bibbo et al. reported excellent results with this method based on a small series of cases. Personal experience confirms that cytologic samples obtained by retrograde brushing under fluoroscopic control may sometimes be informative and contribute in a major way to the diagnosis and localization of radiographically occult high-grade renal pelvic carcinoma (Fig. 23–45). In most space-occupying lesions of the renal pelvis, particularly low-grade tumors, the issues of differential diagnosis may not be solved by this technique.

Cytologic Assessment of Urine from the Ileal Conduit (Ileal Bladder)

Cytologic findings in ileal bladder urine in the absence of cancer were discussed on p. 918.

Examination of urine from ileal bladders is mandatory as a follow-up procedure after radical cystectomy for urothelial tumors. New primary cancers of the renal pelvis or of the ureters following cancer of the bladder may occasionally be diagnosed in this fashion before there is clear-cut clinical evidence of disease. Since hydronephrosis is frequently observed in patients with ileal bladder, radiographic examination in such situations may show only slight changes that would be readily overlooked, were it not for the cytologic report. In one of our early patients, sequential bilateral primary carcinomas of the renal pelves were observed following radical cystectomy for cancer of the bladder (Fig. 23–46). Both kidneys were removed, and the patient was maintained by dialysis for several months pending renal transplant.

Several additional patients with carcinomas of renal pelves or ureters following cystectomy for bladder cancer have been observed (Koss et al., 1977). Similar observations were reported by Malmgren et al. and by Wolinska and Melamed.

Again, it must be stressed that the observer must be familiar with the cytologic appearance of the population of degenerating cells of intestinal (ileal) conduit origin before attempting the diagnosis of carcinoma.

TUMORS OF THE URETHRA

Benign Tumors

Condylomata Acuminata

The most common benign tumors of the urethra in both sexes are condylomata acuminata. As was repeatedly discussed in the preceding pages, the tumors are associated with human papillomavirus (HPV) superinfection, most commonly the types 6 and 11, but occasionally also 16 and 18. In the female, condylomas of the urethra are usually visible lesions, associated with condylomas of external genitalia, a risk factor in cervical neoplastic events (see p. 377).

In the male, condylomas of the urethra occur in two forms: the clinically evident lesions, occupying the tip of the penile urethra at the meatus; and the clinically occult lesions, located within the mem-

(text continues on page 981)

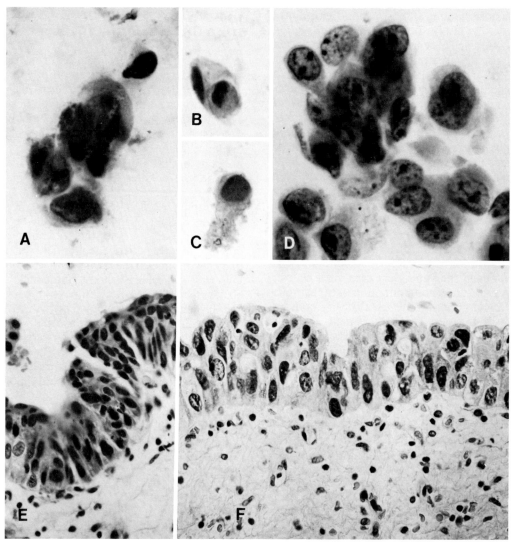

FIGURE 23–44.   Primary radiographically occult, nonpapillary carcinoma in situ of right renal pelvis in an 80-year-old woman: urinary sediment and tissue. (*A, B, C*) Voided urine: urothelial cancer cells are seen singly and in clusters. (*D*) Retrograde catheterization: cluster of cancer cells with large nucleoli. (*E, F*) Two fields of carcinoma in situ. (*A–D* ×1,000; *E, F* ×650. Case courtesy of Dr. Harold Bloch, El Paso, Texas)

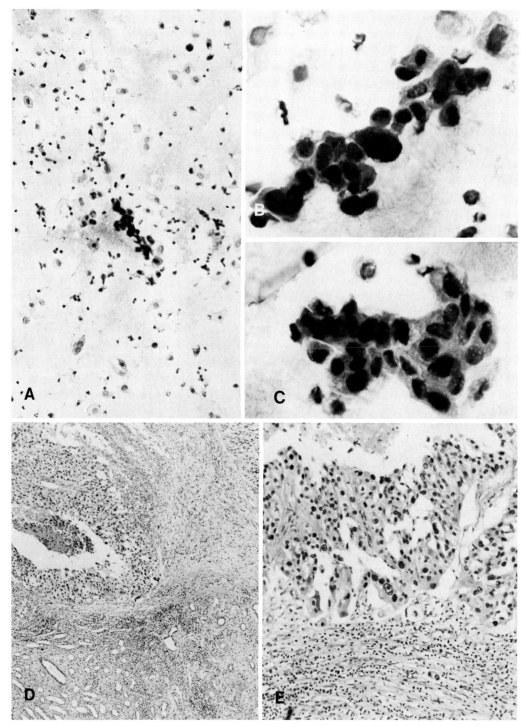

FIGURE 23–45. Radiographically occult grade III carcinoma of renal pelvis in a 38-year-old woman with hematuria. Voided urine contained numerous cancer cells. The lesion was localized to the right renal pelvis by retrograde brushings. (*A*) Brush specimen, low-power view: numerous urothelial cells originating in the renal pelvis and, in the *center*, a cluster of cancer cells; (*B, C*) sheets of cancer cells; (*D*) low-power view of renal pelvic carcinoma; (*E*) higher-power view of the urothelial tumor. (*A, E* ×150; *B, C* ×560; *D* ×50)

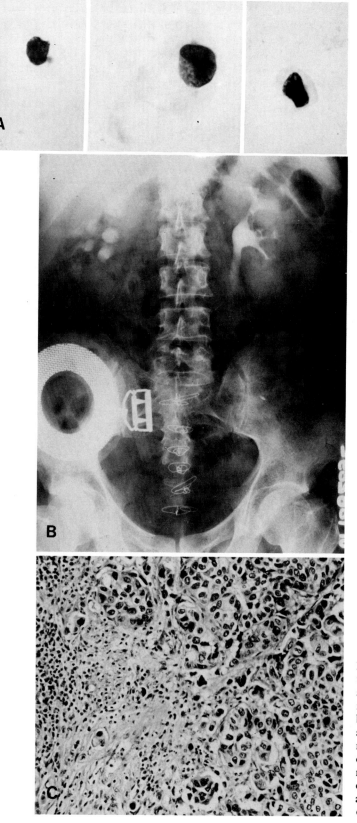

FIGURE 23–46. (*A*) Composite picture of cancer cells found in the urinary sediment from an ileal bladder following radical cystectomy for carcinoma of the bladder. (*B*) Intravenous pyelogram showed only a minimal change in the left renal pelvis. (*C*) Left nephrectomy disclosed a new primary carcinoma of the renal pelvis. Subsequently, the same process affected the right kidney, again heralded by cytologic findings. (*A* ×560; *C* ×150)

branous portion of the penile urethra. The clinically obvious lesions are usually associated with other genital condylomas but may be solitary.

The frequency of occult lesions in the penile urethra is unknown, but there is concern that they may be the source of superinfection of female partners with HPV.

Histologically, the visible papillary lesions are identical with condylomas of the external female genitalia (see Fig. 12–22 and Fig. 23–47*C*). The condylomas of the membranous urethra are generally flat lesions, mimicking cervical epithelial neoplasia (CIN) of low grade and characterized by the presence of koilocytes in upper epithelial layers (see Fig. 23–47*A*). Because of nuclear abnormalities that may be considerable, the lesions are readily mistaken for a carcinoma in situ, as became evident from several consultations. Although the flat condylomas are benign, by definition, and extremely unlikely to invade, all condylomas are difficult to treat because of a high rate of recurrence.

In a series of urethral condylomas in male patients, studied in this laboratory, Del Mistro et al. (1987) observed the lesion in 17 patients, 16 young adults and 1 boy, aged 9, who had an occult lesion. By in situ hybridization, HPV types 6 and 11 were observed in 13 lesions, and types 6 and 18 in 1. In 2 lesions, only type 11 was observed (see Fig. 23–47). One lesion and a recurrence thereof were negative with all probes. Four other recurrent lesions expressed the same type of viral DNA as the original lesion.

Cytologically, koilocytes may be observed in voided urine sediments (see Fig. 23–35). As discussed on p. 969, in the woman, the cells may reflect a cervical or a vaginal lesion, but in the male, they indicate a lesion of the penile urethra or bladder.

Because of concern that occult urethral condylomas may be the male counterpart of cervical lesions and a source of infection, Cecchini et al. (1988) performed brushings of penile urethra in 53 male partners of women with evidence of HPV infection (including CIN). Koilocytes were observed in smears of 26 (49%) of the men and none in the controls.

Cecchini et al. also performed colposcopy on the penile skin ("penoscopy") on the male partners. In five of them, subclinical lesions were observed. Giacomini et al. (1989) also studied the penile urethra, using a specially designed swab.

The issue of subclinical infection of the penile skin and the detection of occult lesions by penile colposcopy was discussed at some length by Sedlacek et al. and by Barrasso et al. (1986). The penile skin lesions are inconspicuous, histologically un-

impressive, and what to do about them is not clear. Treatment by laser has been advocated, as has been protected intercourse until the lesions heal or vanish. At the time of writing (1991), very little is known about the natural history or clinical significance of these lesions.

Malignant Tumors

Female Urethra

Primary carcinoma of the female urethra is an uncommon disease. Occasionally, the lesions occur in urethral diverticula. Over 80% of the lesions are urothelial or epidermoid, whereas 20% are adenocarcinomas. Occasionally, malignant melanomas have been reported. There have been no known attempts to obtain routine smears of the urethra for purposes of early diagnosis. In fully developed cancer, the voided urine sediment may occasionally contain cancer cells (Fig. 23–48). In several instances, personally observed patients with treated carcinoma of the distal urethra were followed by smears obtained by cotton-tipped applicators. Recurrent disease could be diagnosed while still in the stage of carcinoma in situ. The cytologic presentation was similar to that of carcinoma in situ of the cervix or of the vagina, rather than of the urinary bladder. This is in keeping with the epithelium of origin, which in the distal urethra is of the stratified squamous and not the urothelial type.

In a case of malignant melanoma of the urethra, highly abnormal squamous cells were observed in a direct smear, similar to cells observed in primary vaginal melanomas (see p. 652).

Male Urethra

Primary carcinomas of the male urethra not preceded by carcinoma of the bladder are exceedingly uncommon. However, urothelial carcinoma of the male urethra may occur in about 10% of all patients after local treatment or radical cystectomy for carcinoma of the bladder and, rarely, as a sequence of carcinoma of the prostatic ducts. Penile discharge, mucoid, purulent, or hemorrhagic, may be observed on these occasions, and washings of the urethra yield cancer cells similar to those seen in carcinoma of the bladder. Some of the observed lesions were carcinomas in situ or carcinomas in situ with superficial invasion (Figs. 23–49 and 23–50).

Adenocarcinoma of endometrial type, originating in prostatic utricle (uterus masculinus), while very rare (Melicow and Tannenbaum), may have the clinical presentation of a urethral tumor. In one

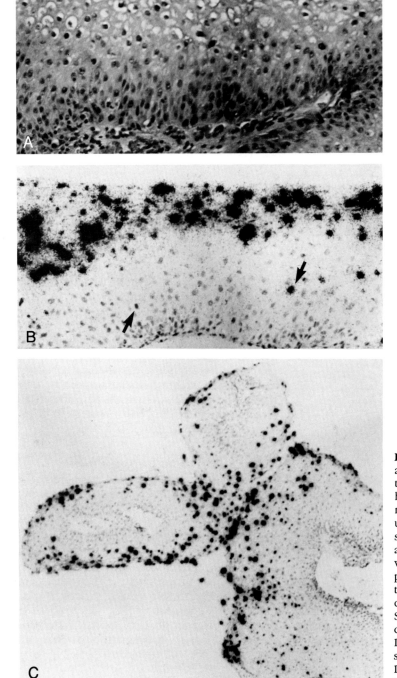

FIGURE 23–47. Primary condyloma acuminatum of penile urethra. (*A*) Histologic section stained with hematoxylin–eosin, showing a flat segment of the lesion with koilocytosis in upper epithelial layers.(*B*) Sequential section of (*A*), hybridized with a radioactive HPV-6 probe and counterstained with hematoxylin, showing a strongly positive reaction (*black nuclei*). Note the presence of positive cells in the deeper epithelial layers (*arrows*) (*C*) Same section as in (*B*) at lower magnification showing the distribution of viral DNA in different areas in the same lesion. (*A, B* ×160; *C* ×64. Modified from Del Mistro et al. Hum. Pathol., *18*:936–940, 1987, with permission)

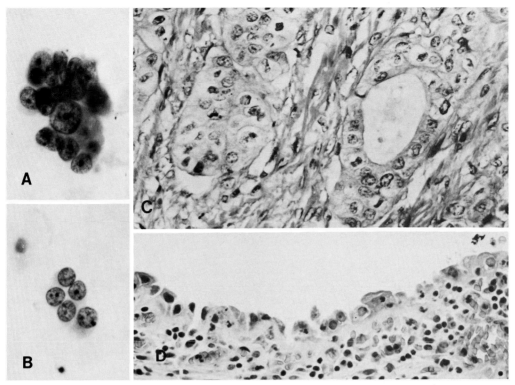

FIGURE 23–48. Adenocarcinoma of urethral diverticulum in a 54-year-old woman: urinary sediment and biopsy. (*A, B*) Clusters of cancer cells suggestive of adenocarcinoma; note papillary configuration, variability of nuclear sizes, and large nucleoli. (*C*) Histologic appearance of tumor. (*D*) Epithelial lining of urethral diverticulum, adjacent to tumor, showing changes consistent with carcinoma in situ. (*A, B* ×560; *C, D* ×350)

such personally observed case there were malignant cells in the urinary sediment and in the washings of the urethra (Fig. 23–51). The tumor proved fatal to the patient.

ACCURACY OF CYTOLOGIC DIAGNOSIS OF CARCINOMA OF THE LOWER URINARY TRACT

The evaluation of the accuracy of urinary cytology depends, to a large extent, on the expectations of the observer. As was discussed above, it is totally unrealistic to expect that well-differentiated papillary urothelial tumors (papillomas and papillary tumors, grade I) will yield diagnostic cells either in voided urine or in specimens obtained by direct sampling (bladder washing or brushing). The only exception to this rule is the finding of fragments of tumor that may be diagnosed by paraffin embed-

ding of sediment, examined by histologic techniques (cell block).

On the other hand, the finding of clearly malignant cells in the urinary sediment or bladder washings calls for a major investigative effort, even in the absence of cystoscopic or radiographic abnormalities. Nonpapillary carcinoma in situ may be present in the bladder, ureter, or renal pelvis in the absence of localizing evidence, as documented in the preceding pages.

The statistical evaluation of performance of urinary cytology published from various sources rarely reflect these elementary observations and thus result in major confusion as to what urinary cytology can and cannot accomplish. In experienced hands (Esposti and Zajicek) carcinoma of the bladder, grade II or above, was accurately identified in 78% of all cases. For high-grade tumors the diagnostic accuracy reached 91%. None of the 52 cases diagnosed as papillomas and papillary carci-

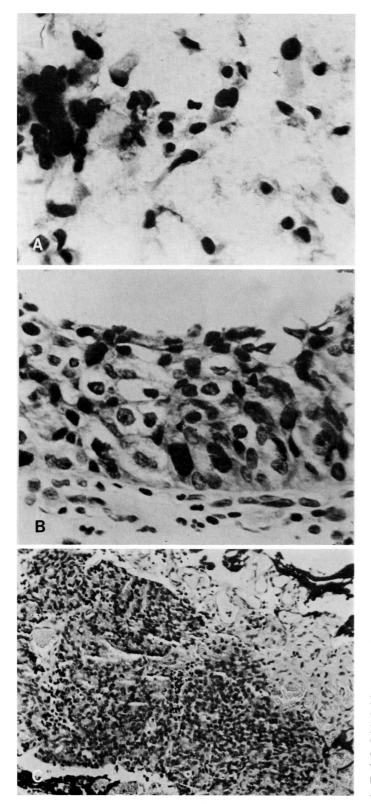

FIGURE 23–49. Carcinoma of the urethra diagnosed cytologically following radical prostatectomy for carcinoma of prostatic ducts. (*A*) A mixture of round and columnar cancer cells. (*B, C*) In the penile urethra, there was a focus of carcinoma in situ (*B*) and a tiny area of infiltrating carcinoma. (*C*). (*A, B* ×560; *C* ×150)

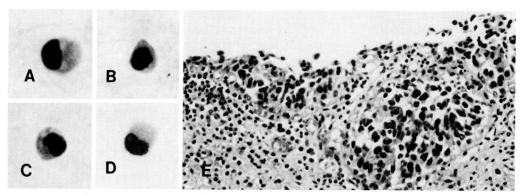

FIGURE 23–50. Carcinoma in situ of penile urethra in a 57-year-old patient with prior multiple transurethral resections of bladder tumors: urethral washings and histologic appearance of resected urethra. (*A, B, C, D*) Small cancer cells observed in urethral washings. Compare with nonpapillary carcinoma in situ of the bladder. (*E*) Section of resected urethra with nonpapillary carcinoma in situ. (*A–D* ×560; *E* ×150)

noma, grade I, could be identified cytologically. Morse and Melamed pointed out that the shedding of cancer cells in the urine is extremely variable. Therefore, three or more specimens must be examined for each patient.

The results of a survey of the diagnostic efficacy of cytology of voided urine based on three samples of urine (Koss et al., 1985) is shown in Table 23–7.

It may be noted that a positive sediment observed in a single case of a papillary tumor grade I was subsequently shown to reflect a flat carcinoma in situ. The results in papillary tumors grade II closely reflected the distribution of the DNA values in this group of tumors (Tribukait, 1985, also see below).

Shenoy et al. (1985) and Murphy (1990) claimed a much higher rate of cytologic diagnosis for grade I tumors. The criteria proposed for recognition of grade I tumors cannot be recommended.

The advantages of bladder washings under cys-

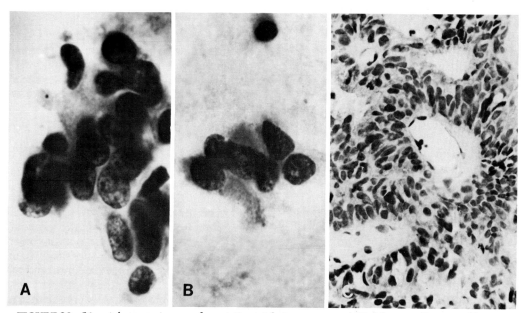

FIGURE 23–51. Adenocarcinoma of prostatic utricle in a man, aged 57: urinary sediment and biopsy section. (*A, B*) Clusters of malignant cells which, because of columnar configuration, are suggestive of adenocarcinoma. (*C*) Histologic appearance of the tumor. (*A, B* ×1,000; *C* ×350)

Table 23–7
Comparison of Highest Cytologic Diagnosis in Three Specimens of Voided Urine with the Highest Grade of Primary Tumor in the Nearest Biopsy in 203 Episodes

Highest Histologic Diagnosis of Primary Tumor	No. of Cases	Highest Cytologic Diagnosis in 3 Specimens of Voided Urine	
		Negative or Atypical	*Suspicious or Positive*
Noninvasive papillary tumors	136	29 (22%)	107 (78%)
Grade I	6	5	1
Grade II	68	20	48
Grade III	62	4	58
Nonpapillary carcinoma *in situ*	14	0	14 (100%)
Invasive carcinoma (all grades)	27	2	25 (92%)
Carcinoma of ureter	4	0	4
Other cancers	2	1	1
No evidence of cancer	20	20	0
Total	203	52	151

(Koss, L.G., et al.: Diagnostic value of cytology of voided urine. Acta Cytol., *29*:810–816, 1985, with permission)

toscopic control as advocated by Harris et al., and Trott and Edwards, among others, are debatable. If cystoscopy, a procedure hardly pleasant to the patient and not without its dangers, is to be performed for the purpose of cytologic examination, the major advantage of urinary cytology, namely the ease with which the examination may be repeatedly performed, no longer applies. Although it is correct that in experienced hands superb specimens may be obtained by washings, the possibility of simultaneous direct biopsies of visible lesions and surrounding epithelium robs this type of sampling of much of its clinical significance. For discussion of bladder washings in DNA analysis see p. 989.

Similar comments apply to carcinomas of the renal pelves and ureters. Eriksson and Johansson, who studied 43 such patients, obtained positive cytologic results in 19 patients, all with tumors grade II or higher. For the later group of poorly differentiated tumors the accuracy of 71% was obtained.

Several important sources of cytologic error, discussed in the preceding pages, must be emphasized: lithiasis, inflammation, infection with human polyomavirus, effects of drugs, and radiotherapy.

The most important accomplishment of cytology of the urinary tract is the diagnosis of clinically unsuspected cases of carcinoma, particularly carci-noma in situ. It has been documented above that this is indeed possible. There is considerable evidence that the salvage of such patients is potentially better than that of patients with advanced cancer, provided that treatment is applied before deep invasion or metastases occur.

Holmquist (1988) observed 12 unsuspected bladder cancers in a survey of urinary sediments in 9,870 routine urinalysis samples (1.2 per 1,000). The initial wet preparations were followed by two routine cytologic procedures whenever there was some suspicion of abnormality (see also comments on routine urinalysis on p. 897).

EVALUATION OF PATIENTS WITH BLADDER TUMORS

A complete evaluation of patients with bladder tumors requires not only a biopsy of the visible lesion, but also an evaluation of the remaining urothelium by cytologic examination of voided urine sediment and by multiple superficial biopsies of the bladder. The recommended minimum workup of such patients calls for cytologic analysis of three voided urine samples on three consecutive days for optimization of results (see p. 896). The biopsies, which should be obtained by special cutting instruments to prevent the loss of the all-important epithelium, should include, besides the visible tumor(s), the trigone of the bladder; the anterior, posterior, and lateral walls; and the dome.

In patients with carcinoma in situ revealed by biopsy or suspected on the basis of cytologic examination, the size and the location of the lesion must be determined by additional multiple biopsies, which *must* include the anterior lobe of the prostate, to rule out an extension of the malignant process into the prostatic ducts or the body of the prostate. In the absence of these measures, a rational mode of treatment cannot be determined. Prevention of invasive cancer is one of the important goals of this evaluation and of further monitoring of patients, outlined on p. 988.

The suggested clinical handling of patients with neoplastic lesions of the bladder is summarized in the list below. The use of cytology and multiple biopsies optimizes the workup of such patients and is also of prognostic value.

Protocol for Handling Primary Neoplastic Lesions of the Bladder

Asymptomatic patients exposed to known carcinogens
Check for hematuria
Urinary cytology $\times$ 3 every 6 months
Cystoscopy and multiple biopsies of bladder if indicated

Symptomatic patients (hematuria, frequency, nocturia, pain, mucous discharge)
Urinary cytology $\times$ 3
Cystoscopy
Multiple biopsies if cytology positive

Lesion (if visible)
Lateral walls
Posterior wall — Each Separately Submitted
Trigone
Dome

Follow-up after removal of localized lesions
Cytology $\times$ 3 every 3 months
Cystoscopy and multiple biopsies if cytologic or cystoscopic abnormalities present

MODALITIES OF TREATMENT AND MONITORING OF UROTHELIAL CANCER

Treatment

Bladder Tumors

Surgical removal and cautery treatment are still the therapeutic methods of choice, particularly for primary and recurrent superficial papillary tumors.

For superficially invasive tumors and for flat carcinomas in situ, not responding to conservative treatment (see below), the therapeutic choices include radical surgery, such as segmental or total cystectomy. Radical cystectomy with the creation of an ileal bladder is curative of nearly all carcinomas in situ and carcinomas in situ with microinvasion. The results of surgery are much less satisfactory for invasive tumors, although cures have been recorded. Radiotherapy has been used in the treatment of advanced invasive tumors, with occasional cure (Whitmore, 1988). For advanced tumors, systemic chemotherapy is usually recommended after primary treatment.

With improved understanding of the pathogenesis of bladder cancer and the recognition that cystoscopically invisible lesions, mainly carcinoma in situ and related epithelial abnormalities (IUN, see p. 940), play an important role in recurrent and invasive tumors, new therapeutic modalities were divised. Two methods of treatment are of major significance in the context of this book: immunotherapy and chemotherapy.

Immunotherapy. Intravesical instillation of the attenuated bovine tuberculosis bacillus (bacillus Calmette-Guérin; BCG), has become a treatment of choice for flat carcinoma in situ and related lesions. A substantial number of papers, based on randomized trials, have documented that, in some patients, long-term remissions, and possibly cures, can be achieved (Pinsky et al., 1985; DeKernion et al., 1985; Brosman, 1985; Herr et al., 1986; Guinan et al., 1987; Herr et al., 1989). A less enthusiastic report was published by Droller and Wash (1985). Although encouraging results for carcinoma in situ with prostatic extension were reported, still 10 of 23 such patients required cystectomy (Bretton et al., 1989). A variant of the method, based on injection of BCG into the tumor was also proposed (Colsini et al., 1987).

The treatment results in formation of microscopic granulomas composed of epithelioid and giant cells of the Langhans' type in the wall of the bladder and in the adjacent prostate, accompanied by a marked inflammatory reaction. The granulomas may show caseation necrosis in their centers, thereby mimicking spontaneously occurring tuberculosis (see p. 906). Although the precise mechanism of effective treatment is still unknown, it is hypothesized that the inflammatory reaction attracts cytotoxic lymphocytes, which, in a manner not clearly understood, help in replacing diseased epithelium by normal mucosa.

Intravesical Chemotherapy. Intravesical instillation of cytotoxic drugs, mainly the alkylating agent thiotepa and the antibiotic mitomycin, have been used in the treatment of papillary tumors to reduce the frequency of recurrences, and in the treatment of carcinoma in situ and resected high-grade tumors to prevent the occurrence of invasive carcinoma (summary in Soloway, 1983, 1985). Therapeutic successes have been reported (Soloway, 1985), but persuasive evidence that these treatment modes are as successful as BCG is not available.

Other Modes of Therapy. Photodynamic therapy of carcinoma in situ and small papillary tumors with hematoporphyrin derivatives has been reported (Hisazumi et al, 1984; Prout et al, 1987). The compound is injected into the patients, localizes in rapidly growing tissues, such as carcinomas, and renders them susceptible to phototherapy by laser. Similar attempts at treatment of carcinoma in situ of the bronchus have been attempted. Although some successes with this mode of treatment were reported, persuasive evidence of its effectiveness is still lacking.

Tumors of Renal Pelvis and Ureter

Nephroureterectomy is the treatment of choice for tumors confined to the organ of origin. In more advanced tumors, radiotherapy and systemic chemotherapy are often used.

Monitoring

Blood Group Antigens

Following the observation by Kovarik et al. (1968) suggesting that the expression of blood group antigens in bladder tumors may be correlated with prognosis, many written reports have accumulated describing a variety of methods and the results of this procedure. The fundamental assumption of these studies was that those epithelial tumors that have retained the ability of normal epithelium to express the blood group antigen of the patient were less likely to recur or progress than tumors that have lost the blood group antigen expression. In the initial studies, erythrocytes of known blood groups were used as markers (Kovarik et al, 1968; Yamase et al., 1981; Weinstein et al., 1981; Limas and Lange, 1982; Flanigan et al., 1983, Cordon-Cardo et al., 1988). Subsequently, serologic methods were developed, and the results were documented by the peroxidase–antiperoxidase sys-

tem (Coon and Weinstein, 1981). Ultrastructural localization of antisera labeled with colloidal gold has also been documented (De Harven et al., 1987).

The concept, while theoretically valid, has been shown to be of limited practical value. The performance of the test, particularly on small bladder biopsies was fraught with technical difficulties. The antibody used in patients with blood group O was a plant extract *(Ulex europeus),* and the expression of blood group antigens in patients with blood group A and B was shown to be related to the secretor status. The application of the method to cytologic samples has not been fully explored, although several successful attempts have been reported (Borgstrøm et al., 1985; Borgstrøm and Wahren, 1986).

Cytogenetics

Following the lead of Falor (1971) and Falor and Ward (1973, 1976), several cytogenetic studies of bladder tumors are on record. Granberg-Oehman et al. (1984) documented that most low-grade non-invasive tumors had a chromosomal component in the normal diploid range and that high-grade tumors had grossly aneuploid karyotypes. Similar observations were reported by Sandberg (see Chap. 7 for further discussion). Such studies may lead to the recognition of specific chromosomal changes in bladder tumors. Because of technical difficulties, however, they have very limited practical applicability for monitoring bladder tumors.

DNA and Gene Analysis

With the development of methods of DNA analysis by cytophotometry, image cytophotometry, and flow cytometry, enumeration of chromosomes could be replaced, to some degree, by measurements of DNA in cell populations. The methods, their accomplishments, and limitations, are described in Chapters 35 and 36. For the purposes of this narrative, the following summary is in order.

Studies of DNA content of bladder tumor, initially conducted by cytophotometry, suggested that low-grade papillary tumors are, for the most part, in the diploid range (i.e., have a DNA content identical or similar to normal tissues). With increasing grade, there was an increasing degree of abnormalities, reaching high aneuploid values for high-grade tumors (Lederer et al., 1972). With the developments in flow cytometry, rapid DNA measurements could be performed in a large number of bladder tumors. As was shown by Wijkstrøm et al. (1984), the DNA values obtained by flow cytometry compared favorably with cytogenetic analysis. Notable contributions to flow cytometric DNA studies of bladder tumors were made, among others, by Tribukait, whose large experience is summarized in Table 23–8.

It may be noted that DNA analysis confirms cytogenetic findings, inasmuch as most noninvasive low-grade tumors have a DNA content in the diploid range. Invasive tumors of high grade, on the other hand, are increasingly aneuploid, as are all cases of flat carcinoma in situ (Tis). This analysis confirms the clinical and pathologic observations on the origin of most high-grade invasive cancers of the urinary bladder from carcinomas in situ by documenting close similarities in DNA content between the two (see p. 938). It is also evident from this analysis that aneuploid noninvasive or superficially invasive tumors are much more likely to progress to invasive cancer than are diploid tumors.

Recently it could be shown that ploidy of bladder tumors could be correlated to some extent with a mutation of the *ras* oncogene (Czerniak et al., 1990). The mutation in position 12 of the gene occured more often in aneuploid than in diploid tumors. Unpublished data from our laboratories also suggest that the expression of the *ras* gene is markedly increased in aneuploid and invasive bladder carcinomas when the mutation of the exon in position 12 is synchronous with an intron muta-

tion. Sidransky et al. (1991) also observed mutations of the p53 inhibitory gene in bladder tumors (for further discussion of these genes see Chap. 2).

Undoubtedly, molecular analysis of tumors of the bladder will continue to provide fragmentary data, until a clear picture of the cascade of genetic abnormalities in bladder tumors will emerge.

DNA Content of Bladder Washings (Barbotage)

Given the premise that the DNA content of the epithelium of the bladder may be predictive of future behavior and, thereby, the prognosis of bladder tumors, DNA measurements on bladder washings were initiated by Melamed et al. (1976). A large number of papers from the Memorial–Sloan Kettering Cancer Center suggested that aneuploid DNA content in the cell suspension obtained, either at the time of cytoscopy or by catheter (barbotage), was predictive of tumor persistence, recurrence, or impending invasion (Klein et al., 1982; Badalament et al., 1986, 1987). The method was shown to be particularly effective in monitoring patients with carcinomas in situ undergoing treatment. As is discussed in Chapter 36, although histograms that are clearly normal or abnormal are easy to interpret, many of the histograms obtained from bladder washings, particularly from patients with low-grade tumors, are not clear-cut, are diffi-

Table 23–8
Distribution of DNA Values in 277 Untreated Bladder Tumors

Grade	No. in Group	Diploid	Aneuploid*
Distribution by Grade			
0	2	2	0
I	30 (100%)	24 (80%)	6 (20%)
II	107 (100%)	56 (52%)	51 (48%)
III	130 (100%)	6 (5%)	124 (95%)
Adenocarcinoma	8	1	7
Total	277	89	188
Distribution by Stage			
T_0	42 (100%)	32 (76%)	10 (24%)
T_1	118 (100%)	50 (42%)	68 (58%)
$T_{2,3,4}$	93 (100%)	7 (7.5%)	86 (92.5%)
Tis†	24 (100%)	0	24 (100%)
TOTAL	277	89	188

*Includes tetraploid–aneuploid tumors.
†Tis, flat carcinoma in situ.
(Modified from Tribukait, B.: Flow cytometry in surgical pathology and cytology of the genito-urinary tract. Koss, L.G., and Coleman, D.V. (eds.): Advances in Clinical Cytology, vol. pp. 163–189. New York, Masson Publishing, 1984)

cult to interpret, and require artificial classification schemes (Koss et al., 1989). Synchronous studies of the DNA content by image analysis and flow cytometry, disclosed that some samples, which were considered normal (diploid) by flow cytometry, could contain small aneuploid cell populations that were revealed by image analysis and were of predictive value for tumor recurrence or progression (Koss et al., 1989). Disregarding the cost of the apparatus and manpower involved in quantitative DNA studies, the expectations that the method would replace cytologic examination of the urinary sediment have not as yet been satisfactorily documented. The methods should be considered as an ancillary procedure.

Attempts to replace bladder washings or barbotage with samples of voided urine for flow cytometric analysis of DNA, as suggested by de Vere White et al. (1988), were not successful in our hands.

Monoclonal Antibodies

Numerous monoclonal antibodies have been tested or are being developed as specific markers for the identification of bladder tumors with invasive potential (Cordon-Cardo et al., 1984; Fradet et al., 1984, 1986, 1987). Some of these monoclonal antibodies may be used in conjunction with flow cytometry to identify subpopulations of cells with particular characteristics or to reveal aneuploidy in subpopulations of cells. Other markers used for these purposes are monoclonal antibodies to keratin filaments, which facilitate the separation of epithelial cells from other cells in bladder washing specimens for DNA measurements. In such studies the DNA can be measured in epithelial cells only (Ramaekers et al., 1984, 1986).

Image Analysis

The principles of image analysis of cells are discussed in Chapter 35. For a number of years our group has attempted to develop a system of objective, computer-based analysis of urothelial cells in voided urine sediments processed by the method of Bales (see Chap. 33 for technical details). The initial results were of interest inasmuch as several subgroups of urothelial cells could be identified with an accuracy surpassing that of the human observer (Sherman et al., 1986). Furthermore, as discussed on p. 949, the "atypical" urothelial cells could be classified into two groups of diagnostic value. Automated processing of 119 specimens of voided urine yielded promising results (Sherman et al., 1984). However, subsequent studies documented several errors in the evaluation system,

which, at the time of this writing (1991), is still being improved. The expectation that image analysis will, in the near future, replace visual examination of cells in the urinary sediment must be considered unlikely, although the technique is interesting.

Morphometry

A number of investigators, particularly a Dutch group headed by Baak, have advocated morphometric measurements of cellular and nuclear features in histologic sections of bladder tumors as a predictor of prognosis (Blomjous et al., 1988, 1989).

The method is interesting, although its major drawback is the need for a subjective selection of the microscopic field to be measured. Similar results were obtained by morphologic classifications of cancer cells in urinary sediment, advocated by Swedish observers many years ago (see p. 944).

Other Markers of Bladder Tumors

Several studies, tangentially related to cytology, have been reported, enhancing still further the concept of two pathways of bladder tumors, described on p. 935. Thus, a study of the density and distribution of nuclear pores (see Fig. 1–22 for description) was shown to correlate with DNA ploidy (Czerniak et al., 1984). The number and density of nuclear pores was significantly higher in aneuploid than in diploid tumors. The expression of a monoclonal antibody Ca1 (epitectine), a presumed marker of surfaces of cancer cells (Ashall et al., 1982), was also shown to be higher in all but one of 12 aneuploid tumors when compared with diploid tumors and normal urothelium (Czerniak and Koss, 1985).

Cytologic Monitoring of Bladder Tumors

In the experience of this writer, the best method of monitoring patients with treated bladder tumors is by cytologic analysis of voided urinary sediment. Each monitoring sequence should be based on three urine samples obtained on consecutive days (see p. 896). The presence of cancer cells, as described in the preceding pages, is always indicative of a recurrence or progression of urothelial carcinoma, regardless of the mode of treatment or presumed clinical status. In fact, in several personally observed cases, urinary sediment that was positive for cancer cells, *in the presence of an apparently good clinical response to treatment,* anticipated an invasive or metastatic cancer that killed the patient. None of the cytotoxic drugs or BCG cause epithelial cell changes that could be confused with cancer. Although minor atypias in the form of cellular and nuclear enlargement may be observed with thiotepa, neither mitomycin or BCG cause any significant cytologic abnormalities, except for nonspecific changes (or granulomatous inflammation in BCG) that may be associated with an inflammatory response. Similar observations were reported by Harving et al. (1988), who documented that cytologic analysis is more sensitive than multiple biopsies in predicting tumor recurrence or progression. The need for cytologic monitoring was also emphasized by Hopkins et al. (1983), who pointed out that a substantial number of patients with seemingly innocuous low-grade tumors may develop an unexpected invasive cancer of the bladder.

After radical cystectomy, the patients must be monitored by periodic cytologic examination of urine from the ileal bladder (see p. 977).

Role of Cytology in the Treatment of Bladder Cancer by Radiation

Changes in benign epithelial cells of the bladder following irradiation were discussed on page 918. Radiotherapy of carcinomas of the bladder results in marked pyknosis and ballooning of the tumor cells (Fig. 23–52*A*), a change often reflected in smears of urinary sediment (see Fig. 23–52*B*). The degree of nuclear abnormality in the cancer cells usually allows an easy differentiation between the irradiated benign and the irradiated malignant cells. However, on occasion the nuclei of irradiated benign cells will display some hyperchromasia that may render the differential diagnosis difficult. In such situations it is advisable to withhold judgment until clear-cut evidence of cancer is obtained on subsequent samples of urine.

The cells of bladder cancer recurring after radiotherapy are in no way different from the cells of the primary tumor (Fig. 23–53). Numerous biopsies or cystotomy often may be required to obtain histologic confirmation of a tumor, especially if there is considerable scarring of the bladder wall.

Cytologic studies of urinary sediment proved to be quite useful in following a group of patients with bladder cancer treated by radiation before undergoing surgery. If preliminary ratiotherapy was successful, it resulted in rapid diminution in the numbers of cancer cells, and, in four cases, in complete disappearance of cancer cells. In these latter cases, histologic studies of totally removed bladders failed to reveal the presence of cancer.

It is of particular interest that in several cases of

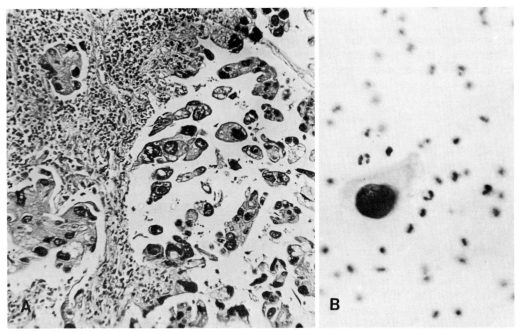

FIGURE 23–52. (*A*) Irradiated urothelial cancer of the bladder. (*B*) Recently irradiated cancer cells from urinary sediment. Note the blown-up appearance of the markedly hyperchromatic nucleus. (*A* ×150; *B* ×560)

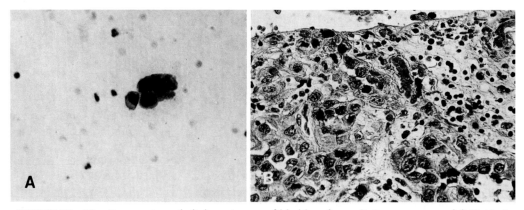

FIGURE 23–53. Recurrent urothelial carcinoma of bladder after radiation treatment. (*A*) Voided urine contained unaffected cancer cells. (*B*) Numerous cytoscopic biopsies of the altered mucosa were negative, but cystotomy disclosed the presence of tumor. (*A, B* approx. ×300)

carcinoma of the bladder treated by radiation, the urinary sediment remained positive in spite of a very favorable clinical response of the tumor to therapy. Subsequent surgical removal of the bladder revealed *residual carcinoma in situ that apparently did not respond to radiation treatment,* whereas the invasive tumor was obliterated (Fig. 23–54). Similar observations were made with carcinoma of the cervix (see p. 669) and in carcinoma of the esophagus (see p. 1035).

Monitoring of Patients with Treated Carcinoma of the Renal Pelvis and Ureter

Because a large proportion of the surviving patients are prone to the development of new carcinomas, either in the opposite renal pelvis and ureter or, most often, in the bladder, the same precautions as described for treated bladder tumors must be observed. Urinary cytology is the primary method of monitoring the occurrence of high-grade tumors. Cystoscopy and examination with computed tomography (CT) serve as monitoring methods for low-grade tumors, not detectable by cytologic techniques.

METASTATIC TUMORS TO THE BLADDER

Malignant epithelial tumors originating in the adjacent organs and, less often, in distant sites may invade the bladder wall and reach the mucosa. Many of these metastatic lesions may be detected

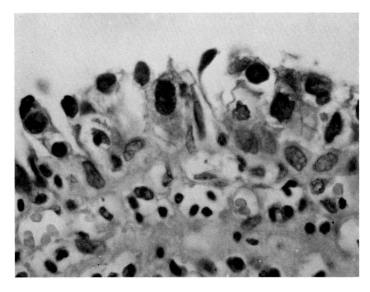

FIGURE 23–54. Carcinoma in situ, urinary bladder. Lesion observed after radiotherapy of bladder tumor with 6,000 R, resulting in eradication of invasive carcinoma. (×650)

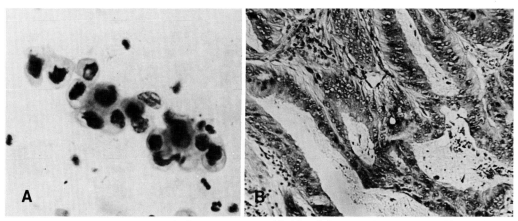

FIGURE 23-55. Metastatic rectal adenocarcinoma to bladder. (*A*) "Signet ring" cancer cells in urinary sediment. Note the vacuolated cytoplasm. (*B*) Biopsy of bladder wall. (*A* ×560; *B* ×150)

cytologically, and their discovery may be of value to the attending physician in the evaluation of the status of the patient. Cancers of the uterine cervix, of the endometrium, and of the large bowel were most frequently diagnosed in this fashion. In some instances of colonic carcinoma, the tumor cells were of signet ring type (Fig. 23–55). In other such cases, columnar cancer cells were observed (Fig. 23–56), akin to the cells of primary adenocarcinoma of the bladder (cf. Fig. 23–31). Occasionally, cancers from more distant primary sites may be seen (Fig. 23–57). Often, it is not possible to determine on cytologic grounds whether the tumor is primary or metastatic.

A notable exception to this last statement is metastatic malignant melanoma. Pigment-containing malignant cells are easily identified (Fig. 23–58). However, as pointed out by Piva and Koss, even this diagnosis is not without is pitfalls. Pigment-containing renal tubular cells may be mistaken for cells of the metastatic tumor (Fig. 23–59). Unless clear-cut nuclear abnormalities are observed, the diagnosis of metastatic melanoma should not be made. A case of melanoma with pigmented casts in the urinary sediment was described by Valente et al. (1985).

Malignant lymphomas may invade the urinary bladder, and malignant cells may be identified in the urine sediment (Fig. 23–60). As is usual, the

(text continues on page 996)

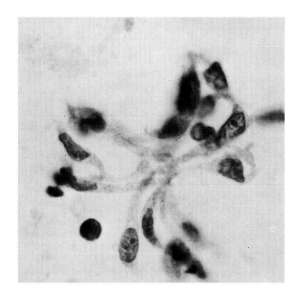

FIGURE 23–56. Urinary sediment. Metastatic colonic carcinoma. Note the columnar configuration of cancer cells. (×1,000)

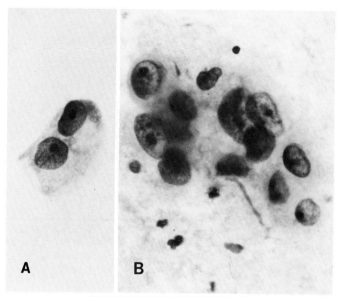

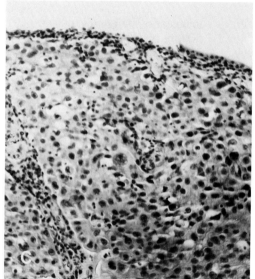

FIGURE 23-57. Bronchogenic carcinoma metastatic to bladder. (*A*) Cells in urinary sediment; (*B*) cells in sputum; (*C*) bladder biopsy disclosed epidermoid carcinoma in subepithelial location. The epithelium was ulcerated elsewhere. (*A, B* ×560; *C* ×150)

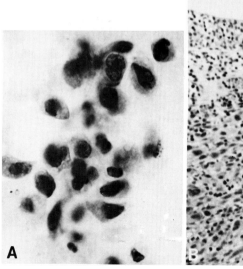

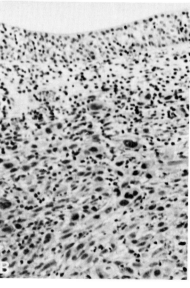

FIGURE 23-58. Malignant melanoma metastatic to urinary bladder. (*A*) Cancer cells with granules of pigment in urinary sediment; (*B*) tumor invading bladder wall. Elsewhere there was ulceration of the epithelium (*A* ×560; *B* ×150. Piva, A., and Koss, L.G.: Cytologic diagnosis of metastatic malignant melanoma in urinary sediment. Acta Cytol., *8*:398–402, 1964)

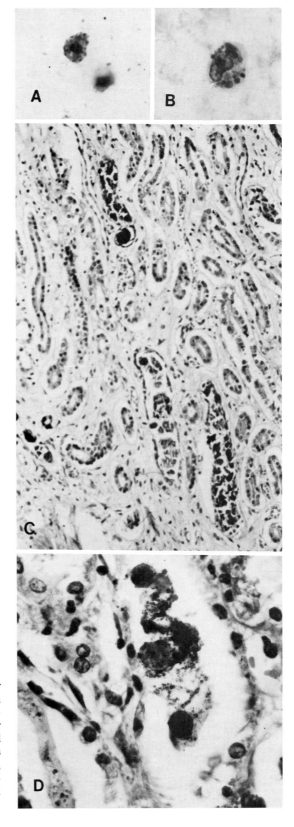

FIGURE 23–59. Pigmented renal tubular cells in urinary sediment. Case of disseminated malignant melanoma with melanuria. (*A, B*) Pigment-containing cells. These were mistaken for cells of melanoma. (*C, D*) Low- and high-power views of the renal tubules (autopsy material). Degenerated pigment-containing cells crowding the tubules. There was no evidence of metastatic melanoma in the urinary tract. (*A, B, D* ×560; *C* ×150. Piva, A., and Koss, L.G.: Cytologic diagnosis of metastatic malignant melanoma in urinary sediment. Acta Cytol., *8*:398–402, 1964)

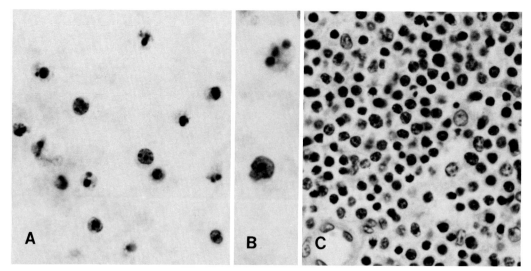

FIGURE 23–60.   Malignant lymphoma involving bladder: urinary sediment and tissue, the latter obtained at postmortem examination. (*A*) Low-power view of urinary sediment showing isolated tumor cells, some showing karyorrhexis. (*B*) The characteristic nuclear protrusion and large nucleolus allow the identification of the tumor type. (*B*) Bladder wall was diffusely infiltrated with a large cell lymphoma. (*A, C* ×350; *B* ×1,000)

tumor cells lie singly, and they sometimes can be identified because of the peculiar nuclear protrusions (nipples) also observed in other fluids (cf. Chap. 26). Acute leukemia may sometimes begin with hematuria. Blast cells may be identified in the urinary sediment (Fig. 23–61).

Unexpected findings may occasionally be observed. A patient with multiple myeloma with renal involvement and impairment (seen through the courtesy of Mr. Arthur Garutti) was shedding bizarre multinucleated cells in his urinary sediment, which could have only represented reactive

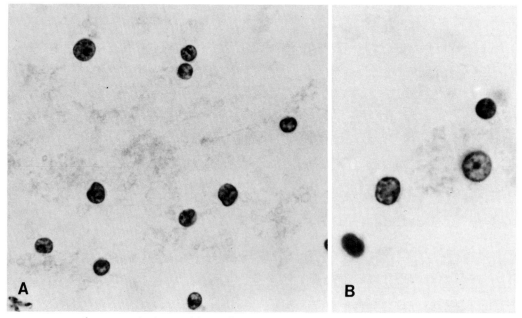

FIGURE 23–61.   Acute leukemia: blast cells in urinary sediment. Note very scanty cytoplasm and prominent nucleoli. (*A* ×560, *B* ×1,000)

renal tubular cells surrounding tubular casts commonly observed in this disease (Fig. 23–62).

URINE CYTOLOGY IN MALIGNANT TUMORS OF THE RENAL PARENCHYMA

Except for the high-grade cancers of the renal pelvis, which offer an excellent chance of cytologic diagnosis, tumors of the kidney and, especially, those originating in the renal parenchyma away from the pelvis offer only a very slim chance of cytologic detection in urinary sediment in the early stages.

Adenocarcinoma of the kidney is a tumor that usually originates in the renal cortex. The most common variety is the clear cell or hypernephroid type of cancer that resembles, by virtue of its large clear cells, the pattern of the adrenal cortex, hence, the old name of "hypernephroma." The tumor cells have distinctly granular or clear cytoplasm and contain both glycogen and lipids. All types of renal cancer, but especially the hypernephroid cancer, have a tendency to invade the renal pelvis and the renal vessels. The penetration into the renal pelvis often brings about hematuria, which is not infrequently the first evidence of the existence of the tumor. Cytologic detection of the tumor is not possible in urine until the cells desquamate into the urinary stream. Concomitant hematuria renders the diagnosis exceedingly difficult. Moreover, renal cancer cells readily undergo degenerative changes, so that, even in the absence of hematuria, it is rare to see cells sufficiently well preserved for an unequivocal diagnosis. The cancer cells are fairly large, with a delicately vacuolated or finely granular cytoplasm, either eosinophilic or basophilic, and with a distinctly abnormal, hyperchromatic large nucleus (Fig. 23–63). Spindly cancer cells may occur. In diagnosing renal carcinoma, one must be certain that the nuclear abnormalities are clearly evident, since cytoplasmic granularity and vacuolization may also be observed in benign cells of urothelial origin, particularly in specimens obtained by retrograde catheterization (cf. p. 899).

The writer has found the urinary sediment to be of questionable value in diagnosing primary renal parenchymal cancers. On only a few occasions were cells from a renal carcinoma unequivocally observed. In most of these cases, the identification of the site of origin of the malignant cells was not possible.

These results are in contradistinction to the experience of other authors who reported a fair measure of success in the diagnosis of renal carcinoma. Umiker (1964) and Meisels (1963) reported between 25% and 50% of renal cancers as diagnosable by cytology. Piscioli et al. (1983) claimed cytologic recognition of renal cancer in 19 or 44 cases. These results could not be duplicated in this laboratory.

Hajdu et al. (1971) suggested the use of fat stain (oil red-O) on cells of the unfixed urinary sediment. Seventeen histologically proved cases of renal carcinoma were studied; in 14 patients, the fat stain was positive in the form of distinct intracytoplasmic granules (Fig. 23–64). Similar cells were observed in cells in direct touch preparations of tumors. The results could not be confirmed by Mount et al. (1973). Kyrkos et al. observed fat-positive cells also in other tumors of the urinary tract. Masin and Masin observed cytoplasmic lipids in

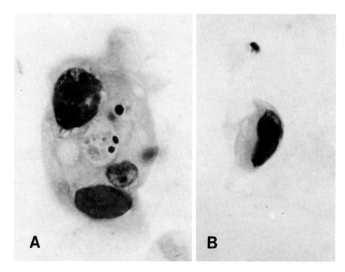

FIGURE 23–62.   (*A, B*) Multiple myeloma with renal impairment: urinary sediment. Bizarre, large cells, very likely of renal tubular origin. (×560. Courtesy Mr. Arthur Garutti, Port Jefferson, New York)

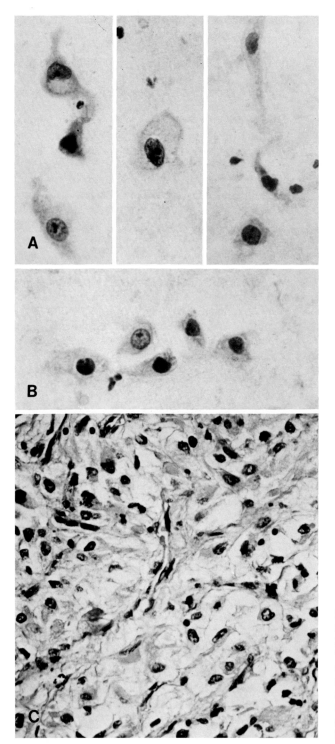

FIGURE 23–63. Renal carcinoma. A case with identifiable cancer cells in urinary sediment. (*A*, *B*) Note the clear cytoplasm and prominent nucleoli. It was not possible from the appearance of the cancer cells to determine the primary site of the tumor. Of note is the spindly appearance of some of the cells corresponding to the focal histologic appearance of the primary tumor (*C*). It is of interest that the spindly appearance of renal carcinoma is a frequent feature in metastatic foci. (*A*, *B* ×560; *C* ×350)

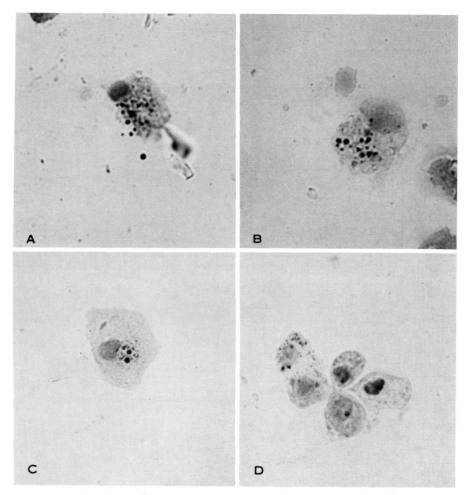

FIGURE 23–64. (*A, B, C*) Coarse intracytoplasmic oil red O-positive (*black*) granules in bizarre large cells in smears prepared from the sediment of unfixed urine of patients with renal cell carcinoma. (*D*) Touch smear of renal cell carcinoma. Note the strikingly similar cells and intracytoplasmic oil red O-positive granules. (*A–D*: Oil red-O ×560. Hajdu, S.I., et al.: Cytologic diagnosis of renal cell carcinoma with the aid of fat stain. Acta Cytol. *15*:31–33, 1971)

benign and in malignant urothelial cells. Hajdu's observation, while not specific, is nevertheless of interest as a screening test. Most renal parenchymal carcinomas are diagnosed today by computed tomography (CT) or angiography, although avascular renal carcinomas do occur.

Sano and Koprowska reported a case of primary *malignant lymphoma* of the kidney diagnosed on urinary sediment.

Several cases of *Wilms' tumor* were observed in urinary sediment. The cancer cells were generally small, elongated, and characteristically in clusters, an appearance that does not occur with either inflammatory cells, leukemias, or lymphomas. When such cells are found in the urinary sediment

of a child, the diagnosis of Wilms' tumor may be entertained (Fig. 23–65). Transcutaneous aspiration of renal tumors is discussed with other abdominal organs in Chapter 29.

THE PROSTATE AND THE SEMINAL VESICLES: VOIDED URINE AND PROSTATIC MASSAGE*

The prostate is a complex gland encased in a heavy shell of fibromuscular tissue (Fig. 23–66*A*). The glands and the ducts are lined by cuboidal to co-

---

Aspiration biopsy of the prostate is discussed in Chap. 29.

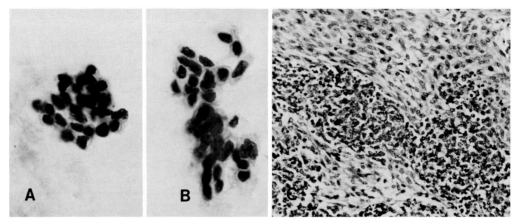

FIGURE 23–65. Urinary sediment and surgical specimen in a 9-year-old boy with an abdominal mass, shown to be a Wilms' tumor. (*A, B*) Clusters of small, tightly packed and elongated malignant cells. (*C*) A histologic field of the tumor mde up of small undifferentiated cells and small spindly cells. (*A, B* ×560; *C* ×150)

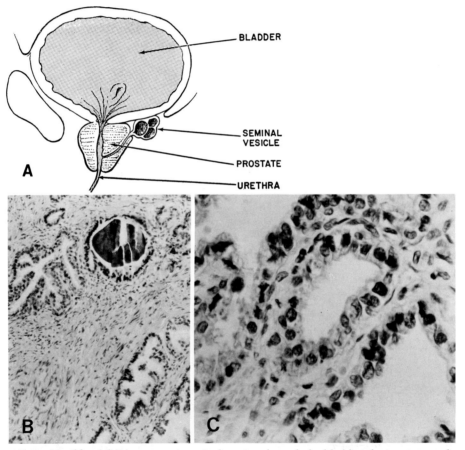

FIGURE 23–66. (*A*) Diagrammatic sagittal section through the bladder, the prostate, and the seminal vesicles. (*B*) Normal prostate. Note the glands and the fibromuscular stroma. (*C*) Seminal vesicle. Complex tubular structure with granules of yellow pigment in the cytoplasm of the glandular cells lining the tubules. Large, hyperchromatic nuclei may be noted in some of the cells. (*B* ×150; *C* ×560)

lumnar epithelium (see Fig. 23–66*B*). Within the lumina of the glands one may frequently observe concretions of prostatic secretions (corpora amylacea) that may undergo calcification and thereby form "prostatic calculi." The sexual apparatus of men also includes two symmetric glandular structures—the seminal vesicles attached to the posterior aspect of the prostate. The seminal vesicles are in close relationship with the spermatic ducts, with which they share a common opening in the prostatic urethra. The seminal vesicles are lined by columnar cells characterized by the accumulation of a yellow pigment in the cytoplasm (see Fig. 23–66*C*). Variability in nuclear sizes and the presence of cells with markedly enlarged, dark nuclei (Arias-Stella and Takano–Moron) characterize the epithelium.

Cells from the prostate and the seminal vesicles are uncommon in spontaneously voided urine. They may be expressed from the prostate by massage and are occasionally seen in ejaculates. They may be observed in vaginal smears (see p. 274).

Cytology of Specimens Obtained by Prostatic Massage

Prostatic massage is commonly used by urologists to obtain samples of prostatic secretions for rapid microscopic analysis. The most common purpose of this procedure is the identification of leukocytes in cases of prostatitis. The experience described here was based on an attempt to diagnose occult prostatic carcinoma in over 2,000 asymptomatic patients aged 50 or older. The cytologic examination of prostatic fluid and, usually of urine sediment after massage, failed to discover occult cancer, but it provided valuable data on prostatic cytology. The method was also used in a group of patients clinically suspected of harboring prostatic cancer.

The cytologic examination of the prostatic fluid and of the urinary sediment obtained after prostatic massage is complicated because cells of four different origins may be present in the specimen: the epithelium of the prostate, the epithelium of the seminal vesicles, the epithelium of the bladder and the urethra, and the sperm or its predecessors expelled from the seminal vesicles.

Normal Prostate

In the absence of disease, cells of the prostatic duct epithelium usually appear in sparse, flat, "honeycomb"-type clusters. The nuclei are round, small, and inconspicuous, and may contain small chromocenters (Fig. 23–67). The cytoplasm of these cells is finely granular or clear and contains demonstrable acid phosphatase and prostate-specific antigen. At the periphery of the clusters the duct cells are cuboidal or columnar. Occasionally, one or two round squamous cells containing yellow deposits of glycogen may be noted. These cells are more commonly seen as a result of estrogen therapy (see p. 1005), but they may also be present in the absence of any treatment. Small, concentric, yellow, but occasionally calcified, prostatic concretions (corpora amylacea) may appear in smears. Cells of prostatic acini are rarely observed in this type of material.

Spermatozoa are readily recognized. The precursor cells of spermatozoa or spermatogonia appear as small cells, about the size of lymphocytes or slightly larger, with a fair amount of somewhat elongated cytoplasm, and peripheral, relatively large, dark nuclei (Fig. 23–68*A*). On occasion, macrophages containing numerous ingested spermatozoa may be noted. Characteristically, the tails of the spermatozoa often remain outside the macrophage (Fig. 23–68*B*).

Cells of the seminal vesicles are relatively uncommon, but when present, may be recognized because of the granules of yellow pigment in the

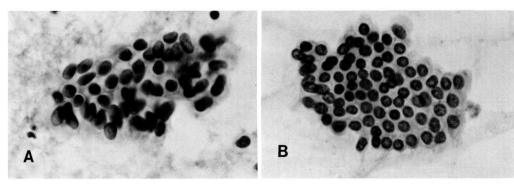

FIGURE 23–67. (*A, B*) Clusters of benign prostatic ductal cell (prostatic massage). (*A, B* ×560)

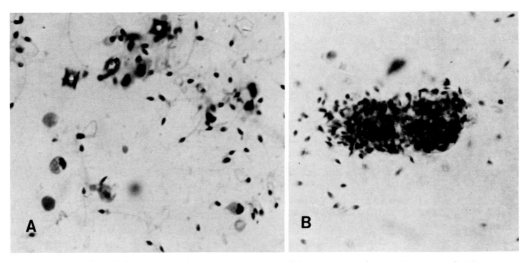

FIGURE 23–68. (*A*) Spermatozoa in various stages of development (prostatic massage). The pear-shaped cells with peripheral dark nuclei represent spermatogonia. (*B*) Macrophages ingesting sper-matozoa. The cells are completely filled and covered by spermatozoa (prostatic massage). (*A, B* ×560)

cytoplasm. The nuclei are usually similar to those of prostatic cells. Occasionally, however, cells with large, dark nuclei may occur. These can be accurately identified by cytoplasmic pigment, but must be recognized as a potential major pitfall of prostatic cytology (Fig. 23–69) (see also comments on p. 1326). Nearly every prostatic massage specimen will contain a few cells very difficult to classify accurately because of the complexity of the participating epithelia.

Benign Prostatic Hypertrophy

A common disease of older men, this disorder is characterized chiefly by an enlargement of the prostate, associated with glandular proliferation with or without an increase in the fibromuscular stroma. The cellular components of a prostatic massage are the same as in normal prostates except for a richer yield of prostatic glandular cells that may appear singly or in clusters. Greenwald et al.,

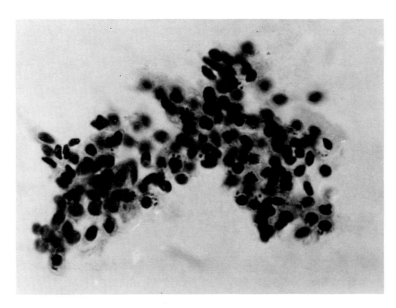

FIGURE 23–69. Cells originating in seminal vesicles (prostatic massage). The cytoplasm contains clearly visible granules of pigment. (×560)

in a major epidemiologic study of prostatic hyperplasia, concluded that such patients are not at an increased risk for prostate cancer.

Carcinoma of the Prostate

Carcinoma of the prostate is one of the most common forms of cancer found at autopsy in the elderly man. It has been variously estimated that between 20% and 80% of all men autopsied at the age of 60 or over may have morphologic evidence of prostate cancer (Peterson, 1986). In a study of clinically unsuspected carcinoma of the prostate, incidentally discovered in prostate chips removed by transurethral resection (TUR), Bauer et al. emphasized that the tumors are not as innocuous as is generally thought. The 5-year survival rate of 55 patients was only 54%. The 10-year survival rate of 24 patients was only 37%. Prostatic cancer ranges histologically from well-differentiated adenocarcinoma to a tumor composed of solid sheets or narrow strands of relatively small cells. The tumor often originates in the posterior lobe of the prostate and has a tendency to invade the perineural spaces. Prostatic adenocarcinoma, as does the normal prostatic gland, has the ability to produce acid phosphatase and prostate-specific antigen, which may be demonstrated in the tumor. An elevation of the specific prostatic antigen in the blood may

often be demonstrated and usually suggests tumor spread beyond the anatomic confines of the prostate. Prostatic cancer may show a dependency on hormones. Estrogens or their chemical substitutes may temporarily arrest the spread of prostatic cancer and bring about subjective and objective improvement.

The attempt by Richardson et al. at cytologic detection of occult prostatic cancer in asymptomatic men over 50 years of age by prostatic massage met with complete failure in the nearly 2,000 patients examined. Well over 99% of the specimens were completely negative, and in the small percentage of cases with slight cellular abnormalities, one could hardly conceive a valid reason for exploring a perfectly asymptomatic patient who was anxious to keep his prostate.

However, in experienced hands cytology of prostatic massage is occasionally helpful in the identification of prostatic cancer in symptomatic patients. The application of thin needle aspiration biopsy technique to the diagnosis of prostatic cancer is discussed in Chapter 29.

Cytology of Prostatic Carcinoma. The presence of cells of prostatic carcinoma in *voided urine* may be noted occasionally, but as a rule, this indicates that the tumor is widespread (Fig. 23–70).

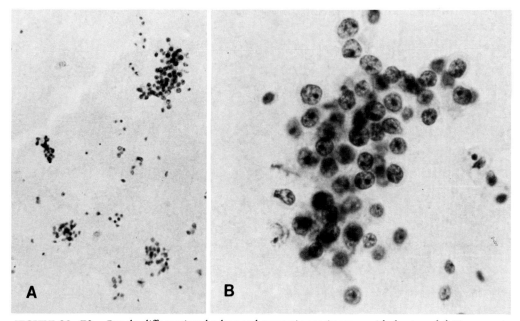

FIGURE 23–70. Poorly differentiated advanced prostatic carcinoma: voided urine. (*A*) Numerous papillary clusters of small cancer cells. (*B*) The cells are characterized by scanty cytoplasm and prominent nucleoli. (*A* ×150; *B* ×560)

The anatomically limited cancer, especially when still confined to the posterior lobe, does not shed cells spontaneously.

In specimens obtained by *prostatic massage* the appearance of cancer cells varies according to the degree of histologic differentiation of the tumor. In poorly differentiated carcinomas, the cancer cells are characterized by relatively large nuclei that vary in size and are provided with pink, large nucleoli (Figs. 23–70 and 23–71).

Well-differentiated prostatic adenocarcinomas often shed tight, papillary clusters of cancer cells (Fig. 23–72), or columnar cancer cells with the well-preserved cytoplasm and nuclear abnormali-

ties customarily encountered in this type of cancer: nuclear enlargement, moderate hyperchromasia, and large irregular nucleoli (Fig. 23–73). Such well-differentiated adenocarcinomas may occur in the anterior lobes of the prostate and may be associated with carcinoma of the bladder.

Material obtained by prostatic massage is rarely optimal and does not compare favorably with material obtained by prostatic aspiration, discussed in detail in Chapter 29. The method is, at best, a substitute that serves to identify an occasional prostatic carcinoma in a patient with prostatic enlargement. In fact, as recently documented, the measurement of prostate-specific antigen in serum

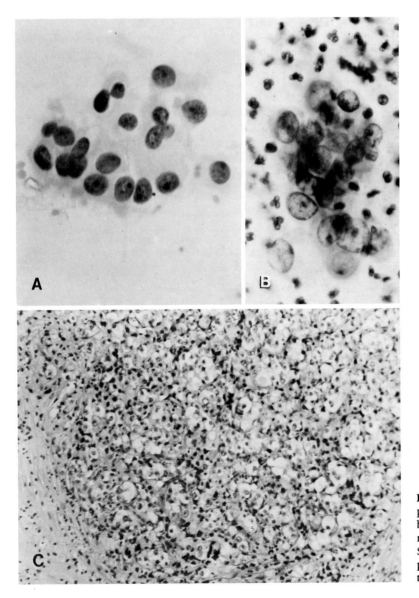

FIGURE 23–71. (*A, B*) Cells from prostatic adenocarcinomas obtained by prostatic massage. Note the large nuclei and prominent nucleoli. (*C*) Section of a poorly differentiated prostatic carcinoma. Same case as that in (*B*). (*A, B* ×560; *C* ×150)

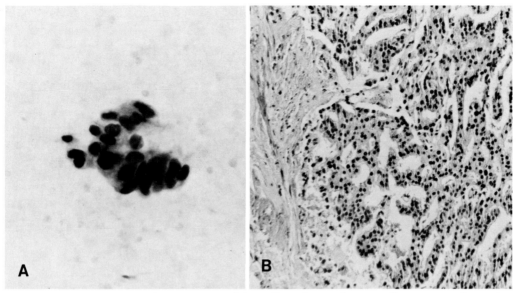

FIGURE 23–72. Prostatic adenocarcinoma. (*A*) Papillary cluster of cancer cells in a smear obtained by prostatic massage; note the flattened peripheral cells. (*B*) Tissue section reveals a well-differentiated adenocarcinoma (*A* ×560; *B* ×150)

may be a much better screening test for this common disease (Catalona et al., 1991).

For comments on the value of DNA measurements in prostatic carcinoma, see Chapter 29.

The Effect of Treatment with Estrogens on Urinary Sediment

Application of estrogens or pharmacologically related compounds in the treatment of prostatic cancer may result in the presence in voided urine of mature squamous cells, many of which contain yellow deposits of glycogen in their cytoplasm (Fig. 23–74*A*). These cells originate in the glands of the cancerous prostate which undergo squamous metaplasia under the impact of estrogens (see Fig. 23–74*B*).

Prostatic Disease and Bladder Cancer

The association of prostatic enlargement, whether due to hyperplasia or to carcinoma, with cancer of the bladder is fairly common. From January 1974 to August 1977 we observed 19 patients, seen primarily because of prostatic disease, whose urinary sediment disclosed urothelial carcinoma, subsequently confirmed by biopsies of the bladder. Barlebo and Sørensen observed two patients with car-

cinoma in situ of the bladder, initially seen because of prostatic hypertrophy. A similar case is recorded in Fig. 23–26.

Further review of the files at Montefiore Hospital for the same period compiled by Dr. Allayne Kahan disclosed 13 patients with coexisting carcinomas of the prostate and of the bladder and 47 patients with benign prostatic hypertrophy and bladder cancer. The 19 patients with occult bladder cancer were among these 60 patients. This observation strongly suggests that all patients with prostatic disease, whether benign or malignant should have the benefit of a cytologic examination of the urinary sediment. Urologists are generally unaware of this association, and the bladder tumors may remain occult unless routine urinary cytology is used and subsequent tissue evidence secured.

A further association of bladder cancer with prostatic disease was reported by Mahadevia et al. (1986) from this laboratory. Mapping of 20 cystoprostatectomy specimens from patients with invasive high-grade bladder cancers or carcinoma in situ, or both, disclosed extension of urothelial tumor to prostatic ducts in 9 of them, all with carcinoma in situ. In fact, this work brought into question the very existence of a primary carcinoma of major prostatic ducts which, if it does exist, must be extremely rare. In the presence of a solid carcinoma of the prostatic ducts (Fig. 23–75), it is man-

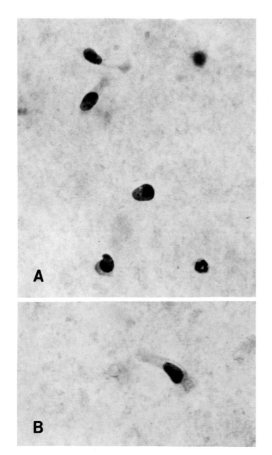

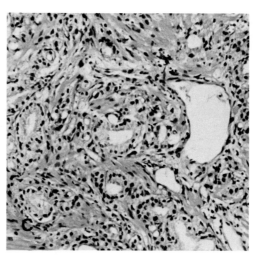

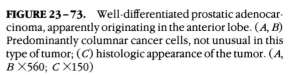

FIGURE 23–73. Well-differentiated prostatic adenocarcinoma, apparently originating in the anterior lobe. (*A, B*) Predominantly columnar cancer cells, not unusual in this type of tumor; (*C*) histologic appearance of the tumor. (*A, B* ×560; *C* ×150)

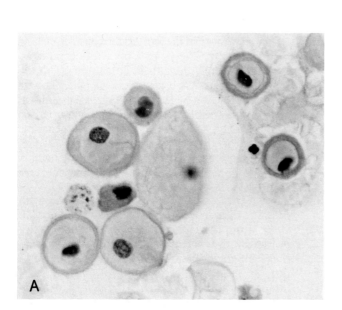

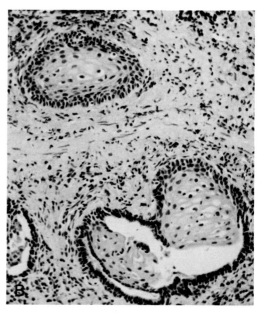

FIGURE 23–74. (*A*) Glycogen-containing squamous cells in the urinary sediment of a patient treated with estrogen-substitutes for cancer of the prostate. The glycogen forms visible yellow particles within the cytoplasm, an appearance more common in old smears than in fresh preparation. (*B*) Squamous metaplasia of cancerous prostatic duct under the influence of estrogen therapy. (*A* ×560; *B* ×150)

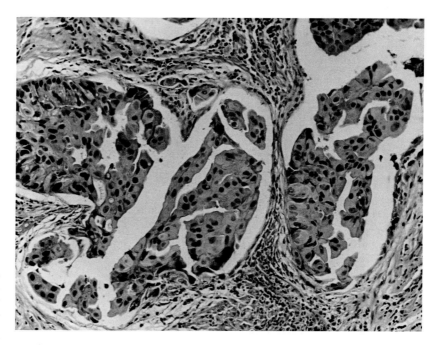

FIGURE 23–75. Urothelial carcinoma in prostatic ducts. The source of origin was an inconspicuous carcinoma in situ in the bladder trigone. (×150)

datory to search for a carcinoma in situ of the bladder by techniques described on p. 986.

Mahadevia's work also confirmed the association of bladder cancer and prostate cancer. The latter was observed in 14 of the 20 patients; only one of these lesions was suspected before cystectomy.

BIBLIOGRAPHY

Tumors of the Bladder (including flat carcinoma in situ)

Allegra, S.R., Broderick, P.A., and Corvese, N.L.: Cytologic and histogenetic observations in well differentiated transitional cell carcinoma of bladder. J. Urol., *107*:777–782, 1972.

Alroy, J., Pauli, B.U., and Weinstein, R.S.: Correlation between numbers of desmosomes and the aggressiveness of transitional cell carcinomas in human urinary bladder. Cancer, *47*:104–112, 1981.

Althausen, A.F., Prout, G.R., Jr., and Daly, J.J.: Noninvasive papillary carcinoma of bladder associated with carcinoma in situ. J. Urol., *116*:575–580, 1976.

Anderstrom, C., Johansson, S., and Nilson, S.: The significance of lamina propria invasion on the prognosis of patients with bladder tumors. J. Urol., *124*:23–26, 1980.

Ashall, F., Bramwell, M.E., and Harris, H.: A new marker for human cancer cells: The Ca antigen and the Ca1 antibody. Lancet, *2*:1–7, 1982.

Atkin, N.B., and Baker, M.C.: Cytogenetic study of ten carcinomas of the bladder: Involvement of chromosomes 1 and 11. Cancer Genet. Cytogenet., *15*:253–268, 1985.

Atkin, N.B., and Petkovic, I.: Variable sex chromatin pattern in an early carcinoma of the bladder. J. Clin. Pathol., *26*:126–129, 1973.

Austen, G.J., and Friedell, G.H.: Observations of local growth patterns of bladder cancer. Trans. Am. Assoc. Genitourin. Surg., *56*:38–43, 1964.

Bales, C.E.: A semi-automated method for preparation of urine sediment for cytologic evaluation. Acta Cytol., *25*:323–326, 1981.

Banigo, O.G., Waisman, J., and Kaufman, J.J.: Papillary (transitional) carcinoma in an ileal conduit. J. Urol., *114*:626–627, 1975.

Barlebo, H., Sorensen, B.L., and Soeberg Ohlsen, A.: Carcinoma in situ of the urinary bladder. Flat intraepithelial neoplasia. Scand. J. Urol. Nephrol., *6*:213–223, 1972.

Barlebo, H., and Sorensen, B.L.: Flat epithelial changes in the urinary bladder in patients with prostatic hypertrophy. Scand. J. Urol. Nephrol., *6*(Suppl 15):121–128, 1972.

Bergkvist, A., Ljunggvist, A., and Moberger, G.: Classification of bladder tumors based on the cellular pattern. Preliminary report of a clinical–pathological study of 300 cases with a minimum follow-up of eight years. Acta Chir. Scand., *130*:371–378, 1965.

Bonser, G.M., Clayson, D.B., Jull, J.W., and Pyrah, L.N.: Carcinogenic properties of 2-amino-1-naphthol hydrochloride and its parent amine 2-naphthylamine. Br. J. Cancer, 6:412–424, 1952.

Boon, M.E., Blomjous, C.E., Zwartendijk, J., Heinhuis, R.J., and Ooms, E.C.M.: Carcinoma in situ of the urinary bladder. Clinical presentation, cytologic pattern, and stromal changes. Acta Cytol., 30:360–366, 1986.

Boyland, E., Harris, J., and Horning, E.S.: Induction of carcinoma of bladder in rats with acetamidofluorene. Br. J. Cancer, 8:647–654, 1954.

Bracken, R.B., and Grabstald, H.: Bladder carcinoma involving the lower abdominal wall. J. Urol., 114:715–721, 1975.

Brawn, P.N.: The origin of invasive carcinoma of the bladder. Cancer, 50:515–519, 1982.

Cifuentes Delatte, L., Oliva, H., and Navarro, V.: Intraepithelial carcinoma of the bladder. Urol. Int., 25:169–186, 1970.

Cole, P., Hoover, R., and Friedell, G.H.: Occupation and cancer of the lower urinary tract. Cancer, 29:1250–1260, 1972.

Cole, P., Monson, R., Haning, H., and Friedell, G.H.: Smoking and cancer of the lower urinary tract. N. Engl. J. Med., 284:129–134, 1971.

Cooper, P.H., Waisman, J., Johnston, W.H., and Skinner, D.G.: Severe atypia of transitional epithelium and carcinoma of the urinary bladder. Cancer, 31:1055–1060, 1973.

Crabbe, J.G.S.: Cytology of voided urine and special reference to "benign" papilloma and some of the problems encountered in the preparation of the smears. Acta Cytol., 5:233–240, 1961.

Crosby, J.H., Allsbrook, W.C., Jr., Koss, L.G., et al.: Cytologic detection of urothelial cancer and other abnormalities in a cohort of workers exposed to aromatic amines. Acta Cytol., 35:263–268, 1991.

Culp, O.S., Utz, D.C., and Harrison, E.G., Jr.: Experience with ureteral carcinoma in situ detected during operations for vesical problems. J. Urol., 97:679–682, 1967.

Cutler, S.J., Heney, N.M., and Friedell, G.H.: Longitudinal study of patients with bladder cancer: Factors associated with disease recurrence and progression. In Bonney, W.W., and Prout, G.R., Jr. (eds.): Bladder Cancer, vol. 1, p. 35. AUA Monographs. Baltimore, Williams & Wilkins, 1982.

Czerniak, B., Deitch, D., Simmons, H., Etkind, P., Herz, F., and Koss, L.G.: Ha-*ras* gene codon 12 mutation and DNA ploidy in urinary bladder carcinoma. Br. J. Cancer, 62:762–763, 1990.

Czerniak, B., and Koss, L.G.: Expression of Ca antigen on human urinary bladder tumors. Cancer, 55:2380–2383, 1985.

Czerniak, B., Koss, L.G., and Sherman, A.: Nuclear pores and DNA ploidy in human bladder carcinomas. Cancer Res., 44:3752–3756, 1984.

Dean, P.J., and Murphy, W.M.: Importance of urinary cytology and future role of flow cytometry. Urology, 26(Suppl.):11–15, 1985.

DeBellis, C.C., and Schumann, G.B.: Cystoscopic biopsy supernate. A new cytologic approach for diagnosing urothelial carcinoma in situ. Acta Cytol., 30:356–359, 1986.

Deden, C.: Cancer cells in urinary sediment. Acta Radiol. [Suppl.], 115:1–75, Figs. 1–36, 1954.

Del Mistro, A., Koss, L.G., Braunstein, J., Bennett, B., Saccomano, G., and Simons, K.M.: Condylomata acuminata of the urinary bladder. Am. J. Surg. Pathol., 12:205–215, 1988.

DeMay, R.M., and Grathwohl, M.A.: Signet-ring-cell (colloid) carcinoma of the urinary bladder. Acta Cytol., 29:132–136, 1985.

deVoogt, H.J., Beyer-Boon, M.E., and Brussee, J.M.: The value of phase contrast microscopy for urinary cytology, reliability and pitfalls. Acta Cytol., 19:542–546, 1975.

deVoogt, H.J., Rathert, P., and Beyer-Boon, M.E.: Urinary Cytology. New York, Springer-Verlag, 1977.

Dimmette, R.M., Sproat, H.F., and Klimt, C.R.: Examination of smears of urinary sediment for detection of neoplasms of bladder; survey of an Egyptian village infested with *Schistosoma hematobium*. Am J. Clin. Pathol., 25:1032–1042, 1955.

Domagala, W., Kahn, A.V., and Koss, L.G.: The ultrastructure of surfaces of positively identified cells in the human urinary sediment: A correlative light and scanning electron microscopic study. Acta Cytol., 23:147–155, 1979.

Droller, M.J.: A rose is a rose is a rose, or is it? [Editorial]. J. Urol., 136:1057–1058, 1986.

Eisenberg, R.B., Roth, R.B., and Schweinsberg, M.H.: Bladder tumors and associated proliferative mucosal lesions. J. Urol., 84:544–550, 1960.

El-Bolkainy, M., and Chu, E.W. (eds.): Detection of bladder cancer associated with schistosomiasis. Cairo, Egypt: National Cancer Institute, Cairo University, Al Ahram Press, 1981.

Elliot, G.B., Moloney, P.L., and Anderson, G.H.: "Denuding cystitis" and in situ urothelial carcinoma. Arch. Pathol., 96:91–94, 1973.

Esposti, P.L., Moberger, G., and Zajicek, J.: The cytologic diagnosis of transitional cell tumors of the urinary bladder and its histologic basis. A study of 567 cases of urinary-tract disorder including 170 untreated and 182 irradiated bladder tumors. Acta Cytol., 14:145–155, 1970.

Esposti, P.L., and Zajicek, J.: Grading of transitional cell neoplasms of the urinary bladder from smears of bladder washings. A critical review of 326 tumors. Acta Cytol., 16:529–537, 1972.

Falor, W.H.: Chromosomes in noninvasive papillary carcinoma of the bladder. JAMA, 216:791–794, 1971.

Falor, W.H., and Ward, R.M.: Cytogenetic analysis: A potential index for recurrence of early carcinoma of the bladder. J. Urol., 115:49–52, 1976.

Falor, W.H., and Ward, R.M.: Fifty-three month persistence of ring chromosome in noninvasive bladder carcinoma. Acta Cytol., 20:271–274, 1976.

Farrow, G.M., Utz, D.C., Rife, C.C., and Greene, L.F.: Clinical observations on 69 cases of in situ carcinoma of the urinary bladder. Cancer Res., 37:2794–2798, 1977.

Farrow, G.M., Utz, D.C., and Rife, C.C.: Morphological and clinical observations in patients with early bladder cancer treated with total cystectomy. Cancer Res., 36:2495–2501, 1976.

Foot, N.C., and Papanicolaou, G.N.: Early renal carcinoma in situ detected by means of smears of fixed urinary sediment. JAMA, 139:356–358, 1949.

Foot, N.C., Papanicolaou, G.N., Holmquist, N.D., and Seybolt, J. F.: Exfoliative cytology of urinary sediments; review of 2,829 cases. Cancer, 11:127–137, 1958.

Forni, A., Ghetti, G., and Armell, G.: Urinary cytology in workers exposed to carcinogenic aromatic amines: A six-year study. Acta Cytol., 16:142–145, 1972.

Fossá, S.D.: Feulgen-DNA-values in transitional cell carcinoma of the human urinary bladder. Beitr. Pathol., 155:44–55, 1975.

Fossá, S.D., and Kaalhus, O.: Nuclear size and chromatin concentration in transitional cell carcinoma of the human urinary bladder. Beitr. Pathol., 157:109–125, 1976.

Fox, A.J., and White, G.C.: Bladder cancer in rubber workers. Do screening and doctors' awareness distort the statistics? Lancet, 1:1009–1011, 1976.

Friedell, G.H., Soloway, M.S., Hilgar, A.G., and Farrow, G.M.: Summary of workshop on carcinoma in situ of the bladder. J. Urol., *136*:1047–1048, 1986.

Garner, J.W., Goldstein, A.M.B., and Cosgrove, M.D.: Histologic appearance of the intestinal urinary conduit. J. Urol., *114*:854–857, 1975.

Grabstald, H.: Carcinoma of ileal bladder stoma. J. Urol., *112*:332–334, 1974.

Grabstald, H., Hilaris, B., Henschke, U., and Whitmore, W.F., Jr.: Cancer of the female urethra. JAMA, *197*:835–842, 1966.

Granberg-Ohman, I., Tribukait, B., and Wijkstrom, H.: Cytogenitic analysis of 62 transitional cell bladder carcinomas. Cancer Genet. Cytogenet., *11*:69–85, 1984.

Grogono, J.L., and Shepheard, B.G.F.: Carcinoma of the urachus. Br. J. Urol., *41*:222–227, 1969.

Harris, M.J., Schwinn, C.P., Morrow, J.W., Gray, R.L., and Browell, B.M.: Exfoliative cytology of the urinary bladder irrigation specimen. Acta Cytol., *15*:385–399, 1971.

Harving, N., Wolf, H., and Melsen, F.: Positive urinary cytology after tumor resection: An indicator for concomitant carcinoma in situ. J. Urol., *140*:495–497, 1988.

Helpap, B., Bodekar, J., and Pfitzenmaier, N.: Histologische under zytologische Aspekte der urotherlialen Atypie (Dysplasie). Pathologe, *6*:292–297, 1985.

Herz, F., Barlebo, H., and Koss, L.G.: Modulation of alkaline phosphatase activity in cell cultures derived from human urinary bladder carcinoma. Cancer, *34*:1934–1943, 1974.

Hirono, I., Shibuya, C., Shimizu, M., and Fushimi, K.: Carcinogenic activity of processed bracken used as human food. JNCI, *48*:1245–1250, 1972.

Houston, W., Koss, L.G., and Melamed, M.R.: Bladder cancer and schistosomiasis: A preliminary cytological study. Trans. R. Soc. Trop. Med. Hyg., *60*:89–91, 1966.

Hueper, W.C.: Occupational and environmental cancers of the urinary system. New Haven, Yale University Press, 1969.

Jacobs, J.B., Arai, M., Cohen, S.M., and Friedell, G.H.: Early lesions in experimental bladder cancer: Scanning electron microscopy of cell surface markers. Cancer Res., *36*:2512–2517, 1976.

Jewett, H.J., Lowell, R.K., and Shelley, W.M.: A study of 364 cases of infiltrating bladder cancer: Relation of certain pathological characteristics to prognosis after extirpation. J. Urol., *92*:668–678, 1964.

Jewett, H.J., and Strong, G.H.: Infiltrating carcinoma of bladder: Relation of depth of penetration of bladder wall to incidence of local extension and metastases. J. Urol., *35*:366–372, 1946.

Jordan, A.M., Weingarten, J., and Murphy, W.M.: Transitional cell neoplasms of the urinary bladder. Can biologic potential be predicted from histologic grading? Cancer, *60*:2766–2774, 1987.

Kakudo, K., Itatani, H., and Uematsu, K.: Non-papillary carcinoma in situ of the urinary bladder. An electron microscopic study. Acta Pathol. Jpn., *34*:345–353, 1984.

Kalnins, Z.A., Rhyne, A.L., Morehead, R.P., and Carter, B.J.: Comparison of cytologic findings in patients with transitional cell carcinoma and benign urologic diseases. Acta Cytol., *14*:743–749, 1970.

Kaye, K.W., and Lange, P.H.: Mode of presentation of invasive bladder cancer: Reassessment of the problem. J. Urol., *128*:31–33, 1982.

Kern, W.H.: The cytology of transitional cell carcinoma of the urinary bladder. Acta Cytol., *19*:420–428, 1975.

Kern, W.H., Bales, C.E., and Webster, W.W.: Cytologic evaluation of transitional cell carcinoma of the bladder. J. Urol., *100*:616–622, 1968.

Knappenberger, S.T., Uson, A.C., and Melicow, M.M.: Primary neoplasms occurring in vesical diverticula: A report of 18 cases. J. Urol., *83*:153–159, 1960.

Koss, L.G.: Some ultrastructural aspects of experimental and human carcinoma of the bladder. Cancer Res., *37*:2824–2835, 1977.

Koss, L.G.: Mapping of the urinary bladder: Its impact on the concepts of bladder cancer. Hum. Pathol., *10*:533–548, 1979.

Koss, L.G.: Environmental carcinogenesis and cytology [Editorial]. Acta Cytol., *24*:281–282, 1980.

Koss, L.G.: Urinary tract cytology. *In* Connolly, J.C. (ed.): Carcinoma of the Bladder. pp. 159–163. New York, Raven Press, 1981.

Koss, L.G.: Evaluation of patients with carcinoma in situ of the bladder. *In* Sommers, C.C., and Rosen, P.P. (eds.): Pathol. Annu. 17 (Part 2):353–359, 1982.

Koss, L.G.: Tumors of the Urinary Bladder. Atlas of Tumor Pathology, 2nd series, fascicle 11. Washington, D.C., Armed Forces Institute of Pathology., 1975 (Supplement, 1985).

Koss, L.G.: The role of cytology in the diagnosis, detection and follow-up bladder cancer. *In* Denis, L., et al. (eds.): Developments in Bladder Cancer. pp. 97–108. New York, Alan R. Liss, 1986.

Koss, L.G.: Precursor lesions of invasive bladder cancer. Eur. Urol., *14*(Suppl.1):4–6, 1988.

Koss, L.G.: Cytologic techniques as a diagnostic and prognostic tool in urologic cancer. *In* O'Reilly, P.H., George, N.J.R., and Weiss, R.M. (eds.): Diagnostic Techniques in Urology. Philadelphia, W.B. Saunders, 1990.

Koss, L.G., Bartels, P.H., Bibbo, M., Freed, S.Z., Sychra, J.J., Taylor, J., and Wied, G.L.: Computer analysis of atypical urothelial cells. I. Classification by supervised learning algorithms. Acta Cytol., *21*:247–260, 1977.

Koss, L.G., Bartels, P.H., Bibbo, M., Freed, S.Z., Taylor, J., and Wied, G.L.: Computer discrimination between benign and malignant urothelial cells. Acta Cytol., *19*:378–391, 1975.

Koss, L.G., Bartels, P.H., Sychra, J.J., and Wied, G.L.: Computer analysis of atypical urothelial cells. II. Classification by unsupervised learning algorithms. Acta Cytol., *21*:261–265, 1977.

Koss, L.G., Deitch, D., Ramanathan, R., and Sherman, A.B.: Diagnostic value of cytology of voided urine. Acta Cytol., *29*:810–816, 1985.

Koss, L.G., and Lavin, P.: Studies of experimental bladder carcinoma in Fischer 344 female rats. I. Induction of tumors with diet low in vitamin B_6 containing *N*-2-fluorenylacetamide after single dose of cyclophosphamide. JNCI, *46*:585–595, 1971.

Koss, L.G., Melamed, M.R., and Kelly, R.E.: Further cytologic and histologic studies of bladder lesions in workers exposed to *para*-aminodiphenyl: Progress report. JNCI, *43*:233–243, 1969.

Koss, L.G., Melamed, M.R., Ricci, A., Melick, W.F., and Kelly, R.E.: Carcinogenesis in the human urinary bladder. Observations after exposure to *para-aminodiphenyl*. N. Engl. J. Med., *272*:767–770, 1965.

Koss, L.G., Nakanishi, I., and Freed, S.Z.: Nonpapillary carcinoma in situ and atypical hyperplasia in cancerous bladders. Further studies of surgically removed bladders by mapping. Urology, *9*:442–455, 1977.

Koss, L.G., Tiamson, E.M., and Robbins, M.A.: Mapping cancerous and precancerous bladder changes. A study of the urothelium in ten surgically removed bladders. JAMA, *227*:281–286, 1974.

Lange, P.H., and Limas, C.: Molecular markers in the diagnosis and prognosis of bladder cancer. J. Urol., *23S*:46, 1984.

Laursen, B.: Cancer of the bladder in patients treated with chlornaphazine. Br. Med. J., *3*:684–685, 1970.

Lederer, B., Mikuz, G., Gütter, W., and zur Neiden, G.: Zyto-photometrische Untersuchungen von Tumoren des Uber-gangsepithels der Harnblase. Vergleich zytophotome-trischer Untersuchungsergebnisse mit dem histologischen Grading. Beitr. Pathol., *147*:379–389, 1972.

Lerman, R.I., Hutter, R.V., and Whitmore, W.F., Jr.: Papilloma of the urinary bladder. Cancer, *25*:333–342, 1970.

Levi, P.E., Cooper, E.H., Anderson, C.K., and Williams, R.E.: Analysis of DNA content, nuclear size and cell proliferation of transitional cell carcinoma in man. Cancer, *23*:1074–1085, 1969.

Limas, C., and Lange, P.P: T-antigen in normal and neoplastic urothelium. Cancer, *58*:1236–1245, 1986.

Linker, D.G., and Whitmore, W.F.: Ureteral carcinoma in situ. J. Urol., *113*:777–780, 1975.

Mahadevia, P.S., Koss, L.G., and Tar, I.J.: Prostatic involvement in bladder cancer: Prostate mapping in 20 cystoprostatectomy specimens. Cancer, *58*:2096–2102, 1986.

Marshall, V.V.: Current clinical problems regarding bladder tumors. Cancer, *9*:543–550, 1956.

Meisels, A.: Cytology of carcinoma of kidney. Acta Cytol., *7*:239–244, 1963.

Melamed, M.R., Grabstald, H., and Whitmore, W.F., Jr.: Carcinoma in situ of bladder: Clinico-pathologic study of case with suggested approach to detection. J. Urol., *96*:466–471, 1966.

Melamed, M.R., and Koss, L.G.: Developments in cytological diagnosis of cancer. Med. Clin. North Am., *50*:651–666, 1966.

Melamed, M.R., Koss, L.G., Ricci, A., and Whitmore, W.F. Jr.: Cytohistological observations on developing carcinoma of urinary bladder in man. Cancer, *13*:67–74, 1960.

Melamed, M.R., Traganos, F., Sharpless, T., and Darzynkiewica, Z.: Urinary cytology automation. Preliminary studies with acridine orange stain and flow-through cytofluorometry. Invest. Urol., *13*:331–338, 1976.

Melamed, M.R., Voutsa, N.G., and Grabstald, H.: Natural history and clinical behavior of in situ carcinoma of the human urinary bladder. Cancer, *17*:1533–1545, 1964.

Melick, W.F., Escue, H.M., Naryka, J.J., Mezera, R.A., and Wheeler, E.P.: First reported cases of human bladder tumors due to new carcinogen xenylamine. J. Urol., *74*:760–766, 1955.

Melicow, M.M.: Histological study of vesical urothelium intervening between gross neoplasms in total cystectomy. J. Urol., *68*:261–278, 1952.

Melicow, M.M.: Tumors of the bladder: A multifaceted problem. J. Urol., *112*:467–478, 1974.

Melicow, M.M.: Carcinoma in situ: An historical perspective. Urol. Clin. North Am. *3*:5–11, 1976.

Melicow, M.M., and Hollowell, J.W.: Intraurothelial cancer: Carcinoma in situ, Bowen's disease of the urinary system: Discussion of thirty cases. J. Urol., *68*:763–772, 1952.

Morse, N., and Melamed, M.R.: Differential counts of cell populations in urinary sediment smears from patients with primary epidermoid carcinoma of bladder. Acta Cytol., *18*:312–315, 1974.

Mostofi, F.K.: Pathological aspects and spread of carcinoma of the bladder. JAMA, *206*:1764–1769, 1968.

Mostofi, F.K.: Pathology and spread of carcinoma of the urinary bladder. *In* Johnson, D.E., and Samuels, M.L. (eds.): Cancer of the Genitourinary Tract. p. 303. New York, Raven Press, 1979.

Mostofi, F.K., Thomson, R.V., and Dean, A.L., Jr.: Mucous adenocarcinoma of urinary bladder. Cancer, *8*:741–758, 1955.

Murphy, W.M., and Soloway, M.S.: Developing carcinoma (dysplasia) of the urinary bladder. Pathol. Annu., *17*(Pt.1):197–217, 1982.

Murphy, W.M., and Soloway, M.S.: Urothelial dysplasia. Urol., *127*:849–854, 1982.

Murphy, W.M., Soloway, M.S., Jukkola, A.F., Grabtree, W.N., and Ford, K.S.: Urinary cytology and bladder cancer. The cellular features of transitional cell neoplasms. Cancer, *53*:1555–1565, 1984.

Pamukcu, A.M., Gorsoy, S.K., and Price, J.M.: Urinary bladder neoplasms induced by feeding bracken fern (*Pteris aquilina*) to cows. Cancer Res., *27*:917–924, 1964.

Papanicolaou, G.N., and Marshall, V.F.: Urine sediment smears as diagnostic procedure in cancers of urinary tract. Science, *101*:519–520, 1945.

Pedersen-Bjergaard, J., Ersboli, J., Hansen, V.L., Sorensen, B.L., Christoffersen, K., Hou-Jensen, K., Nissen, N.I., Knudsen, J.B., and Hansen, M.M.: Carcinoma of the urinary bladder after treatment with cyclophosphamide for non-Hodgkin's lymphoma. N. Engl. J. Med., *318*:1028–1032, 1988.

Pettersson, S., Hansson, G., and Blohme, I.: Condyloma acuminatum of the bladder. J. Urol., *115*:535–536, 1976.

Piper, J.M., Tonascia, J., and Matanoski, G.M.: Heavy phenacetin use and bladder cancer in women aged 20 to 49 years. N. Engl. J. Med., *313*:292–295, 1985.

Prout, G.K., Jr.: Current concepts: Bladder carcinoma. N. Engl. J. Med., *287*:86–90, 1972.

Prout, G.R., Griffin, P.P., and Daly, J.J.: The outcome of conservative treatment of carcinoma in situ of the bladder. J. Urol., *138*:766–770, 1987.

Prout, G.R., Griffin, P.P., Daly, J.J., and Heney, N.M.: Carcinoma in situ of the urinary bladder with and without associated neoplasms. Cancer, *52*:524–532, 1983.

Pugh, R.C.B.: The pathology of bladder tumours. *In* Wallace, D.M. (ed.): Neoplastic Disease at Various Sites: Tumours of the Bladder. pp. 116–156. Edinburgh, E. & S. Livingstone, 1959.

Pugh, R.C.B.: The pathology of cancer of the bladder. An editorial overview. Cancer, *32*:1267–1274, 1973.

Rehn, L.: Blasengeschwuelste bei Anilinarbeitern. Arch. Klin. Chir., *50*:588–600, 1895.

Rehn, L.: Blasengeschwuelste bei Fuchsinarbeitern. Arch. Klin. Chir., *53*:383–392, 1896.

Reichborn-Kjennerud, S., and Hoeg, K.: The value of urine cytology in the diagnosis of recurrent bladder tumors. A preliminary report. Acta Cytol., *16*:269–272, 1972.

Roland, S.I., and Marshall, V.F.: Reliability of Papanicolaou technique when cancer cells are found in urine. Surg. Gynecol. Obstet., *104*:41–44, 1957.

Rosa, B., Cazin, M., and Dalian, G.: Urinary cytology for carcinoma in situ of the urinary bladder. Acta Cytol., *29*:117–124, 1985.

Rosenkilde, O.P., Wolf, H., Schroeder, T., Fischer, A., and Hjgaard, K.: Urothelial atypia and survival rate of 500 unselected patients with primary transitional-cell tumor of the urinary bladder. Scand. J. Urol., Nephrol., *22*:257–263, 1988.

Sarnacki, C.T., McCormack, L.J., Kiser, W.S., Hazard, J.R., McLaughlin, T.C., and Belovich, D.M.: Urinary cytology and clinical diagnosis of urinary tract malignancy: A clinicopathologic study of 1,400 patients. J. Urol., *106*:761–764, 1971.

Schade, R.O.K., Serck-Hanssen, A., and Swinney, J.: Morphological changes in the ureter in cases of bladder carcinoma. Cancer, *27*:1267–1272, 1971.

Schade, R.O.K., and Swinney, J.: Precancerous changes in bladder epithelium. Lancet, *2*:943–946, 1968.

Schade, R.O.K., and Swinney, J.: The association of urothelial atypism with neoplasia: Its importance in treatment and prognosis. J. Urol., *109*:619–622, 1973.

Schulte, P.A., Ringen, K.N., Hemstreet, G.P., et al.: Risk assessment of a cohort exposed to aromatic amines. Initial results. J. Occup. Med., *27*:115–121, 1985.

Schulte, P.A., Ringen, K., Hemstreet, G.P., et al.: Risk factors of bladder cancer in a cohort exposed to aromatic amines. Cancer, *58*:2156–2162, 1986.

Seemayer, T.A., Knaack, J., Thelmo, W.L., Wang, N.-S., and Ahmed, M.N.: Further observations on carcinoma in situ of the urinary bladder: Silent but extensive intraprostatic involvement. Cancer, *36*:514–520, 1975.

Sherman, A., Koss, L.G., Adams, S., Schreiber, K., Moussouris, H.F., Fred, S.Z., Bartels, P.H., and Wied, G.L.: Bladder cancer diagnosis by image analysis of cells in voided urine using a small computer. Anal. Quant. Cytol., *3*:239–249, 1981.

Sidransky, D., Von Eschenbach, A., Tsai, Y.C., Jones, P., Summerhayes, I., Marshall, F., Paul, M., Green, P., Hamilton, S.R., Frost, P., and Vogelstein, B.: Identification of p53 gene mutations in bladder cancers and urine samples. Science, *252*:706–709, 1991.

Simon, W., Cordonnier, J.J., and Snordgrass, W.T.: The pathogenesis of bladder carcinoma. J. Urol., *88*:797–802, 1962.

Skinner, D.G., Richie, J.P., Cooper, P.H., Waisman, J., and Kaufman, J.J.: The clinical significance of carcinoma in situ of the bladder and its association with overt carcinoma. J. Urol., *112*:68–71, 1974.

Smith, A.F.: An ultrastructural and morphometric study of bladder tumours. Virchows Arch. [A], *406*:7–16, 1985.

Starklint, H., Jensen, N.K., and Thybo, E.: The extent of carcinoma in situ in urinary bladders with primary carcinoma. Acta Pathol. Microbiol. Scand. [A], *84*:130–136, 1976.

Starklint, H., Kjaergaard, J., and Jensen, N.K.: Types of metaplasia in forty urothelial bladder carcinomas. A systematic histological investigation. Acta Pathol. Microbiol. Scand., *84*:137–142, 1976.

Suprun, H., and Bitterman, W.: A correlative cytohistologic study on the interrelationship between exfoliated urinary bladder carcinoma cell types and the staging and grading of these tumors. Acta Cytol., *19*:265–273, 1975.

Temkin, I.S.: Industrial Bladder Carcinogenesis. New York, Pergamon Press, 1963.

Thelmo, W.L., Seemayer, T.A., Madarnas, P., Mount, B.M.M., and Mackinnon, K.J.: Carcinoma in situ of the bladder with associated prostatic involvement. J. Urol., *111*:491–494, 1974.

Travis, L.B., Cutis, R.E., Boice, J.D., Jr., and Fraumeni, J.F., Jr.: Bladder cancer after chemotherapy for non-Hodgkin's lymphoma. N. Engl. J. Med., *321*:544–545, 1989.

Trott, P.A., and Edwards, L.: Comparison of bladder washings and urine cytology in the diagnosis of bladder cancer. J. Urol., *110*:664–666, 1973.

Umiker, W.: Accuracy of cytologic diagnosis of cancer of the urinary tract. Acta Cytol., *8*:186–193, 1964.

Umiker, W., Lapides, J., and Soureene, R.: Exfoliative cytology of papillomas and intraepithelial carcinomas of the urinary bladder. Acta Cytol., *6*:255–266, 1962.

Utz, D.C., Hanash, K.A., and Farrow, G.M.: The plight of the patient with carcinoma in situ of the bladder. J. Urol., *103*:160–164, 1970.

Utz, D.C., Schmitz, S.E., Fugelso, P.D., and Farrow, G.M.: A clinicopathologic evaluation of partial cystectomy for carcinoma of the urinary bladder. Cancer, *32*:1075–1077, 1973.

Utz, D.C., and Zincke, H.: The masquerade of bladder cancer in situ as interstitial cystitis. Trans. Am. Assoc. Genitourin. Surg., *75*:64–65, 1973.

Videbaek, A.: Chlornaphazin (Erysan) may induce cancer of the urinary bladder. Acta Med. Scand., *176*:45–50, 1964.

Voutsa, N.G., and Melamed, M.R.: Cytology of in situ carcinoma of the human urinary bladder. Cancer, *16*:1307–1316, 1963.

Wallace, D.: Cancer of the bladder. Am. J. Roentgenol. Radium Ther. Nucl. Med., *102*:581–586, 1968.

Ward, E., Halperin, W., Thun, M., Grossman, H.B., Fink, B., Koss, L.G., Osorio, A.M., and Schulte, P.: Bladder tumors in two young males occupationally exposed to MBOCA. Am. J. Ind. Med., *14*:267–272, 1988.

Webber, M.M.: A study of malignant bladder mucosa using autoradiography of exfoliated epithelial cells. Acta Cytol., *13*:128–132, 1969.

Weinstein, R.S.: Changes in plasma membrane structure associated with malignant transformation in human urinary bladder epithelium. Cancer Res., *36*:2518–2524, 1976.

Weinstein, R.S., Coon, J.S., Schwartz, D., Miller, A.W. III, and Pauli, B.U.: Pathology of superficial bladder cancer with emphasis on carcinoma in situ. Urology, *26*(Suppl.):2–10, 1985.

Wheeler, J.D., and Hill, W.T.: Adenocarcinoma involving urinary bladder. Cancer, *7*:119–135, 1954.

Whitmore, W.F., Jr.: Bladder cancer: An overview. CA *38*:213–223, 1988.

Widran, J., Sanchez, R., and Gruhn, J.: Squamous metaplasia of the bladder: A study of 450 patients. J. Urol., *112*:479–482, 1974.

Wiggishoff, C.C., and McDonald, J.H.: Urinary exfoliative cytology in the diagnosis of bladder tumors. Acta Cytol., *16*:139–141, 1972.

Wolf, H., and Hjøgaard, K.: Urothelial dysplasia concomitant with bladder tumours as a determinant factor for future new occurrences. Lancet, *2*:134–136, 1983.

Wolinska, W.H., Melamed, M.R., and Klein, F.A.: Cytology of bladder papilloma. Acta Cytol., *29*:817, 1985.

Wynder, E.L., and Goldsmith, R.: The epidemiology of bladder cancer. A second look. Cancer, *40*:1246–1268, 1977.

Wynder, E.L., Onderdonk, J., and Mantel, N.: An epidemiologic investigation of cancer of the bladder. Cancer, *16*:1388–1407, 1963.

Yamada, T., Masawa, N., Honma, K., Yokogawa, M., Fukui, I., and Mitani, G.: Nonpapillary intraepithelial and/or early invasive cancer arisen in the urinary bladder—their developmental and advancing courses. Dokkyo J. Med. Sci., *11*:51–69, 1984.

Yamada, T., Yokogawa, M., Mitani, G., Inada, T., Ohwada, F., and Fukui, I.: Two different types of cancer development in the urothelium of the human urinary bladder with different prognosis. Jpn. J. Clin. Oncol., *5*:77–90, 1975.

Yates-Bell, A.J.: Carcinoma in situ of the bladder. Br. J. Surg., *58*:359–364, 1971.

Zincke, H., Utz, D.C., and Farrow, G.M.: Review of Mayo Clinic experience with carcinoma in situ. Urology, *26*(Suppl. 4):39–46, 1985.

Bladder Tumor Treatment: New Developments

Bretton, P.R., Herr, H.W., Whitmore, W.F., Jr., Badalament, R.A., Kimmel, M., Provet, J., Oettgen, H.F., Melamed, M.R., and Fair, W.R.: Intravesical bacillus Calmette-

Guérin therapy for in situ transitional cell carcinoma involving the prostatic urethra. J. Urol., *141*:853–856, 1989.

Brosman, S.A.: The use of bacillus Calmette-Guérin in the therapy of bladder carcinoma in situ. J. Urol., *134*:36–39, 1985.

Calsini, P., Scapicchi, G., Scapicchi, G., Melone, F., Aulisi, A., Pellegrini, G., Fabris, N., and Provinciali, M.: Immunotherapy of bladder cancer with intralesional injection with BCG. J. Exp. Pathol., *3*:579–586, 1987.

DeKernion, J.B., Haung, M.-Y., Linder, A., Smith, R.B., and Kaufman, J.J.: The management of superficial bladder tumors and carcinoma in situ with intravesical bacillus Calmette-Guérin. J. Urol., *133*:598–601, 1985.

Droller, M.J., and Walsh, P.C.: Intensive intravesical chemotherapy in the treatment of flat carcinoma in situ: Is it safe? J. Urol., *134*:1115–1117, 1985.

Guinan, P., Crispen, R., and Rubenstein, M.: BCG management of superficial bladder cancer. Urology, *30*:515–519, 1987.

Herr, H.W.: Immunobiology of human bladder cancer. J. Urol., *115*:1976.

Herr, H.W., Badalament, R.A., Amato, D.A., Laudone, V.P., Fair, W.R., and Whitmore, W.F., Jr.: Superficial bladder cancer treated with bacillus Calmette-Guérin: A multivariate analysis of factors affecting tumor progression. J. Urol., *141*:22–29, 1989.

Herr, H.W., Laudone, V.P., Badalament, R.A., Oettgen, H.F., Sogani, P.C., Freedman, B.D., Melamed, M.R., and Whitmore, W.F., Jr.: Bacillus Calmette-Guérin therapy alters the progression of superficial bladder cancer. J. Clin. Oncol., *6*:1450–1455, 1988.

Herr, H.W., Pinsky, C.M., Whitmore, W.F., Jr., Sogani, P.C., Oettgen, H.F., and Melamed, M.R.: Long-term effect of intravesical bacillus Calmette-Guérin on flat carcinoma in situ of the bladder. J. Urol., *135*:265–267, 1986.

Hisazumi, H., Miyoshi, N., Naito, K., and Misaki, T.: Whole bladder wall photoradiation therapy for carcinoma in situ of the bladder: A preliminary report. J. Urol., *131*:884–887, 1984.

Oates, R.D., Stilmant, M.M., Freedlund, M.C., and Siroky, M.B.: Granulomatous prostatitis following bacillus Calmette-Guérin immunotherapy of bladder cancer. J. Urol., *140*:751–754, 1988.

Pinsky, C.M., Camacho, F., Kerr, D., Geller, N.L., Klein, F.A., Herr, H.A., Whitmore, W.F., Jr., and Oettgen, H.F.: Intravesical administration of bacillus Calmette-Guérin in patients with recurrent superficial carcinoma of the urinary bladder: Report of a prospective randomized trial. Cancer Treat. Rep., *69*:47–53, 1985.

Prout, G.R., Lin, C-W., Benson, R., Jr., et. al.: Photodynamic therapy with hematoporphyrin derivative in the treatment of superficial transitional-cell carcinoma of the bladder. N. Engl. J. Med., *317*:1251–1255, 1987.

Schellhammer, P.F., Ladaga, L.E., and Fillion, M.B.: Bacillus Calmette-Guérin for superficial transitional cell carcinoma of the bladder. J. Urol., *135*:261–264, 1986.

Siref, L.E., and Zincke, H.: Radical cystectomy for historical and pathologic T1,N0,M0 (stage A) transitional cell cancer. Need for adjuvant systemic chemotherapy? Urology, *31*:309–311, 1988.

Soloway, M.S.: Surgery and intravesical chemotherapy in the management of superficial bladder cancer. Semin. Urol., *1*:23, 1983.

Soloway, M.S.: Treatment of superficial bladder cancer with intravesical mitomycin C: Analysis of immediate and long-term response in 70 patients. J. Urol., *134*:1107–1109, 1985.

Whitmore, W.F., Jr., Bush, I.M., and Esquivel, E.: Tetracycline ultraviolet fluorescence in the bladder carcinoma. Cancer, *17*:1528–1532, 1964.

Whitmore, W.F., Whitmore, W.F., Jr., Grabstald, H., and Mackenzie, A.R.: Preoperative irradiation with cystectomy in the management of bladder cancer. Am. J. Roentgenol. Radium. Ther. Nucle. Med., *102*:570–576, 1968.

Bladder Tumors: New Methods of Analysis

Badalament, R.A., Fair, W.R., Whitmore, W.F., Jr., and Melamed, M.R.: The relative value of cytometry and cytology in the management of bladder cancer: The Memorial Sloan–Kettering Cancer Center experience. Semin. Urol., *6*:22–30, 1988.

Badalament, R.A., Gary, H., Whitmore, W.F., Jr., et al.: Monitoring intravesical bacillus Calmette-Guérin treatment of superficial bladder carcinoma by serial flow cytometry. Cancer, *58*:2751–2757, 1986.

Badalament, R.A., Hermansen, D.K., Kimmel, M., et al.: The sensitivity of bladder wash flow cytometry, bladder wash cytology, and voided cytology in the detection of bladder carcinoma. Cancer, *60*:1423–1427, 1987.

Blomjous, C.E., Schipper, N.W., Baak, J.P., van Galen, E.M., de Voogt, H.J., and Meyer, C.J.: Retrospective study of prognostic importance of DNA flow cytometry of urinary bladder carcinoma. J. Clin. Pathol., *41*:21–25, 1988.

Blomjous, E.C., Schipper, N.W., Baak, J.P., Vos, W., De Voogt, H.J., and Meijer, C.J.: The value of morphometry and DNA flow cytometry in addition to classic prognosticators in superficial urinary bladder carcinoma. Am. J. Clin. Pathol., *91*:243–248, 1989.

Borgstrøm, E., and Wahren, B.: Clinical significance of A, B, H isoantigen deletion of urothelial cells in bladder carcinoma. Cancer, *58*:2428–2434, 1986.

Borgstrøm, E., Wahren, B., and Gustafson, H.: Fluorescence methods for measuring the A, B, and H isoantigens on cytological material from bladder carcinoma. Urol. Res., *13*:43–45, 1985.

Collste, L.G., Devonec, M., Darzynkiewicz. Z., Traganos, F., Sharpless, T.K., Whitmore, W.F., Jr., and Melamed, M.R.: Bladder cancer diagnosis by flow cytometry. Correlation between cell samples from biopsy and bladder irrigation fluid. Cancer, *45*:2389–2394, 1980.

Coon, J.S., and Weinstein, R.S.: Detection of A,B,H tissue isoantigens by immunoperoxidase methods in normal and neoplastic urothelium. Comparison with the erythrocyte adherence method. Am. J. Clin. Pathol., *76*:163–171, 1981.

Cordon-Cardo, C., Reuter, V.E., Lloyd, K.O., Sheinfeld, J., Fair, W.R., Old, L.J., and Melamed, M.R.: Blood group-related antigens in human urothelium: Enhanced expression of precursor, Le[x], and Le[y] determinants in urothelial carcinoma. Cancer Res., *48*:4113–4120, 1988.

Czerniak, B., Deitch, D., Simmons, H., Etkind, P., Herz, F., and Koss, L.G.: Ha-*ras* gene codon 12 mutation and DNA ploidy in bladder carcinoma. Br. J. Cancer, *62*:762–763, 1990.

Czerniak, B., and Koss, L.G.: Expression of Ca antigen on human urinary bladder tumors. Cancer, *55*:2380–2383, 1985.

Czerniak, B., Koss, L.G., and Sherman, A.: Nuclear pores and DNA ploidy in human bladder carcinomas. Cancer Res., *44*:3752–3756, 1984.

Dean, P.J., and Murphy, W.M.: Importance of urinary cytology and future role of flow cytometry. Urology, *26*(Suppl.):11–15, 1985.

DeHarven, E., He, S., Hanna, W., Bootsma, G., and Connolly, J.G.: Phenotypically heterogeneous deletion of the A,B,H antigen from the transformed bladder urothelium. A scanning electron microscope study. J. Submicrosc. Cytol., *19*:639–649, 1987.

deVere White, R.W., Olsson, C.A., and Deitch, A.D.: Flow cytometry: Role in monitoring transitional cell carcinoma of bladder. Urology, *28*:15–20, 1986.

deVere White, R.W., Deitch, A.D., Baker, W.C., Jr., and Strand, M.A.: Urine: A suitable sample for deoxyribonucleic acid flow cytometry studies in patients with bladder cancer. J. Urol., *139*:926–928, 1988.

Devonec, M., Darzynkiewicz, Z., Whitmore, W.F., and Melamed, M.R.: Flow cytometry for followup examinations of conservatively treated low stage bladder tumors. J. Urol., *126*:166–170, 1981.

Falor, W.H., and Ward, R.M.: Cytogenetic analysis: A potential index for recurrence of early carcinoma of the bladder. J. Urol., *115*:49–52, 1976.

Falor, W.H., and Ward, R.M.: DNA banding patterns in carcinoma of the bladder. JAMA, *226*:1322, 1973.

Farsund, T.: Selective sampling of cells for morphological and quantitative cytology of bladder epithelium. J. Urol., *128*:267–271, 1982.

Flanigan, R.C., King, C.T., Clark, T.D., Cash, J.B., Greenfield, B.J., Sniecinski, I.J., and Primus, F.J.: Immunohistochemical demonstration of blood group antigens in neoplastic and normal human urothelium: A comparison with standard red cell adherence. J. Urol., *130*:499–503, 1983.

Fosså, S.D.: Feulgen-DNA-values in transitional cell carcinoma of the human urinary bladder. Beitr. Pathol., *155*:44–55, 1975.

Fradet, Y., Cordon-Cardo, C., Thomson, T., Daly, M.E., Whitmore, W.F., Jr., Lloyd, K.O., Melamed, M.R., and Old, L.J.: Cell monoclonal antibodies. Proc. Natl. Acad. Sci. USA, *81*:224–228, 1984.

Fradet, Y., Cordon-Cardo, C., Whitmore, W.F., Melamed, M.R., and Old, L.: Cell surface antigens of human bladder tumors: Definition of tumor subsets by monoclonal antibodies and correlation with growth characteristics. Cancer Res., *46*:5183–5188, 1986.

Granberg-Ohman, I., Tribukait, B., and Wijkstrom, H.: Cytogenitc analysis of 62 transitional cell bladder carcinomas. Cancer Genet. Cytogenet., *11*:69–85, 1984.

Harving, N., Wolf, H., and Melsen, F.: Positive urinary cytology after tumor resection: An indicator for concomitant carcinoma in situ. J. Urol., *140*:495–497, 1988.

Hopkins, S., Ford, K.S., and Soloway, M.S.: Invasive bladder cancer: Support for screening. J. Urol., *130*:61–64, 1983.

Klein, F.A., Herr, H.W., Whitmore, W.F., Sogani, P.C., and Melamed, M.R.: An evaluation of automated flow cytometry (FCM) in detection of carcinoma in situ of the urinary bladder. Cancer, *50*:1003–1008, 1982.

Koss, L.G., Bartels, P.H., Bibbo, M., Freed, S.Z., Sychra, J.J. Taylor, J., and Wied, G.L.: Computer analysis of atypical urothelial cells. I. Classification by supervised learning algorithms. Acta Cytol., *21*:247–260, 1977.

Koss, L.G., Bartels, P.H., Bibbo, M., Freed, S.Z., Taylor, J., and Wied, G.L.: Computer discrimination between benign and malignant urothelial cells. Acta Cytol., *19*:378–391, 1975.

Koss, L.G., Bartels, P.H., Sherman, A., Sychra, J.J., Schreiber, K., Moussouris, H.S., and Wied, G.L.: Computer identification of degenerated urothelial cells. Anal. Quant. Cytol., *2*:107–111, 1980.

Koss, L.G., Bartels, P.H., Sychra, J.J., and Wied, G.L.: Computer analysis of atypical urothelial cells. II. Classification by unsupervised learning algorithms. Acta Cytol., *21*:261–265, 1977.

Koss, L.G., Bartels, P., and Wied, G.L.: Computer-based diagnostic analysis of cells in the urinary sediment. J. Urol., *123*:846–849, 1980.

Koss, L.G., Wersto, R.P., Simmons, D.A., Deitch, D., Herz, F., and Freed, S.Z.: Predictive value of DNA measurements in bladder washings. Comparison of flow cytometry, image cytophotometry, and cytology in patients with a past history of urothelial tumors. Cancer, *64*:916–924, 1989.

Kovarik, S., Davidsohn, I., and Stejkal, R.: ABO antigen in cancer: Detection with the mixed cell agglutination reaction. Arch. Pathol., *86*:12–21, 1968.

Lange, P.H., and Limas, C.: Molecular markers in the diagnosis and prognosis of bladder cancer. J. Urol., *23S*:46, 1984.

Lederer, B., Mikuz, G., Gütter, W., and zur Neiden, G.: Zytophotometrische Untersuchungen von Tumoren des Ubergangsepithels der Harnblase. Vergleich zytophotometrischer Untersuchungsergebnisse mit dem histologischen Grading. Beitr. Pathol., *147*:379–389, 1972.

Levi, P.E., Cooper, E.H. Anderson, C.K., and Williams, R.E.: Analysis of DNA content, nuclear size and cell proliferation of transitional cell carcinoma in man. Cancer, *23*:1074–1085, 1069.

Limas, C., and Lange, P.: A, B, H antigen detectability in normal and neoplastic urothelium. Influence of methodologic factors. Cancer, *49*:2476–2484, 1982.

Limas, C., and Lange, P.: Lewis antigens in normal and neoplastic urothelium. Am. J. Pathol., *121*:176–183, 1985.

Limas, C., and Lange, P.: T-antigen in normal and neoplastic urothelium. Cancer, *58*:1236–1245, 1986.

Melamed, M.R., and Klein, F.A.: Flow cytometry of urinary bladder irrigation specimens. Hum. Pathol., *15*:302–395, 1984.

Melamed, M.R., Traganos, F., Sharpless, T., and Darznkiewicz, Z.: Urinary cytology automation: Preliminary studies with acridine orange stain and flow-through cytofluorometry. Invest. Urol., *13*:333–338, 1976.

Melder, K.K., and Koss, L.G.: Automated image analysis in the diagnosis of bladder cancer. Appl. Opt., *26*:3367–3372, 1987.

Sherman, A.B., Koss, L.G., and Adams, S.E.: Interobserver and intraobserver differences in the diagnosis of urothelial cells. Comparison with classification by computer. Anal. Quant. Cytol., *6*:112–120, 1984.

Sherman, A., Koss, L.G., Adams, S., Schreiber, K., Moussouris, H.F., Fred, S.Z., Bartels, P.H., and Wied, G.L.: Bladder cancer diagnosis by image analysis of cells in voided urine using a small computer. Anal. Quant. Cytol., *3*:239–249, 1981.

Sherman, A.B., Koss, L.G., Wyschogrod, D., Melder, K.H., Eppich, E.M., and Bales, C.E.: Bladder cancer diagnosis by computer image analysis of cells in the sediment of voided urine using a video scanning system. Anal. Quant. Cytol. Histol., *8*:177–186, 1986.

Spooner, M.E., and Cooper, E.H.: Chromosome constitution of transitional cell carcinoma of the urinary bladder. Cancer, *29*:1401–1412, 1972.

Tribukait, B.: Flow cytometry in surgical pathology and cytology of tumors of the genito-urinary tract. *In* Koss, L.G., and Coleman, D.V. (eds.): Advances in Clinical Cytology, vol. 2. pp. 163–189. New York, Masson Publishing, 1984.

Tribukait, B.: Flow cytometry in assessing the clinical aggressiveness of genito-urinary neoplasms. World J. Urol., *5*:108–122, 1987.

Tribukait, B., Gustafson, H., and Esposti, M.D.: Ploidy and

proliferation of human bladder tumors as measured by flow-cytofluorometric DNA-analysis and its relations to histopathology and cytology. Cancer, 43:1742–1751, 1979.

Weinstein, R.S., Coon, J., Alroy, J., and Davidsohn, I.: Tissue-associated blood group antigens in human tumors. *In* De-Lellis, R.A. (ed.): Diagnostic Immunohistochemistry. pp. 239–261. New York, Masson Publishing, 1981.

Wied, G.L., Bartels, P.H., Bahr, G.F., and Oldfield, D.G.: Taxonomic intracellular analytic system (TICAS) for cell identification. Acta Cytol., 12:180–204, 1968.

Wijkstrom, H., Granberg-Ohman, I., and Tribukait, B.: Chromosomal and DNA patterns in transitional cell bladder carcinoma. A comparative cytogenetic and flow-cytofluorometric DNA study. Cancer, 53:1718–1723, 1984.

Yamase, H.T., Powell, G.T., and Koss, L.G.: A simplified method of preparing permanent tissue sections for the erythrocyte adherence test. Am. J. Clin. Pathol., 75:178–181, 1981.

Rare and Metastatic Bladder Tumors

Ainsworth, A.M., Clark, W.H., Jr., Mastrangelo, M., and Conger, K.B.: Primary malignant melanoma of the urinary bladder. Cancer, 37:1928–1936, 1976.

Auvert, J., Boureau, M., and Weisberger, G.: Embryonal sarcoma of the lower urinary tract in children: 5-year survival in two cases after radical treatment. J. Urol., 112:396–401, 1974.

Auvigne, R., Auvigne, J., and Kerneis, J.: Un cas de plasmocytome de la vessie. J. Urol., 62:85–90, 1956.

Bhansali, S.K., and Cameron, K.M.: Primary malignant lymphoma of the bladder. Br. J. Urol., 32:440–454, 1960.

Brinton, J.A., Ito, Y., and Olsen, B.S.: Carcinosarcoma of the urinary bladder. Cancer, 25:1183–1186, 1970.

Cheson, B.D., Schumann, G.B., and Johnston, J.L.: Urinary cytodiagnosis of renal involvement in disseminated histiocytic lymphoma. Acta Cytol., 28:148–152, 1984.

Crane, A.R., and Tremblay, R.G.: Primary osteogenic sarcoma of the bladder. Ann. Surg., 118:887–896, 1943.

Del Mistro, A., Koss, L.G., Braunstein, J., Bennett, B., Saccomano, G., and Simons, K.M.: Condylomata acuminata of the urinary bladder. Am. J. Surg. Pathol., 12:205–215, 1988.

Foote, J.W., Seemayer, T.A., and Duignan, J.P.: Desmoid tumor involving the bladder: Case report. J. Urol., 114:147–149, 1975.

Fromowitz, F.B., Bard, R.H., and Koss, L.G.: The epithelial origin of a malignant mesodermal mixed tumor of the bladder: Report of case with long-term survival. J. Urol., 132:2385–2389, 1984.

Ganem, E.J., and Batal, J.T.: Secondary malignant tumors of the urinary bladder metastatic from primary foci in distant organs. J. Urol., 75:965–972, 1956.

Holtz, F., Fox, J.E., and Abell, M.R.: Carcinosarcoma of the urinary bladder. Cancer, 29:294–304, 1972.

Jao, W., Soto, J.M., and Gould, V.E.: Squamous carcinoma of bladder with pseudosarcomatous stroma. Arch. Pathol., 100:461–466, 1975.

Klinger, M.E.: Secondary tumors of the genitourinary tract. J. Urol., 65:144–153, 1951.

Koss, L.G.: Tumors of the Urinary Bladder. Atlas of Tumor Pathology, 2nd series, fascicle 11. Washington, D.C., Armed Forces Institute of Pathology, 1975 (Supplement 1985).

Krumerman, M.S., and Katatikaru, V.: Rhabdomyosarcoma

of the urinary bladder with intraepithelial spread in an adult. Arch. Pathol. Lab. Med., 100:395–397, 1976.

MacKenzie, A.R., Sharma, T.C., Whitmore, W.F., Jr., and Melamed, M.R.: Non-extirpative treatment of myosarcomas of the bladder and prostate. Cancer, 28:329–334, 1971.

MacKenzie, A.R., Whitmore, W.F., Jr., and Melamed, M.R.: Myosarcomas of the bladder and prostate. Cancer, 22:833–843, 1968.

Obe, J.A., Rosen, N., and Koss, L.G.: Primary choriocarcinoma of the urinary bladder. Report of a case with probable epithelial origin. Cancer, 52:1405–1409, 1983.

Pang, S.-C.: Bony and cartilaginous tumours of the urinary bladder. J Pathol. Bacteriol., 76:357–377, 1958.

Parton, I.: Primary lymphosarcoma of the bladder. Br. J. Urol., 34:221–223, 1962.

Pettersson, S., Hansson, G., and Blohme, I.: Condyloma acuminatum of the bladder. J. Urol., 115:535–536, 1976.

Peven, D.R., and Hidvegi, D.F.: Clear-cell adenocarcinoma of the female urethra. Acta Cytol, 29:142–146, 1985.

Piva, A., and Koss, L.G.: Cytologic diagnosis of metastatic malignant melanoma in urinary sediment. Acta Cytol., 8:398–402, 1964.

Pringle, J.P., Graham, R.C., and Bernier, G.M.: Detection of myeloma cells in the urine sediment. Blood, 43:137–143, 1974.

Sano, M.E., and Koprowska, I.: Primary cytologic diagnosis of a malignant renal lymphoma. Acta Cytol., 9:194–196, 1965.

Santino, A.M., Shumaker, E.J., and Garces, J.: Primary malignant lymphoma of the bladder. J. Urol., 103:310–313, 1970.

Stitt, R.B., and Colapinto, V.: Multiple simultaneous bladder malignancies: primary lymphosarcoma and adenocarcinoma. J. Urol., 96:733–736, 1966.

Su, C., and Prince, C.L.: Melanoma of the bladder. J. Urol., 87:365–367, 1962.

Valente, P.T., Atkinson, B.F., and Guerry, D.: Melanuria. Acta Cytol., 29:1026–1028, 1985.

Wang, C.C., Scully, R.E., and Leadbetter, W.F.: Primary malignant lymphoma of the urinary bladder. Cancer, 24:772–776, 1969.

Weinberg, T.: Primary chorionepithelioma of the urinary bladder in a male. Report of a case. Am. J. Pathol., 15:783–795, 1939.

Tumors of Kidney and Ureter: Urinary Sediment

Baird, S.S., Bush, L., and Livingstone, A.G.: Urethrectomy subsequent to total cystectomy for papillary carcinoma of the bladder. Case reports. J. Urol., 74:621–625, 1955.

Bibbo, M., Gill, W.B., Harris, M.J., Lu, C.-T., Thomsen, S., and Wied, G.L.: Retrograde brushing as a diagnostic procedure of ureteral, renal pelvic and renal calyceal lesions. A preliminary report. Acta Cytol., 18:137–141, 1974.

Chasko, S.B., Gray, G.F., and McCarron, J.P.: Urothelial neoplasia of the upper urinary tract. *In* Sommers, S.C., and Rosen, P.P. (eds). Pathol. Annu., 16(part 2):123–127, 1981.

Cordonnier, J.J., and Spjut, H.J.: Urethral occurrence of bladder carcinoma following cystectomy. J. Urol., 87:398–403, 1962.

Cullen, T.H., Popham, R.R., and Voss, H.J.: Urine cytology and primary carcinoma of the renal pelvis and ureter. Aust. N. Z. J. Surg., 41:230–236, 1972.

Culp, O.S., Utz, D.C., and Harrison, E.G., Jr.: Experiences with ureteral carcinoma in situ detected during operations for vesical neoplasms. J. Urol., *97*:679–682, 1967.

Eriksson, O., and Johansson, S.: Urothelial neoplasms of the upper urinary tract. A correlation between cytologic and histologic findings in 43 patients with urothelial neoplasma of the renal pelvis or ureter. Acta Cytol., *20*:20–25, 1976.

Foot, N.C., and Papanicolaou, G.N.: Early renal carcinoma in situ detected by means of smears of fixed urinary sediment. JAMA, *139*:356–358, 1949.

Framowitz, F.B., Steinbook, M.L., Lautin, E.M., et al.: Inverted papilloma of the ureter. J. Urol., *126*:113–116, 1981.

Gill, W.B., Lu, C.T., and Thomsen, D.: Retrograde brushing: A new technique for obtaining histologic and cytologic material from ureteral, renal pelvic, and renal calyceal lesions. J. Urol., *109*:573–578, 1973.

Gillenwater, J.Y., and Burros, H.M.: Unusual tumors of the female urethra. Obstet. Gynecol., *31*:617–620, 1968.

Hajdu, S.I.: Exfoliative cytology or primary and metastatic Wilms' tumors. Acta Cytol., *15*:339–342, 1971.

Hajdu, S.I., Savino, A., Hajdu, E.O., and Koss, L.G.: Cytologic diagnosis of renal cell carcinoma with the aid of fat stain. Acta Cytol., *15*:31–33, 1971.

Johansson, S., Angervall, L., Bengtson, U., and Wahlquist, L.: Uroepithelial tumors of the renal pelvis associated with abuse of phenacetin-containing analgesics. Cancer, *33*: 743–753, 1974.

Johnson, D.E., and Guinn, G.A.: Surgical management of urethral carcinoma occurring after cystectomy. J. Urol., *103*:314–316, 1970.

Kakizoe, T., Fujita, J., Murase, T., Matsumoto, K., and Kishi, K.: Transitional cell carcinoma of the bladder in patients with renal pelvic and ureteral cancer. J. Urol., *124*:17–19, 1980.

Khan, A.U., Farrow, G.M., Zincke, H., Utz, D.C., and Greene, L.F.: Primary carcinoma in situ of the ureter and renal pelvis. J. Urol., *121*:681–, 1979.

Kobayashi, S., Ohmori, M., Miki, H., Hirata, K., and Shimada, K.: Exfoliative cytology of a primary carcinoma of the renal pelvis. A case report. Acta Cytol., *29*:1021–1025, 1985.

Koss, L.G.; Tumors of the Urinary Bladder. Atlas of Tumor Pathology, 2nd series, fascicle 11. Washington, D.C., Armed Forces Institute of Pathology, 1975, Supplement 1985.

Koss, L.G., Nakanishi, I., and Freed, S.: Nonpapillary carcinoma in situ and atypical hyperplasia in cancerous bladders. Further studies of surgically removed bladders by mapping. Urology, *9*:442–455, 1977.

Linker, D.G., and Whitmore, W.F.: Ureteral carcinoma in situ. J. Urol., *113*:777–780, 1975.

Liwnicz, B.H., Lepow, H., Schutte, H., Fernandez, R., and Caberwal, D.: Mucinous adenocarcinoma of the renal pelvis: Discussion of possible pathogenesis. J. Urol., *114*:306–310, 1975.

Lomax-Smith, J.D., and Seymour, A.E.: Neoplasia in analgesic nephropathy. A urothelial field change. Am. J. Surg. Pathol., *4*:565–572, 1980.

Mahadevia, P.S., Karwa, G.L., and Koss, L.G.: Mapping of urothelium in carcinomas of the renal pelvis and ureter. A report of nine cases. Cancer, *51*:890–897, 1983.

Malmgren, R.A., Soloway, M.S., Chu, E.W., DelVecchio, P.R., and Ketcham, A.S.: Cytology of ileal conduit urine. Acta Cytol., *15*:506–509, 1971.

Mancilla-Jimenez, R., Stanley, R.J., and Blath, R.A.: Papillary renal cell carcinoma. A clinical, radiologic, and pathologic study of 34 cases. Cancer, *38*:2469–2480, 1976.

Melicow, M.M., and Tannenbaum, M.: Endometrial carcinoma of uterus masculinus (prostatic utricle). Report of 6 cases. J. Urol., *106*:892–902, 1971.

Mount, B.M., Curtis, M., Marshall, K., and Husk, M.: Cytologic diagnosis of renal cell carcinoma. Urology, *2*:421–425, 1973.

Murphy, W.M., von Buedinger, R.P., and Poley, R.W.: Primary carcinoma in situ of the renal pelvis and urethra. Cancer, *34*:1126–1130, 1974.

Naib, Z.M.: Exfoliative cytology of renal pelvic lesions. Cancer, *14*:1085–1087, 1961.

Ohkawa, M., Sugata, T., Hisazumi, H., Ishikawa, Y., and Mukawa, A.: Primary carcinoma in situ of the ureter: A case report. J. Urol., *132*:1184–1185, 1984.

Piscioli, F., Detassis, C., Polla, E., Pusiol, T., Reich, A., and Luciani, L.: Cytologic presentation of renal adenocarcinoma in urinary sediment. Acta Cytol., *27*:383–390, 1983.

Potts, I.F., and Hirst, E.: Inverted papilloma of the bladder. J. Urol., *90*:175–179, 1963.

Schade, R.O.K., Serck-Hanssen, A., and Swinney, J.: Morphological changes in the ureter in cases of bladder carcinoma. Cancer, *27*:1267–1272, 1971.

Schellhammer, P.F., and Whitmore, W.F., Jr.: Urethral meatal carcinoma following cystourethrectomy for bladder carcinoma. J. Urol., *115*:61–64, 1976.

Sharma, T.C., Melamed, M.R., and Whitmore, W.F.: Carcinoma in situ of the ureter in patients with bladder carcinoma treated by cystectomy. Cancer, *26*:583–587, 1970.

Sherwood, T.: Upper urinary tract tumours following bladder carcinoma: Natural history of urothelial neoplastic disease. Br. J. Radiol., *44*:137–141, 1971.

Smart, J.G.: Renal and ureteric tumours in association with bladder tumours. Br. J. Urol., *36*:380–390, 1964.

Sternheimer, R.: A supravital cytodiagnostic stain for urinary sediments. JAMA, *231*:826–832, 1975.

Stragier, M., Desmet, R., Denys, H., Vergison, R., and Vanvuchelen, J.: Primary carcinoma in situ of renal pelvis and ureter. Br. J. Urol., *52*:401, 1980.

Sylora, H.O., Diamond, H.M., Kaufman, M., Straus, F., and Lyon, E.S.: Primary carcinoid tumor of the urethra. J. Urol., *114*:150–153, 1975.

Wagle, D.G., Moore, R.H., and Murphy, G.P.: Primary carcinoma of the renal pelvis. Cancer, *33*:1642–1648, 1974.

Wallace, D.: Cancer of the bladder. Am. J. Roentgenol. Radium. Ther. Nucl. Med., *102*:581–586, 1968.

Wolinska, W.H., and Melamed, M.R.: Urinary conduit cytology. Cancer, *32*:1000–1006, 1973.

Tumors of the Urethra

Barrasso, R., De Brux, J., Croissant, O., and Orth, G.: High prevalence of papillomavirus-associated penile intraepithelial neoplasia in sexual partners of women with cervical intraepithelial neoplasia. N. Engl. J. Med., *317*:916–923, 1987.

Bretton, P.R., Herr, H.W., Whitmore, W.F., Jr., Badalament, R.A., Kimmel, M., Provet, J., Oettgen, H.F., Melamed, M.R., and Fair, W.R.: Intravesical bacillus Calmette-Guérin therapy for in situ transitional cell carcinoma involving the prostatic urethra. J. Urol., *141*:853–856, 1989.

Giacomini, G., Bianchi, G., and Moretti, D.: Detection of sexually transmitted diseases by urethral cytology, the ignored male counterpart of cervical cytology. Acta Cytol., *33*:11–15, 1989.

Gillenwater, J.Y., and Burros, H.M.: Unusual tumors of the female urethra. Obstet. Gynecol., *31*:617–620, 1968.

Gowing, N.F.: Urethral carcinoma associated with cancer of the bladder. Br. J. Urol., *32*:428–438, 1960.

Grabstald, H.: Tumors of the urethra in men and women. Cancer, *32*:1235–1236, 1973.

Grabstald, H., Hilaris, B., Henschke, U., and Whitmore, W.F., Jr.: Cancer of the female urethra. JAMA, *197*:835–842, 1966.

Grussendorf-Conen, E.-I., Deutz, F.J., and de Villers, E.M.: Detection of human papillomavirus-6 in primary carcinoma of the urethra in men. Cancer, *60*:1832–1835, 1987.

Katz, J.I., and Grabstald, H.: Primary malignant melanoma of the female urethra. J. Urol., *116*:454–457, 1976.

Murphy, M.W., Fu, Y.S., Lancaster, W.D., and Jenson, A.B.: Papillomavirus structural antigen in condyloma acuminatum of the male urethra. J. Urol., *130*:84–85, 1983.

Murphy, W.M., von Buedinger, R.P., and Poley, R.W.: Primary carcinoma in situ of the renal pelvis and urethra. Cancer, *34*:1126–1130, 1974.

Peven, D.R., and Hidvegi, D.F.: Clear-cell adenocarcinoma of the female urethra. Acta Cytol., *29*:142–146, 1985.

Richie, J.P., and Skinner, D.G.: Carcinoma in situ of the urethra associated with bladder carcinoma: The role of urethrectomy. J. Urol., *119*:80–81, 1978.

Sacks, S.A., Waisman, J., Apfelbaum, H.B., Lake, P., and Goodwin, W.E.: Urethral adenocarcinoma (possibly originating in the glands of the Littré). J. Urol., *113*:50–55, 1975.

Schellhammer, P.F., and Whitmore, W.F., Jr.: Transitional cell carcinoma of the urethra in men having cystectomy for bladder cancer. J. Urol., *115*:56–60, 1976.

Sylsora, H.O., Diamond, H.M., Kaufman, M., Straus, F., and Lyon, E.S.: Primary carcinoid tumor of the urethra. J. Urol., *114*:150–153, 1975.

Tyler, D.E.: Stratified squamous epithelium in the vesical trigone and urethra: Findings correlated with the menstrual cycle and age. Am. J. Anat., *111*:319–325, 1962.

Wolinska, W.H., Melamed, M.R., Schellhammer, P.F., and Whitmore, J.W.F.: Urethral cytology following cystectomy for bladder carcinoma. Am. J. Surg. Pathol., *1*:225–234, 1977.

Tumors of Prostate: Urinary Sediment

Arias-Stella, J., and Takano-Moron, J.: Atypical epithelial changes in the seminal vesicle. Arch. Pathol., *66*:761–766, 1958.

Bamforth, J.: Cytological diagnosis of prostatic carcinoma. Ann. R. Coll. Surg. Engl., *23*:248–264, 1958.

Barlebo, S., and Sorensen, B.L.: Flat epithelial changes in the urinary bladder in patients with prostatic hypertrophy. Scand. J. Urol. Nephrol., *6*(Suppl. 15):121–128, 1972.

Bauer, W.C., McGavran, M.H., and Carlin, M.R.: Unsuspected carcinoma of prostate in suprapubic prostatectomy specimens; clinicopathological study of 55 consecutive cases. Cancer, *13*:370–378, 1960.

Catalona, W.J., Smith, D.S., Ratlif, T.L. et al.: Measurement of prostate-specific antigen in serum as a screening test for prostate concern. N. Engl. J. Med., *324*:1156–1161, 1991.

Clarke, B.G., and Bamford, S.B.: Cytology of prostate gland in diagnosis of cancer. JAMA, *172*:1750–1753, 1960.

Couture, M.L., Freund, M., and Katubig, C.P., Jr.: The isolation and identification of exfoliated prostate cells from human semen. Acta Cytol., *24*:262–267, 1980.

Edwards, C.N., Steinhorsson, E., and Nicholson, D.: Autopsy study of latent prostatic cancer. Cancer, *6*:531–554, 1953.

Foti, A.G., Cooper, J.F., Herschman, H., and Malvaez, R.R.: Detection of prostatic cancer by solid-phase radioimmunoassay of serum prostatic acid phosphatase. N. Engl. J. Med., *297*:1357–1361, 1977.

Frank, I.N.: Cytologic evaluation of prostatic smear in carcinoma of prostate. J. Urol., *73*:128–138, 1955.

Frank, I.N., Benjamin, J.A., and Sergerson, J.E.: Cytologic examination of semen. Fertil. Steril., *5*:217–226, 1954.

Frank, I.N., and Scott, W.W.: Cytodiagnosis of prostatic carcinoma; follow-up study. J. Urol., *79*:983–988, 1958.

Gardner, W.A., Culberson, D.E., and Bennett, B.D.: *Trichomonas vaginalis* in the prostate gland. Arch. Pathol. Lab. Med., *110*:430–432, 1986.

Garret, M., and Jassie, M.: Cytologic examination of post prostatic massage specimens as an aid in diagnosis of carcinoma of the prostate. Acta Cytol., *20*:126–131, 1976.

Gray, G.F., Jr., and Marshall, V.F.: Squamous carcinoma of the prostate. J. Urol., *113*:736, 738, 1975.

Greenebaum, E.: Megakaryocytes and ganglion cells mimicking cancer in fine needle aspiration of the prostate. Acta Cytol., *32*:504–508, 1988.

Greenwald, P., Damon, A., Kirmss, V., and Polan, A.K.: Physical and demographic features of men before developing cancer of the prostate. JNCI, *53*:341–346, 1974.

Greenwald, P., Kirmss, V., Polan, A.K., and Dick, V.S.: Cancer of prostate among men with benign prostatic hyperplasia. JNCI, *53*:335–340, 1974.

Harbitz, T.B.: Endocrine disturbances in men with benign hyperplasia and carcinoma of the prostate. Acta Pathol. Microbiol. Scand. [A], 244:1–13, 1974.

Kaufman, J.J., Rosenthal, M., and Goodwin, W.E.: Methods of diagnosis of carcinoma of the prostate: A comparison of clinical impression, prostatic smear, needle biopsy, open perineal biopsy and transurethral biopsy. J. Urol., *72*:450–465, 1954.

Koivuniemi, A., and Tyrkko, J.: Seminal vesicle epithelium in fine needle aspiration biopsies of the prostate as a pitfall in the cytologic diagnosis of carcinoma. Acta Cytol., *20*:116–119, 1976.

Koss, L.G.: The puzzle of prostatic carcinoma. Mayo Clin. Proc., *63*:193–197, 1988.

Koss, L.G., Woyke, S., Schreiber, K., Kohlberg, W., and Freed, S.Z.: Thin-needle aspiration of the prostate. Urol. Clin. North Am. *11*:237–251, 1984.

MacKenzie, A.R., Sharma, T.C., Whitmore, W.F., Jr., and Melamed, M.R.: Non-extirpative treatment of myosarcomas of the bladder and prostate. Cancer, *28*:329–334, 1971.

MacKenzie, A.R., Whitmore, W.F., Jr., and Melamed, M.R.: Myosarcomas of the bladder and prostate. Cancer, *22*:833–843, 1968.

Mahadevia, P.S., Koss, L.G., and Tar, I.J.: Prostatic involvement in bladder cancer: Prostate mapping in 20 cystoprostatectomy specimens. Cancer, *58*:2096–2102, 1986.

Melicow, M.M., and Tannenbaum, M.: Endometrial carcinoma of uterus masculinus (prostatic utricle). Report of 6 cases. J. Urol., *106*:892–902, 1971.

Mostofi, F.K.: Grading of prostatic carcinoma. Cancer Chemother. Rep. *59*:111–117, 1975.

Nowels, K., Kent, E., Rinsho, K., and Oyasu, R.: Prostate specific antigen and acid phosphatase-reactive cells in cystitis cystica and glandularis. Arch. Pathol. Lab. Med., *112*:734–737, 1988.

Peterson, R.O.: Urologic Pathology. pp. 613–638. Philadelphia, J. B. Lippincott, 1986.

Ramzy, I., and Larson, V.: Prostatic duct carcinoma: Exfoliative cytology. Acta Cytol., *21*:417–420, 1977.

Razvi, M., Firfer, R., and Berkson, B.: Occult transitional cell carcinoma of the prostate presenting as skin metastasis. J. Urol., *113*:734–735, 1975.

Riaboff, P.J.: Detection of early prostatic and urinary tract cancer in asymptomatic patients 50 years of age and over; preliminary report. J. Urol., *72*:62–66, 1954.

Richardson, H.L., Durfee, G.R., Day, E., and Papanicolaou, G.N.: Role of cytology in detection of early prostatic cancer. In Homburger, F., and Fishman, W.H. (eds.): The Laboratory Diagnosis of Cancer of the Prostate, pp. 14–17. Boston, Tufts Medical School, 1954.

Tanner, F.H., and McDonald, J.R.: Granulomatous prostatitis: Histologic study of a group of granulomatous lesions collected from prostate glands. Arch. Pathol., *36*:358–370, 1943.

Vihko, P., Kontturi, M., Lukkarinen, O., Ervasti, J., and Vihko, R.: Screening for carcinoma of the prostate: Rectal examination, and enzymatic and radioimmunologic measurements of serum acid phosphatase compared. Cancer, *56*:173–177, 1985.

24

The Gastrointestinal Tract

The parts of the gastrointestinal tract that are accessible to cytologic investigation are the esophagus, the stomach, the duodenum (including samples from the biliary and the pancreatic ducts), and the colon (Fig. 24–1).

METHODS

The introduction of flexible fiberoptic instruments that allow brushing and washing of lesions under direct visual control has greatly expanded the usefulness and precision of gastrointestinal cytology. Thanks to these instruments the diagnostic procedures leading to cytologic sampling and to biopsies are now significantly less tedious to the patients than in the recent past.

"Salvage cytology" is a technique introduced by Graham et al. (1978) that consists of washing the channel of the endoscopic instrument with saline and collecting the fluid for cytologic analysis into a suction trap. Initially, the technique was intended for use after biopsies (Graham and Spjut, 1979), but Caos et al. (1986) reported its successful application even without biopsies.

Washings of the esophagus or stomach without endoscopic control are still occasionally used (Drake, 1985). The function and use of the esophageal balloon technique are described on p. 1025.

Methods of cytologic investigation of the colon and rectum are described on p. 1067. Cytologic evaluation of other abdominal organs by aspiration biopsy is discussed in Chapter 29.

THE ESOPHAGUS

Anatomy

The esophagus is a tubular structure with muscular walls. It extends from the pharynx across the diaphragm to the cardia of the stomach. The esophagus is in close proximity to many vital structures. In the neck, the larynx and the trachea are immediately anterior; the recurrent nerves run along the lateral walls of the esophagus, and the vagus nerves descend along its anterior and posterior walls. In the upper thorax the esophagus comes into contact with the bifurcation of the trachea and with the aorta. At the level of the heart, the left auricle is in close proximity. Thus, cancers of the esophagus not only may obstruct its narrow lumen, but also may invade and damage several vital organs.

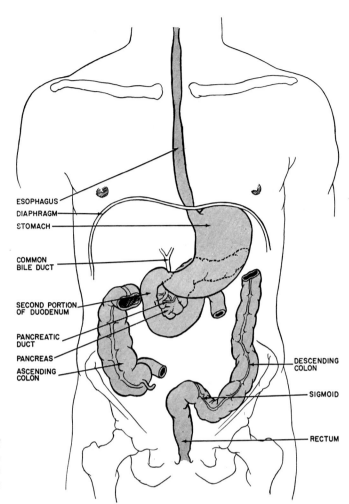

FIGURE 24-1. Schematic representation of portions of the gastrointestinal tract accessible to cytologic investigation. The transverse colon is omitted, to demonstrate the pancreas and the duodenum.

Labels in figure: ESOPHAGUS, DIAPHRAGM, STOMACH, COMMON BILE DUCT, SECOND PORTION OF DUODENUM, PANCREATIC DUCT, PANCREAS, ASCENDING COLON, DESCENDING COLON, SIGMOID, RECTUM

Histology and Normal Cytology

The esophagus is lined by nonhornifying squamous epithelium (Fig. 24-2). Islands of gastric epithelium may be found in the areas immediately adjacent to the cardia and, rarely, elsewhere within the esophagus. Small, mucus-producing glands are found in the submucosa.

The ultrastructure of the squamous epithelium of the esophagus is that of a stratified, nonkeratinizing squamous epithelium, without distinguishing features.

The cytology of the esophageal aspirates, brushings, and washings in the absence of disease is extremely simple. The smears are composed essentially of superficial squamous cells identical with those observed in sputum samples (see p. 694 and Fig. 19-6). Less commonly, smaller, deeper squamous cells with relatively larger nuclei, and occa-

sionally squamous "pearls" may be noted. It is not unusual to find swallowed cells of respiratory origin, such as dust-containing macrophages and ciliated bronchial cells (Fig. 24-3A). Also, gastric epithelial cells, singly or in clusters, may occur (see Fig. 24-3B). Foreign material, especially plant cells, may be present if there is an obstruction of the esophageal lumen.

Noncancerous Diseases

Acute and Chronic Esophagitis

This group of diseases of varying etiology is very important from the point of view of diagnostic cytology, since it produces cells that may be readily confused with cancer. Ulcerative esophagitis may be primary and due to trauma or herpes, or secondary to such diseases as cardiospasm of long stand-

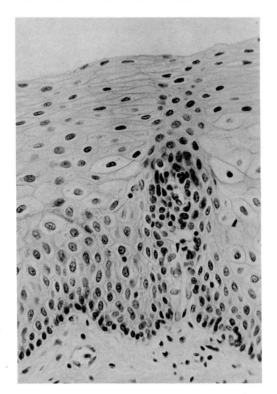

FIGURE 24 – 2.   The squamous epithelium of the esophagus. (×300)

ing, Plummer – Vinson syndrome, some forms of avitaminosis, scleroderma, and hiatus hernia. A rare, sometimes fatal disorder of unknown etiology is chronic erosive esophagitis.

The histologic lesion in esophagitis is mucosal ulceration of varying depth and configuration. There is a moderate infiltration of the stroma with inflammatory cells. The surface of the lesion may be covered with fibrin. Chronic erosive esophagitis is characterized by loss of superficial epithelial layers (mucosal erosions) (Fig. 24 – 4A). Squamous metaplasia of the submucosal glands may occur (see Fig. 24 – 4B).

Cells desquamating from the eroded epithelium are essentially of the same size as small squamous or parabasal cells. The most outstanding features of the comparatively large nuclei are large isolated clumps of chromatin and, occasionally, large nucleoli (Fig. 24 – 5). However, there is no significant hyperchromasia. The cytoplasm is evenly distributed, and the cells do not vary much in size. In clusters, there is good adherence of the cells to each other. Careful attention to cellular detail helps in the correct interpretation of the cytologic findings. The cells seen in erosive esophagitis are similar to those observed in pemphigus (see Fig. 21 – 6).

Herpetic Esophagitis

Many years ago Berg emphasized the occurrence of this disease in cancer patients who, in the course of treatment, sustained a surgical or radiation injury to the esophagus. Immunosuppressive therapy and the use of cytotoxic anticancer drugs have contributed to an increased frequency of this disease. Herpetic esophagitis produces extensive, although superficial, ulcerations of the esophageal mucosa. Intranuclear eosinophilic inclusions within the epithelial cells are observed in histologic material. The use of cytology resulted in the primary clinical diagnosis of several such cases. Surprisingly, in some patients, there was no past history of immune deficiency or immunosuppression. It is, therefore, likely that the disease is more common than hitherto anticipated. Most patients observed had vague complaints referable to the esophagus, such as retrosternal pain or mild dysphagia. Apparent simultaneous involvement of the esophagus and the bronchial tree has been noted. The disease may be diagnosed in sputum or in material obtained from the esophagus by aspiration, washings, or brushing. The cytologic findings are identical with those observed in the material from the female genital tract (see p. 351 and Fig. 10 – 49, and the respiratory tract (see p. 733 and Fig. 19 – 62). Multinucleated cells with molded "ground-glass," opaque nuclei, and cells with intranuclear eosinophilic inclusions are observed (Fig. 24 – 6).

Esophageal Infections in Acquired Immunodeficiency Syndrome

Esophagitis is a common early manifestation of the acquired immunodeficiency syndrome (AIDS). Candidiasis (moniliasis), (see Fig. 10 – 36), cytomegalovirus infection (see Fig. 22 – 26), herpetic esophagitis (see above), and other infectious agents may be identified in cytologic samples obtained during esophagoscopy.

Esophageal Diverticula

Distended diverticula may produce symptoms of esophageal obstruction similar to those of cancer. Also, cancers originating within the diverticula may be diagnosed cytologically (see p. 1027).

Barrett's Syndrome

The syndrome, first described by Barrett in 1950, consists of an extensive replacement of the esophageal squamous epithelium by columnar epithelium of gastric or intestinal type, associated with hiatus hernia and, quite often, esophageal stricture

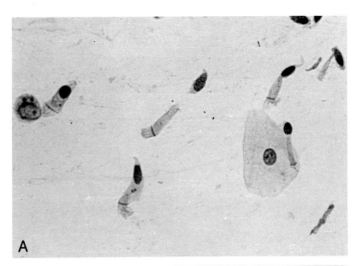

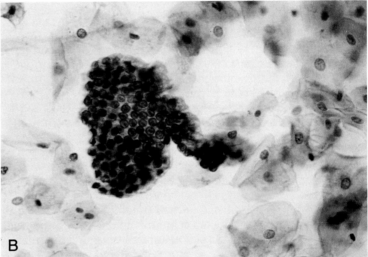

FIGURE 24–3. Esophageal washings in absence of disease. (*A*) The cellular components include squamous cells (which usually are the dominant component), ciliated cells, and an alveolar macrophage of respiratory tract origin. (*B*) Squamous cells and a fragment of benign gastric epithelium. (*A, B* ×500. Greenebaum, E., et al.: Use of esophageal balloon in the diagnosis of carcinomas of the head, neck, and upper intestinal tract. Acta Cytol., *28*:9–15, 1984)

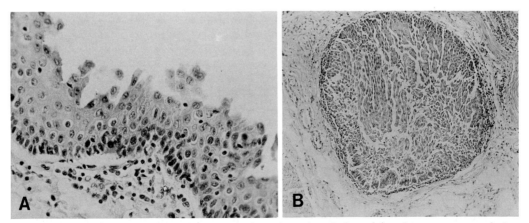

FIGURE 24–4. Erosion of superficial layers of esophageal epithelium (*A*) and squamous metaplasia of a submucosal gland (*B*) from a fatal case of chronic erosive esophagitis of unknown etiology. Note cellular atypia. (*A* ×300; *B* ×75. Johnson, W. D., et al.: Cytology of esophageal washings; evaluation of 364 cases. Cancer, *8*:951–957, 1955)

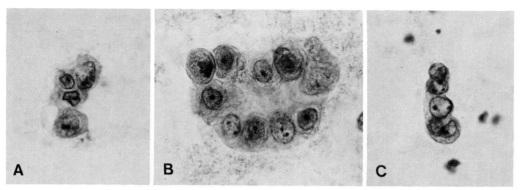

FIGURE 24 – 5. (*A, B, C*) Clusters of atypical cells from cases of chronic erosive esophagitis (cluster in *A*, from case shown in Fig. 24 – 4). Note prominent granularity of the nuclei, scanty cytoplasm, and some variability in cell size. Large nucleoli may be present. Absence of hyperchromasia as well as good adhesion of cells in clusters are of importance in differentiating this lesion from cancer. (×600. Johnson, W. D., et al.: Cytology of esophageal washings; evaluation of 364 cases. Cancer, *8*:951–957, 1955)

(Mossberg; Burgess et al.). Peptic ulcer and adenocarcinoma of gastric type may occur within the affected area of the esophagus (see below). The symptoms associated with Barrett's syndrome are dysphagia, regurgitation, heartburn, and pain. Episodes of acute obstruction may occur (Fig. 24 – 7). Radiographic examination may reveal a stricture that may mimic to perfection the appearance of an esophageal carcinoma (see Fig. 24 – 7*A*), although there is usually a preservation of esophageal peristalsis above and below. Histologic findings show an abrupt transition from the normal squamous epithelium to mucus-producing columnar epithelium (see Fig. 24 – 7*C*). Cytologic examination of gastric aspirates, washings, or brush specimens may contribute in a major way to the accurate diagnosis. The smears contain goblet cells and

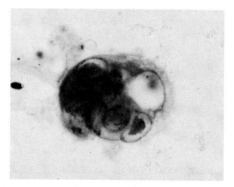

FIGURE 24 – 6. Esophagus washings: herpetic esophagitis. A characteristic multinucleated cell with nuclear molding and eosinophilic nuclear inclusions is shown. (×560)

mucus-producing benign columnar cells, usually in clusters, characteristic of mucus-producing epithelium (see Fig. 24 – 7*B*).

Because adenocarcinoma may occur in Barrett's esophagus (although the frequency of this event is disputed) and because the esophagus can be closely monitored by endoscopic techniques, this disorder became a subject of intense scientific interest (summary in Spechler and Goyal, 1986). The sequence of morphologic events in the genesis of adenocarcinoma became the subject of numerous scientific communications. Briefly summarized, morphologic precancerous abnormalities in columnar epithelium (named *dysplasia,* rather than carcinoma in situ) precede carcinoma (Smith et al., 1984; Lee, 1985). The lesion known as dysplasia consists of nuclear enlargement and hyperchromasia, occasionally with branching of the affected glands and a marked increased in abnormal mitoses (Rubio and Riddell, 1989). The lesions are very similar to precancerous abnormalities and carcinoma in situ of the gastric epithelium, shown in Figs. 24 – 34, 24 – 35, and 24 – 37. Prospective studies of patients with Barrett's dysplasia indicate a very high level of progression to carcinoma (Lee, 1985; Spechler and Goyal, 1986). Carcinomas occurring in Barrett's mucosa are nearly always adenocarcinomas of the gastrointestinal type (Smith et al., 1984). Other variants of gastrointestinal cancers may also occur (adenosquamous carcinoma, etc.).

Patients with Barrett's syndrome are monitored by endoscopic biopsies and, to some extent, by cytologic studies. Nuclear abnormalities were observed in columnar cells in a case of dysplasia

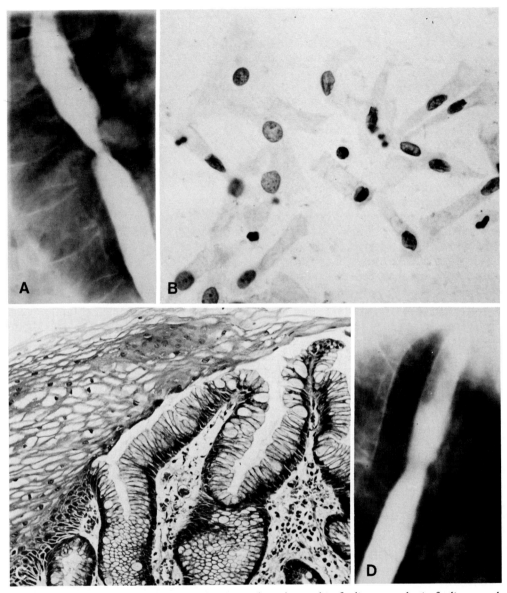

FIGURE 24-7. Barrett's syndrome, man age 54. Radiographic findings, cytologic findings, and biopsy specimen. (*A*) Esophageal narrowing shown in a barium swallow after an episode of acute esophageal obstruction. The similarity to esophageal carcinoma is evident. (*B*) Columnar, mucus-producing benign cells and goblet cells in esophageal washings. (*C*) Esophageal biopsy specimen showing replacement of a portion of esophageal lining by hyperplastic mucus-producing epithelium made up of columnar and goblet cells. (*D*) Radiographic findings 15 months later: the lumen of the esophagus is almost normal after conservative antiulcer therapy. (*B* ×560; *C* ×150)

(Robey et al., 1988). The monitoring of epithelial DNA content by flow cytometry disclosed abnormal, aneuploid DNA histograms in dysplasias and in carcinomas (Haggitt et al., 1988). Although Barrett's esophagus presents a tempting target of investigations because of its accessibility to monitoring and sampling, the disease is uncommon, and the new information has not modified the approaches to treatment which, in esophageal carcinoma, requires surgery.

Benign Tumors

In 1982 Syrjänen et al. described a rare lesion of the esophagus, akin to a condyloma acuminatum, and postulated that human papillomavirus (HPV) may be a factor in the genesis of this tumor. Winkler et al. (1985) confirmed this hypothesis by documenting the presence of HPV antigen in two such lesions and in 11 of 73 "focal hyperplasias," some of which resembled "flat condylomas" with significant koilocytosis and nuclear abnormalities. Apparently, none of these lesions progressed to cancer. It is of note, though, that Syrjänen (1982) observed "flat condylomas" at the periphery of invasive esophageal cancers. There is no known cytologic presentation of these lesions.

Koilocytes were not observed by the Chinese observers in the detection studies of early esophageal cancer. Also note the recent observations on the presence of HPV DNA in esophageal carcinomas, summarized below (Chang et al., 1990).

Cancer of the Esophagus

Epidermoid carcinoma of the esophagus has an interesting geographic distribution. The disease is quite common in northeastern Iran, in northern China and among Chinese in Singapore, among Africans in parts of southern Africa, and in Brittany (France). The disease is more common in males than in females. Epidemiologic data suggest that intake of hot beverages, cigarette smoking, or alcohol intake may in part account for it, although a recent study in China failed to reveal any risk factors (Li et al., 1989). Auerbach et al. demonstrated a high frequency of epidermoid carcinoma in situ of the esophagus among smokers. Adenocarcinoma occurring in Barrett's esophagus was discussed above.

Invariably, as with all squamous cancers, the question of human papillomavirus (HPV) as a factor in the genesis of this tumor was raised (Syrjänen, 1987). Except for squamous papilloma (see above), the evidence of HPV presence in esophageal cancer was initially limited to one paper (Kulski et al., 1986) in which the presence of HPV DNA was observed in five invasive cancers. More recently, work on invasive esophageal carcinoma based on biopsy material from 51 Chinese patients revealed the presence of HPV in 25 of them (49%). In 16 of these 25 specimens, HPV types 16 and 18 were documented by in situ hybridization. Other types of HPV were observed in the remaining 7 patients (Chang et al., 1990). In the same study, in 80 cytologic preparations, also from Chinese patients from a high-risk area, there were 53 samples positive for HPV by filter in situ hybridization. It was of note that HPV was detected in 2 of 9 patients without cytologic abnormalities, in 3 of 6 patients with mild dysplasia, in 25 of 31 patients with moderate dysplasia, in 19 of 28 patients with severe dysplasia, and in 4 of 6 patients with invasive carcinoma. Since a person-to-person transmission of HPV is unlikely in these patients, an activation of the latent viral infection is a more likely explanation of these findings.

Histology

Epidermoid carcinoma is by far the most common type of esophageal cancer. The disease may affect any part of the esophagus, but occurs most frequently in areas where the esophagus is slightly narrowed: at the level of the thyroid cartilage, at the level of the bifurcation of the trachea, and at the level of the diaphragm. The degree of differentiation may vary from highly keratinized (verrucous) types to poorly differentiated small-cell carcinomas (Bogomoletz et al., 1989). Approximately 3% esophageal cancers are adenocarcinomas. The latter usually originate in islands of gastric mucosa, but they may also arise in the submucosal glands. When such lesions occur in Barrett's esophagus, they are sometimes referred to as Dawson's syndrome. Most adenocarcinomas of the esophagus occur in the area of the cardia and are histologically indistinguishable from gastric cancers. Focal glandular features may be observed in a substantial proporation of epidermoid carcinomas (Kuwano et al., 1988). As a general rule, esophageal cancers cause obstruction of the esophagus, resulting in difficulties of swallowing and dysphagia.

Uncommonly, epidermoid carcinomas of the esophagus (but also of the larynx and pharynx) develop into rather bulky tumors, the surface of which is formed by a well-differentiated epidermoid carcinoma, sometimes in situ. The bulk of the tumor is composed of elongated spindly cells, occasionally accompanied by bizarre giant cells. Experience with these lesions suggests that the spindle and giant cell components represent a peculiar metaplasia of epidermoid carcinoma and not a benign "pseudosarcoma," as was originally suggested by Stout and Lattes. Still, the latter term is often used to describe this lesion. It must be stressed that in spite of its ominous appearance the pseudosarcoma appears to offer a much better prognosis than ordinary esophageal carcinoma.

Among very rare neoplastic diseases of the

esophagus that may become targets of cytologic examination, one must mention squamous papillomas, small-cell (oat cell) type of carcinoma first described by Rosen et al. (1975), and primary melanomas.

Precursor Lesions of Epidermoid Carcinoma and Their Detection

In the 1961 and 1968 editions of this book, it was anticipated that carcinoma of the esophagus must be preceded by precancerous epithelial changes, such as carcinoma in situ and related abnormalities.

These speculations were confirmed by extensive cytologic and histologic studies of esophageal cancer conducted by Chinese investigators. The stimulus for these studies was the very high prevalence rate of esophageal cancer in certain areas of central and northern China (Shu, 1984, 1985). It is of incidental interest that, in the same areas of China, chickens are susceptible to a cancerlike tumor of the gullet.

The purpose of the Chinese studies was to detect by cytologic means precancerous states, such as carcinoma in situ, in asymptomatic, high-risk populations, with the hope that early surgical intervention will prevent invasive esophageal cancer that carries with it a very high mortality rate. The instrument used in these investigations, devised by the Chinese scholars, was a small, inflatable plastic balloon with abrasive surface (Fig. 24–8). The balloon was attached to a narrow-caliber tube with color markers to indicate the position of the balloon in the esophagus. The balloon could be easily swallowed in deflated state, moved by peristalsis to the cardia, inflated, and slowly withdrawn to the level of cricoid cartilage. At this point, the balloon was deflated and withdrawn. The abrasive surfaces of the balloon, which contained cells scraped from the esophageal epithelium, were examined in the form of smears. The method causes trivial discomfort to the patients and was well accepted.

The first results of the population survey were presented in the Fourth International Cancer Congress in Florence, Italy in 1974 by an anonymous group representing the Chinese Academy of Medical Sciences. Because of a very high rate of esophageal cancer in Henan Province in northern China, a cytologic survey of 17,471 persons over 30 years of age was conducted. Dysplasia of the esophageal epithelium was observed in 276 patients, mostly below the age of 40, whereas invasive carcinoma in this population usually occurs in patients older than 40. Follow-up study of these 276 patients,

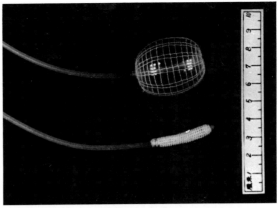

FIGURE 24–8. Esophageal balloon, collapsed (*bottom*) and distended with air (*top*). Note the rugosity of the surface that serves to obtain cell samples from the esophagus. The balloon is connected to a plastic tube with markers to indicate the position of the balloon in the esophagus. (Courtesy of Dr. Yi-Jing Shu)

some over a period of 7 to 10 years, disclosed that 30.3% of them developed esophageal carcinoma, in 27.3% the lesion persisted unchanged, and in 42.4% the changes either regressed to mild dysplasia or reverted to normal. In histologic studies of 67 patients, progression of mild and marked dysplasia to carcinoma in situ could be observed in many specimens. It was the conclusion of this study that marked dysplasia must be considered a precancerous lesion.

During the intervening years and changing political conditions in China, the names of the investigators became known (summary in Shu, 1984, 1985; Shen, 1984), and the results of several surveys became available.

Briefly, based on cytologic and histologic criteria, the Chinese investigators divided the precancerous lesions into two groups: dysplasia and carcinoma in situ. The criteria were derived from the now obsolete classification of precancerous lesions of the uterine cervix (see Chaps. 11 and 12). Lesions with more orderly epithelial growth, surface differentiation, and relatively minor nuclear abnormalities were classified as *dysplasia* and lesions with more significant atypia were classed as *carcinoma in situ* (Fig. 24–9).

The dysplasias were further subdivided into mild, moderate, and severe, based mainly on cytologic criteria (see below). The true significance of dysplasia is not clear, but there is no doubt that, in a substantial number of untreated patients with this disorder, invasive cancer of the esophagus devel-

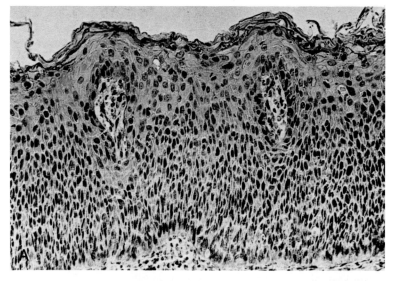

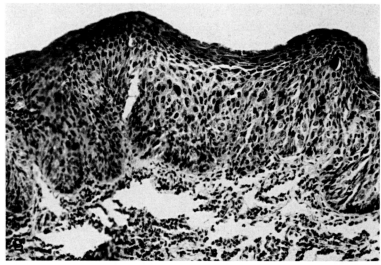

FIGURE 24–9. Precancerous lesions of the esophagus. (*A*) Low-grade lesion or "dysplasia," (*B*) carcinoma in situ. Although the two photographs are not fully comparable, the increased degree of nuclear abnormalities in (*B*) is evident. (×150. Courtesy of Dr. Yi-Jing Shu)

oped subsequently. It appears though, that in some patients, the lesions either failed to progress or even regressed (Shu, 1984, 1985). In any event, the precancerous lesions of the esophagus and subsequent events appear to have a remarkable similarity to lesions of the uterine cervix.

The accuracy of balloon sampling was tested on several large hospital populations with overt esophageal cancer, documented by biopsy, totaling 1,861 patients. The accuracy varied in a number of studies from 87.2% to 99%, averaging 94.9% (summary in Shu, 1984, 1985).

For the diagnosis of carcinoma in situ and early invasive cancer, the cytologic sampling proved to

be much superior to either endoscopy or radiologic examination (Shu, 1984).

The accomplishments of the Chinese scholars soon found several imitators. Thus, Berry et al. (1981) attempted a similar project in South Africa (where the rate of esophageal cancer is very high among some black populations), resulting in the discovery of 15 occult invasive carcinomas and carcinomas in situ in 500 patients. Dysplasia was illustrated, but the clinical significance of the lesion was not discussed. Jaskiewicz et al. (1984) used a small sponge, attached to a string and packaged in an easy-to-swallow gelatin capsule, to study a high-risk rural population in Transkei (South Africa) with similar results. In five patients, dysplastic changes progressed to invasive cancer. Greenebaum et al. (1984) used the balloon technique in 96 high-risk Montefiore hospital patients in New York City with the unexpected finding of 3 occult recurrent oropharyngeal cancers and one carcinoma in situ of the esophagus.

In the Western world, the knowledge of precancerous lesions of the esophagus is scarce. There are many cases on record in which carcinoma in situ and related lesions have been observed as incidental findings (Auerbach et al.; Ushigama et al.) or as a lesion accompanying invasive carcinoma (Suckow et al.; O'Gara and Horn; Kuwano et al.).

Cytology

PRECURSOR LESIONS

Much of the current knowledge of cytology of precursor lesions comes from Chinese sources (summaries in Shu, 1984, 1985; Shen, 1984). There is a remarkable similarity between the cytologic presentation of carcinoma in situ and related lesions of the esophagus and those of the uterine cervix (see Chap. 12).

Lower-grade lesions of the esophagus (dysplasia, see Fig. 24–9A) are characterized by well-dif-

ferentiated superficial and intermediate squamous cells with marked nuclear enlargement and hyperchromasia (Fig. 24–10). The resemblance of these cells to dyskaryosis of cervical squamous cells is remarkable (cf. Fig. 12–2).

The squamous cancer cells derived from high-grade lesions, such as carcinoma in situ (see Fig. 24–9B), are of the smaller parabasal variety. Although the nuclear abnormalities are approximately the same as in low-grade lesions, the cytoplasm is scanty, reflecting a lesser degree of surface maturation (Figs. 24–11 and 24–12). Cell clustering is common as shown in Figs. 24–11B and 24–12B. Shu (1984, 1985) illustrated several examples of progression of dysplasias to carcinoma in situ over a period of 2 to 4 years and, in some cases, to invasive carcinomas. One wonders to what extent the accuracy of balloon sampling may have influenced these results.

There are very few cases of carcinoma in situ diagnosed by cytology in the Western world.

One case of carcinoma in situ of the esophagus diagnosed by cytology was reported by Imbriglia and Lopusniak, and one case of a lesion approaching carcinoma in situ was personally observed in a 59-year-old man with a diverticulum. The washings were obtained because of symptoms of ob-

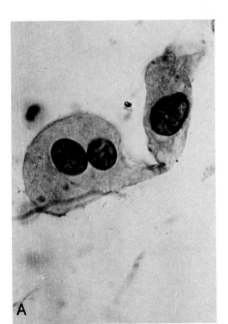 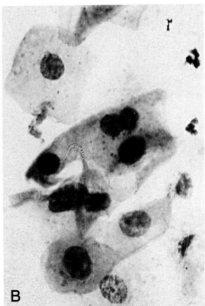

FIGURE 24–10. (*A, B*) Abnormal, well-differentiated, superficial and intermediate squamous cells ("dyskaryosis") derived from a low-grade neoplastic lesion of the esophagus (dysplasia). Note the abundant cytoplasm and the markedly enlarged, hyperchromatic nuclei. (× approx. 800. Courtesy of Dr. Yi-Jing Shu)

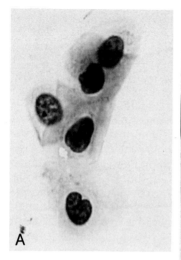
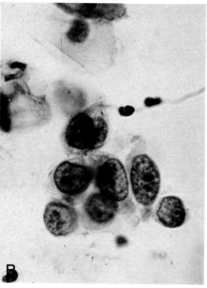

FIGURE 24–11. (*A, B*) Small epidermoid cancer cells of parabasal type, characteristic of carcinoma in situ of the esophagus. Note enlarged, hyperchromatic nuclei and scanty cytoplasm. The clustering of cells is shown in (*B*). (*A, B* × approx. 800. Courtesy of Dr. Yi-Jing Shu)

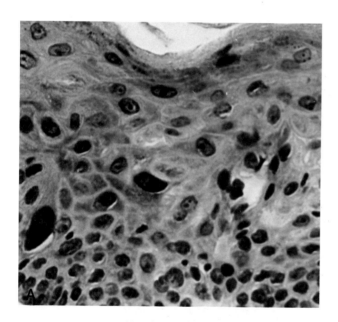

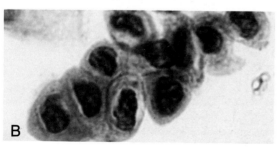

FIGURE 24–12. Another example of esophageal carcinoma in situ, comparing the tissue obtained at surgery (*A*) with a cell sample obtained by balloon (*B*). A cluster of small cancer cells is shown in (*B*). (*A* × approx. 350; *B* × approx. 800. Courtesy of Dr. Yi-Jing Shu)

struction. The biopsies, which unfortunately were obtained after an initial short course of radiotherapy, localized the lesion to the diverticulum, which was subsequently resected successfully. Cytologically, the lesion was characterized by well-differentiated superficial and parabasal squamous cells with abnormal, enlarged, and hyperchromatic nuclei, quite similar to the squamous dyskaryotic cells in the cervix. The histologic appearance of the epithelium disclosed nuclear abnormalities and some degree of disarrangement of the component cells.

RESULTS OF SCREENING

There is no doubt that mass screening for esophageal carcinoma in high-risk areas of China had a major beneficial effect. Before screening was instituted, the diagnosis of carcinoma in situ or early invasive carcinoma was 2 per 1000 in low-risk areas and 10 per 1000 in high-risk areas, where physicians and surgeons were alerted to this possibility. Screening of 81,187 asymptomatic people over the age of 30 in the high-risk Henan Province resulted in the discovery of 880 esophageal cancers (1%!), of which 649 (73.7%) were early and treatable by surgery (Shu, 1984). Less is known about survival of these patients, but Dr. Shu assured me that most of the treated patients survived 5 years or longer with a good quality of life. This information must be compared with a survival of 5% or fewer patients with invasive cancer of the esophagus commonly observed in the United States.

The Chinese experience has not been duplicated in the Western countries, except for the work in this laboratory reported above (Greenebaum et al., 1984). In this study, one case of presumed carcinoma in situ of the esophagus was observed in a man with prior history of squamous carcinoma of the larynx (Fig. 24–13). The biopsy of the esophagus disclosed fragments of squamous cancer in the absence of radiologic abnormalities.

The question of screening of patients in Western countries by the esophageal balloon technique must remain open. The experience from this laboratory (Greenebaum et al., 1984) suggests that in high-risk patients (i.e., patients with prior cancers of the larynx and pharynx, alcoholics who are also heavy cigarette smokers, etc.) a larger survey may be worthwhile. Clearly, in geographic areas at high risk for esophageal cancer, a major effort at balloon screening may be indicated.

INVASIVE EPIDERMOID CARCINOMA

These tumors may occur in a variety of grades and degrees of differentiation, ranging from a keratinizing, pearl-forming squamous cancer to anaplastic small-cell epidermoid carcinoma. The cytologic findings in esophageal washings closely reflect these structural varieties.

The squamous carcinoma produces highly keratinized abnormal cells with either completely pyknotic, hyperchromatic nuclei, or with nuclear shadows, much in the manner described for squamous carcinoma of the bronchus (Fig. 24–14A). The epidermoid cancers are characterized by smaller and less well-differentiated cells, frequently with very scanty basophilic cytoplasm (Figs. 24–14B and 24–15). Here the diagnosis of tumor type depends largely on the finding of cancer cells with eosinophilic cytoplasm. These may be very few. The most anaplastic varieties of epidermoid cancer produce cells that often are very small, with abnormally large nuclei and very scanty cytoplasm (Fig. 24–16). All of the epidermoid cancers are characterized by marked nuclear abnormalities, especially hyperchromasia and, frequently, large prominent nucleoli. Horai et al. (1978) described several examples of a small-cell anaplastic carcinoma.

Carcinomas of the distal end of the esophagus may extend into the cardia and fail to produce radiographic abnormalities of cancer. In such situations cytologic examination may be of critical diagnostic importance (Fig. 24–17).

The cytologic evidence of cancer is often scanty. More often than not, careful screening is required. Cell blocks of sediment remaining after preparation of smears are occasionally useful in the diagnosis of cases in which the smears were inadequate for definitive conclusions.

OTHER CANCERS OF THE ESOPHAGUS

Adenocarcinoma and Mucoepidermoid Carcinoma. These tumors occur most often in the lowest portion of the esophagus.

Adenocarcinomas of the esophagus usually resemble gastric adenocarcinomas (see p. 1044 for further discussion). Occasionally, however, papillary adenocarcinomas composed of large, columnar cancer cells, may be observed (Fig. 24–18). These uncommon cases may be related to Barrett's esophagus, wherein precancerous lesions of a similar histologic and cytologic type have been observed (Belladonna et al., 1974). For further discussion of Barrett's esophagus, see p. 1020.

Of interest is the presence of pagetoid change that has been observed in the esophageal epithelium adjacent to areas of carcinoma (Fig. 24–19).

(text continues on page 1034)

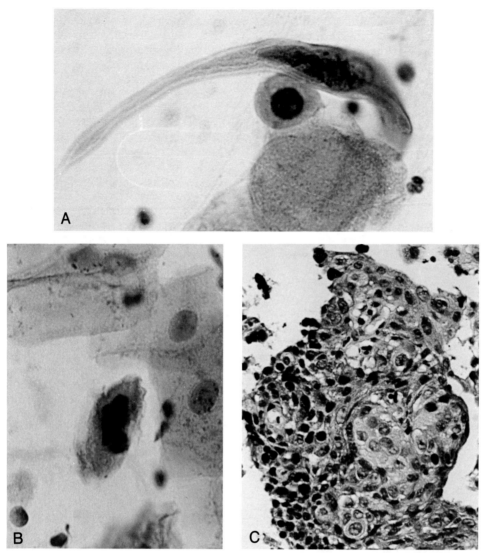

FIGURE 24-13.   Occult carcinoma of the esophagus discovered by balloon technique in a patient with past history of laryngeal carcinoma, successfully treated by radiotherapy nearly 5 years before this episode. (*A, B*) Squamous cancer cells; (*C*) esophageal biopsy section: fragment of squamous carcinoma, presumably still in situ. (*A* ×1,120; *B* ×800; *C* ×350. Greenebaum E., et al.: Use of esophageal balloon in the diagnosis of carcinoma of the head, neck, and upper intestinal tract. Acta Cytol., *28*:9–15, 1984)

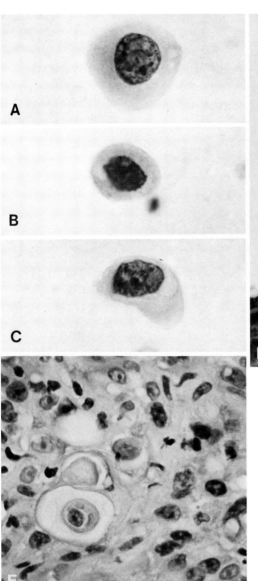

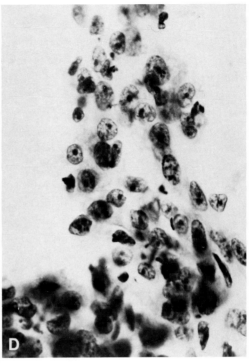

FIGURE 24–14. Keratinizing (squamous) carcinoma of esophagus. Comparison of esophageal washing, brush specimen, and biopsy section. (*A, B, C*) Esophageal washing. Classic cells of keratinizing squamous carcinoma. (*D*) Esophageal brush specimen: cancer cells removed from deep portions of the growing tumor do not have the cytoplasmic or nuclear characteristics of squamous cancer and are characterized by prominent nucleoli and scanty cytoplasm. (*E*) Biopsy specimen of tumor showing focal keratin formation and small cancer cells. (*A, B, C* ×1,000; *D, E* ×560)

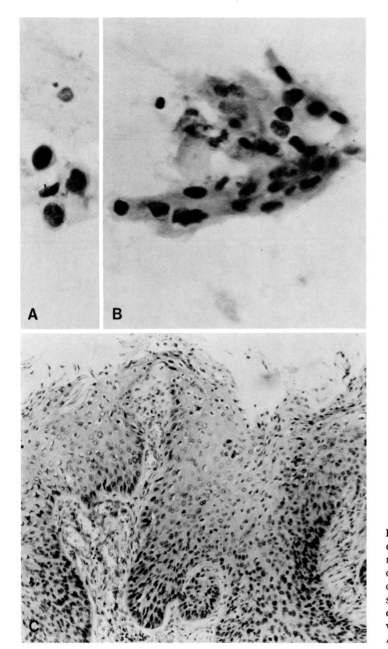

FIGURE 24–15. Epidermoid carcinoma of esophagus. The cells (*A, B*) show hyperchromatic, irregular nuclei. On gross inspection of the mucosa of the surgical specimen no obvious lesion could be found. Histologic sections (*C*) revealed invasive cancer of esophagus originating from an extensive, well-differentiated carcinoma in situ. (*A, B* ×560; *C* ×150)

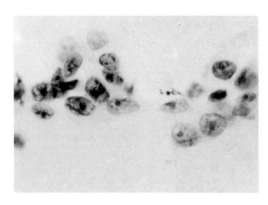

FIGURE 24–16. Cells from an anaplastic epidermoid carcinoma of esophagus (esophageal washings). Note prominent nucleoli. (×560)

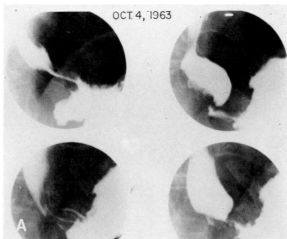

FIGURE 24–17. Epidermoid carcinoma of lower end of esophagus in a 67-year-old woman with dysphagia. Primary diagnosis by cytology. (*A*) Radiographic appearance of the lower end of esophagus reported as showing slight abnormalities, possibly due to a hiatus hernia, but no evidence of cancer. (*B*) Gastric washing. Clusters of malignant cells suggestive of epidermoid carcinoma. (*C*) Histologic section of surgically removed lower esophagus and adjacent stomach, showing epidermoid carcinoma invading gastric mucosa. (*D*) Carcinoma in situ in adjacent esophagus. (*B* ×560; *C, D* ×150)

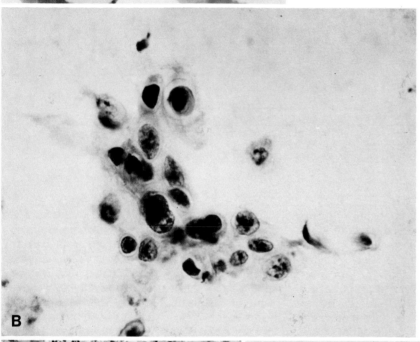

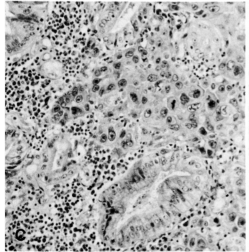

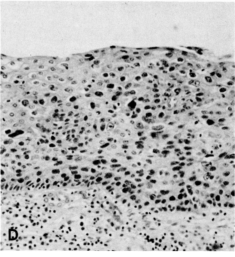

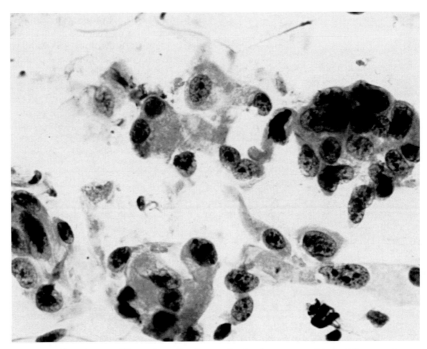

FIGURE 24-18.   Papillary adenocarcinoma in the lower one-third of the esophagus in a 28-year-old man. Note the columnar cancer cells with granular, hyperchromatic nuclei and prominent, sometimes multiple, nucleoli. A rounded "papillary" cluster of cancer cells may be noted. The tumor was large and destructive of the esophagus, hence, the origin of this tumor in Barrett's esophagus could not be confirmed. (×560)

The invasion of the squamous epithelium by cells of adjacent carcinoma resulted in this readily identifiable histologic pattern, similar to that occurring in the epithelium of the nipple in Paget's disease (cf. p. 1226). In the case illustrated here, the cancer cells shed from the pagetoid area were round and occasionally arranged in the cell-in-cell pattern (see Fig. 24-19B), whereas the cells from the main bulk of the tumor were poorly differentiated (see Fig. 24-19A). This observation appears to be unique (Yates and Koss).

As frequently happens in areas of the body where two different types of mucosa meet, tumors that may have the properties of glandular and squamous epithelium may occur in the lower esophagus. These cancers may be best classified as mucoepidermoid. There is no evidence that their behavior is in any way different from the behavior of pure epidermoid or pure mucus-producing varieties of cancer.

Melanoma.   One of these very infrequent tumors of the esophagus was diagnosed cytologically as cancer, but, in the absence of pigment, it was thought to be an epidermoid carcinoma. Several additional case reports of primary esophageal melanoma appeared within recent years (Basque et al.; Bullock et al.; Chaput et al.), occasionally associated with melanosis (De la Pava et al.; Piccone et al.). Recent summaries of the subject were presented by Mills and Cooper (1983) and by Kanavaros et al. (1989). Broderick et al. reported a case of esophageal melanoma with cytologic diagnosis. The malignant cells were clearly pigmented and, accordingly, the accurate diagnosis could be readily established. A similar case was reported by Aldovini et al. (1983).

CYTOLOGY IN DETERMINATION OF THE SPREAD OF ESOPHAGEAL EPIDERMOID CANCER TO THE RESPIRATORY TRACT

On numerous occasions attempts have been made to determine preoperatively, by aspiration of the tracheobronchial tree, whether or not cancer of the esophagus had invaded the respiratory tract. These attempts failed in my experience. Thus, in several cases, the washings of the trachea were positive in the absence of a tumor anatomically, and

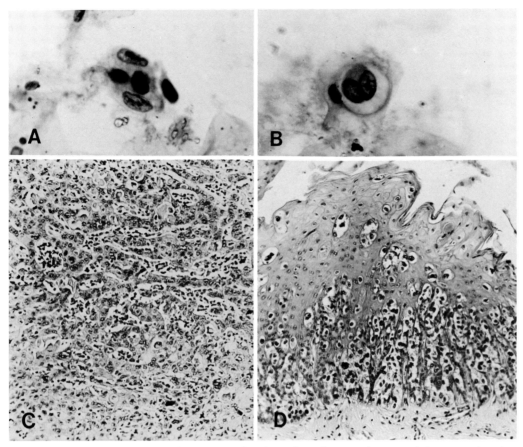

FIGURE 24–19. Carcinoma at the junction of cardia and esophagus with pagetoid changes in the adjacent esophageal epithelium. (*A*) Cluster of poorly differentiated cancer cells (esophageal washings). (*B*) Elsewhere in the smear isolated, large cancer cells with clear cytoplasm were noted. (*C*) The surgical specimen disclosed a carcinoma of the cardia extending into the esophagus. (*D*) The squamous epithelium of esophagus at the edge of the tumor disclosed a typical pagetoid change with large cells with clear cytoplasm. (*A, B* ×560; *C, D* ×150)

vice versa, the washings were occasionally negative in the presence of tumor spread eventually proved by biopsy. The cancer cells from the esophagus may undoubtedly be regurgitated, reach the trachea, and be aspirated by the bronchoscope. The decision on the operability of an esophageal cancer can gain no support from cytology.

CYTOLOGY IN THE FOLLOW-UP STUDY OF PATIENTS WITH ESOPHAGEAL CANCER TREATED BY RADIOTHERAPY OR CHEMOTHERAPY

The customary treatment of invasive carcinoma of the esophagus is either by radiotherapy alone or by radiotherapy followed by an attempt at surgical removal of the lesion. In several cases so treated, the observation has been made that, in spite of the remarkable clinical improvement following radiotherapy, the smears remained positive. In several of the surgically removed esophagi, there was disappearance of much of the invasive tumor, but areas of carcinoma in situ were not affected by therapy. This situation is reminiscent of the results of radiation treatment of carcinoma of the bladder, discussed on page 992.

Radiation changes observed in esophageal cytologic material are closely similar to those described for the uterine cervix (see p. 666) and the respiratory tract (see p. 749). The changes may affect both benign and malignant cells (Cabré-Fiol). The diagnosis of persisting or residual carcinoma should be made only on cells showing no significant alterations from radiation.

Radiomimetic changes in esophageal epithe-

Table 24–1
Results of Cytologic Examination of the Esophagus

	Total Cases	Cytology		
		Pos.	Susp.	Neg. or Insuff.
Malignant tumors primary in esophagus	148 (100%)	103 (70%)	18	27
No malignant tumor	135	3*	7	125

*Three cases of esophagitis. See discussion on page 1020.
(Johnson, W.D., et al.: Cytology of esophageal washings, evaluation of 364 cases. Cancer, 8:951–957, 1955)

lium were described by O'Morchoe et al. (1983) in patients receiving cytotoxic drug therapy. Some of these patients also had herpetic esophagitis and infections with fungi of the *Candida* species.

EFFECTIVENESS OF CYTOLOGY IN THE DIAGNOSIS OF ESOPHAGEAL CANCER

The effectiveness of balloon cytology in the detection of precancerous lesions of the esophagus has been documented in the studies from the People's Republic of China, cited on page 1026.

The contributions of cytology in symptomatic patients are best assessed by comparison with other diagnostic techniques: a few cases of esophageal carcinoma with negative radiographic findings were observed in this laboratory (cf. Fig. 24–17). Raskin et al. (1959) reported their results from 69 patients with carcinoma of the esophagus. Radiographic examination was suggestive or diagnostic of cancer in 55 cases, whereas cytology was positive in 66 cases (95%). Although this may represent an exceptionally high level of accomplishment obtained by a team of unsurpassed skill, the results were no less interesting when reported from my laboratory and Papanicolaou's laboratory by Johnson et al. in 1955. The cytologic results in 148 cases of esophageal cancer and 135 controls are outlined in Tables 24–1 and 24–2.

In a significant percentage of cases (12%), cytology yielded positive results, whereas the biopsy was either negative or impossible to obtain. This result alone fully justifies the use of cytology in investigation of patients with possible or probable cancers of the esophagus.

Other studies (Prolla and Kirsner; Cabré-Fiol) also show a very high rate of accuracy in the diagnosis of esophageal carcinoma, between 90% and 95%. Summary of more recent findings was compiled by Drake (1985). It is of interest that the introduction of fiberoptics and of direct brushing resulted in only slight improvement in the accu-

racy of cytologic diagnoses of esophageal cancer, when compared with the simpler methods of washings and aspirations. This is in marked contrast with results in gastric cytology, which were greatly improved with the introduction of the new instruments.

THE STOMACH

Anatomy

The stomach is a pouch situated between the esophagus and the duodenum, immediately below the diaphragm; it forms a reservoir of variable capacity within which the preliminary stages of digestion take place. The stomach is divided anatomically into several regions: the cardia (the orifice between the stomach and the esophagus and the adjacent area of stomach), the fundus, the body, and the pyloric area. The pyloric area is separated from the duodenum by a powerful ring of smooth muscle, the pylorus. Obstruction of the gastric

Table 24–2
Comparison of Results of Cytologic Examination With Results of Biopsy in 148 Primary Cancers of Esophagus

	Total Cases	Cytology		
		Pos.	Susp.	Neg.
Biopsy				
Positive	117	85	14	18
Negative	18	11	2	5
Impossible to obtain	13	7	2	4
	148			

(Johnson, W. D., et al.: Cytology of esophageal washings; evaluation of 364 cases. Cancer, 8: 951–957, 1955)

lumen may occur at both ends of the stomach—the cardia and the pylorus (see Fig. 24-1).

Histology of Gastric Mucosa

The gastric mucosa is composed of simple tubular glands. The lining of the glands of the fundus and the body of the stomach is complex: the surface and the necks of the glands are lined by mucus-producing cells. The deeper portions of the glands contain pepsin-producing chief cells and the eosinophilic parietal cells that produce hydrochloric acid (Fig. 24-20A). The hydrochloric acid is excreted through microscopic canaliculi passing between the chief cells. The gastric glands of the pyloric area are fairly uniformly lined by mucus-producing cells (see Fig. 24-20B).

Electron microscopic studies revealed distinct differences between the cells lining the gastric surface and those lining the neck of the glands. Both cells are mucus-producing, but they differ in the type of secretory granules, thus probably performing somewhat different functions. The ultrastructure of the parietal cell fails to reveal any secretory activity. Accordingly, the Golgi complex is small. The pepsin-producing chief cells resemble somewhat the exocrine pancreatic and salivary gland cells (cf. Fig. 1-17) inasmuch as they contain secretory granules and an abundant rough-surfaced reticulum. Argentaffin cells containing dense cytoplasmic granules may be observed in some of the crypts.

Cytology of the Normal Stomach

The makeup of the specimens varies according to the method used to collect the material. In brush specimens, cohesive fragments of epithelium are usually observed. If the fixation is not optimal, the cellular details are often deficient. On close inspection, uniformity and small size of the nuclei in the component cells may be recognized. In specimens that are better fixed, the appearance of the epithelial fragments is the same as in lavage specimens.

Gastric epithelium is scanty in lavage specimens obtained from stomachs showing no evidence of disease. The most common presentation of normal gastric epithelium in well-preserved cytologic specimens is in clusters of mucus-producing columnar cells (Fig. 24-21A), originating from the gastric surface. The centers of the clusters display the characteristic honeycomb appearance of central cells. The peripheral cells are flattened on one side, corresponding to the flat surface of the gastric lining. The relatively uncommon single cells display an abundant cytoplasm and have one flattened surface, whereas the opposite end usually tapers off in the form of a tail. Although the cytoplasm is rich in mucus, the nuclei assume a position closer to the center of the cell than is the case with goblet cells.

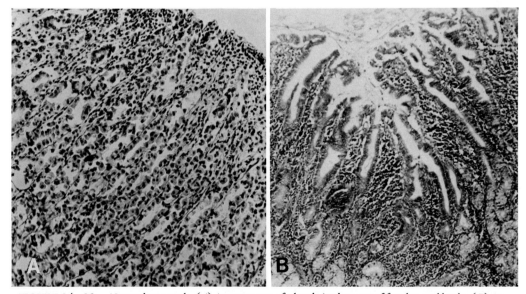

FIGURE 24-20. Normal stomach. (*A*) Appearance of glands in the area of fundus and body. (*B*) Appearance of glands at the pylorus. (*A, B* ×75)

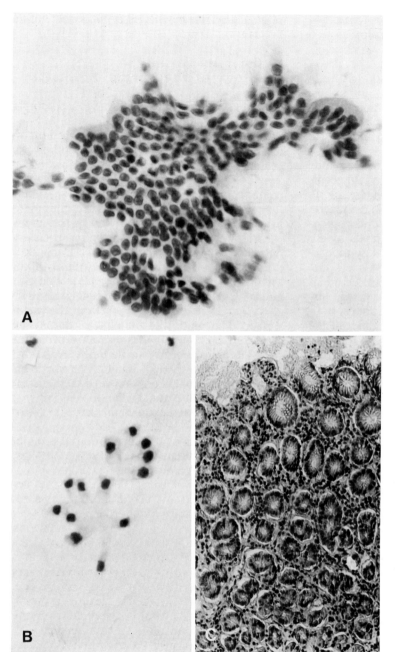

FIGURE 24–21. Gastric epithelium in smears and cell block (gastric washings). (*A*) Typical cluster of benign superficial gastric epithelial cells. Note the even size of the small nuclei. The "honeycomb" appearance of the central portion of the cluster may be contrasted with the peripheral columnar cells forming the flat surface of gastric lining. (*B*) Gastric cells display the not uncommon "wheel-spokes" arrangement. (*C*) Fragment of gastric mucosa observed in a cell block preparation. (*A, B* ×560; *C* ×150)

The nucleus is usually round, somewhat opaque, and contains a few granules of chromatin and occasionally a noticeable, very small pink nucleolus. A "wheel-spokes" arrangement of single cells, their "tails" toward the center (see Fig. 24–21*B*), may be observed. Occasionally, the cytoplasm of the gastric cells is destroyed in the processing of specimens, and "naked" nuclei or nuclei surrounded by cytoplasmic shreds may be quite abundant. In cell blocks, small fragments of gastric epithelium may be identified occasionally (see Fig. 24–21*C*). Raskin et al. (1961) pointed out that the cells from the area of the pyloric antrum have a more abundant cytoplasm containing droplets of mucus. The nucleus in such cells may be displaced toward the narrow, distal end of the cell.

In our experience, using rapidly fixed material and Papanicolaou stain, we have not been able to identify with certainty the parietal and the zymogenic (chief) cells in the smears of gastric specimens. However, Henning and Witte, using air-dried specimens and Pappenheim stain, demonstrated these cells very nicely; chief cells were described as plump and containing numerous coarse basophilic granules in the cytoplasm; the parietal cells were described as small cylindrical cells with a very marked vacuolization of the cytoplasm.

Nieburgs and Glass, using a gastric brush, identified chief cells as "darkly stained cells of intermediate size." Granules were not demonstrated in Papanicolaou stain. The parietal cells were identified by the same authors as "large, pale, round or triangular cells," and thus their description is at variance with that given by Henning and Witte, but more in keeping with the histologic appearance of these cells. Takeda (1983) also described the parietal cells as triangular cells with granular cytoplasm.

In gastric specimens obtained by aspiration or washings, swallowed cells of the respiratory and the upper alimentary tract are often present. Ciliated respiratory cells, dust-containing macrophages, and squamous cells of buccal and esophageal origin are represented. Also, food particles and, in particular, plant (vegetable) cells may contaminate the specimen, occasionally rendering it totally useless (see Chap. 19 for detailed description).

Other cells present in gastric specimens include polymorphonuclear leukocytes and lymphocytes in varying numbers. Recognizable macrophages may be noted. The parasite *Giardia lamblia* may occasionally be observed (Fig. 24–22).

Previously rarely identified, *Giardia lamblia* has now been recognized as a rather common cause of gastrointestinal disturbances. Bloch et al. (1987) observed the parasite in the peritoneal fluid of a patient with severe infestation. Trophozoites

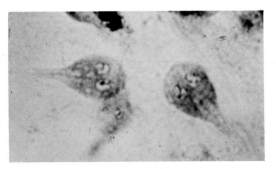

FIGURE 24–22. *Giardia lamblia* in gastric washings. Note the characteristic two nuclei. (Courtesy of Dr. Elizabeth McGrew, Chicago, Illinois)

of the *Acanthamoeba* species, probably a contaminant, were observed by Hoffler and Rubel.

Inflammatory Disorders

Gastric Ulcer and Acute Gastrites (Type B Gastritis)

Until a few years ago the causes of acute gastritis and of gastric or duodenal ulcer were not clearly understood. In 1983, an anonymous observation was reported in the journal *Lancet,* suggesting that a not-further-identified bacterium may be associated with gastritis. The bacterium, now known as *Helicobacter pylori* (previously known as *Campylobacter pylori*), has now been shown to be closely associated with acute gastritis and gastric ulcer (Goodwin et al., 1986; Blaser, 1987). In asymptomatic persons the bacterium is also associated with clinically occult gastritis (Dooley et al., 1989). The bacterium is a gram-negative spiral or curved bacillus that can be cultured and identified in tissue and in cytologic samples by silver or Giemsa stains (Taylor et al., 1987). The bacterium is fairly common, but it is now thought that it may be the cause of acute gastritis (also known as pyloric or type B gastritis), ulcer disease, and colitis. The precise mechanisms of interaction of the bacterium with gastric epithelium are not yet known.

Gastric ulcerations are the prime target of endoscopic and cytologic studies. When these lesions are small and superficial, the clinical and radiographic differential diagnosis between a gastric carcinoma and a chronic peptic ulcer may be extremely difficult (Cantrell; Prolla et al., 1971; Prolla and Kistner, 1972.) Histologic findings in chronic peptic ulcers show an inflammatory defect in the gastric epithelium extending for a variable depth into the submucosa. Occasionally, the ulcer may penetrate into the muscularis and beyond. Depending on the chronicity of the disease, the tissues surrounding the ulcer bed may show varying degrees of chronic inflammation and fibrosis. Occasionally, large aggregates of lymphocytes and plasma cells may be noted. The epithelium surrounding the ulcer shows various degrees of hyperplasia and regeneration. In the latter case, marked mitotic activity and atypia may be present (Fig. 24–23*A*). There is considerable debate over whether gastric carcinoma can originate in such atypical epithelium. Cases do occur wherein this possibility is strongly suggested by histologic findings. In view of these complex histologic data, it is not surprising that the interpretation of cytologic findings may be occasionally extremely difficult.

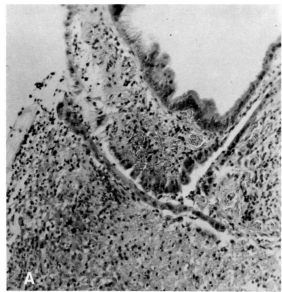

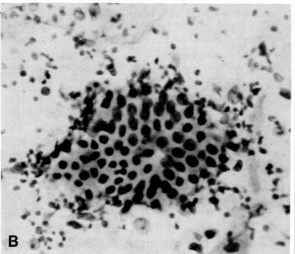

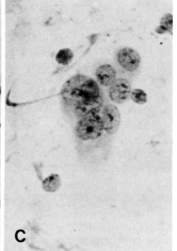

FIGURE 24–23.   (*A*) Tissue pattern from the edge of gastric peptic ulcer (same case as that in *C*) showing reactive proliferation and atypia of gastric epithelium. (*B, C*) Cluster of gastric epithelial cells from two cases of gastric peptic ulcer (gastric washings). (*B*) Cluster displays some measure of variation in nuclear sizes, but is still comparable with the cluster of gastric cells in the absence of disease (cf. Fig. 24–21 *A*). Note the background of necrosis and inflammation. (*C*) Nuclear enlargement and granularity is noted in this cluster. Also, "naked nuclei" of gastric cells are seen. Note enlarged nucleoli and the regular nuclear membrane. Compare with the jagged edges of nuclei of cancer cells (see Fig. 24–29B). (*A* ×150; *B, C* ×560)

Gastric cytology and the endoscopic biopsy are the prime methods of differential diagnosis between benign ulcer and carcinoma. The cytologic sample may be obtained by gastric lavage with a gastric tube, or it may be obtained during the gastroscopic procedure with a fiberoptic instrument either by direct washing or by a gastric brush. Regardless of the technique used, the specimens are usually cellular and contain many clusters of gastric epithelial cells. Necrotic material and inflammatory cells are usually present in the background, although their proportion varies from one specimen to another.

In peptic ulceration and the acute or subacute gastritis that usually accompanies it, the changes in the gastric epithelial cells are important to identify. It may be stated in general terms that in inflammatory gastric disease *the cells desquamate in clusters, single cells are few, and usually show only inconspicuous abnormalities*. The cell clusters are usually flat, the cells are arranged side by side without being superimposed (see Fig. 24–23B). Admittedly, in brush specimens, this important relationship of cells to each other cannot always be fully appreciated because the cell clusters may be thick and unfit for detailed visual analysis. Such clusters are best disregarded for purposes of diagnosis.

It has been repeatedly stated in the writings on this subject that in inflammatory gastric disease the nuclei of gastric epithelial cells are enlarged. This is generally not true, and most nuclei are of normal size (see Fig. 24–23*B*). However, occasional nuclei may be enlarged, as shown in Figure 24–23*C*. On the other hand, the gastric epithelial cells in inflammatory disease may be polyhedral rather than columnar in configuration, and their overall size may be somewhat smaller than that of normal cells. This may suggest nuclear enlargement because of a change in the nucleocytoplasmic ratio. Drake (1985) stressed nuclear enlargement as a common feature of epithelial cells in chronic gastric ulcer. In my view, however, this observation pertains to only some of the cells.

The nuclear changes may range from slight to conspicuous. Slight changes consist of the presence of small, single or double nucleoli in a finely granular background. More conspicuous changes consist of enlarged nucleoli and some variability in nuclear sizes (see Fig. 24–23*C*). In rare instances, very large nucleoli and a measure of nuclear hyperchromasia may be observed. If this latter change is also present in isolated epithelial cells, the differential diagnosis between gastric carcinoma and inflammatory disease becomes exceedingly difficult, as in any type of "repair." Absence of significant variability in nuclear sizes and regular, smooth border speak in favor of inflammatory disease, but this criterion is not always helpful. Miyoke et al. (cited by Prolla et al., 1971) concluded that intranucleolar vacuolization occurs only in carcinoma cells, whereas the nucleoli in inflammatory lesions are compact. Unfortunately, electron microscopy is required to establish this point of differential diagnosis, which, therefore, is of little practical value. It must also be pointed out that occasional gastric carcinomas may shed cancer cells with only modest nuclear abnormalities, thus compounding the problem of differential diagnosis. In such, fortunately uncommon, cases, the degree of histologic abnormality in a biopsy may also present a diagnostic dilemma that is best solved by additional sampling and closer observation of the patient.

As a testimonial to the degree of epithelial fragility in inflammatory disease, cell debris and isolated ("naked") nuclei may be abundant within the inflammatory background or fibrin in smears. This feature is not at all helpful in the differential diagnosis from carcinoma. Diagnostic misinterpretation in extreme cases of inflammatory atypia occurs even among observers who combine clinical and laboratory experience and thus are best placed to avoid such mistakes. Prolla and Kistner cite 5 such mistakes among 2,196 patients with benign gastric disease (1.8%), and Foushee et al. observed suspicious cells in 17 of 509 patients with inflammatory gastric or duodenal disorders. Cell changes similar to those in chronic ulcer may occur in "aspirin gastritis."

Aspirin Gastritis. Some users of aspirin and similar analgesics are prone to erosions of gastric mucosa, with episodes of hematemesis. Patients with rheumatoid arthritis appear to be at significant risk, presumably because of long-term use of large doses of these drugs. In fortuitous biopsies of the gastric erosions, there is a partial loss of the surface epithelium and a marked disruption of the glandular pattern (Fig. 24–24*A*). The glands, particularly in the deeper portion of the epithelium, show very marked nuclear abnormalities, with enlargement, hyperchromasia, and mitotic activity, undoubtedly as a function of regeneration or "repair" (Fig. 24–24*B*).

Cell samples obtained by brushing may show conspicuous abnormalities (see Fig. 24–24*C*–*F*). The gastric epithelial cells may form clusters or strips wherein there is a variability of nuclear sizes and hyperchromasia of individual nuclei (see Fig. 24–24*C*). Some cells may contain large nucleoli. Such clusters naturally suggest a gastric carcinoma. The examination of dispersed single cells usually confirms the presence of nuclear abnormalities. The cells may be columnar or cuboidal in shape and contain somewhat hyperchromatic nuclei with visible nucleoli (see Fig. 24–24*D,E*). Perhaps the most disturbing cytologic finding is the presence of clusters of dark nuclei, stripped of cytoplasm (see Fig. 24–24*F*).

An accurate clinical history of analgesic intake may prevent the faulty diagnosis of gastric carcinoma. This is particularly important because, within a few weeks after discontinuation of analgesics, the gastric epithelium recovers (see Fig. 24–24*G*).

In a prior edition of this book (1979), this writer felt that the differential diagnosis of aspirin gastritis from carcinoma was not possible in the absence of history. This view may be somewhat modified today. Although cell clusters may strongly suggest a malignant tumor (see Fig. 24–24*C,F*), the abnormalities in the single cells, essential to confirm the diagnosis, do not quite measure up to cancer. The degree of nuclear changes and the size and variability of the nucleoli are less conspicuous than in cancer, but, admittedly, these may be personal perceptions, not easily duplicated.

Gastric Atypias in Hepatic Artery Infusion. Infusion chemotherapy for metastatic tumors in

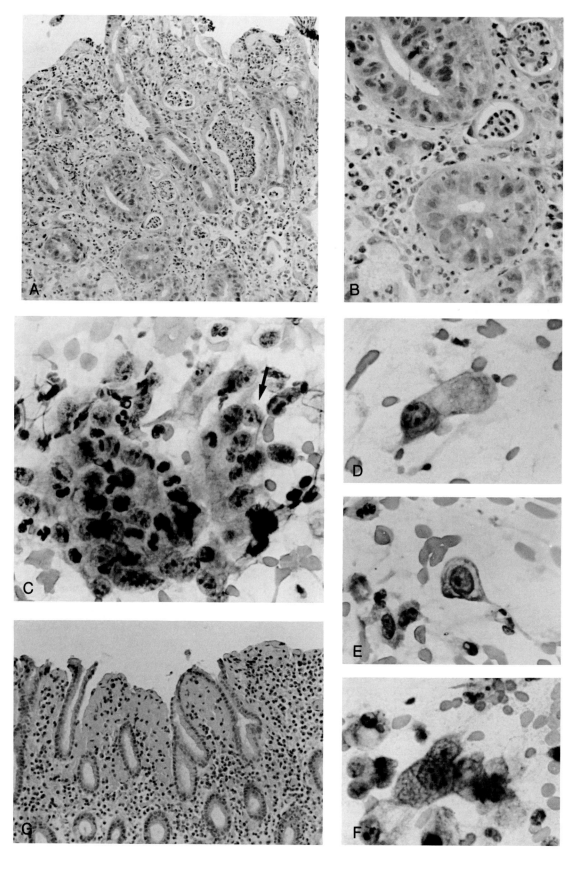

the liver affects gastric epithelium, causing a radiomimetic effect (Becker et al., 1986). Cell enlargement, with preservation of the normal nucleocytoplasmic ratio, binucleation, and multinucleation of gastric epithelial cells in gastric brushing material and biopsies, were reported in six patients with secondary gastric ulceration.

Chronic Gastritis (Type A Gastritis) and Intestinalization of the Gastric Mucosa

The replacement of normal gastric epithelium by cells akin to those of the mucus-producing epithelium lining the large intestine, is known as intestinal metaplasia or intestinalization (Fig. 24-25A). This may be observed in a variety of chronic inflammatory conditions and in pernicious anemia. Such changes usually affect the corpus of the stomach, but are uncommon in the pyloric region.

The intestinal metaplasia consists of mucus-producing cells, which are often referred to as goblet cells but are morphologically somewhat different (see below), and Paneth cells with granular and eosinophilic cytoplasm, which cannot be identified in cytologic material. Rubio and Antonioli (1988) reported rare cases of intestinal metaplasia with cilia.

The significance of intestinal metaplasia as a precancerous event has been studied morphologically (Morson, 1955) and by epidemiologic analysis of gastric cancer-prone populations (Correa, 1982; Rubio et al., 1987). The consensus has developed that, in populations with a high rate of intestinal metaplasia, there is also a high rate of gastric carcinoma of intestinal type (see below).

The condition may be recognized occasionally in cytologic material, which may contain columnar epithelial cells larger than the normal gastric cells and provided with an abundant, somewhat opaque, cytoplasm (see Fig. 24-25B). The nuclei are round and even, but are frequently larger than normal and dark. These cells are more slender than

the goblet cells, but closely resemble normal columnar cells desquamating from the colonic mucosa (cf. Fig. 24-48B).

Ménétrier's Disease. Ménétrier's disease is a disorder of gastric epithelium in which gastric rugae are markedly thickened ("hypertophic gastritis"). This disorder has no known cytologic counterpart but may be associated with gastric polyps and carcinoma (Appleman, 1984; Wood et al., 1983).

Gastric Syphilis. Ulcerative gastric lesions may occur in secondary and tertiary syphilis. Prolla et al. (1970) described the cytologic findings in two such cases. Atypical cells, presumably atypical macrophages or epithelioid cells with large nuclei and prominent nucleoli, were observed. Langhans' type giant cells were also noted.

Other Granulomatous Inflammatory Lesions of the Stomach. Markedly atypical giant cells were observed by Bennington et al. (1968) in a case of sarcoidosis. The cytologic findings in nonspecific granulomatous gastritis, Crohn's disease involving stomach, gastric tuberculosis, and sarcoid may be similar to those described for syphilis (Raskin et al., 1961). Drake (1985) described epithelioid cells and multinucleated giant cells in gastric brushings of a patient with Crohn's disease.

Malacoplakia of the stomach has been described (summary in Flint and Murad, 1984). Cytologic presentation of this rare disorder is discussed on p. 917.

Benign Gastric Polyps

Benign gastric polyps cannot be recognized cytologically unless small fragments of such tumors are present in the exfoliated material processed as a cell block. In this case, the interpretation is that of a

---

FIGURE 24-24. Aspirin gastritis in a 63-year-old woman with rheumatoid arthritis and daily intake of large doses of aspirin-containing analgesics. Gastric biopsies and brushings were obtained after an episode of hematemesis. (*A*) Low-power view of the original biopsy section showing marked inflammation, loss of surface epithelium (an erosion on gastroscopy), and a marked disruption of the glandular pattern. (*B*) Conspicuous abnormalities of deeper glands consisted of multilayered cuboidal epithelium, variability in nuclear sizes, nuclear hyperchromasia, and mitotic activity (last not shown), consistent with active regeneration. (*C*) A cluster (*left*) and a strip (*right*) of glandular epithelium with nuclear hyperchromasia. A cell with two prominent nucleoli is marked by an *arrow*. (*D, E*). Abnormalities of individual epithelial cells. Note the prominent nucleoli. (*F*) A cluster of "stripped" large, hyperchromatic nuclei. (*G*) Gastric biopsy specimen obtained 6 weeks after discontinuation of drugs shows a gastric epithelium nearly restored to normal: the gland pattern was nearly normal and parts of the surface epithelium have regrown. Chronic inflammation persisted. (*A, G* ×150; *B* ×350; *C-F* ×560)

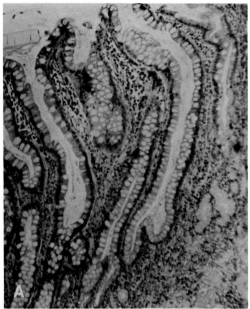

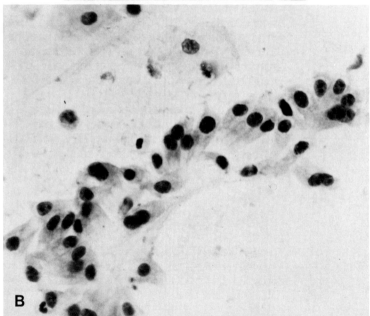

FIGURE 24-25. (A) Intestinalization of gastric mucosa. Note the replacement of gland lining by numerous mucus-producing cells. (*B*) A cluster of cells of gastric epithelium from a case of intestinalization of gastric mucosa (gastric washings). Note the large cell sizes, prominent nuclei and clear columnar cytoplasm. Note also that the cells differ from ordinary goblet cells. (*A* ×150; *B* ×560)

biopsy specimen. Occasionally, atypical (adenomatous) polyps may cause the same diagnostic problems as described for gastric ulcer. Polypoid carcinomas, on the other hand, have the same cytologic presentation as other forms of gastric cancer.

Carcinoma of the Stomach

Gastric carcinoma is exceedingly common in Japan, Korea, certain other areas in Asia, South America, and in Eastern Europe. Its incidence has been declining sharply in the Western world, also among people of Japanese ancestry living in Hawaii and the continental United States (Haenszel et al.). It is generally assumed that dietary factors are responsible, although the exact cause–effect relationship between nutrients and gastric cancer has not been successfully established.

Because of the interest in gastric carcinoma in Japan, a major national effort has been mounted to improve the dismal mortality statistics. This effort was remarkably successful and resulted in the development of new diagnostic approaches by fiber-optic gastroscopy associated with cytology and biopsies (Kasugi et al.). Discovery of gastric cancer in the early stage, notably as superficial carcinoma and as carcinoma in situ, has become the rule, rather than the exception, and the mortality statistics have been significantly improved. The techniques of gastric cancer diagnosis have now achieved worldwide dissemination.

Fiberoptic gastroscopy may be adapted to the collection of cytologic material by means of a directed jet wash or by means of a brush. In this fashion, direct sampling of visible mucosal abnormalities may be obtained.

In spite of this progress, the older and well-tolerated technique of gastric lavage still has its place as a means of gastric cancer detection in high-risk patients without any suspicion of malignant gastric disease, for example, in patients with pernicious anemia or those with minimal symptoms referrable to the upper gastrointestinal tract. This simple technique allowed Schade to lay down the principles of cytologic detection of early gastric cancer (summary in Schade, 1960).

Clinical Presentation and Classification

Gastric carcinomas most often assume the form of defects of gastric epithelium and thus mimic benign gastric ulcers. Polypoid or flat lesions may also occur. A form of gastric cancer with diffuse infiltration of gastric wall (leather bottle stomach) is well known. The gastroscopic appearance of early (superficial) gastric cancer is discussed below.

In 1965, Lauren classified gastric carcinomas into two groups: the *intestinal type* and the *diffuse type.* Lauren documented that the behavior, hence the prognosis, of the two types of tumor were different. The intestinal type of carcinoma is usually associated with intestinal metaplasia, which undergoes a transformation to an intramucosal carcinoma (carcinoma in situ), whence generally bulky, readily visible tumors are derived. Intestinal carcinomas are usually well-differentiated adenocarcinomas, composed of large, mucus-producing cells, and generally have a better prognosis. The less common diffuse type of gastric carcinoma (sometimes also called the *gastric type*) is derived from glandular crypts and is not accompanied by either intestinal metaplasia or intramucosal carcinoma. The diffuse type of gastric carcinoma is composed of small cancer cells (including the signet ring cell types) and tends to infiltrate the gastric wall early and deeply; hence, it usually appears as a flat or ulcerated lesion, with poor prognosis. A diagram in Fig. 24–26 summarizes these events.

The confirmatory evidence of this classification scheme was provided by Japanese investigators who studied small, early gastric cancers discovered as a part of the cancer detection effort. The genesis of the two types of cancer could be confirmed by these studies (summary in Takeda, 1983, 1984). There is other supporting evidence for this concept. In a study of distribution of H-*ras* oncogene product, protein p21 (see p. 79), it was documented by Czerniak et al. (1989) that, in the intestinal type of gastric cancer, the product was expressed in the areas of intestinal metaplasia and adjacent carcinoma in situ. In the diffuse type, the *ras* product expression was confined to morphologically normal mucosa, apparently the source of cancer (Fig. 24–27). Needless to say, there are cases of gastric cancer wherein both types of disease occur in the same stomach.

The concept of the two types of gastric cancer is not only of theoretical, but also of practical diagnostic and prognostic value and is reflected in histology and cytology of gastric carcinoma. Carcinomas of the intestinal type shed large, readily recognizable cancer cells, whereas carcinomas of the diffuse type are characterized by smaller, sometimes inconspicuous cancer cells. There are no differences in abnormal DNA values in these two tumor types (Czerniak et al., 1989).

Pilotti et al. (1977) tested this type of classification of gastric carcinoma by gastric cytology in 78 patients with considerable success. Takeda et al. (1981) also successfully tested this classification in 119 cases of early gastric carcinoma in gastric cytologic material.

Cytology of Invasive Gastric Carcinoma

In gastric lavage specimens, the background of smears often contains evidence of inflammation and necrosis that may obscure the cytologic features. Direct brush specimens, particularly if obtained from the surface of the lesion, may also contain a great deal of necrotic material. Perhaps the easiest to interpret are lavage specimens obtained by means of a jet of fluid under direct gastroscopic control.

In all types of gastric cancer the presence of single cancer cells with identifiable malignant features is an important diagnostic prerequisite.

Cytology of Gastric Adenocarcinoma of Intestinal Type

The intestinal-type tumors form distinct cancerous glands (Fig. 24–28E and see 24–30C) that are usually composed of large cancer cells of cuboidal or columnar configuration, often recognizable in

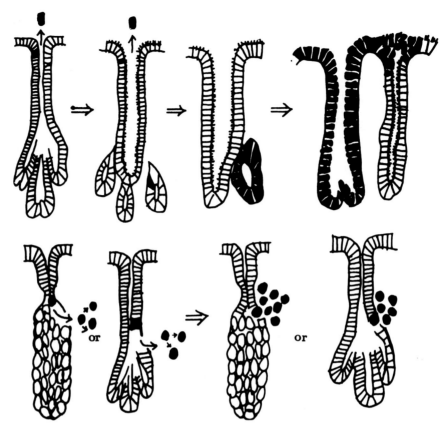

FIGURE 24 – 26. Diagrammatic representation of the events in the two types of gastric carcinoma, as suggested by Hattori and Fujita (cited by Takeda, 1984). *Top row*: Events in carcinoma of the intestinal type starting with a single cell transformation (*black cell*), the process involves gastric glands leading to an intramucosal carcinoma (carcinoma in situ), whence bulky, generally well-differentiated gastric cancers are derived. *Bottom row*: Events in carcinoma of diffuse type: the cancer cells, usually small and poorly differentiated (*black*) originate in glandular crypts and infiltrate the adjacent gastric wall without forming a carcinoma in situ. (Modified from Takeda, M.: Gastric cytology— recent developments. *In* Koss, L.G., and Colman, O.V. (eds.): Advances in Clinical Cytology, Vol. 2. pp. 49–65. New York, Masson, 1984, with permission)

smears. The fragile cytoplasm may be stripped or damaged, leaving behind the characteristic enlarged, pale or translucent nuclei with a prominent nuclear membrane that is often jagged or indented. Within the nuclei, there are single or multiple spherical or irregular, comma-shaped nucleoli (Figs. 24–28*C,D*, 24–29, and also see 24–35, 24–36). The size of the cancer cells may be variable, but extreme size differences are rare. The cancer cells are dispersed or form loosely structured, tridimensional clusters, sometimes of papillary configuration, which may be compared with tightly knit, honeycomb-type flat clusters of benign gastric cells, often observed in the same smears (see Fig.

24–28*A,B,C*). Cell clusters are more common in brush specimens than in lavage specimens. Nuclear hyperchromasia, or at least coarse granularity of the chromatin and opaque appearance of the nuclei, may be observed (see Fig. 24–29*A*), but this feature is not as dominant as nuclear enlargement, distorted nuclear contour, and abnormal nucleoli. Truly hyperchromatic cancer cells may be occasionally observed in gastric washings (Fig. 24–30), most likely representing dead cells removed from the surface of the tumor. Multinucleated giant cancer cells are uncommon.

The differential diagnosis of gastric adenocarcinoma is mainly with chronic peptic ulcer (see p.

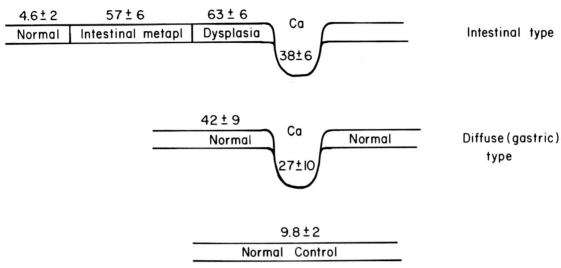

Semiquantitative Distribution of <u>ras</u> Oncogene p21 Protein
in Early Gastric Cancer and Adjacent Epithelium
(% of "positive" cells)

FIGURE 24–27. Differences in the distribution of *ras* oncogene product, protein p21, in two types of gastric cancer. It may be noted that the levels of expression of this protein are higher in the precancerous lesions surrounding the invasive carcinoma (Ca) than in the cancer itself, in keeping with the assumed role of p21 as a factor in the development of cancer. (Based on data from Czerniak, B., et al.: Cancer, *64*: 1467–1473, 1989)

1039) and regenerating gastric epithelium, as observed in aspirin gastritis (see p. 1041). In most instances, the abundance of the characteristic cancer cells in the cytologic specimen is sufficiently persuasive for the diagnosis of cancer to be made. If the evidence is scanty, however, the knowledge of clinical history and roentgenologic findings is of significant assistance in avoiding errors.

Cytology of Gastric Adenocarcinoma of Diffuse ("Gastric") Type

The diffuse-type adenocarcinomas are generally poorly differentiated tumors, composed either of small or medium-sized cancer cells without distinguishing morphologic characteristics, or of signet ring cancer cells, characterized by spherical cells with a large, mucus-containing cytoplasmic vacuole, pushing the nucleus to the side. Gland formation may occur, but it is usually an inconspicuous feature of these tumors.

In cytologic material, the cancer cells are generally smaller than in carcinoma of the intestinal type and rarely assume the columnar or cuboidal configuration. The nucleocytoplasmic ratio is usually high. Small clusters of cells, sometimes of oval or spherical (papillary) configuration may be observed (see Figs. 24–31, 24–33).

Signet ring-type cells are recognized by their large cytoplasmic vacuoles. Before making this diagnosis, it is important, however, to ascertain that the cell is malignant because of its nuclear characteristics: enlarged clear nuclei with irregularly shaped nuclear membrane and large, irregular nucleoli (Fig. 24–31) or large, hyperchromatic nuclei (Fig. 24–32*B*). Similarly structured benign cells without nuclear abnormalities may also occur.

Anaplastic carcinomas are characterized by densely packed clusters of small cancer cells, with very scanty cytoplasm and irregularly shaped, hyperchromatin nuclei (Fig. 24–33). Binucleated cells may occur (see Fig. 24–32*A*). Single cells of a similar type are invariably present. The configuration of cancer cells in such rare cases is reminiscent of an oat cell carcinoma (see p. 785) because of the small cell size and nuclear molding (see Fig. 24–33).

The differential diagnosis in tumors of this type

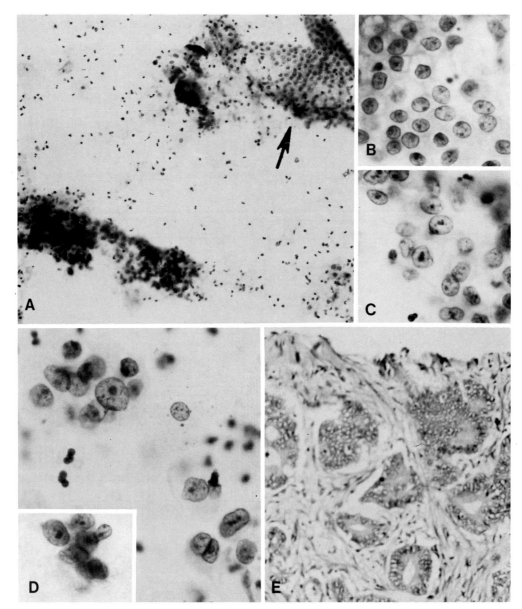

FIGURE 24–28. Gastric adenocarcinomas of intestinal type: brush specimens. (*A–C*) Superficial gastric carcinoma with metastases. (*A*) A low-power view of the smear with a flat cluster of benign gastric epithelial cells (*top, arrow*) and a thick, dense cluster of superimposed cancer cells (*bottom, left*). (*B*) A higher magnification of benign epithelial cells shows good adhesiveness and small, uniform monotonous nuclei, some with small chromocenters. (*C*) A higher magnification of cancer cells shows loose arrangement of the cluster, which is "falling apart." The individual nuclei vary in size and several show very large, irregular nucleoli. (*D, E*) Infiltrating gastric adenocarcinoma: (*D*) and *inset* show nuclear features of malignant cells, variability in sizes, and large nucleoli, corresponding to the tumor shown in (*E*). (*A, E* ×150; *B–D*, and *inset*, ×560)

also comprises chronic gastric ulcer and regenerative gastric epithelium (see above). In anaplastic carcinomas, metastatic (or swallowed) cells of bronchogenic oat cell carcinoma and a malignant lymphoma must be considered. Clustering and molding of cells, however, usually precludes the diagnosis of lymphoma (see p. 1058).

(text continues on page 1051)

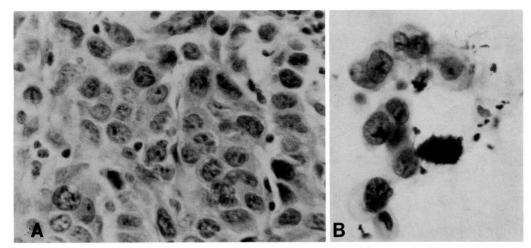

FIGURE 24–29. Case of gastric adenocarcinoma of intestinal type. (*A*) Focus of metastatic adenocarcinoma of the stomach to omentum. (*B*) Cancer cells from gastric washings. Note large size of cells and nuclear abnormalities. The lacy, faintly vacuolated cytoplasm is commonly observed in well-preserved cancer cells of this type. The dark object in the center of the photograph is a contaminant. (*A, B* ×560)

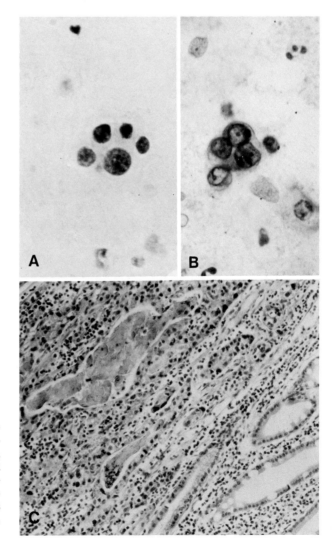

FIGURE 24–30. Gastric adenocarcinoma of intestinal type. (*A, B*) Gastric washings: cells of gastric adenocarcinoma. Note nuclear abnormalities and scanty, poorly preserved cytoplasm. (*C*) The tissue pattern in this case discloses a poorly differentiated adenocarcinoma partly replacing the gastric epithelium. A portion of benign gastric mucosa with intestinalization is shown in the *lower right corner* of the photograph. (*A, B* ×560: *C* ×150)

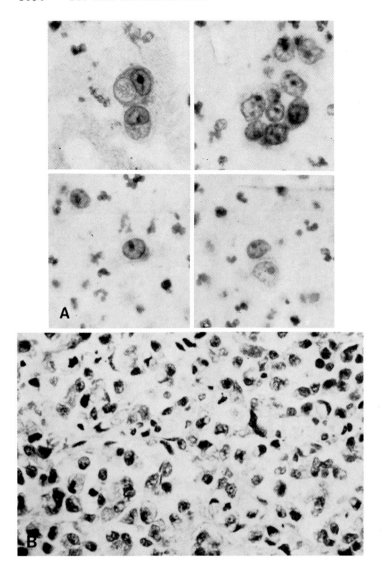

FIGURE 24–31. Gastric adenocarcinoma of diffuse type. (*A*) Composite picture of cells and cell clusters from gastric washings. Note irregular nuclear outline and large, irregular nucleoli. The cluster displays the papillary grouping of cells commonly observed in these tumors. The cells in the *top left* photograph are signet ring cancer cells, with a large, mucus-containing cytoplasmic vacuole, pushing the nucleus to the side. (*B*) Histologic section of the same tumor. Scattered signet ring cells may be observed. (*A* ×560; *B* ×350)

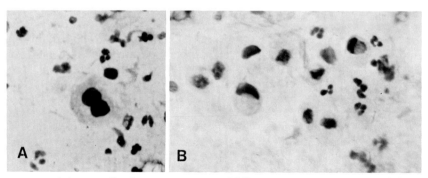

FIGURE 24–32. Cells of gastric carcinoma of diffuse type in gastric washings. (*A*) An example of a binucleated cancer cell. (*B*) Signet-ring cancer. Mucus pushes the hyperchromatic nucleus to one side. (*A, B* ×560)

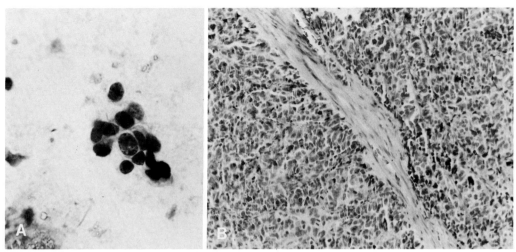

FIGURE 24–33. (*A*) Clutter of tumor cells from a highly anaplastic adenocarcinoma of the stomach of diffuse type. Note nuclear molding, the scanty cytoplasm, and the papillary arrangement of cells (gastric washings). (*B*) Tissue pattern from this case. The similarity to an "oat cell" carcinoma is striking. (*A* ×560; *B* ×150)

Mixed Types of Gastric Carcinomas

Rarely, the intestinal and diffuse type of gastric carcinoma may occur simultaneously. Pilotti et al. (1977) identified only 2 such cases in 78 patients with gastric cancer. The cytologic presentation combined the features of the intestinal and diffuse carcinomas.

Rare Types of Gastric Carcinoma

Epidermoid carcinoma or a mixture of epidermoid and adenocarcinoma (adenosquamous carcinoma) may occur in the area of the cardia and is similar to esophageal carcinoma of the same type (see Fig. 24–17). Keratin-forming, true squamous cancers can occur but are rare. In these latter cases, swallowed cancer cells from a tumor of the respiratory tract or esophagus must be considered in the differential diagnosis.

Rare malignant tumors comprising features of an adenocarcinoma and of a carcinoid have been recognized in cytologic material (Wheeless et al., 1984). Large, columnar cells of an adenocarcinoma and small, monotonous cells of a carcinoid (see Fig. 20–61) were observed side by side in the same gastric brush smear.

Gastric carcinomas have been observed in Ménétrier's disease (Wood et al., 1983, see also p. 1043). A rare instance of association of gas cysts of the stomach (pneumatosis cystoides intestinorum; summary in Koss, 1952), with gastric cancer was reported by Bhathal et al. (1985). The cysts are often lined by flattened, multinucleated giant cells of foreign body type. Such cells were observed in smears next to malignant cells.

Early Superficial Carcinoma

The extensive Japanese experience in the detection of early gastric cancer has led to the formulation of new concepts of this disease. Because of special anatomic features of the stomach, the term *carcinoma in situ* was replaced by the term *superficial or surface carcinoma*. It is well recognized that carcinoma confined to the gastric epithelium (true carcinoma in situ) does exist. However, even very superficial extension of these lesions into the submucosa may occasionally be associated with metastases to the regional lymph nodes. Hence, it is considered more prudent to speak of superficial carcinoma and to treat it accordingly.

Special attention has been paid in Japan to the endoscopic appearance of early (superficial) gastric carcinoma. The lesions have been divided into three principal types. Type I is a polypoid lesion, elevated above the normal level of the epithelium; type II, a flat lesion, either slightly elevated above the level of the epithelium or slightly depressed; type III is a superficially ulcerated lesion (Fig. 24–34). A combination of the three types is sometimes observed.

The type I and II abnormalities, by far the most common, usually reflect carcinomas of the intestinal type. Type III abnormality usually reflects a

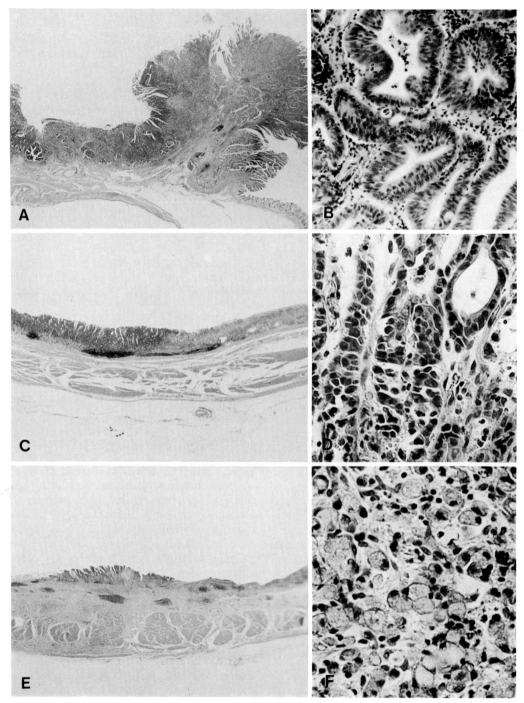

FIGURE 24–34. Superficial gastric carcinomas. (*A, B*) Type I, polypoid lesion; well-differentiated intestinal type of adenocarcinoma. (*C, D*) Type II, flat lesion; moderately well-differentiated adenocarcinoma of intestinal type. (*E, F*) Type III, ulcerated lesion; signet-ring carcinoma of diffuse type. (*A, C, E* approx. ×4; *B, D, F* approx. ×300. Cases courtesy of Prof. S. Shida, Dokkyo University, Mibu, Japan)

carcinoma of the diffuse type that may already be invasive at the time of discovery. This classification is helpful in the optical identification of small carcinoma, but has limited bearing on the rate of successful identification by cytology or by biopsies (Kobayashi et al.; Kasugai and Kobayashi).

The pioneering work in cytologic detection of superficial gastric carcinoma was done by Dr. R. O. K. Schade, formerly of Newcastle-on-Tyne. Schade applied gastric cytology in a systematic fashion to a group of patients with vague clinical complaints referable to the gastrointestinal tract. His method of obtaining cytologic specimens consisted of washing the stomach with saline on 3 consecutive days. Within 5 years (1954–1959), Schade was able to diagnose cytologically 41 cases of very superficially invasive or preinvasive cancer of the stomach, of which 16 were in entirely asymptomatic patients (Fig. 24–35). Pernicious anemia patients were the chief target of Schade's investigation, since they would seem to represent the group most susceptible to the development of gastric cancer. In common with early cancers of other organs, the cases of gastric carcinoma in situ examined by Schade shed cancer cells easily and in abundance. Extensive necrosis, so often complicating the problem of cytologic diagnosis of advanced and ulcerated gastric cancers, was virtually nonexistent.

The lesions observed by Schade were mainly of the intestinal type. The cancer cells were large, cuboidal, and contained large, somewhat hyperchromatic nuclei of variable sizes, with prominent multiple nucleoli (see Fig. 24–35A). The tissue abnormality disclosed a disorderly array of glands of irregular shape and variable sizes, lined by cancer cells (see Fig. 24–35B).

The work of Schade found a following primarily in Japan, where gastric carcinoma is a national scourge. There the lavage cytologic techniques were supplemented with fiberoptic gastroscopy and gastric camera, the latter permitting taking short sequences of color photographs of the gastric mucosa. Major pioneering work on gastric cancer detection by numerous investigators (for summary see Inokuchi; Yamada et al.; Kasugai and Kobayashi) resulted in the diagnosis of literally hundreds of cases of superficial gastric carcinoma. The accomplishments of the Japanese scientists have radically altered the outlook on the diagnosis and prognosis of gastric carcinoma. Thus Inokuchi reported on a long-term follow-up study of 82 treated patients with superficial gastric carcinoma diagnosed by the methods outlined above. There were only three recurrences, 9, 7, and 3 years after the original diagnosis. Two of those three patients were still alive after treatment for 11 and 14 years following the initial diagnosis. This represents a 5-year cure rate of over 90%, a figure that could not have been attained were it not for the painstaking work of gastric cancer detection. Muto et al. compared the survival rates for Japanese patients with gastric cancer for the years 1961 to 1965 and documented a statistically significant improvement of survival rates for the years 1963 to 1965, corresponding to the introduction of fibergastroscopy and cytology.

In a recent review of the Japanese experience (Yamazaki et al., 1989), the survival of 509 treated patients with early gastric cancer detected by radiologic techniques was close to 100%. By contrast, about one-half of 18 patients with this disorder, who were not treated for various reasons, died of gastric cancer after 5 years. The comparative survival of 350 patients with occult, but advanced, gastric cancer, treated by curative surgical resection, was 72% after 5 years and 65% after 10 years. On the other hand, all 127 patients with advanced cancer who, for various reasons, were not treated for cure, died within 3 years. This study clearly demonstrates the benefits of screening for gastric cancer, particularly the early stages of the disease.

It is still not clear how much time is required for the progression of untreated carcinoma in situ of gastric mucosa to invasive carcinoma. The progression is likely to be much slower in the intestinal than in the diffuse type of lesions. The evidence at hand strongly suggests, however, that superficial gastric cancers, particularly of the diffuse type, are potentially highly dangerous and must be treated.

Cytologic Observations in Superficial Gastric Cancers. Schade's observations, cited above, that cytologic preparations from superficial carcinomas are easier to interpret than similar preparations from advanced gastric cancers have received ample confirmation from Japanese sources and are also in keeping with personal experience. The specimens are usually free of extensive necrosis and debris and the cancer cells are well preserved (Figs. 24–35A, 24–36). The essential characteristics of gastric cancer cells described above are still applicable here. However, in well-differentiated, superficial gastric adenocarcinomas of intestinal type, the cells tend to form more compact clusters than in more advanced cancers. This is particularly evident in brush specimens. The nuclear and nucleolar abnormalities, particularly the latter, become, therefore, of paramount diagnostic significance. Superficial diffuse carcinomas of signet ring type

(text continues on page 1056)

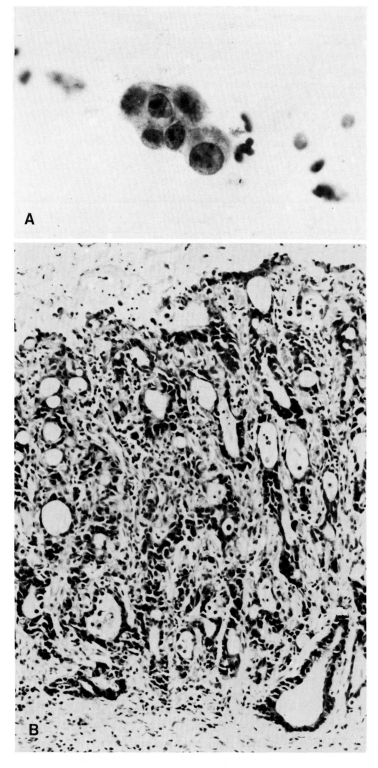

FIGURE 24–35. Cluster of cancer cells (*A*) and tissue section (*B*) from a case of asymptomatic carcinoma in situ of the stomach diagnosed by gastric washings. (*A* approx. ×600; *B* approx. ×300. Courtesy of Dr. R. O. K. Shade, Newcastle-upon-Tyne, England)

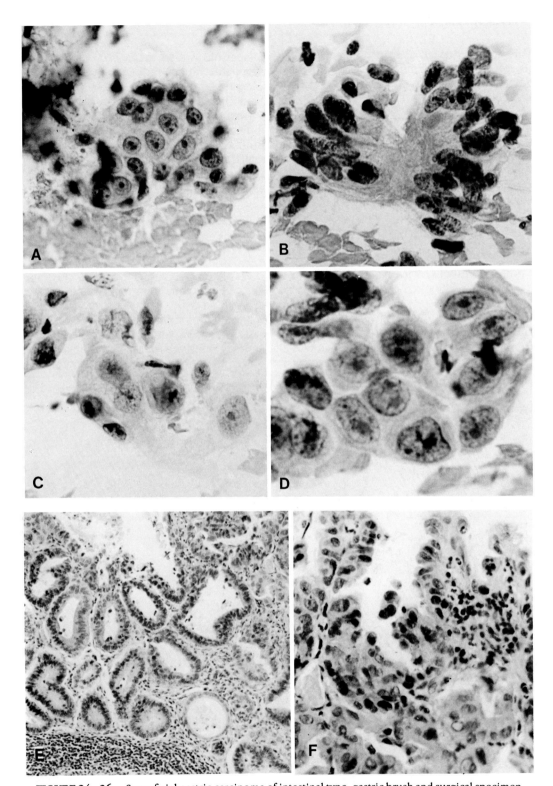

FIGURE 24–36. Superficial gastric carcinoma of intestinal type: gastric brush and surgical specimen. (*A, B*) Arrangement of cancer cells in cohesive clusters. In cluster *A* very large nucleoli may be observed. Cluster *B* shows a rosette-like arrangement of large cancer cells, with hyperchromatic nuclei. The cells are joined to each other by their cytoplasmic processes, with nuclei ranged at the periphery. (*C, D*) Details of nuclear structure of gastric cancer cells. Note coarse texture of nuclear chromatin and very large nucleoli of irregular configuration. (*E, F*) Low and high- power view of a well-differentiated carcinoma, confined to the gastric epithelium. (*A, B* ×560; *C, D* ×1,000; *E* ×150; *F* ×350. Case courtesy of Prof. S. Shida, Dokkyo University, Mibu, Japan)

also shed better preserved cancer cells in which the presence of mucus-containing vacuoles and the morphologic abnormalities of the eccentric nucleus are well evident.

Precancerous States

Borderline Lesions. Regardless of the diagnostic sophistication of the observer, gastric cytology occasionally poses major diagnostic dilemmas. The difficulties of differential diagnosis between gastric epithelium surrounding chronic gastric ulcers and aspirin gastritis have been discussed above (see pp. 1039 and 1041). Occasionally, however, in the absence of an ulcer, epithelial abnormalities may occur that are clearly on the border of cancerous changes. The exact clinical significance of such changes is not clearly understood, and the therapeutic dilemma is often resolved by surgical intervention that is dictated by prudence, rather than by biologic facts. The case recorded below is an illustration of such a dilemma. The patient, a 54-year-old white man, had vague abdominal complaints, but no radiographic lesion of note. Cytologic examination of a gastric specimen (Fig. 24–37) revealed numerous clusters of highly abnormal large cells with hyperchromatic nuclei and abnormal chromatin patterns. The histologic examination of the resected sleeve of the stomach revealed an atrophic gastritis with good preservation of the glandular pattern (Fig. 24–38*A*), but with significant nuclear abnormalities within the glands (Fig. 24–38*B*). Similar lesions were classified by others as "dysplasia" of gastric epithelium (Morson et al., 1980, Jass 1983). The lesions must be considered precursors of gastric cancer.

Pernicious Anemia as a Precancerous State. Pernicious anemia is often associated with atrophic gastritis. Therefore, gastric cancer is a well-known complication of this disease.

It is of special interest to note here that Schade denies the existence of any specific cytologic or histologic alterations of the gastric mucosa in perni-

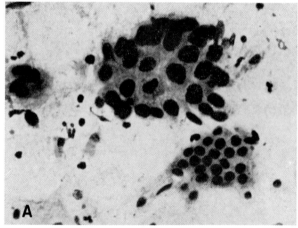

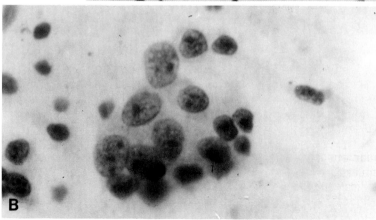

FIGURE 24–37. Cytologic abnormalities observed in a specimen of gastric washings (referred to in the text). (*A*) A cluster of small benign gastric cells (*bottom*) next to a cluster of significantly enlarged abnormal gastric cells. The latter display marked nuclear hyperchromasia and irregularity. (*B*) Note the very prominent large nucleoli, quite comparable with those seen in cancer. Compare this figure with the histologic pattern of gastric mucosa in this case (Fig. 24–38, *opposite*). (*A, B* ×560)

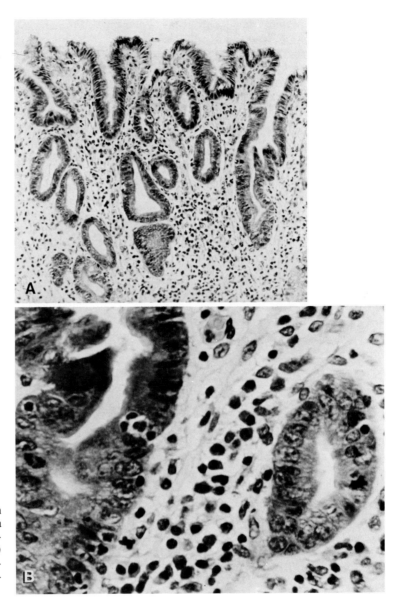

FIGURE 24-38. Tissue pattern from the case shown in Fig. 24-37 discloses a good preservation of glandular structure (*A*), but in high magnification (*B*) crowding of cells and nuclear abnormalities are really noted. There are also numerous mitoses. (*A* ×150; *B* ×560)

cious anemia. Intestinalization of gastric mucosa (or atrophic gastritis) is, in Schade's experience, a common background of cancers developing in the presence or the absence of the hematologic disorder (cf. Fig. 26-13). Graham and Rheault, Massey and Rubin and others have observed in patients with pernicious anemia gastric and squamous cells with abnormally enlarged nuclei, similar to dyskaryotic cells. Personal experience indicates that slightly atypical squamous cells with enlarged nuclei occur quite often in gastric washings. A hema-

tologic investigation of several such patients failed to reveal a relationship between these cell changes and a disease state. It is entirely possible that the intubation of the esophagus or, for that matter, a number of dietary deficiencies—such as vitamin B_{12} or folic acid deficiency—may account for these abnormalities. Takeda (1983) illustrated three clusters of enlarged, bland, empty-looking nuclei in gastric cells in pernicious anemia. Drake (1985) also speaks of "active" gastric cells, with visible nucleoli, in pernicious anemia. The specificity or, for that matter, diagnostic value, of such changes is in doubt (see also the discussion of this problem on p. 356).

Cytology in the Diagnosis of Recurrent Gastric Cancer

After partial gastectomy for gastric cancer, it may occasionally be possible to diagnose recurring tumor by means of gastric washings (Figs. 24–39). The matter is more often than not of theoretic value only, since in most such cases metastases are present. Offerhaus et al. (1984) observed that "dysplasia" of the residual gastric stump after resection for gastric carcinoma was a precursor lesion of recurrent gastric cancer. Unfortunately, the study did not include a cytologic component.

Gastric Sarcomas

Malignant Lymphomas and Pseudolymphomas

Classification of malignant lymphomas is discussed in Chapter 29. Nearly all gastric lymphomas are of non-Hodgkin's type. Hodgkin's disease may involve the gastric wall, by spreading from the gastric lymphnodes. Primary gastric Hodgkin's disease is very rare. Hodgkin's disease involving the

stomach may be observed occasionally in the exfoliated material. The few abnormal cells were clearly malignant and polyhedral, simulating an epithelial tumor (Fig. 24–40). The nuclei were hyperchromatic and occasionally double. Contrary to the experiences of Rubin and of Raskin, who observed Reed–Sternberg cells in gastric cytologic material, it has not been possible to establish the specific diagnosis of Hodgkin's disease in our experience.

Large-cell malignant lymphoma of various subtypes is the most frequent form of gastric lymphoma (Weingrad et al., 1982). The disease is intramural, but may be diagnosed cytologically if the mucosa is involved or if there is an ulcerative lesion. In the example shown in Fig. 24–41, medium-sized malignant cells with very scanty cytoplasm were observed in gastric brushings. The cells formed loosely structured clusters and occurred singly, as is characteristic of malignant lymphoma (see pp. 1057 and 1284). Large, prominent, often multiple nucleoli were noted within the granular nuclei. Other cytologic features of large-cell gastric malignant lymphoma are similar to those seen in effusions (see p. 1057). Thus, nuclear protrusions, nuclear cleavage (Fig. 24–42), and karyorrhexis may be observed. Lozowski and Hajdu (1984), in an exhaustive cytologic study of 29 cases of primary lymphomas of the gastrointestinal tract (in-

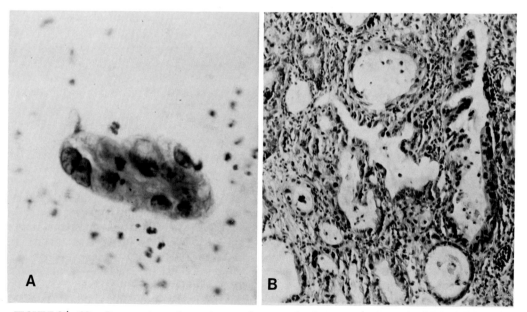

FIGURE 24–39. Recurrent gastric carcinoma after partial gastrectomy. The lesion, recurring in the region of the cardia, was first diagnosed by washings (*A*) and confirmed by a biopsy (*B*). (*A* ×560; *B* ×150)

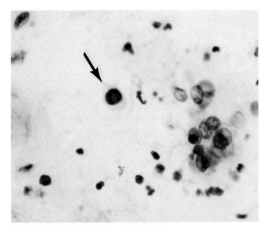

FIGURE 24–40. A single abnormal cell (*arrow*) from a case of Hodgkin's disease involving the stomach (gastric washings). Note the resemblance to an epithelial cancer cell. On the right-hand side of the photograph there is a cluster of degenerating gastric cells. (×560)

cluding 24 primary gastric lymphomas), stressed the presence of single cells in brush smears. In the more common, large-cell lymphoma, the nuclei were large (two to three times the size of normal lymphocytes) and there was some variability of nuclear sizes. Nuclear protrusions, indentations, and nucleoli were evident. Primary cytologic diagnosis was rendered in 5 of 24 gastric lymphomas, 1 of 2 lymphomas of small bowel, and all 3 colonic lymphomas.

The differential diagnosis of large-cell lymphoma is with small-cell anaplastic carcinoma. In the latter, cell clustering and molding is a dominant feature (see Fig. 24–33). Lack of tight cell clusters and the nuclear features described above are characteristic of malignant lymphoma.

Because of the presence of necrotic material and debris in ulcerated lesions, the diagnosis of lymphoma is difficult in gastric lavage (see Fig. 24–42). Brush specimens, however, usually show a nearly pure population of malignant cells with little debris (see Fig. 24–41).

The cytologic diagnosis of small-cell lymphosarcoma (well-differentiated lymphocytic lymphoma) is exceedingly difficult in my experience. On the one hand, the presence of lymphocytes is a common finding in the presence of chronic gastritis or gastric ulcer. On the other hand, the cellular and nuclear characteristics of the very small malignant cells are rarely sufficiently clear to establish this diagnosis. Furthermore, it must be noted that malignant lymphomas develop *beneath* the gastric epithelium, which must become ulcerated for the malignant cells to reach the gastric lumen. This explains the relatively poor experience with cytologic diagnosis of these lesions reported by Katz et al. On the other hand, Kline and Goldstein reported successful cytologic identification in nine of ten patients with this group of diseases. Prolla, Kobayashi, and Kirsner identified 30 such lesions in 46 patients.

A further diagnostic complication is the so-called *gastric pseudolymphoma.* In this presumably benign disease, large collections of lymphocytes may be observed in the gastric wall.

Through the courtesy of Dr. Misao Takeda from Jefferson Medical College in Philadelphia, I had the opportunity to study the gastric washings in one such case and found the differential diagnosis between a lymphosarcoma and a pseudolymphoma impossible to achieve (Fig. 24–43). The presence of nucleoli in the lymphocytes was particularly disturbing. Prolla and Kirsner apparently shared this experience. The presence of plasma cells, which Prolla and Kirsner considered in favor of pseudolymphoma, is not sufficiently characteristic to be relied upon in the differential diagnosis. Clinical data and radiographic or gastroscopic appearance, or even biopsies of the lesion are generally not helpful, and in the final analysis, the diagnosis is usually made on the gastrectomy specimen. However, the problems of differential diagnosis between a lymphoma and pseudolymphoma may also extend to the tissue. Fortunately, the pseudolymphoma is a very uncommon lesion.

In the presence of lymphoma, gastric epithelial cells may disclose considerable atypia, similar to that seen in peptic ulcers and probably caused by nonspecific ulcerative changes in the mucosa (see Fig. 24–43).

Leiomyosarcomas

Cabré-Fiol and his associates observed three cases of leiomyosarcoma in gastric brush specimens. They observed the characteristic elongated, spindle-shaped, malignant cells, sometimes with very long cytoplasm next to large malignant cells without distinguishing features. Similar cases were described by Qizilbash et al. (1980) and by Drake (1985). Prolla and Kirsner observed similar elongated malignant cells in bundles *after* gastric biopsies. It must be noted that leiomyosarcomas, as lymphosarcomas, develop beneath the gastric epithelium, which must become ulcerated before the cancer cells can reach the gastric lumen.

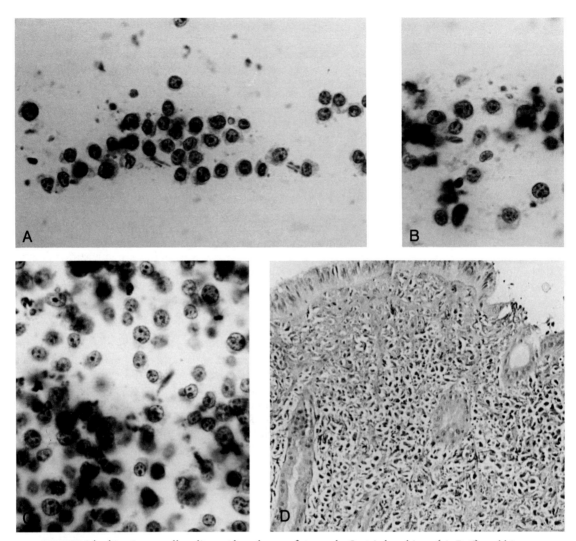

FIGURE 24–41. Large-cell malignant lymphoma of stomach. Gastric brushings (*A, B, C*) and histologic section of tumor (*D*). (*A*) The field shows very loosely structured cluster and dispersed malignant cells of monotonous sizes. The nuclei are large and are surrounded by a small rim of cytoplasm. (*B, C*) Higher-power view of the dispersed malignant cells. The spherical or oval nuclei are provided with one to three conspicuous nucleoli. An occasional nucleus is cleaved. The cytoplasm, if present, is scanty. (*D*) Histologic section of a gastric biopsy shows a large-cell lymphoma infiltrating the gastric wall. In this area the surface epithelium was intact. Elsewhere it was ulcerated. (*A* ×350; *B, C* ×560; *D* ×150)

Other Malignant Tumors Involving the Stomach

A case of primary gastric melanoma, with a contributory diagnosis by cytology, was reported by Reed et al. Pigmented malignant cells were observed. Undoubtedly, contribution of cytology to the diagnosis of other rare gastric neoplasms will be published from time to time. Contrary to primary gastric carcinoma and lymphoma, most of these malignant tumors are not, as a rule, accessible to cytologic sampling.

Metastatic tumors to the stomach may occasionally be diagnosed by gastric washings. Such was the case in a few instances of mammary carcinoma observed in this laboratory. It should be noted that patients with mammary carcinoma treated by steroids are prone to gastric metastases.

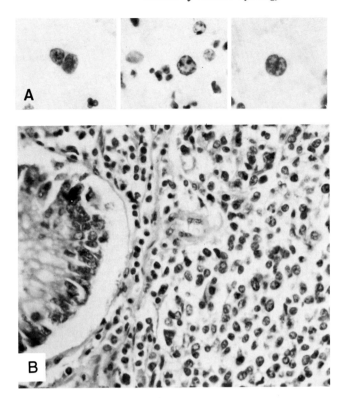

FIGURE 24–42. Large-cell malignant lymphoma in gastric lavage specimen. (*A*) Composite picture of scattered small malignant cell nuclei, with prominent nucleoli and, in one cell, nuclear cleavage (*right*). (*B*) Histologic section of the resected stomach showing tumor in the submucosa. (*A* ×560; *B* ×350)

Somewhat more frequently, *swallowed cancer cells* of esophageal, laryngeal, and pulmonary origin may be observed in gastric specimens (cf. p. 1051). This is an important potential source of diagnostic error that may result in an unnecessary laparotomy or even gastric resection.

RESULTS OF GASTRIC CYTOLOGY

Specialized laboratories report very high percentages of gastric cancers diagnosed by cytology. Some of the outstanding results are summarized in Table 24-3.

In the published series erroneous diagnoses of cancer were reported, varying from 0% to 4.3%. Personal work in gastric cytology was summarized by McNeer in Table 24–4.

Tables 24–3 and 24–4 do not adequately reflect the progress that has been made in the diagnosis of gastric diseases, both benign and malignant, since the introduction of fiberoptic instruments in the 1960s. The progress has been mainly in the discovery of early gastric carcinomas (superficial or surface lesions) that offer significantly better therapeutic options than more advanced gastric

cancer. A comparison of the routine lavage method and direct vision methods of cell collection was documented by early data published by Kasugai and Kobayashi (1974) (Table 24–5).

The same authors emphasize that the overall accuracy of direct vision biopsy in gastric cancer is 92.8%. With the use of multiple biopsies the diagnosis of *early* gastric cancer may be achieved in 98.3% of lesions.

Another, perhaps less tangible, advantage of these methods has been the reduction in the number and scope of radiographic examinations to which gastric cancer suspects have been previously exposed. The fiberoptic methods have now achieved worldwide dissemination and significantly enhanced the art of diagnosis of gastric cancer. Still, there is some controversy in reference to the value of brush cytology when compared with direct biopsy of gastric lesion. Thus, Cook et al. (1988) suggested that the brushings add very little to biopsies and are a source of "false-positive" errors. In Qizilbash's hands (1980) the brush specimen was positive in about 89% of the cases, the biopsy in 93%, and the combination of the two methods in over 95% of the cases. A more optimistic evaluation was offered by Gupta and Rogers

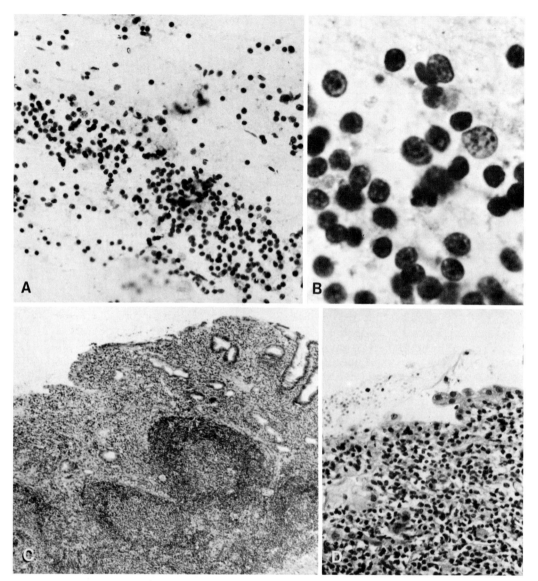

FIGURE 24–43. Gastric pseudolymphoma in a young woman, presenting as a bulky gastric lesion. There was no evidence of disease 5 years after surgical resection. Gastric lavage and surgical specimen. (*A*) Low-power view of gastric smear containing numerous lymphocytes in loosely arranged aggregates. (*B*) High-power view of the gastric smear. Numerous lymphocytes with multiple nucleoli of various sizes and follicle center cells with large, clear nuclei. (*C*) Low-power view of resected stomach showing large lymph follicles in the submucosa. The gastric epithelium is partly atrophic and focally ulcerated. (*D*) High-power view of ulcerated gastric epithelium with a dense lymphocytic infiltration of submucosa. Note atypia of epithelial cells. (*A* ×250; *B* ×1,000; *C* ×60; *D* ×250. Courtesy of Dr. Misao Takeda, Philadelphia, Pennsylvania)

(1983), who diagnosed, by brush cytology, 21 carcinomas that initially could not be documented by other means. The cost of this achievement was, however, 9 unproved, presumably false-positive cases.

In reviewing the accumulated data, it appears that the most important aspect of gastric cytology is the false-positive rate, the principal sources of error being regenerating gastric epithelium, as in chronic peptic ulcer or aspirin gastritis (see above).

Table 24-3
Gastric Cancers Diagnosed by Cytology

Author and Year	Number of Cancers Investigated	Positive Diagnoses (%)
Rubin et al., 1953, 1957	54	89
Seybolt and Papanicolaou, 1957	77	66
Raskin et al., 1961	152	88
Brandborg et al., 1961	103	90
Reece, et al., 1961	115	64
Yamada et al., 1964	147	81
Prolla and Kirsner, 1972	379	77
Cabré-Fiol, 1970	354	89

Table 24-4
Radiographic and Cytologic Contribution to the Diagnosis of 105 Consecutive Gastric Cancers Confirmed by Histologic Examination (Memorial Hospital for Cancer and Allied Diseases, 1959-1962)

	Number of Cases
Radiographic examination positive	92
Cytology positive in the absence of conclusive radiographic diagnosis*	13

*Radiographic examination was completely negative in four cases and inconclusive in nine cases. There were no erroneous cytologic diagnoses of cancer in this series.

The accuracy of the diagnoses obviously depends on quality of the specimens, their technical handling, and the competence and experience of the observer. The most important application of gastric cytology is the detection of early, occult cancers and, to some extent, in a differential diagnosis of space-occupying lesions. For clinically obvious cases of gastric cancer, brushing cytology adds comparatively little to other means of diagnosis.

THE DUODENUM, BILIARY, AND PANCREATIC DUCTS

Anatomy and Histology

The duodenum is the portion of the small bowel between the pylorus and the jejunum. The duodenum is divided into four segments, the last of which is in continuity with the jejunum. Of special interest in cytology is the second or descending segment of the duodenum. The openings of the main bile duct and the pancreatic ducts are found here. The main bile duct (ductus choledochus) carries bile from the liver into the duodenum. The terminal portion of the bile duct forms a dilatation (the ampulla of Vater) just prior to its entry into the duodenum. The main pancreatic duct (duct of Wirsung) usually opens into the ampulla of Vater, but may have a separate outlet into the duodenum. An accessory pancreatic duct usually opens into the second duodenal segment, independently of the main duct.

The duodenum is lined by a mucosa quite similar to that of the pyloric portion of the stomach. The main bile duct and the main pancreatic ducts are lined by a single layer of cylindrical epithelium, which may be ciliated.

Table 24-5
Comparison of Cytologic Results in the Diagnosis of Gastric Cancer

	Number of Cases of Gastric Carcinoma	Cytology Positive	Diagnostic Accuracy
Routine lavage	136	110	80.9%
Direct vision lavage			
Early Carcinoma	128	122	95.3%
Advanced Carcinoma	384	372	96.9%
Direct vision brushing	21	20	95.5%

(Modified from Kasugai, T., and Kobayashi, S.: Evaluation of biopsy and cytology in the diagnosis of gastric cancer. Am. J. Gastroenterol., 62: 199-203, 1974)

Methods of Investigation

In skilled hands, cytology may contribute in a significant fashion to the diagnosis of cancer of the pancreas and of the biliary tree, including the ampulla of Vater. Increased sophistication in the use of fiberoptic instruments and a combination of cytology with pancreatic function study and radiologic techniques have been shown to yield important diagnostic results. Cytologic samples are generally obtained from the duodenum. Direct sampling of bile and of pancreatic juice has also been recorded. An elaborate method of collection of duodenal content was described by Yamada et al. (1984). The goal of these investigations is early diagnosis of cancer of these organs, which may contribute to the improvement of the currently dismal therapeutic results. As a consequence of these efforts in numerous institutions, the knowledge of normal and abnormal cytology of the pancreaticoduodenal area has increased appreciably within the recent years. Transcutaneous aspiration cytology of abdominal organs is discussed in Chapter 29.

Normal Cytology of Duodenal Aspirates

In the absence of disease, the duodenal and pancreatic samples usually contain very few cells. The cells from duodenal lining cannot be clearly differentiated from cells of pancreatic or biliary duct ori-

gin. All such cells occur singly or in clusters and have a columnar configuration, with a striated, occasionally ciliated, flat luminal surface. The cells are large and may measure 50 μm in length. The nuclei, often provided with a small nucleolus, are round and clear and are usually placed toward the basal portion of the cell (Fig. 24–44). When seen in flat clusters, the cells assume a honeycomb appearance with the nucleus centrally located within the clear cytoplasmic areas. The cytoplasm is generally opaque, sometimes finely vacuolated, and is either acidophilic or cyanophilic. Goblet cells may also occur. They are of approximately the same size and have the characteristic cyanophilic and finely granular cytoplasm and peripheral nucleus. In the absence of disease, the epithelial cells are usually well preserved. The smears contain very few leukocytes or macrophages.

Inflammatory Changes

In the presence of inflammatory changes due to duodenitis, duodenal peptic ulcer, or pancreatitis, there is usually a marked increase in the number of cells present in smears. The preservation of the epithelial cells is usually poor and numerous stripped or "naked" nuclei may appear. Orell and Ohlsen identified two patterns of smears: in pattern *A* the smears contained mainly small, rounded, poorly preserved epithelial cells with granular or vacuolated cytoplasm and degenerated nuclei showing chromatin clumping or karyor-

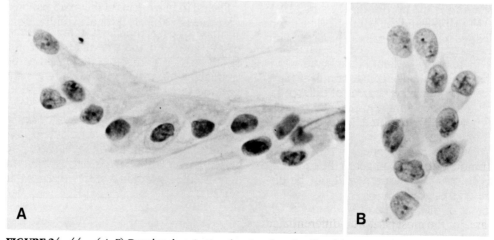

FIGURE 24–44. (*A, B*) Duodenal aspiration: benign ductal cells of the bile duct or pancreatic duct origin. Note columnar shape of cells, finely granular, opaque cytoplasms, and nuclei of even sizes and configuration. There is a slight variation in the degree of nuclear staining. Tiny nucleoli may be observed. (*A, B* ×560)

rhexis. Occasionally, such smears contained a large number of leukocytes. In pattern *B* the smears contained, in addition, a large number of stripped nuclei. Pattern *B* was observed mainly in patients with chronic pancreatitis, whereas no specific diagnostic significance could be attributed to pattern *A*. Cheli et al. observed an increase of goblet cells in chronic duodenitis. *Giardia lamblia* (see Fig. 24–22) may be occasionally observed in duodenal aspirates.

Carcinomas of the Pancreaticoduodenal Area in Duodenal Samples

Histology and Natural History

The most common tumors of this area are of pancreatic origin. There is statistical evidence strongly suggesting that pancreatic carcinoma is on the increase in the United States. Most patients with pancreatic carcinoma are symptomatic when first seen. The most favorable outlook is that for patients with carcinoma of the head of the pancreas that has invaded and obstructed the ampulla of Vater and caused clinical jaundice early in the course of the disease. Some of these tumors may be surgically resected. Virtually all other carcinomas of the pancreas are fatal to the patient. Yet, as a study by Cubilla and Fitzgerald has shown, there is good evidence that carcinoma of the pancreatic ducts, which is the most common form of pancreatic cancer, originates from an abnormal duct epithelium identified as atypical papillary hyperplasia or as carcinoma in situ. These findings suggest that the option of cytologic diagnosis of carcinoma in situ of pancreatic ducts remains open, although, to the best of my knowledge, not a single case has been diagnosed in a living patient. Pancreatic carcinomas, whether of ductal or acinar origin, are adenocarcinomas with varying degrees of differentiation. Highly anaplastic pancreatic cancers, akin to pulmonary oat cell carcinoma, have been described (Corrin et al.). Tumors of the islets of Langerhans, the endocrine component of the pancreas (islet cell tumors), do not connect to the excretory pancreatic ducts and, therefore, will not be discussed here (see Chap. 29).

Carcinomas of the ampulla of Vater and of the bile ducts are, for the most part, well-differentiated adenocarcinomas that may be mucus-producing. Occasionally, squamous carcinomas or carcinomas of mixed adenosquamous type have been recorded.

Cytology

Duodenal Samples. Cytologic presentation of all carcinomas of the pancreaticoduodenal area is very similar, and it is virtually impossible to determine the organ of primary origin on cytologic evidence obtained by aspiration of the duodenum.

The smears usually contain necrotic material, cell debris, and leukocytes. Yet, individual cancer cells are sometimes very well preserved. As a general rule, the cancer cells are large and appear singly or in clusters of variable size. The nuclear features dominate. The nuclei are large, hyperchromatic, and often have large, prominent, often multiple, irregularly shaped nucleoli (Fig. 24–45). In the better-differentiated adenocarcinoma, the cytoplasm is fairly abundant and of irregular, sometimes columnar, configuration. Papillary arrangement of cells in clusters is occasionally observed. Vacuolated cytoplasm may be noted on occasion. Examination of the bile either during the minilap procedure or by direct cannulation of the common bile duct may also yield cells of diagnostic value (see below).

Results. The pioneering efforts of Raskin et al. in this area of cytology are summarized in Table 24–6. With the exception of Dreiling et al. and Goldstein and Ventzke, who achieved cytologic diagnoses in about 75% of tumors, the results of duodenal aspiration remain within the limits reported by Raskin. However, a combination of cytologic with biochemical studies of pancreatic function after secretion injection appears to yield significant additional data (Prolla and Kirsner; Bourke et al.; Cabré-Fiol and Vilardell). Good diagnostic results have been recorded by direct aspiration of pancreatic duct at laparotomy (Rosen et al.) and with the use of duodenal fiberscope (Endo et al.). Yamada et al. (1984) achieved remarkable diagnostic results with a painstaking method for collection of duodenal juice after appropriate stimulation of secretions. Several very small cancers of the head of the pancreas and of the biliary tract were diagnosed on cytologic samples.

To a large extent, the duodenal aspiration technique has now been replaced by transcutaneous thin-needle aspiration biopsies, discussed in Chapter 29.

Cytology of Bile

It is not customary to think of bile as a diagnostic medium for cytologic diagnosis. Usually the bile is

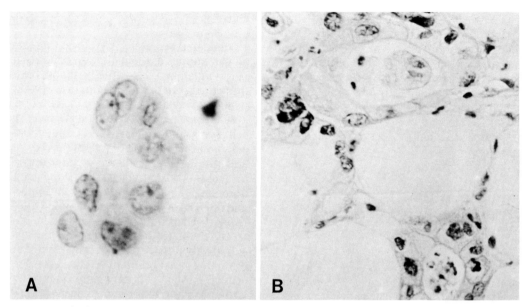

FIGURE 24–45. Pancreatic carcinoma in duodenal aspirate. Group of malignant cells (*A*) and tissue section (*B*) of a well-differentiated ductal adenocarcinoma. (Raskin, H. F., et al.: Gastrointestinal cancer; definitive diagnosis by exfoliative cytology. Arch. Surg., 76:507–516, 1958)

studied for its chemical components, such as cholesterol crystals and bilirubinate granules. Prolla and Kirsner observed that the cholesterol crystals are usually *absent* in patients with diseases of the liver or the pancreas, such as cirrhosis, pancreatitis, or pancreatic carcinoma. Cholesterol crystals were *present* in nearly all patients with a variety of disorders of the biliary tree, such as cholelithiasis or cholecystitis. No specific diagnostic significance could be attributed to bilirubinate granules. Prolla and Kirsner suggest that these findings are a helpful

Table 24–6
Location of 95 Cancers of the Duodenal Area and Results of Cytologic Examination of Duodenal Aspirates and Pancreatic Function Tests

Site	Cytology Negative	Cytology Positive
Pancreas	34	37
Bile duct	5	5
Gall bladder	6	3
Duodenum — primary	0	2
Duodenum — metastatic	0	3
	45	50

(Data from Dr. H. Raskin, Baltimore, Md.)

complementary diagnostic procedure, particularly in the differential diagnosis of jaundice.

Perhaps the first observers to comment on the diagnostic value of bile cytology were Wertlake and Del Guercio in 1976. These authors found it advantageous to examine bile obtained at the time of the so-called minilap procedure. This approach combines a transhepatic cholangiogram, liver biopsy, and an omentoportography for evaluation of liver function in hepatic disorders. It is usually performed on ambulatory patients. Cytologic study of the bile contributed additional diagnoses of metastatic carcinoma in two of five patients.

Bile may also be obtained at the time of surgical exploration of the biliary tree. Personal experience is based on this latter procedure.

The preservation of cells in the bile is usually excellent, although the background of smears contains numerous particles of bilirubinate. The normal cell population is similar to the cells derived from pancreatic duct (see Fig. 24–44). Cohesive sheets of large epithelial cells of bile duct origin are readily identified against the granular background. The cells are cuboidal or columnar, and are provided with granular nuclei with tiny nucleoli of monotonous size. Occasional cytoplasmic vacuoles may be noted (Fig. 24–46).

Cancer cells of bile duct origin are usually *smaller*, and occur either in clusters or singly. The

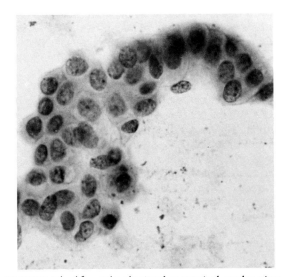

FIGURE 24-46. Bile obtained at surgical exploration. Benign cells from bile duct epithelium. Note a cohesive, flat cluster of large cuboidal–columnar cells with a flat surface, suggestive of origin in epithelial lining. The nuclei are granular, of monotonous size, and are provided with tiny nucleoli. The cytoplasm shows occasional vacuoles. Smear background contains granules of bilirubinate. (×560)

clusters are either loosely structured or show piling up and superposition of cells of variable sizes. Single cancer cells may show a cell-in-cell configuration. Nuclear abnormalities, particularly in well-differentiated carcinoma, need not be striking; increase in the size and number of nucleoli is common. In single cells marked nuclear hyperchromasia may be noted (Fig. 24–47).

With the passage of time, the value of bile in the diagnosis of carcinoma of the biliary tree and the pancreas was confirmed by several observers (Coble and Floyd, 1985; Ishikawa et al., 1988). The methods of securing the bile vary among observers and the reader is referred to the original work for a detailed description.

Aspiration biopsy of abdominal organs is discussed in Chapter 29.

THE RECTUM AND COLON

Methods of Investigation

Carcinoma of the colon is second in frequency only to lung cancer in men and to breast cancer in women. The results of treatment remain unsatisfactory and, therefore, a major diagnostic effort is afoot to diagnose the disease in earlier stages.

For many years the colon has been the target of

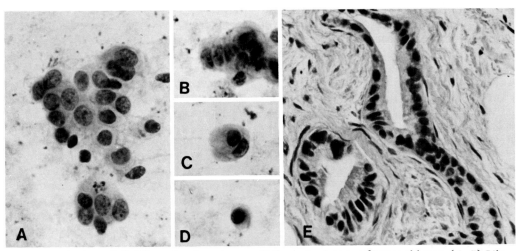

FIGURE 24-47. Well-differentiated carcinoma of bile duct origin in a 60-year-old man. (*A–D*) Bile obtained at surgical exploration. The cancer cells are smaller than benign ductal cells shown in Fig. 24–46. Smear background contains bilirubinate granules. (*A*) Loosely arranged cluster of cancer cells of variable size. A few nuclei are hyperchromatic. (*B*) Cluster showing superposition and, at one end, flattening of cancer cells of uneven size. (*C*) Small cancer cells showing a cell-in-cell arrangement. (*D*) A single cancer cell with a hyperchromatic nucleus. (*E*) Biopsy specimen of bile duct wall showing a well-differentiated adenocarcinoma. (*A–D* ×560; *E* ×350)

cytologic investigations for detection or early diagnosis of colonic cancer. Bader and Papanicolaou (1952) used a rectal-washing apparatus devised by Loeb (Loeb and Scapier, 1951), to obtain samples from the rectum and lower sigmoid, and colon washing for lesions located in descending colon. The target of the study was the cytologic diagnosis of carcinomas in clinically suspect situations.

The concept of colonic lavage for the diagnosis of occult colonic carcinomas was subsequently advocated by Raskin and Pleticka (1964, 1971), who achieved remarkable diagnostic results in selected patients who had clinical symptoms, but no radiologic evidence of abnormalities on barium enema. The technique of lavage consisted of an enema with 500 to 1,000 ml of warm Ringer's solution applied after appropriate preparation of the patient.

Several other lavage techniques were advocated (De Luca et al., 1974; Katz et al., 1974, 1977). Casts of colon obtained by injecting a soft plastic (Spjut et al., 1963), and even sponges packed in soluble capsules (Cromanty, 1977) were used to secure cellular samples from the colon. The effort has not been abandoned: new isotonic colon lavage solutions taken by mouth, and used for bowel cleansing before colonoscopy may also serve as a cell-collecting fluid (Rozen et al., 1990). A similar experiment was conducted on 12 patients before colonoscopy by Grunebaum and Brand at Montefiore Hospital. Cytologic examination failed to add any information of note (unpublished data).

Whether these techniques will become established to supplement radiologic and endoscopic techniques remains to be seen. Still, because of a great need for a reliable means of colon cancer detection, it is likely that the efforts will continue until a better approach is found.

For rectal cancer within the reach of the examiner's finger, Linehan et al. (1983) advocated the preparation of a smear from the surface of the glove. The method was successful in the diagnosis of several adenocarcinomas and squamous cancers.

The main thrust of colon cancer detection is based on the detection of occult blood in stool by means of commercially available slidelike devices. The presence of blood is indicated by a change in color of the slide in contact with a small sample of stool. The test is of low specificity, and the presence of blood in stool must be further clarified by additional procedures (Gnauck, 1977). With the widespread use of colonoscopy (recent review in Shinya, 1982), direct brushing techniques have become an important application of cytology. Colorectal cytology is primarily useful in the identifica-tion of cancer in high-risk patients (patients with familial polyposis of colon, ulcerative colitis, or patients previously treated for colon cancer) and for the clarification of obscure radiographic or colonoscopic findings.

Bardawil et al. (1990) reviewed their large experience with colonoscopic brush cytology. These authors stressed the prospective value of a positive or suspicious cytologic diagnosis in high-risk patients, even in the absence of initial histologic evidence of carcinoma. The diagnosis was ultimately confirmed in all but 1 patient with a "positive" diagnosis and in 29 of 34 patients with "suspicious" cytologic findings.

Histology and Normal Cytology

The mucosa of the large bowel is composed of a single or a double layer of columnar cells, arranged in simple tubular glands (Fig. 3–6). There are numerous goblet cells within the mucosa. The intervening columnar cells have an opaque cytoplasm.

Electron microscopic studies have confirmed the existence of two types of cells in the mucosa of the large intestine. The surface-lining cells are columnar with striated border; the mucus-producing cells are of the goblet cell type.

The cytologic features of rectal and sigmoid washings in the absence of disease are quite simple. Scanty columnar cells, goblet cells, macrophages, leukocytes, some squamous cells of anal origin and, almost invariably, debris form the cytologic picture (Fig. 24–48). In brushings and jet washings, the benign colonic cells appear in tightly knit clusters (see Fig. 24–52A). One of the most difficult tasks in obtaining cytologic specimens from this area is to limit the amount of debris to ensure a clean smear.

Inflammatory Diseases

The presence of an extensive inflammatory process involving the large bowel may render vain all attempts at the cytologic diagnosis of cancer. Such disorders as amebic colitis, or acute diverticulitis, may result in smears so rich in debris and inflammatory exudate that no intact epithelial cells may be observed (Fig. 24–49).

Unless specific causative agents (such as *Amoeba histolytica* or ova of *Schistosoma*) are identified, the cytologic diagnosis of colitis must remain nonspecific.

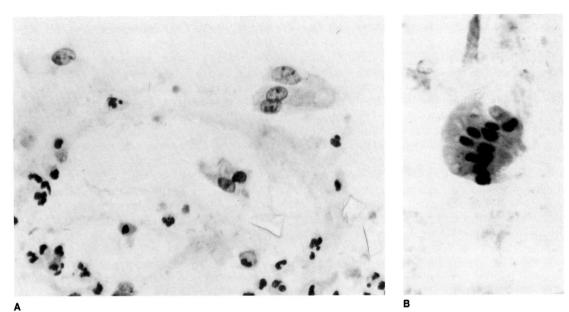

A   B

FIGURE 24–48. (*A*) Colonic washings. Benign columnar cells of colonic mucosa accompanied by mucus, numerous polymorphonuclear leukocytes, and detritus. A characteristic cytologic picture. (*B*) A cluster of benign columnar colonic epithelial cells in effluent, secured by isotonic oral solution before colonoscopy. (*A, B* ×560. *B* Courtesy of Dr. Ellen Greenebaum)

Chronic Ulcerative Colitis

Chronic ulcerative colitis is a disease that quite often presents a major diagnostic challenge. Patients with this disorder are particularly prone to the development of colonic adenocarcinoma (Cook et al.). The cytologic findings, particularly during the acute stage of the disease, are often very difficult to interpret. Galambos et al. and Boddington and Truelove emphasized some of the diagnostic problems. Galambos described two types of abnormal epithelial cells: the *bland* cells and the *active* cells. The bland cells are larger than normal colonic cells and have large, clear, pale nuclei. The

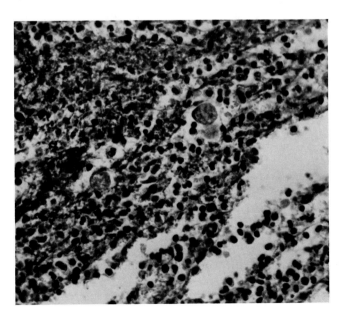

FIGURE 24–49. Amebic colitis, rectal washing. The material is a dense plaque of cellular material, composed mainly of leukocytes. Several spherical trophozoites of *Entamoeba histolytica* containing ingested erythrocytes may be observed. (×560)

active cells are also larger than normal, and their nuclei are characterized by the presence of large, sometimes irregularly shaped nucleoli. If the active cells also display variability in size, the differential diagnosis between active chronic ulcerative colitis and incipient colonic carcinoma may prove extremely difficult, if not impossible. Predictably, the small diagnostic dilemma may occur in the interpretation of biopsies. Similar difficulties were emphasized by Raskin and Pleticka (1964) and by Prolla and Kirsner. The latter authors also reported the presence of atypical cells of the lymphoid series, which may complicate the cytologic picture still further. Katz et al. advocated segmental lavage of areas of colon showing strictures, grossly distorted mucosa, or endoscopically inaccessible areas for purposes of cytologic diagnosis of occult cancer.

Festa et al. (1985) studied multiple cytologic samples obtained by colonic lavage and brushings from 41 patients with ulcerative colitis and also observed a wide spectrum of cytologic abnormalities, ranging from mild atypia, to severe atypia, to carcinoma. These observers found that the morphologic differences between "severe atypia" and carcinoma were difficult to ascertain. The same problem of interpretation apparently occurred with corresponding biopsies. Six carcinomas of the colon (including two in situ carcinomas) were accurately diagnosed. In the absence of long-term follow-up, the significance of the severe atypias cannot be ascertained, but it is presumably a high-risk lesion, akin to the dysplasia of other observers.

Flat precancerous abnormalities of colonic epithelium, akin to flat carcinoma in situ (colonic dysplasia) may occur in ulcerative colitis. Such patients are at high risk for the development of colonic cancer. These lesions may be identified by selective brushing and biopsies of the suspect areas during colonoscopy. Melville et al. (1988) suggested that colonic "dysplasia" could be identified as such when compared with cells of colonic carcinoma. The evidence in support of this view was not persuasive. In my judgment, all these lesions have the appearance of cancer cells (see below).

Benign Polyps

In my experience, benign polyps of the colonic mucosa cannot be identified as such with certainty. Occasionally, small fragments too thick for proper microscopic evaluation may be present in washings. The diagnosis can sometimes be made in cell blocks of the sediment.

Thabet and Macfarlane emphasize the presence of slender, elongated "needle" cells and of columnar, fan-shaped cells as characteristic of benign colonic polyps.

Brush cytology of adenomatous polyps during sigmoidoscopy or colonoscopy, prior to biopsy or removal, may contribute to the discovery of small foci of carcinoma.

Carcinoma

Histology

The frequency of colonic carcinoma and the serious threat that this disease presents to the societies in developed countries has been alluded to before. It is the belief of many epidemiologists that dietary factors are responsible for the frequency of this disease. An inherited disorder, polyposis of the colon, is known to carry with it a very high risk of carcinoma. Yet, as has been emphasized by Lane, not all polypoid lesions may be considered precursor lesions of colonic cancer. Polypoid hyperplasia (hyperplastic polyps), lined by well-differentiated mucus-producing colonic epithelium, are not considered precancerous. Adenomatous polyps, lined by epithelium crowded with cells showing nuclear enlargement, must be considered precancerous. Another polypoid lesion, villous papilloma, characterized by long, delicate stalks, may become malignant in a high proportion of cases (Takolander).

Colonic carcinomas are mucus-producing adenocarcinomas of varying levels of differentiation, ranging from well-defined, glandular structures, to solidly growing, anaplastic cancers. Signet ring adenocarcinoma is well known. Brekkan et al. observed a small series of colonic carcinomas developing at the site of prior ureterosigmoidostomy. Squamous cancers are occasionally observed (Lundquest et al., 1988), as are very rare cancers of other types.

Colonic carcinoids originate in the deep layers of the epithelium and are generally not identified in cytologic preparations.

Raskin and Pleticka (1964) believe that up to 20% of malignant lesions of the colon cannot be definitely identified on the initial radiographic examination. These same authors presented an impressive array of figures based on 569 cytologic examinations of the colon to support the claim that over 80% of *all* colonic carcinomas may be diagnosed by cytology by a skilled team. Among those were many not identified on radiographic examination.

To a large extent, prior concerns about the adequacy of radiologic examination of the colon in suspect patients have been resolved by colonoscopy. Hence, the role of cytology has been diminished and confined to high-risk patients, such as those with colonic polyposis, ulcerative colitis, or patients with prior local resection of colonic carcinoma who are at risk for recurrence. There is some evidence that surgical removal of adenomatous polyps discovered on colonoscopy or double-contrast barium enema may prevent, or at least significantly reduce, the occurrence of colonic cancer. It is not known whether these procedures are applicable to a large-scale colon cancer detection effort.

Cytology

The cells obtained from adenocarcinomas of the colon do not differ significantly from cells of other tumors of the gastrointestinal tract of a similar histologic structure. Large hyperchromatic nuclei with prominent nucleoli are characteristic (Figs. 24–50, 24–51, 24–52). The cytoplasm varies in amount and is often poorly preserved. The diagnosis is based on nuclear abnormalities. In cell blocks of effluents, fragments of colonic cancer may be observed (Fig. 24–53).

The difficulties of differential diagnosis between carcinoma and chronic ulcerative colitis have been emphasized above.

DeLuca et al. emphasized the usefulness of colonic cytology in the diagnosis of recurrent carcinoma after segmental resection of the bowel. It is of note that cells of colonic carcinoma may express the product of the oncogene Ha-*ras*, which may facilitate their recognition in difficult diagnostic situations (Czerniak et al., 1984).

Results. The results of some of the older reported series of cases of colonic carcinoma are recorded in Table 24–7. It must be emphasized that some of the highly satisfactory results contain a mixture of lesions both within and beyond the reach of the rigid sigmoidoscope. Obviously, cytology is a superfluous luxury if a visible and suspicious lesion can be biopsied, as is often the case with the use of a flexible colonoscope. The value of colonic cytology is primarily in the evaluation of lesions not accessible to biopsy, without clear-cut endoscopic or radiographic findings, and in monitoring high-risk patients.

(text continues on page 1074)

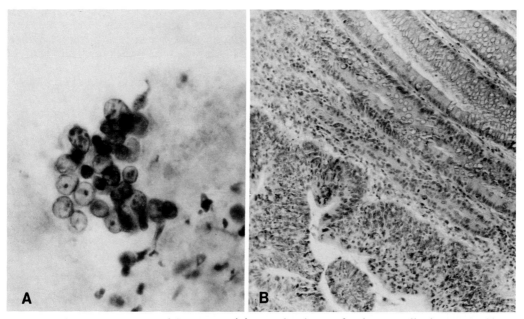

FIGURE 24–50. Carcinoma of the rectum. (*A*) Note the cluster of malignant cells characterized by very prominent nucleoli (colonic washings). The tissue section (*B*) discloses an orderly adenocarcinoma (*bottom*), next to benign mucosa. (*A* ×560; *B* ×150)

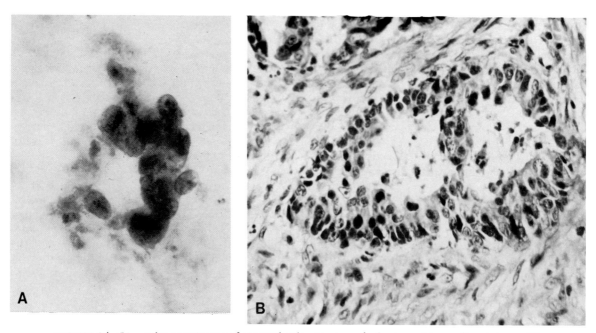

FIGURE 24–51.   Adenocarcinoma of sigmoid colon in smear (colonic washings; *A*) and tissue (*B*). Note papillary arrangement of cells and nuclear abnormalities. (*A* ×560; *B* ×350)

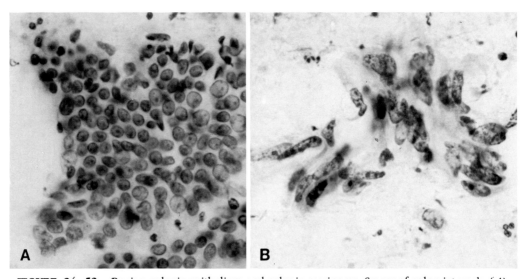

FIGURE 24–52.   Benign colonic epithelium and colonic carcinoma. Smear of colon jet wash. (*A*) Fragment of benign colonic epithelium. Note the cohesive cluster of orderly cells with small nuclei of monotonous sizes. (*B*) Cells of colonic adenocarcinoma. Clusters of elongated cells with large nuclei of uneven size and configuration. Note large nucleoli. (×560. Courtesy of Dr. S. Katz, Great Neck, L.I., New York)

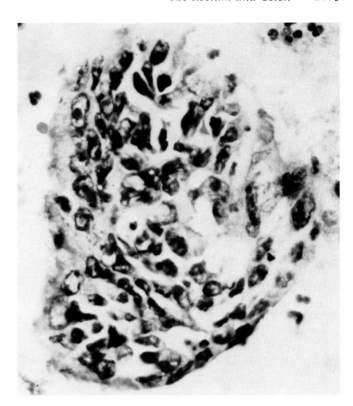

FIGURE 24-53. A fragment of colonic carcinoma observed in effluent prior to colonoscopy (for method see text). (×560. Courtesy of Dr. Ellen Greenebaum)

Table 24-7
Effectiveness of Cytology in the Diagnosis of Colonic Carcinoma

Author	Method	Number of Patients With Colonic Carcinoma	Number of Positive Results	Positive Cytology (%)
Raskin and Pleticka, 1971	Enema	94	70	74
Katz et al., 1972	Jet Wash	24*	12	50
Kline and Yum, 1976	Colonoscopy lavage	34	24	70
Bemvenuti et al., 1974	Colonoscopy brush	19	16	84
DeLuca et al., 1974	Enema	79	41	52

*Lesions beyond the reach of rigid sigmoidoscope.

BIBLIOGRAPHY

Esophagus

Benign Disorders

Berg, J.W.: Esophageal herpes; complication of cancer therapy. Cancer, *8*:731–740, 1955.

Brandborg, L.L., Taniguchi, L., and Rubin, C.E.: Exfoliative cytology of nonmalignant conditions of the upper intestinal tract. Acta Cytol., *5*:187–190, 1961.

Drake, M.: Gastro-Esophageal Cytology. Basel, S. Karger, 1985.

Greenebaum, E., Schreiber, K., Shu, Y.-J., and Koss, L.G.: Use of esophageal balloon in the diagnosis of carcinomas of the head, neck, and upper gastrointestinal tract. Acta Cytol., *28*:9–15, 1984.

Henning, N., and Witte, S.: Atlas der Gastroenterologischen Cytodiagnostik. Stuttgart, Georg Thieme, 1957.

Johnson,W.D., Koss, L.G., Papanicolaou, G.N., and Seybolt, J.F.: Cytology of esophageal washings; evaluation of 364 cases. Cancer, *8*:951–957, 1955.

Kobayashi, S., Prolla, J.C., and Kirsner, J.B.: Brushing cytology of the esophagus and stomach under direct vision by fiberscopes. Acta Cytol., *14*:219–223, 1970.

Lodge, K.V.: Pathology of non-specific oesophagitis. J. Pathol. Bacteriol., *69*:17–24, 1955.

O'Morchoe, P.J., Lee, D.C., and Kozak, C.A.: Esophageal cytology in patients receiving cytotoxic drug therapy. Acta Cytol., *27*:630–634, 1983.

Palmer, E.D.: The esophagus and its diseases. New York, Paul B. Hoeber, 1952.

Panico, F.G.: Cytologic patterns in benign and malignant gastric and esophageal lesions. Surg. Gynecol. Obstet., *94*:733–742, 1952.

Prolla, J.C., and Kirsner, J.B.: Handbook and Atlas of Gastrointestinal Exfoliative Cytology. Chicago, University of Chicago Press, 1972.

Weiden, P.L., and Schuffler, M.D.: Herpes esophagitis complicating Hodgkin's disease. Cancer, *33*:1100–1102, 1974. *See also Chapter 31 (AIDS).*

Barrett's Esophagus

Adler, R.H.: The lower esophagus lined by columnar epithelium: its association with hiatal hernia, ulcer, stricture, and tumor. J. Thorac. Cardiovasc. Surg., *45*:13–34, 1963.

Barrett, N.R.: Chronic peptic ulcer of the esophagus and esophagitis. Br. J. Surg., *38*:175–182, 1950.

Burgess, J.N., Payne, W.S., Andersen, H.A., Weiland, L.H., and Carlson, H.C.: Barrett esophagus. The columnar-epithelial-lined lower esophagus. Mayo Clin. Proc., *46*:728–734, 1971.

Cameron, A.J., Ott, B.J., and Payne, W.S.: The incidence of adenocarcinoma in columnar-lined (Barrett's) esophagus. N. Engl. J. Med., *313*:857–859, 1985.

Haggitt, R.C., Reid, B.J., Rabinovitch, P.S., and Rubin, C.E.: Barrett's esophagus—correlation between mucin histochemisty, flow cytometry, and histologic diagnosis for predicting increased cancer risk. Am. J. Pathol., *131*:53–61, 1988.

Hawe, A., Payne, W.S., and Weiland, L.H., et al: Adenocarcinoma in the columnar epithelial lined lower (Barrett) oesophagus. Thorax, *28*:511–514, 1973.

Jernstrom, P., and Brewer, L.A. III.: Primary adenocarcinoma of the mid-esophagus arising in ectopic gastric mucosa with associated hiatal hernia and reflux esophagitis (Dawson's syndrome). Cancer, *26*:1343–1348, 1970.

Lee, R.G.: Dysplasia in Barrett's esophagus. Am. J. Surg. Pathol., *9*:845–852, 1985.

Mossberg, S.M.: The columnar-lined esophagus (Barrett syndrome)—an acquired condition? Gastroenterology, *50*:671–676, 1966.

Robey, S.S., Hamilton, S.R., Gupta, P.K., and Erozan, Y.S.: Diagnostic value of cytopathology in Barrett esophagus and associated carcinoma. Am. J. Clin. Pathol., *89*:493–498, 1988.

Rubio, C.A., and Riddell, R.H.: Atypical mitoses in dysplasias of the Barrett's mucosa. Pathol. Res. Pract., *184*:1–5, 1989.

Rubio, C.A., and Riddell, R.: Musculo-fibrous anomaly in Barrett's mucosa with dysplasia. Am. J. Surg. Pathol., *12*:885–889, 1988.

Skinner, D.B., Walther, B.C., Riddell, R.H., Schmidt, H., Iascone, C., and DeMeester, T.R.: Barrett's esophagus: comparison of benign and malignant cases. Ann. Surg., *198*:554–565, 1983.

Smith, R.R.L., Hamilton, S.R., Boitnott, J.K., and Rogers, E.L.: The spectrum of carcinoma arising in Barrett's esophagus. Am. J. Surg. Pathol., *8*:563–573, 1984.

Spechler, S.J., and Goyal, R.K.: Barrett's Esophagus—Pathophysiology, Diagnosis, and Management. New York, Elsevier, 1985.

Spechler, S.J., and Goyal, R.K.: Barrett's esophagus. N. Engl. J. Med., *315*:362–371, 1986.

Veen, V.D.A.H., Dees, J., Blankenstein, J.D., and Blankenstein, V.M.: Adenocarcinoma in Barrett's oesophagus: an overrated risk. Gut, *30*:14–18, 1989.

Carcinoma

Andersen, H.A., McDonald, J.R., and Olsen, A.M.: Cytologic diagnosis of carcinoma of esophagus and cardia of stomach. Proc. Mayo Clin., *24*:245–253, 1949.

Appelman, H.D.: Pathology of the Esophagus, Stomach, and Duodenum. pp. 70–119. New York, Churchill Livingstone, 1984.

Auerback, O., Stout, A.P., Hammond, E.C., and Garfinkel, L.: Histologic changes in esophagus in relation to smoking habits. Arch. Environ. Health, *14*:4–15, 1965.

Barge, J., Molas, G., Maillard, J.N., Fekete, F., Bogomoletz, W.V., and Potet, F.: Superficial oesophageal carcinoma: an oesophageal counterpart of early gastric cancer. Histopathology, *5*:499–510, 1981.

Basque, G.J., Boline, J.E., and Holyoke, J.B.: Malignant melanoma of the esophagus; first reported case in a child. Am. J. Clin. Pathol., *53*:609–611, 1970.

Belladonna, J.A., Hajdu, S.I., Bains, M.S., and Winawer, S.J.: Adenocarcinoma in situ of Barrett's esophagus diagnosed by endoscopic cytology. N. Engl. J. Med., *291*:895–896, 1974.

Berry, A.V., Baskind, A.F., and Hamilton, D.G.: Cytologic screening for esophageal cancer. Acta Cytol., *25*:135–141, 1981.

Bogomoletz, W.V., Molas, G., Gayet, B., and Potet, F.: Superficial squamous cell carcinoma of the esophagus. A report of 76 cases and review of the literature. Am. J. Surg. Pathol., *13*:535–546, 1989.

Bullock, W.K., and Snyder, E.N.: Carcinoma in situ occurring in pharyngeal diverticulum. Cancer, *5*:737–739, 1952.

Cabré-Fiol, V.: Cytologic diagnosis of esophageal and gastric cancer. *In* Advances in gastrointestinal Endosopy. Proc. 2nd World Congress of Gastroint. Endoscopy. pp. 219–225. July 1–11, 1970.

Carrie, A.: Adenocarcinoma of the upper end of the esophagus arising from ectopic gastric epithelium. Br. J. Surg., *37*:474, 1950.

Chang, F., Syrjanen, S., Shen, Q., Ji, H., and Syrjanen, K.: Human papillomavirus (HPV) DNA in esophageal precancer lesions and squamous cell carcinoma from China. Abstr. 351. Papilloma Virus Workshop, Heidelberg, 1990.

Dawson, J.L.: Adenocarcinoma of the middle oesophagus arising in an oesophagus lined by gastric (parietal) epithelium. Br. J. Surg., *51*:940–942, 1964.

Enrile, F.T., DeJesus, P.O., Bakst, A.A., and Baluyot, R.: Pseudosarcoma of the esophagus (polypoid carcinoma of esophagus with pseudosarcomatous features). Cancer, *31*:1197–1202, 1973.

Fraser, G.M., and Kinley, C.E.: Pseudosarcoma with carcinoma of the esophagus. A report of 2 cases. Arch. Pathol., *85*:325–330, 1968.

Greenebaum, E., Schreiber, K., Shu, Y.-J., and Koss, L.G.: Use of the esophgeal balloon in the diagnosis of carcinomas of the head, neck and upper gastrointestinal tract. Acta Cytol., *28*:9–15, 1984.

Gupta, R.K., and Rogers, K.E.: Endoscopic cytology and biopsy in the diagnosis of gastroesophageal malignancy. Acta Cytol., *27*:17–22, 1983.

Henning, N., and Witte, S.: Atlas der Gastroenterologischen Cytodiagnostik. Stuttgart, Georg Thieme, 1957.

Hishon, S., Lovell, D., Gummer, J.W.P., Smithies, A., Shawdon, H., and Blendis, L.M.: Cytology in the diagnosis of oesophageal cancer. Lancet, *1*:296–297, 1976.

Horai, T., Kobayashi, A., Takeishi, R., Wada, A., Taniguchi, H., Taniguchi, K., Sano, M., and Tamura, H.: A cytologic study on small cell carcinoma of the esophagus. Cancer, *41*:1890–1878, 1978.

Huang, G.J., and K'ai W.Y.: Carcinoma of the Esophagus and Gastric Cardia. pp. 156–190. New York, Springer-Verlag, 1984.

Hughes, J.H., and Cruickshank, A.H.: Pseudosarcoma of the oesophagus. Br. J. Surg., *56*:72–76, 1969.

Imbriglia, J.E., and Lopusniak, M.S.: Cytologic examination of sediment from esophagus in case of intra-epidermal carcinoma of esophagus. Gastroenterology, *13*:457–463, 1949.

Jaskiewicz, K., Venter, F.S., and Marasas, W.F.: Cytopathology of the esophagus in Transkei. JNCI, *79*:961–967, 1987.

Johnson, W.D., Koss, L.G., Papanicolaou, G.N., and Seybolt, J.F.: Cytology of esophageal washings; evaluation of 364 cases. Cancer, *8*:951–957, 1955.

Kobayashi, S., Prolla, J.C., and Kirsner, J.B.: Brushing cytology of the esophagus and stomach under direct vision by fiberscopes. Acta Cytol., *14*:219–223, 1970.

Kuwano, H., Nagamatsu, M., Ohno, S., Matsuda, H., Mori, M., and Sugimachi, K.: Coexistence of intraepithelial carcinoma and glandular differentiation in esophageal squamous cell carcinoma. Cancer, *62*:1568–1572, 1988.

Maimon, H.N., Dreskin, R.B., and Cocco, A.E.: Positive esophageal cytology without detectable neoplasm. Gastrointest. Endosc., *20*:156–159, 1974.

Messelt, O.T.: Cytological diagnosis of esophagus cancer. Acta Chir. Scand., *103*:440–441, 1952.

Mori, M., Matsukuma, A., Adachi, Y., Miyagahara, T., Matsuda, H., Kuwano, H., Sugimachi, K., and Enjoji, M.: Small cell carcinoma of the esophagus. Cancer, *63*:564–573, 1989.

Morson, B.C., and Belcher, J.R.: Adenocarcinoma of oesophagus and ectopic gastric mucosa. Br. J. Cancer, *6*:127–130, 1952.

Palmer, E.D.: The Esophagus and Its Diseases. New York, Paul B. Hoeber, 1952.

Panico, F.G.: Cytologic patterns in benign and malignant gastric and esophageal lesions. Surg. Gynecol. Obstet., *94*:733–742, 1952.

Pour, P., and Ghadirian, P.: Familial cancer of the esophagus in Iran. Cancer, *33*:1649–1652, 1974.

Prolla, J.C., and Kirsner, J.B.: Handbook and Atlas of Gastrointestinal Exfoliative Cytology. Chicago, University of Chicago Press, 1972.

Prolla, J.C., Reilly, R.W., Kirsner, J.B., and Cockerham, L.: Direct-vision endoscopic cytology and biopsy in the diagnosis of esophageal and gastric tumors: current experience. Acta Cytol., *21*:399–402, 1977.

Prolla, J.C., Yoshi, Y., Xavier, R.G., and Kirsner, J.B.: Further experience with direct vision brushing cytology of malignant tumors of upper gastrointestional tract; histopathologic correlation with biopsy. Acta Cytol., *15*:375–378, 1971.

Raskin, H.R., Kirsner, J.B., and Palmer, W.L.: Role of exfoliative cytology in the diagnosis of cancer of the digestive tract. JAMA, *169*:789–791, 1959.

Riberi, A., Battersby, J.S., and Vellios, F.: Epidermoid carcinoma occurring in pharyngoesophageal diverticulum. Cancer, *8*:727–730, 1955.

Rosen, Y., Moon, S., and Kim, B.: Small cell epidermoid carcinoma of the esophagus. An oat-cell-like carcinoma. Cancer, *36*:1042–1049, 1975.

Rubin, C.E., Massey, B.E., Kirsner, J.B., Palmer, W.L., and Stonecypher, D.D.: Clinical value of gastrointestinal cytologic diagnosis. Gastroenterology, *25*:119–138, 1953.

Rubin, P., Wynder, E., Mabuchi, K., Wiot, J.W., Felson, B., Morrisey, J.F., and Prolla, J.C.: Cancer of the gastrointestinal tract. I. Esophagus: detection and diagnosis. JAMA, *226*:1544–1588, 1973.

Rubio, C.A., Auer, G.U., Kato, Y., and Liu, F.S.: DNA profiles in dysplasia and carcinoma of the human esophagus. Anal. Quant. Cytol. Histol., *3*:207–210, 1988.

Shu, Y.J.: Cytopathology of Esophageal Cancer. New York, Masson Publishing, 1985.

Souquet, J.C., Berger, F., Bonvoisin, S., Partensky, C., Boulez, J., Descos, F., and Lambert, R.: Esophageal squamous cell carcinoma associated with gastric adenocarcinoma. Cancer, *63*:786–790, 1989.

Steiner, P.E.: Etiology and histogenesis of carcinoma of esophagus. Cancer, *9*:436–452, 1956.

Stout, A.P., and Lattes, R.: Tumors of the Esophagus; Atlas of Tumor Pathology, sect. 5, fasc. 20. Washington, D.C., Armed Forces Institute of Pathology, 1957.

Suckow, E.E., Yokoo, H., and Brock, D.R.: Intraepithelial carcinoma concomitant with esophageal carcinoma. Cancer, 15:733–740, 1962.

Turnbull, A.D.M., and Goodner, J.T.: Primary adenocarcinoma of the esophagus. Cancer, 22:915–918, 1968.

Ushigome, S., Spjut, H.J., and Noon, G.P.: Extensive dysplasia and carcinoma in situ of esophageal epithelium. Cancer, 20:1023–1029, 1967.

Yates, D.R., and Koss, L.G.: Paget's disease of the esophageal epithelium. Report of first case. Arch. Pathol., 86:447–452, 1968.

Cancer Screening

Chinese Academy of Sciences and Honan Province: Coordinating group for research on esophageal carcinoma. Studies on the relationship of dysplasia to carcinoma of the esophagus. Abstr. Proc. 4th Int. Cancer Congr., 4:472, 1974.

Greenebaum, E., Schreiber, K., Shu, Y.-J., and Koss, L.G.: Use of esophageal balloon in the diagnosis of carcinomas of the head, neck, and upper gastrointestinal tract. Acta Cytol., 28:9–15, 1984.

Jaskiewicz, K., Venter, F.S., and Marasas, W.F.: Cytopathology of the esophagaus in Transkei. JNCI, 79:961–967, 1987.

Li, J.-Y., Ershow, A.G., Chen, Z.-J., Wacholder, S., Li, G.-Y., Guo, W., Li, B., and Blot, W.J.: A case–control study of cancer of the esophagus and gastric cardia in Linxian. Int. J. Cancer, 43:755–761, 1989.

Shu, Y.-J.: Cytopathology of the esophagus. An overview of esophageal cytopathology in China. Acta Cytol., 27:7–16, 1983.

Shu, Y.-J.: Detection of esophageal carcinoma by the balloon technique in the People's Republic of China. In Koss, L.G., and Coleman, D.V. (eds.): Advances in Clinical Cytology. vol. 2, pp. 67–102. New York, Masson Publishing, 1984.

Rare Tumors

Aldovini, D., Detassis, DC., and Piscioli, d.: Primary malignant melanoma of the esophagus. Brush cytology and histogenesis. Acta Cytol., 27:65–68, 1983.

Boyd, D.P., Meissner, W.A., Velkoff, C.L., and Gladding, T.C.: Primary melanocarcinoma of esophagus: report of a case. Cancer, 7:266–270, 1954.

Broderick, P.A., Allegra, S.R., and Corvese, N.: Primary malignant melanoma of the esophagus: a case report. Acta Cytol., 16:159–164, 1972.

Bullock, W.K., Thompson, H.L., and Gregory, G.: Primary melanocarcinoma of the esophagus. Cancer, 6:578–580, 1953.

Chaput, J.D., Gourdier, S., Martin, E., Larriev, H., and Etienne, J.-P.: Naevocarcinome primitif de l'oesophage. Sem. Hop. Paris, 50:151–157, 1974.

De la Pava, S., Nigogsyan, G., Pickeren, J.W., and Cabrera, A.: Melanosis of the esophagus. Cancer, 16:48–50, 1963.

Enrile, F.T., DeJesus, P.O., Bakst, A.A., and Baluyot, R.: Pseudosarcoma of the esophagus (polypoid carcinoma of esophagus with pseudosarcomatous features). Cancer, 31:1197–1202, 1973.

Fraser, G.M., and Kinley, C.E.: Pseudosarcoma with carcinoma of the esophagus. A report of 2 cases. Arch. Pathol., 85:325–330, 1968.

Garfinkle, J.M., and Cahan, W.G.: Primary melanocarcinoma of esophagus; first histologically proved case. Cancer, 5:921–926, 1952.

Hughes, J.H., and Cruickshank, A.H.: Pseudosarcoma of the oesophagus. Br. J. Surg., 56:72–76, 1969.

Kanavaros, P., Galian, A., Periac, P., Dayan, S., Licht, H., and Lavergne, A.: Melanome malin primitif de l'oesophage developpe sur une melanose. Ann. Pathol., 1:57–61, 1989.

Mills, S.E., and Cooper, P.H.: Malignant melanoma of the digestive system. Pathol. Annu., 18:1–26, 1983.

Minwalla, S.P., and Parry, W.R.: A case of primary malignant melanoma of the esophagus. Br. J. Surg., 48:461–462, 1961.

Piccone, V.A., Klopstock, R., LeVeen, N.H., and Sika, J.P.: Primary malignant melanoma of the esophagus associated with melanosis of the entire esophagus. J. Thorac. Cardiovasc. Surg., 59:864–870, 1970.

Waken, J.K., and Bullock, W.K.: Primary melanocarcinoma of the esophagaus. Am. J. Clin. Pathol., 38:415–421, 1962.

Yates, D.R., and Koss, L.G.: Paget's disease of the esophageal epithelium. Report of first case. Arch. Pathol., 86:447–452, 1968.

Stomach

Benign Disorders

Anonymous: Unidentified curved bacilli on gastric epithelium in active chronic gastritis [Editorial]. Lancet, 1:1273–1275, 1983.

Appelman, H.D.: Pathology of the Esophagus, Stomach, and Duodenum. pp. 70–119. New York: Churchill Livingstone, 1984.

Arnold, W.T., Hampton, J., Olin, W., Glass, H., and Carruth, C.: Gastric lesions, including exfoliative cytology. A diagnostic approach. JAMA, 173:1117–1120, 1960.

Ayre, J.E., and Oren, B.G.: New rapid method for stomach-cancer diagnosis; gastric brush. Cancer, 6:1177–1181, 1953.

Becker, S.N., Sass, M.A., Petras, R.E., and Hart, W.R.: Bizarre atypia in gastric brushings associated with hepatic artery infusion chemotherapy. Acta Cytol., 30:347–350, 1986.

Bennington, J.L., Porus, R., Ferguson, B., and Hannon, G.: Cytology of gastric sarcoid. Report of a case. Acta Cytol., 12:30–36, 1968.

Blaser, M.J.: Gastric campylobacter-like organisms, gastritis, and peptic ulcer disease. Gastroenterology, 93:371–383, 1987.

Bloch, T., Davis, T.E., Jr., and Schwenk, G.R., Jr.: Giardia lamblia in peritoneal fluid. Acta Cytol., 31:783–784, 1987.

Boddington, M.M., and Spriggs, A.I.: The epithelial cells in megaloblastic anemias. J. Clin. Pathol., 12:228–234, 1959.

Boen, S.T.: Changes in nuclei of squamous epithelial cells in pernicious anemia. Acta Med. Scand., 159:425–431, 1957.

Boon, T.H., Schade, R.O.K., Middleton, G.D., and Reece, M.F.: An attempt at presymptomatic diagnosis of gastric carcinoma in pernicious anaemia. Gut, 5:269–270, 1964.

Bultz, W.C.: Giant hypertrophic gastritis: a report of fourteen cases. Gastroenterology, 39:183–190, 1960.

Correa, P.: Precursors of gastric and esophageal cancer. Cancer, 50:2554–2565, 1982.

Dooley, C.P., Cohen, H., Fitzgibbons, P.L., Bauer, M., Appleman, M.D., Perez-Perez, G.I., and Blaser, M.J.: Prevalence of Helicobacter pylori infection and histologic gastritis in asymptomatic persons. N. Engl. J. Med., 321:1562–1566, 1989.

Drake, M.: Gastro-Esophageal Cytology. Basel, S. Karger, 1985.

colonic cytology: A simplified method of collection and initial results. Acta Cytol., *34*:627–631, 1990.

Sharkey, F.E., Clark, R.L., and Gray, G.F.: Perianal Paget's disease: report of 2 cases. Dis. Colon Rectum, *18*:245–248, 1975.

Shinya, H.: Colonoscopy: Diagnosis and Treatment of Colonic Diseases. New York, Igaku-Shoin, 1982.

Spjut, H.J., Margulis, A.R., and Cook, G.B.: The silicone-foam enema: a source for exfoliative cytological specimens. Acta Cytol., *7*:79–84, 1963.

Takolander, R.J.: Villous papilloma of the colon and rectum. Part I. A clinical study of 213 patients. Ann. Chir. Gynaecol., *64*:257–264, 1975.

Thabet, R.J., Knoernschild, H.E., and Hausner, J.L.: Millipore filtration technique for colon washings. Cytol. Newslett., *2*:2–3, 1960.

Thabet, R.J., and Macfarlane, E.W.E.: Cytological field patterns and nuclear morphology in the diagnosis of colon pathology. Acta Cytol., *6*:325–331, 1962.

van der Heide, H., Lantink, J.A., Wiltink, E., and Tytgat, G.N.J.: Comparison of whole-gut irrigation with GoLYTELY (GOL) and with a balanced electrolyte solution (BES) as a preparation for colonoscopy. Endoscopy, *18*:182–184, 1986.

Williams, S.L., Rogers, L.W., and Quan, H.Q.: Perianal Paget's disease: report of seven cases. Dis. Colon Rectum, *19*:30–40, 1976.

Wisseman, C.L., Jr., Lemon, H.M., and Lawrence, K.B.: Cytologic diagnosis of cancer of descending colon and rectum. Surg. Gynecol. Obstet., *89*:24–30, 1949.

Wolff, W.I., and Shinya, H.: Earlier diagnosis of cancer of the colon through colonic endoscopy (colonoscopy). Cancer, *34*:1974.

Biliary and Pancreatic Ducts

Aka, E., and Garret, M.: Diagnosis of the pancreatic carcinoma by cytologic examination of pancreatic duct aspiration fluid during surgery. Ann. Surg., *167*:427–432, 1968.

Cabre-Fiol, V., and Vilardell, F.: Diagnostic cytologique du cancer du pancreas. Med. Chir. Dig., *4*:277–282, 1975.

Cheli, R., Astet, H., Nicolo, G., and Ciancomerla, G.: Cytological findings in chronic non-specific duodenitis. Endoscopy, *6*:110–115, 1974.

Cobb, C.J., and Floyd, W.N.: Usefulness of bile cytology in the diagnostic management of patients with biliary tract obstruction. Acta Cytol., *29*:93–100, 1985.

Cubilla, A.L., and Fitzgerald, P.J.: Morphological lesions associated with human primary invasive nonendocrine pancreas cancer. Cancer Res., *36*:2690–2698, 1976.

Drieling, D.A., Nieburgs, H.E., and Janowitz, H.D.: The combined secretion and cytology test in the diagnosis of pancreatic and biliary tract cancer. Med. Clin. North Am., *44*:801–815, 1960.

Goldstein, H., and Ventzke, L.E.: Value of exfoliative cytology in pancreatic carcinoma. Gut, *9*:316–318, 1968.

Hatfield, A.R.W., Whittaker, R., and Gibbs, D.D.: The collection of pancreatic fluid for cytodiagnosis using a duodenoscope. Gut, *15*:305–307, 1974.

Ishikawa, O., Ohhigashi, H., Sasaki, Y., Imaoka, S., Iwanaga, T., Wada, A., Ishiguro, S., Tateishi, R., Kishigami, Y., and Sone, H.: The usefulness of saline-irrigated bile for the intraoperative cytologic diagnosis of tumors and tumorlike lesions of the gallbladder. Acta Cytol., *32*:475–481, 1988.

McNeer, G., and Ewing, J.H.: Exfoliated pancreatic cancer cells in duodenal drainage; case report. Cancer, *2*:643–645, 1949.

Nieburgs, H.E., Dreiling, M.D., Rubio, C., and Reisman, H.: The morphology of cells in duodenal-drainage smears: histologic origin and pathologic significance. Am. J. Dig. Dis., *7*:489–505, 1967.

Orell, S.R., and Ohlsen, P.: Normal and post-pancreatic cytologic patterns of the duodenal juice. Acta Cytol., *16*:165–171, 1972.

Raskin, H.F., Moseley, R.D., Jr., Kirsner, J.B., and Palmer, W.L.: Cancer of the pancreas, biliary tract and liver. CA, *11*:137–148, 166–181, 1961.

Raskin, H.F., Wenger, J., Sklar, M., Pleticka, S., and Yarema, W.: Diagnosis of cancer of pancreas, biliary tract, and duodenum by combined cytologic and secretory methods. I. Exfoliative cytology and description of rapid method of duodenal intubation. Gastroenterology, *34*:996–1008, 1958.

Rosen, R.C., Garret, M., and Aka, E.: Cytologic diagnosis of pancreatic cancer by ductal aspiration. Ann. Surg., *167*:427–432, 1968.

Smithies, A., Hatfield, A.R.W., and Brown, B.E.: The cytodiagnostic aspects of pure pancreatic juice obtained at the time of endoscopic retrograde cholangiopancreatography (ERCP). Acta Cytol., *21*:191–195, 1977.

Strack, P.R., Newman, H.K., Lerner, A.C., Green, S.H., Meng, C., and DelGuercio, L.R.M.: Integrated procedure for the rapid diagnosis of biliary obstruction, portal hypertension and liver disease of uncertain etiology. N. Engl. J. Med., *285*:1225–1231, 1971.

Wasastjerna, C., and Ekelung, P.: The amino acid napthylamidase reaction of the bile canaliculi in liver smears. Acta Cytol., *18*:23–29, 1974.

Wasastjerna, C., Kekelung, P., and Haltia, K.: The bile canaliculi in cytological aspiration biopsy from patients with liver disorders. Scand. J. Gastroenterol., *5*:327–331, 1970.

Wenger, J., and Raskin, H.F.: Diagnosis of cancer of pancreas, biliary tract, and duodenum by combined cytologic and secretory methods. II. Secretion test. Gastroenterology, *34*:1009–1017, 1958.

Weretlake, P.T., and Del Guercio, L.R.M.: Cytopathology of intrahepatic bile as component of integrated procedure ("minilap") for hepatobiliary disorders. Acta Cytol., *20*:42–45, 1976.

Yamada, T., Murohisa, B., Muto, Y., Okamoto, K., Doi, K., and Tsuchia, R.: Cytologic detection of small pancreaticoduodenal and biliary cancers in the early developmental stage. Acta Cytol., *28*:435–442, 1984.

25

Effusions in the Absence of Cancer

ANATOMY AND HISTOLOGY OF THE PLEURAL, THE PERITONEAL, AND THE PERICARDIAL CAVITIES

These three cavities, generally designated as body cavities, have a common embryologic origin in the mesenchymal embryonal layer. The pleura encloses the lungs; the peritoneum, the intestinal tract; and the pericardium, the heart (Fig. 25–1; see also Fig. 3–8). Structurally, all three cavities are quite similar, inasmuch as they are formed by a thin membrane that forms a double layer of protection. The layer covering the organs contained within the cavity is referred to as the *visceral layer*, whereas that which lines the outer walls of the respective cavity is called the *parietal layer*. The visceral and the parietal layers in continuity with each other form a cavity that normally is self-contained and not in contact with the outside world.

The body cavities are lined by a single layer of flat cells—the *mesothelium*, supported by connective tissue and an appropriate vascular and nervous apparatus (Fig. 25–2). Under favorable circumstances of perfect fixation and gentle processing, a brush border may be observed on the luminal surface of the cells (Fig. 25–3). In the absence of disease, the parietal and the visceral layers of the mesothelium are separated by a thin layer of lubricating fluid that facilitates the movements of the two membranes against each other. Therefore, the cavities are not true cavities but *virtual* cavities, a fact of considerable importance in the proper functioning of the organs contained therein.

Transmission electron microscopic studies of the mesothelium reveal a continuous single layer of cells with microvilli extending toward the body cavity and a number of pinocytotic vesicles (Fig. 25–4). Scanning electron microscopy confirmed that the mesothelial cells lining the surface are provided with short, even microvilli. The flow of fluids lubricating the mesothelial surfaces is regulated by cells.

BODY CAVITIES UNDER PATHOLOGIC CONDITIONS

The presence of gases or fluids in the body cavities will change them into true cavities. The presence of gas constitutes, respectively, a *pneumothorax*, a

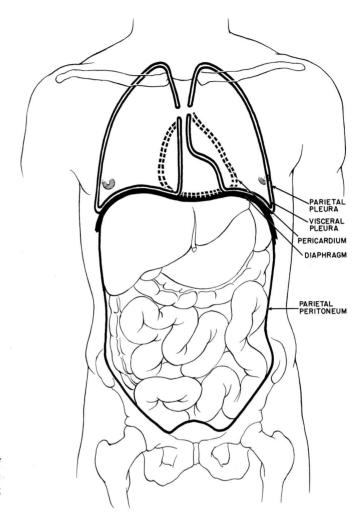

FIGURE 25–1. Schematic representation of the three body cavities. The visceral layer of the peritoneum is identical with the serosal lining of the intestinal tract.

pneumoperitoneum, or a *pneumopericardium.* The presence of fluid constitutes an *effusion,* which in the abdomen is often called *ascites.*

The fluids or effusions may be classified as transudates or exudates.

Transudates

The transudates are fluids characterized by a low protein content (usually below 3 g/100 ml) and a low specific gravity, often below 1.015. The accu-

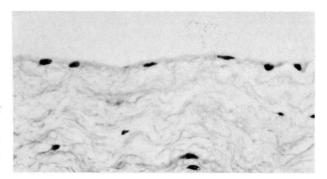

FIGURE 25–2. Mesothelial lining: single layer of flat cells on the surface of supporting connective tissue (epicardium). (×350)

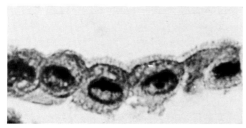

FIGURE 25–3. Brush border, mesothelial cells (pericardial sac aspiration). (Oil immersion, ×1,400)

mulation of transudates with body cavities appears to be due to filtration of blood serum across the physically intact vascular wall—for example, in hypoproteinemia resulting from malnutrition, in cirrhosis of the liver, and in certain diseases of the kidney or the heart. Two mechanisms explain the occurrence of transudates: either reduced intravascular osmotic pressure, as in hypoproteinemia, or increased filtration pressure, as in heart failure.

The scanty cellular components of transudates are mesothelial cells and a few leukocytes. When the cytologic components of an effusion are more complex, it is in all likelihood an exudate.

Exudates

The exudates result from an accumulation of fluid within the body cavities, associated with damage to the walls of the capillaries. The exudates are characterized by a relatively high protein content (usually above 3 g/100 ml) and, therefore, a high specific gravity (usually above 1.015). The exudates are rich in fibrin and may coagulate on standing. There are several causes of exudates.

Exudates Caused by Infections

Such exudates may be acute or chronic and may be primary within the body cavities or, more often, secondary to inflammatory processes of the organs contained therein. The main causes of infectious exudates in the three cavities are as follows:

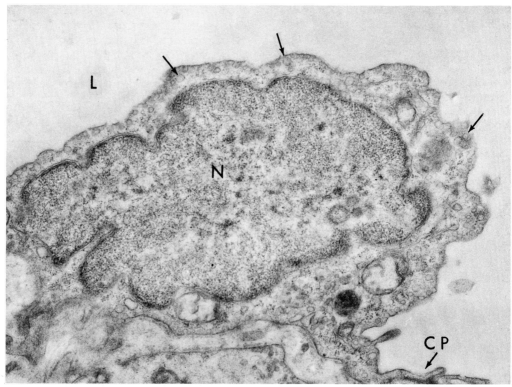

FIGURE 25–4. Electron micrograph of a mesothelial cell, rat peritoneum. A cytoplasmic process (CP) with a few microvilli may be noted. Such processes form much of the peritoneal covering. Note the comparatively large nucleus (N). Numerous pinocytotic vesicles (*arrows*) may be noted in the cytoplasm. L, lumen of peritoneal cavity. (×17,000)

Pleura. The exudates may be caused by pleurisy secondary to pneumonia or abscess of the lungs, tuberculosis, or bacterial or fungal infection.

Peritoneum. The exudates may result from peritonitis secondary to a visceral injury or pathologic perforation, tuberculosis, primary bacterial peritonitis (rarely seen except in children), or, in women, peritonitis secondary to inflammatory processes within the genital tract.

Pericardium. These may result from bacterial pericarditis or tuberculosis.

Exudates Caused by Tumors

The tumors producing exudates are rarely benign or primary, but are commonly malignant and metastatic. Experimental studies by Siegler and Koprowska on the mechanism of ascites formation in mice in the presence of cancer cells indicated the following sequence of events: within 24 hours after intraperitoneal inoculation, cancer cells penetrated through the mesothelium and established colonies within the subperitoneal tissue. At 48 hours solid tumor growth was established, associated with local capillary rupture. The flow of cancer cells in the direction of the peritoneal cavity, accompanied by a leakage of plasma from the injured capillaries and lymphatics began on the third day. Thus, in this experimental setting, the formation of ascites, containing malignant cells, was conditioned by damage to the capillaries and lymphatics by colonies of cancer cells. It is likely that a similar mechanism is operative in humans.

Other Causes of Exudates

Exudates may occur in a variety of diseases and disease states other than infection or tumors. Thus, rheumatoid arthritis, uremia, lupus erythematosus, lung infarct, etc., may be associated with exudates. Exudates may also be induced by certain drugs and may occur in disease states of still unknown etiology, such as eosinophilic pleural effusion. These disorders and their cytologic manifestations will be discussed below.

Hemothorax, Hemoperitoneum, and Hemopericardium

These terms denote the presence of bloody fluid in one of the body cavities. The hemorrhagic component may either be due to trauma or to the rupture of a viscus. In such instances, gases are also present within the body cavity. Also, tuberculosis and, especially, *metastatic tumors* may be associated with a bloody effusion.

METHODS OF INVESTIGATION OF EFFUSIONS

The customary methods of investigation of causes of effusions are cytologic examination of the fluid and biopsy of the pleura, pericardium, or peritoneum, supplemented by biochemical and bacteriologic investigation. Storey et al. stated that cytologic examination and determination of protein levels were the most useful methods of assessment of pleural effusions. In the great majority of cancer patients the effusions had protein levels of 3 g/100 ml or more. Protein values of less than 3 g/100 ml encompassed most patients with congestive heart failure, the principal cause of chronic effusions in the absence of cancer.

A number of biochemical methods is also used in the evaluation of effusions. Thus, the level of lactic dehydrogenase and other enzymes, several antigens (human chorionic gonadotrophin [hCG], carcinoembryonic antigen [CEA, CA-125— useful in ovarian carcinoma]) are often measured. The value of these procedures is still being debated. They sometimes supplement, but rarely replace, the cytologic examination.

Several immunocytologic procedures have also been proposed to identify cancer cells, effusions being a common target (Coleman and Ormerod, 1984; Johnston, 1987). The subtyping of lymphocytes in effusions has also been reported (Guzman et al., 1988) (see Chap. 34 for further discussion).

The value of biopsies when compared with cytologic examination is discussed on page 1177.

CELL POPULATIONS IN EFFUSIONS

Effusions as a Tissue Culture Medium

In the absence of disease, the fluids within the body cavities are limited to an insignificant lubricating layer that cannot be aspirated. Therefore, the mere presence of a fluid in any of the body cavities and, especially, a quantity of fluid sufficient for aspiration, indicates a pathologic process. Although the main purpose of cytologic investigation in such cases is to determine the presence or the absence of tumors, the diagnosis of many other conditions may be accomplished.

The body fluids constitute an ideal natural tissue culture medium wherein desquamated cells, benign and malignant, may proliferate freely. The temperature, the supply of nutrients, the oxygen and carbon dioxide are provided by the body of the patient and regulated by much finer homeostatic mechanisms than is possible in vitro. The morphology of cells growing in tissue culture is usually quite different from the cells of origin (see Fig. 1–1). Specifically, in actively growing tissue cultures the morphologic differentiation of benign from malignant cells is often very difficult. For this reason, the morphology of free-floating, and often proliferating, cells in effusions may be at considerable variance with that of cells of similar origin removed directly from the tissue. This accounts for some of the problems of morphologic cell identification and diagnosis. It also offers the benefit of study of these cells and their interrelationships in their natural setting. Many of the established human cell lines used for in vitro studies have their origin in human effusions, rather than in solid tissues. Apparently, the ability of these cells to proliferate in the effusion enhances the chances of successful growth in the laboratory. Thus, the study of fluids constitutes a precious scientific resource which is barely beginning to be explored.

The principal cell types encountered in the absence of cancer are: *mesothelial cells, macrophages* (histiocytes), *leukocytes,* and *other benign cells.* These are described in the following pages.

Mesothelial Cells

An effusion within the body cavities brings about separation of the two mesothelial layers and, as a consequence, the mesothelial lining cells become cuboidal. In the presence of an inflammatory process, and sometimes under other circumstances,

the orderly arrangement of the mesothelial cells is disturbed. There may be extensive proliferation both in thickness and in depth, with the formation of several layers of mesothelial cells and sinuses and channels in continuity with the surface (Fig. 25–5). The cuboidal mesothelial cells desquamate from the surface and may accumulate or even proliferate in the body fluids.

When mesothelial cells are scraped or aspirated by a needle from the surface of the pleural or abdominal cavity, they appear as tightly fitting sheets of polygonal cells, about 20 μm in diameter, with delicate, yet sharply demarcated, cyanophilic or eosinophilic cytoplasm and round or oval nuclei. The nuclei, generally located in the center of the cell, are of even size, sharply demarcated, slightly granular, and contain one or two, centrally located, readily visible chromocenters or nucleoli. Occasionally, a central fold may appear in the nucleus (Figs. 25–6 and 25–7).

Free-floating mesothelial cells in fluids appear singly and in clusters. On the basis of scanning and transmission electron microscopy, it is quite certain that many single cells hitherto thought to be of mesothelial origin are in reality macrophages (histiocytes), as will be set forth below. Nevertheless, the general guidelines for the identification of the mesothelial cells can be given.

Single mesothelial cells in body fluids are usually round or oval and measure between 10 and 20 μm in diameter. The cyanophilic or faintly eosinophilic cytoplasm is sharply demarcated (Fig. 25–8). It is not uncommon to recognize two cytoplasmic zones: a perinuclear, denser zone, and a peripheral, clear zone. The difference is due to accumulation of cell organelles in the perinuclear area. Spriggs and Meek pointed out that free-float-

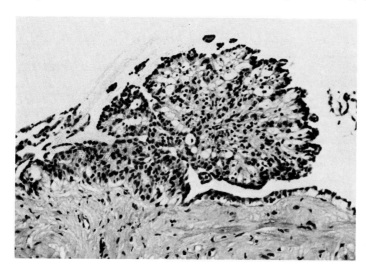

FIGURE 25–5. Benign proliferation of mesothelial cells, wall of hydrocele. This degree of proliferation is unusual. ($\times$140)

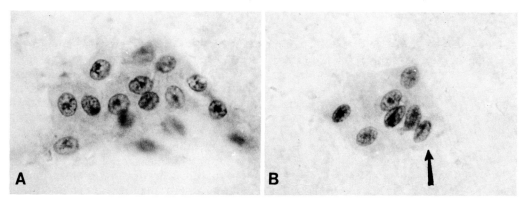

FIGURE 25-6. (*A, B*) Two sheets of mesothelial cells removed by scraping from the parietal pleura. Note tightly fitting arrangement of polygonal cells. The individual cell boundaries cannot be well identified. The nuclei are uniform in size and configuration, with a single, usually centrally located chromocenter or nucleolus. In some of the nuclei a longitudinal fold may be noted (*arrow*). (*A, B* ×560)

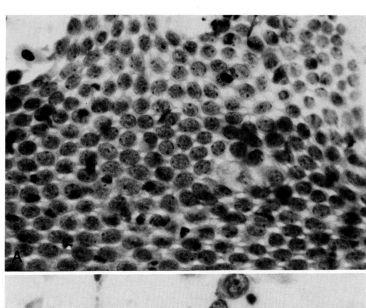

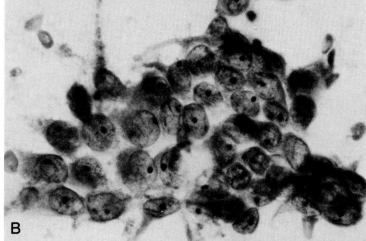

FIGURE 25-7. Sheets of mesothelial cells of pleura in a thin-needle aspirate. The relationship of the cells is well shown in (*A*). The cell borders are clearly outlined. Narrow gaps or "windows" separate cells from each other. The nuclei are of monotonous, equal sizes; each is provided with a prominent, but exceedingly regular, spherical nucleolus, better seen in (*B*). (*A* ×500; *B* ×800. Modified from Koss, L.G., et al.: Aspiration Biopsy: Cytologic Interpretation and Histologic Bases. New York, Igaku-Shoin, 1984, with permission)

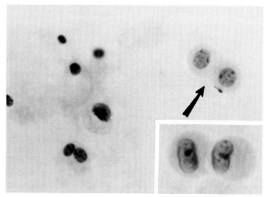

FIGURE 25-8. Pleural effusion. Mesothelial cells and macrophages (histiocytes). Two mesothelial cells (*arrow*) attached to each other may be contrasted with macrophages. The latter have a cytoplasm studded with fine vacuoles and a peripheral nucleus. The cell size and nuclear characteristics of single cells are very similar for both cell types. (*Inset*) High magnification of two mesothelial cells. Note the indentation in the cell membrane of one cell to accommodate the convexity of the adjacent cell, which has a kidney-shaped nucleus. The two cells appear to be separated by a narrow clear space, or a "window." A sex chromatin body may be seen in one of the cells. (×560; *inset* ×1,000)

ing mesothelial cells in effusions may show a narrow brush border that may be observed both in light and electron microscopic preparations (see Fig. 25-3). In light microscopy the mesothelial cells often show a clear zone surrounding the cell

membrane, probably corresponding to a poorly preserved brush border.

The nuclei of free-floating mesothelial cells are large and occupy about half of the cell diameter. The nucleus is usually centrally located within the cell. The morphologic characteristics of the nucleus are of great diagnostic importance. The nuclear membrane is prominent. The chromatin net is fine and rather inconspicuous, with a few small, but sharply defined, chromocenters and occasionally one or two small, round nucleoli. In female patients a single sex chromatin body may occasionally be observed (see Fig. 25-8).

Mesothelial cells in fluids are more readily identified in clusters. The clusters may be large and composed of several dozen cells or, more often, are made up of a smaller number of cells. In general, clusters of mesothelial cells are flat and consist of a single layer of uniform cells adhering well to each other (Figs. 25-9 and 25-10). The uniformity of the nuclei speaks strongly in favor of their mesothelial origin, even if the details of nuclear structure are obscured. In smaller clusters, the mesothelial cells often display a molding of cell surfaces (Fig. 25-11). Sometimes adjacent molded mesothelial cells appear to be separated from each other by a narrow, regular, slitlike clear space that is occasionally referred to as a "window" (Figs. 3-8, 25-8, and 25-12). The nature of this clear space is not definitely known, but it may represent surface structures (microvilli or blebs) observed on mesothelial cells by scanning electron microscopy (see Fig. 25-16). The flat clusters may contain two,

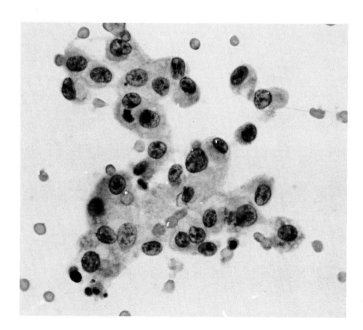

FIGURE 25-9. A sheet of mesothelial cells from pleural fluid: no evidence of cancer. The relationship of the cells, although not as clear as in aspirated material (see Fig. 25-7) may still be recognized. The cell borders are well defined, although the clear gaps (windows) are not seen in this photograph. The spherical or ovoid nuclei are of approximately equal size and contain one or two small chromocenters or nucleoli. (×560)

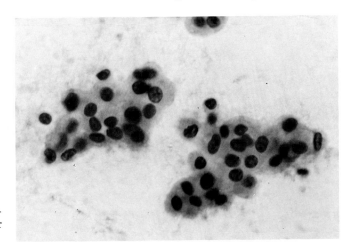

FIGURE 25-10. Pericardial tap; papillary clusters of uniform mesothelial cells. The nuclear structure is obscured in this material. (×560)

three, four, or more cells, which sometimes are arranged in short chains (see Fig. 25-11 and 25-12). The nuclear features are essentially similar to those seen in tissue scrapes (see Fig. 25-6), although occasionally the nuclei stain more intensely with hematoxylin, especially in fluids aspirated after a long period of accumulation in a body cavity. The nuclear structure in the latter cells cannot be studied, but the cell size and nuclear configuration are comparable with those of better-preserved cells (see Fig. 25-12). The mesothelial cells may also form much larger clusters, wherein the monolayer arrangement of tightly fitting cells may no longer be seen (see Fig. 25-9). Such large clusters often occur as a consequence of abnormal proliferation of mesothelial surfaces, such as shown in Fig. 25-3, and often contain visible nucleoli (Fig. 25-13). The identification of such clusters as mesothelial in origin is based primarily on the uniformity of nuclear size and lack of significant variation in nuclear structure. Occasionally, mesothelial cells form papillary or rosettelike arrangements characterized by small, uniform nuclei (Fig. 25-14A,B). These usually differ by nuclear features from similar cell clusters occurring in malignant tumors (see p. 1132). In extreme cases, however, such as the one described by Spriggs and Jerrome in 1979, "tumor-ball"-like structures may be formed by mesothelial cells. In such rare cases, the diagnosis of "benign cells" may be impossible.

There is excellent evidence that mesothelial cells are capable of multiplying while free-floating in effusions (see Fig. 25-14C). The mitotic figures are usually of normal configuration, but, on very rare occasion, an atypical mitosis may be observed (see Fig. 25-28). A cell-in-cell arrangement in which one mesothelial cell appears to be engulfed by another may occur, although this is more commonly a function of macrophages (see Fig. 25-19, 25-28A, and 25-31).

In the absence of rapid processing or proper fixation, the mesothelial cells may become ballooned up with a concomitant loss of the details of nuclear structure (Fig. 25-15), making identification difficult.

For special comments on pericardial fluid see p. 1112.

Special Stains in Identification of Mesothelial Cells. In 1959, Nathan Chandler Foot examined the specificity of the periodic acid-Schiff reagent (PAS) for the mesothelial cell. He found, as did Ceelen, that the cytoplasm of most mesothelial cells contains PAS-positive granules concentrated at the periphery and representing, in all likelihood, neutral mucopolysaccharides. Although the cytoplasm of some of the cancer cells also takes the dye,

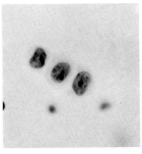

FIGURE 25-11. A chain composed of three tightly fitting mesothelial cells. The cell and nuclear characteristics are the same as in Fig. 25-6. (×560)

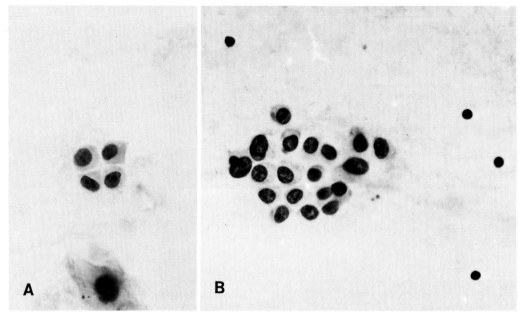

FIGURE 25-12. Pleural fluids—first taps—no evidence of cancer. Two clusters of benign cells with dark, somewhat hyperchromatic nuclei of even size. (*A*) The mesothelial origin of the cells is secure because of the molding of cell surfaces and the presence of slitlike clear areas (windows) separating the cells. In (*B*), which also contains normal lymphocytes, the nuclear characteristics of the clustered cells are the same, but the cells are rounded and their cytoplasmic border is not crisp. It cannot be stated with complete certainty whether these are mesothelial cells or macrophages. (*A, B* ×560)

the red color is diffuse and not confined to the granules. Foot recommended Mowry's stain for the differential diagnostic staining.

Mavrommatis, also using Mowry's technique, generally confirmed the observations of Foot, but suggested caution in the interpretation of results.

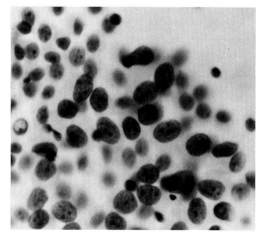

FIGURE 25-13. Sheets of mesothelial cells. Chronic pleurisy. Note small nucleoli and striking uniformity of nuclei. (×560).

Pfitzer, using alcian–PAS-staining technique, observed bright scarlet granules in benign mesothelial cells (and in cells from a case of malignant mesothelioma) and also in other malignant cells. Pfitzer denied any diagnostic value in the use of PAS technique. In my experience, the PAS method is rarely of diagnostic assistance in a critical morphologic situation. Of greater use are stains identifying mucin, such as mucicarmine. Mucicarmine-positive granules have never been observed in this laboratory in mesothelial cells. Their presence in an appropriately controlled setting invariably indicates a mucin-producing carcinoma.

Many attempts have been made to identify cancer cells in effusions by the use of oncofetal antigens and monoclonal antibodies (MAb) (see p. 1136 and Chap. 34). A monoclonal antibody recognizing mesothelial cells, developed by Singh, was used by us in the identification of a mesothelioma of the tunica vaginalis of the testis (Japko et al., 1982). The applicability of this MAb to routine cytologic targets was not tested.

Macrophages (Histiocytes)

Studies based on scanning and transmission electron microscopy of fluids disclosed that many cells

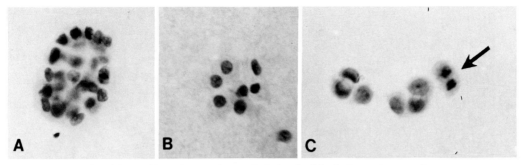

FIGURE 25–14. (*A*) Papillary cluster of mesothelial cells (alcoholic cirrhosis with massive ascites, proved by autopsy). Note the three-dimensional structure of the cluster, with many cells out of focus. Note also the small size of the cells and the uniformity of the small nuclei. For differential diagnosis with similarly structured clusters of malignant tumors, see text. (*B*) Rosettelike grouping of mesothelial cells. Ascites in Laennec's cirrhosis of the liver. (*C*) Group of mesothelial cells; one is in mitosis (*arrow*). (*A, B, C* ×560)

that have been hitherto classified as of mesothelial origin belong to the family of macrophages (Domagala and Woyke; Murad; Domagala and Koss). The surface configuration of the two cell types in scanning electron microscopy discloses major differences. The mesothelial cells are characterized by the presence of regular short microvilli or a mixture of microvilli with bleblike surface structures, the latter characterizing older cells. The macrophages have a very characteristic surface configuration, wherein the cell membrane forms folds or ridges (Fig. 25–16). The features of macrophages in transmission electron microscopy are discussed in Chapter 3. Although mesothelial cells contain some lysosomes (Cotran and Karnovsky), they do not possess the elaborate lysosomal apparatus characterizing the macrophages.

The macrophages are of bone marrow origin and represent transformed monocytes. Occasionally, however, mesothelial cells may acquire phagocytic properties and morphologic features that make the differentiation between these two cell types extremely difficult by light microscopy. Efrati and Nir observed ultrastructural cell changes in pleural and peritoneal effusions that they interpreted as evidence of transition between mesothelial cells and macrophages. These observations are insecure because the criteria for the light microscopic identification of the two cell types were not given. The issue is rarely of diagnostic significance.

In effusions, the macrophages appear as monto onucleated cells similar in size to mesothelial cells (10 to 20 μm in diameter). They usually occur singly or in loosely arranged clusters and never show

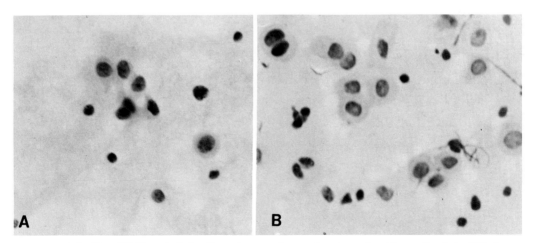

FIGURE 25–15. (*A*) Mesothelial cells and macrophages. Specimen fixed immediately in 50% alcohol. (*B*) Same specimen; no fixative added for several hours preceding the processing of smears. Note the blown-up cells and hazy appearance of the nuclei. (*A, B* ×560)

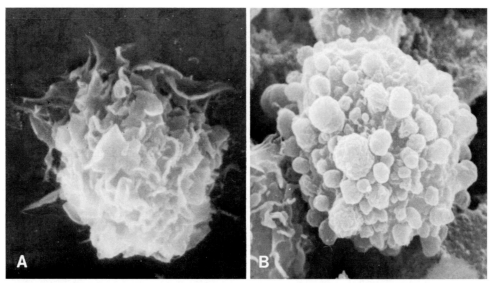

FIGURE 25–16.   Pleural fluid. Scanning electron microscopy of two cells of approximately equal size (10 μm in diameter) and similar light microscopic configuration. Cell (*A*) shows a surface arrangement of folds and ridges, identifying it as a macrophage. Cell (*B*) shows short microvilli and blebs on its surface, identifying it as a mesothelial cell. (*A* ×5,500; *B* ×4,600. Courtesy of Dr. W. Domagala)

cytoplasmic molding. The macrophages are characterized by a foamy cytoplasm, studded with minute vacuoles, and a cell border that readily blends with smear background, in contrast with the sharply demarcated mesothelial cells (see Fig. 25–8). The nuclei of macrophages are usually peripheral and sometimes stain somewhat denser than the nuclei of mesothelial cells present in the same field (Figs. 25–17 and 25–18). Kidney-shaped nuclei may be observed in both cell types. The nuclear configuration or staining properties are of limited value in the separation of macrophages from mesothelial cells.

The cytoplasm of the macrophages may become markedly distended with large vacuoles (Fig. 25–19). Bi- and multinucleated macrophages may occasionally be observed (Fig. 25–20). The latter cells are large and in no way differ from foreign

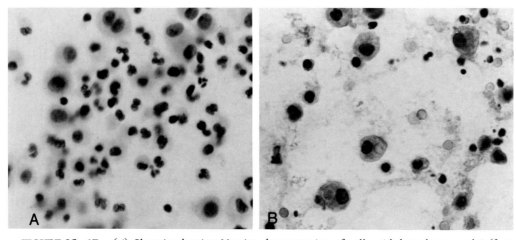

FIGURE 25–17.   (*A*) Chronic pleurisy. Massive desquamation of cells with hazy large nuclei (first tap). Numerous mesothelial cells, leukocytes, and macrophages are present. (*B*) Pleural effusion in pneumonia caused by *Legionella*, as proved by culture. The dominant cells are macrophages and lymphocytes. (*A*, *B* ×560).

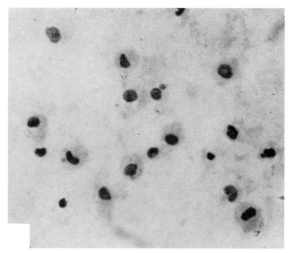

FIGURE 25–18. Sheets of macrophages in ascites. Numerous granules of ingested material are readily noticeable in the phagocytic cells. (×560)

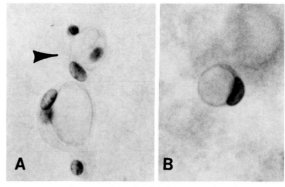

FIGURE 25–19. Pleural fluid. Vacuolated macrophages. Note the displacement of the nucleus to the periphery of the cells. Also shown in (*A*) is a macrophage wherein the vacuole contains a phagocytized cell (*arrowhead*). There is also a small, nonvacuolated macrophage in this field. (*A* ×560; *B* ×1,000)

body giant cells, Langhans' cells, or other polykaryons (see p. 1094). They are usually observed in fluids after introduction of foreign material during surgery or after another stimulus, such as radiotherapy (Figs. 25–20 and 25–21).

Phagocytic activity and lysosomal activity are characteristic functions of macrophages. These features may be used to good advantage in the identification of these cells in light microscopy.

Particle or cell engulfment by macrophages (see Figs. 25–18 and 25–19) may be observed. The use of stain for iron may disclose phagocytized particles of hemosiderin. Iron stain may be of particular value in chronic hemorrhagic pleurisy or pericarditis, wherein large hemosiderin deposits in macrophages may obscure their nuclei and may mimic malignant melanoma. Stains for enzymes, such as acid phosphatase or esterases, may document the

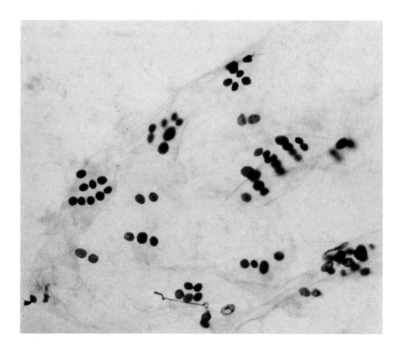

FIGURE 25–20. Ascitic fluid. Numerous multinucleated giant macrophages, observed after surgery and radiotherapy for ovarian carcinoma. (×350)

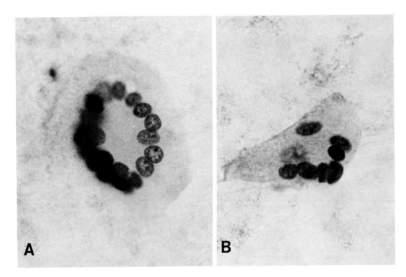

FIGURE 25–21. (*A*, *B*) Forms of multinucleated macrophages (polykaryons). Note the similarity of the cells in (*A*) to a Langhans' giant cell. (×560)

intense lysosomal activity. None of these functions is normally observed in mesothelial cells. Bakalos et al. advocated the use of the Sudan black-B stain for positive identification of macrophages and other phagocytic cells.

Macrophages in effusion smears may also be identified by supravital staining with neutral red or Janus green (reported by Hazard and by Foot and Holmquist). The method allows for differentiation between leukocytes and macrophages that accept the stain and mesothelial and cancer cells that do not.

In the past, it had been thought that the presence of macrophages reflected a chronic inflammatory process. Current evidence strongly suggests that macrophages are ubiquitous cells that appear in effusions not only as a consequence of inflamma-

tion, but also in the presence of cancer and, presumably, under other circumstances as well. The relationship of macrophages to cancer cells is discussed on p. 1136.

In some infectious effusions, notably in *Legionella micdadei* infection, the macrophages may be the dominant cell population (see Fig. 25–17*B*).

Leukocytes

Leukocytes in effusions are extremely common. In cases of long-standing effusion, lymphocytes may be predominant (Fig. 25–22). If they are numerous—and especially if no other leukocytes are present—the possibility of tuberculosis, lymphocytic leukemia, or lymphosarcoma should be investigated. Typing and enumeration of B and T

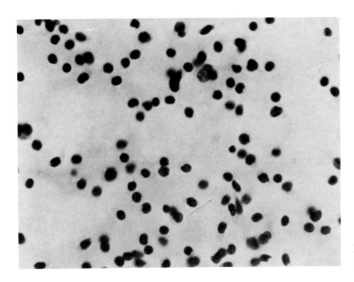

FIGURE 25–22. Tuberculous pleural effusion. Numerous lymphocytes are present. (×560)

lymphocytes and their subtypes may be of diagnostic value. The implications of this observation in reference to cancer is discussed on p. 1137.

Polymorphonuclear neutrophilic leukocytes invariably indicate an inflammatory process, which may be secondary to cancer or to other disorders. Eosinophilic leukocytes may be seen in eosinophilic pleural effusions (see below) and in a variety of inflammatory processes. They are not uncommon in tuberculosis, but are rarely seen in cases of Hodgkins' disease.

Plasma cells may be noted in chronic inflammatory processes in multiple myeloma, and in Hodgkin's disease (see p. 1161). *In the presence of an extensive inflammatory process, for reasons emphasized on page 1097, the diagnosis of cancer should not be made, except on the strength of irrefutable evidence.*

Other Benign Cells Encountered in Effusions

Cells similar to *Anitschkow's myocytes*, with their very characteristic central bar of chromatin, from which radiate numerous short lateral processes, have been noted in a rare case of effusion of long standing and of unknown etiology (Fig. 25–23). *Liver cells*, singly or in sheets, may be observed if this organ is penetrated accidentally while fluids are aspirated from the right pleural cavity (Fig. 25–24). The identification is quite easy because of the large size of the cells and their abundant, faintly vacuolated cytoplasm surrounding large single or double nuclei. Characteristically, tiny, green-staining intracytoplasmic bile deposits may be observed in the fresh preparations. In older preparations, the bile forms amorphous masses.

Readily recognizable ciliated *respiratory cells* and dust-containing macrophages in pleural fluid

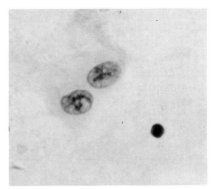

FIGURE 25–23. Cells resembling Anitschkow's myocytes in pleural fluid. Case of chronic pleural effusion of unknown etiology in a 46-year-old man. There was no evidence of cancer. (Approx. ×600)

may be the result of traumatic injury to lung tissue or may suggest a bronchopleural fistula or a teratoma.

Squamous Cells. In general, the presence of squamous cells in effusions suggests a squamous carcinoma (see p. 1138). In a case described by Cobb et al. (1985), benign squamous cells, anucleated squames, and hair shafts were observed in pleural fluid in a boy with ruptured benign cystic teratoma (dermoid cyst) of the anterior mediastinum. Squamous cells derived from the epidermis of the skin are virtually never seen in effusions.

Megakaryocytes and Other Hematopoetic Cells. Calle (1968) was the first to observe these cells in abdominal fluid of a female patient with myeloid metaplasia (see Fig. 19–19). Extramedullary hematopoesis appears to be the common de-

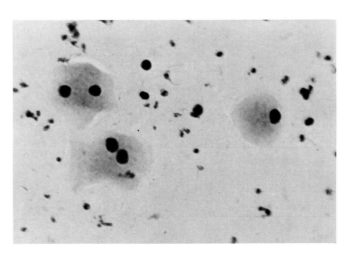

FIGURE 25–24. Mono- and binucleated large liver cells in fluid aspirated from right pleural cavity. (×560)

nominator of cases reported by others (Vilaseca et al., 1981; Pedio et al., 1985; Silverman, 1985). Bartziota and Naylor (1986) observed megakaryocytes in a bloody pleural effusion in a patient with overdose of an anticoagulant.

Fat cells and striated muscle originating in subcutaneous fat and muscle, may be noted occasionally. They indicate accidental inclusions in the course of tapping.

Acellular Components in Effusions

Curschmann's Spirals. Curschmann's spirals are commonly observed in sputum as protein casts derived from bronchioles. Similar structures have now been observed in effusions. Wahl (1986) observed these structures in nine peritoneal washings, two pleural fluids, and in a peritoneal dialysis fluid. Wahl hypothesized that the spirals were possibly of connective tissue origin. Naylor (personal communication, 1989) confirmed Wahl's observation in three pleural and two peritoneal fluids. In two of the cases, Curschmann's spirals were associated with mucus-producing adenocarcinoma, in one patient with pseudomyxoma peritonei, and in two patients with inflammation.

The spirals were very similar to those seen in the respiratory tract, except for their smaller size (Fig. 25–25). Naylor suggested that some of the spirals could be the product of mucus-producing cancer cells and, in inflammatory processes, be derived from connective tissue mucins. It may be, of course, that the spirals are an artifact of processing and protein precipitation.

Immunoglobulin Crystals. Martin et al. (1987) observed spindle-shaped, extracellular crystals and crystalline inclusions in macrophages in ascitic fluid from a patient with cryoglobulinemia. The authors postulated that the crystals (confirmed by electron microscopy) represented crystallized immunoglobulin in a patient with plasma cell dyscrasia.

Charcot–Leyden Crystals. These spindle-shaped crystals have a close relationship with eosinophils, whence they are derived (see Fig. 19–17). Krishnan et al. (1983) observed Charcot–Leyden crystals in pleural fluid rich in eosinophils in a young patient with a benign cystic teratoma. Naylor and Novak (1985) observed the crystals in eight patients with eosinophilic pleural effusion, two of which were "idiopathic" and six associated with other disorders (for description of eosinophilic pleural effusion, see p. 1099).

Hemoglobin Crystals. These crystals, phagocytized by polymorphonuclear leukocytes in pleural and cerebrospinal fluid, were reported by Zaharopoulos and Wong (1987), the result of polymerization of hemoglobin molecules occurring for unknown reasons.

Oxalate Crystals. Such crystals were observed in pleural fluid by Reyes et al. (1979) in a case of aspergillosis.

Cholesterol Crystals. These crystals may be observed in chronic effusions of long duration.

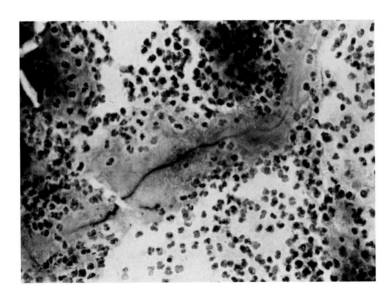

FIGURE 25–25. A Curschmann's spiral in pleural fluid in a 52-year-old man with empyema. Note the condensed central core and fuzzy coat. Numerous polymorphonuclear leukocytes, characteristic of empyema, surround the spiral. (×208. Courtesy of Dr. Bernard Naylor, Ann Arbor, Michigan)

Naylor (1990) reported such crystals in effusions in rheumatoid arthritis.

CELLULAR PATTERNS OF EFFUSIONS IN VARIOUS NONCANCEROUS DISEASES

Guidelines in the Interpretation of Chronic Effusions

Regardless of cause, effusions of long standing are often characterized by an accumulation of poorly preserved cells of mesothelial type and of macrophages that cannot always be accurately identified and are often very numerous (see Fig. 25–17). This is particularly important in the first tap, which may yield large, blown-up mesothelial cells with enlarged, hyperchromatic nuclei (see Fig. 25–15). It is likely that such mesothelial cells are old or dead, and that their enlargement is due to the loss of selective permeability of the cellular membrane. In some such instances, an erroneous diagnosis of cancer is readily made if the clinical history is not taken into account. In general, well-fixed and well-prepared material that is not subjected to excessive handling in the laboratory is easier to interpret and lends itself less to an erroneous diagnosis of cancer.

Nevertheless, for reasons that are not clear, the mesothelial cells and macrophages may occasionally assume a very abnormal appearance that makes their differentiation from cells of metastatic tumors exceedingly difficult. These abnormalities may affect individual cells or the grouping of cells and, fortunately, are quite rare.

As a rule a thumb, the association of cancer cells with a severe inflammatory reaction in an effusion is uncommon; this would usually indicate perforation of a viscus by a malignant process and result in a critical clinical situation. On the other hand, such inflammatory processes as tuberculosis usually persist for a considerable time before the patient comes to the hospital. Thus, if cancer is suspected, but the fluid shows massive evidence of an inflammatory process, it is advisable to interpret the material with caution and with knowledge of the clinical setting.

The clinical history is of paramount importance in evaluating fluid specimens of a borderline nature. If there is the slightest suspicion that the abnormal cells may be benign, the diagnosis of cancer should not be made. Only too often a patient with an erroneous diagnosis of metastatic carcinoma to a body cavity may be deprived of effective treatment for a treatable disease.

General diagnostic guidelines that help to avoid diagnostic mistakes, and especially the erroneous diagnosis of cancer, are as follows:

1. An accurate clinical history must be obtained.
2. Protein determination must be made. If the protein is less than 3 g/100 ml, the presence of cancer is much less likely than if protein is above 3 g/100 ml.
3. Cytologic diagnosis of cancer should be *avoided* if: (*a*) the morphology of cells is not optimal; (*b*) the cells and nuclear sizes are monotonous and within upper limits of normal (25 μm in diameter), and the nuclei do not appear significantly enlarged for size of cells; (*c*) there are no obvious structural nuclear abnormalities; or (*d*) there is evidence of an inflammatory process with numerous polymorphonuclear leukocytes, macrophages, and cell necrosis.

Occasionally, the diagnostic dilemmas are solved on the second tap, which will display the morphology of the cells in fluids to a better advantage.

The availability of well-fixed material and technically satisfactory preparations is particularly important in these difficult diagnostic situations. Most of the errors are made on technically inadequate material, such as thick, overstained smears, poorly prepared and stained filter preparations, and inadequate evidence in cell blocks. It must be pointed out that the packaging of centrifuged material in paraffin for cell block preparation may create artifacts of cell configuration, such as clustering, that may sometimes be misleading to an inexperienced observer.

Specific Nonmalignant Disease States Associated with Effusions

General and Circulatory Disorders

Hypoproteinemia. Low protein levels in the blood may cause accumulation of fluids in all three body cavities and generalized edema (anasarca). The causes are various and comprise inadequate nutrition and various renal diseases. Fluids may occasionally be submitted for cytologic examination. These are classic transudates, with a low protein level and low cell content that do not cause any diagnostic dilemmas.

Congestive Heart Failure. Congestive heart failure is perhaps the most common cause of chronic pleural effusion not due to cancer. Accumulation of pericardial and ascitic fluid may also occur. Although it is frequently stated that the right pleural cavity is more commonly affected, in my experience, the distribution of effusions is about equilateral. The fluids often have a low protein content and scant cellularity; hence, they correspond to the classic transudates. They rarely cause any particular diagnostic dilemma except in an occasional case of heart failure associated with inflammatory changes, wherein numerous polymorphonuclear leukocytes accompany poorly preserved macrophages and mesothelial cells in sheets or clusters. Heart failure in rheumatic heart disease is the common background of such findings, but similar observations can be made in congestive heart failure associated with pneumonia or pulmonary infarction. The reader is referred to the general discussion above for the guidelines in the diagnostic interpretation of this type of material.

Pleural Effusion in Pulmonary Infarcts. Embolization of pulmonary vessels need not necessarily be associated with pulmonary infarcts. Acute infarction does not usually result in an immediate effusion, but, as the infarct becomes organized, a marked pleural reaction may set in and result in a chronic pleural effusion, which may be tapped for relief of the patient or for diagnostic study. It is evident from Fig. 25–26 that in such fluids proliferation of mesothelial cells may be very marked and

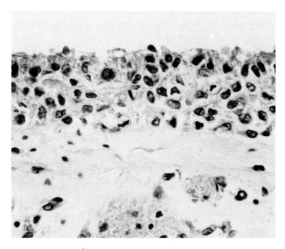

FIGURE 25–26. Pulmonary infarct. Pleural reaction overlying a healing pulmonary infarct. Note the hyperplastic and multilayered mesothelial lining with considerable nuclear variability, the source of atypical mesothelial cells in pleural fluids from such patients. (×650. Courtesy of Dr. B. S. Bhagavan, Baltimore, Maryland)

may cause major diagnostic problems if sheets and clusters of mesothelial cells are present (cf. Fig. 25–9).

Inflammatory Processes

Acute Inflammatory Processes. Acute bacterial pneumonia, lung abscess, acute pleurisy, pericarditis, peritonitis, and postsurgical states are frequently associated with accumulation of fluid in one or more of the body cavities. Such fluids rarely present a diagnostic dilemma because they are composed of purulent exudate, containing numerous polymorphonuclear leukocytes and necrotic material. As has been mentioned above, it is not prudent to make a diagnosis of cancer under these circumstances except in the presence of overwhelming evidence.

The cell population differs in *legionnaires' disease* and in *viral pneumonia*. Therein the cell content of pleural effusions is dominated by lymphocytes and macrophages (see Fig. 25–17*B*).

Chronic Inflammatory Processes. Chronic pneumonia, pericarditis, and peritonitis of various causes may also cause accumulation of fluid in body cavities. The cytologic interpretation of this material may cause some of the principal difficulties outlined above. The classic example of such difficulties is tuberculosis.

Tuberculous Effusions. Pleural effusions in pulmonary tuberculosis wherein the pleura is not directly involved are characterized by predominance of lymphocytes (see Fig. 25–22). Few macrophages or mesothelial cells are present. The differential diagnosis comprises leukemias and malignant lymphomas (see p. 1094) and, occasionally, viral pneumonia.

Direct involvement of the body cavities by the tuberculous process (tuberculous pleurisy, pericarditis, and peritonitis) may result in a major diagnostic dilemma because of a marked proliferation of mesothelial cells in sheets and clusters, many of which may assume papillary configuration (Fig. 25–27). The presence of marked inflammation and necrosis in smear background may prevent the erroneous diagnosis of cancer by an alert observer.

In general, the specific diagnosis of tuberculosis cannot be made on the basis of fluid cytology. The presence of Langhans' giant cells is not specific (see Fig. 25–21). Granulomas may be observed on pleural or peritoneal biopsies which should be a part of proper workup of patients. While microbiologic studies of fluids are usually of limited yield

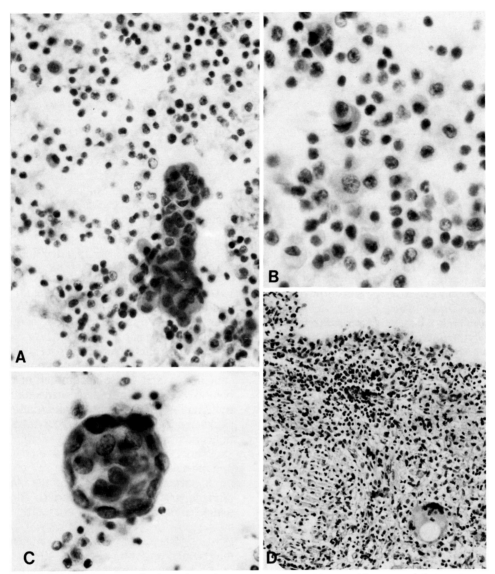

FIGURE 25–27. Ascitic fluid in tuberculous peritonitis in a 23-year-old woman. (*A*) Low-power view of the material showing the presence of large papillary clusters of mesothelial cells against a background of a marked inflammatory reaction. (*B*, *C*) Details of mesothelial cell structure and arrangement. In (*B*) a cell-in-cell is noted; in (*C*), a papillary cluster that could not be distinguished from that of a papillary carcinoma. The nuclei are uniform in size and fail to show large nucleoli. (*D*) Histologic section of peritoneal biopsy showing granulomatous inflammation. There was a bacteriologic confirmation of tuberculosis. (*A* ×350; *B*, *C* ×560; *D* ×140. Case courtesy of Dr. Lucy Feiner, Queens General Hospital, New York, New York)

(Storey et al.), the diagnosis must still be confirmed by culture.

Nonspecific Chronic Inflammatory Processes. Such processes may occasionally produce major abnormalities of mesothelial cells, such as cell engulfment and, on rare occasion, abnormal mitotic figures (Fig. 25–28). Under these circumstances an erroneous diagnosis of cancer is virtually unavoidable. For further comments on abnormal mitotic figures in fluids see p. 1132.

Eosinophilic Pleural Effusion. The exact etiology of this ill-defined group of diseases is not

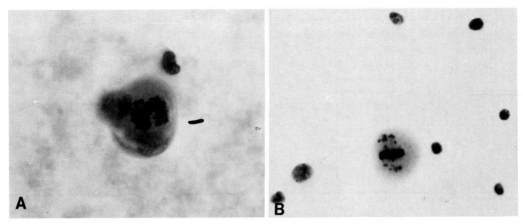

FIGURE 25 – 28. (*A*) Pleural fluid. Chronic pleurisy of inflammatory etiology; no evidence of cancer. An atypical mitotic figure in a mesothelial cell, engulfed by another mesothelial cell or macrophage, an extremely rare event. (*B*) Atypical mitosis, apparently of a mesothelial cell, in the absence of tumor. A marked chromosomal lag is observed. (*A* ×1,000; *B* ×600. *B* from Melamed, M. R.: The cytologic presentation of malignant lymphomas and related diseases in effusions. Cancer *16*:413–431, 1963)

clearly understood. There is lack of universal agreement about when an effusion should be so designated; the majority of authors suggest 10% of eosinophils as an acceptable criterion and others (Robertson) raise this to 50%. In my experience 10% of eosinophils is sufficient to designate a fluid as belonging to this group of diseases with their uniquely favorable prognosis. A number of factors, including allergy and hypersensitivity to drugs, trauma to the chest (Contino and Vance; Nanar et al.), pneumothorax (Spriggs) and asbestosis (Adelman et al. 1984), have been implicated in the pathogenesis of eosinophilic pleural effusion. Yet, in a substantial proportion of such cases, no clear-cut evidence of a sensitizing factor can be identified

and the term *idiopathic eosinophilic pleural effusion* is suggested for such cases. Synchronous eosinophilia in the peripheral blood is rare; hence, the effusion presumably reflects a local event confined to the pleura.

Kokkola and Valta studied 78 patients with pleural fluid containing 10% or more eosinophils. In 42 patients the effusion was idiopathic (i.e., not associated with any other disease state). Sixteen patients had some form of ill-defined "collagen disease" not confirmed by clinical data, 6 had cancer, and 14 had tuberculosis.

Of particular interest is the *idiopathic eosinophilic pleural effusion* (Fig. 25 – 29). The disease is usually unilateral, although bilateral effusion has

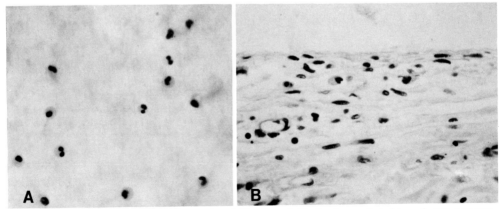

FIGURE 25 – 29. So-called idiopathic eosinophilic pleural effusion in a male in his early 50s. Approximately 50% of cells in the smear were eosinophilic polymorphonuclear leukocytes (*A*). An exploratory thoracotomy revealed only a nonspecific pleurisy (*B*). The peripheral blood picture was normal. No clinical reason for eosinophilic effusion was ever found, and the patient was in good health several years later. (*A, B* ×350)

been observed. It is not infrequent to observe it in young, otherwise healthy people whose sole complaints are referable to a long-standing accumulation of pleural fluid. Occasionally, the disease is totally disabling because of dyspnea. Veress, Schreiber, and Koss reviewed the data on 30 patients with eosinophilic pleural effusion observed at Montefiore Hospital between May 1974 and January 1977. There were 11 patients younger than 50 and 19 patients older than 50, reflecting the hospital population. Six patients had a past history of cancer. Four patients had a history of asthma and 8 of thoracic trauma. The summary of the key laboratory observations is given in Table 25–1.

It may be seen that eosinophilia in pleural fluid was accompanied by lymphocytosis. The fluids had a high specific gravity and high protein content, indicating that they were exudates. Lactic dehydrogenase (LDH) activity was within normal limits, in contrast with the observations in cancerous effusions (see p. 1176). The findings in the pleural fluid did not correlate with the findings in the peripheral blood. Only 4 of the 30 patients had blood eosinophilia of 10% or more.

On cytologic examination of the sediment, the key feature is the presence of numerous bilobate eosinophils, accompanied by lymphocytes, scarce mesothelial cells, which may be quite atypical, macrophages, and occasional plasma cells (Fig. 25–30). Pleural biopsies show either fibrosis of the pleura (see Fig. 25–29B) or chronic inflammation with deposition of fibrin (see Fig. 25–30). Eosinophils may be also observed in about 25% of all pleural biopsies. Naylor and Novak (1985) observed Charcot–Leyden crystals in several such cases (see above).

Regardless of the etiology and pathogenesis of the eosinophilic pleural effusion, it is usually self-limiting and has an excellent prognosis, although its course may be protracted, sometimes lasting 2 years. Twenty-eight of the 30 Montefiore Hosptial patients had adequate follow-up. Six patients died of myocardial infarction. In the remaining 22 patients, including the 6 patients with past history of cancer, the effusion cleared up without specific treatment.

Cirrhosis of the Liver

The cytologic investigation of ascitic fluid in patients with liver insufficiency is often of crucial clinical diagnostic importance. The clinical differential diagnosis usually comprises cirrhosis of the liver and various forms of primary or metastatic cancer.

In most patients the ascitic fluid in cirrhosis of the liver does not present a diagnostic challenge. The cell population is clearly identified as mesothelial cells or macrophages, and there is no inflammatory component. Occasionally, however, marked proliferation of mesothelial cells in the form of papillary clusters may be noted (see Fig. 25–14A,B).

In the presence of active cirrhosis with liver necrosis and jaundice, very atypical mesothelial cells in clusters may be observed (Fig. 25–31). Cell-in-cell, papillary, or rosettelike arrangement of mesothelial cells may be noted, accompanied by nuclear hyperchromasia and slight nuclear irregularities and enlargement. Such clusters may be accompanied by multinucleated macrophages that may suggest to an uninitiated observer giant cancer cells. In fact, the presence of such macrophages is most unusual in untreated cancer and should be construed as a clue to the benign nature of the lesion. The mesothelial cell nuclei, although enlarged and often hyperchromatic, are generally of

Table 25–1
Montefiore Medical Center: Summary of Some Important Laboratory Data in 30 Patients with Eosinophilic Pleural Effusion

	Blood		**Pleural Effusion**	
	Range	*Mean*	*Range*	*Mean*
Eosinophils (%)	0–50	7.17	12–85	38 (*n* = 43)*
Lymphocytes (%)	7–48	20.2	5–73	34 (*n* = 43)
Total protein g./dl.	5.2–8.3	6.9	2–5.9	4.19 (*n* = 33)
LDH (IU)†	124–1240	331	71–600	267 (*n* = 32)
Specific gravity			1.016–1.037	1.027 (*n* = 16)

* *n*, number of patients.
†LDH (IU), lactic dehydrogenase in international units per liter.

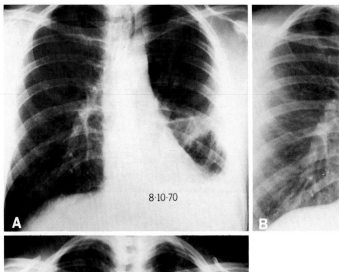

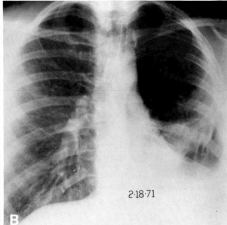

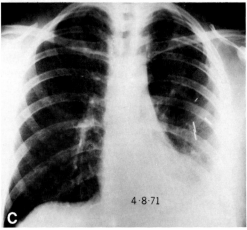

FIGURE 25–30. Idiopathic eosinophilic effusion, left pleural cavity, in a young physician otherwise completely free of disease. (*A, B, C*) Three dated chest radiographs show the chronic character of the disease. The radiograph dated 4-8-71 shows surgical clips after an exploratory thoracotomy that disclosed only thickened pleura, shown below. The patient recovered completely.

(continued)

fairly monotonous, even size when compared with nuclei of cancer cells (cf. Fig. 26 – 36C) — another feature that calls for diagnostic caution.

It is of interest here that To et al. (1981) observed major chromosomal abnormalities in cultures and direct spreads of mesothelial cells from ascitic fluid of five patients with alcoholic cirrhosis of the liver. After colchicine treatment, metaphase spreads with over 70 chromosomes, clones of abnormal cells with marker chromosomes, and other major cytogenetic abnormalities were observed. The authors suggested that these startling findings represented an alcohol-induced transformation of mesothelial cells. A confirmation of this apparently unique observation would be desirable because, in practice, mitotic abnormalities in effusions are extremely rare in the absence of cancer. The possibility that the highly abnormal mesothelial cells, such as are shown in Figs. 25 – 31 and 25 – 32, are trans-

formed cells with an abnormal chromosomal component cannot be ruled out.

Occasionally, in a very active cirrhotic process with extensive necrosis of the liver associated with clinical jaundice, strikingly abnormal single cells may be noted. Some of these cells appear to be mesothelial in origin and have a large nucleolus, whereas others are large and have large dark nuclei. The thought that at least the largest of these abnormal cells represent necrotic cells of hepatic origin is a tempting one, but is by no means proved (Fig. 25 – 32). It should be pointed out that some of the most ominous-appearing nuclei (see Fig. 25 – 32B, C) have in reality little in their internal structure to suggest an abnormal chromatin pattern. They are merely blown-up and dark. However, this affords only limited comfort when the very difficult diagnostic decision has to be reached in these fortunately very uncommon cases. For further dis-

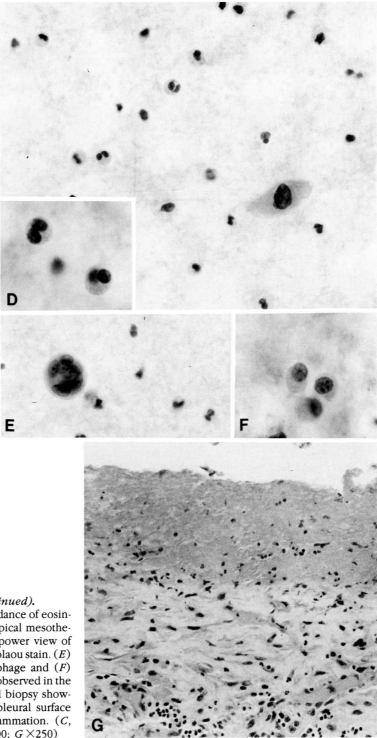

FIGURE 25–30 *(Continued).*
(*D*) Pleural fluid: abundance of eosin-ophils and a single atypical mesothe-lial cell. (*Inset*) High-power view of eosinophils in Papanicolaou stain. (*E*) Multinucleated macrophage and (*F*) cluster of plasma cells observed in the same fluid. (*G*) Pleural biopsy show-ing fibrin deposit on pleural surface and mild chronic inflammation. (*C*, *E* ×500; *inset*, *F* ×1,000; *G* ×250)

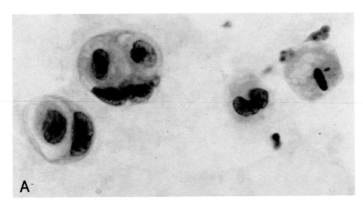

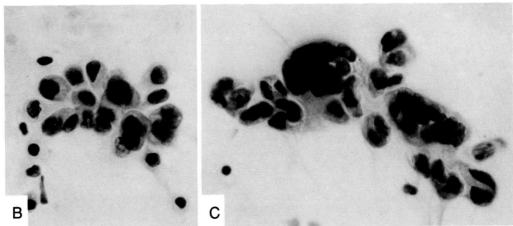

FIGURE 25–31. Atypical, large mesothelial cells in ascitic fluid in advanced alcoholic cirrhosis of the liver. (*A*) Two cell-in-cell clusters of mesothelial cells. Note the enlarged and somewhat irregular nuclei. To the right, there is one macrophage with a phagocytized particle of foreign material, next to a multinucleated smaller macrophage. (*B*) A papillary cluster of mesothelial cells with somewhat hyperchromatic, predominantly spherical or oval, nuclei. Binucleated cells mimic nuclear enlargement. (*C*) Same case as *B*; multinucleated macrophages next to two clusters of atypical mesothelial cells, similar to those shown in *B*. The presence of the multinucleated macrophages suggests that the atypia may be the consequence of prior abdominal taps resulting in a macrophage reaction. In both cases, advanced cirrhosis was proved by autopsy. (*A, B, C* ×560. *B, C* courtesy of Dr. Vincent Palladino, Nassau County Medical Center, East Meadow, New York)

cussion of cytogenetic findings in effusions see p. 1134.

Pancreatitis

The effects of acute or chronic pancreatitis are usually limited to the abdominal cavity. Direct transcutaneous thin-needle aspirations of the pancreas may occasionally cause diagnostic problems (see Chap. 29). Ascitic fluid that may be observed in pancreatitis is very rarely aspirated after the clinical diagnosis has been established. Kutty et al. (1981) pointed out that pleural fluid accumulations that may be sometimes observed in pancrea-

titis may contain modified mesothelial cells mimicking a malignant tumor. The changes described and illustrated were very similar to those shown in Fig. 25–33 in uremia.

Renal Diseases

It is uncommon to associate renal diseases with cytology of effusions. Such links, however, do exist as, for example, in hypoproteinemia (see p. 1097), uremia, and dialysis ascites.

Uremia. Uremic pericarditis has long been recognized as a frequent and ominous feature of

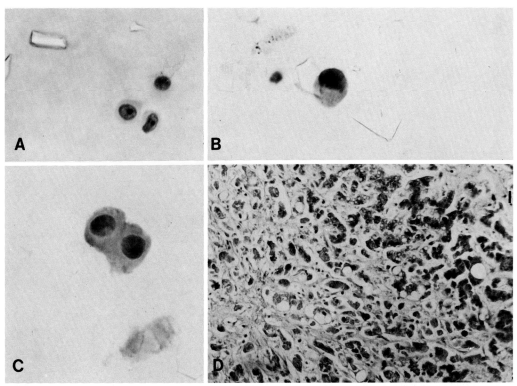

FIGURE 25–32. Cells from ascitic fluid and tissue from a case of very active cirrhosis of the liver with extensive necrotic component, proved by autopsy. Prominent nucleoli (*A*), enlarged, hyperchromatic nuclei (*B*), and cells suggesting degenerated liver cells (*C*) may be noted. Of interest is the absence of internal structure within the degenerated dark nuclei. The tissue section of the liver is shown in (*D*). (*A, B, C* ×560; *D* ×150)

uremia. The cytology of uremic pericarditis is unknown because the fluid is virtually never aspirated. On occasion, uremic pleurisy may develop, and the pleural fluid may contain numerous atypical mesothelial cells. In exceptional cases, such as the one illustrated in Figure 25–33, highly abnormal mono- and multinucleated mesothelial cells, occasionally with markedly enlarged nuclei and multiple, irregularly shaped nucleoli, may be observed. These cells were unequivocally classified as malignant, but a careful postmortem examination revealed only an abnormal proliferation of the mesothelium. Although this case seems exceptional, occasional mistakes due to abnormal proliferation of mesothelial cells in uremia seem unavoidable.

Dialysis Ascites. Some patients receiving peritoneal dialysis or hemodialysis develop a nearly intractable chronic accumulation of ascitic fluid. The ascites disappears after surgical removal of the kidneys. In seven cases of dialysis ascites personally studied, the only cytologic observation of note was the presence of erythrophagocytosis (Fig. 25–34). It is not known by what mechanism the red blood cells become sensitized and ingested; nor is it known whether the cells containing ingested erythrocytes are mesothelial or macrophages. Biopsies of peritoneum in dialysis ascites disclose fibrinous peritonitis, with a slight to moderate proliferation of mesothelial cells.

Collagen Diseases

Pleural effusions and occasionally ascites are not uncommon in the ill-defined group of diseases that have in common changes in tissues derived from the embryonal mesenchyme. Necrosis of small blood vessels and inflammatory perivascular changes are some of the common morphologic denominators of this group of disorders that otherwise have diverse clinical manifestations.

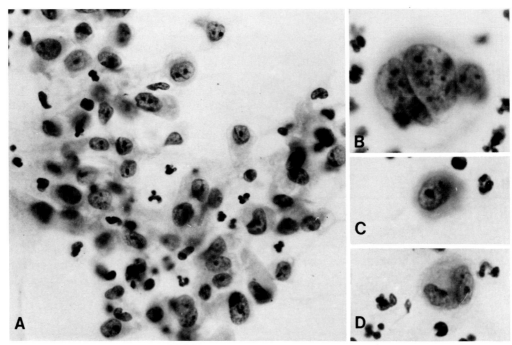

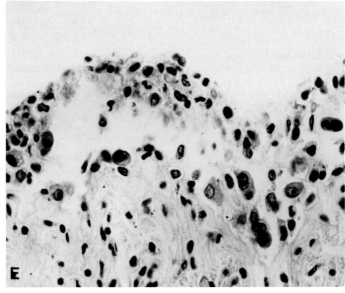

FIGURE 25 – 33. Uremic pleurisy in a 60-year-old man with renal failure caused by arteriosclerotic renal disease. (*A*) Large cluster of mesothelial cells with irregular nuclei and multiple, prominent nucleoli. (*B, C, D*) High-power view of single abnormal mesothelial cells. Note large, irregular, and in (*B*) and (*D*), multiple nuclei. Particularly striking is the large size, number, and irregular configuration of the nucleoli. These cells were mistaken for cancer cells. (*E*) Section of pleura from a most carefully conducted postmortem examination. Note the disorderly proliferation of the mesothelial cells. (*A, E* ×650; *B, C, D* ×1,000)

Systemic Lupus Erythematosus. The finding of a degenerated nucleus of a leukocyte phagocytized by another leukocyte, the so-called lupus erythematosus (LE) cell, is, with the exception of a few drug-induced disorders, virtually pathognomonic of this disease. Such cells may be produced in vitro by incubating patient's blood at 37°C. It is, therefore, not surprising that in effusions, which offer optimal conditions for incubation, LE cells will occasionally be observed (Fig. 25 – 35). Such cells have been observed in pleural, ascitic, and synovial fluids of patients with lupus erythematosus (Pandya; Metzger et al.; Hunder and Pierre; Reda and Baigelman). Kaplan et al. reported the presence of LE cells in the pleural fluid of an elderly patient with lupus induced by procainamide hydrochloride.

Kelley et al. described large atypical cells, akin

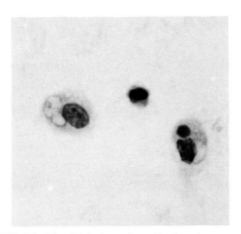

FIGURE 25–34. Dialysis ascites. Erythrophagocytosis observed in ascitic fluid of a 34-year-old man with end-stage glomerulonephritis receiving hemodialysis. The biopsy of the peritoneum in the same case disclosed fibrinous peritonitis with a moderate proliferation of mesothelial cells. (×1,000)

to plasma cells, in pleural fluids in eight of ten patients with systemic lupus. These authors considered these cells of great diagnostic significance for early diagnosis of this disease.

Carr et al. pointed out that in the majority of patients with lupus the pleural effusions had a high protein content (over 3 g/100 ml) and a glucose content of more than 55 mg/100 ml. This latter value is in contradistinction to rheumatoid arthritis wherein pleural effusions usually have glucose levels of less than 20 mg/100 ml of fluid.

Rheumatoid Arthritis. In 1968 Nosanchuk and Naylor described a characteristic cytologic

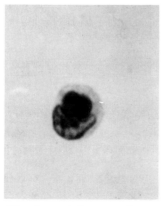

FIGURE 25–35. Systemic lupus erythematosus; LE cell in pleural fluid. Note the degenerated basophilic nucleus ingested by a leukocyte. (×1,000)

picture in pleural effusions in five of ten patients with rheumatoid arthritis. The principal feature is the background of smears, made up of granular, amorphous, particulate material or debris of various hues. The material is sometimes eosinophilic, sometimes more cyanophilic, or even green, in Papanicolaou stain. Within this background there are elongated, fibroblastlike cells (epithelioid cells) and numerous multinucleated, often elongated, giant cells and degenerating leukocytes. The combination of the debris, spindle cells, and multinucleated giant cells in fluids is pathognomonic for rheumatoid arthritis (Fig. 25–36). The origin of these cells is from the rheumatoid nodules involving the pleural cavity. The granular material originates in the necrotic part of the nodule. The spindle and giant cells originate in the characteristic "palisading" epithelioid cell lining the periphery of rheumatoid nodules. It is of note that glucose content in fluids showing this cytologic picture is generally below 20 mg/100 ml (Carr et al.). Naylor (1990) also observed cholesterol crystals in pleural effusions of several patients.

It must be added that the characteristic findings are present only in those patients whose pleura contains rheumatoid nodules. Patients with rheumatoid arthritis may also develop pleural effusion that does not show this extremely characteristic picture.

Boddington et al. pointed out that the effusion associated with rheumatoid arthritis occurs more often in males than statistically warranted and that it may occur at any time during the course of the primary disease and even as the first manifestation of rheumatoid arthritis. These observations were confirmed by Naylor (1990). Boddington et al. pointed out that the presence of the amorphous material alone is also diagnostic of rheumatoid effusion. They further reported that the amorphous material fluoresced with anti-gamma globulin antisera, a reaction that was not observed in control fluids.

Ragocytes, or RE cells, first described in synovial fluid of patients with rheumatoid arthritis are neutrophilic polymorphonuclear leukocytes with cytoplasmic inclusions resembling seeds of grapes (*rago* = (Greek) = grape). For further description of these cells, see p. 1206. Naylor (1990) observed such cells in effusions in rheumatoid pleurisy, but did not consider them to be of diagnostic value.

Scleroderma. Mesothelial cells with markedly hyperchromatic, enlarged nuclei were observed in a case of generalized scleroderma (Fig. 25–37).

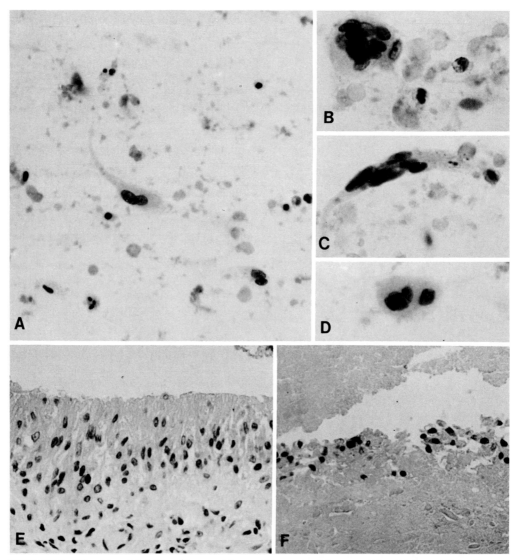

FIGURE 25 – 36.   Pleural fluid in a 63-year-old man. Diagnosis of rheumatoid arthritis established by cytology. (*A*) Low-power view showing the characteristic background of granular debris and a binucleated spindle cell in center. (*B, C, D*) Various forms of multinucleated giant cells. Note the granular, amorphous particles in background. (*E*) Pleural biopsy: fragment of a rheumatoid nodule. Note the palisading of the epithelioid cells lining the periphery of the nodule. (*F*) Other areas of the same pleural biopsy. Note the necrotic core of the rheumatoid nodule and the residual fragments of the palisading cells. (*A, E, F* ×350; *B, C, D* ×560)

The origin of the cells could be traced to a abnormal peritoneal lining.

Miscellaneous Cytologic Abnormalities

Effects of Radiotherapy.   Acute radiation effect on mesothelial cells has not been extensively studied. Enlargement and vacuolization of mesothelial cells have been observed in fluids after intrapleural instillation of radioactive phosphorous (^{32}P).

Abnormally shaped mesothelial cells with considerable nuclear hyperchromasia and distortion were observed in a patient who received 5,000 rad to the abdomen for an inoperable leiomyosarcoma of the duodenum (Fig. 25–38). Two years after

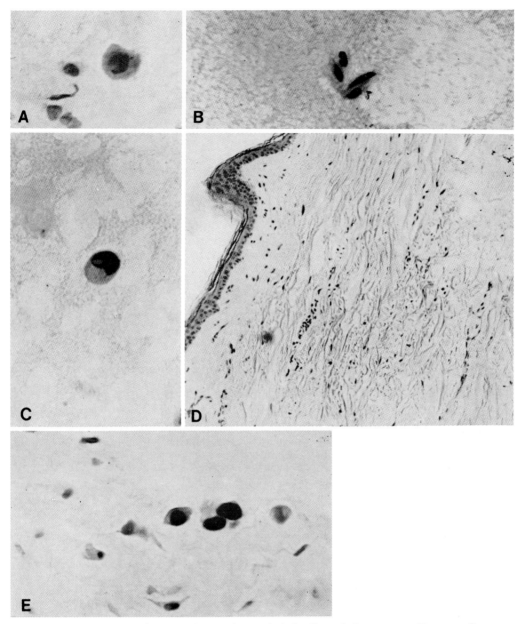

FIGURE 25–37. (*A, B, C*) Highly abnormal mesothelial cells in chylous ascites of long standing, associated with diffuse scleroderma. The markedly enlarged, hyperchromatic nuclei strongly suggest malignant cells. (*D*) Skin showing changes of scleroderma. (*E*) High-power view of the serosal lining of the small bowel in the same case. The origin of the abnormal cells in the serosa is clearly demonstrated. (*A–C, E* ×560; *D* ×150)

treatment the patient died with jaundice and a considerable ascites. At autopsy no tumor was found, but the peritoneal lining was histologically abnormal (see Fig. 25–28*C*), while the liver displayed unusual necrotic changes, possibly a late result of radiation (see Fig. 25–38*D*).

Amyloidosis. In a most unusual case of generalized amyloidosis, clusters of mesothelial cells had a strikingly abnormal pattern of chromatin with prominent nucleoli (Fig. 25–39). The differentiation of such cells from tumor cells was difficult.

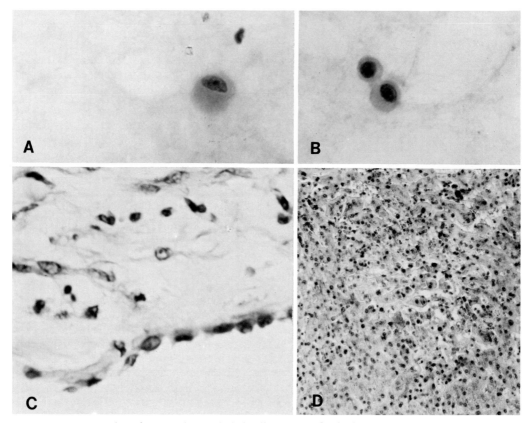

FIGURE 25–38.   (*A–D*) Atypical mesothelial cells in ascitic fluid. The patient received 5,000 *r* to the upper abdomen for leiomyosarcoma of duodenum and lived subsequently for over 2 years. Prior to death, liver failure and ascites were noted. The mesothelial lining of the stomach (*C*) was atypical. The liver (*D*) showed unusual changes, perhaps radiation necrosis. (*A, B, C* ×560; *D* ×150)

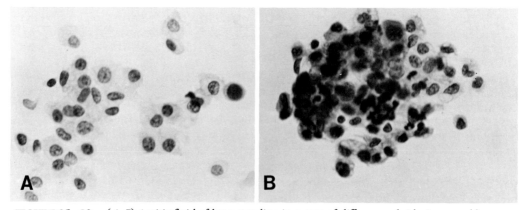

FIGURE 25–39.   (*A, B*) Ascitic fluid of long standing in a case of diffuse amyloidosis proved by autopsy. Note the clustering of cells and striking hyperchromasia of nuclei of individual mesothelial cells. (*A, B* slightly reduced from ×560. Courtesy of Drs. David Jones and Eleanor Bechtold, Syracuse, New York)

Endometriosis. A case of endometriosis of the lung and pleura with diagnosis by aspiration biopsy was recorded by Granberg and Willems. Subsequently, Zaatari et al. (1982) reported on two cases of pleural endometriosis with the characteristic recurrent hemorrhagic effusion. Endometrial cells of columnar configuration, singly and in clusters, derived from the lining of the endometrial cyst, were described as characteristic of the disease process. The fluids also contained hemosiderin-laden macrophages and clusters of smaller epithelial cells showing intercellular molding. Somewhat similar findings were reported by Kumar and Esfahani (1988) in ascitic fluid in two patients with ruptured endometriotic ovarian cysts. However, besides the columnar epithelial cells described by Zaatari et al., clusters of typical endometrial and stromal cells were observed. The endometrial gland cells formed flat sheets and glands, similar to those observed in direct endometrial samples (see p. 561). Spindly stromal cells were also noted. The Kumar and Esfahani observations were of significant diagnostic value because both their patients were initially thought to have ruptured malignant tumors of ovary. Cytologic findings in aspirates of endometriosis are also described and illustrated in Chapter 29.

Erythrophagocytosis. Ingestion of the patient's own erythrocytes by cells in pleural or ascitic fluids may be occasionally observed, for example, in dialysis ascites (see p. 1105). Several other examples have been observed under a variety of circumstances (Fig. 25–40). It is not known whether the erythrocyte surface has to be modified for these cells to be phagocytosed. Nor is it known whether the phagocytes are mesothelial cells or macrophages, although the latter seems a more likely candidate for this function. It must be pointed out that in a rare disorder, Chediak–Higashi syndrome, erythrophagocytosis has been observed (Valenzuela et al.).

Sickle Cell Anemia. Dekker et al. (1975) identified erythrocyte sickling in a patient with sickle cell crisis and pleural effusion. These authors point out the potential diagnostic significance of this observation.

"Yellow Nail" Syndrome. "Yellow nail" syndrome is a rare, apparently reversible disorder characterized by yellow color, slow growth and absence of cuticles in finger- and toenails. The syndrome, first described by Sammon and White (1964), is often associated with lymphedema and

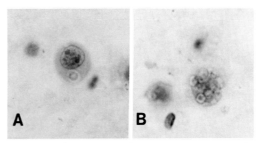

FIGURE 25–40. Erythrophagocytosis in pleural fluid. Phagocytosis of a single red blood cell (*A*) and many red blood cells (*B*) by macrophages, in a 76-year-old woman who received a transthoracic cardiac massage because of cardiac arrest. Fluid obtained 3 days after this event. (*A, B* ×560)

pleural effusion (Dilley et al., 1968; Dwek and Greenberg, 1973). It may be occasionally associated with cancer (Guin and Elleman, 1979) and a broad variety of other disorders, such as thyroid disease, rheumatoid arthritis, and immune deficiencies (review in DeCoste et al., 1990).

Information on the cytologic makeup of the effusions in this disease is very limited. In a case brought to my attention by Mr. Allan Olschewski, the pleural fluid contained a rich population of active lymphocytes, lymphoblasts, and eosinophiles. Pleural biopsies disclosed lymphocytic infiltration of the submesothelial connective tissue. The presence of atypical lymphocytes in the fluid led to a negative work-up of the patient for a malignant lymphoma.

Parasites

As in other diagnostic cytologic media, a variety of parasites may be observed in fluids. Thus, microfilariae of *Mansonella ozzardi* were observed in ascitic fluid by Figueroa (Fig. 25–41) and the ova of the lung fluke *Paragonimus kellicotti* by McCallum.

Strongyloides stercoralis larvae (see p. 743 and Fig. 19–80) were observed in ascitic fluid by Avagnina et al. (1980) in an immunosuppressed renal transplant patient. The authors postulated that the larvae penetrated the wall of the bowel in a patient whose infestation was confirmed at autopsy.

Giardia lamblia (see p. 1039 and Fig. 24–22) cysts and trophozoites were observed in peritoneal fluid after a blunt trauma to the abdomen (Bloch et al., 1987).

Jacobson described a case of echinococcosis diagnosed on pleural fluid. The characteristic sco-

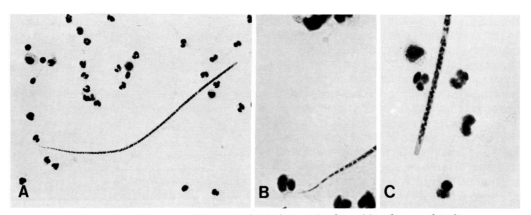

FIGURE 25 – 41.   Filaria (*M. ozzardi*) in ascitic fluid of a San Blas (Republic of Panama) Indian woman with metastatic ovarian carcinoma. (*A*) The entire worm. (*B, C*) High-power view of both extremities, which allows the classification of filaria. (*A* ×400; *B, C* ×1,000. Courtesy of Mr. Jesus Figueroa, Gorgas Hospital, Canal Zone, Panama)

lex and hooklets of *Echinococcus granulosus* were readily observed (Fig. 25 – 42). It must be noted that the fluid of echinococcal cysts is highly antigenic and, when aspirated, may cause a severe anaphylactic reaction in the patient. Thus, no deliberate attempt at fluid aspiration in a case of suspected echinococcosis should be made.

PERICARDIAL FLUID

In my experience, the cytologic findings in benign pericardial fluids present an important diagnostic challenge. The mesothelial cells in pericardial fluids may form large sheets with a spherical, hence, "papillary" configuration (see Fig. 25 – 10). Furthermore, it is not uncommon to see rather prominent nucleoli in such cells (Fig. 25 – 43). The reasons for the high frequency of these findings is unclear and is probably related to some special features of pericardial mesothelium about which nothing is known.

The aspiration of the pericardial fluid is not as simple a procedure as the aspiration of the pleural or ascitic fluid. Because of the danger of myocardial perforation, the procedure is not undertaken lightly and only in patients in whom the diagnosis of pericardial effusion is a major dilemma or for

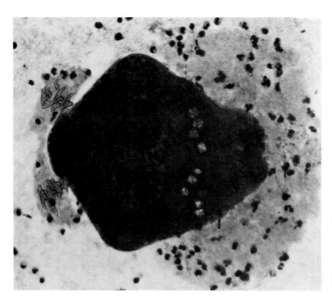

FIGURE 25 – 42.   Pleural fluid. Scolex of *E. granulosus* with the characteristic hooklets. A hepatic echinococcus cyst ruptured into the pleural cavity. (Jacobson, E.S.: A case of echinococcosis diagnosed by cytologic examination of pleural fluid and needle biopsy of pleura. Acta Cytol., *17:*76, 1973)

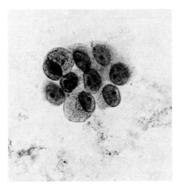

FIGURE 25–43. Pericardial fluid. Chronic pericarditis of unknown etiology in a 30-year-old woman. A cluster of atypical mesothelial cells. Note the even size of nuclei, each containing a prominent single round nucleolus. (×650)

whom a pericardial "window" must be established to prevent cardiac tamponade. The differential diagnosis often comprises a metastatic or a primary tumor of the heart or of the mediastinum (a lymphoma, a thymoma, a seminoma, or a malignant teratoma; see p. 1336) or a chronic inflammatory process, such as a rheumatic pericarditis or postinfarction pericarditis. All of the benign disorders cause atypias of mesothelial cells described above.

Other rare nonmalignant disorders causing pericardial effusion include *Histoplasma capsulatum* pericarditis (Kaplan and Sherwood, 1963) and tuberculous pericarditis (Kapoor et al., 1973). For description of cytologic findings in tuberculosis see p. 1098.

A major source of diagnostic error may be chronic hemorrhagic pericarditis, with accumulation of massive amounts of hemosiderin in macrophages, mimicking a malignant melanoma. Iron stain may clarify the nature of the accumulated pigment.

BIBLIOGRAPHY

Structure and function of the mesothelium
Effusions in the absence of cancer

Structure and Function of the Mesothelium

Andrews, P., and Porter, K.L.: The ultrastructural morphology and possible functional significance of mesothelial microvilli. Anat. Rec., *177*:408–426, 1973.

Carr, I., Clarke, J.A., and Salsbury, A.J.: The surface structure of mouse peritoneal cells—a study with the scanning electron microscope. J. Microsc., *89*:105–111, 1969.

Cotran, R.S., and Karnovsky, M.J.: Ultrastructural studies on the permeability of the mesothelium to horseradish peroxidase. J. Cell Biol., *37*:123–137, 1968.

Felix, M.D.: Observations on the surface cells of the mouse omentum as studied with the phase-contrast and electron microscopes. JNCI, *27*:713–745, 1961.

Felix, M.D., and Dalton, A.J.: A comparison of mesothelial cells and macrophages in mice after the intraperitoneal inoculation of melanin granules. J. Biophys. Biochem. Cytol., *2* (Suppl.):109–114, 1956.

LaRocca, P.L., and Rheinwald, J.G.: Coexpression of single epithelial keratins and vimentin by human mesothelium and mesothelioma in vivo and in culture. Cancer Res., *44*:2991–2999, 1984.

Nicosia, S.V., and Nicosia, R.F.: Neoplasms of the ovarian mesothelium. *In* Azar, H.A. (ed.): Pathology of Human Neoplasms. An Atlas of Diagnostic Electron Microscopy and Immunohistochemistry. pp. 435–486. New York, Raven Press, 1988.

Odor, D.L.: Observations of the rat mesothelium with the electron and phase microscopes. Am. J. Anat., *95*:433–466, 1954.

Odor, D.L.: Uptake and transfer of particulate matter from the peritoneal cavity of the rat. J. Biophys. Biochem. Cytol. *2* (Suppl.):105–108, 1956.

Policard, A., Collet, A., and Giltaire-Ralyte, L.: Bordure superficielle de pseudopodes au niveau des cellules mésotheliales du révêtement peritonéal chez les mammifères. Experientia, *11*:152, 1955.

Ramsey, S.J., Tweeddale, D.N., Bryant, L.R., and Braunstein, H.: Cytologic features of pericardial mesothelium. Acta Cytol., *14*:283–290, 1970.

Stranbesand, J., and Schmidt, W.: Zur Histophysiologie des Herzbeutels. I. Elektronenmikroskopische Beobachtungen an den Deckzellen des Peri-und Epikards. Z. Zellforsch., *53*:55–68, 1960.

Vogel, A.: Zur Struktur des Peritoneal-Mesothels. Experientia, *13*:54–55, 1957.

Effusions in the Absence of Cancer

Adelman, M., Albelda, M.S., Gottlieb, J., and Haponik, F.E.: Diagnostic utility of pleural fluid eosinophilia. Am. J. Med., *77*:915–920, 1984.

Alarcon-Segovia, D.: Drug-induced lupus syndromes. Mayo Clin. Proc., *44*:664–681, 1969.

Arismendi, G.S., Isard, M.W., Hampton, W.R., and Maher, J.R.: The clinical spectrum of ascites associated with maintenance hemodialysis. Am. J. Med., *60*:46–51, 1976.

Avagnina, M.A., Eisner, B., Iotti, R.M., and Re, R.: *Strongyloides stercoralis* in Papanicolaou-stained smears of ascitic fluid. Acta Cytol., *24*:36–39, 1980.

Balachandran, I., Jones, D.B., and Humphrey, D.M.: A case of *Pneumocystis carinii* in pleural fluid with cytologic, histologic and ultrastructural documentation. Acta Cytol., *34*:486–490, 1990.

Barziota, E.V., and Naylor, B.: Megakaryocytes in a hemorrhagic pleural effusion caused by anticoagulant overdose. Acta Cytol., *30*:163–165, 1986.

Block, T., Davis, T.E., Jr., and Schwenk, G.R., Jr.: *Giardia lamblia* in peritoneal fluid. Acta Cytol., *31*:783–784, 1987.

Boddington, M.M., Spriggs, A.I., Morton, J.A., and Mowat,

A.G.: Cytodiagnosis of rheumatoid pleural effusions. J. Clin. Pathol., *24*:95–106, 1971.

Calle, S.: Megakaryocytes in an abdominal fluid. Acta Cytol., *12*:78–80, 1968.

Campbell, G.D., and Webb, W.R.: Eosinophilic pleural effusion: a review with the presentation of seven new cases. Am. Rev. Respir. Dis., *90*:194–201, 1964.

Cobb, C.J., Wynn, J., Cobb, S.R., and Duane, G.B.: Cytologic findings in an effusion caused by rupture of a benign cystic teratoma of the mediastinum into a serous cavity. Acta Cytol., *29*:1015–1020, 1985.

Contino, C.A., and Vance, J.W.: Eosinophilic pleural effusion. N. Y. State J. Med., *66*:2044–2048, 1966.

Covell, J.L., Lowry, E.H., Jr., and Feldman, P.S.: Cytologic diagnosis of blastomycosis in pleural fluid. Acta Cytol., *26*:833–836, 1982.

Curran, W.S., and Williams, A.W.: Eosinophilic pleural effusion. A clue in differential diagnosis. Arch. Intern. Med., *111*:809–813, 1963.

DeCoste, S.D., Imber, M.J., and Baden, H.P.: Yellow nail syndrome. J. Am. Acad. Dermatol., *22*:608–611, 1990.

Dekker, A., Graham, T., and Bupp, P.A.: The occurrence of sickle cells in pleural fluid: report of a patient with sickle cell disease. Acta Cytol., *19*:251–254, 1975.

Dilley, J.J., Keirland, R.R., Randall, R.V., and Shick, R.M.: Lymphedema associated with yellow nails and pleural effusion. JAMA, *204*:670–673, 1968.

Domagala, W., Emeson, E., and Koss, L.G.: T and B lymphocyte enumeration in in the diagnosis of lymphocyte-rich plural fluids. Acta Cytol., *25*:108–110, 1981.

Domagala, W., and Koss, L.G.: Configuration of surfaces of human cancer cell in effusions. A scanning electron microscope study of microvilli. Virchows Arch. [B], *26*:27–42, 1977.

Domagala, W., and Woyke, S.: Transmission and scanning electron microscopic studies of cells in effusions. Acta Cytol., *19*:214–224, 1975.

Dwek, J.H. and Greenberg, G.M.: Yellow nails, lymphedema and pleural effusion. N.Y. State J. Med. *73*:1093–1097, 1973.

Efrati, P., and Nir, E.: Morphological and cytochemical investigation of human mesothelial cells from pleural and peritoneal effusions. A light and electron microscopy study. Isr. J. Med. Sci., *12*:662–673, 1976.

Feingold, L.N., Gutman, R.A., Walsh, F.X., and Gunnells, J.C.: Control of cachexia and ascites in hemodialysis patients by binephrectomy. Arch. Intern. Med., *134*:989–997, 1974.

Figueroa, J.M.: Presence of microfiliariae of *Mansonella ozzardi* in ascitic fluid. Acta Cytol., *17*:73–75, 1973.

Foot, N.C.: The identification of mesothelial cells in sediments of serous effusions. Cancer, *12*:429–437, 1959.

Foot, N.C., and Holmquist, N.D.: Supravital staining of sediments of serous effusions. A simple technique for rapid cytological diagnosis. Cancer, *11*:151–157, 1958.

Gartmann, J.: Rationale Diagnostik bei pleuraler Ergussbildung. Schweiz. Med. Wochenschr., *116*:1699–1708, 1986.

Gotloib, L., and Servadio, C.: Ascites in patients undergoing maintenance hemodialysis. Report of six cases and physiopathologic approach. Am. J. Med., *61*:465–470, 1976.

Granberg, I., and Willems, J.S.: Endometriosis of lung and pleura diagnosed by aspiration biopsy. Acta Cytol., *21*:295–297, 1977.

Guhl, R.: Uber pleurale Eosinophilie, die sogenannte "Eosinophile Pleuritis." Schweiz. Med. Wochenschr., *87*:838–842, 1957.

Guin, J.D., and Elleman, J.H.: Yellow nail syndrome. Possible association with malignancy. Arch. Dermatol., *115*:734–735, 1979.

Gutch, C.F., Mahony, J.F., Pingerra, W., Holmes, J.H., Ramirez, G., and Ogden, D.A.: Refractory ascites in chronic dialysis patients. Clin. Nephrol., *2*:59–62, 1974.

Hunder, G.G., and Pierre, R.V.: In vivo LE cell formation in synovial fluid. Arthritis Rheum., *13*:448–451, 1970.

Hurwitz, P.A. and Pinels, D.J.: Pleural effusion in chronic hereditary lymphedema. Radiology, *82*:246–248, 1964.

Jacobson, E.S.: A case of secondary echinococcosis diagnosed by cytologic examination of pleural fluid and needle biopsy of pleura. Acta Cytol., *17*:76–79, 1973.

Jarvi, O.H., Kunnas, R.J., Laitio, M.T., and Tyrkko, J.E.S.: The accuracy and significance of cytologic cancer diagnosis of pleural effusions. (A follow-up study of 338 patients). Acta Cytol., *16*:152–157, 1972.

Kaplan, A.I., Zakher, F., and Sabin, S.: Drug-induced lupus erythematosus with in vivo lupus erythematosus cells in pleural fluid. Chest, *78*:875–876, 1978.

Kelley, S., McGarry, P., and Hutson, Y.: Atypical cells in pleural fluid characteristic of systemic lupus erythematosus. Acta Cytol., *15*:357–362, 1971.

Kokkola, K., and Valta, R.: Aetiology and findings in eosinophilic pleural effusion. Scand. J. Respir. Dis. [Suppl.], *89*:161–165, 1974.

Koss, L.G., and Domagala, W.: Configuration of surfaces of human cancer cells in effusions. A review. Scan. Electron Microsc., *3*:89–100, 1980.

Krishnan, S., Statsinger, A.L., Kleinman, M., Bertoni, M.A., and Sharman, P.: Eosinophilic pleural effusion with Charcot–Leyden crystals. Acta Cytol., *27*:529–532, 1983.

Kumar, N., Varkey, B., and Mathai, G.: Post-traumatic pleural fluid and blood eosinophilia. JAMA, *234*:625–626, 1975.

Kumar, P.V., and Esfahani, F.N.: Cytopathology of peritoneal endometriosis caused by ruptured ovarian cysts. Acta Cytol., *32*:523–526, 1988.

Kumar, S., Seshadri, S.M., Koshi, G., and John, J.T.: Diagnosing tuberculous pleural effusion: comparative sensitivity of mycobacterial culture and histopathology. Br. Med. J., *283*:20–22, 1981.

Kutty, C.P.K., Remeniuk, E., and Verkey, B.: Malignant-appearing cells in pleural effusion due to pancreatitis. Case report and literature review. Acta Cytol., *25*:412–416, 1981.

MacMurray, F.G., Katz, S., and Zimmerman, H.J.: Pleural-fluid eosinophilia. N. Engl. J. Med., *243*:330–334, 1950.

Marcel, B.R., Koss, R.S., and Cho, S.I.: Ascites following renal transplantation. Am. J. Dig. Dis., *22*:137–139, 1977.

Martin, A.W., Carsten, P.H.B., and Yam, L.T.: Crystalline deposits in ascites in a case of cryoglobulinemia. Acta Cytol., *31*:631–636, 1987.

Mavrommatis, F.S.: Some morphologic features of cells containing PAS positive intracytoplasmic granules in smears of serous effusions. Acta Cytol., *8*:426–430, 1964.

Metzger, A.L., Coyne, M., Lee, S., and Kramer, L.S.: In vivo LE cell formation in peritonitis due to SLE. J. Rheumatol., *1*:130–133, 1974.

Murad, T.M.: Electron microscopic studies of cells in pleural and peritoneal effusions. Acta Cytol., *17*:401–409, 1973.

Naylor, B.: Curschmann's spirals in pleural and peritoneal effusions. Acta Cytol., *34*:474–478, 1990.

Naylor, B.: The pathognomonic cytologic picture of rheumatoid pleuritis. The 1989 Maurice Goldblatt Cytology Award Lecture. Acta Cytol., *34*:465–473, 1990.

Naylor, B., and Novak, P.M.: Charcot–Leyden crystals in pleural fluids. Acta Cytol., *29*:781–784, 1985.

Nosanchuk, J.S., and Naylor, B.: A unique cytologic picture in pleural fluid from patients with rheumatoid arthritis. Am. J. Clin. Pathol., *50*:330–335, 1968.

Pandya, M.: In vivo LE phenomenon in pleural fluid. Arthritis Rheum., *19*:962–963, 1976.

Pedio, G., Krause, M., and Jansova, I.: Megakaryocytes in ascitic fluid in a case of agnogenic myeloid metaplasia [Letter]. Acta Cytol., *29*:89–90, 1985.

Pfitzer, P.: Alcian–PAS positive granules in mesothelioma and mesothelial cells. Acta Cytol., *10*:205–213, 1966.

Quensel, U.: Zur Frage der Zytodiagnostik der Ergusse seröser Höhlen. Acta Med. Scand, *68*:427–457, 1928.

Ramsey, S.J., Tweeddale, D.N., Byrant, L.R., and Braunstein, H.: Cytologic features of pericardial mesothelium. Acta Cytol., *14*:283–290, 1970.

Reda, M.G., and Baigelman, W.: Pleural effusion in systemic lupus erythematosus. Acta Cytol., *24*:553–557, 1980.

Rhodes, J.M., Birch-Andersen, A., and Ravn, H.: The effect of cyclophosphamide, methotrexate and x-irradiation on the ultrastructure and endocytic capacity of murine peritoneal macrophages. Acta Pathol. Microbiol. Scand. [A], *83*:443–453, 1975.

Robertson, R.F.: Pleural eosinophilia. Br. J. Tuberc., *48*:111–119, 1954.

Rodriguez, H.J., Walls, J., Slatopolsky, E., and Klahr, S.: Recurrent ascites following peritoneal dialysis. A new syndrome? Arch. Intern. Med., *134*:283–287, 1974.

Sammon, P.D. and White, W.F.: The "yellow nail" syndrome. Brit. J. Dermat. *76*:153–157, 1964.

Silverman, F.J.: Extramedullary hematopoietic ascitic fluid cytology in myelofibrosis. Am. J. Clin. Pathol., *84*:125–128, 1985.

Soendergaard, K.: On the interpretation of atypical cells in pleural and peritoneal effusions. Acta Cytol., *21*:413–416, 1977.

Spieler, P.: The cytologic diagnosis of tuberculosis in pleural effusions. Acta Cytol., *23*:374–379, 1979.

Spriggs, A.I.: Eosinophilic pleural effusion is often due to pneumothorax. Acta Cytol., *23*:425, 1979.

Spriggs, A.I.: The architecture of tumor cell clusters in serous effusions. *In* Koss, L.G., and Coleman, D.V. (eds.): Advances in Clinical Cytology, vol. *2*. pp. 267–290. New York, Masson Publishing, 1984.

Spriggs, A.I., and Jerrome, D.W.: Benign mesothelial proliferation with collagen formation in pericardial fluid. Acta Cytol., *23*:428–430, 1979.

Storey, D.D., Dines, D.E. and Coles, D.T.: Pleural effusion. A diagnostic dilemma. JAMA, *236*:2183–2186, 1976.

To, A., Boyo-Ekwueme, H.T., Posnansky, M.C., and Coleman, D.V.: Chromosomal abnormalities in ascitic fluid from patients with alcoholic cirrhosis. Br. Med. J., *282*:1659–1660, 1981.

Veress, J., Schreiber, K., and Koss, L.G.: Eosinophilic pleural effusion. Report of 30 cases. Acta Cytol., *23*:1979.

Vilaseca, J., Arnau J.M., Talladam, N., and Salas, A.: Megakaryocytes in serous effusions. Am. J. Clin. Pathol., *34*:939, 1981.

Wahl, W.R.: Curschmann's spirals in pleural and peritoneal fluids. Acta Cytol., *34*:147–151, 1986.

Wang, F., Pillay, V.K., Ing, T.S., Armbruster, K.F., and Rosenberg, J.C.: Ascites in patients treated with maintenance hemodialysis. Nephron, *12*:105–113, 1974.

Watts, K.C., To, A., Posnansky, M.C., Boyo-Ekwueme, H., and Coleman, D.V.: Chromosome studies of cells cultured from serous effusions: use in routine cytological practice. Acta Cytol., *27*:38–44, 1983.

Zaatari, G.S., Gupta, P.K., Bhagavan, B.S., and Jarboe, R.R.: Cytopathology of pleural endometriosis. Acta Cytol., *26*:227–232, 1982.

Zaharopoulos, P.: Hemoglobin crystals in fluid specimens from confined body spaces. Acta Cytol., *31*:777–782, 1987.

26

Effusions in the Presence of Cancer

PRIMARY TUMORS OF BODY CAVITIES

Mesotheliomas

Primary tumors of the mesothelium and of its supporting connective tissue, although still rare, are seen with increasing frequency. The incidence of the tumors was estimated at 2.8:1 million males and at 0.7:1 million females in North America for the year 1972 (McDonald et al., 1980). The most common primary site of these tumors is the pleura, followed by the peritoneum and, occasionally, the pericardium (Sytman). Simultaneous or sequential involvement of two or all three body cavities by these malignant tumors is relatively common. Benign proliferation of the mesothelium and, very rarely, primary mesotheliomas, may also occur in hernia sacs and in the lining of the tunica vaginalis testis (see p. 1119). Mesotheliomas of primary origin in ovarian lining have also been recorded (Parmly and Woodruff). It is of interest that spontaneous peritoneal mesotheliomas, apparently of viral etiology, occur in the golden hamster (Mehnert et al.)

In humans, exposure to asbestos has been shown to be an important etiologic factor in the genesis of mesotheliomas and of lung cancer (see also p. 769). Not all types of asbestos fibers have the same pathogenetic significance. Long, thin crocidolite and amosite fibers, mined in South Africa, have a high level of association with mesotheliomas. The association is low with chrysotile fibers mined in North America (reviews in McDonald et al., 1980; Craighead and Mossman, 1982; Pisani et al., 1988; Mossman et al., 1990). Because the asbestos fibers are ubiquitous (see p. 830), their mere presence in lung tissue or the mesothelium does not necessarily lead to tumor formation. Benign pleural fibrous plaques containing asbestos fibers are found with greater frequency than mesotheliomas (Roberts; Rous et al.).

Malignant mesotheliomas are, to some extent, an occupational disease in people with a high level of exposure to carcinogenic asbestos. Thus, miners of high-risk asbestos, insulation workers, and shipyard workers may develop the disease. Still, in a substantial proportion of patients, probably close to 50%, no occupational hazard could be identified

(McDonald et al., 1980). Most people develop mesotheliomas in the sixth decade of life or later, but a case was described in an infant (Chu et al., 1989) and several in childhood (Ground and Miller, 1972; Kovalikover and Motovic, 1985). There is also a known familial occurrence of this tumor (review in Hammar et al., 1989).

The classification of tumors of mesothelial origin has been greatly influenced by a single tissue culture study reported by Stout and Murray in 1942. These authors reported that a fragment of a solitary fibrous pleural tumor grew cells similar to mesothelial cells. To the best of my knowledge, there has been no further confirmation of this observation, which is contrary to electron microscopic observations on mesothelial structure and should undergo a further critical investigation. Pending such an investigation, it appears more reasonable to assume, as did Klemperer and Rabin in 1931, that most tumors involving mesothelial surfaces may be either of mesothelial cell or of connective tissue origin, although mixed forms may occur. For obvious reasons the tumors of the mesothelial lining have a supporting connective tissue stroma, as do all other epithelial tumors. Also, tumors of connective tissue will at times encompass portions of the mesothelial lining, which may proliferate, lining various interstitial spaces and giving rise to papillary and tubular structures.

The following simple classification is proposed, based on prior study of material from the Memorial Hospital for Cancer and Allied Diseases, and also adopted by Ratzer et al.

Classification of Tumors of Mesothelial Origin

Tumors of mesothelial lining cells
    Benign: papillary mesothelioma
    Malignant: carcinomatous mesothelioma
                cystic peritoneal mesothelioma
Tumors of supporting connective tissue
    Benign: fibromas (cellular or hyalinized) (often referred to as fibrous mesotheliomas) and other rare tumors. Fibrous pleural plaques.
    Malignant: fibrosarcomatous mesothelioma
Mixed tumor types: synoviomalike mesothelioma

Pleural effusion was not observed in any of the patients with benign pleural tumors seen at the Memorial Hospital (Ratzer et al.). Only 1 of the 18 patients with benign mesothelioma of the pleura reported by Foster and Ackerman had pleural effusion. Most of these tumors were observed on chest radiographs, and cytology had little to contribute

to their diagnosis. Pleural plaques do not cause effusions as a rule.

Pleural or pericardial effusion and ascites are a common first manifestation of carcinomatous mesotheliomas but, in my experience, *are rare as the first manifestation of sarcomatous tumors.* Only one of the five sarcomatous mesotheliomas produced effusion in a series presented by Klima et al., and 8 of 15 such cases discussed by Ratzer et al. In the latter series, in most patients the effusions occurred late in the disease.

An accurate cytologic diagnosis of a malignant mesothelioma early in the disease may perhaps contribute to salvage of these patients, whose outlook at this time is not favorable, although some therapeutic successes were reported with small peritoneal mesotheliomas (Antman et al., 1985).

Carcinomatous Mesothelioma

Histology. The most characteristic histologic trait of these tumors is the formation of delicate papillary structures in which a central thin, branching core of connective tissue is lined with a single or double layer of oval, round, or slightly elongated eosinophilic cells of variable size (Fig. 26–1). Regardless of whether the bulk of the tumor is solid, forms glandular spaces or tubular structures, the identification of the "Christmas-tree"–like papillae is helpful in the differentiation of the carcinomatous mesothelioma from metastatic adenocarcinomas. Another point of diagnostic assistance is the search for mesothelial changes in situ, confined to the single layer of mesothelial cells lining an organ. The cancerous cells, often arranged in a palisade, are larger than normal mesothelial cells, are frequently elongated or club-shaped, and are attached by the narrow end to the surface of the organ. Their nuclei are large and contain distinct, often multiple nucleoli (Fig. 26–2). Transitions between the in situ changes and the papillary structures are frequent. In the gland-forming and tubular forms of carcinomatous mesothelioma, a negative mucicarmine stain will often permit differentiation from a pulmonary adenocarcinoma, or an adenocarcinoma metastatic from a distant site.

With the introduction of immunocytologic techniques, large batteries of special stains were tested to refine the separation of carcinomatous mesotheliomas from primary or metastatic adenocarcinomas. Aside from being expensive and time-consuming, the results of these studies were, at best, equivocal. Carcinoembryonic antigen (CEA) and monoclonal antibodies to epithelial mem-

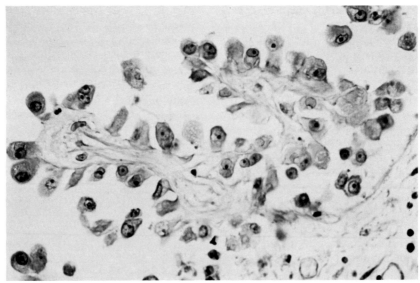

FIGURE 26–1. Carcinomatous mesothelioma, papillary component of the tumor. (×350)

brane antigen (EMA) are usually expressed in metastatic tumors, but not in mesothelioma (Battifora and Kopinski, 1985; Dewar et al., 1987). On the other hand, Walz and Koch (1990) documented positive staining with EMA and CEA in 8 of 43 mesotheliomas. In my experience, the inexpensive mucin stains are irreplaceable and, when appropriately controlled, are as reliable as any complex staining procedure in separating cells of metastatic adenocarcinomas, which usually contain mucin, from carcinomatous mesothelioma, which does not. A monoclonal antibody to mesothelial cells, provided by Dr. G. Singh, has been successfully used by us in one case (see Fig. 26–10), but its widespread usefulness has not been documented. (See also Chap. 34.)

Ultrastructural studies may disclose differences between primary pulmonary adenocarcinoma and carcinomatous mesothelioma. Features of Clara cell or pneumocytes type II origin (see p. 793) are not seen in mesotheliomas. The latter are provided with abundant, long anastomosing surface microvilli of irregular configuration (see Figs. 26–10 and 26–11) that may make contact with collagen fibers across the defective basement membrane (Valente and Corrin, 1987). These features are usually less marked in metastatic carcinomas, but exceptions may occur, and the diagnostic value of microvilli remains in doubt.

Of special interest in the differential diagnosis is a peripheral form of pulmonary adenocarcinoma with pleural fibrosis described by Harwood et al. as a pseudomesotheliomatous carcinoma. In most such cases the pleural fluid does not contain any malignant cells.

Cytology. An accurate assessment of effusions, which are often the first evidence of disease,

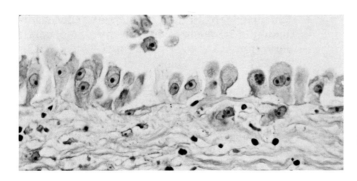

FIGURE 26–2. Carcinomatous mesothelioma in situ. Surface of spleen in an abdominal tumor. Same case as that in Fig. 26–1. (×350)

is of paramount importance in the diagnosis of carcinomatous mesothelioma.

The tumors often, but not always, shed abundant malignant cells, singly and in clusters (Fig. 26–3*A*). The presence of *numerous* mulberry-shaped papillary clusters of cells in an effusion of a patient *without a known primary cancer* should direct one's attention toward the possibility of a primary carcinomatous mesothelioma. The clusters, sometimes referred to as "morulae," are occasionally larger and more complex than any clusters of benign mesothelial cells observed in this laboratory (Figs. 26–3*D*, 26–4*A*, 26–5, 26–6, and see 26–8). Cancer cells appearing either in clusters or singly may closely resemble benign mesothelial cells because of abundant, occasionally faintly vacuolated cytoplasm, often with a distinct, clear cell border and denser perinuclear area, provided with a comparatively small, somewhat hyperchromatic nucleus (see Fig. 26–3*B–D*, 26–6, and 26–8). The presence of large, irregular nucleoli is not frequent. The difficulty of differentiating such cells from benign mesothelial cells has been emphasized by other observers, notably Klempman, Naylor, and Benge and Gröntoft.

However, in virtually every case of carcinomatous mesothelioma, one sees at least a few and occasionally many cells with nuclear and cytoplasmic abnormalities of a sufficient degree to make the diagnosis of a malignant tumor possible. Bizarre cell forms, nuclear irregularities and large nucleoli, abnormal mitoses, glandlike structures, and peculiar multinucleated cells may be observed (see Figs. 26–3*B–D*, 26–6*D*, and 26–8*D*). Calcified bodies similar to psammoma bodies were seen on several occasions (see Fig. 26–8*C*). Yet even in the presence of evidence clearly indicating a malignant process, the exact identity of the underlying cancer may remain obscure for fear that one is dealing with a metastatic carcinoma, either masquerading as a mesothelioma, or associated with an unusual, but benign, proliferation of mesothelial cells. In a prior review of the diagnostic performance from my laboratory (Ratzer et al.), the diagnosis of cancer was established in 9 of 11 cases of carcinomatous pleural mesothelioma. The suspicion that the cancer was in fact a carcinomatous mesothelioma was expressed in a few cases, but before 1963 not a single case was unequivocally diagnosed on cytologic grounds alone. With additional experience, it was possible to establish the diagnosis of a primary mesothelioma in several personally observed cases. In one of them, early diagnosis led to a major and apparently successful surgical resection of the lesion (see Fig. 26–6). In another

case, the disease was primarily in the pericardium (Fig. 26–7). In yet another instance, the diagnosis, based on a study of pleural fluid, was established 1 year before tissue confirmation could be obtained. It is of interest that Becker et al. (1976) reported a case of an apparently benign mesothelial papillary lesion of the pericardium with a cytologic pattern suggestive of a carcinomatous mesothelioma.

Differences Between Carcinomatous Mesotheliomas of the Pleura and the Peritoneum. In 1982, Boon et al. compared the cytologic presentation of carcinomatous mesotheliomas occurring as either primary pleural or peritoneal tumors. She noted in air-dried, Giemsa-stained smears that the cytoplasm of the pleural mesothelioma cells was smaller and contained few cytoplasmic vacuoles. Many of the cells of the peritoneal mesotheliomas were larger and characterized by numerous perinuclear vacuoles. Other features, such as cluster (morulae) formation were similar for both tumor types. Further analysis of the cytoplasmic vacuoles was provided by Boon et al. in 1984. The vacuoles in malignant mesothelioma cells stained for fat, but not for mucin, contrary to vacuoles in metastatic cancer. It was also acknowledged that the vacuolated appearance of mesothelioma cells was much easier to observe in air-dried, Giemsa-stained material than in fixed, Papanicolaou-stained smears. The features described by Boon et al. were observed by us in a case of a mesothelioma of tunica vaginalis testis (see below and Fig. 26–8).

Other Presentations of Mesothelioma. Spriggs and Grunze (1983) described three cases of *pleural* mesothelioma with foamy, macrophage-like cells and vacuolated cells, not unlike those attributed by Boon et al. to abdominal lesions. A similar case of a malignant pleural mesothelioma with macrophages and vacuolated signet ring-type cells was described by Gaffanti and Falen (1985).

It is quite evident, therefore, that the cytologic presentation of malignant mesotheliomas may occasionally differ from the classic type. The presence of vacuolated cell forms may render the differential diagnosis from metastatic cancer (including the very rare signet ring-type lymphomas) very difficult. In such cases, a surgical biopsy occasionally may be helpful.

Carcinomatous Mesothelioma of Tunica Vaginalis Testis. A primary cytologic diagnosis of a malignant carcinomatous mesothelioma of tunica vaginalis testis was reported by Japko et al. (1982). The cytologic presentation of hydrocele fluid in a
(text continues on page 1123)

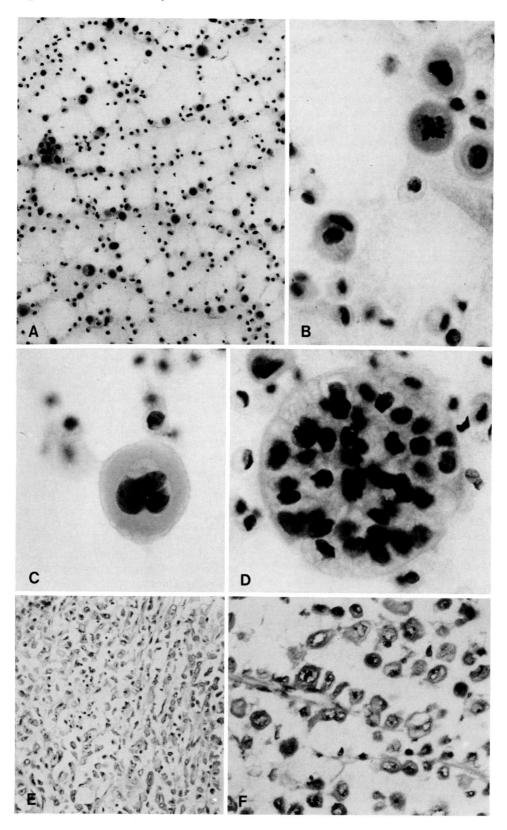

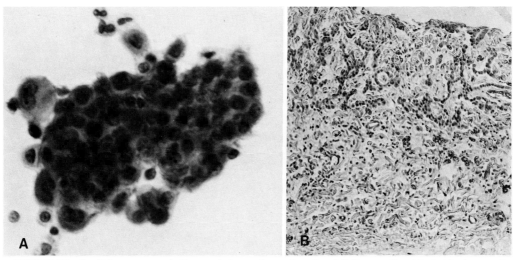

FIGURE 26–4. Primary mesothelioma of the peritoneal cavity. (*A*) Smear of ascitic fluid; cluster of cancer cells. Note the resemblance of some of the peripheral cells to benign mesothelial cells. (*B*) Section of the peritoneal surface. (*A* ×560; *B* ×150. Courtesy of Dr. Leopold Reiner, New York, New York).

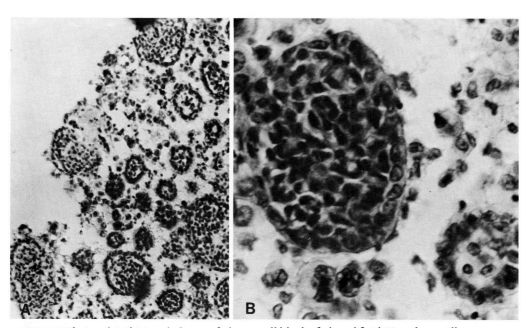

FIGURE 26–5. (*A, B*) Mesothelioma of pleura; cell block of pleural fluid. Note the papillary appearance of clusters of cancer cells. Mitoses are numerous. (*A* ×150; *B* ×560. Courtesy Drs. Karl Menk and John W. Todd, Staunton, Virginia)

FIGURE 26–3. Primary peritoneal mesothelioma in a 43-year-old man; ascitic fluid. (*A*) Low-power view of the smear shows a very marked cellularity. The small cells in the background are mainly macrophages. (*B, C, D*) Some details of the tumor cells: in (*B*) an abnormal mitosis is evident; in (*C*) a large, multinucleated cancer cell; and in (*D*) an unusual papillary cluster. Note striking similarity of the tumor cells to normal mesothelial cells. In (*C*) a peripheral zone, probably a brush border, may be seen. (*E, F*) Histologic section of tumor. (*A, E* ×150; *B, C, D* ×560; *F* ×350)

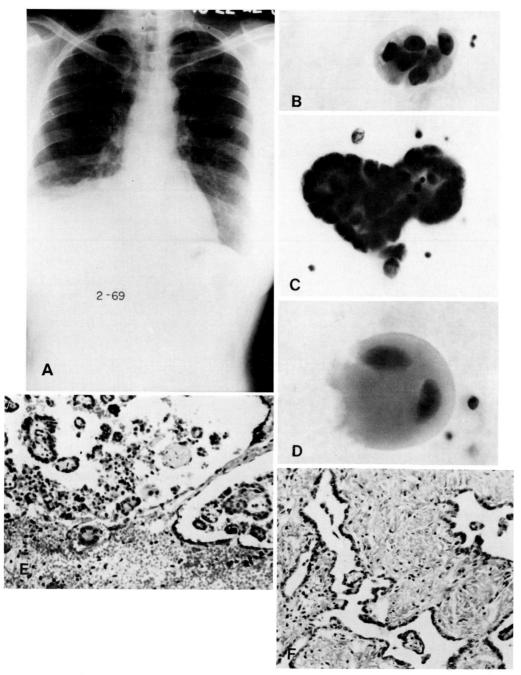

FIGURE 26–6. Carcinomatous mesothelioma of pleura extending to diaphragm in a 55-year-old patient. Apparent surgical cure (5 years). Primary diagnosis by cytology. (*A*) Chest radiograph 5 months after onset of chest pain. Note effusion on right. Two prior chest radiographs were negative. (*B, C*) Representative examples of numerous papillary clusters (morulae) observed in pleural fluid. Some of the clusters could not be differentiated from benign mesothelial cells (*B*). Other clusters (*C*) were three-dimensional and made up of a very large number of cells, an appearance practically never seen in benign fluids. The diagnosis was clinched by the finding of isolated large, clearly malignant cells (*D*). (*E, F*) The resected tumor of the pleura had a papillary configuration (*E*) and invaded the adjacent diaphragm (*F*). (*B, C, D* ×560, *E, F* ×150)

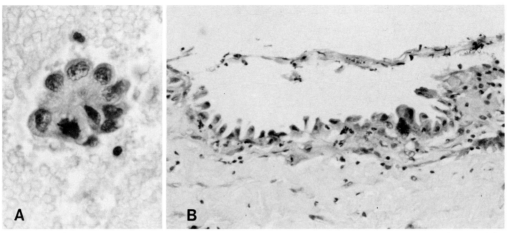

FIGURE 26–7.   Carcinomatous mesothelioma of pericardium with massive pericardial effusion. (*A*) Pericardial fluid: characteristic papillary cluster of malignant cells (cell block). (*B*) Pericardial biopsy section: view of parietal pericardium, showing mesothelioma in situ. Note the characteristic palisading of malignant cells. Elsewhere the tumor formed marked proliferative pattern. (*A* ×650; *B* ×250. Case courtesy of Dr. Larry Palileo, Fort Harrison, Montana)

30-year-old man with a history of exposure to asbestos was a paradigm of this disease (Fig. 26–8). Numerous spherical, mulberry-shaped cell clusters (morulae) were noted (Fig. 26–8*A*). On closer scrutiny they were composed of atypical cells of mesothelial type (Fig. 26–8*B*). Isolated malignant cells of mesothelial type with obvious nuclear abnormalities were also present (Fig. 26–8*D*). It may be noted that the cytoplasm of the cancer cells contained numerous small perinuclear vacuoles, in keeping with Boon's observations pertaining to malignant mesothelioma of peritoneal origin (see above). Numerous calcified psammoma bodies were present in some of the cell clusters (see Fig. 26–8*C*).

Histologic examination of the resected tumor documented papillary growth on the surface of the tumor (Fig. 26–9*A*) with solid growth areas (see Fig. 26–9*B,E*). Transition of normal mesothelium to abnormal mesothelium was observed (Fig. 26–9*C*) as was the presence of calcified bodies (Fig. 26–9*E*). Invasion of lymphatics was also observed (Fig. 26–9*D*). The tumor gave a positive immunoreaction with a monoclonal antibody to mesothelial cells (Fig. 26–10*A,B*). On electron microscopic examination numerous long surface microvilli were observed on tumor cells (see Fig. 26–10*C*).

Tufts of long microvilli may be also observed in light microscopy on surfaces of mesothelioma cells in fluids (Fig. 26–11).

RARE TYPES OF EPITHELIAL MESOTHELIOMAS

Multicystic Peritoneal Mesothelioma.   Several cases of this very rare disorder have been reported (summary in Alvarez-Fernandez et al., 1989). The disease must be differentiated from other cystic tumors of the abdominal cavity, notably of ovarian and vascular origin. The neoplasm appears to be of low grade, capable of recurrence, but consistent with long-term survival. In a case reported by Baddoura and Varma (1990), large sheets of benign mesothelial cells were observed in fluid drained from the cysts. The patient remained well for 7 years after the onset of symptoms.

Ovarian Mesotheliomas.   These rare tumors have a histologic and cytologic presentation of carcinomatous mesothelioma, except for their primary presentation on the ovarian surface (Nicosia and Nicosia, 1988). In a few personally observed tumors of ovary with ascites, the diagnosis of mesothelioma could be suggested on cytologic grounds and confirmed by histology. Interestingly, the ovarian mesotheliomas do not invade the ovary, but envelop its surface and metastasize to the peritoneum. A mesothelioma in situ can be observed on the ovarian surface. Whether the very rare primary papillary peritoneal neoplasia is a form of mesothelioma or of metastatic ovarian cancer is not clear (Lindeque et al., 1985).

(text continues on page 1127)

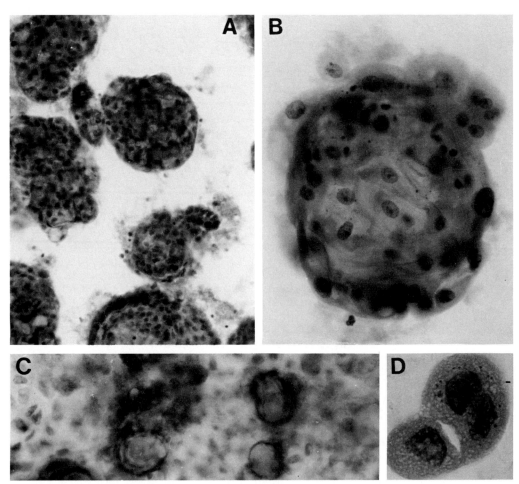

FIGURE 26–8. Malignant mesothelioma of tunica vaginalis testis in a 30-year-old man: the same case as Figs. 26–9 and 26–10. Primary diagnosis by cytologic examination of hydrocele fluid. (*A*) Low-power view of spherical clusters of cells. (*B*) Higher magnification of a mulberry-shaped cell cluster. Note several enlarged and hyperchromatic nuclei at the periphery of the cluster. (*C*) Calcified structures (psammoma bodies) within a cell cluster; (*D*) two malignant cells separated from each other by a clear space ("window"). Note the fine cytoplasmic vacuoles in perinuclear location, consistent with Boon's observations in peritoneal mesotheliomas. (*A* ×140; *B, C* ×350; *D* ×560. Japko, L., et al.: Malignant mesothelioma of the tunica vaginalis testis; report of first case with preoperative diagnosis. Cancer, *49*: 119–127, 1982)

FIGURE 26–9. Histologic appearance of malignant mesothelioma: same case as Figs. 26–8 and 26–10. (*A*) Low-power view showing exophytic, papillary proliferations protruding into the lumen of the tunica vaginalis; (*B*) detail of the tumor with an abnormal mitotic figure; (*C*) gradual transition between normal mesothelial cells and tumor. Note superficial extension of the tumor into the connective tissue stroma (*arrow*). (*D*) Plug of tumor in a lymphatic vessel; (*E*) area of solidly growing tumor with psammoma bodies. (*A, C, D* ×140; *B* ×560; *E* ×350. Japko, L., et al.: Malignant mesothelioma of the tunica vaginalis testis; report of first case with preoperative diagnosis. Cancer, *49*: 119–127, 1982)

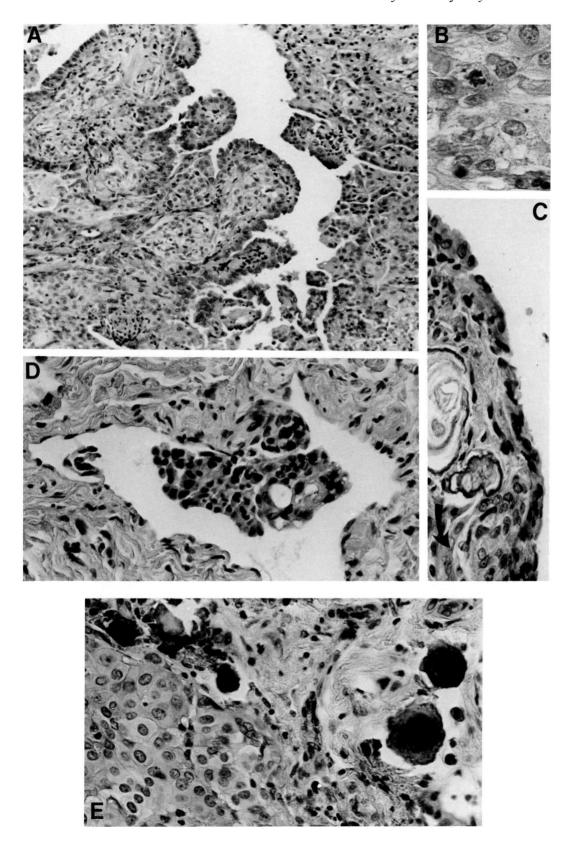

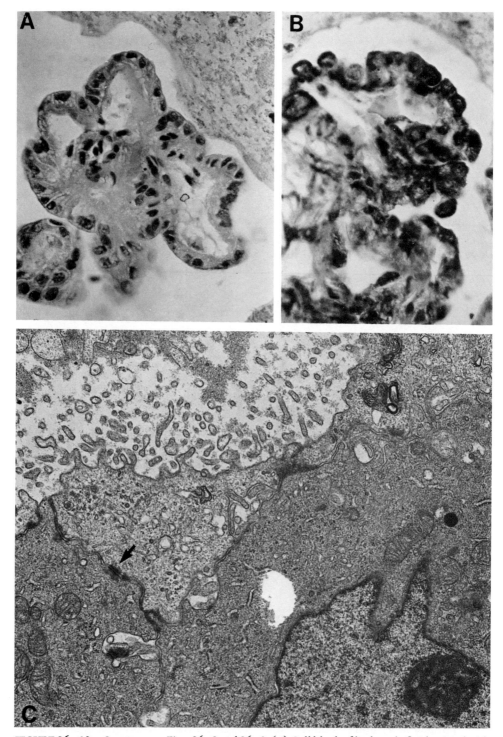

FIGURE 26–10. Same case as Figs. 26–8 and 26–9. (*A*) Cell block of hydrocele fluid stained with hematoxylin and eosin and (*B*) with monoclonal antibody to mesothelial cells provided by Dr. G. Singh of the University of Pittsburgh (peroxidase–antiperoxidase staining). (*C*) Electron micrograph of tumor cells showing numerous, often swollen microvilli on cell surfaces. The tumor cells were bound to each other by desmosomes (*arrow*). (*A, B* ×350; *C* ×12,400. Japko, L., et al.: Malignant mesothelioma of the tunica vaginalis testis; report of first case with preoperative diagnosis. Cancer, *49*:119–127, 1982)

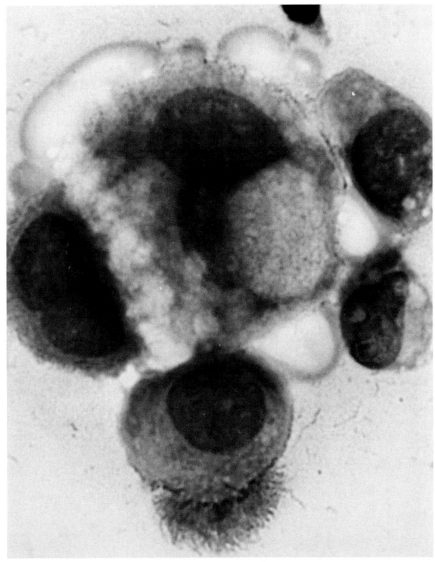

FIGURE 26–11.   Cluster of cells in a malignant mesothelioma of tunica vaginalis testis in a 21-year-old man. A tuft of long microvilli may be observed on one of the cells. (×2,000. Courtesy of Dr. Arthur Spriggs, Oxford, England)

Fibrosarcomatous Mesotheliomas

Histology.   These are malignant tumors, in many ways resembling other fibrosarcomas. Bundles of elongated, malignant, but sometimes deceptively benign-looking spindly cells are usually observed. In contrast with carcinomatous mesothelioma, this author has never observed a mesothelioma in situ associated with one of the fibrosarcomas. As has been emphasized above, this type of tumor is almost never associated with a primary effusion. Furthermore, if effusion does occur, it rarely contains cancer cells. In most instances the diagnosis of sarcomatous mesothelioma has been established on direct needle aspiration of pleural lesions or on tissue biopsy. A spindle cell malignant tumor of the diaphragm in an asbestos worker has been reported as a leiomyosarcoma by Dionne et al.

It is still a matter for debate whether circumscribed, solitary fibrous pleural mesotheliomas, some of which may display a histologic pattern of sarcoma, are benign or malignant. Briselli et al. (1981) reviewed a large series of those cases. The mortality was 12%, regardless of histologic pattern. Effusions are extremely rare as the first manifestation of these tumors. It is of note, though, that hypoglycemia may be the primary clinical event in about 4% of these patients (summary in Roncalli et al., 1981).

Cytology. In sarcomatous mesotheliomas there is usually none of the diagnostic difficulty encountered with carcinomatous mesothelioma. In material aspirated directly from the tumors, the cancer cells are spindly, often forming sheets or whorls (Figs. 26–12 and 26–13), and usually have the classic nuclear abnormalities of cancer.

Mixed Type of Malignant Mesotheliomas

The mixed variety of mesotheliomas, resembling malignant synovioma, is deserving of special mention. These tumors are composed of solid sheets of small, spindly cells with slitlike cavities lined by cuboidal cells. In my opinion, this is possibly the only primary tumor of mesothelial surfaces in which a simultaneous participation of the epithelial and the connective tissue components may be reasonably proposed.

With this tumor type, effusions containing malignant cells have been observed. The cancer cells are usually spindly in configuration and are often accompanied by markedly atypical, but not clearly malignant, mesothelial cells (Fig. 26–14).

Other Primary Malignant Tumors of Mesothelial Surfaces

Such tumors are exceedingly rare. Through the courtesy of Dr. M. Wilson Toll, this writer had the opportunity to observe a primary squamous carcinoma of the pleura developing in a tuberculous patient with an induced pneumothorax of many years' duration. The cytologic presentation was that of a classic keratinizing squamous carcinoma, with formation of squamous "pearls" and many anucleated squamae. At the time of autopsy, the tumor was present in the pleura and had metastasized to the liver (Fig. 26–15).

METASTATIC CANCERS

The frequently emphasized difficulty in the diagnosis of metastatic neoplasms in body fluids is due to two factors: *(1)* abnormal mesothelial cells or macrophages may simulate a malignant tumor, or may conceal the presence of tumor cells; and *(2)* the body fluids constitute a natural and hitherto inadequately explored medium of tissue culture, wherein the tumor cells may proliferate free of the

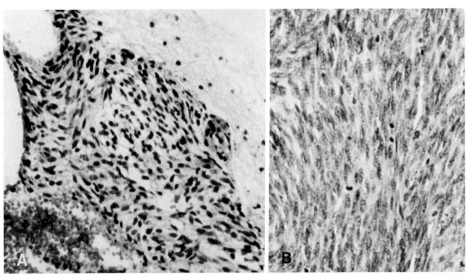

FIGURE 26–12. Fibrosarcomatous mesothelioma, pleura. (*A*) Fragment of a spindle cell malignant tumor in cell block of pleural fluid. (*B*) Histologic section of the same tumor. (*A, B* ×150)

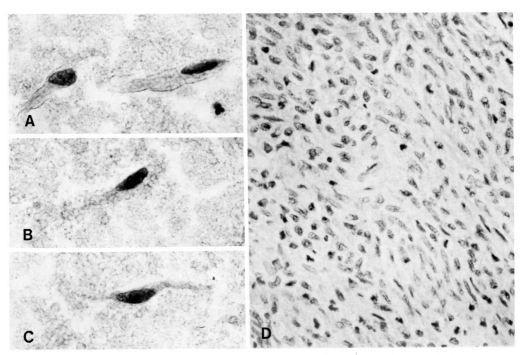

FIGURE 26–13. Fibrosarcomatous mesothelioma. (*A, B, C*) Aspiration biopsy of pleura. Note spindly cancer cells. (*D*) Histologic appearance of tumor that metastasized widely. (*A, B, C* ×560; *D* ×350. Case courtesy of Dr. Vincent Palladino, Meadowbrook Hospital, East Meadow, New York)

boundaries imposed upon them by the framework of organs and tissues. It is known to all students of experimental tissue culture in vitro that morphologic identification of benign versus malignant cultured cells may be fraught with considerable difficulty. Similarly, the characteristic features of human cancer cells, as described for the various organs, may undergo substantial modifications when these cells are capable of unrestricted proliferation in an effusion. The abnormal cell shapes that often help in the identification of exfoliated or aspirated cancer cells may no longer be present in a fluid wherein the cancer cells may assume a neutral, round appearance. Nuclear hyperchromasia is another feature that may sometimes be difficult to identify in cancer cells in fluids. One must also keep in mind that proliferating mesothelial cells and macrophages may show nuclear features that may render the differential diagnosis with cancer cells difficult (see Chap. 25).

In spite of these words of caution, it is entirely possible in the vast majority of effusions to identify cancer cells accurately, often to identify tumor type, and, sometimes, to suggest the primary tumor of origin, even in the absence of accurate clinical history.

Identification of Cells of Metastatic Cancer in Effusions

The diagnosis of metastatic cancer in a pleural, pericardial, or peritoneal fluid is of capital importance for the patient and the attending physician or surgeon. In most such instances the rapid fatal outcome of the disease may be anticipated. However, with the use of appropriate therapy, some metastatic tumors offer a much better prognosis than others. For example, metastatic mammary carcinoma may be controlled, often for a period of several years, by means of hormonal manipulation and chemotherapy. Malignant lymphomas and some of the malignant tumors in children (neuroblastoma, embryonal rhabdomyosarcoma) may also respond to energetic therapeutic measures. Therefore, the responsibility of the pathologist is twofold: *(1)* to identify cancer cells accurately, and *(2)* to identify tumor type and, if possible, the site of primary origin. The latter task is greatly facilitated by review of prior histologic material, if available, and by an accurate clinical history.

As a general rule, it is better to exercise diagnostic caution than to "stamp" a patient as having metastatic carcinoma on insufficient evidence and

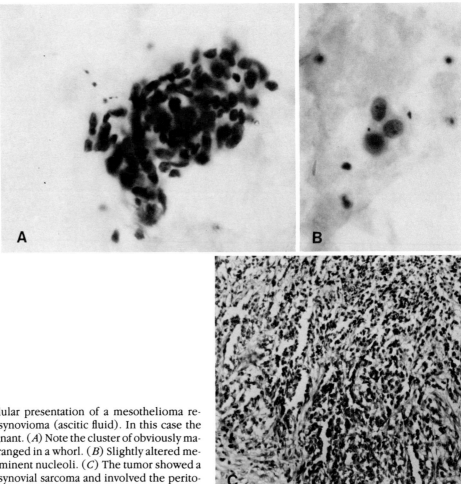

FIGURE 26–14. Cellular presentation of a mesothelioma resembling a malignant synovioma (ascitic fluid). In this case the tumor was highly malignant. (*A*) Note the cluster of obviously malignant spindly cells arranged in a whorl. (*B*) Slightly altered mesothelial cells with prominent nucleoli. (*C*) The tumor showed a striking similarity to a synovial sarcoma and involved the peritoneal as well as pleural surfaces. (*A, B* ×560; *C* ×150)

thereby possibly neglect further investigation and treatment. Satisfactory evidence of cancer is as necessary in effusions as in any other type of material before the diagnosis with all its potentially tragic consequences is made.

Techniques

The use of impeccable technical preparations is of utmost importance in ensuring diagnostic accuracy. The laboratory techniques are discussed in detail in Chapter 33. There are three types of preparation in general use: smears, filter preparations, and histologic sections of the sediment (cell block technique).

In my experience the cytologic diagnosis of cancer in effusions is easier in smears and cell blocks than in filter preparations. Cellular distor-

tions caused by improper use of filters may constitute an important source of error. Rapid fixation of material (unless processed without any delay) is also important.

General Characteristics of Cancer Cells in Effusions

Cell Size

Cell size in metastatic tumors may vary greatly according to tumor type. The comparison must be made with identifiable cell types in smears, such as erythrocytes, lymphocytes, polymorphonuclear leukocytes, and with mesothelial cells. Generally speaking, metastatic malignant tumors in effu-

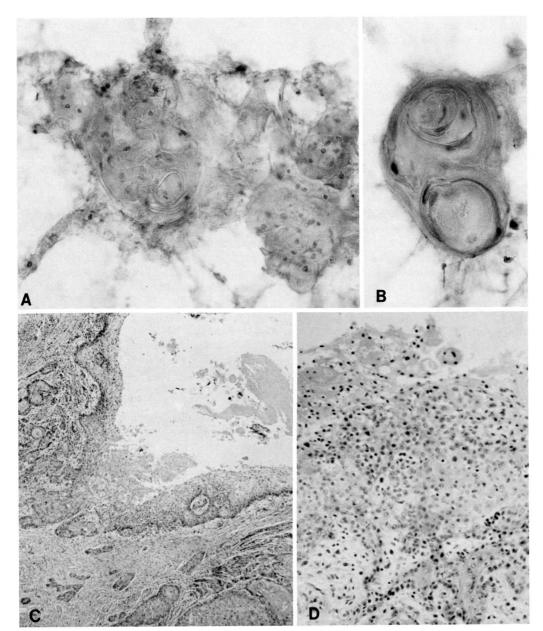

FIGURE 26–15.   Pleura: primary squamous (keratinizing) cell carcinoma originating in squamous metaplasia of pleura. Tuberculous patient with pneumothorax maintained for many years. (*A, B*) Pleural fluid. Low- and high-power views of the keratin "pearl" forming tumor. This presentation in fluids is diagnostic of squamous cancer. The search for more "classic" cancer cells is usually futile. (*C*) Low-power view of pleural lining showing squamous metaplasia and carcinoma derived therefrom. (*D*) Higher-power view of carcinoma in situ with foci of invasive carcinoma. (*C, D* from autopsy sections.) (*A* ×250; *B* ×500; *C* ×40; *D* ×150. Case courtesy of Dr. M. Wilson Toll, Baltimore, Maryland)

sions may be classed in three groups, made up of large, small, and medium cells.

Large-Cell Types.   The cells are significantly larger than mesothelial cells. Many metastatic epidermoid and adenocarcinomas, malignant melanoma, and many sarcomas belong in this group. When combined with abnormal nuclear features, to be described below, the identification of such tumors is easy (see Fig. 26–21*A*).

Small-Cell Types.   The tumors are made up of cells much smaller than mesothelial cells. Most malignant lymphomas, many of the malignant tumors of childhood (neuroblastoma, Wilms' tumor) and certain carcinomas (small-cell carcinoma of the breast, oat cell carcinoma) belong here. Close attention must be paid to nuclear features and interrelationship of cells for accurate identification (see Figs. 26–32 and 26–37).

Medium-Cell Types.   The cells are approximately of the same size as mesothelial cells. A variety of carcinomas of mammary, gastric, pancreatic, or lung origin belong here. This is perhaps the most difficult group of tumors to identify and the most important source of diagnostic error (see Figs. 26–30 and 26–31).

Nuclear Abnormalities

Nuclear Size and Shape.   Most malignant cells in fluids have enlarged nuclei. The change in the nucleocytoplasmic (N/C) ratio varies according to tumor type. In some of the mucus-producing cancer cells and keratinizing squamous cancers the cytoplasm may remain abundant, and the nucleocytoplasmic ratio may not be conspicuously changed. In most other tumors, however, the nucleocytoplasmic ratio is larger than in mesothelial cells (see Fig. 26–21*A*).

The nuclear shapes of cells of metastatic carcinomas in fluids are rarely abnormal. Most such cells display round or oval nuclei with smooth borders. Occasionally, on closer scrutiny, an irregular nuclear outline may be observed and is of diagnostic assistance when associated with other features, such as hyperchromasia (see Figs. 26–30*D*, and 26–31*C,D*).

In sarcomas and mainly in malignant lymphomas, abnormalities of nuclear shape, sometimes in the form of nipplelike protrusions, are of major diagnostic significance (see p. 1157).

Nuclear Hyperchromasia and Nuclear Texture.   In most, although not all, malignant tumors, the cancer cells in effusions have enlarged, markedly hyperchromatic nuclei. In rare instances, the nuclei are homogeneous and opaque. In most cancer cells the chromatin appears granular, and its texture is often much denser than in mesothelial cells and macrophages (see Figs. 26–21*A* and 26–22). Very rarely, clear, transparent nuclei may be observed.

Nucleoli.   Except in keratinizing squamous carcinomas, large, irregularly shaped, single or multiple nucleoli may be frequently observed. On the rarest occasion, similar nucleolar abnormalities may occur in mesothelial cells (see p. 1104 and Fig. 25–33), thereby constituting an important source of error. As a matter of practical importance, other abnormal features are usually present in cancer cells, and these must be recognized before the diagnosis of cancer is rendered (see Fig. 26–24).

Abnormal Mitoses.   Abnormal mitotic figures, such as multipolar mitoses or chromosomal lag (see p. 142), are among the most reliable identifying features of cancer cells in effusions. However, I encountered, in a few cases, morphologically atypical mitoses in pleural fluid when surgical exploration of the pleural space revealed no cancer (Fig. 25–28). Papanicolaou in his *Atlas* also mentioned two similar cases. It may be stated safely that such occurrences are extraordinarily rare and should not detract from the diagnostic value of abnormal mitotic figures, which very strongly suggest a malignant process (see Fig. 26–27). It is conceivable that chromosomal abnormalities observed in ascites with cirrhosis of the liver and exceptionally in other disorders may account for the rare mitotic abnormalities observed in benign effusions (see p. 1102). Occasionally, the nuclear membrane is missing or defective and the nuclear area is filled with chromatin granules. These images, suggestive of a mitotic prophase, are uncommon in benign cells.

Multiple Sex Chromatin Bodies.   In cancers occurring in female patients a scrutiny of sex chromatin bodies may be of diagnostic assistance. Two or more sex chromatin bodies are virtually diagnostic of cancer cells. This observation is particularly helpful in the diagnosis of mammary and ovarian carcinoma, wherein the morphologic abnormalities of malignant cells are not pronounced (see Fig. 26–28). Mesothelial cells and histiocytes have a single sex chromatin body, except in the very rare superfemales (karyotype 47, XXX).

Nuclear Cytoplasmic Inclusions. Clear areas within the nucleus, corresponding to cytoplasmic invaginations, have been observed in a variety of cancer cells, such as cells of metastatic melanomas, pulmonary adenocarcinomas, and thyroid cancers (see Fig. 26–65). I have never observed this feature in benign cells in effusions.

Cell Shape

Bizarre- or spindle-shaped cells almost always suggest a metastatic malignant tumor, often one of unusual makeup. Many sarcomas have this appearance (see Fig. 26–59). Other cell configurations may also be noted, for example, columnar cells or cells resembling bronchial lining cells (see Figs. 26–36 and 26–42). Because benign cells in fluids virtually never assume this appearance, unusual cell shapes are very helpful in identifying cancer. The only exceptions may occur when the needle used for aspiration of fluid penetrates into adjacent or underlying organ. Liver cells, bronchial lining cells, and, very rarely, benign fibroblasts, may be observed in such fluids (see Chap. 25).

Cell Aggregates

Although mesothelial cells may form cell aggregates, as described on p. 1088, these are usually few, and rarely, they are made up of a large number of cells. When such aggregates are numerous, the possibility of a malignant mesothelioma must be considered (see p. 1119).

Many malignant tumors, principally adenocarcinomas of various primary origin, may form cell aggregates, often composed of a very large number of cells (see Figs. 26–23*A* and 26–29). Such aggregates are three-dimensional (i.e., made up of several superimposed cell layers that cannot be brought into a single focus). Round aggregates corresponding to papillary projections, or aggregates forming glandlike structures with a central lumen (see Fig. 26–24) are particularly helpful in identifying malignant tumors.

Spriggs (1984), in a detailed light and electron microscopic study of cell aggregates in effusions, pointed out that these commonly encountered cell clusters are actually elaborate, organized three-dimensional structures. Spriggs divided the structures into three groups: papillary, tubulopapillary, and acinar (Fig. 26–16). On cross section the cells composing the clusters surround a lumen, form cell junctions, and often contain collagen fibers as supporting structures. The papillary and tubulopapillary clusters are provided with microvilli on their outer surfaces, whereas the acinar structures contain microvilli on the surface facing the lumen. Thus the cell clusters, far from being haphazard accumulations of epithelial cells, are, in fact, organized, growing fragments of mesothelial cells (benign or malignant) and of epithelial cancer cells.

There is no need to resort to electron microscopy to appreciate the elaborate structure of such cell aggregates: synchronous use of the cell-block technique is often very helpful in revealing the true nature of the clusters (Fig. 26–17).

Cell Products

Products of metabolic activity of cells, such as mucus (demonstrated by means of special stains), melanin pigment, psammoma bodies, cytoplasmic cross-striations, and keratin, are never produced by benign cells in effusions. Hence, their identification is diagnostic of a metastatic tumor.

Calcified, concentrically laminated, round or oval bodies, 20 to 50 μm in size, usually referred to

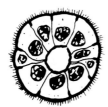
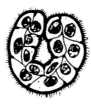
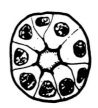

Papillary   **Tubulo-papillary**   **Acinar**

FIGURE 26–16. Spriggs' representation of cell clusters in effusions. The clusters are organized structures that may be either papillary with microvilli on the outer surface; tubulopapillary with microvilli on both surfaces; or acinar, with microvilli on the inner luminal aspect of the cluster. (Spriggs, A.I.: The architecture of tumor cell clusters in serous effusions. *In* Koss, L.G., and Coleman, D.V. (eds.): Advances in Clinical Cytology, Vol. 2. New York, Masson, 1984)

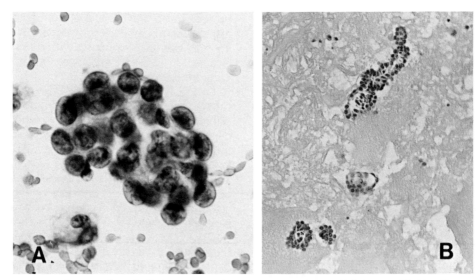

FIGURE 26–17. Pleural effusion, metastatic mammary carcinoma. (*A*) Smear of fluid sediment with a large aggregate of cancer cells. (*B*) Cell block section of the same sediment: acinar and tubular structure of cell clusters is documented. (*A* ×560; *B* ×150).

as *psammoma bodies*, are most commonly observed in metastatic tumors of ovarian origin (see Fig. 26–38), but may also be produced by carcinomatous mesotheliomas, bronchogenic adenocarcinoma, thyroid cancer (see Fig. 26–47; rarely observed in effusions), and sometimes by other metastatic tumors. Metastatic pancreatic carcinoma, carcinoma of the renal pelvis, endometrial carcinoma, and mammary carcinoma with psammoma bodies have been personally observed.

It must be noted that the presence of calcified bodies is of limited diagnostic value in material aspirated from cul-de-sac through the vagina or in pelvic washings (see p. 630).

Cell Surfaces

Spriggs and Meek observed the presence of peculiar surface structures in some malignant cells in pleural and peritoneal effusions: tufts of hairlike processes were noted, often covering the entire cell; these were particularly striking in certain cases of metastatic ovarian carcinoma. Similar structures may be observed in carcinomatous mesotheliomas (see Fig. 26–11). Electron microscopic studies revealed cytoplasmic processes similar to elongated microvilli, which the authors considered as a possible attempt to form intercellular contacts. Similarly, Ebner and Schneider observed "ciliated malignant cells" in carcinoma of the ovary.

Domagala and Woyke, and subsequently Domagala and Koss, using scanning electron microscopy, demonstrated that the surfaces of cancer cells in effusions were covered by innumerable microvilli of variable shape and configuration (Fig. 26–18). These observations were made on malignant cells of various primary origins, comprising adeno- and epidermoid carcinomas. It was further documented by Domagala and Koss that when some cancer cells settle on a hard surface, such as glass, the microvilli are capable of forming extensions of considerable length, not unlike cells cultured on hard surfaces in vitro (Fig. 26–19). The scanning electron microscopic appearance of the surfaces of cancer cells was markedly different from surface configuration of histiocytes and mesothelial cells, described on p. 1091. The significance of microvilli, also observed in other malignant processes in humans, (see p. 140) is not understood at the time of this writing. Nevertheless, this feature appears promising for the identification of cancer cells in effusions.

Cytogenetic Features

The finding of cells with abnormal chromosomal numbers and configuration has been shown to be diagnostic of cancer cells in effusions (Goodlin; Ishihara and Sandberg; Jackson). The apparent exceptions to this rule are the observations by To et

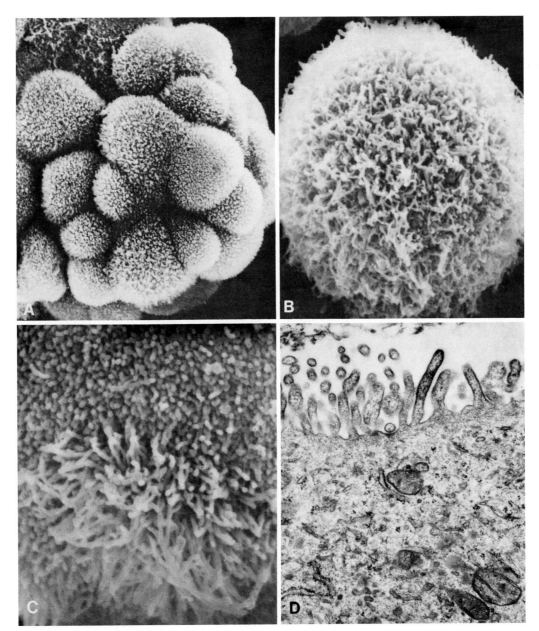

FIGURE 26–18.   Scanning and transmission electron microscopy (TEM) of cancer cells in effusions. (*A*) Cluster of cancer cells from a metastatic ovarian carcinoma. Note innumerable microvilli on the surfaces of cancer cells. (*B*) Breast cancer cell. Note shaggy appearance due to numerous slender microvilli. (*C*) Lung cancer cell (adenocarcinoma). Short stubby microvilli are adjacent to long slender microvilli. (*D*) Cell of ovarian carcinoma in TEM. Note innumerable microvilli of uneven size and configuration on the cell surface. (*A* ×2,300; *B* ×4,600; *C* ×6,000; *D* ×18,600. Courtesy of Dr. W. Domagala, Montefiore Hospital)

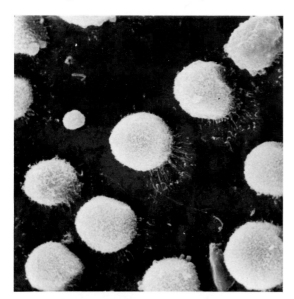

FIGURE 26–19. Scanning electron microscopy of cells of breast cancer settling on glass prior to fixation. The cell surfaces are covered by microvilli. Fan-shaped extensions of microvilli on glass may be observed, (×1,000. Courtesy of Dr. W. Domagala, Montefiore Hospital)

al. (1981) and by Watts et al. (1983) who observed abnormal mitotic figures in several ascitic fluids associated with liver cirrhosis and in one pleural effusion associated with pneumonia (see also p. 1102). Apparently, other disorders such as rheumatoid arthritis or pulmonary embolus may occasionally be associated with chromosomal abnormalities (summary in Watts et al., 1983). These studies did not include chromosomal banding. It would be of great interest to confirm these observations by contemporary cytogenetic techniques. Benedict et al. pointed out that a long acrocentric chromosome was often associated with metastatic malignant tumors, regardless of primary origin and histologic type. Miles and Wolinska compared the sensitivity of cytogenetic studies with light microscopic diagnoses in 58 cancer patients. In 38 patients routine cytology disclosed cancer, whereas cytogenetic studies were positive in only 24 of these patients. In 2 patients chromosome analysis disclosed an aneuploid chromosomal component, whereas routine cytology was negative. Cytogenetic studies in this group of patients may have been handicapped by prior treatment. In general a large population of dividing cancer cells is required for a successful direct chromosomal analysis. Watts et al. (1983) documented the successful use of a cell culture technique for cytogenetic study of effusions.

DNA Measurements in Effusions as Tumor Markers

Freni et al. (1971) and Krvinkova et al. (1976) were apparently the first groups of investigators to recognize the diagnostic value of DNA measurements by cytophotometry in the identification of malignant cells in effusions. With the introduction of flow cytometers, the DNA measurements became more rapid, and several groups of investigators have reported abnormal DNA histograms in fluids containing malignant cells (Evans et al., 1983; Unger et al., 1983; Katz et al., 1985; Croonen et al., 1988). In a study from this laboratory, Schneller et al. (1987) pointed out that flow cytometry does not always show aneuploidy in the presence of cancer cells. With use of cytophotometry as a second mode of analysis, aneuploid DNA values were observed in a number of effusions containing malignant cells, in the absence of flow cytometric abnormalities. For further discussion of cytophotometry and flow cytometry, see Chapters 35 and 36.

Immunocytochemistry (see also Chap. 34)

Cells in effusions are the favored target of immunocytochemical investigations because of abundant cell populations and the ease with which multiple samples can be obtained in the form of smears, cytocentrifuge preparations (cytospins), and cell blocks (buttons). A multiple-well technique, which permits synchronous testing of several aliquots of cells with several monoclonal antibodies, was described by Guzman et al. (1988).

The number of reagents and monoclonal antibodies tested on effusions is very large and the principal observations are discussed in Chapter 34. Hence, only a brief summary is presented in Table 26–1.

Regardless of results, the immunocytochemical observations must be considered a secondary mode of cancer cell identification that may sometimes enhance, but never replace, morphologic observations.

Immunologic Features

Another approach of current interest in the study of effusions is the relationship of various cell populations engaged in immune responses to cancer cells in effusions.

Scanning electron microscopic studies by Domagala and Koss strongly suggested that cell contacts between lymphocytes and macrophages and between macrophages and cancer cells may occur in effusions. The latter relationship has since been confirmed in light microscopy. Cancer cells in

Table 26–1
*Principal Reagents Tested on Effusions and Their Principal Characteristics**

Reagent	Discrimination Between Benign and Malignant Cells	Discrimination Among Tumor Types
Common Reagents		
Mucicarmine, Periodic acid-Schiff (PAS)	Occasionally	Positive in many adenocarcinomas, negative in mesotheliomas
Complex Reagents		
Epithelial membrane antigen (EMA) (Coleman and Omerod, 1984)	Questionable; many normal epithelial surfaces give positive stain	Many carcinomas (over 75%) stain with EMA. Mesothelioma: weak stain
Carcinoembryonic antigen (CEA) (Coleman and Omerod, 1984)	Yes, few exceptions	Many adenocarcinomas stain with CEA; mesotheliomas, see p. 1117
B72.3 monoclonal antibody (Johnston et al., 1986)	Endometrium and benign apocrine cells stain with reagent	Many tumor types stain. No stain in oat cell carcinomas and melanomas
Antibodies to intermediate filaments (see p. 42 and Chap. 34)	No	No (except lymphomas)
Lymphocyte markers (summary in Guzman et al., 1988, and Chap. 34)	No (in lymphoid cells)	Yes: identification of lymphomas
CA 1 antibody (epitectin) (summary in Czerniak, et al., 1985)	Usually	Most carcinomas stain with CA 1
Various monoclonal antibodies raised against malignant cells of various origins (CA 125, MBr1, MOv2) (Menard et al., 1985)	Generally, yes	Enhances the recognition of some malignant cells

*See also Chap. 34.

contact with variable numbers of macrophages have been repeatedly observed (Fig. 26–20).

Domagala et al. (1978, 1981) also studied the distribution of B and T lymphocytes in the peripheral blood and in effusions of patients with metastatic carcinoma of various primary origins. In most cases there was a statistically significant increase of T lymphocytes in fluids. Similar observations have been made by Djeu et al. It appears that a selective migration of T lymphocytes to the effusions may be taking place in cancer patients. These observations suggest that some immune mechanisms of unknown significance may be operative even in the terminal stages of cancer. The exception to this rule is the T-cell lymphoma.

With use of a panel of monoclonal antibodies, Guzman et al. (1988) studied the distributions of subtypes of lymphocytes in treated and untreated patients with ascites due to serous papillary ovarian cancer. The differences were not significant, except for an increase in cells expressing interleukin-2 receptors in treated patients. The method of multiple aliquots of cells placed in wells is worthy of consideration in future studies of this type.

Identification of Common Patterns of Tumors

Diagnosis of patterns of tumor growth is occasionally much more difficult in body fluids than in other cytologic media because of the exuberant proliferation of cells that may take place within the fluid. The best chances of identification of tumor

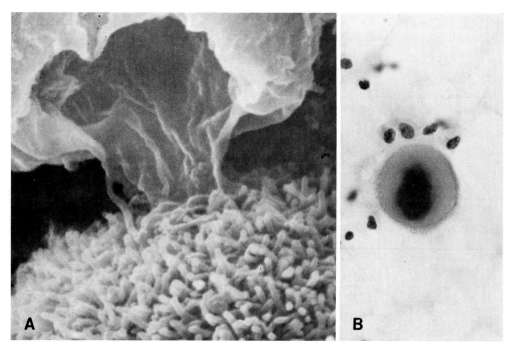

FIGURE 26–20.   Contacts between macrophages and cancer cells. (*A*) Scanning electron micrograph showing an extension of the cytoplasm of a macrophage onto the surface of a cancer cell identified by microvilli. (*B*) Pleural fluid showing a large squamous cancer cell of lung origin surrounded by several macrophages. (*A* ×14,000; *B* ×1,000. *A* Courtesy of Dr. W. Domagala, Montefiore Hospital)

type occur when cancer cells form multicellular structures akin to those observed in tissues, for example, glands or acini. The other identification options are based on cell relationships and identification of cell products. Adenocarcinomas are often relatively easy to identify and so too are occasionally keratin-forming, squamous cancers. Nonkeratinizing epidermoid carcinomas may cause problems in identification. The unique cytologic features of metastatic malignant lymphomas and the special features of other metastatic tumors are discussed below.

Nonkeratinizing Epidermoid Carcinoma

Identification of tumor type in metastatic nonkeratinizing epidermoid carcinoma in effusions is often difficult. The tumor cells may vary greatly in size and may occur singly or in clusters. The tumor cells are characterized by abnormal, often hyperchromatic nuclei, but the cytoplasmic eosinophilia characteristic of this tumor type in other diagnostic media is often absent (Fig. 26–21*A*). It should be emphasized that cytoplasmic eosinophilia may occasionally be observed in other tumor types, as well as in mesothelial cells. Clumps of

tumor cells, either in smears or in cell blocks, are not especially helpful in establishing the diagnosis of epidermoid carcinoma.

The differential diagnosis comprises a variety of carcinomas of other histologic types, mainly poorly differentiated metastatic adenocarcinomas, which may have an identical cytologic presentation.

Keratinizing Squamous Carcinoma

Well-differentiated, keratin-producing squamous cancers are rarely observed in effusions. The reasons for this are not clear. Spriggs (1954), in discussing effusions in lung cancer, also pointed out the rarity of identifiable squamous carcinoma. Nevertheless, when such tumors metastasize and grow in effusions, their identification is relatively easy. The cells are, as a rule, very heavy keratin producers. This results in the presence of anucleated squames of odd shapes and sizes. Nucleated cancer cells are comparatively few, and in such cells the classic nuclear abnormalities of size and shape and hyperchromasia are infrequent. Occasionally, the cells resemble normal squamous cells. More commonly, the nuclei appear necrotic, shadowy, and

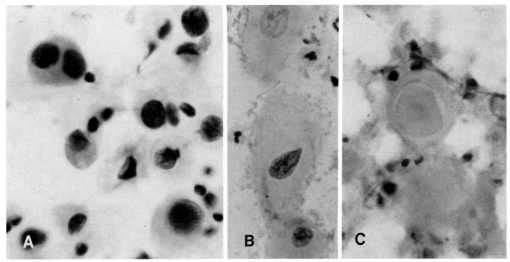

FIGURE 26-21. (*A*) This is a common presentation of epidermoid bronchogenic cancer in body fluids. There is an abundant proliferation of large cancer cells, with no distinguishing features (pleural fluid). The nuclei are hyperchromatic and large. (*B, C*) Bronchogenic squamous carcinoma in pleural fluid. There is keratinization of cancer cells (*B*) and pearl formation (*C*). (*A, B, C* ×560)

pale (see Fig. 26-21*B*). Pearl formation, when present, is absolutely diagnostic of this type of cancer (see Figs. 26-21*C* and 26-15).

As a rule of thumb, the presence of numerous squamous cells in an effusion, regardless of the status of nuclear abnormalities, is for all practical purposes diagnostic of metastatic squamous carcinoma. Contamination with squamous cells of the epidermis removed during the aspiration procedure is very rare, and then it results in only a few such cells. The one exception to this rule, cited on p. 1095, was a ruptured benign dermoid cyst of the mediastinum.

Adenocarcinoma

Metastatic adenocarcinomas are generally easier to identify in fluids than the two tumor types discussed above. This identification is helped if the cells form multi-layered, round or oval cell clusters suggestive of papillary growth (Figs. 26-7, 26-22, and 26-23). To differentiate such clusters from similar clusters of benign mesothelial cells, nuclear abnormalities must be identified. Usually, in cancer cells, there is marked nuclear enlargement, some hyperchromasia, and clearly abnormal, large nucleoli. Also helpful in the identification of adenocarcinomas is the presence of glandlike structures formed by abnormal cells (Fig. 26-24). In paraffin-embedded (cell block) material, glandular

features of adenocarcinoma may be sometimes identified with ease (Figs. 26-17 and 26-25), provided that nuclear abnormalities are present.

When metastatic adenocarcinomas do not form such structures, but occur as single cells, their iden-

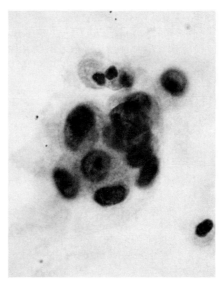

FIGURE 26-22. Metastatic ovarian carcinoma in pleural fluid. Note the clustering and superposition of cancer cells with large, hyperchromatic nuclei and large nucleoli, characteristic of papillary tumors. (×560)

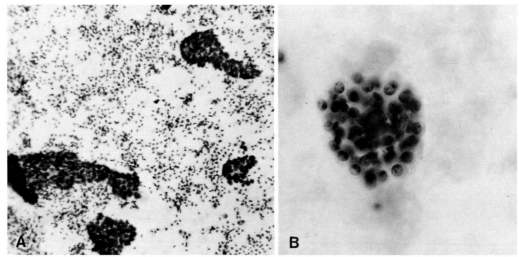

FIGURE 26–23. (*A*) Papillary adenocarcinoma of ovary in pleural fluid (same case as that in Fig. 26–22). Low-power view of numerous papillary clusters of tumor. Note the crowding and superposition of cells, also visible in the high-power photograph (Fig. 26–22). (*B*) Gastric adenocarcinoma in ascitic fluid (same case as that in Fig. 26–41*A*). Note a typical papillary cluster characteristic of adenocarcinoma. (*A* ×150; *B* approx. ×300)

tification is more difficult. If mucus production by cancer cells can be documented by special stains, the diagnosis is secure. Other special cell features may identify tumors of various specific origins (see below). However, there will always remain a group of metastatic adenocarcinomas in which a specific identification of tumor type will prove impossible. *It is particularly important to reemphasize that the mere presence of cytoplasmic vacuoles is not diagnostic of adenocarcinoma. The vacuoles may occur in tumor cells of other types, but also in benign cells such as macrophages and mesothelial cells (see p. 1092 and Fig. 25–19).*

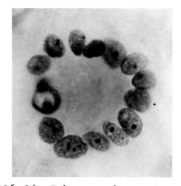

FIGURE 26–24. Pulmonary adenocarcinoma. Smear of pleural fluid. Note glandular arrangement of cells with product of secretion (mucin?) in the central lumen. Prominent nucleoli are well in evidence. (×560)

Cytologic Presentation of Frequently Observed Metastatic Carcinomas

Carcinoma of the Breast

Mammary carcinoma is by far the most common tumor associated with pleural effusions in women. It may also cause ascites and, occasionally, pericardial effusions. The identification of the primary origin of tumor may be of considerable prognostic value because in many instances effusions resulting from breast cancer may be controlled by hormonal manipulation, chemotherapy, and radiotherapy.

The cytologic presentation of mammary carcinoma depends to a significant extent on histologic tumor type and is quite variable. Cell size may vary from very large to very small. The large tumor cells correspond to carcinomas of duct origin and the less common medullary carcinomas, papillary carcinomas, and colloid carcinomas. The metastases from infiltrating duct carcinoma with fibrous stroma (scirrhous carcinoma) usually produce medium-sized- or small-cell cancer. Infiltrating lobular carcinomas generally are made up of small-cell cancer cells, which may occasionally be mucus-producing and resemble signet ring cell carcinoma (see below).

Breast carcinomas of the *large-cell type* in effusions usually have the classic features of metastatic

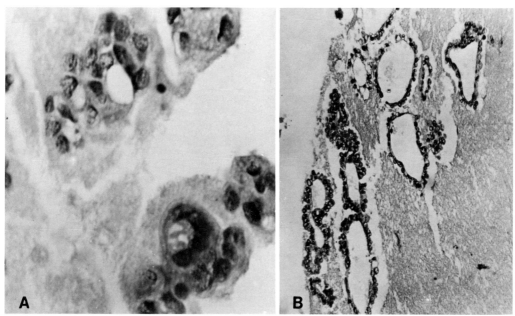

FIGURE 26-25. (*A*) Breast cancer. Formation of glandular structures in cell block of pleural fluid. Note that the abnormal nuclei and the complex arrangement of abnormal cells rule out a centrifugation artifact. (*B*) Ovarian adenocarcinoma. Cell block of ascitic fluid disclosing the nature of the tumor. (*A* ×560; *B* ×150)

adenocarcinomas and form large, three-dimensional clusters of round, oval, or irregular configuration, wherein the cells are superimposed on each other (Fig. 26-26). Single cancer cells are also commonly observed. The nuclear features of cancer are usually classic and comprise abnormal mitoses (Fig. 26-27), nuclear enlargement, and prominent nucleoli. The degree of hyperchromasia is variable. It is of great interest that sex chromatin bodies, single or multiple, may be readily identified in some of the cancer cells (Fig. 26-28). *Multiple sex chromatin bodies in a cell nucleus practically assure the diagnosis of cancer, most likely of mammary origin, regardless of other cell features.* Mesothelial cells have only one sex chromatin body, unless the patient has an abnormal karyotype, which is an extremely rare event (see p. 1132). (For further discussion of sex chromatin bodies in breast cancer see Chap. 28). Tissue culture pattern with abundant proliferation of cancer cells may also occur (Fig. 26-29). Occasionally, the cancer cells are arranged in Indian file (see below).

The diagnostic difficulty with breast cancer in fluids occurs with the *medium- and small-cell type,* when the cancer cells cannot readily be distinguished by size from mesothelial cells and macrophages. The cancer cells are often arranged in single file (Indian file), a pattern that reproduces the arrangement of cancer cells in tissues (Fig. 26-30).

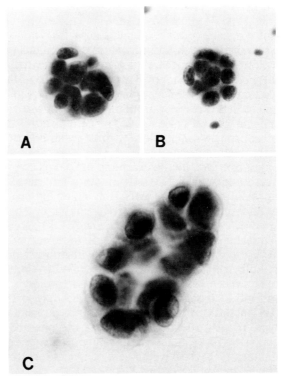

FIGURE 26-26. (*A, B, C*) Metastatic breast cancer, duct cell type, pleural fluid. Papillary clusters of cancer cells with large hyperchromatic nuclei and scanty cytoplasm. The clusters are three-dimensional (i.e., not all the cells are in the plane of the photograph) (*A, B* ×650; *C* ×1,000)

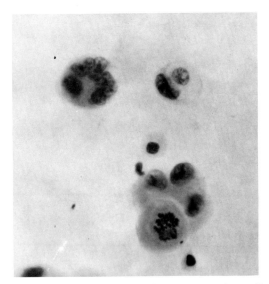

FIGURE 26–27. Metastatic breast cancer, duct cell type, in pleural fluid. Mitosis with abnormal spread of chromosomes, a multinucleated cancer cell, a cell-in-cell arrangement, and other nuclear abnormalities may be noted. (×560)

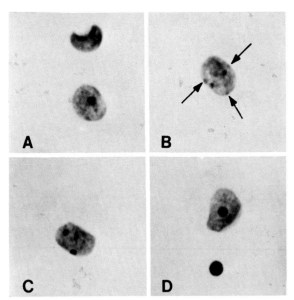

FIGURE 26–28. (*A–D*) Metastatic breast cancer, duct cell type, pleural fluid. Nuclear features of isolated cancer cells. The focus of the photographs was on the nuclei, and the cytoplasm cannot be seen except as a faint outline. Note granular nuclear texture, large nucleoli, and, in one cell, multiple sex chromatin bodies (*arrows*). (×1,000)

This is of great diagnostic value. Long chains of cancer cells arranged in single file are virtually diagnostic of carcinoma of the breast (Fig. 26–31). Mesothelial cells may occasionally form short chains that very rarely are composed of more than three to four cells (see Fig. 25–11). Cancer cells of other primary origin may also form a chainlike arrangement, but the cells are usually larger than in breast cancer, with the exception of oat cell carcinoma (see below). The recognition of nuclear abnormalities in the cells within the Indian file, such as nuclear enlargement, hyperchromasia, or a peculiar square configuration (see Fig. 26–30), is essential for the diagnosis of cancer. In the absence of such abnormalities, the differential diagnosis with mesothelial cells may prove very difficult. Mammary cancers of small-cell type may also proliferate to form a "tissue culture" pattern and may form clusters similar to those described for the large-cell type. If such cells occur singly the diagnosis becomes very difficult unless clear-cut nuclear abnormalities or excessive numbers of sex chromatin bodies are observed (Fig. 26–32).

Spriggs and Jerrome were the first to point out that in some breast cancers in effusions signet ring-like cells may be noted. The cytoplasm was distended by large, mucus-containing vacuoles with a central eosinophilic inclusion. The inclusion was shown by electron microscopy to be an amorphous mass, presumably inspissated secretions, located within a cytoplasmic space lined by microvilli (Fig. 26–33). This ultrastructural presentation corresponds to the light microscopic appearance that is occasionally observed in mammary carcinoma.

The small cancer cells have large cytoplasmic vacuoles displacing the nuclei, thus resembling somewhat the signet ring cells. Within the cytoplasmic vacuoles, there are single central "inclusions" (Fig. 26–34). The inclusions give a strongly positive stain with mucicarmin and, accordingly, are composed of mucin. This appearance of cancer cells, whether seen in direct aspiration biopsy material or in effusions is uniquely characteristic of primary or metastatic mammary carcinoma of lobular type.

Effusions caused by metastatic mammary carcinoma in males are extremely rare. In a personally observed case the cells in the pleural effusion were of large-cell type.

Carcinoma of the Lung

Lung cancer is the most frequently observed cause of pleural effusions caused by malignant disease in men. A rapid increase in the incidence of this dis-

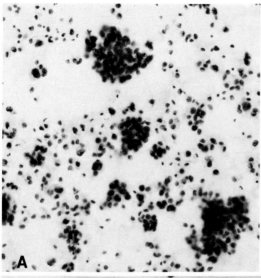

FIGURE 26-29. Pleural fluid; metastatic mammary carcinoma, duct cell type. (*A*) Tissue culture effect with innumerable cancer cells singly and in clusters. (*B*) Clusters of large cancer cells. (*C*) Tissue section of the primary infiltrating duct carcinoma. (*A, C* ×150; *B* ×560)

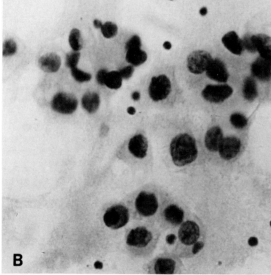

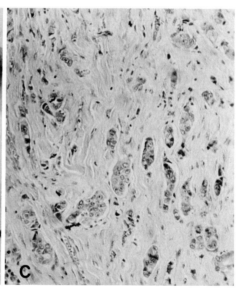

ease in women has been documented. Pericardial effusions and ascites associated with lung cancer are much less frequent. The cytologic presentation depends on tumor type.

Keratinizing Epidermoid (Squamous) Carcinoma. The cytologic presentation in effusions is described on p. 1138 (see Figs. 26–15 and 26–21*B,C*). The finding of squamous cells or anucleated squamae is diagnostic of the disease, even in the absence of nuclear abnormalities. This tumor type is relatively infrequently seen in effusions, presumably because only viable cells survive and these have little tendency to keratin formation.

Epidermoid Carcinoma, Large-Cell Type. The features of the cytoplasm that are very helpful in identifying this tumor in sputum are usually absent in fluids. The cytoplasm is thin, delicate, and transparent, and the nuclei are hyperchromatic and large. The cells occur singly or in small clusters. The exact identification of tumor type is rarely possible in fluids, except occasionally in cell blocks (Figs. 26–21*A* and 26–35).

Adenocarcinoma. This has become by far the most common type of lung cancer in effusions. It is characterized by large cancer cells, usually forming

(text continues on page 1147)

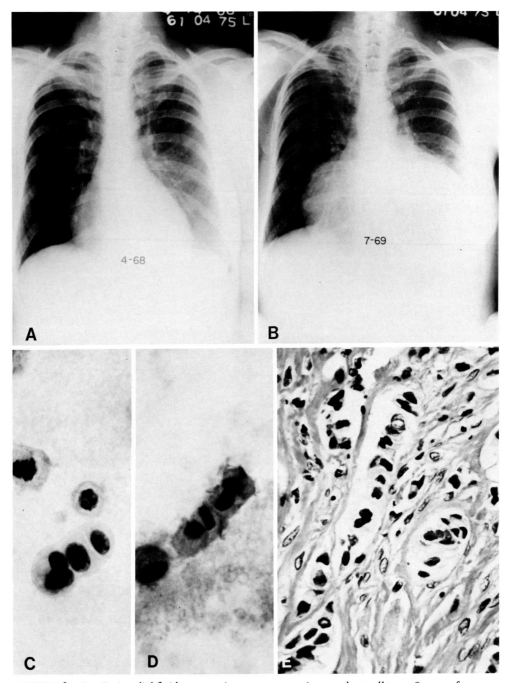

FIGURE 26–30.   Pericardial fluid: metastatic mammary carcinoma, duct cell type, 8 years after mastectomy. Dramatic remission after radiotherapy. (*A*) Normal control chest radiograph in April 1968. (*B*) Chest radiograph obtained because of dyspnea in July, 1969 shows a massive pericardial effusion. (*C*) Abnormal cells in pericardial fluid. Except for nuclear hyperchromasia, the identification of these cells as malignant is very difficult. (*D*) Indian file of cancer cells—note abnormal nuclear shapes. (*E*) Area of original infiltrating duct carcinoma with Indian file arrangement of cells. (*C, D* ×560; *E* ×350)

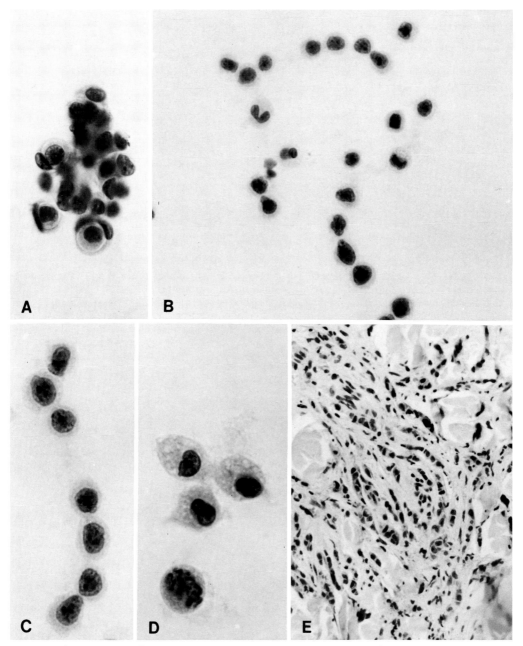

FIGURE 26–31.   Pleural fluid. Metastatic mammary carcinoma, ductal type (small cell). (*A*) Papillary cluster of small cancer cells. Note the three cell-in-cell arrangements at the periphery of the cluster. Although this may also occur with mesothelial cells and macrophages, it would be most unusual to see three such images in one field. Note also nuclear hyperchromasia. (*B*) Very long Indian file of cancer cells. This length of cell file is practically never seen in the absence of cancer. (*C*) Detail of cells shown in (*B*). It may be noted that such nuclear features as hyperchromasia, irregular border, and large nucleoli are strongly suggestive of cancer. (*D*) Elsewhere in the same smear there were clearly malignant cells with atypical mitoses. (*E*) Histologic section of the original infiltrating duct carcinoma (scirrhous carcinoma) of the breast. Note the characteristic arrangement of cancer cells in Indian file. (*A, B* ×650; *C, D* ×1,000; *E* ×250)

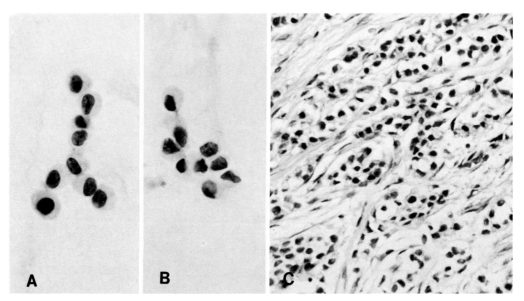

FIGURE 26–32. Ascitic fluid. Metastatic mammary carcinoma, lobular type. (*A, B*) Two clusters of small cancer cells. In cluster (*A*) the Indian file may be readily mistaken for mesothelial cells, except that the cell chain is somewhat longer than customarily seen with mesothelial cells. There is also some nuclear hyperchromasia. Cluster (*B*) shows abnormalities of nuclear shape and a dense nuclear texture not usually observed in mesothelial cells or macrophages. The diagnosis of breast cancer in this setting is very difficult. (*C*) Infiltrating lobular carcinoma removed 1 year before effusion occurred. (*A, B* ×560; *C* ×350)

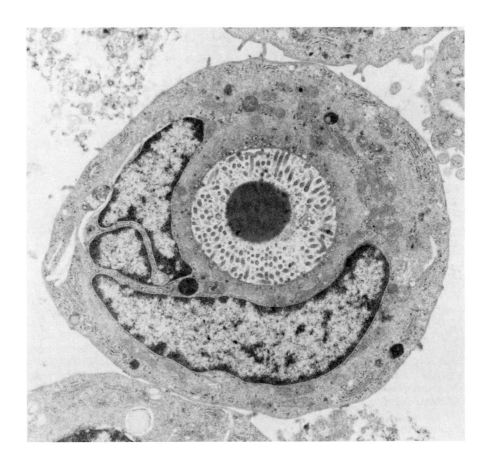

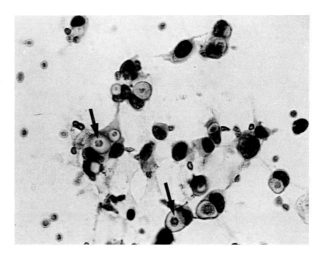

FIGURE 26 – 34. Lobular carcinoma of breast, aspiration biopsy. Small cancer cells with large cytoplasmic vacuoles, pushing the nucleus to the side and giving the cells the "signet ring" appearance. Within the vacuoles there are condensations of mucus (*arrows*) giving the vacuoles a "bull's-eye" appearance. Compare with the electronmicrograph of an identical cell shown in Fig. 26–33. Such cells, whether observed in effusions or in aspiration biopsies from the breast or various other body sites, are nearly always diagnostic of mammary carcinoma of lobular type. (×450. Modified from Koss, L.G., et al.: Aspiration Biopsy. Cytologic Interpretation and Histologic Bases. New York, Igaku-Shoin, 1984, with permission)

distinct multilayered clusters, sometimes with a round, papillary configuration. Glandlike structures can be noted (see Fig. 26–24). In women, these tumors may be confused with breast cancer of large-cell type. When cancer cells occur singly the tumor type can rarely be identified. Occasionally, however, the tumor cells assume a configuration suggestive of bronchial cell origin, with a terminal plate and suggestion of cilia formation (Fig. 26–36). The nuclei have very large nucleoli and are usually somewhat less hyperchromatic than cells of epidermoid carcinoma. Cell blocks often reveal gland formation.

Oat Cell Carcinoma. In effusions, these tumors are made up of small cells with hyperchromatic nuclei and scanty cytoplasm. Salhadin et al., using fixed material stained with Papanicolaou stain, and Spriggs and Boddington, using air-dried smears and May-Grünwald or Giemsa stain, nearly simultaneously reported on the specificity of the cytologic presentation of this tumor type in effusions. The small malignant cells usually form clusters of variable size. Although most cancer cells are round, elongated cells may also be noted (Fig. 26–37). Considerable cell molding with cell-in-cell configuration may occur.

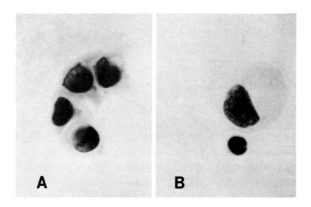

FIGURE 26 – 35. Pleural fluid. Lung, epidermoid carcinomas in two adult male patients. Two somewhat different aspects of similar tumors. (*A*) Cluster of large cancer cells in a chainlike arrangement. (*B*) Similar cell, lying singly. Nuclear hyperchromasia is evident and a large nucleolus is seen in (*B*). The histologic type of cancer cannot be identified because of absence of any distinct cytoplasmic characteristics. (*A, B* ×1,000)

FIGURE 26 – 33. Pleural fluid: metastatic mammary carcinoma. Electron micrograph of a cell showing an intracytoplasmic space lined by microvilli. Within the space a round, dense inclusion gives a positive stain for mucus. This appearance, both in light and electron microscopy, is very characteristic of mammary carcinoma, usually of lobular type. (Spriggs, A., and Jerrome, D.W.: Intracellular mucous inclusions. A feature of malignant cells in the serous cavities, particularly due to carcinoma of the breast. J. Clin. Pathol., *28*:929–936, 1975)

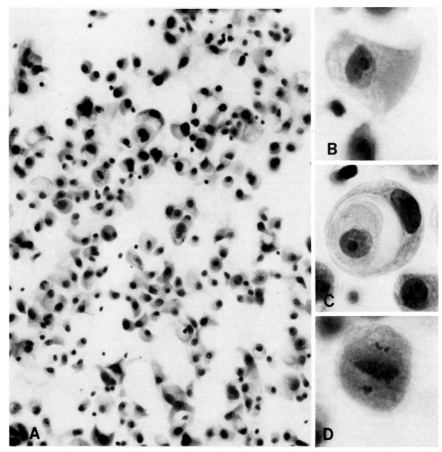

FIGURE 26–36. Pleural fluid. Metastatic bronchogenic adenocarcinoma, man, aged 60. (*A*) Abundant growth of cancer cells forming tissue culture pattern. (*B*) Note extraordinary resemblance of a metastatic malignant cell to bronchial epithelial cells. Note a terminal plate and, possibly, cilia on one surface. The nuclear abnormalities, especially the huge nucleoli, are clearly those of cancer. (*C, D*) Other details of malignant cells: a cell-in-cell arrangement (*C*), and an atypical mitosis with chromosomal lag (*D*). Compare *C* with cell-in-cell arrangement of mesothelial cells in cirrhosis, shown in Fig. 25–31A. (*A* ×250; *B, C, D* ×1,000)

Perhaps the most characteristic feature of cells of oat cell carcinoma in effusions is the formation of strings or chains made up of flattened cancer cells of various sizes. These resemble a pile of coins of various denominations or a string of flat beads. Salhadin compared this last presentation to the arrangement of vertebrae in spinal column, a most appropriate comparison (see Fig. 26–37). This arrangement of cells of oat cell carcinoma is similar to the Indian files observed in small-cell mammary carcinoma. Cytologically, the two tumors may be confused. However, mammary carcinoma is practically never seen in male patients, whereas oat cell carcinoma is more common in men than in women.

Because of the small size of cancer cells in oat cell carcinoma, another important point of differential diagnosis is malignant lymphoma. The latter never forms elongated cells or tightly fitting cell clusters. Yet sometimes the cells of oat cell carcinoma may be completely dissociated and appear singly, resulting in a diagnostic dilemma that cannot be solved in the absence of clinical data.

Carcinoma of the Ovary

Following breast cancer, ovarian cancer is the second most frequent malignant tumor in women that gives rise to effusions. Ascites is by far the more frequent effusion in ovarian cancer, but pleural ef-

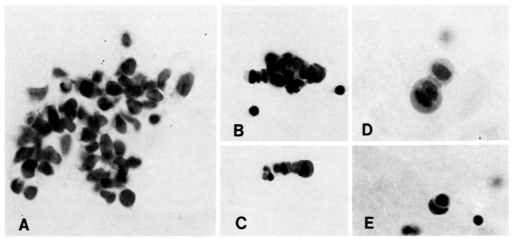

FIGURE 26–37. Metastatic oat cell carcinoma, pleural fluid. (*A*) Loose cluster of small cancer cells, some of elongated configuration. (*B*) Another, tightly packed cluster of cancer cells. At the periphery of the cluster, the cells are arranged in sequence resembling a string of flat beads or coins. (*C*) The tight cluster of flat, small cancer cells resembles the arrangement of vertebrae in the spine or a rouleau of erythrocytes. (*D, E*) Small cancer cells arranged in a short file (*D*) and showing cell-in-cell configuration (*E*). (*A–E* ×560)

fusions may also occur. The exact identification of tumor type may occasionally be possible, depending on the histologic type.

Serous Type of Ovarian Carcinoma. The cytological presentation of this tumor is usually that of a papillary adenocarcinoma made up of large cells and often accompanied by psammoma bodies (Figs. 26–22, 26–23*A* and 26–38). This presentation is sometimes sufficiently characteristic in ascitic fluid to allow specific organ diagnosis. In the pleural fluid the differential diagnosis includes bronchogenic carcinoma, carcinomatous mesothelioma, and thyroid carcinoma, all of which may have a similar cytologic configuration and occasionally form psammoma bodies. However, it is unusual for ovarian cancer to produce pleural effusions without clinical evidence of abdominal disease. Thus, an accurate clinical history is helpful in the differential diagnosis. Other metastatic tumors that occasionally produce psammoma bodies in ascitic fluid are endometrial carcinomas and renal carcinomas. The uncommon low-grade (borderline) ovarian carcinomas, the so-called endosalpingiomas, have a rather characteristic cytologic presentation and produce large sheets of fairly uniform cells (Fig. 26–39).

Mucinous Ovarian Tumors. Such tumors, whether cytologically benign or malignant, have a propensity to spread on the peritoneal surfaces and produce mucus. Mucus production results in formation of *pseudomyxoma peritonei*, which may lead to enormous abdominal distention. The gross and cytologic presentation of pseudomyxoma peritonei is quite characteristic. The material obtained from the abdominal cavity is a viscous, whitish or yellowish fluid. On microscopic examination there are very few cells, and the customary population of macrophages, mesothelial cells, and leukocytes is absent. Well-differentiated columnar cells with small, even nuclei, occurring singly and in small clusters floating in thick mucus, are characteristic of this disease (Fig. 26–40). Nuclear abnormalities may occur in the histologically more malignant variants of the tumor, but the essential cell features, as described, apply to all histologic grades. Occasionally, only acellular thick mucus is observed. This, in conjunction with clinical history, may suggest pseudomyxoma peritonei. Unfortunately, this relatively benign cytologic appearance does not correspond to the clinical course of the disease. The mucus-producing cells are most difficult to eradicate, and the patients usually die of intestinal obstruction. Pseudomyxoma peritonei may also occur as a complication of a ruptured mucocele of the appendix or Meckel's diverticulum. In the latter situations the disease may occur also in males.

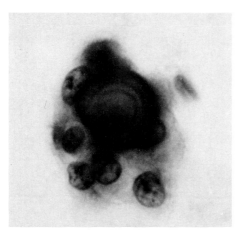

FIGURE 26–38. Ascitic fluid. Metastatic serous ovarian carcinoma with a psammoma body. Note the laminated structure of the latter, surrounded by a cluster of cancer cells. (×1,000)

Endometrioid Carcinoma. The third important subgroup of malignant ovarian tumors, histologically similar to endometrial cancer, may produce ascites or pleural effusion due to metastases. The cytologic presentation has few characteristic features beyond those of adenocarcinomas, as described above. Psammoma bodies may occasionally be observed. Metastatic endometrial carcinoma and endometrial type of carcinomas developing in foci of endometriosis in various locations cannot be differentiated from the ovarian variant (for review see Labay and Feiner).

Mixed Types of Carcinomas. Occasionally, metastatic ovarian tumors in effusions may produce a mixed population of cancer cells, combining the features of a serous carcinoma with mucus-producing cancer cells of signet ring type (cf. Fig. 26–43). Histologically, such tumors are usually predominantly of the serous type containing foci of mucus-producing cells.

Other Ovarian Tumors. In young girls and women embryonal carcinomas of the ovary and dysgerminomas may occasionally be observed. The tumor cells are readily recognized as malignant. Yolk-sac tumors, sometimes referred to as endodermal sinus tumors, may form papillary clusters of tumor cells. Cells of dysgerminoma are usually single or form small clusters. The nuclei are usually provided with large nucleoli. Multinucleated giant cells may occur. It is of interest that cells shed from dysgerminoma do not necessarily indicate a hopeless prognosis and, with vigorous treatment, recovery is possible. Metastatic seminomas of testicular or of mediastinal origin have a cytologic presentation identical with ovarian dysgerminoma (see Fig. 27–31).

An ovarian yolk-sac tumor was identified in ascitic fluid by Roncalli et al. (1988). In the cell block of the sediment the characteristic periodic acid-Schiff (PAS)-positive hyaline globules also stained with an antiserum to alpha-fetoprotein.

Occasionally primary squamous carcinomas originating in benign teratomas (dermoid cysts) of

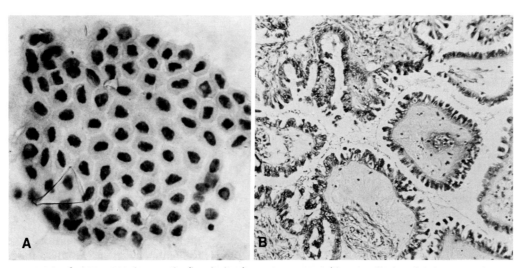

FIGURE 26–39. Very low-grade (borderline) ovarian cancer (the so-called endosalpingioma) in ascitic fluid (*A*) and in a section from the ovary (*B*). The cytologic presentation in plaques is quite characteristic. (*A* ×560; *B* ×150)

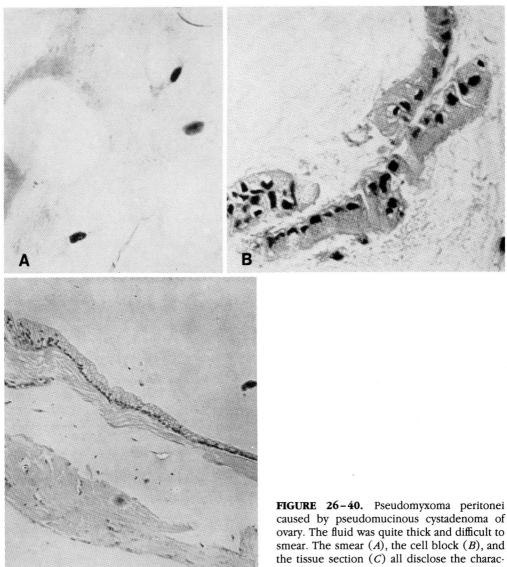

FIGURE 26–40. Pseudomyxoma peritonei caused by pseudomucinous cystadenoma of ovary. The fluid was quite thick and difficult to smear. The smear (*A*), the cell block (*B*), and the tissue section (*C*) all disclose the characteristic mucus-producing columnar cells. (*A*, *B* ×560; *C* ×150)

the ovary may form metastases leading to peritoneal effusion.

Cul-de-Sac Washings. The evaluation of fluid in the posteroinferior abdominal recess of the peritoneum, known as the cul-de-sac, is an important part of assessment of ovarian and other gynecologic tumors at the time of surgery. If the tumor is grossly still confined to the ovaries, the presence of tumor cells in fluid aspirated from the cul-de-sac, or in washings obtained therefrom, is of unfavorable, but by no means hopeless, prognostic signifi-

cance. The principal point of differential diagnosis is sheets of poorly preserved mesothelial cells that may suggest tumor cells to an inexperienced eye (for an extensive discussion, see Chap. 16).

Carcinoma of the Gastrointestinal Tract

Most tumors of gastric or colonic origin are mucus-producing adenocarcinomas, most commonly observed in ascitic fluid. The cytologic presentation is often that of an adenocarcinoma, either in the form of single cells (Fig. 26–41) or in the

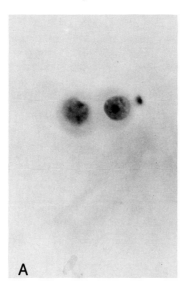
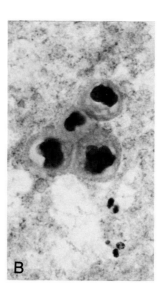

FIGURE 26–41.   Cells of metastatic gastric carcinoma. (*A*) Ascitic fluid; note the presence of large nucleoli and only slight nuclear granularity (cfr. Fig. 26–23*B*, same case). (*B*) Pericardial fluid; the nuclei are multiple, large, irregular, and hyperchromatic (in contrast with *A*), probably because of cell degeneration owing to fluid accumulation of long standing. (*A, B* ×560).

form of papillary clusters (see Fig. 26–23*B*). Well-preserved cells of gastric carcinoma are often approximately spherical, have large nucleoli and granular nuclei, with a low level of hyperchromasia (see Fig. 26–41*A*). Similar cells obtained from a fluid of long standing (in this example a pericardial effusion) may show marked nuclear hyperchromasia and multinucleation, presumably a degenerative phenomenon (see Fig. 26–41*B*).

There are two cytologic presentations that are strongly suggestive, although not fully diagnostic,

of metastatic adenocarcinoma of gastrointestinal tract origin. The presence of large, columnar cancer cells strongly suggests metastatic colonic carcinoma (Fig. 26–42). Signet ring-type cells derived from mucus-producing adenocarcinomas are large, round, or oval, with markedly abnormal, usually hyperchromatic, eccentric nuclei. The cytoplasm of these cells gives a positive stain for mucus (Fig. 26–43). The signet ring cancer cells must be differentiated from vacuolated macrophages (see Fig. 25–19) which may be of similar

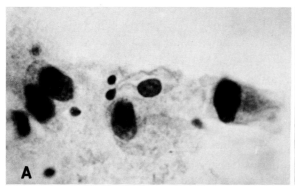
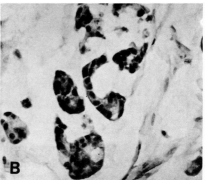

FIGURE 26–42.   Ascitic fluid: metastatic colonic carcinoma. (*A*) Note the columnar configuration of some of the large cancer cells and the finely granular, opaque cytoplasm in others. (*B*) Cell block of the same fluid showing a mucus-producing carcinoma. (*A* ×1,000; *B* ×250)

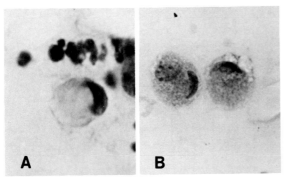

FIGURE 26–43. Ascitic fluid: metastatic colonic carcinoma—signet-ring type. (*A*) Note the large size of the hyperchromatic, peripheral nucleus and the opaque cytoplasm. (*B*) Mucicarmine stain. Positive, gray, in reality red, stain of the cytoplasmic contents. (*A*, *B* ×1,000)

size and have similar general configuration, except for the absence of nuclear abnormalities. Occasionally, lobular carcinoma of the breast may have a similar presentation, but the malignant cells are much smaller (see Fig. 26–34).

Pozalaky et al. (1983) pointed out that cancer cells of colorectal origin in effusions have a characteristic electron microscopic feature that facilitates their recognition. The presence of microvilli, with dense cores of microfilaments that extend deeply into the cytoplasm ("cytoplasmic rootlets"), was observed in cells of colorectal origin (Fig. 26–44), but not in pulmonary adenocarcinoma. Rootlets were also absent in cells of ovarian carcinoma (see Fig. 26–18*D*).

Epidermoid carcinomas of the esophagus or gastric cardia have a similar presentation to that of lung cancers of the same histologic type (see p. 1138). Dr. Jeffie Roszell pointed out that keratinizing squamous carcinomas of the stomach may occur in horses and produce metastases made up of perfectly well-differentiated squamous cells, which can be identified in ascitic fluid (Fig. 26–45).

Metastatic Pancreatic Carcinomas. Such carcinomas have no distinguishing features in fluids. The large cancer cells, easily recognizable, usually have large nucleoli and, occasionally, a makeup suggestive of adenocarcinoma.

Contrary to some statements in the literature that primary *hepatocellular carcinomas* cannot be identified in ascitic fluid, several such cases have been observed personally and by others. The cancer cells, usually of moderate size, but occasionally large, either occur singly (Fig. 26–46) or in clusters suggestive of adenocarcinoma. Specific cytoplasmic features, such as bilelike material and formation of bile canaliculi, were identified by ultrastructural studies (Woyke et al.)

Other Carcinomas

Accurate identification of specific patterns of less common metastatic, malignant epithelial tumors is occasionally possible.

Thyroid carcinomas may form psammoma bodies (Fig. 26–47), but so can other cancers, as discussed on p. 1134. In general, however, the cells of thyroid carcinoma are smaller than those of most other cancers that form psammoma bodies. Cells of metastatic papillary carcinomas (or of the follicular variant thereof) may also contain intranuclear cytoplasmic inclusions ("nuclear holes") commonly observed in this tumor type, but by no means limited to it (see below, malignant melanoma). However, the combination of papillary cell clusters, psammoma bodies, *and* intranuclear cytoplasmic inclusions is *diagnostic* of metastatic papillary carcinoma of the thyroid (Fig. 26–48).

Renal carcinomas have few distinguishing features. The cell size and configuration and finely vacuolated cytoplasm may render the differential diagnosis with mesothelial cells and macrophages very difficult (Fig. 26–49).

Urothelial carcinomas or *adenocarcinomas of the lower urinary tract* origin can rarely be identified as to site of origin. Occasionally, however, better-differentiated urothelial carcinomas may form cells similar to umbrella cells (see Chap. 23). Keratinizing squamous cancers of these organs usually show the features diagnostic of this tumor type. *Prostatic carcinomas* appear as adenocarcinomas. They may be identified by immunocytologic staining for prostatic antigen (see Chap. 34). *Endometrial carcinomas* usually appear as papillary adenocarcinomas. Occasionally, however, they have the pattern of a poorly differentiated tumor. Psammoma bodies may occur in these tumors.

Cytologic Presentation of Malignant Disorders of Lymphoid and Hematogenous Origin

Malignant Lymphoma

The cytologic diagnosis of malignant lymphoma in effusions may be made in most cases. Such a diagnosis is not merely a theoretical nicety, but often is of significant therapeutic and prognostic value. Malignant lymphomas can be treated suc-

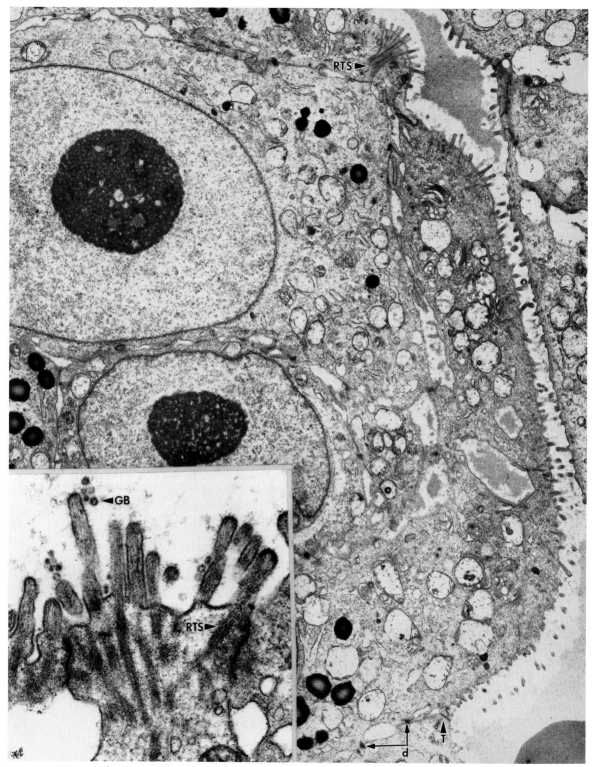

FIGURE 26–44. Electron micrograph of a cluster of metastatic cancer cells of rectal origin in pleural fluid. Note the numerous microvilli on cell surface with deep "cytoplasmic rootlets" (RTS). *Inset*: The dense filamentous core of the microvilli and the rootlets extending deeply into the cytoplasm are shown. (d, desmosomes; GB, glycocalyceal bodies; RTS, rootlets; T, tight junction). (×9,000; *inset* × 36,000, reduced 81%. Pozalaky Z., et al.: Electron microscopic identification of the colorectal origins of tumor cells in pleural fluid. Acta Cytol., *27*:45–48, 1983)

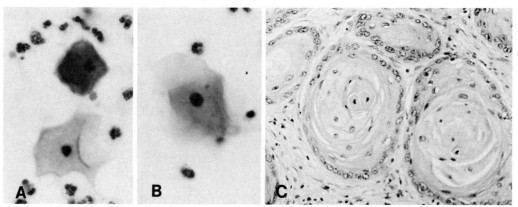

FIGURE 26–45. Ascitic fluid; metastatic squamous carcinoma of stomach in a horse. (*A, B*) Extremely well-differentiated squamous cancer cells. (*C*) Metastatic, very well-differentiated squamous carcinoma in omentum. (*A, B* ×560; *C* ×150. Courtesy of Dr. Jeffie Roszell, Tulsa, Oklahoma)

cessfully by numerous means: thus, the identification of malignant lymphoma in an effusion is not tantamount to a hopeless situation, as is true with many other metastatic cancers. A rapid identification of the disease may lead to aggressive treatment and may be compatible with many years of useful life.

The experience in my laboratory, based on the study of 200 consecutive patients with malignant lymphoma and related diseases who had pleural effusion or ascites, was summarized by Melamed (Table 26–2).

Within recent years the histologic terminology of various types of malignant lymphoma has been repeatedly modified, notably by Rappaport and by Lukes.

For the purposes of cytologic recognition in effusions, four groups of malignant lymphomas may be recognized.

1. Large-cell lymphomas
2. Small-cell lymphomas
3. Hodgkin's disease
4. Miscellaneous lymphoproliferative and hematologic disorders, including rare types of lymphomas, plasma cell myelomas, and leukemias

This classification is for morphologic purposes only. Classification of malignant lymphomas into B- and T-cell types and further immunologic classification of this group of disorders are discussed in Chapters 29 and 34.

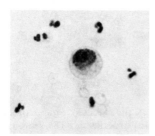

FIGURE 26–46. Ascitic fluid; metastatic hepatocellular carcinoma. The small cancer cell is not diagnostic of the tumor type. (×560)

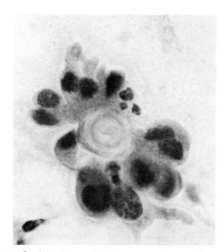

FIGURE 26–47. Pleural fluid; metastatic papillary carcinoma of thyroid. Cancer cells surround a centrally located psammoma body. (×1,000)

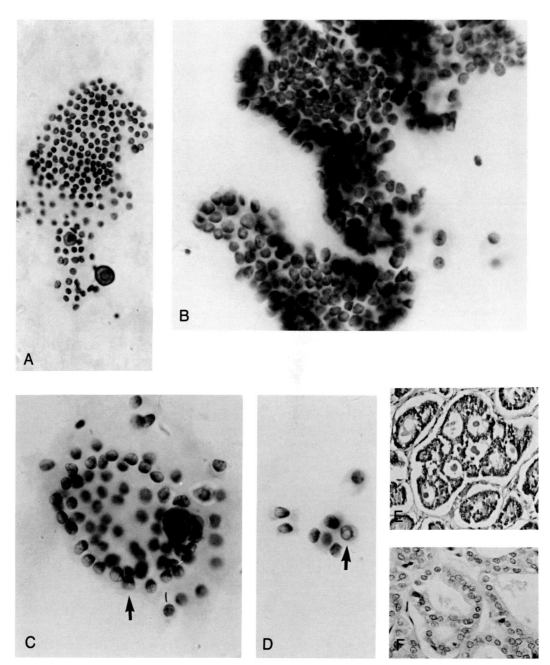

FIGURE 26–48.   Metastatic papillary carcinoma (follicular variant) of thyroid in pleural fluid of a 54-year-old woman. (*A–D*) Pleural fluid: (*A*) Low-power view of a cluster of small, monotonous cancer cells with two psammoma bodies. (*B*) Elsewhere the small tumor cells formed large papillary clusters. (*C*) Another cluster with psammoma body and an intranuclear cytoplasmic inclusion (*arrow*), not well focused. (*D*) Another cluster of small tumor cells with focus on the intranuclear cytoplasmic inclusion (*arrow*). (*E*) Biopsy of the metastatic cancer in lung. The pattern is that of a follicular variant of papillary carcinoma. (*F*) Brain metastasis at postmortem examination. The characteristic opaque nuclear configuration in the acini is consistent with the follicular variant of a papillary thyroid carcinoma. (*A*, *F* ×150; *B*, *C*, *D* ×560; *E* ×350. Courtesy of Dr. Myron R. Melamed, New York, New York)

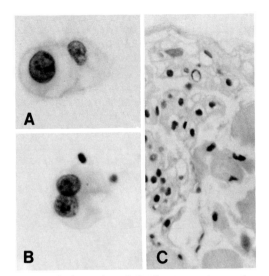

FIGURE 26–49. Pleural fluid. Metastatic renal carcinoma, clear cell type. The malignant cells (*A, B*), although large, show few classic features of cancer. The nuclei are granular and contain small nucleoli. Pleural biopsy (*C*) shows a focus of metastatic cancer in striated muscle. (*A, B* ×560; *C* ×150)

General Characteristics of Malignant Lymphomas in Effusions. Regardless of the type of malignant lymphoma, the cancer cells from such cases *virtually never form cohesive aggregates or clumps of cells.* The cancer cells *lie singly,* and it is permissible to state that, in effusions, any malignant tumor characterized by cell clusters, which are not an artifact of preparatory techniques, is *not* a malignant lymphoma, regardless of the size and makeup of individual cells. The diagnosis of malignant lymphoma is made as much on the pattern of smears as on individual cell abnormalities. The latter are described in some detail according to predominant tumor type.

Large Cell Lymphoma. This group comprises B- and T-cell lymphomas, with or without cleaved nuclei, including the immunoblastic and lymphoblastic types (National Cancer Institute classification of 1982). Malignant lymphomas of large-cell type are the easiest to diagnose cytologically, because the cell abnormalities are usually well evident, and the number of malignant cells in fluids is frequently large. The cells of large-cell lymphomas vary in size but nearly always some large cancer cells are observed. There is usually considerable variation in shapes of cells, some of which may be very bizarre. However, the most significant abnormalities pertain to the nuclei. The nuclei, rarely round or oval, have more often a very irregular contour. Sometimes indentations or cleavage may be observed. *Nuclear protrusions* in the form of small, tonguelike projections, single or multiple, are characteristic of malignant lymphoma cells and are uncommon in other malignant tumors

Table 26–2
Incidence of Malignant Cells in Effusion According to Histologic Type of Malignant Lymphoma

Histological Diagnosis	Cytologic Evidence of Cancer				
	Total No. Pt.	Present No. Pt.	Present % Pt.	Susp., No. Pt.	Not Pres., No. Pt.
Reticulum cell sarcoma (Large-cell lymphoma)	71	53	75	7	11
Lymphosarcoma					
Diffuse	32	19	59	6	7
Nodular	16	9	56	3	4
Hodgkin's disease	56	14	25	6	36
Acute leukemia	10	5		3	2
Chronic leukemia	6	4		1	1
Leukolymphosarcoma	4	4		..	..
Plasmacytic myeloma	3	2		1	..
Letterer–Siwe disease	2	1		1	

(Modified from Melamed, M. R.: The cytological presentation of malignant lymphomas and related diseases in effusions. Cancer, *16*:413–431, 1963)

(Fig. 26–50). Atkin and Baker observed nuclear protrusions in an ovarian carcinoma in ascitic fluid and attributed the protrusion to an abnormally long marker chromosome. It is of interest that an early analysis of chromosomal makeup of malignant lymphomas by Miles (1966) yielded several tumors with long marker chromosomes. Whether the nuclear protrusions observed so often in cells of large-cell lymphoma in effusions are due to marker chromosomes remains to be determined. For further comments on cytogenetics of malignant lymphomas see Chapter 7.

Nucleolar abnormalities are frequent and often striking in large-cell lymphomas. The nucleoli are large, irregular in shape, and often multiple. The author has never observed a larger-cell lymphoma without obvious nucleolar abnormalities. Usually, there is some relationship between the size of the nucleus and the size of the nucleolus: larger tumor cells have larger (and sometimes more numerous) nucleoli than smaller tumor cells (see Fig. 26–50B,D and 26–51). Prominent chromocenters may also be present. Abnormal mitoses are fairly common (see Fig. 26–51B).

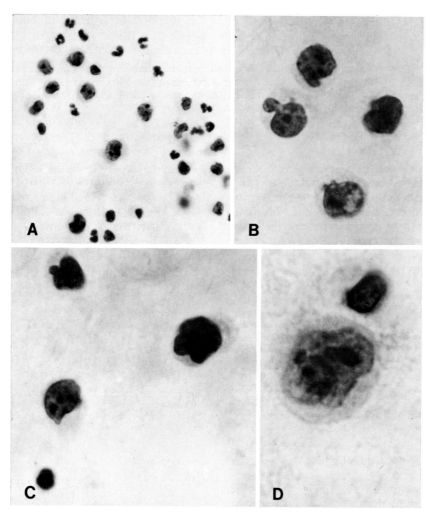

FIGURE 26–50. Cytologic presentation of a large-cell lymphoma in effusion. (*A*) Low-power view showing large malignant cells intermixed with polymorphonuclear leukocytes. (*B, C, D*) Details of cell structure. Note irregular nuclei with protrusion, well seen in (*B*) and (*C*). Large, irregular nucleoli may be observed in (*B*) and (*D*). (*A* ×560; *B, C* ×1,425; *D* ×2,000, oil immersion. Melamed, M.R.: The cytologic presentation of malignant lymphomas and related diseases in effusions. Cancer, *16*:413–431, 1963)

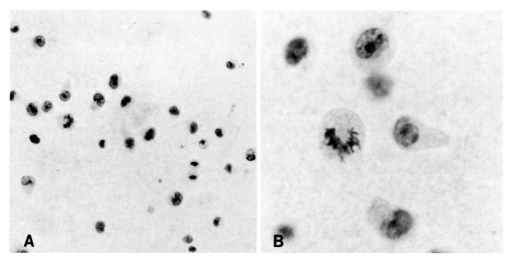

FIGURE 26–51. Pleural fluid. Metastatic large-cell lymphoma imitating metastatic carcinoma. (*A*) Tissue culture pattern with a marked proliferation of malignant cells lying singly. Note extensive mitotic activity. (*B*) High-power view of cancer cells shows abundant cytoplasm and marked nuclear abnormalities. Note an abnormal mitosis. (*A* ×150; *B* ×1,000)

The cytoplasm of cells of large-cell lymphoma is usually scanty, faintly basophilic and delicate, and is rarely well preserved. When the cytoplasm is intact, faint vacuolization may be noted. The contrast between this delicate cytoplasm and the large, abnormal nucleus is usually very marked. Occasionally, however, the cytoplasm may be surprisingly abundant and the malignant cells may mimic a metastatic carcinoma (see Fig. 26–51).

In a classic case, the diagnosis of large-cell lymphoma in effusions presents comparatively little difficulty both for the presence of malignant disease and the identification of the tumor type (see Fig. 26–50). At both ends of the spectrum diagnostic difficulties may arise. If the tumors are composed of small, fairly uniform cells, the differentiation from a small-cell lymphoma may be a matter of individual opinion, as is also found with histologic material.

The differential diagnosis between the cells of a large-cell lymphoma with abundant cytoplasm, such as shown in Fig. 26–51, and metastatic carcinoma with dispersed cells (cf. Fig. 26–41, as an example) may require the use of common lymphocyte antigen and other immunostaining techniques to establish the diagnosis (see Chap. 34). It is rare, though, for a carcinoma not to show a few organized cell clusters, a helpful feature in determining tumor type. As always, an accurate clinical history and review of previous histologic material is a key to diagnostic accuracy.

Small-Cell Lymphoma. This type of malignant lymphoma is usually characterized in exudates by small malignant cells 6 to 12 μm in diameter, rarely larger. The most common diagnostic presentation is "the variable lymphocytic type" (Melamed, 1963). The cells are usually round or oval, with very scanty, barely visible cytoplasm. There is a significant variation in the size of these cells—hence, the name (Figs. 26–52 and 26–53). The nuclei are

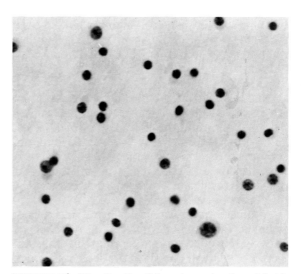

FIGURE 26–52. Small-cell lymphoma in pleural fluid. Note the variation in size of cells. Nucleoli are visible in the large cells. (×560)

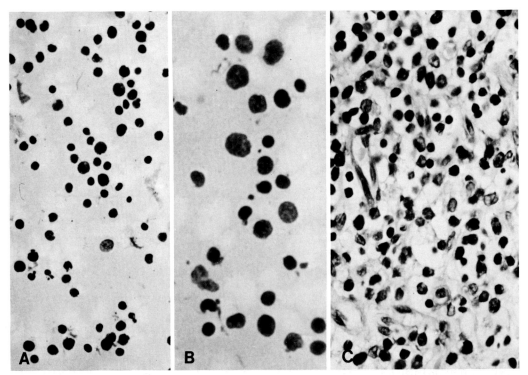

FIGURE 26–53. Variable lymphocyte type of malignant lymphoma in effusions. (*A*) The variation in cell size characteristic of malignant lymphoma is seen in low-power view. The cells have virtually no cytoplasm, but the nuclei are round and the nucleoli less prominent than in large-cell lymphoma (cf. Fig. 26–50). (*B*) Note small nuclear protrusions. Corresponding tissue section is seen in (*C*). (*A*, *C* ×560; *B* ×1,140. Melamed, M.R.: The cytological presentation of malignant lymphomas and related diseases in effusions. Cancer, *16*:413–431, 1963)

hyperchromatic, occasionally cleaved or somewhat irregular in shape, but mainly round or oval. Nucleoli are present in many of the cells, but they do not stand out as in large-cell lymphomas. Nuclear protrusions may be observed (see Fig. 26–53*B*).

Nuclear fragmentation in the form of massive karyorrhexis of nuclei may occur (Fig. 26–54). This may represent the effect of treatment (see p. 1174), but has been repeatedly observed in the absence of any history of treatment. Massive karyorrhexis has not been observed by me in any tumors other than malignant lymphoma and appears to be diagnostic of this group of diseases.

Another helpful feature in identifying cells of lymphocytic lymphoma (and chronic lymphocytic leukemia) in effusions is the granularity of the nuclei. The feature was first described by Spriggs and Vanhegan (1981) as *cellules grumelées* or "lumpy cells," characterized by numerous coarse aggregates of chromatin in otherwise spherical nu-

clei (see Fig. 27–19*A*). Seidel and Garbes (1985) reviewed the diagnostic value of this feature and found it to be a useful fixation artifact that occurred only in malignant disorders, but not in benign lymphocytes.

The characteristic cytologic presentation of small-cell lymphoma is virtually never confused with other cancers, but not infrequently it is mistaken for an inflammatory reaction. A technically impeccable preparation is required for diagnosis, which cannot be made with the help of various filter devices or other technical shortcuts. The differentiation between cells of small-cell lymphoma or chronic lymphocytic leukemia and normal lymphocytes may be difficult or impossible without clinical information and immunologic analysis (see Chap. 34).

Cardiac Malignant Lymphomas. The rare primary cardiac lymphomas cause pericardial effusions and, accordingly, are amenable to primary

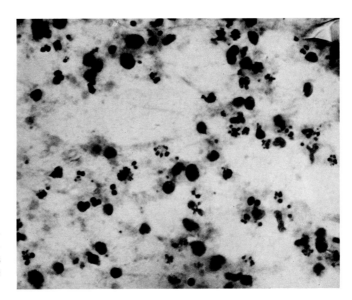

FIGURE 26–54. Karyorrhexis in small-cell malignant lymphoma. This event may occur spontaneously or may be secondary to treatment and is diagnostic of the disease. In this example, the agent was nitrogen mustard. (Approx. ×300)

diagnosis by cytology. Cases of this type were reported by Pozniak et al. (1986) and Castelli et al. (1989).

Primary lymphomas also may develop in heart transplant patients and may also cause pericardial effusions. We observed a case of large-cell lymphoma, first diagnosed by cytology in a 52-year-old man with a heart transplant.

Hodgkin's Disease. The diagnosis of Hodgkin's disease in effusions can be made only if Reed–Sternberg cells are identified. Although mononucleated cells with large nucleoli (Hodgkin's cells) may also be noted, it is safer to confine this diagnosis to cells with two or more nuclei (Fig. 26–55). In the binucleated cells the two nuclei may form mirror images of each other (Fig. 26–56A).

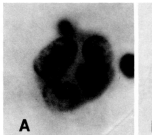 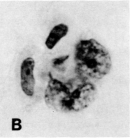

FIGURE 26–55. Pleural fluids; two examples of Reed–Sternberg cells in metastatic Hodgkin's disease. (A) Cell with four nuclei, each containing a very large nucleolus. (B) A cell with two very large and two small nuclei, suggestive of uneven division of nuclear material. Note large nucleoli in the two large nuclei. (A, B ×1,000)

More often the nuclei are oval and separated by a band of cytoplasm. Regardless of the nuclear shape, very large, usually single nucleoli are present. It is of note that phagocytized small particles may often be observed in the cytoplasm of such cells.

Accompanying the Reed–Sternberg cells are mononucleated cells of the type described for large-cell lymphoma, or lymphocytic cells of various types. Plasma cells are occasionally observed (see Fig. 26–56B). Eosinophilic leukocytes are scarce. Of all forms of malignant lymphoma, the diagnosis of Hodgkin's disease is by far the most difficult. Differentiation of Reed–Sternberg cells from atypical mesothelial cells, on the one hand, and from cancer cells of epithelial origin, on the other, may be the source of substantial difficulty. The differentiation of Hodgkin's disease from a large-cell lymphoma may prove impossible.

Differentiation of Malignant Lymphoma from Nonmalignant Disorders. The differentiation of malignant lymphoma from other malignant tumors has been discussed above. It must be stressed that abundant lymphocytes may be present in a variety of effusions caused by infectious diseases, primarily tuberculosis. However, the latter may be accompanied by a very marked mesothelial proliferation that is rarely conspicuous in malignant lymphoma, except in Hodgkin's disease.

Nevertheless, noncancerous disease occasionally will have a cytologic presentation similar to that of a malignant lymphoma. One such example,

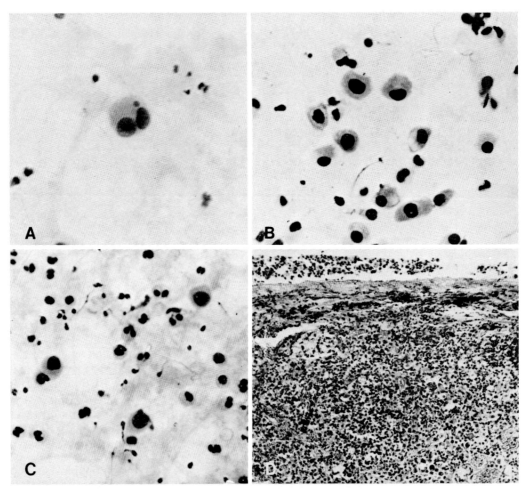

FIGURE 26–56. (*A*) Hodgkin's disease in pleural fluid. Characteristic Reed–Sternberg cell. Note the large nucleoli. A particle of phagocytized material is present in the cytoplasm. (*B*) Hodgkin's disease in abdominal fluid, presenting clinically as a chronic chyloperitoneum caused by obstruction of cisterna magna by tumor. Note the numerous plasma cell-like cells. All the cells are somewhat overstained, and no definite tumor cells may be seen in this field. (*C, D*) Hodgkin's disease involving pleura (same case as that in Fig. 20–80). The cytologic presentation suggests a large-cell lymphoma. Tissue section of pleura (*D*) shows Hodgkin's disease. (*A, B, C* ×560; *D* ×150)

quoted by Melamed, was in ascitic fluid from a child with giant cell hepatitis and extensive extramedullary hematopoiesis. Leukemoid reactions of various types, accompanied by effusions, may also result in confusing cellular patterns.

In the final analysis, the cytologic diagnosis of malignant lymphoma in debatable cases should be supported by clinical and immunologic evidence, as is the case with histologic material.

The effects of therapy on cells of malignant lymphoma are discussed on page 1174.

Very Rare Types of Malignant Lymphoma. Young and Crocker (1984) reported a case of lymphoplasmacytoid lymphoma. The tumor cells in pleural fluid contained conspicuous intracytoplasmic immunoglobulin inclusions. The case was thought to be a variant of vacuolated B-cell lymphoma (Kim et al., 1978; Harris et al., 1981). The cells shown were somewhat similar to the cells of metastatic lobular carcinoma (cf. Fig. 26–34), except for the absence of the central mucinous inclusion or cell clustering. The rare Ki lymphomas may mimic metastatic carcinoma (see Chap. 29).

Miller et al. (1987) described a case of multilobated lymphoma in pleural fluid. The highly malignant tumor was characterized by multilobated tumor cells, each nucleus provided with a nucleolus. The tumor was shown to be a B-cell lymphoma, although in its original description by Pincus et al. (1979), the neoplasm was thought to be of T-cell derivation. I observed an identical case in cerebrospinal fluid (see Chap. 27).

Vernon and Rosenthal (1979) described the presence of Sézary cells in ascitic fluid in a patient with disseminated mycosis fungoides, a cutaneous form of T-cell lymphoma. The large malignant cells are characterized by complex nuclear convolutions ("serpentine or cerebriform nuclei") and scanty cytoplasm (see also p. 1286 and Fig. 29–53).

Effusions in Leukemias

Chronic lymphocytic leukemia gives a fairly uniform cytologic pattern of lymphocytes; its differentiation from an inflammatory exudate rich in lymphocytes or from metastatic well-differentiated small-cell lymphoma may be extremely difficult and must usually rest on clinical and hematologic evidence except for the presence of "lumpy cells" (see above).

Other leukemic cells may often be identified in effusions. Acute myeloid and monocytic leukemias may be confused with large-cell lymphoma. Effusions in chronic myelogenous leukemia must be differentiated from inflammatory reactions. Yam (1985) described an unusual case of granulocytic sarcoma (tumor manifestation of chronic granulocytic leukemia) in pleural fluid. The cells were identified as granulocytic precursors by a battery of cytochemical studies. It is exceedingly rare for patients with leukemia to develop effusions in the absence of prior clinical diagnosis. Hence, the cytopathologist will rarely have the opportunity to establish the primary diagnosis of the disease in effusions. Rather, he will be requested to help delineate the extent of the disease for purposes of treatment (see also Spinal Fluid, p. 1201).

Plasma Cell Myeloma

Disseminated plasma cell myeloma (multiple myeloma) may be associated with pleural effusion or ascites. In several such cases a surprisingly uniform population of readily identifiable plasma cells was observed (Fig. 26–57). In several personally observed cases the *primary* diagnosis of plasma cell myeloma was made in effusions before any clinical evidence of skeletal disease. In two instances, one of pleural and the other of ascitic* fluid, a pure pop-

---

*Case courtesy of Ms. Carol Bales.

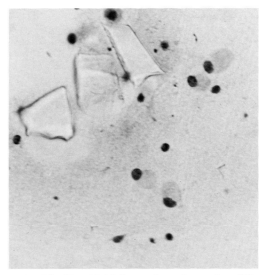

FIGURE 26–57. Multiple myeloma becoming diffuse; pleural fluid. Note clearly identifiable plasma cells with peripheral nuclei. The crystals represent a condensation of the mounting medium and are not related to the disease. (×560)

ulation of well-differentiated plasma cells was observed (Fig. 26–58). In one of the cases a pleural biopsy disclosed an infiltration with plasma cells and immunoelectrophoresis of the pleural fluid disclosed an abnormal globulin pattern. In both cases, subsequent evidence of inconspicuous skeletal lesions was obtained, followed by fatal outcome of the disease. Again, it must be stressed that isolated plasma cells may be observed in lymphomas, especially in Hodgkin's disease and in chronic inflammatory processes.

Cytologic Presentation of Sarcomas and Other Less Common Cancers

Sarcomas of Soft Tissues and Bone

A large variety of metastatic sarcomas may produce effusions wherein cancer cells may be identified. The subject has been extensively discussed by Hajdu and Hajdu. All sarcomas of soft tissues tend to form unusual, large, and bizarre tumor cells. In general, the exact identification of type of tumor is rarely possible in fluids, although there are occasional exceptions. Since it is most unusual for sarcomas to produce effusions as the first manifestation of disease, knowledge of past history and review of prior histologic material is very helpful in

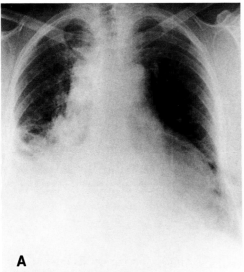

A

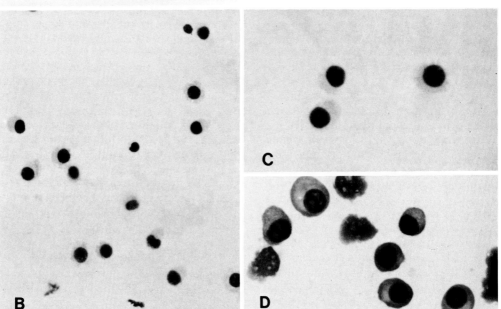

B   C   D

FIGURE 26–58. Plasma cell myeloma in a 54-year-old woman. Primary diagnosis on pleural fluid. The patient died of disseminated myeloma 12 months later. (*A*) Chest radiograph showing right pleural effusion. (*B, C*) Pleural fluid showing numerous mature plasma cells (Papanicolaou stain). (*D*) The same fluid: air-dried sediment stained with Wright's stain. The classic configuration of plasma cells with a peripheral nucleus and "cartwheel" arrangement of chromatin is well shown. (*B* ×560; *C, D* ×1,000)

the determination of tumor type. It must be stressed that the exact classification of many spindle cell sarcomas is often the subject of considerable debate, even on ample histologic material. Hence, it would be unlikely that such difficult diagnostic problems could be solved on examination of a handful of cells in a fluid.

Spindle Cell Sarcomas. Sarcomas of connective tissue, nerve, muscle, vascular, synovial, or bone origin are either composed of, or have a large component of, spindle cells. Kaposi's sarcomas cause bloody effusions wherein fibroblast-like cells can be observed.

When seen in fluids, the tumor cells are often large, bizarre, and multinucleated. The nuclei are usually very large, hyperchromatic, and provided with multiple, large nucleoli; thus the identification of malignant disease is usually easy (Fig. 26–59).

Further classification of these tumors in fluids is sometimes possible.

Rhabdomyosarcomas. These tumors are characterized by the presence of large, bizarre, often multinucleated tumor cells (Hajdu and Koss) (Fig. 26–60). The diagnosis may be established with complete certainty if cytoplasmic cross-striations

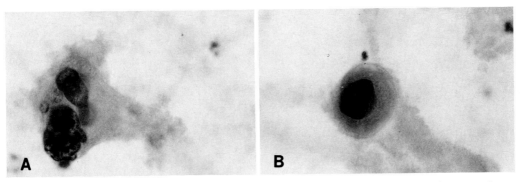

FIGURE 26–59. (*A, B*) Pleural fluid. Metastatic stromal sarcoma of breast. Note large, bizarre malignant cells. (*A, B* ×500)

are present. This may occur with metastatic rhabdomyosarcomas or with mesodermal mixed tumors that contain an element of rhabdomyosarcoma (Fig. 26–61).

Embryonal Rhabdomyosarcoma. See below, Effusions in Children.

Leiomyosarcoma. The cancer cells in fluids rarely retain the elongated form observed in tissue or in gynecologic material (see p. 643). The cells are few, round or oval, with abnormal nuclei, surrounded by scanty, poorly demarcated cytoplasm. Giant cells are very rarely seen (Hajdu and Koss). In the absence of past history and histologic material, the precise diagnosis of leiomyosarcoma is rarely possible in fluids.

Sarcomas of Bone. Metastatic osteogenic sarcomas may produce effusions, usually in the pleural cavity in association with pulmonary metastases. Although occasionally bizarre cancer cells are noted, formation of osteoid tissue by these cells has not been observed; thus, the exact diagnosis of these tumors in effusions is virtually impossible. It is of interest, however, that huge, multinucleated giant cells with regular, even nuclei, provided with small nucleoli, have been observed in such effusions. Similar cells have been noted in material from recurrent giant cell tumors of bone and, consequently, it may be assumed that these cells belong to the family of osteoclasts (Fig. 26–62; see also Fig. 27–29). These cells are much larger than multinucleated macrophages or megakaryocytes, and thus, their presence may prove of diagnostic value. Cytochemical demonstration of alkaline phosphatase in tumor cells is also diagnostic of osteogenic sarcoma (Fig. 26–63).

Malignant Melanomas

Malignant melanomas, usually of cutaneous or ocular origin and of highly unpredictable behavior,

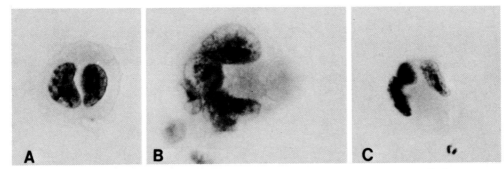

FIGURE 26–60. Metastatic rhabdomyosarcoma. Large, multinucleated tumor giant cells from metastatic rhabdomyosarcoma in pleural (*A, B*) and ascitic fluid (*C*). Striking nuclear abnormalities are evident, thus securing the diagnosis of cancer. The exact determination of tumor type on this evidence is difficult, although not impossible. (*A, B, C* ×560, Hajdu, S.I., and Koss, L.G.: Cytologic diagnosis of metastatic myosarcoma. Acta Cytol., *13*:545–551, 1969)

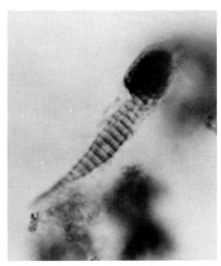

FIGURE 26–61. Ascites; metastatic mesodermal mixed tumor of ovary. Rhabdomyoblast with cytoplasmic cross-striations in ascitic fluid of a woman with mesodermal mixed tumor of ovary, growing chiefly as rhabdomyosarcoma. This cell type is fully diagnostic of rhabdomyosarcoma. (Oil immersion. Courtesy of Dr. Misao Takeda, Philadelphia, Pennsylvania)

are frequently associated with effusions. Contrary to most other malignant tumors for which clinical evidence of metastatic disease usually precedes the accumulation of fluid, effusions in malignant melanoma may occur as the primary evidence of me-

tastases, sometimes many years after the treatment of the primary tumor. Thus, the identification of this tumor type may be of considerable diagnostic importance.

Metastatic malignant melanomas in fluids usually form a rich population of clearly malignant, sometimes bizarre, cells of variable size and configuration. Cytoplasmic granules of brown or black melanin pigment, if present, are diagnostic of the disease. Most cancer cells occur singly, but small cell clusters are common. The cells, which are either mono-, bi-, or multinucleated, are often characterized by a peripheral location of the nuclei (Fig. 26–64). Yamada et al., and subsequently Hajdu and Savino, pointed out that the presence of clear zones or "holes" within the nucleus (nuclear cytoplasmic inclusions) is a frequent event in cells of malignant melanoma (Fig. 26–65). The nuclear inclusions represent intranuclear cytoplasmic invaginations that may be differentiated from very large nucleoli by careful focusing up and down under the high-power lens of the microscope. It will be seen that the inclusions have an irregular contour, vary in size, depending on the depth of focus, and are present at all levels of the nucleus. The nucleoli, on the other hand, occupy only a single band of nuclear thickness and are out of focus as soon as the lens is focused above or below them. The nuclear inclusions occur in a number of normal tissues and in other malignant tumors. Thyroid carcinomas (see Fig. 26–48) and bronchogenic ad-

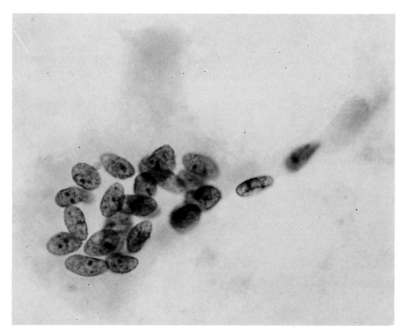

FIGURE 26–62. Osteoclastlike giant cells from pleural fluid of a patient with metastatic osteogenic sarcoma to the lung. (×1,000)

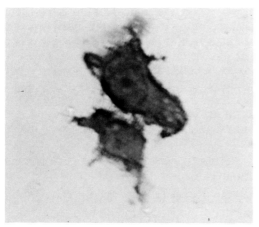

FIGURE 26-63. Metastatic osteogenic sarcoma. Alkaline phosphatase in the form of black precipitate is present in tumor cells. (Approx. ×600)

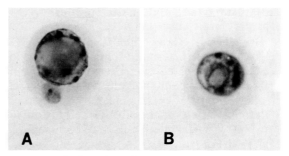

FIGURE 26-65. (*A, B*) Metastatic malignant melanoma: pleural fluid. Cells with intranuclear cytoplasmic inclusions. (*A, B* ×1,000)

enocarcinomas (see Fig. 20-35), among others, form such inclusions. Another common feature of cells of malignant melanoma is the presence of very large single or multiple nucleoli, which sometimes may occupy a substantial portion of the nucleus. Phagocytic cell images (cell-in-cell) are also frequent.

The melanin pigment that is the principal identifying feature of cells of malignant melanoma is not a constant feature. Hajdu and Savino used ferric ferricyanide stain to demonstrate melanin in tumor cells in effusions. Immunocytochemistry may also be used to confirm the diagnosis (see Chap. 34). It is of interest that if the same patient is studied by repeated taps, the presence of pigment

may vary from sample to sample. In some melanomas, the pigment is present in virtually every cell; in others, pigment formation is confined to a few cells or may be completely absent. Nevertheless, the identification of melanoma with a modest margin of error is possible if the other cell features are noted. Few other metastatic tumors in fluids have this variegated appearance.

Hemosiderosis, or accumulation of hemosiderin in macrophages in chronic hemorrhagic effusions is the most important source of diagnostic error. The macrophages may be of abnormal shapes, and their nuclear structure may appear abnormal, although partly concealed by pigment, mimicking a metastatic melanoma. Therefore, it is suggested that a simple stain for iron be included as a part of the workup of samples containing brown pigment, before the diagnosis of metastatic malignant melanoma is made (for further discussion, see p. 1113).

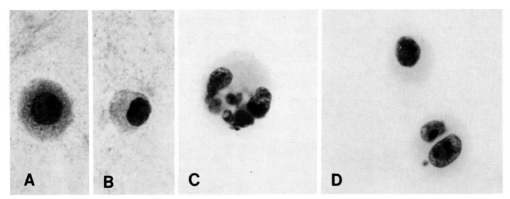

FIGURE 26-64. Pleural fluids; cells of metastatic malignant melanoma. (*A, B*) Cells with cytoplasmic pigment. Note peripheral location of the nucleus in (*B*). (*C*) Multinucleated cancer cell; (*D*) binucleated cancer cell with large nucleoli. (*A-D* ×560)

Other Metastatic Malignant Tumors

Mesodermal Mixed Tumors of the Uterus. Uterine mesodermal mixed tumors may produce ascites or pleural effusion. Very bizarre tumor cells, sometimes combining the features of carcinoma and spindle cell sarcoma, may be observed. If the metastatic tumor has features of rhabdomyosarcoma, striated cancer cells may be noted (see Fig. 26–61).

Testicular Tumors.   The most common testicular tumors capable of forming metastases and effusions are seminomas, malignant teratomas, and, in the older man, malignant lymphomas. Metastatic seminomas are characterized by a population of large malignant cells, often accompanied by numerous lymphocytes (see Fig. 27–31). Malignant teratomas are most often identified in fluids as embryonal carcinomas (see below). The rare malignant lymphomas of testicular origin have a cytologic presentation similar to that of other malignant lymphomas (see p. 1153).

Miscellaneous Tumors.   It is virtually impossible to mention, let alone describe, the cytologic presentation of a multitude of other metastatic malignant tumors, of a variety of origins that may occasionally form effusions. In such rare instances the knowledge of clinical history and a review of histologic material may help in the identification of tumor type.

Some of these very rare events were described. A case of thymoma causing pleural effusion was reported by Zirkin (1985). Pleural effusion caused by a rupture of a benign cystic mediastinal teratoma was described by Cobb et al. (1985). The fluid contained benign squamous cells and hair shafts documenting the dermoid nature of the tumor (see p. 1095).

Of the very rare tumors, a metastatic olfactory neuroblastoma (esthesioneuroblastoma) was reported by Jobst et al. (1983). A Merkel cell carcinoma of the skin causing pleural effusion was described by Watson and Friedman (1985). Peritoneal implants of an endodermal sinus tumor via a ventricular shunt were reported by Kimura et al. (1984).

EFFUSIONS IN CHILDREN

The variety of malignant tumors in young children, capable of producing effusions, is relatively limited. It is unusual for such tumors to produce effusions before the clinical diagnosis has been established, but occasionally this has been noted. Most malignant tumors of childhood are made up of small cells and thus resemble malignant lymphomas and other small-cell tumors. These points have to be kept in mind in the differential diagnosis, *which must always include lymphomas and leukemias.* The aspiration biopsy findings in this group of childhood tumors are discussed in Chapter 29.

Wilms' Tumor

These malignant teratoid renal tumors comprise elements of adenocarcinoma and sarcomas, the latter most commonly a rhabdomyosarcoma. The cytologic patterns in effusions are usually characterized by small, round cancer cells arranged in small balls or clusters, suggestive of an embryonal carcinoma (Fig. 26–66). Occasionally one may also observe elongated malignant cells suggestive of a spindle cell sarcoma, side by side with the small, round cells. The diagnosis rests on this mixture of cell types which, in a child, is uniquely characteristic of Wilms' tumor (Fig. 26–67).

Neuroblastoma

These tumors of neural crest origin, usually primary in the adrenal medulla, are characterized by small, round cells, occasionally forming small aggregates with a central lumen or the so-called rosettes. In fluids, the cells of neuroblastoma resemble the round, small cells observed in Wilms' tumor, described above and shown in Fig. 26–66A. The formation of rosettes, which is diagnostic of these tumors, is very infrequently observed in fluids. *Ewing's sarcoma of bone* has a histologic and cytologic presentation very similar to that of a neuroblastoma (see Fig. 29–133). For comments on the cytogenetic differences between these two tumors, see Chapter 7.

Embryonal Rhabdomyosarcomas

Three anatomic sites of these muscle-derived sarcomas are seen almost exclusively in childhood: tumors of the vagina in girls, tumors of the prostate in boys, and tumors of bladder in children of both sexes. In all these organs the tumor may assume a grapelike configuration, hence the name "botryoid sarcoma" (see also p. 645). Embryonal rhabdomyosarcomas of soft parts, derived from peripheral muscle, may be seen in children and in adults.

The tumors are characterized by proliferation of small to medium-sized malignant cells, occasion-

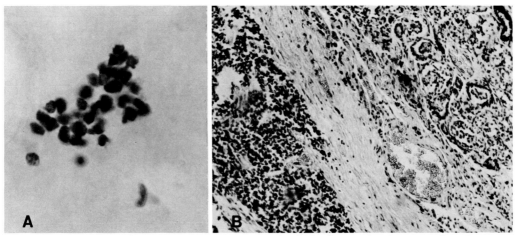

FIGURE 26–66. (*A, B*) Metastatic Wilms' tumor in pleural fluid. Note the clustering of small tumor cells around a lumen, resembling a rosette. Tissue section of the pleura (*B*) discloses the formation of glomeruluslike structures by tumor. (*A* ×560; *B* ×150)

ally assuming an organoid pattern (alveolar rhabdomyosarcoma). Cross-striations diagnostic of this tumor are not readily observed, and often one must rely on the finding of myoglobin deposits in the cytoplasm of the tumor cells or on immunocytochemistry for diagnosis.

In effusions, the most commonly observed pattern is that of elongated tumor cells (Fig. 26–68). Sometimes the tumor cells are larger and resemble the adult type of rhabdomyosarcoma (Fig. 26–69).

Embryonal Carcinomas and Endodermal Sinus Tumors

These tumors of various primary anatomic origin (ovary, testis, anterior mediastinum, sacrococcygeal region) are seen predominantly in childhood or early adolescence, but they also may occur in adults. Quite often these tumors represent a unilateral development of complex malignant teratomas; for example, in the testis or in the mediasti-

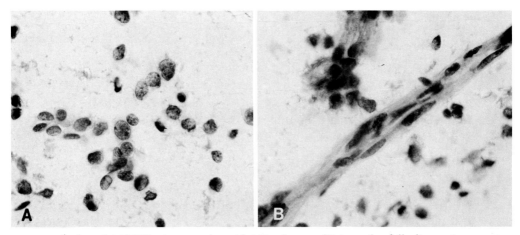

FIGURE 26–67. (*A, B*) Wilms' tumor, pleural fluid in a boy aged 9. A rare, but fully diagnostic presentation, combining small cancer cells in cluster (*A*) with malignant spindly cells (*B*). (*A, B* ×500)

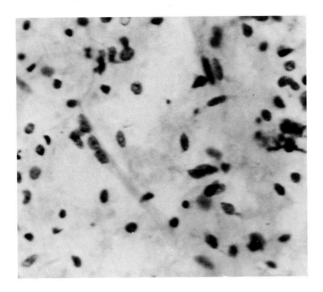

FIGURE 26–68. Metastatic embryonal rhabdomyosarcoma to the pleura. Note the markedly elongated cells —an appearance practically never seen in benign cells. (×560)

num. The cytologic presentation of these tumors in fluids is the same, regardless of anatomic origin. Tumor cells of moderate sizes, often of monotonous appearance, occur in papillary clusters or singly. The nuclei are provided with conspicuously large, irregular nucleoli (Fig. 26–70). This cytologic configuration, essentially suggestive of an adenocarcinoma, when seen in a young patient strongly suggests an embryonal carcinoma. For comments on yolk-sac tumors see p. 1150.

Malignant Lymphomas and Leukemia

Malignant lymphomas and leukemia are the most common group of malignant tumors in childhood responsible for effusions. The cytologic presentation is similar to that observed in other age groups (see p. 1153). It must be pointed out, however, that children with immune disorders and such genetic abnormalities as Down's syndrome are more susceptible to the development of malignant diseases than normal children (Fig. 26–71; see Chap. 6).

Rare Tumors of Childhood

In one case of Letterer–Siwe disease it was possible to identify the tumor cells in the pleural fluid as belonging to the class of histiocytes because of their striking morphologic similarities to normal histiocytic elements and their phagocytic activity (Fig.

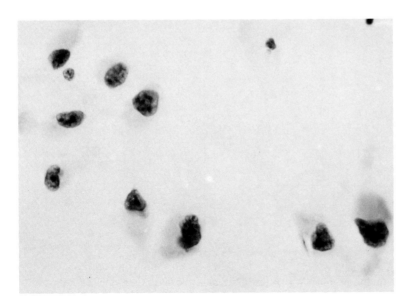

FIGURE 26–69. Embryonal rhabdomyosarcoma, pleural fluid. The cytologic presentation in this case is similar to rhabdomyosarcoma, adult type (cf. Fig. 26–60) and is characterized by large, bizarre, malignant cells. (×560)

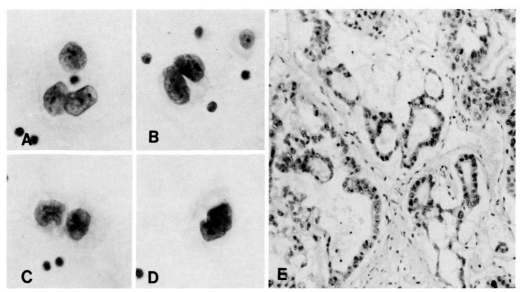

FIGURE 26–70. Testicular embryonal carcinoma metastatic to pleura in a boy aged 9 months. Pleural fluid and primary tumor. (*A–D*) Malignant epithelial cells in small clusters. (*E*) Testicular tumor showing formation of glandular spaces, somewhat resembling embryonal structures. (*A–D* ×560; *E* ×150)

26–72). In one instance, cells of a malignant teratoma of the pericardium growing chiefly as embryonal adenocarcinoma (Fig. 26–73) were identified by us in pericardial fluid.

With improved survival, metastases of osteo-genic sarcoma are now observed with increasing frequency in effusions in adolescents (Geisinger et al., 1984; see pp. 1165 and 1375 for comments on cytologic presentations of these tumors).

McCollum (1988) described an unusual event:

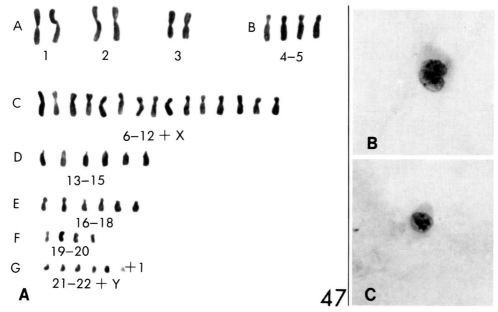

FIGURE 26–71. Hodgkin's disease with pleural effusion in an 8-year-old child with Down syndrome. (*A*) Karyotype showing 47 chromosomes with an extra chromosome in the G group (trisomy 21, see Chap. 6). (*B, C*) Reed–Sternberg cells in pleural fluid. (*B, C* ×560)

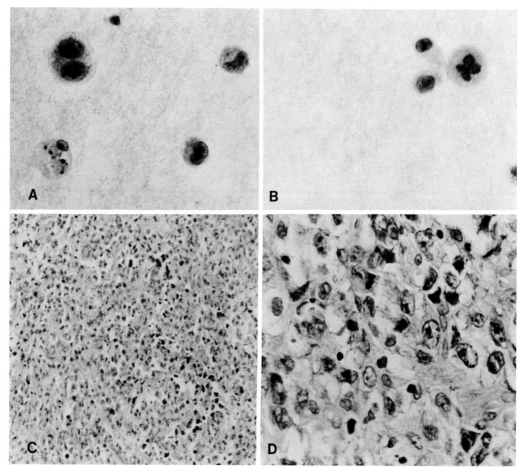

FIGURE 26–72. (*A, B*) Pleural fluid from a 3-year-old child. Note bizarre, large tumor cells, and an abnormal mitosis in (*B*). The phagocytic activity of some of the tumor cells suggested a malignant process of the reticuloendothelial system. (*C, D*) Tissue section of lymph node interpreted as malignant reticuloendotheliosis (Letterer–Siwe disease). (*A, B, D* ×560; *C* ×150)

peritoneal metastases of a choroid plexus carcinoma of the brain in a 5-year-old boy with a ventricular–peritoneal shunt. The tumor cells were identified in the ascitic fluid. Kimura et al. (1984) described peritoneal implants of an endodermal sinus tumor of the pineal region, also in a patient with a shunt.

PERICARDIAL CAVITY

Besides the primary cardiac lymphomas, described on p. 1160, pericardial effusions may occur as a consequence of metastatic cancer and under a number of other circumstances.

Yazdi et al. (1980) reviewed cytologic findings in 72 patients with positive pericardial effusions to establish the frequency of primary tumor sites as a source of pericardial metastases. Lung and breast cancer were the most common carcinomas; lymphomas and leukemias the most common nonepithelial tumors, with mesothelioma a close third. Unfortunately, the results were not presented according to the sex of patients.

In my experience, the primary sites appear to be the same as for the pleural effusions both in men and in women, and numerous examples of metastatic carcinomas of mammary (Figs. 26–30 and 26–74), lung, or gastric origin (see Fig. 26–41*B*) have been observed. The cytologic presentation of these effusions is the same as for other body fluids and need not be repeated here.

Occasionally, very unusual events may lead to pericardial effusion. Thus, Venegas and Sun

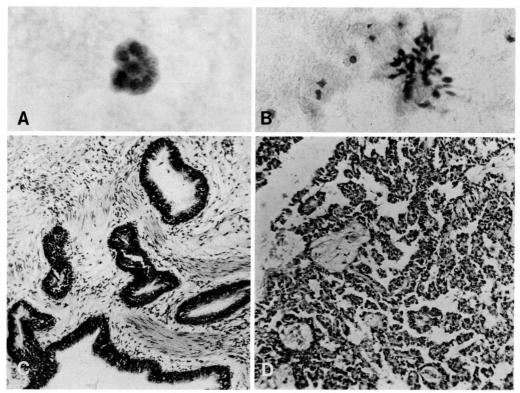

FIGURE 26–73. Malignant teratoma of pericardium in a child 4 years of age, with primary diagnosis by cytology (pericardial tap). (*A*) Rosette of tumor cells suggestive of adenocarcinoma. (*B*) Cluster of small ciliated cells of respiratory type on the same smear. (*C, D*) Tissue sections, disclosing the bronchial component of the tumor (*C*) and the embryonal carcinoma in adjoining areas (*D*). (*A, B* ×560; *C, D* ×150)

(1988) reported a case of a malignant thymoma causing cardiac tamponade.

Postinfarction chronic hemorrhagic pericarditis may also constitute a source of diagnostic error because the hemosiderin-laden macrophages may be mistaken for cells of malignant melanoma, as happened in one of our patients. It is a wise precaution to perform an iron stain whenever metastatic melanoma is suspected.

It must be noted that accumulation of pericardial fluid due to a metastatic tumor may be an acute threat to the life of the patient because of possible interference with cardiac function or because of cardiac tamponade. Thus, rapid diagnosis and aggressive treatment may prove lifesaving.

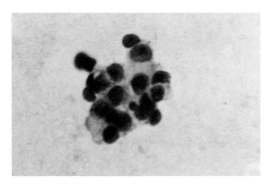

FIGURE 26–74. Metastatic breast cancer in pericardial fluid. (×560)

FREQUENCY OF METASTASES FROM TUMORS OF VARIOUS SITES

Many a malignant tumor manifests itself primarily as an effusion. The primary site frequently remains hidden, and there are no statistics available that would be at once comprehensive and accurate concerning the relative frequency with which various tumors metastasize to the various body cavities. However, in the experience of the author, the most commonly observed metastatic tumors are listed in order of frequency in Tables 26–3, 26–4,

Table 26–3
Relative Frequency of Origin of Common, Effusion-Forming, Metastatic Malignant Tumors in Body Cavities in Adult Women

Pleural Fluid	Peritoneal Fluid (Ascites)
1. Breast	Ovary
2. Ovary	Breast
3. Gastrointestinal tract (stomach, esophagus, colon)	Gastrointestinal tract (colon, stomach, pancreas)
4. Lung	
5. Malignant lymphoma	Malignant lymphoma

and 26–5. In the absence of clinical history, these tables offer some guidance to the most likely origin of malignant cells.

APPLICATION OF CYTOLOGY OF BODY FLUIDS AS AN INDEX OF RESPONSE OF CANCERS TO THERAPY

Since ascitic tumors in animals had long been utilized as a tool in the evaluation of chemotherapeutic agents, it was logical that a correlation of the response of tumor cells in human body fluids with the effectiveness of therapeutic anticancer agents should be attempted.

A sustained, long-term major study of the response of various tumors to radiation and chemotherapeutic agents has not yet been performed. However, some information on this topic is available.

The cells of malignant lymphomas in effusions react to either radiation or alkylating agents with karyorrhexis (see Fig. 26–54). This effect may be so striking that Melamed considered it as diagnostic of malignant lymphomas and named it the "nuclear fragmentation pattern." This pattern may occur regardless of the type of lymphoma or the therapeutic mode used and may also be observed in the absence of therapy (see p. 1160). It appears inherent in the nature of the tumor. The reasons for this type of response are not clear.

Personal experience has shown that those carcinomas presenting a marked tissue culture pattern, or a diffuse proliferation of relatively uniform cancer cells, responded better to systematically administered chemotherapeutic agents than tumors with different patterns of growth. Among the poor responders were tumors growing in clusters of papillary or glandular type.

A remarkable response has been observed in a case of widespread ovarian carcinoma treated with floxuridine (5-fluorodeoxyuridine; FUDR). This compound was injected directly into the pleura and the peritoneum and produced striking mitotic abnormalities of cancer cells in fluids, resulting in the formation of gigantic, grotesque cell forms (Fig. 26–75). These cytologic changes preceded a sustained clinical remission.

This observation clearly requires additional confirmatory research.

Table 26–4
Relative Frequency of Origin of Common, Effusion-Forming, Metastatic Malignant Tumors in Body Cavities in Adult Men

Pleural Fluid	Peritoneal Fluid (Ascites)
1. Lung	Gastrointestinal tract (colon, pancreas, stomach)
2. Gastrointestinal tract (esophagus, stomach, colon)	
3. Malignant lymphoma	Malignant lymphoma

Table 26-5
Relative Frequency of Origin of Metastatic Malignant Tumors in Children

Pleural or Peritoneal Fluid

1. Leukemia–lymphoma
2. Wilms' tumor
3. Neuroblastoma
4. Embryonal rhabdomyosarcoma
5. Ewing's tumor

Effects of Radiation and Radiomimetic Drugs

The effects of radiation may be observed following either an intracavitary application of radioactive phosphorus or external irradiation treatment. The effects, both on mesothelial cells and on cancer cells, are in essence similar to those observed in other organs and tissue (cf. pp. 666 and 1108). Ballooning of cells, cytoplasmic vacuolization, and nuclear enlargement may be noted in the mesothe-

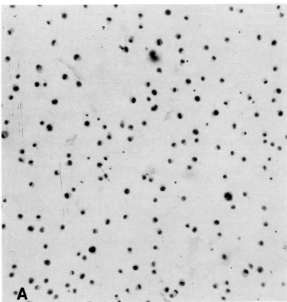

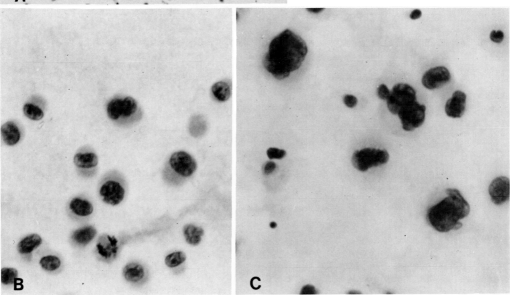

FIGURE 26-75. Effect of floxuridine (FUDR) administered intrapleurally in a case of metastatic ovarian carcinoma. (*A*) Tissue culture effect in fluid before treatment. (*B*) High-power view of the same to emphasize the uniformity of tumor cells. (*C*) Appearance of fluid 9 days after treatment: most cells are multinucleated giant cells, suggesting that the drug interfered with mitotic activity. (*A* ×150; *B*, *C* ×560)

lial cells and the cancer cells (Figs. 25–38 and 26–76). Karyorrhexis observed in malignant lymphomas has been mentioned above. It is rarely observed in other tumors.

Among the radiomimetic drugs, alkylating agents must be singled out. Their effect on some cancer cells may be identified with that of radiation, resulting in ballooning of cells and nuclear enlargement or degeneration.

CANCER CELLS IN EFFUSIONS AS A TARGET OF BIOLOGIC INVESTIGATIONS

From a great many points of view, effusions caused by cancer are eminently suitable as a medium of study of cancer cells. Malignant cells in effusions may proliferate and thereby form naturally occurring cultures of cancer cells. Koller, Ishihara and Sandberg, Miles, and others have utilized effusions as a means of determining the chromosomal constitution (or its DNA equivalent) of cancer cells.

In addition to attempts at differential staining of mesothelial cells in effusions, several cytochemical techniques may be used to advantage in cells from body fluids. (see Table 26–1, p. 1137). Stains for organ-specific cell products, such as acid and alkaline phosphatases, may be demonstrated in cells originating in prostatic carcinoma and osteogenic sarcoma, respectively (see Fig. 26–63). Some of the techniques used to demonstrate enzyme systems by means of tetrazolium salts may be applied. Thus, lactic dehydrogenase and other enzymes could be demonstrated in tumor cells in effusions (Fig. 26–77). Effusions have been a common tar-

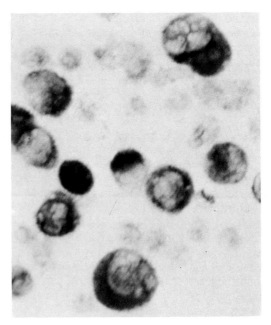

FIGURE 26–77.   Same case as that in Fig. 26–75. Ovarian carcinoma in pleural fluid. Lactic dehydrogenase in the cytoplasm of tumor cells. Note the dark precipitate of tetrazolium salts. (×560. Courtesy of Dr. Myron R. Melamed, New York, New York)

get for testing of the specificity and staining reactions of various monoclonal antibodies (see Chap. 34).

Human effusions can be used for the study of ultrastructural configuration of cancer cells and other cells and their mutual relationship (see p. 1134). Immunologic and biochemical studies of these naturally occurring tissue culture media are only in their beginnings. Human effusions can also serve as a target for the investigation of effects of various therapeutic agents in a manner similar to that applied in experimental systems (Rhodes et al.). Finally, cancer cells in effusions may also serve to establish human cancer cell lines in vitro. This is a useful tool for the study of biologic aspects of human cancer and its response to chemotherapeutic agents (Cailleau et al.; Soule et al.).

EVALUATION OF DIAGNOSTIC RESULTS IN EFFUSIONS

This area of application of diagnostic cytology is among the most difficult to evaluate objectively. There are several reasons for this, the most impor-

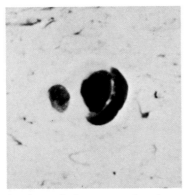

FIGURE 26–76.   Cells from an irradiated ovarian carcinoma. Note the ballooning of the malignant cells and an adjacent smaller cell, presumably a macrophage. (×1,000)

tant one being the occurrence of effusions in patients *with* cancer *but not caused by cancer.* Even the comparison of cytologic results with autopsy material may be misleading unless there is no significant delay between the two procedures. Otherwise, in a cancer patient metastases may develop that did not exist at the time of tapping of the fluid.

In effusions the avoidance of an erroneous diagnosis of cancer appears as important as the determination of the presence of cancer cells. With the exception of malignant lymphomas, breast cancer, and a few other tumors, the diagnosis of a cancerous effusion is tantamount to a sentence of death. Rarely is the patient investigated further, and the treatment is usually palliative. An error of this type should be avoided at all costs. Consequently, the measure of a good laboratory in this area is not so much the largest possible number of cancers correctly diagnosed, but the smallest number of cancers incorrectly diagnosed.

Grunze (1964), in a thorough review of this topic, reported correct positive results from various sources ranging from 50% (Graham et al.) to 90% (von Haam). The widely acknowledged work of Saphir resulted in 80% correct positive diagnoses. It is much more difficult to assess the number of errors. Ceelen (1964) states that no such errors were made in the evaluation of 667 cases — a most commendable performance. Grunze (1964) records three positive errors in 140 patients without cancer whose clinical findings and history were known to him. Results from my laboratories are summarized in Tables 26 – 6 to 26 – 9.

In cancer hospitals it is very difficult to determine the overall accuracy of cytologic diagnosis

Table 26 – 6

Comparison of Diagnostic Results of Pleural Biopsies and Cytology of Pleural Fluid

Patients Studied

Patients with cancer		72
Patients with cancer and malignant effusion	46	
Patients with cancer and benign effusion	26	
Patients without cancer		90
TOTAL		162

(Frist, B., et al.: Comparison of diagnostic values of biopsies of the pleura and cytologic evaluation of pleural fluids. Am. J. Clin. Pathol., 72:48–51, 1979)

with reference to the presence or absence of cancer because very few patients with effusions caused by nonneoplastic diseases are admitted.

A better assessment of performance can be obtained by a simultaneous study of pleural biopsies and fluid cytology, summarized in Tables 26 – 6 to 26 – 9, based on work performed at Montefiore Hospital by Dr. B. Frist.

These results clearly document that in malignant disease the cytologic examination of fluid is by far more accurate than a pleural biopsy. In infectious diseases, however, particularly in such granulomatous diseases as tuberculosis, the pleural biopsy is superior to cytologic examination in establishing the etiology of this disorder. Similar data have been provided by Von Hoff and Livolsi.

Table 26 – 7

Comparison of Diagnostic Results of Pleural Biopsies and Cytology of Pleural Fluid — Clinical Data

Patients With Known Cancer	Number	Female	Male
Clinical suspicion of metastatic carcinoma to pleura	61	39	22
No clinical suspicion of metastases (CHF, obstr. lung disease and other medical problems)	11	4	7
TOTAL	72	43	29
Patients with microscopic evidence of metastatic cancer	44	32	12

(Frist, B., et al.: Comparison of diagnostic values of biopsies of the pleura and cytologic evaluation of pleural fluids. Am. J. Clin. Pathol., 72:48–51, 1979)

Table 26–8

Comparison of Diagnostic Results of Pleural Biopsies and Cytology of Pleural Fluid

Cases of Proven Metastatic Cancer

Cytology positive, biopsy positive	15
Cytology positive, biopsy negative	28
Biopsy positive, cytology negative (on review cytology suspicious)	1
TOTAL	44

(Frist, B., et al: Comparison of diagnostic values of biopsies of the pleura and cytologic evaluation of pleural fluids. Am. J. Clin. Pathol., 72:48–51, 1979.)

Table 26–9

Comparison of Diagnostic Results of Pleural Biopsies and Cytology of Pleural Fluid

Benign Causes of Pleural Effusion in Patients With Known History of Cancer

Pneumonia	12 cases
Congestive heart failure	18 cases
Low serum albumin	2 cases

(Frist, B., et al.: Comparison of diagnostic values of biopsies of the pleura and cytologic evaluation of pleural fluids. Am. J. Clin. Pathol., 72: 48–51, 1979)

BIBLIOGRAPHY

Tumors of the mesothelium
Metastatic cancer
Malignant lymphoma
Tumor markers

Tumors of the Mesothelium

Alvarez-Fernandez, E., Rabano, A., Barros-Malvar, J.L., and Sanabia-Valdez, J.: Multicystic peritoneal mesothelioma: a case report. Histopathology, 14:199–208, 1989.

Anderson, K.A., Hurley, W.C., Hurley, B.T., and Ohrt, D.W.: Malignant pleural mesothelioma following radiotherapy in a 16-year-old boy. Cancer, 56:273–276, 1985.

Antman, K.H., Klegar, K.L., Promfret, E.A., Osteen, R.T., Amato, D.A., Larson, D.A., and Corson, J.M.: Early peritoneal mesothelioma: a treatable malignancy. Lancet, 2:977–981, 1985.

Baddoura, F.K., and Varma, V.A.: Cytologic findings in multicystic peritoneal mesothelioma. Acta Cytol., 34:524–528, 1990.

Battifora, H., and Kopinski, M.I.: Distinction of mesothelioma from adenocarcinoma: an immunohistochemical approach. Cancer, 55:1679–1685, 1985.

Becker, S.N., Papin, D.W., and Rosenthal, D.L.: Mesothelial papilloma: a case of mistaken identity in a pericardial effusion. Acta Cytol., 20:266–268, 1976.

Benge, T., and Grontoft, O.: Cytologic diagnosis of malignant pleural mesothelioma. Acta Cytol., 9:207–212, 1964.

Boon, M.E., Kwee, W.S., Alons, C.L., Morawetz, F., and Veldhuizen, R.W.: Discrimination between primary pleural and primary peritoneal mesotheliomas by morphometry and analysis of the vacuolization pattern of the exfoliated mesothelial cells. Acta Cytol., 26:103–108, 1982.

Boon, M.E., Veldhuizen, R.W., Ruinaard, C., Snieders, M.W., and Kwee, W.S.: Quantitative distinctive differences between the vacuoles of mesothelioma cells and cells from metastatic carcinoma exfoliated in pleural fluid. Acta Cytol., 28:443–449, 1984.

Borow, M., Conston, A., Livornese, L., and Schalet, N.: Mesothelioma following exposure to asbestos. A review of 72 cases. Chest, 5:641–646, 1973.

Brenner, J., Sordillo, P.P., Magill, G.B., and Golbey, R.B.: Malignant mesothelioma of the pleura. Review of 123 patients. Cancer, 49:2431–2435, 1982.

Briselli, M.B., Mark, E.J., and Dickersin, G.R.: Solitary fibrous tumors of the pleura: eight new cases and review of 360 cases in the literature. Cancer, 47:2678–2689, 1981.

Chu, L.M., Lee, Y.-J., and Ho, M.Y.: Malignant mesothelioma in infancy. Arch. Pathol. Lab. Med., 113:409–411, 1989.

Craighead, J.E., and Mossman, B.T.: The pathogenesis of asbestos-associated diseases. N. Engl. J. Med., 306:1446–1455, 1982.

Dewar, A., Valente, M., Ring, N.P., and Corrin, B.: Pleural mesothelioma of epithelial type and pulmonary adenocarcinoma: an ultrastructural and cytochemical comparison. J. Pathol., 152:309–316, 1987.

Dionne, G.P., Beland, J.E., and Wang, N.-S.: Primary leiomyosarcoma of the diaphragm of an asbestos worker. Arch. Pathol. Lab. Med., 100:398, 1976.

Donaldson, J.C., Kaminsky, D.B., Elliott, R.C., Walsh, T.E., and Newby, J.G.: Psammoma bodies in pleural fluid associated with a mesothelioma: case report. Milit. Med., 144:476–479, 1979.

Duggan, M.A., Masters, C.B., and Alexander, F.: Immunohistochemical differentiation of malignant mesothelioma, mesothelial hyperplasia and metastatic adenocarcinoma in serous effusions, utilizing staining for carcinoembryonic antigen, keratin and vimentin. Acta Cytol., 31:807–814, 1987.

Epstein, J.I., and Budin, R.E.: Keratin and epithelial membrane antigen immunoreactivity in nonneoplastic fibrous pleural lesions: implications for the diagnosis of desmoplastic mesothelioma. Hum. Pathol., 17:514–519, 1986.

Foster, E.A., and Ackerman, L.V.: Localized mesotheliomas of the pleura. The pathologic evaluation of 18 cases. Am. J. Clin. Pathol., 34:349–364, 1960.

Gaffanti, M.C., and Falen, M.L.: Benign-appearing mesothelioma cells in a serous effusion. Acta Cytol., 29:90–92, 1985.

Gibbs, A.R., Harach, R., Wagner, J.C., and Jasani, B.: Comparison of tumor markers in malignant mesothelioma and pulmonary adenocarcinoma. Thorax, 40:91–95, 1985.

Godwin, M.C.: Diffuse mesotheliomas with comment on their relation to localized fibrous mesotheliomas. Cancer, 10:298–319, 1957.

Grund, G.W., and Miller, R.W.: Malignant mesothelioma in childhood: report of 13 cases. Cancer, 30:1216–1218, 1972.

Guzman, J., Bross, K.J.B., Wurtemberger, G., and Costabel,

U.: Immunocytology in malignant pleural mesothelioma. Expression of tumor markers and distribution of lymphocyte subsets. Chest, *95*:590–595, 1989.

Hammar, S.P., Bockus, D., Remington, F., Freidman, S., and LaZerte, G.: Familial mesothelioma: a report of two families. Hum. Pathol., *20*:107–122, 1989.

Harrington, J.S., Gilson, J.C., and Wagner, J.C.: Asbestos and mesothelioma in man. Nature, *232*:54–55, 1971.

Harwood, T.R., Gracey, D.R., and Yokoo, H.: Pseudomesotheliomatous carcinoma of the lung: a variant of peripheral lung cancer. Am. J. Clin. Pathol., *65*:159–167, 1976.

Henderson, D.W.: Asbestos-related pleuropulmonary diseases: asbestosis, mesothelioma and lung cancer. Pathology, *14*:239–243, 1982.

Japko, L., Horta, A.A., Schreiber, K., Mitsudo, S., Singh, G., and Koss, L.G.: Malignant mesothelioma of the tunica vaginalis testis; report of first case with preoperative diagnosis. Cancer, *49*:119–127, 1982.

Klemperer, P., and Rabin, C.B.: Primary neoplasms of the pleura. Arch. Pathol., *11*:385–412, 1931.

Klempman, S.: The exfoliative cytology of diffuse pleural mesothelioma. Cancer, *15*:691–704, 1962.

Klima, M., Spjut, H.J., and Seybold, W.D.: Diffuse malignant mesothelioma. Am. J. Clin. Pathol., *65*:583–600, 1976.

Kobzik, L., Antman, K.H., and Warhol, M.J.: The distinction of mesothelioma from adenocarcinoma in malignant effusions by electron microscopy. Acta Cytol., *29*:219–225, 1985.

Kovalivker, M., and Motovic, A.: Malignant peritoneal mesothelioma in children: description of two cases and review of the literature. J. Pediatr. Surg., *20*:274–275, 1985.

Laurini, R.N.: Diffuse pleural mesothelioma with distant bone metastasis. Acta Pathol. Microbiol. Scand., *82*:296–298, 1974.

Lindeque, B.G., Cronje, H.S., and Deale, C.J.: Prevalence of primary papillary peritoneal neoplasia in patients with ovarian carcinomas. S. Afr. Med. J., *67*:1005–1007, 1985.

McCaughey, W.T.E., Wade, O.L., and Elmes, P.C.: Exposure to asbestos dust and diffuse pleural mesotheliomas. Br. Med. J., *2*:1397, 1962.

McDonald, A.D., and McDonald, J.C.: Malignant mesothelioma in North America. Cancer, *46*:1650–1656, 1980.

Morawetz, F.: Die Zytodiagnostik der primaeren malignen Mesotheliome des Peritoneums. Internist. Prax., *17*:631–641, 1977.

Mossman, B.T., Bignon, J., Corn, M., Seaton, A., and Gee, J.B.L.: Asbestos: scientific developments and implications for public policy. Science, *247*:294–301, 1990.

Naylor, B.: The exfoliative cytology of diffuse malignant mesothelioma. J. Pathol. Bacteriol., *86*:293–298, 1963.

Nicosia, S.V., and Nicosia, R.F.: Neoplasms of the ovarian mesothelium. *In* Azar, H.A. (ed.): Pathology of Human Neoplasms. An Atlas of Diagnostic Electron Microscopy and Immunohistochemistry. pp. 435–486. New York, Raven Press, 1988.

O'Donnell, R.H., Mann, R.H., and Grosh, J.L.: Asbestos, an extrinsic factor in the pathogenesis of bronchogenic carcinoma and mesothelioma. Cancer, *19*:1143–1148, 1966.

Obers, V.J., Leiman, G., Girdwood, R.W., and Spiro, F.I.: Primary malignant pleural tumors (mesotheliomas) presenting as localized masses. Fine needle aspiration cytologic findings, clinical and radiologic features and review of the literature. Acta Cytol., *32*:567–574, 1988.

Parmley, T.H., and Woodruff, J.D.: The ovarian mesothelioma. Am. J. Obstet. Gynecol., *120*:234–241, 1974.

Pinto, M.M., Bernstein, L.H., Brogan, D.A., and Crisculo,

E.M.: Carcinoembryonic antigen in effusions. A diagnostic adjunct to cytology. Acta Cytol., *31*:113–118, 1987.

Pisani, R.J., Colby, T.V., and Williams, D.E.: Malignant mesothelioma of the pleura. Mayo Clin. Proc., *63*:1234–1244, 1988.

Ratzer, E.R., Pool, J.L., and Melamed, M.R.: Pleural mesotheliomas. Clinical experiences with thirty-seven patients. Am. J. Roentgenol. Radium. Ther. Nucl. Med., *99*:863–880, 1967.

Rous, V., and Studeny, J.: Aetiology of pleural plaques. Thorax, *25*:270–284, 1970.

Schneller, J., Eppich, E., Greenebaum, E., Elequin, F., Sherman, A., Wersto, R., and Koss, L.G.: Flow cytometry and Feulgen cytophotometry in evaluation of effusions. Cancer, *59*:1307–1313, 1987.

Selikoff, J.J., Churg, J., and Hammond, E.C.: Relation between exposure to asbestos and mesotheliomata. N. Engl. J. Med., *272*:560–565, 1965.

Spriggs, A.I., and Grunze, H.: An unusual cytologic presentation of mesothelioma in serous effusions. Acta Cytol., *27*:288–292, 1983.

Stout, A.P., and Murray, M.: Localized pleural mesothelioma. Arch. Pathol., *34*:951–964, 1942.

Sytman, A.L., and MacAlpin, R.N.: Primary pericardial mesothelioma: report of 2 cases and review of the literature. Am. Heart J., *81*:760–769, 1971.

Triol, J.H., Conston, A.S., and Chandler, S.V.: Malignant mesothelioma. Cytopathology of 75 cases seen in a New Jersey community hospital. Acta Cytol., *28*:37–45, 1984.

Walters, J.K.L., and Martinez, A.J.: Malignant fibrous mesothelioma metastatic to brain and liver. Acta Neuropathol. (Berl.), *33*:173–177, 1975.

Walz, R., and Koch, H.K.: Malignant pleural mesothelioma: some aspects of epidemiology, differential diagnosis and prognosis. Pathol. Res. Pract., *186*:124–134, 1990.

Whitewell, F., and Rawcliffe, R.M.: Diffuse malignant pleural mesothelioma and asbestos exposure. Thorax, *26*:6–22, 1971.

Yoon, I.L.: Malignant mesothelioma of the peritoneum. Report of a case and review of the literature. JAMA, *181*:1107–1110, 1962.

Metastatic Cancer

Ashton, P.R., Hollingsworth, A.S., Jr., and Johnston, W.W.: The cytopathology of metastatic breast cancer. Acta Cytol., *19*:1–6, 1975.

Atkin, N.B., and Baker, M.C.: A nuclear protrusion in a human tumor associated with an abnormal chromosome. Acta Cytol., *8*:431–433, 1964.

Backman, A., and Pasila, M.: Pleural biopsy in the diagnosis of pleural effusion. Scand. J. Respir. Dis. [Suppl.], *89*:155–157, 1974.

Bakalos, D., Constantakis, N., and Tsicricas, T.: Recognition of malignant cells in pleural and peritoneal effusions. Acta Cytol., *18*:118–121, 1974.

Benedict, W.F., Brown, C.D., and Porter, I.H.: Long acrocentric marker chromosomes in malignant effusions and solid tumors. N.Y. State J. Med., *71*:952–955, 1971.

Benedict, W.F., and Porter, I.H.: The cytogenetic diagnosis of malignancy in effusions. Acta Cytol., *16*:304–306, 1972.

Bierman, H.R., Marshall, G.J., Kelly, K.H., and Alexander, M.J.: Method for evaluation of chemotherapeutic agents in man. Cancer, *13*:328–333, 1960.

Boon, M.E., Veldhuizen, R.W., Ruinaard, C., Snieders, M.W.,

and Kwee, W.S.: Quantitative distinctive differences between the vacuoles of mesothelioma cells and cells from metastatic carcinoma exfoliated in pleural fluid. Acta Cytol., *28*:443–449, 1984.

Cabin, H.S., Costello, R.M., Vasudevan, G., Maron, B.J., and Roberts, W.C.: Cardiac lymphoma mimicking hypertrophic cardiomyopathy. Am. Heart J., *102*:466–468, 1981.

Cailleau, R., Young, R., Olive, M., and Reeves, W.J., Jr.: Breast tumor cell lines from pleural effusions. JNCI, *53*:661–674, 1974.

Castelli, M.J., Mihalov, M.L., Posniak, H.V., and Gattuso, P.: Primary cardiac lymphoma initially diagnosed by routine cytology: case report and literature review. Acta Cytol., *33*:355–358, 1989.

Ceelen, G.H.: The cytological diagnosis of ascitic fluid. Acta Cytol., *8*:175–185, 1964.

Chou, S.-T., Arkles, L.B., Gill, G.D., Pinkus, N., Parkin, A., and Hicks, J.D.: Primary lymphoma of the heart: a case report. Cancer, *52*:744–747, 1983.

Clarkson, B., Ota, K., Ohkita, T., and O'Connor, A.: Kinetics of proliferation of cancer cells in neoplastic effusions in man. Cancer, *18*:1189–1213, 1965.

Cobb, C.J., Wynn, J., Cobb, S.R., and Duane, G.B.: Cytologic findings in an effusion caused by rupture of a benign cystic teratoma of the mediastinum into a serous cavity. Acta Cytol., *29*:1015–1020, 1985.

Croonen, A.M., van der Valk, H.C.J., and Lindeman, J.: Cytology, immunology and flow cytometry in the diagnosis of pleural and peritoneal effusions. Lab. Invest., *58*:725–731, 1988.

Czerniak, B., Papenhausen, P.R., Herz, F., and Koss, L.G.: Flow cytometric identification of cancer cells in effusions with Ca1 monoclonal antibody. Cancer, *55*:2783–2788, 1985.

Danner, D.E., and Gmelich, J.T.: A comparative study of tumor cells from metastatic carcinoma of the breast in effusions. Acta Cytol., *19*:509–518, 1975.

Djeu, J.Y., McCoy, J.L., Cannon, G.B., Reeves, W.J., West, W.H., and Herberman, R.B.: Lymphocytes forming rosettes with sheep erythrocytes in metastatic pleural effusion. JNCI, *56*:1051–1052, 1976.

Domagala, W., Emeson, E.E., Greenwald, E., and Koss, L.G.: A scanning electron microscopic and immunologic study of B-cell lymphosarcoma cells in cerebrospinal fluid. Cancer, *40*:716–720, 1977.

Domagala, W., Emeson, E.E., and Koss, L.G.: Distribution of T lymphocytes and B lymphocytes in peripheral blood and effusions of patients with cancer. JNCI, *61*:285–300, 1978.

Domagala, W., Emeson, E.E., and Koss, L.G.: T and B lymphocyte enumeration in the diagnosis of lymphocyte-rich pleural fluids. Acta Cytol., *25*:108–110, 1981.

Domagala, W., and Koss, L.G.: Configuration of surfaces of human cancer cells in effusions. A scanning electron microscopic study of microvilli. Virchows Arch. [B], *26*:27–42, 1977.

Domagala, W., and Woyke, S.: Transmission and scanning electron microscopic studies of cells in effusions. Acta Cytol., *19*:214–224, 1975.

Duggan, M.A., Masters, C.B., and Alexander, F.: Immunohistochemical differentiation of malignant mesothelioma, mesothelial hyperplasia and metastatic adenocarcinoma in serous effusions, utilizing staining for carcinoembryonic antigen, keratin and vimentin. Acta Cytol., *31*:807–814, 1987.

Ebner, H.J.: Untersuchungen zur Cytologie und Cytochemie cilioepithelialer Tumorzellen im Punktat seröser Ovarial-

cystome und Cystadenocarcinome. Z. Krebsforsch., *59*:581–593, 1954.

Ebner, H.J., and Schneider, W.: Zur Zytologie eines menschlichen Aszitestumor. Zentralbl. Gynakol., *78*:1486–1494, 1956.

Farr, G.H., and Hajdu, S.I.: Exfoliative cytology of metastatic neuroblastoma. Acta Cytol., *16*:203–206, 1972.

Freni, S.C., James, J., and Prop, F.J.A.: Tumor diagnosis in pleural and ascitic effusions based on DNA cytophotometry. Acta Cytol., *15*:154–162, 1971.

Frist, B., Kahan, A.V., and Koss, L.G.: Comparison of diagnostic values of biopsies of the pleura and cytologic evaluation of pleural fluids. Am. J. Clin. Pathol., *72*:48–51, 1979.

Geisinger, K.R., Hajdu, S.I., and Helson, L.: Exfoliative cytology of nonlymphoreticular neoplasms in children. Acta Cytol., *28*:16–28, 1984.

Ghosh, A.K., Spriggs, A.I., and Mason, D.Y.: Immunocytochemical staining of T and B lymphocytes in serous effusions. J. Clin. Pathol., *38*:608–612, 1985.

Goodlin, R.C.: Utilization of cell chromosome number for diagnosis of cancer cells in effusions. Nature, *197*:507, 1961.

Green, N., Gancedo, H., Smith, R., and Bernett, G.: Pseudomyxoma peritonei—nonoperative management and biomedical findings. A case report. Cancer, *36*:1834–1837, 1975.

Grunze, H.: The comparative diagnostic accuracy, efficiency and specificity of cytologic technics used in the diagnosis of malignant neoplasm in serous effusions of the pleural and pericardial cavities. Acta Cytol., *8*:150–163, 1964.

Grunze, H.: Cytologic studies of pleural fluid. Acta Unio. Int. Contra Cancrum, *14*:504–507, 1958.

Guzman, J., Bross, K.J., and Costabel, U.: Malignant pleural effusions due to small cell carcinoma of the lung. An immunocytochemical cell-surface analysis of lymphocytes and tumor cells. Acta Cytol., *34*:497–501, 1990.

Guzman, J., Costabel, U., Bross, K.J., Wiehle, U., Grunert, F., and Schaefer, H.E.: The value of the immunoperoxidase slide assay in the diagnosis of malignant pleural effusions in breast cancer. Acta Cytol., *32*:188–192, 1988.

Guzman, J., Hilgarth, M., Bross, K.J., Wiehle, U., Ross, A., Kresin, V., and Costabel, U.: Lymphocyte subpopulations in malignant ascites of serous papillary ovarian adenocarcinoma: an immunocytochemical study. Acta Cytol., *32*:811–815, 1988.

Hajdu, S.I., and Hajdu, E.O.: Cytopathology of Sarcomas and Other Nonepithelial Malignant Tumors. Philadelphia, W.B. Saunders, 1976.

Hajdu, S.I., and Koss, L.G.: Cytologic diagnosis of metastatic myosarcomas. Acta Cytol., *13*:545–551, 1969.

Hajdu, S.I., and Nolan, M.A.: Exfoliative cytology of malignant germ cell tumors. Acta Cytol., *19*:255–260, 1975.

Hajdu, S.I., and Savino, A.: Cytologic diagnosis of malignant melanoma. Acta Cytol., *17*:320–327, 1973.

Hanna, W., and Kahn, H.J.: The ultrastructure of metastatic adenocarcinoma in serous fluids. An aid in identification of the primary site of the neoplasm. Acta Cytol., *29*:202–210, 1985.

Hazard, J.B.: Cytologic studies of cell suspensions with special reference to neoplasms. Lab. Invest., *3*:315–336, 1954.

Hollander, D.H., and Brogaonkar, D.S.: The quinacrine fluorescence method of Y-chromosome identification. Acta Cytol., *15*:452–454, 1971.

Holland, W.W., Doll, R., and Carter, C.O.: The mortality from leukaemia and other cancers among patients with Down's syndrome (mongols) and among their parents. Br. J. Cancer, *16*:178–186, 1962.

Ishihara, T., and Sandberg, A.A.: Chromosome constitution of diploid and pseudodiploid cells in effusions of cancer patients. Cancer, *16*:885–895, 1963.

Jackson, J.F.: Chromosome analysis of cells in effusions from cancer patients. Cancer, *20*:537–540, 1967.

Jobst, S.B., Ljung, B.-M., Gilkey, F.N., and Rosenthal, D.L.: Cytologic diagnosis of olfactory neuroblastoma. Report of a case with multiple diagnostic parameters. Acta Cytol., *27*:299–308, 1983.

Johnston, W.W., Szpak, C.A., Lottich, S.C., Thor, A., and Schlom, J.: A monoclonal antibody (B72.3) as a novel immunohistochemical adjuvant for the diagnosis of carcinoma in fine needle aspiration biopsy specimens. Hum. Pathol., *17*:501–513, 1986.

Johnston, W.W., Szpak, C.A., Thor, A., and Schlom, J.: Use of a monoclonal antibody as an immunocytochemical adjunct to diagnosis of adenocarcinoma in human effusions. Cancer, *45*:1894–1900, 1985.

Kapadia, S.B.: Cytological diagnosis of malignant pleural effusion in myeloma. Arch. Pathol. Lab. Med., *101*:534–535, 1977.

Kaplan, M.M., and Sherwood, L.M.: Acute pericarditis due to *Histoplasma capsulatum.* Ann. Intern. Med., *58*:862–867, 1963.

Kapoor, O.P., Mascarenhas, E., Rananaware, M.M., and Gadgil, R.K.: Tuberculoma of the heart: report of 9 cases. Am. Heart J., *86*:334–340, 1973.

Keettel, W.C., Pixley, E.E., and Buchsbaum, H.J.: Experience with peritoneal cytology in the management of gynecologic malignancies. Am. J. Obstet. Gynecol., *120*:174–182, 1974.

Kimura, N., Namiki, T., Wada, T., and Sasano, N.: Peritoneal implantation of endodermal sinus tumor of the pineal region via a ventricular shunt. Acta Cytol., *28*:143–147, 1984.

Kmetz, D.R., and Newton, W.A., Jr.: The role of clinical cytology in a pediatric institution. Acta Cytol., *7*:207–210, 1963.

Kobzik, L., Antman, K.H., and Warhol, M.J.: The distinction of mesothelioma from adenocarcinoma in malignant effusions by electron microscopy. Acta Cytol, *29*:219–225, 1985.

Koller, P.C.: Cytologic variability in human carcinomatosis. Ann. N. Y. Acad. Sci., *63*:793–817, 1956.

Koprowska, I.: Exfoliative cytology in study of ascites tumors. Ann. N. Y. Acad. Sci., *63*:738–747, 1956.

Koss, L.G.: Examination of effusions (pleural, ascitic and pericardial fluids). *In* Wied, G.L., Koss, L.G., and Readan, J.W. (eds.): Compendium on Diagnostic Cytology, 7th ed. Tutorials of Cytology. Chicago, 1988.

Krivinkova, H., Ponten, J., and Blondai, T.: The diagnosis of cancer from body fluids. A comparison of cytology, DNA measurement, tissue culture, scanning and transmission microscopy. Acta Pathol. Microbiol. Scand. [A], *84*:455–467, 1976.

Labay, G.R., and Feiner, F.: Malignant pleural endometriosis. Am. J. Obstet. Gynecol., *110*:478–480, 1971.

Li, C.-Y., Lazcano-Villareal, O., Pierre, R.V., and Yam, L.T.: Immunocytochemical identification of cells in serous effusions. Am. J. Clin. Pathol., *88*:696–705, 1987.

Lopes-Cardozo, E., and Harting, M.C.: On the function of lymphocytes in malignant effusions. Acta Cytol., *16*:307–313, 1972.

Lozowski, W., Hajdu, S.I., and Melamed, M.R.: Cytomorphology of carcinoid tumors. Acta Cytol., *23*:360–365, 1979.

Luettges, J., Neumann, K., Pflueger, K.-H., and Schmitz-Moorman, P.: Differentialzytologie von Ergussfluessigkeiten unter Anwendung von monoklonalen Antikoerpern. Pathologe, *9*:137–142, 1988.

Luse, S.A., and Reagan, J.W.: Histocytologic and electron microscopic study of effusions associated with malignant disease. Ann. N. Y. Acad. Sci., *63*:1331–1347, 1956.

Martini, N., Freiman, A.H., Watson, R.C., and Hilaris, B.S.: Malignant pericardial effusion. N. Y. State J. Med., *76*:719–721, 1976.

McCallum, S., Cooper, K., and Franks, D.N.: Choroid plexus carcinoma: cytologic identification of malignant cells in ascitic fluid. Acta Cytol., *32*:263–266, 1984.

Melamed, M.R.: The cytological presentation of malignant lymphomas and related diseases in effusions. Cancer, *16*:413–431, 1963.

Menard, S., Rilke, F., Della Torre, G., Mariani-Constantini, R., Regazzoni, M., Tagliabue, E., Alasio, L., and Colnaghi, M.I.: Sensitivity enhancement of the cytologic detection of cancer cells in effusions by monoclonal antibodies. Am. J. Clin. Pathol., *83*:571–576, 1985.

Miles, C.P., Geller, W., and O'Neill, F.: Chromosomes in Hodgkin's disease and other malignant lymphomas. Cancer, *19*:1103–1116, 1966.

Miles, C.P., and Wolinska, W.: A comparative analysis of chromosomes and diagnostic cytology in effusions from 58 cancer patients. Cancer, *32*:1458–1469, 1973.

Miller, A.J.: Some observations concerning pericardial effusions and their relationship to the venous and lymphatic circulation of the heart. Lymphology, *3*:76–78, 1970.

Miner, R.W.(ed.): Ascites tumors as tools in quantitative oncology. Ann. N. Y. Acad. Sci., *63*:637–1030, 1956.

Monte, S.A., Ehya, H., and Lang, W.R.: Positive effusion cytology as the initial presentation of malignancy. Acta Cytol., *31*:448–451, 1987.

Perou, M.L., and Littman, M.S.: Diagnostic study of serous effusions with emphasis on some unusual findings. Am. J. Clin. Pathol., *25*:467–479, 1955.

Peterson, C.D., Robinson, W.A., and Jurnick, J.E.: Involvement of the heart and pericardium in the malignant lymphomas. Am. J. Med. Sci., *272*:161–165, 1976.

Pinto, M.M., Bernstein, L.H., Brogan, D.A., and Crisculo, E.M.: Carcinoembryonic antigen in effusions. A diagnostic adjunct to cytology. Acta Cytol., *31*:113–118, 1987.

Pozalaky, Z., McGinley, D., and Pozalaky, I.P.: Electron microscopic identification of the colorectal origins of tumor cells in pleural fluid. Acta Cytol., *27*:45–48, 1983.

Pozniak, A.L., Thomas, R.D., Hobbs, C.B., and Lever, J.V.: Primary malignant lymphoma of the heart. Antemortem cytologic diagnosis. Acta Cytol., *30*:662–664, 1986.

Rhodes, J.M., Birch-Andersen, A., and Ravn, H.: The effect of cyclophosphamide, methotrexate and x-irradiation on the ultrastructure and endocytic capacity of murine peritoneal macrophages. Acta Pathol. Microbiol. Scand. [A], *83*:443–453, 1975.

Robey, S.S., Cafferty, L.L., Beschorner, W., and Gupta, P.K.: Value of lymphocyte marker studies in diagnostic cytopathology. Acta Cytol., *31*:453–459, 1987.

Rodriguez, L.I., Casal, I.L., Carballo, C., and Lado, L.F.: Pleuropericardial effusion as the initial manifestation of malignant thymoma. Med. Clin. (Barc.), *84*:377–378, 1985.

Roh, L.S., and Paparo, G.P.: Primary malignant lymphoma of the heart in sudden unexpected death. J. Forensic Sci., *27*:718–722, 1982.

Rona, A., Marshall, K., and Raymont, E.: The cytological diagnosis of an ovarian mucinous cystoma from a virtually acellular specimen of abdominal fluid. Acta Cytol., *13*:672–674, 1969.

Roncalli, M., Gribaudi, G., Simoncelli, D., and Servida, E.: Cytology of yolk-sac tumor of the ovary in ascitic fluid. Acta Cytol., *32*:113–116, 1988.

Safa, A.M., and Van Orstrand, H.S.: Pleural effusion due to myeloma. Chest, *64*:246–248, 1973.

Salhadin, A., Nasiell, M., Nasiell, K., Silfversward, C., Hjerpe, A., Wadas, A.-M., and Enstad, I.: The unique cytologic picture of oat cell carcinoma in effusions. Acta Cytol., *20*:298–302, 1976.

Sano, M.E.: Diagnostic value of tissue culture studies of pleural effusions; 5 year follow-up of cases. Surg. Gynecol. Obstet., *97*:665–676, 1953.

Saphir, O.: Cytologic diagnosis of cancer from pleural and peritoneal fluids. Am. J. Clin. Pathol., *19*:309–314, 1949.

Sasser, R.L., Yam, L.T., and Li, C.Y.: Myeloma with involvement of the serous cavities. Cytologic and immunochemical diagnosis and literature review. Acta Cytol., *34*:479–485, 1990.

Sears, D., and Hajdu, S.I.: The cytologic diagnosis of malignant neoplasms in pleural and peritoneal effusions. Acta Cytol., *31*:85–97, 1987.

Siegler, R., and Koprowska, I.: Mechanism of ascites tumor formation. Cancer Res., *22*:1273–1277, 1962.

Singer, S., Boddington, M.M., and Hudson, E.A.: Immunocytochemical reaction of Ca1 and HMFG2 monoclonal antibodies with cells from serous effusions. J. Clin. Pathol., *38*:180–184, 1985.

Söderström, N., and Biorklund, A.: Intranuclear cytoplasmic inclusions in some types of thyroid cancer. Acta Cytol., *17*:191–197, 1973.

Spieler, P., and Gloor, F.: Identification of types and primary sites of malignant tumors by examination of exfoliated tumor cells in serous fluids. Comparison with diagnostic accuracy on small histologic biopsies. Acta Cytol., *29*:753–767, 1985.

Spieler, P., Kradolfer, D., and Schmidt, U.: Immunocytochemical characterization of lymphocytes in benign and malignant lymphocyte-rich serous effusions. Virchows Arch. [A], *409*:211–221, 1986.

Spriggs, A.I.: The architecture of tumor cell clusters in serous effusions. *In* Koss, L.G., and Coleman, D.V. (eds.): Advances in Clinical Cytology, vol. 2. pp. 267–290. New York, Masson Publishing, 1984.

Spriggs, A.I.: The Cytology of Effusions in the Pleural Pericardial and Peritoneal Cavities, 2nd ed. London, William Heinemann, 1972.

Spriggs, A.I.: Malignant cells in serous effusions complicating bronchial carcinoma. Thorax, *9*:26–34, 1954.

Spriggs, A.I., and Boddington, M.M.: Oat-cell bronchial carcinoma. Identification of cells in pleural fluid. Acta Cytol., *20*:525–529, 1976.

Spriggs, A.I., and Jerrome, D.W.: Intracellular mucous inclusions. A feature of malignant cells in effusions in the serous cavities, particularly due to carcinoma of the breast. J. Clin. Pathol., *28*:929–936, 1975.

Spriggs, A.I., and Meek, G.A.: Surface specializations of free tumor cells in effusions. J. Pathol. Bacteriol., *82*:151–159, 1961.

Spring-Mills, E., and Elias, J.J.: Cell surface differences in ducts from cancerous and noncancerous human breasts. Science, *188*:947–949, 1975.

Strum, S.B., and Rappaport, H.: Hodgkin's disease in the first decade of life. Pediatrics, *46*:748–759, 1970.

Szpak, C.A., Johnston, W.W., Roggli, V., Kolbeck, J., Lottich, S.C., Volmer, R., Thor, A., and Schlom, J.: The diagnostic distinction between malignant mesothelioma of the pleura and adenocarcinoma of the lung as defined by a monoclonal antibody. Am. J. Pathol., *122*:252–260, 1986.

Takagi, F.: Studies on tumor cells in serous effusion. Am. J. Clin. Pathol., *24*:663–675, 1954.

To, A., Boyo-Ekwueme, H.T., Posnansky, M.C., and Coleman, D.V.: Chromosomal abnormalities in ascitic fluid from patients with alcoholic cirrhosis. Br. Med. J., *282*:1659–1660, 1981.

Venegas, R.J., and Sun, N.C.J.: Cardiac tamponade as a presentation of malignant thymoma. Acta Cytol., *32*:257–262, 1988.

von Haam, E.: A comparative study of the accuracy of cancer cell detection by cytological methods. Acta Cytol., *6*:508–518, 1962.

Von Hoff, D.D., and LiVolsi, V.: Diagnostic reliability of needle biopsy of the parietal pleura, a review of 272 biopsies. Am. J. Clin. Pathol., *64*:200–203, 1975.

Wanebo, H.J., Martini, N., Melamed, M.R., Hilaris, B., and Beattie, E.J., Jr.: Pleural mesothelioma. Cancer, *38*:2481–2488, 1976.

Weick, J.F., Kiely, J.M., Harrison, E.G., Carr, D.T., and Scanlon, P.W.: Pleural effusion in lymphoma. Cancer, *31*:848–853, 1973.

Wilson, L.M., and Kinnier Draper, G.J.: Neuroblastoma, its natural history and prognosis: a study of 487 cases. Br. Med. J., *3*:301–307, 1974.

Witte, S.: Cytodiagnostik mit Hilfe einer Fluorochromierung in vivo. Verh. Dtsch. Ges. Inn. Med., *61*:254–256, 1955.

Woyke, S., and Czerniak, B.: The morphology of cells in effusions settled on glass. Acta Cytol., *21*:508–513, 1977.

Woyke, S., and Czerniak, B.: The surface coat of the human effusion cells. Acta Cytol., *21*:447–454, 1977.

Woyke, S., Domagala, W., and Olszewski, W.: Alveolar cell carcinoma of the lung: an ultrastructural study of the cancer cells detected in the pleural fluid. Acta Cytol., *16*:63–69, 1972.

Woyke, S., Domagala, W., and Olszewski, W.: Ultrastructure of hepatoma cells detected in peritoneal fluid. Acta Cytol., *18*:130–136, 1974.

Wroblewski, F.: Significance of alterations in lactic dehydrogenase activity of body fluids in diagnosis of malignant tumors. Cancer, *12*:27–39, 1959.

Wroblewski, F., and Wroblewski, R.: Clinical significance of lactic dehydrogenase activity of serous effusions. Ann. Intern. Med., *48*:813–822, 1958.

Yamada, T., Itou, U., Watanabe, Y., and Ohashi, S.: Cytologic diagnosis of malignant melanoma. Acta Cytol., *16*:70–76, 1972.

Yamagishi, K., Tajima, M., Suzuki, A., and Kimura, K.: Relation between cell composition of pleural effusions in patients with pulmonary carcinomas and their clinical courses. Acta Cytol., *20*:537–541, 1976.

Yazdi, H., Hajdu, S.I., and Melamed, M.R.: Cytopathology of pericardial effusion. Acta Cytol., *24*:401–412, 1980.

Zemanski, A.P., Jr.: Examination of fluids for tumor cells; analysis of 113 cases checked against subsequent examination of tissue. Am. J. Med. Sci., *175*:489–504, 1928.

Zirkin, H.J.: Pleural fluid cytology of invasive thymoma. Acta Cytol., *29*:1011–1014, 1985.

Malignant Lymphomas

Cabin, H.S., Costello, R.M., Vasudevan, G., Maron, B.J., and Roberts, W.C.: Cardiac lymphoma mimicking hypertrophic cardiomyopathy. Am. Heart J., *102*:466–468, 1981.

Castelli, M.J., Mihalov, M.L., Posniak, H.V., and Gattuso, P.: Primary cardiac lymphoma initially diagnosed by routine cytology: case report and literature review. Acta Cytol., *33*:355–358, 1989.

Chou, S.-T., Arkles, L.B., Gill, G.D., Pinkus, N., Parkin, A., and Hicks, J.D.: Primary lymphoma of the heart: a case report. Cancer, *52*:744–747, 1983.

Domagala, W., Emeson, E.E., Greenwald, E., and Koss, L.G.: A scanning electron microscopic and immunologic study of B-cell lymphosarcoma cells in cerebrospinal fluid. Cancer, *40*:716–720, 1977.

Domagala, W., Emeson, E., and Koss, L.G.: T and B lymphocyte enumeration in the diagnosis of lymphocyte-rich plural fluids. Acta Cytol., *25*:108–110, 1981.

Geisinger, K.R., Buss, D.H., Kawamoto, E.H., and Ahl, E.T., Jr.: Multiple myeloma. The diagnostic role and prognostic significance of exfoliative cytology. Acta Cytol., *30*:334–340, 1986.

Ghosh, A.K., Spriggs, A.I., and Mason, D.Y.: Immunocytochemical staining of T and B lymphocytes in serous effusions. J. Clin. Pathol., *75*:53–60, 1985.

Hajdu, S.I., and Hajdu, E.O.: Cytopathology of Sarcomas and Other Nonepithelial Malignant Tumors. Philadelphia, W. B. Saunders, 1975.

Harris, M., Eyden, B., and Reed, G.: Signet ring lymphoma: a rare variant of follicular lymphoma. J. Clin. Pathol., *34*:884–891, 1981.

Holland, W.W., Doll, R., and Carter, C.O.: The mortality from leukaemia and other cancers among patients with Down's syndrome (mongols) and among their parents. Br. J. Cancer, *16*:178–186, 1962.

Janckila, A.J., Yam, L.T., and Li C-Y.: Immunocytochemical diagnosis of acute leukemia with pleural involvment. Acta Cytol., *29*:67–72, 1985.

Kapadia, S.B.: Cytological diagnosis of malignant pleural effusion in myeloma. Arch. Pathol. Lab. Med., *101*:534–535, 1977.

Kim, H., Dofman, R.F., and Rappaport, H.: Signet ring lymphoma. A rare morphologic and functional expression of nodular (follicular) lymphoma. Am. J. Surg. Pathol., *2*:119–132, 1978.

Melamed, M.R.: The cytological presentation of malignant lymphomas and related diseases in effusions. Cancer, *16*:413–431, 1963.

Miller, R.T., Baker, K.I., and Moga, D.: Multilobated B-cell lymphoma. Report of a case with immunocytologic diagnosis in pleural fluid. Acta Cytol., *31*:785–790, 1987.

Peterson, C.D., Robinson, W.A., and Jurnick, J.E.: Involvement of the heart and pericardium in the malignant lymphomas. Am. J. Med. Sci., *272*:161–165, 1976.

Pincus, G.S., Said, J.W., and Hargreaves, H.: Malignant lymphoma, T-cell type: a distinct morphologic variant with large, multilobated nuclei, with a report of four cases. Am. J. Clin. Pathol., *72*:540–550, 1979.

Pozniak, A.L., Thomas, R.D., Hobbs, C.B. and Lever, J.V.: Primary malignant lymphoma of the heart. Antemortem cytologic diagnosis. Acta Cytol., *30*:662–664, 1986.

Roh, L.S., and Paparo, G.P.: Primary malignant lymphoma of the heart in sudden unexpected death. J. Forensic Sci., *27*:718–722, 1982.

Safa, A.M., and Van Orstrand, H.S.: Pleural effusion due to myeloma. Chest, *64*:246–248, 1973.

Sasser, R.L., Yam, L.T., and Li, C.Y.: Myeloma with involvement of the serous cavities. Cytologic and immunochemical diagnosis and literature review. Acta Cytol., *34*:479–485, 1990.

Seidel, T.A., and Garbes, A.D.: Cellules grumelées: old terminology revisited; regarding the cytologic diagnosis of chronic lymphocytic leukemia and well-differentiated lymphocytic lymphoma in pleural effusions. Acta Cytol., *29*:775–780, 1985.

Spieler, P., Kradolfer, D., and Schmidt, U.: Immunocytochemical characterization of lymphocytes in benign and malignant lymphocyte-rich serous effusions. Virchows Arch. [A], *409*:211–221, 1986.

Spriggs, A.I., and Vanhegan, R.I.: Cytologic diagnosis of lymphoma in serous effusions. J. Clin. Pathol., *34*:1311–1325, 1981.

Vernon, S.E., and Rosenthal, D.L.: Sézary cells in ascitic fluid. Acta Cytol., *23*:408–411, 1979.

Wilson, M.S., Theil, K.S., Goodwin, R.A., and Brandt, J.T.: Comparison of Papanicolaou's and Wright–Giemsa stains in the examination of body fluids for Hodgkin's disease. Arch. Pathol. Lab. Med., *112*:612–615, 1988.

Yam, L.T.: Granulocytic sarcoma with pleural involvment. Identification of neoplastic cells with cytochemistry. Acta Cytol., *29*:63–66, 1985.

Young, J.A. and Crocker, J.: Pleural fluid cytology in lymphoplasmacytoid lymphoma with numerous intracytoplasmic immunoglobulin inclusions. A case report with immunocytochemistry. Acta Cytol., *28*:419–424, 1984.

Tumor Markers (see also Chap. 34)

Coleman, D.V., and Ormerod, M.B.: Tumor markers in cytology. *In* Koss, L.G., and Coleman, D.V. (eds.): Advances in Clinical Cytology, vol. 2. pp. 33–48. New York, Masson Publishing, 1984.

Croonen, A.M., van der Valk, H.C.J., and Lindeman, J.: Cytology, immunology and flow cytometry in the diagnosis of pleural and peritoneal effusions. Lab. Invest., *58*:725–731, 1988.

Czerniak, B., Papenhausen, P.R., Herz, F., and Koss, L.G.: Flow cytometric identification of cancer cells in effusions with Cal monoclonal antibody. Cancer, *55*:2783–2788, 1985.

Dalquen, P., Bittel, D., Gudat, F., Overbeck, J.V., and Heitz, P.U.: Combined immunoreaction and Papanicolaou's stain on cytological smears. Pathol. Res. Pract., *181*:50–54, 1986.

Domagala, W., and Koss, L.G.: Configuration of surfaces of cells in effusions by scanning electron microscopy. *In* Koss, L.G., and Coleman, D.V. (eds.): Advances in Clinical Cytology. pp. 270–313. London, Butterworths, 1981.

Freni, S.C., James, J., and Prop, F.J.A.: Tumor diagnosis in pleural and ascitic effusions based on DNA cytophotometry. Acta Cytol., *15*:154–162, 1971.

Goodlin, R.C.: Utilization of cell chromosome number for diagnosis of cancer cells in effusions. Nature, *197*:507, 1961.

Guzman, J., Bross, K.J., and Costabel, U.: Malignant pleural effusions due to small cell carcinoma of the lung. An immunocytochemical cell-surface analysis of lymphocytes and tumor cells. Acta Cytol., *34*:497–501, 1990.

Guzman, J., Costabel, U., Bross, K.J., Wiehle, U., Grunert, F., and Schaefer, H.E.: The value of the immunoperoxidase slide assay in the diagnosis of malignant pleural effusions in breast cancer. Acta Cytol., *32*:188–192, 1988.

Guzman, J., Hilgarth, M., Bross, K.J., Wiehle, U., Ross, A., Kresin, V., and Costabel, U.: Lymphocyte subpopulations in malignant ascites of serous papillary ovarian adenocarcinoma: an immunocytochemical study. Acta Cytol., *32*:811–815, 1988.

Johnston, W.W., Szpak, C.A., Lottich, S.C., Thor, A., and Schlom, J.: A monoclonal antibody (B72.3) as a novel immunohistochemical adjuvant for the diagnosis of carcinoma in fine needle aspiration biopsy specimens. Hum. Pathol., *17*:501–513, 1986.

Johnston, W.W., Szpak, C.A., Thor, A., and Schlom, J.: Use of a monoclonal antibody as an immunocytochemical adjunct to diagnosis of adenocarcinoma in human effusions. Cancer, *45*:1894–1900, 1985.

Krivinkova, H., Pontén, J., and Blondai, T.: The diagnosis of cancer from body fluids. A comparison of cytology, DNA measurement, tissue culture, scanning and transmission microscopy. Acta Pathol. Microbiol. Scand. [A], *84*:455–467, 1976.

Li, C.-Y., Lazcano-Villareal, O., Pierre, R.V., and Yam, L.T.: Immunocytochemical identification of cells in serous effusions. Am. J. Clin. Pathol., *88*:696–705, 1987.

Lindeque, B.G., Cronje, H.S., and Deale, C.J.: Prevalence of primary papillary peritoneal neoplasia in patients with ovarian carcinomas. S. Afr. Med. J., *67*:1005–1007, 1985.

Luettges, J., Neumann, K., Pflueger, K.-H., and Schmitz-Moorman, P.: Differentialzytologie von Ergussfluessigkeiten unter Anwendung von monoklonalen Antikoerpern. Pathologe, *9*:137–142, 1988.

Menard, S., Rilke, F., Della Torre, G., Mariani-Costantini, R., Regazzoni, M., Tagliabue, E., Alasio, L., and Colnaghi, M.I.: Sensitivity enhancement of the cytologic detection of cancer cells in effusions by monoclonal antibodies. Am. J. Clin. Pathol., *83*:571–576, 1985.

Miles, C.P., and Wolinska, W.: A comparative analysis of chromosomes and diagnostic cytology in effusions from 58 cancer patients. Cancer, *32*:1458–1469, 1973.

Orell, S.R., and Dowling, K.D.: Oncofetal antigens as tumor markers in the cytologic diagnosis of effusions. Acta Cytol., *27*:625–629, 1983.

Pinto, M.M., Bernstein, L.H., Brogan, D.A., and Crisculo, E.M.: Carcinoembryonic antigen in effusions. A diagnostic adjunct to cytology. Acta Cytol., *31*:113–118, 1987.

Robey, S.S., Cafferty, L.L., Beschorner, W., and Gupta, P.K.: Value of lymphocyte marker studies in diagnostic cytopathology. Acta Cytol., *31*:453–459, 1987.

Schneller, J., Eppich, E., Greenebaum, E., Elequin, F., Sherman, A., Wersto, R., and Koss, L.G.: Flow cytometry and Feulgen cytophotometry in evaluation of effusions. Cancer, *59*:1307–1313, 1987.

Singer, S., Boddington, M.M., and Hudson, E.A.: Immunocytochemical reaction of Ca1 and HMFG2 monoclonal antibodies with cells from serous effusions. J. Clin. Pathol., *38*:180–184, 1985.

Sloane, J.P., and Ormerod, M.G.: Distribution of epithelial membrane antigen in normal and neoplastic tissues and its value in diagnostic tumor pathology. Cancer, *47*:1786–1795, 1981.

Spieler, P., Kradolfer, D., and Schmidt, U.: Immunocytochemical characterization of lymphocytes in benign and malignant lymphocyte-rich serous effusions. Virchows Arch. [A] *409*:211–221, 1986.

Szpak, C.A., Johnston, W.W., Roggli, V., Kolbeck, J., Lottich, S.C., Volmer, R., Thor, A., and Schlom, J.: The diagnostic distinction between malignant mesothelioma of the pleura and adenocarcinoma of the lung as defined by a monoclonal antibody. Am. J. Pathol., *122*:252–260, 1986.

Unger, K.M., Rabes, M., Bedrossian, C.W.M., Stein, D.A., and Barlogie, B.: Analysis of pleural effusions using automated flow cytometry. Cancer, *52*:873–877, 1983.

27

Cerebrospinal Fluid, Miscellaneous Fluids; Exfoliative Cytology of the Eye and the Skin

CEREBROSPINAL FLUID

Anatomic and Physiologic Considerations

The cerebrospinal fluid (CSF) is formed from circulating blood by a complex epithelial organ, the *choroid plexus,* located within the ventricular system of the brain.

The normal choroid plexus is a highly selective filter that regulates the chemical makeup of the CSF and maintains it at a constant level, independently of variations in the blood serum. The choroid plexus does not allow the passage of most toxic substances or blood cells, except for an occasional mononucleated cell, a monocyte, or a lymphocyte. The choroid plexus, therefore, constitutes a highly effective blood–brain barrier, ensuring for the brain the optimal working conditions. Normal CSF is a crystal clear liquid containing only very few mononucleated blood cells and lower levels of glucose and proteins than the blood.

The CSF bathes the entire internal ventricular system of the brain, its external surfaces, the cerebellum, and the spinal cord. The extracerebral CSF is contained between two epithelial meningeal membranes, the pia (lining the brain) and the arachnoid (lining the dura). Occasionally, cells derived from the choroid plexus, the pia, and the arachnoid may desquamate into the CSF. Normally, there are very few of these cells, and they are difficult to identify.

Any increase in the number of cells in the CSF or changes in the glucose and protein content invariably indicate a pathologic process. Enumeration and cytologic examination of the cells in the spinal fluid serve to clarify the nature of the disease.

Cytologic examination of the CSF has become

an important part of a complete neurologic evaluation, particularly of cancer patients with clinical evidence or suspicion of central nervous system involvement and in patients with the acquired immunodeficiency syndrome (AIDS). Also patients with space-occupying lesions of unknown nature in the central nervous system discovered by new radiographic techniques such as computed tomographic scanning (CT) or magnetic resonance imaging (MRI) should have the benefit of this examination. Cytologic evaluation of CSF has become an essential step in the follow-up of patients with certain malignant diseases, particularly lymphoma and leukemia. The approach to the therapy of leukemia, particularly in children, and of some small-cell tumors (oat cell carcinoma), has been revolutionized by these procedures. Other applications of cytology comprise the diagnosis of infectious processes of obscure etiology.

Impeccable laboratory techniques are essential if the cytologic evaluation of the fluid is to be successful. The various technical approaches are discussed in Chapter 33. Regardless of the method used, cell loss must be avoided. The use of hematologic techniques of cell preparation and staining is useful in lymphomas and leukemias.

An obvious condition for a successful cytologic diagnosis of a primary or a metastatic tumor is the seeding of tumor cells into the subarachnoid space or into the cerebral ventricles. Even if the lesion is in contact with CSF, the number of malignant cells observed may be very small; the diagnosis may have to rest on the presence of a dozen or, sometimes, fewer malignant cells. However, in this particular setting, even a single abnormal cell should be most carefully evaluated. The sources of error are relatively few and rarely of importance.

The presence of abundant cancer cells in the cerebrospinal fluid almost invariably indicates extensive involvement of leptomeninges.

Cells in Normal Cerebrospinal Fluid

With the cell collection techniques used in this laboratory, notably cytocentrigation (see Chap. 33), only a very few small inactive lymphocytes and monocytes are observed in the CSF of adults. The monocytes have a somewhat larger, more open, sometimes indented nucleus and a slightly larger rim of cytoplasm. Thus, only two types of cells and two nuclear forms are normally observed (Fig. 27 – 1). By using a careful cell collection technique, Dyken (1975) found that the cell count is higher in neonates (less than 1 month in age) than in older

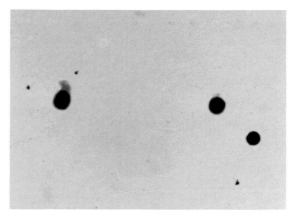

FIGURE 27–1. Cerebrospinal fluid, cytocentrifuge preparation: one lymphocyte and two larger mononucleated cells. In this photograph the nuclear structure cannot be seen. (×560)

persons. For the neonates the average count was 10.17 ± 8.45 cells per cubic millimeter, and for older persons 2.59 ± 1.73 cells per cubic millimeter. There were also some differences in the differential counts: monocytes were the most prevalent cell in neonates, whereas in older persons lymphocytes were most commonly observed.

In a subsequent study, Dalens et al. (1982) confirmed the original observations; additionally, cells of the choroid plexus and the arachnoid were noted as a transient phenomenon during the first week of life. These changes are probably due to the slight brain trauma sustained at birth.

The identification of choroid plexus, ependymal, and meningeal cells is extremely difficult in adult patients. Kline (1962) and Naylor (1961, 1964) described ependymal cells as small cuboidal cells arranged in rows or clusters. In the author's laboratories, such cells have been very rarely observed; their occurrence may be expected only in fluid aspirated directly from the cerebral ventricles or the cysterna magna, mainly in neonates. Elongated cells described by Kline as originating from meningeal lining have not been observed by us in the spinal fluid of patients without disease. Koelmel (1976) observed such cells after pneumoencephalography.

Wertlake et al. observed in ventricular fluid occasional pia–arachnoid cells, resembling mesothelial cells, rare cuboidal or columnar cells interpreted as cells of ependymal origin, and, occasionally, cells interpreted as astrocytes. The cytologic–histologic correlation of these very rare cells has been carried out by McGarry et al. (1969). Oehmichen (1976) used CSF for characterization of mononuclear phagocytes with membrane markers. The use of other markers will be described below, as needed.

Changes in Benign Cell Populations in Cerebrospinal Fluid

Under pathologic conditions several changes in the benign cell population of the CSF may take place.

Transformation of Lymphocytes and Monocytes. The lymphocytes may increase in number and may undergo a transformation that increases substantially the variety of cell and nuclear sizes. Cells resembling immunoblasts, with a clear nucleus and large nucleolus, may occur, but only as a small subpopulation of transformed lymphocytes. The monocytes may also be transformed into macrophages and may assume a phagocytic activity (Fig. 27–2). This response is not specific and may occur under a broad variety of circumstances, such as viral meningoencephalitis and some forms of chronic inflammation, such as tuberculous meningitis.

Effects of Myelograms. The injection of a radiopaque medium into the spinal canal results in activation of monocytes into macrophages. The large cells with round or kidney-shaped nuclei and vacuolated cytoplasm increase in number, become quite conspicuous, and often contain phagocytized yellow deposits of the radiopaque material.

Invasion of Cerebrospinal Fluid by Neutrophilic Polymorphonuclear Leukocytes. These cells normally do not cross the blood–brain barrier; hence, they must be considered as invaders of the CSF. The presence of polymorphonuclear leukocytes in CSF *always* indicates an acute inflammatory process, such as bacterial meningitis, brain abscess, or an acute inflammatory process of another etiology. The cells most likely are derived directly from damaged blood capillaries located within the brain or the meninges.

Eosinophils may occur in CSF as a consequence of a parasitic infection of the central nervous system (*Cysticercus cellulosae* cysts, see below), in chronic inflammations, or as a reaction to a trauma. The condition is extremely rare in my ex-

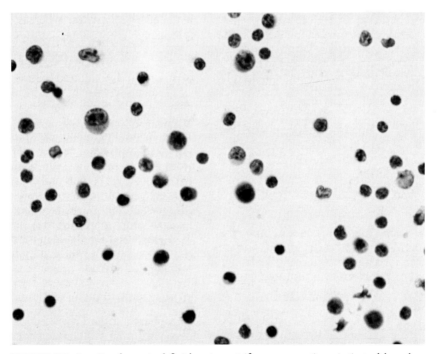

FIGURE 27–2. Cerebrospinal fluid, cytocentrifuge preparation: Activated lymphocytes in recovery stage of tuberculous meningitis. Note the variability in the cell population, ranging from the small, inactive lymphocytes with condensed nuclei, to large immunoblasts with visible nucleoli. Cells of intermediate sizes represents intermediate stages in lymphocyte activation. Compare with acute stage of the disease in Fig. 27–6. (×560)

perience. Conrad (1986) observed eosinophils in metastatic cancer and in children with a shunt.

Red Blood Cells and Hemosiderin. Erythrocytes do not normally cross the blood–brain barrier. The most common source of erythrocytes in CSF is a traumatic tap, a surgical intervention, or a trauma. The presence of hemosiderin-laden macrophages, on the other hand, indicates a previous hemorrhagic event. This may be a cerebral or subdural acute or chronic hemorrhage or the presence of a tumor. Bernad and Taft (1980) documented that the presence of numerous hemosiderin-bearing macrophages was consistent with an intraventricular hemorrhage in a neonate. An iron stain should be performed to differentiate hemosiderin from melanin pigment. Benign cells containing melanin have been observed in melanosis of the meninges (Rosenthal, 1984). These must be differentiated from cells of primary or metastatic malignant melanoma (see below) and from hemosiderin-bearing cells.

Other Cells
Plasma Cells. The presence of plasma cells always indicates an important abnormality in CSF. This may be a neurologic disease, a chronic inflammatory event, or a multiple myeloma (see below).

Bone Marrow Cells. These may be observed when the tap needle inadvertently enters a vertebral body. Megakaryocytes are usually a conspicuous component of such faulty taps.

Cartilage Cells. Chondrocytes occur when the tap needle incidentally enters the intervertebral cartilage (Bigner and Johnston, 1981; Takeda et al., 1981). Notochordal cells from nucleus pulposus have been observed in an infant (Takeda et al., 1981).

Squamous Cells and Anucleated Squamae. These are usually of skin origin. An important point of differential diagnosis is a ruptured benign squamous cyst of the brain or a ruptured craniopharyngioma. Both conditions are usually recognized clinically.

Acellular Components. Corpora amylacea, spherical proteinaceous structures, commonly seen in the brain of the elderly, may occasionally occur in the CSF (Bigner and Johnston, 1981). They may be occasionally calcified and mimic a psammoma body or a fungus (Preisig and Buhaug 1978).

Fragments of myelinated nerves have been observed by us in a case of multiple sclerosis, during a severe, debilitating relapse of the disease in a young woman (Fig. 27–3).

Powder Crystals. Cerebrospinal fluid may be contaminated by starch granules from powder used on surgical gloves. In a personally observed case, seen in consultation, the approximately spherical crystals were mistaken for *Cryptococcus neoformans* (Fig. 27–4). Such particles may be phagocytized, as reported by Reinharz et al. (1978). In polarized light, the starch particles form a Maltese cross but this may also occur with *Cryptococcus*. In general starch particles are larger than *Cryptococcus*, fail to show spores or mucous capsule, and often contain a central density.

Cytology of Cerebrospinal Fluid in Nonmalignant Disorders

Acute Bacterial Meningitis

Cerebrospinal fluid in meningitis caused by *Neisseria meningitidis, Haemophilus influenzae,* pneumococci, or sometimes other organisms, is characterized by the dominance of numerous neutrophilic polymorphonuclear leukocytes (Fig. 27–5). The glucose content of CSF is reduced, and the protein level is markedly elevated.

"Aseptic" Viral Meningitis and Meningoencephalitis

Viral (aspetic) meningitis may be due to a variety of RNA viruses. The cytologic findings are characterizd by a population of activated lymphocytes, with resulting variability in cell population of lymphocytic derivation (see above, p. 1187). Polymorphonuclear leukocytes and macrophages are either absent or few. The glucose content is nearly normal, and the protein level only slightly increased. The picture of viral meningitis may cause problems in the differential diagnosis of malignant lymphoma (see below).

Herpes Simplex

Encephalitis caused by infection with herpes simplex virus type I is characterized by hemorrhagic necrosis of the brain. Type II herpesvirus may also cause meningitis. Gupta et al. (1972) were the first to observe the characteristic virus-induced inclusions in CSF. For the descriptions of the herpesvirus-induced cellular changes see Chapter 10, p. 351.

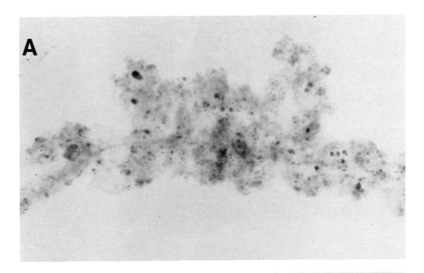

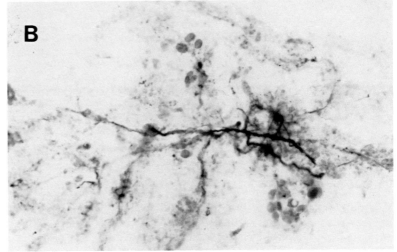

FIGURE 27–3. Cerebrospinal fluid, cytocentrifuge preparation. Multiple sclerosis in a woman, aged 39. (*A*) Fragment of a degenerated neural matter, Papanicolaou stain. The threadlike structure within the fragment is a nerve. The nature of the dark particles is not known. (*B*) Bodian stain, documenting the presence of a myelinated nerve within another fragment of neural matter. (*A, B* ×350)

FIGURE 27–4. Cerebrospinal fluid in a 7-year-old child. Starch granules from surgical powder after surgery for a medulloblastoma, mistaken for *Cryptococcus neoformans* (cf. Fig. 27–6). The large size of the granule, its configuration, and the presence of a dark center are characteristic of starch. Another granule with angular configuration is also shown. A small lymphocyte in the same field gives a good idea of the size of the granules. (×560)

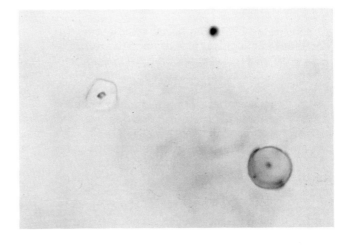

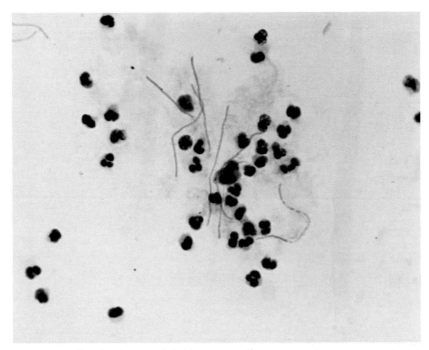

FIGURE 27–5. Cerebrospinal fluid; cytocentrifuge preparation: acute meningitis caused by *Klebsiella* species in a patient with AIDS. The dominant cell population is polymorphonuclear neutrophilic leukocytes. The nature of the filamentous organism was confirmed by culture. (×350)

Chemical Meningitis

Chemical meningitis is due to chemical substances, such as chemotherapeutic agents, injected into the CSF. Under these circumstances the CSF is rarely examined by cytologic methods. In an occasional case, polymorphonuclear leukocytes and activated macrophages can be observed.

Chronic Meningitis

Tuberculosis. After a lull of several years, tuberculous meningitis is seen again with increasing frequency, in part because of the AIDS epidemic.

The cytologic picture depends on the stage of the disease. In early stages, the CSF is very rich in cells and presents a panorama of transformed lymphocytes, plasma cells, activated macrophages, and polymorphonuclear leukocytes (Fig. 27–6). With therapy, the cytologic picture changes: the polymorphonuclear leukocytes are markedly reduced, and there is a dominance of transformed lymphocytes, monocytoid cells, and macrophages (see Fig. 27–2; also Jeren and Beus, 1982). The presence of multinucleated giant cells has been noted (Kolmel,

1976). This finding is nonspecific. For example, Bigner et al. (1985) observed multinucleated giant cells in CSF as a reaction to foreign material introduced during surgery and in a patient with sarcoidosis.

Fungal Meningitis. The most common fungus causing meningitis, particularly in immunocompromised or debilitated patients, is *Cryptococcus neoformans*. The round or oval yeast organisms, measuring from 4 to 10 μm in diameter, are provided with a thick, mucoid capsule that can be easily visualized by lowering the stage of the microscope. The diagnosis can be confirmed by a number of mucus stains [mucicarmin, periodic acid-Schiff (PAS)], by a silver stain, or an India ink preparation (Fig. 27–7). The microscopic diagnosis is comparatively easy, the only possible source of confusion being the grains of powder derived from surgical gloves (see above and Fig. 27–4).

Meningeal cryptococcosis causes only a minimal cytologic reaction in CSF—the organisms are accompanied by a scattering of mature lymphocytes and an occasional macrophage.

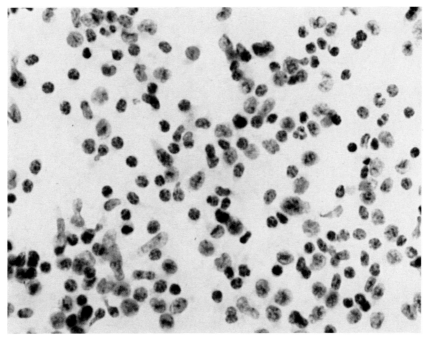

FIGURE 27–6. Cerebrospinal fluid, cytocentrifuge preparation: tuberculous meningitis, acute stage. A very rich population of mononuclear cells of lymphocytic and monocytic derivation. Occasional polymorphonuclear leukocyte may be noted. (×560)

In immunocompromised hosts, such as patients with AIDS or patients undergoing intensive chemotherapy, meningitis caused by other fungi can be observed. Thus *Candida albicans* (moniliasis), mucormycosis (zygomycosis, phycomycosis), and aspergillosis have been observed. Undoubtedly, other fungi as well will be observed with the passage of time. For the description of the fungi, see Chapter 19.

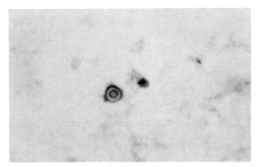

FIGURE 27–7. Spinal fluid sediment: *Cryptococcus neoformans (hominis).* Periodic acid-Schiff stain, which brings out the thick capsule characterizing the fungus. (×560)

Rare Forms of Meningitis

Lyme Disease. Lyme disease, an ubiquitous infection with the tick-transmitted spirochete *Borrelia burgdorferi*, may cause meningitis. The CSF may show marked hypercellularity, with activated lymphocytes in all stages, plasma cells, and macrophages (Steere et al., 1983; Benach et al., 1983; Razavi-Eucha et al., 1987).

Mollaret's Meningitis. This exceedingly rare form of periodically recurrent aseptic meningitis of unknown etiology has a very characteristic cytologic presentation in CSF (Mollaret, 1977; Gledhill et al., 1975; Lowe, 1982). During the attack, the CSF has a very high and variegated cellular content, with numerous polymorphonuclear leukocytes, monocytes, plasma cells, and lymphocytes. The dominant cell, however, is a large mononucleated (monocytoid) cell with abundant cytoplasm and peculiar nuclei, resembling footprints in the sand (Fig. 27–8A, B). These cells disappear rapidly from the CSF; hence, they are considered to be fragile. Mollaret throught that these cells were possibly of endothelial origin, but their derivation is most likely from transformed monocytes, capa-

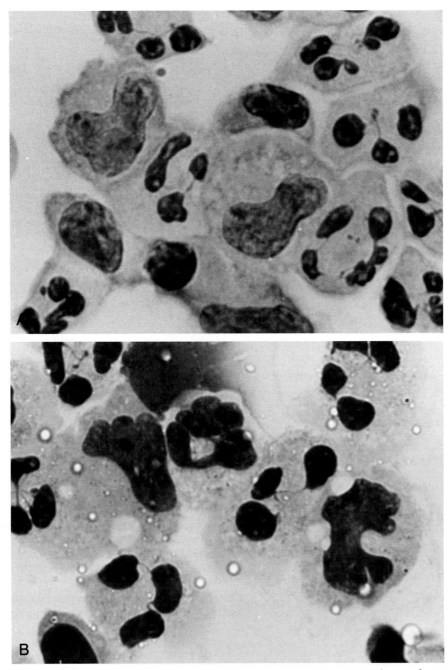

FIGURE 27-8.   Mollaret's meningitis in a 48-year-old man with recurrent bouts of transient meningitis: cerebrospinal fluid. (*A*) Papanicolaou-stained sediment characterized mainly by the large, mononucleated (monocytoid) cells, with peculiar nuclei of uneven width, resembling footprints. (*B*) The footprint image is enhanced in air-dried smears, stained with May–Grünwald–Giemsa stain.

(continued)

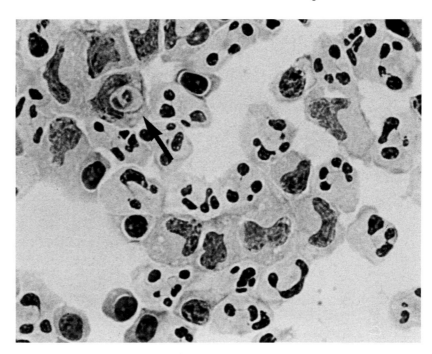

FIGURE 27–8 *(Continued).*
(*C*) The monocytoid cells are capable of engulfing other cells (*arrow*), hence of phagocytic activity. Numerous polymorphonuclear leukocytes, lymphocytes, and plasma cells complete the cytologic picture. (*A, B* approx. ×1,000; *C,* approx. ×400. Courtesy of Dr. D. N. Ferguson, from Lowe, E.: Mollaret's meningitis. A case report. Acta Cytol., *26*:338–340, 1982, with permission)

ble of phagocytosis (see Fig. 27–8*C*) (Gledhill et al., 1975; Lowe, 1982). The presence of herpesvirus simplex DNA has been documented in this disease by polymerase chain reaction (Yamamoto et al., 1991).

Other Rare Forms of Meningitis. Sporadic case reports of unusual cytologic findings in CSF in secondary involvement of the central nervous system (CNS) in systemic disorders appear from time to time in the literature. Thus Jaeckle (1982) described the presence of numerous macrophages phagocytosing hemosiderin in a case of systemic lupus erythematosus with transient blindness (Anton's syndrome).

De la Monte et al. (1985) observed a polymorphous cell population (transformed lymphocytes, plasma cells, large atypical mononuclear cells) in patients with Sjögren's syndrome with CNS involvement.

Lowe (1982) discussed the differential diagnosis of Mollaret's meningitis in CSF by citing the findings in a number of very uncommon systemic disorders with incidental meningitis (Behçet's, Vogt–Koyanagi, and Harada's syndromes). The reader is referred to specialized sources for further discussion of these very rare events (Hermans et al., 1972).

Guillain-Barré Syndrome. This is an acute, progressive form of neuropathy of unknown etiology. The CSF is characterized by an increase in proteins in the absence of an increase in cell population. Nyland and Ness (1978) observed an occasional increase in CSF lymphocytes.

Parasites

Cysticercosis. Cystic larvae of the tape worm *Taenia solium* may affect the brain (and other organs). The cysts are usually identified by a CT scan. Aspiration biopsy of one of the brain cysts may yield anucleated squames and, sometimes, hooklets from the scolex or the head of the larva, not unlike the hooklets in ecchinococcal cysts (see p. 1112 and Fig. 29–104). There is no documented evidence that CSF can serve as a diagnostic medium in this infection.

Toxoplasmosis. *Toxoplasma gondii* is an ubiquitous coccidian parasite that hitherto has been observed mainly in newborn children whose eyes and brain are chiefly affected. With the onset of AIDS and immunosuppressive therapy, the cerebral form of the infection in adults has become much more common. The tachyzoites (nucleated form of the parasite) have been identified in direct aspirates from the brain (Fig. 27–9). So far, there are no case reports of parasite identification in CSF, but this possibility may be anticipated with the spread of AIDS.

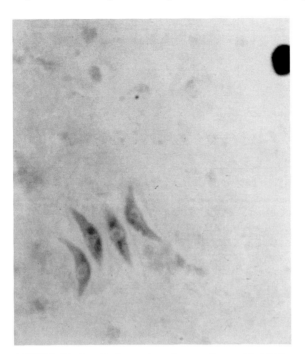

FIGURE 27–9. Brain aspirate in a patient with AIDS. Spindle-shaped tachyzoites (nucleated forms) of *Toxoplasma gondii.* The size of the organism may be compared with a lymphocyte in the same field. (×1,800)

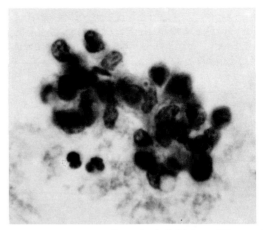

FIGURE 27–10. Cerebrospinal fluid in a 32-year-old woman with a history of debilitating headaches at the times of menstrual bleeding. Bloody tap, containing clusters of typical endometrial glandular cells, consistent with endometriosis of the meninges. (×560)

It may also be anticipated that other blood and tissue protozoa (malaria, trypanosomiasis, leishmaniasis, etc.) will be identified in CSF in AIDS patients.

Other Rare Benign Conditions

Endometriosis. In a personally observed case, periodic headaches in a 32-year-old woman were due to a focus of meningeal endometriosis. A cluster of typical endometrial glandular cells was observed in CSF. The tap also contained red blood cells and hemosiderin-laden macrophages (Fig. 27–10).

Syringomyelia. Highly atypical cells of unknown origin or significance were observed in a case of syringomyelia (Fig. 27–11).

Fluid From Ventricular Shunts

The use of cerebroabdominal shunts has gained popularity as a means of alleviating intracranial pressure and reducing hydrocephalus. Bigner et al. (1985) described the cytologic finding in the CSF in three patients. Foreign body giant cells, papillary

fronds derived from the choroid plexus and, in one case, tumor cells from a malignant pineal germinoma were observed. In one ascitic fluid sample, fragments of choroid plexus were noted. McCallum et al. (1988) also identified cells of the rare choroid plexus carcinoma in ascitic fluid of a 5-year-old child with a shunt. Kimura et al. (1984) described peritoneal implants of an endodermal sinus tumor of pineal origin (see Chap. 26).

Primary Tumors of the Central Nervous System

The introduction of stereotactic computed roentgenologic equipment has permitted direct thin-

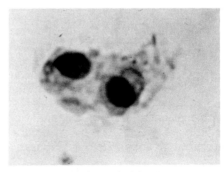

FIGURE 27–11. Cerebrospinal fluid in a case of syringomyelia. Bizarre cells of unknown origin. (Approx. ×800)

needle aspirations and tissue core biopsies of brain lesions, with a very high degree of diagnostic accuracy. Several reviews of the cytologic findings in aspirates or touch preparations are available (Barnard, 1981; Liwnicz and Rodirguez, 1984; Chandrasoma and Apuzzo, 1989; see also Chap. 29). On the rarest occasions high-grade astrocytomas may metastasize to extracranial lymph nodes and meninges. Pasquier et al. (1980) described two such cases and summarized over 70 similar cases from the literature. Thus, with the notable exception of medulloblastomas and related tumors, the CSF is rarely studied as a means of primary diagnosis of brain tumors, and the cytologic observations may be considered as incidental. In fact, much of the writing on this subject is based on touch preparations of tumor fragments or on CSF obtained after surgery or another type of intervention, such as a cysternal tap. Nonetheless, there are occasionally situations when an unexpected diagnosis of a primary brain tumor can be suggested (or confirmed) on cytologic examination of the CSF, and this is the purpose of this brief synopsis.

Several major reviews of this subject are available, notably by Kline, Naylor, Gondos and King, Watson and Hajdu and, more recently, by Bigner and Johnston (1981).

The recognition of cells originating in the primary neoplasms of the central nervous system in CSF depends on two factors: anatomic location and degree of differentiation. Tumors located within the depths of the brain or the spinal cord and thus not bathed by CSF cannot be recognized except by direct sampling. Well-differentiated glial tumors (astrocytomas grade I and II) do not shed cells readily when compared with poorly differentiated neoplasms such as astrocytoma grade III and IV (high-grade gliomas and glioblastoma multiforme). Furthermore, the recognition of the cells from well-differentiated neoplasms may be fraught with difficulties, as these tumors are often made up of cells with benign appearance. For example, cells from ependymomas usually appear as benign cuboidal or columnar cells. The recognition of the tumor, therefore, hinges on the finding in the CSF of "foreign" cells (i.e., cells that are not normally observed). Naylor's data suggest that the fluid from cerebral ventricles or the cisterna magna is a better medium of diagnosis than spinal tap. The cytologic presentation of the most common primary tumors of the central nervous system in CSF is as follows.

Low-Grade Astrocytomas, Grades I and II

These tumors of glia shed very few cells into the CSF. The cells appear epithelial, although occa-sionally stellate cytoplasm may be observed. The nuclei appear pale, not enlarged, and cannot be recognized as malignant. In fact, Bigner and Johnston pointed out that identical cells may be observed in benign destructive processes.

High-Grade Astrocytomas, Grades III and IV (Glioblastoma Multiforme)

The CSF may contain a few cells with nuclear enlargement and hyperchromasia. Multinucleated giant tumor cells, so characteristic of this tumor in tissue, are very rarely seen in CSF. When observed they are strongly suggestive of this neoplasm.

An important caveat is in order here: the presence of conspicuous cancer cells in CSF is much more likely to represent a metastatic tumor than a high-grade glioma. Thus, the diagnosis of a primary high-grade brain tumor should be made only in the presence of confirmatory clinical and roentgenologic evidence.

Oligodendroglioma

Watson and Hajdu described the cytology of this tumor as made up of uniformly round cells with round and eccentric nuclei provided with nucleoli. This is the appearance of these cells in touch preparations seen in our laboratories.

Midline Tumors

This large group of tumors, of diverse origin and histologic presentation, occupy the area surrounding the midbrain (diencephalon). The group includes tumors of the pituitary, the pineal, and craniopharyngiomas. The tumors are generally accessible to an aspiration biopsy and, except for the malignant tumors of the pineal region, are very rarely recognized in CSF.

The tumors of the pineal region may be benign or malignant. They occur in several forms: as benign or malignant pinealomas, benign dermoid cysts, malignant teratomas, and germinomas. Germinomas occur predominantly in adolescent boys and are of special interest here because they can be recognized in CSF. Thus, Ginhorst and Tskahara (1979) described a case of recurrent pineal germinoma with pulmonary metastases. Large tumor cells were recognized in CSF and in sputum. Of note was the elevation of the beta subunit of human chorionic gonadotropin in the spinal fluid. Several additional cases of pineal germinoma with cells in CSF have been described (Zaharopoulos and Wong, 1980; Bigner and Johnston, 1981; Geisinger et al., 1984).

Medulloblastomas and Related Tumors (Intracranial Neuroblastoma, Retinoblastoma)

This family of tumors is characterized by tumor cells resembling primitive neurons, often arranged in rosettes around a central lumenlike area filled with neurofilaments. These highly malignant tumors, occurring mainly in children, are capable of metastases, and are the only tumors of the central nervous system that *consistently* shed cells into the CSF and thus may be identified cytologically in a high proportion of cases. In CSF, the cancer cells are usually numerous and readily identified as malignant. The cells vary in size. They are larger in some tumors than in others but, within each tumor, remain fairly monotonous (cfr. Figs. 27–12 and 27–13). The nuclei are hyperchromatic and contain visible nucleoli. The cytoplasm is scanty, readily visible, and is sometimes elongated.

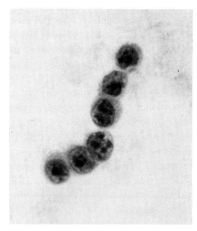

FIGURE 27–12.   Cerebrospinal fluid from a case of medulloblastoma. Note a chain of malignant cells with prominent nucleoli. The cancer cells were larger than average in this tumor (cfr. Fig. 27–13*A*). (×560. Case courtesy of Dr. Lucy Feiner, New York, New York)

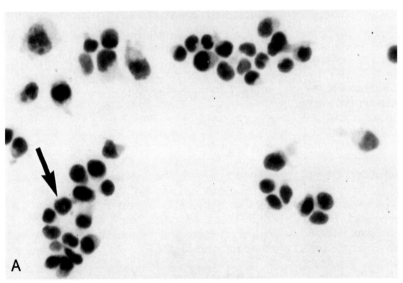

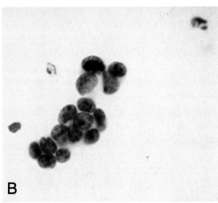

FIGURE 27–13.   (*A*) Cerebrospinal fluid in a child with medulloblastoma. Numerous clusters of cancer cells, one with a central lumen suggestive of a rosette formation (*arrow*). Scattered single larger tumor cells, some of nearly columnar shape, may be noted. The preparation was slightly overstained and nuclear structure is not well seen. (*B*) Cerebrospinal fluid in a child with an ocular retinoblastoma. A cluster of small tumor cells with prominent nucleoli is shown. Rosette formation is not evident. (*A, B* ×560)

The cancer cells may occur in small clusters (Fig. 27–12) or singly (Fig. 27–13) and may form rosettes (Fig. 27–13*A*). Prominent nucleoli are extremely characteristic in well-fixed and well-stained material (see Fig. 27–13*B*). Such cancer cells cannot be distinguished from cells of metastatic neuroblastoma and may also mimic a malignant lymphoma (see below and Fig. 27–18). At least some tumors identified as medulloblastomas are probably variants of primary malignant lymphomas of the brain, which have a more favorable response to radiotherapy than medulloblastomas (Zimmerman).

Sarcomas of the Central Nervous System

Occasionally, spindle cell sarcoma of the brain may be observed. Such tumors are difficult to classify, yet are highly malignant. Obvious cancer cells may be observed in CSF in such cases, in the presence of the primary or recurrent tumor (Fig. 27–14).

Primary Meningeal Sarcomas

These are exceedingly rare tumors. In a personally observed case numerous large malignant cells, single and in clusters, were seen in the CSF in a young man (Fig. 27–15). Although the diagnosis of a malignant tumor involving the subarachnoid space was evident on cytologic material, only a complete autopsy established the final diagnosis. A nearly identical case was described by Garbos (1984).

Other Rare Central Nervous System Tumors

Sporadic case reports describe CSF cytology in a variety of uncommon malignant tumors.

Primary melanoma of meninges is a rare disorder that may occasionally be diagnosed by cytology of the CSF before any space-occupying lesions may be observed on a CT scan (Aichner and Schuler, 1982). Schmidt et al. (1988) also described such a case and reviewed the literature, noting seven prior cases diagnosed by cytology of the CSF.

The cytologic presentation may vary. In Aichner and Schuler's case the morphologic appearance of the cancer cells was inconspicuous, and the melanin pigment was scanty. The diagnosis was confirmed by ultrastructural studies that disclosed numerous melanosomes in tumor cells. In the case described by Schmidt et al., the huge cancer cells had abundant melanin pigment that obscured the cellular morphology; the diagnosis was confirmed on autopsy. Metastatic melanoma, particularly of ocular origin, must be considered in the differential diagnosis of these rare cases.

A case of primary intracranial squamous carcinoma, derived from an epidermoid cyst at the base of the brain, with keratinized cancer cells in CSF was described by Bondeson and Falt (1984).

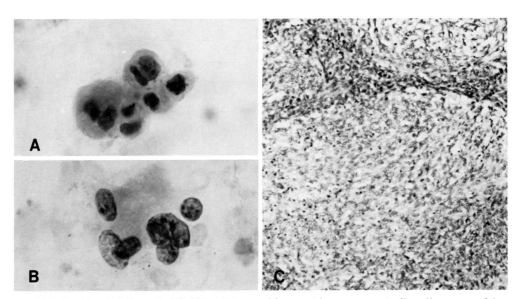

FIGURE 27–14. Cerebrospinal fluid in a 27-year-old man with recurrent spindle cell sarcoma of the cerebellum, previously treated by surgery and radiotherapy. (*A, B*) Clusters of obvious, large cancer cells in CSF. The configuration of the clusters is more suggestive of a carcinoma than a sarcoma. (*C*) Biopsy section of primary tumor showing a spindle cell sarcoma. (*A, B* ×560; *C* ×150)

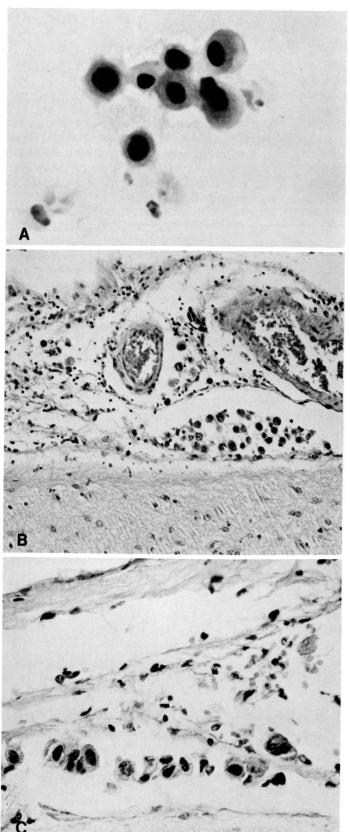

FIGURE 27–15. Primary meningeal sarcoma in a 33-year-old man. (*A*) Spinal fluid. One of the numerous clusters of malignant cells suggestive of a metastatic carcinoma with meningeal involvement. (*B, C*) Sections of subarachnoid space obtained at time of autopsy. The tumor is growing in loose clusters, with single cells apparently originating from endothelial lining. There was no evidence of another primary tumor. The tumor fits the classification of primary meningeal endothelial sarcoma. (*A* ×560; *B* ×150; *C* ×350. Case courtesy of Dr. Sol Teitelbaum, Beaumont, Texas)

A primary neuroblastoma of a cerebral hemisphere was described by Gandolf (1980).

Primary malignant lymphomas of the brain are seen with increased frequency in AIDS patients (Hautzer et al., 1987; review in Bonnin, 1987). The cytologic presentation of these tumors is described with other lymphomas (see below).

The extremely rare *choroid plexus papillomas* and *carcinomas* may also be identified in CSF. The papillomas shed cohesive clusters of epithelial cells in papillary arrangements. The cells of carcinomas have the features of any adenocarcinoma, with large nuclei and prominent, large nucleoli (Bigner and Johnston, 1981; Kim et al., 1985). As always, when confronted with large cancer cells in CSF, the question of metastatic cancer must be raised. Clinical and roentgenologic data may be essential in the interpretation.

Results of Cytologic Examination of Cerebrospinal Fluid Patients With Primary Tumors of the Central Nervous System

On the average about 25% of tumors of the central nervous system will yield diagnostic cells in well-prepared CSF. The data from two surveys are summarized in Table 27–1.

Special Diagnostic Procedures. Kajikawa et al. used CSF to establish primay short-term tissue cultures of various primary tumors of the central nervous system. The procedure was successful in a number of instances, and the identification of tumor type was easier in the culture than in the original CSF.

Metastatic Tumors to the Central Nervous System

Next to the identification of infectious processes, discussed in the opening pages of this chapter, the recognition of metastatic malignant tumors, particularly leukemias and lymphomas, but also solid tumors, is the most important task of cytologic assessment of the CSF. This has lately assumed an even greater significance for several reasons: first, the epidemic of AIDS, wherein the development of a meningeal or cerebral lymphoma is a feared and common complication; second, because the aggressive chemotherapy of leukemias, lymphomas, and some carcinomas, particularly bronchogenic carcinomas of small-cell type, may result in cerebromeningeal metastases. Malignant lymphomas are also seen with increasing frequency in organ transplant recipients, with attendant immunosuppression; such tumors may invade the central nervous system.

The prevention or early recognition of these metastases is critical in deciding on further therapeutic measures that may significantly alter the course of the disease.

Leukemia

The examination of CSF for the presence of leukemic cells, initiated by the writer around 1960, has become a routine procedure, especially in acute leukemia in children. It has been shown that leukemic cells may be present in CSF for some time before there are clinical manifestations of meningeal involvement, and that prophylactic therapy to the

Table 27–1
Cerebrospinal Fluid: Diagnostic Results With Some Primary Tumors of the Central Nervous System Expressed as Percentage of Positive Results

Diagnosis	Gondos and King (%)	Watson and Hajdu (%)
Astrocytoma, grades I and II	25	30*
Astrocytoma, grades III and IV	28.6	42†
Medulloblastoma	61.9	72
Ependymoma	23.1	
Meningioma	0.0	

*Grade I through III.
†Grade IV only.
(Data from Gondos, B., and King, E.B.: Cerebrospinal fluid cytology: Diagnostic accuracy and comparison of different techniques. Acta Cytol., 20:542–547, 1976; Watson, C.W., and Hajdu, S.I.: Cytology of primary neoplasms of the central nervous system. Acta Cytol., 21:4–47, 1977)

central nervous system has a beneficial effect on the survival rate and even cure of such patients.

A simple increase in the number of cells of the lymphocytic series in CSF under the appropriate clinical circumstances must be considered as a major warning and calls for a careful evaluation of the cytologic evidence. In acute leukemia or in chronic leukemia in crisis, the blast cells in the CSF may be readily identified in Papanicolaou stain because of their usually large size (two to four times larger than normal lymphocytes) and two characteristic nuclear features: the presence of nucleoli and of nuclear protrusions (Fig. 27–16). The protrusions vary in size and usually have the shape of a nipple. Whether the protrusions represent an abnormal chromosomal component or an artifact is immaterial, because of their major diagnostic value. Although similar nuclear protrusions may be observed in solid malignant lymphomas (see below), for all practical purposes, they are never observed in normal lymphocytes. The nuclei are surrounded by a thin rim of delicate transparent cytoplasm. Hematologic stains can also be used on air-dried CSF sediment. The nucleoli are usually easier to observe in such preparations.

The diagnosis is much more difficult in the rare instances of CSF involvement by chronic lymphocytic leukemia (and corresponding lymphomas). If the cell population is monotonous and composed exclusively of well-differentiated small lymphocytes, the diagnosis is fairly secure, especially if the chromatin of the lymphocytes is "lumpy" (cellules grumelées, see Fig. 27–19*A* and p. 1160), and it is supported by clinical data. If, however, the cell population is polymorphous, the possibility of one of the meningitic processes, described above, occurring in or with lymphomas must be considered, since the two disease processes are not mutually exclusive. The resolution rests on careful analysis of cytologic and clinical data.

Cerebrospinal fluid involvement in chronic myelogenous leukemia is very uncommon in my experience. When it does happen, the cell population is heterogeneous, with all stages of granulocyte precursors represented. The possibility of a granulocytic sarcoma (chloroma), with involvement of the brain or meninges, must be considered if a population of granulocyte precursors is observed in CSF in the absence of clinical leukemia. At all times, a contamination of CSF by leukemic cells from peripheral blood may occur.

As has been mentioned above, one of the principal goals of cytology of the CSF in leukemia is to monitor the effects of treatment, particularly in children. Involvement of the central nervous system or meninges may occur surreptitiously in asymptomatic patients, whose peripheral blood and bone marrow may show good response to ther-

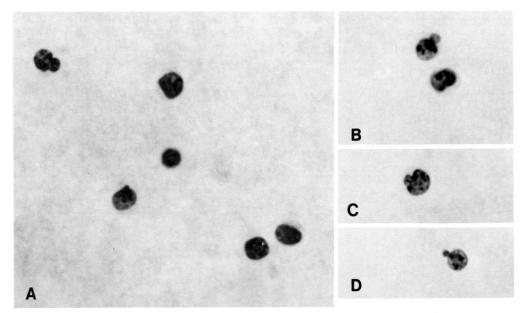

FIGURE 27–16. (*A–D*) Spinal fluid in a 10-year-old boy with acute blastic leukemia (cytocentrifuge preparation). In this example, the leukemic cells are small (averaging 8 μm in diameter) and are characterized by very scanty, delicate cytoplasm. The nuclei contain nucleoli and show the extremely characteristic nuclear protrusions. (*A–D* ×1,000)

apy. Another occult site of residual or recurrent leukemia in boys is the testis. In such cases, prophylactic radio- or chemotherapy to the brain and the meninges or testes has been shown to be an essential step in cure, which can now be achieved in a substantial proportion of young patients.

The effects of therapy on the CSF cytology in leukemia has been studied by Aaronson et al. (1975). It was shown that, with the onset of therapy, there is a rapid and marked reduction of blast cells in CSF, leading to the their complete disappearance.

Malignant Lymphoma

Meningeal and cerebral involvement in malignant non-Hodgkin's lymphoma is sufficiently frequent to warrant the examination of CSF even if there is only a slight clinical suspicion of central nervous system involvement. The identification of the malignant cells in CSF is similar to that described for effusions (see p. 1157), with special emphasis on the presence of nucleoli and nuclear protrusions (Figs. 27–17 and 27–18). Occasionally, a lumpy chromatin pattern may be observed (cellules grumelées, see above) (Fig. 27–19*A*).

Cerebrospinal fluid can be used for the identification of B or T origin of malignant lymphocytes, and for such other studies as scanning electron microscopy (Domagala et al.) (Fig. 27–19).

Malignant lymphoma, usually of the large-cell type, is a fairly frequent complication of AIDS, particularly in children, who nearly all die of it. The principles of cytologic diagnosis in CSF (and in effusions, for that matter) remain the same. On occasion, the malignant lymphoma may be pri-

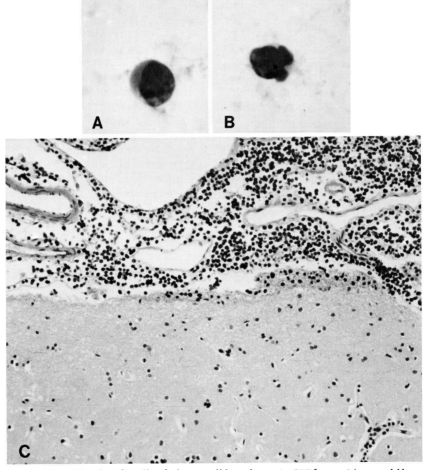

FIGURE 27–17. (*A, B*) Cells of a large-cell lymphoma in CSF from a 14-year-old boy with history of bowel resection for intussusception. (*C*) At autopsy the tumor was found to involve the subarachnoid space. (*A* approx. ×1,000; *B* ×150)

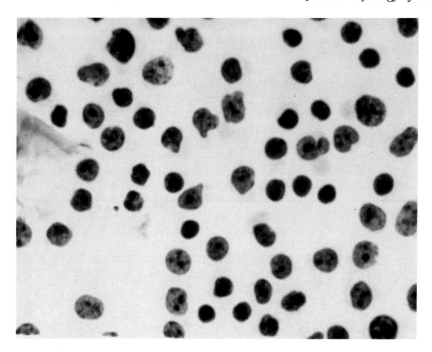

FIGURE 27–18. Cerebrospinal fluid, cytocentrifuge preparation. Metastatic large cell lymphoma: note dispersed, large tumor cells with nuclear protrusions. In a few cells single or multiple large nucleoli may be seen. (×560)

mary in the brain (reviews in Hautzer et al., 1987; Bonnin, 1987), and the initial diagnosis may have to be rendered on CSF in the absence of peripheral disease and only slight roentgenologic abnormalities.

Borowitz et al. (1981) discussed several pitfalls in the diagnosis of leukemia and lymphoma in CSF. Ten "false-positive" diagnoses were observed among 34 specimens diagnosed as "leukemia–lymphoma." Several sources of error were identified: viral and fungal meningitis, viral encephalitis, possible contamination with peripheral blood in cases of known leukemia, and a postsurgical reaction. Even though the authors attempted to identify the cytologic differences between the true-positive and false-positive cases, the evidence presented was not fully persuasive. Many of the "benign" cells illustrated had the characteristics of a malignant lymphoma with nuclear protrusions. The paper should serve as a warning that pitfalls may occur and great care is required for diagnosis.

Sequential samples of CSF may be used to monitor the effects of treatment (Mayer and Watson, 1980).

Rare Forms of Malignant Lymphoma

Malignant Histiocytosis (Histiocytic Medullary Reticulosis). This rare form of lymphoma, characterized by erythrophagocytosis and a rapid, unfavorable clinical course, may occasionally be ob-

served in CSF. A case of "histiocytosis," primary in the brain and meninges in a young girl, was described by Wolfson (1979). Large, abnormal cells with vacuolated cytoplasm were observed in the CSF. Five cases of this type were described by Hamilton et al. (1982). In four of them erythrophagocytosis by abnormal histiocytes was observed in CSF. The question of precise classification of the diseases in this group of patients was presented, but the final diagnosis in some of them was insecure. A case of metastatic malignant histiocytosis was described by Carbone and Volpe (1980).

A case of *multilobate lymphoma* with a bizarre clinical course was observed by us (Fig. 27–20). The multilobate cells contained numerous nuclei, each provided with a large nucleolus. The patient died after intensive therapy, and there was no residual evidence of disease at autopsy.

Cases of *mycosis fungoides* (T-cell lymphoma of the skin) with involvement of the CNS was described by Gobel (1976) and by Bodenstein (1982). The characteristic Sézary cells, with convoluted (cerebriform) nuclei, were observed in CSF (see also Chap. 29, p. 1286, and Fig. 29–53).

Plasmocytoma. The finding of plasma cells in CSF as a part of a heterogeneous population of inflammatory cells is frequent in chronic inflammatory processes. If, however, the plasma cells are the sole population of cells in CSF sediment, the diag-

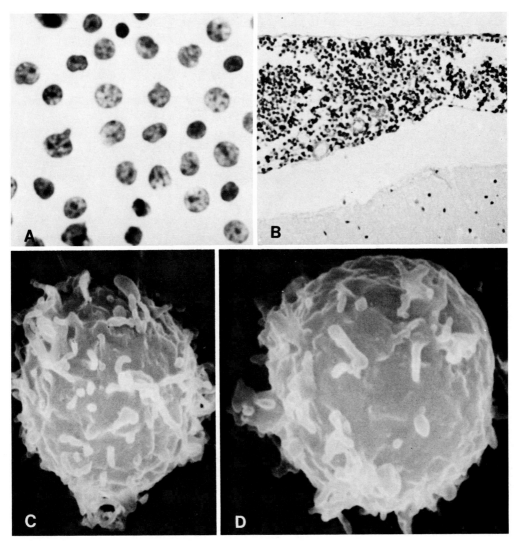

FIGURE 27–19. Cerebrospinal fluid in a 65-year-old woman with meningeal involvement by lymphosarcoma. (*A*) Cytocentrifuge preparation showing numerous malignant cells with prominent nucleoli and nuclear protrusions characteristic of malignant lymphoma. Note also the "lumpy" chromatin (cellules grumelée of Spriggs), another characteristic feature of lymphoma and leukemia (see p. 1160). Nearly all the cells in the fluid were shown to be B lymphocytes by immunologic techniques. Autopsy disclosed extensive involvement of meninges by lymphosarcoma (*B*). Scanning electron microscopy demonstrated considerable variability in surface configuration of the malignant cells (*C, D*). (*A* ×1,000; *B* ×150; *C, D* approx. ×6,000. *C, D* courtesy of Dr. W. Domagala)

nosis of plasma cell myeloma must be considered. This may be a direct extension of a vertebral or skull lesion into the subarachnoid space or, most uncommonly, an actual metastasis to the meninges. For further description and illustrations of cells of plasma cell myeloma in fluids, see Chapter 26 and Figs. 26–57 and 26–58.

Epithelial Tumors

Central nervous system involvement by metastatic epithelial tumors carries with it an abysmal prognosis. With the emergence of multidrug intensive chemotherapeutic regimens in the 1970s, the clinical behavior of some small-cell cancers, such as the

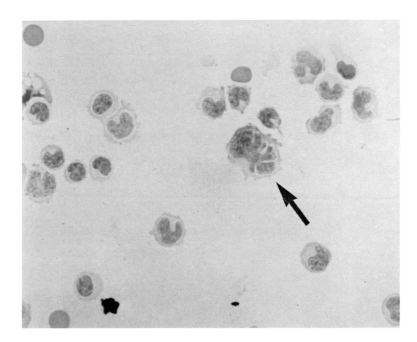

FIGURE   27-20. Cerebrospinal fluid: malignant lymphoma with bizarre, multilobate cells (*arrow*).

oat cell carcinoma of the lung, has been drastically altered. Good response of the primary tumor and local metastases to treatment failed to prevent cerebral and meningeal involvement (Aisner et al., 1979). In other words, these tumors, previously virtually incurable, began to behave in a fashion similar to leukemias or malignant lymphomas. Thus, cytologic detection of tumor cells in CSF at an early stage of CNS involvement acquired therapeutic implications and led to regimens of preventive treatment.

For some other carcinomas, such as mammary carcinomas, new therapeutic options also altered the short-term prognosis. Although cure of these cancers after involvement of the CNS is, at this time (1991), still impossible, short remissions with a good quality of life now can occur. Consequently, the identification of cells of metastatic carcinoma has acquired, in some cases, new significance beyond diagnosis.

The most commonly identified metastatic carcinomas in CSF are of mammary and bronchogenic origin. The cytologic presentation depends on the type of metastases and type of tumor. Nodular metastases usually shed single cells or cell clusters. Massive cytologic evidence usually indicates a diffuse involvement of the subarachnoid space, or *meningeal carcinomatosis.*

Cancer cells may be accompanied by reactive lymphocytosis and by macrophages. As a general rule, cells of metastatic carcinomas, even of small size, are larger than transformed lymphocytes, although, on a very rare occasion, very small carcinoma cells may be observed. In general, the recognition of metastatic carcinoma in CSF is comparatively easy in good preparations.

Mammary Carcinoma. Small-cell carcinomas, usually of lobular type, shed scattered small cancer cells, sometimes of signet ring-type configuration (Fig. 27-21). Occasionally, short chains of cancer cells are noted (Fig. 27-22), although this cell arrangement is not specific for mammary carcinoma, as it may also be observed in other tumors (see Fig. 27-12).

The ductal type of mammary carcinoma sheds large, readily recognizable cancer cells that may sometimes show peripheral cytoplasmic protrusions (Fig. 27-23). In other cases, cancer cells with large nuclei and nucleoli may be recognized. Mitotic figures may occur (Fig. 27-24). Intrathecal treatment with methotrexate may produce cytoplasmic vacuolization of cancer cells, but this rarely interferes with their recognition.

Lung Cancer. In general, the cytologic presentation of lung cancer in CSF follows the pattern seen in effusions. Adenocarcinomas and epidermoid carcinomas shed large cancer cells, often in small clusters (see Figs. 26-21 and 26-24). Oat cell carcinoma sheds small cancer cells, often singly, often in clusters, sometimes arranged in short

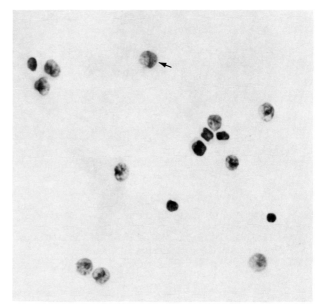

FIGURE 27–21. Spinal fluid: metastatic mammary carcinoma, lobular type. Cytocentrifuge preparation. Numerous small cancer cells may be identified. Note large nucleoli and, in one cell (*arrow*), a signet ring-like appearance. (×560)

chains with nuclear molding, resembling a string of vertebrae (see Fig. 26–37).

Other Carcinomas. Carcinomas of virtually every origin may occasionally metastasize to the CNS and be recognized as cancers in CSF. Thus, bladder and prostate cancer are seen with a fair frequency (Eyha et al., 1981).

Other Tumors

In children, neuroblastomas were seen with a fair frequency before the introduction of contempo-

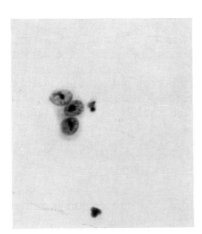

FIGURE 27–22. Metastatic mammary carcinoma. Note the cohesive chain of cells with prominent nucleoli. (Spinal fluid, ×560)

rary therapy (Fig. 27–25). Contrary to the presentation in aspiration biopsies and sometimes in effusion, rosettes were virtually never observed, and only single cancer cells were noted.

Of special interest in adults is *metastatic melanoma*, which may affect the central nervous system as the only metastatic site, sometimes many years after removal of the primary tumor (Fig. 27–26). The malignant cells are often remarkably well preserved (Fig. 27–27), although, in the absence of pigment formation, the exact identification of the tumor type may prove difficult.

Spinal Fluid in Assessment of Effect of Treatment

Samples of spinal fluid repeatedly obtained while the patient is under treatment for metastatic involvement of the meninges or the central nervous system may yield information on the response of the tumor to therapy. In leukemia and malignant lymphoma, karyorrhexis in tumor cells may be noted. In epithelial tumors, cells changes in the form of enlargement and vacuolization of the nucleus and cytoplasm may be brought about by radio- or chemotherapy.

SYNOVIAL FLUID

Normal synovial fluid contains a small number of leukocytes, macrophages, and synovial lining cells,

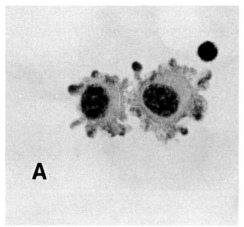
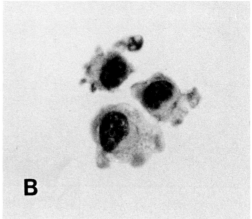

FIGURE 27–23.   Cerebrospinal fluid: metastatic mammary carcinoma, ductal type. Large cancer cells with cytoplasmic protrusions. (×560)

the latter resembling mesothelial cells (cf. p. 1086). During the acute stage of inflammatory disorders the number of cells is greatly increased, the majority being polymorphonuclear leukocytes. In chronic inflammatory disorders, the synovial fluid greatly resembles other effusions (Fig. 27–28): synovial (mesothelial) cells, leukocytes, and histiocytes are evident.

Naib pointed out that, in traumatic arthritis, degenerated cartilage cells may be observed singly and in sheets. Cartilage cells and fragments may be also present in degenerative joint diseases (osteoarthritis) of various etiologies.

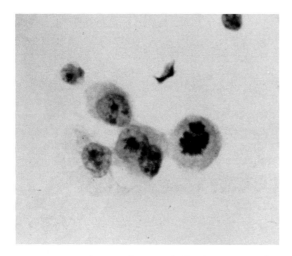

FIGURE 27–24.   Cerebrospinal fluid, cytocentrifuge preparation: metastatic mammary carcinoma, large-cell ductal type. Note large nucleoli and a mitotic figure. (×560)

Cytology in Nonmalignant Disorders

Villonodular Synovitis

In villonodular synovitis brown inclusions of hemosiderin may be observed in macrophages, side by side with multinucleated giant cells (cf. Fig. 27–29). The latter may be observed also in other forms of synovitis and in giant cell tumors of bone, involving joints (see below).

Rheumatoid Arthritis

This disease, of unknown etiology, may affect patients of all ages, and it is usually diagnosed by clinical and laboratory data other than cytology. However, students of this disease, notably Hollander et al., pointed out the existence of the synovial fluid of neutrophilic polymorphonuclear leukocytes containing in their cytoplasm from 2 to 15 dark, basophilic, round inclusions. Delbarre named such cells *ragocytes*, and the name has generally been accepted. It has been postulated (Fallet) that the inclusions represent an accumulation of abnormal immunoglobulins. Naib has observed such cells in other diseases, for example, in rheumatic arthritis, and considers ragocytes specific for rheumatoid arthritis only if found in excess of 10% of cell population of the synovial fluid.

Gout and Pseudogout

Naib and Suprun and Mansoor reported the presence of uric acid crystals in synovial fluids. The crystals are needle-shaped and either lie freely in fluid or are phagocytosed by polymorphonuclear

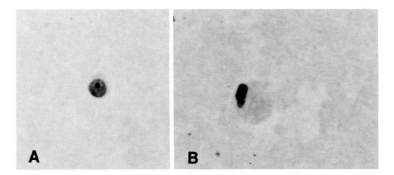

FIGURE 27–25. Metastatic neuroblastoma in spinal fluid. Tumor cells (*A*) were accompanied by numerous large macrophages (histiocytes) (*B*), some containing hemosiderin. (*A, B* ×560)

leukocytes. The birefringent crystals are diagnostic of gout.

Pseudogout is an inflammatory, often hereditary, joint disease, caused by deposition of calcium salt crystals. Zaharopoulos and Wong (1980) observed calcium pyrophosphate dehydrate crystals in fresh joint fluids, in the form of rod-shaped or rhomboid structures. In other forms of arthritis, noncrystalline deposits of calcium were occasionally noted. Other crystals, such as cholesterol crystals, can occasionally be observed (Schumacher, 1966).

Cytology in Malignant Tumors Involving Joints

It is most uncommon to establish the diagnosis of a malignant tumor of synovial membranes or adjacent bone or cartilage on aspirated synovial fluid. Hence, the recorded cases are very few. Meisels and Berebichez reported three cases of osteogenic sarcoma diagnosed on synovial fluid, two from the lower extremities and one from the shoulder. Naib reported two cases of synovial sarcoma and four of metastatic tumors to the joints. Generally, malignant tumors involving joints are uncommon, and accumulation of synovial fluid as the first evidence of disease is extremely rare.

Figure 27–29 shows a recurrent giant cell tumor of bone in synovial fluid.

HYDROCELE FLUIDS

Aspiration of fluids accumulating in hydroceles is a common procedure. Usually the fluids are nearly acellular, but occasionally, sheets of markedly

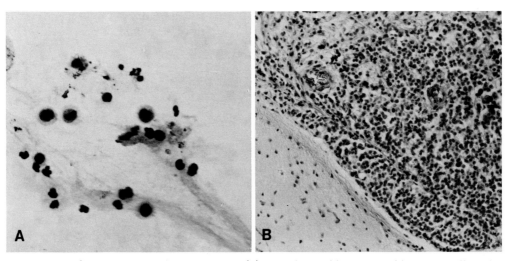

FIGURE 27–26. Metastatic melanoma in CSF. (*A*) Note the readily recognizable cancer cells with granules of pigment. (*B*) The histologic section through the subarachnoid space reveals melanoma. (*A, B* ×150. Case courtesy of Dr. R.V.P. Hutter, New York, New York, and Mr. W. Kennedy, Norfolk, Virginia)

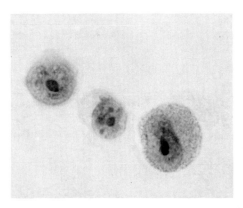

FIGURE 27–27. Spinal fluid: cells of metastatic malignant melanoma. Note excellent preservation of nuclear and cytoplasmic features. The cytoplasm was pigmented in the largest of the three cells. Huge nuclei and nucleoli are present. (×1,000)

atypical mesothelial cells may be observed therein (Fig. 27–30). These may constitute an important source of diagnostic error. Similar observations were reported by Piscioli et al. (1983). Rare primary mesotheliomas have been observed in hydroceles and in hernia sacs (Tang et al.). A case of primary malignant mesothelioma of the tunica vaginalis testis is illustrated in Figs. 26–8, 26–9, and 26–10. Nodular, but benign, proliferation of mesothelial lining may also occur. The differential diagnosis between benign and malignant mesothelial proliferation may be difficult (for further discussion of this topic, see p. 1086).

Occasionally, a malignant testicular tumor may be observed in hydrocele fluid (Fig. 27–31).

AMNIOTIC FLUID

Amniocentesis, or aspiration of amniotic fluid, usually past the 16th week of pregnancy, is performed under ultrasound guidance for the identification of congenital abnormalities in the fetus and for the determination of fetal sex.

Although the principal tool in the study of amniotic fluid is a cytogenetic analysis, the morphology of the cells in the fluid is occasionally of interest. A detailed analysis of the cells found in amniotic fluid with histologic correlation has been reported by Morris and Bennett (1974), Casadei et al. (1973), Schnage et al. (1982), and Blekinsopp et al. (1984). The cells of fetal origin are:

Anucleated squamae of buccal or skin origin
Nucleated squamous cells
    Superficial and intermediate type, of skin, vaginal, and buccal origin, and parabasal type, probably of amniotic origin
Amniotic cells
    Isolated
    In sheets and clusters of various types

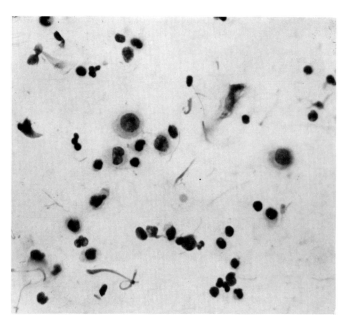

FIGURE 27–28. Synovial fluid, chronic synovitis, knee joint. Single mesothelial cells and leukocytes, mainly lymphocytes, may be noted. (×560)

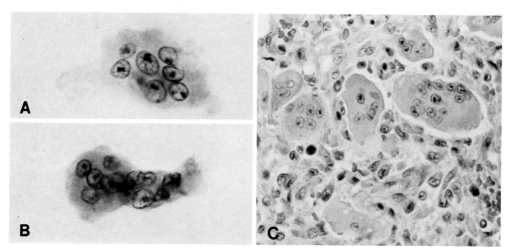

FIGURE 27–29. Aspiration smear of right wrist joint: recurrent giant cell tumor of radius, 2 years after surgical treatment. (*A, B*) Large multinucleated giant cells similar to those observed in osteogenic sarcoma (cf. 26–62). (*C*) Biopsy of recurrent tumor. (*A, B* ×560; *C* ×350)

Fragments of chorionic villi
Macrophages

Blekinsopp et al. (1984) analyzed the proportion of various cell components in amniotic fluid from 480 patients, 16- to 20-weeks pregnant. Actual cell counts were performed in cytocentrifuge preparations of 50 normal fluids. Squamous cells of superficial and intermediate type formed 80% of the cell population in the samples. The recognition of these cells presented no difficulties, as their morphology was identical with similar cells of female genital tract or respiratory tract origin.

Amnion cells, singly and in sheets, constituted 12% of the cell population. The cells were about the size of small parabasal squamous cells, with central small nuclei, and were distinguished by a marked peripheral thickening of the cytoplasm. Occasionally, the nuclei of the amnion cells were peripheral.

Small macrophages, always occurring singly, formed about 2% of the cell population. The cells had a vacuolated cytoplasm. Some of the macrophages had an elongated cytoplasmic tail, and were thought to represent similar cells known as Hofbauer cells of the placenta.

The remainder of the cell population was represented by fetal cells, mainly nucleated erythrocytes, somewhat larger than mature erthrocytes.

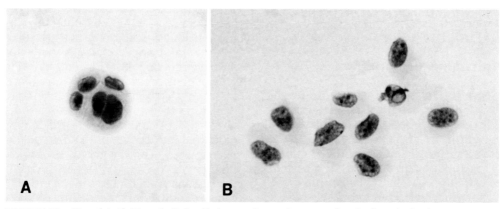

FIGURE 27–30. (*A, B*) Mesothelial cell clusters from a long-standing hydrocele fluid. Note the enlarged, hyperchromatic nuclei in both photographs. The cluster in (*A*) has a papillary arrangement imitating adenocarcinoma. In the surgical specimen there was proliferation of mesothelium, similar to that shown in Fig. 25–4, but no evidence of malignant tumor. (*A, B* ×560)

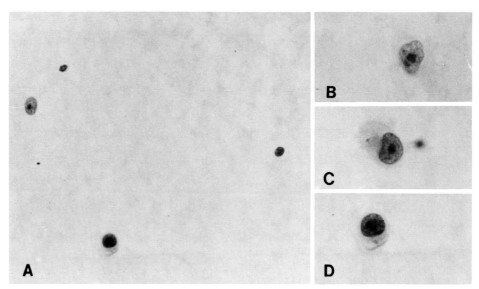

FIGURE 27–31. Hydrocele fluid with cells of testicular seminoma. (*A*) Low-power view to show cancer cells and lymphocytes. (*B, C, D*) Higher-power view of small cancer cells with marked nuclear abnormalities, notably large nucleoli and moderately abundant cytoplasm. (*A* ×350; *B, C, D* ×560)

Small lymphocytes and neutrophils were observed. Tips of chorionic villi, represented by cohesive clusters of small, tightly bound cells, usually with sharply demarcated clear cytoplasmic borders, were observed in 16% of the normal specimens. Placental cytotrophoblasts were identified as small, usually cuboidal basophilic cells, with somewhat hyperchromatic nuclei with a coarse chromatin pattern.

Schrage et al. (1982) also identified superficial urothelial "umbrella" cells in amniotic fluid (see p. 892).

Determination of Fetal Sex

Next to cytogenetic studies, the most reliable methods for determination of fetal sex are the count of sex chromatin bodies and identification of Y chromosomes. In female fetuses, the sex chromatin bodies are usually found in 20% or more of squamous cells. It is of interest that a low percentage of cells with sex chromatin bodies (up to 4%) may be observed in male fetuses, probably because of contamination with maternal cells. The identification of the male Y chromosome by quinacrine fluorescence (see p. 134) appears to be very reliable. Generally 60% of the cells in males contain the fluorescent Y chromosome. Errors are very few and usually pertain to a very small Y chromosome or a laboratory error (Adams et al.). If both procedures are performed simultaneously (i.e., sex chromatin count and Y chromosome fluorescence), the chances of error are remote. Because the size of the Y chromosome is an inherited characteristic, Adams et al. (1973) recommend a simultaneous examination of the father's Y fluorescence to determine the size of the Y chromosome.

Much less reliable is the count of cyanophilic squamous cells or the determination of the karyopyknotic index in amniotic fluids stained with Papanicolaou method, although both approaches have their proponents. Hudson and Arendzen and Huisjes consider a count of 30% or more of cyanophilic cells per cubic millimeter of fluid reliably diagnostic of female sex. Hudson also reported a negative correlation between the karyopyknotic index and estrogen levels in amniotic fluids in female fetuses. With the fall in estrogen concentration before delivery, the karyopyknotic index increased in female fetuses in a statistically significant fashion. Male fetuses did not display the same effect. Because the determination of fetal sex by karyotyping or by the identification of male and female sex chromosomes is consistently reliable, these are the methods of choice.

Estimation of Gestational Age

The estimation of lipid-containing cells stained with Nile blue sulfate as an index of fetal maturity was discussed by Johannsen (1974). This paper contains a summary of reported data and records an accuracy of ± 1 week in 72% of 106 women studied. The method is cited for historical reasons, as the gestational age can now be determined with great accuracy by ultrasound examination.

Estimation of Fetal Death

The finding of necrotic cells, ciliated cells of respiratory tract origin, bacteria, fungi, or intranuclear inclusions consistent with a viral infection are strongly suggestive of fetal death in utero. The reader is referred to the book by Barcellos for a detailed analysis of findings.

Identification of Congenital Abnormalities

The principal reason for amniocentesis is the recognition of congenital abnormalities. Amniocentesis or the equivalent sampling (biopsy) of chorionic villi (CVS; see below) should be performed on women with a high risk for an abnormal pregnancy because of age or other factors. Because there is a small risk (about 0.5%) of inducing an abortion, the procedures should not be used routinely. Cytogenetic techniques in licensed and appropriately supervised laboratories offer nearly fool-proof evidence of almost all major chromosomal disorders. Each cytogenetic examination must be performed twice, on two samples of the same fluid, to ensure the highest possible level of accuracy. The cells from the amniotic fluid are cultured, treated with colchicine to arrest mitotic division at the metaphase stage, and the chromosomes analyzed for number and morphology, using the Giemsa (G)-banding technique (for further details see Chap. 6).

The most commonly encountered karyotypic abnormality is Down's syndrome (trisomy 21) with other abnormalities being much less frequent (for further discussions see Chap. 6).

Chorionic Villi Sampling

In skilled hands, amniocentesis may be replaced by a cytogenetic analysis of tissue obtained by a direct biopsy of placental chorionic villi, preferably under ultrasound guidance (Horwell et al., 1983;

Simoni et al., 1983). There is one clear advantage to this method: the analysis may be performed from the eighth week of pregnancy on, when a termination of pregnancy, if desired, is much easier than after the 16th week. The disadvantage of the method is the difficulty with obtaining adequate chromosomal spreads. The chromosomes tend to be "fuzzy," and the cytogenetic analysis is more difficult than in amniotic fluids. A short-term culture of the trophoblastic tissue improves the quality of the preparations. The fetal wastage (induced abortions) is about 1% of pregnancies, apparently somewhat higher than for amniocentesis (Rhoads et al., 1989; Doran, 1990).

Neural Tube Closure Defects

Neural tube closure defects may result in a broad range of congenital abnormalities, ranging from anencephaly, which is not compatible with survival, to spina bifida. At the time of this writing (1991) the recognition of these abnormalities is based on ultrasound examination of the fetus, supported by elevation of alpha-fetoprotein levels in the amniotic fluid. However, before this technology was perfected, a cytologic analysis of the amniotic fluid was diagnostic of anencephaly, with a high level of accuracy in experienced hands (Chapman et al., 1981; Blenkinsopp et al., 1984). Lesser degrees of neural tube closure defect, such as spina bifida, could not be identified by cytologic methods.

Anencephaly was characterized by the presence of numerous primitive neural cells and large, pigmented macrophages. The neural cells were small, about 5 to 6 μm in diameter, with barely visible cytoplasm and densely staining nuclei. The cells occurred singly and in loosely structured clusters, some of which, in the view of this writer, resembled rosettes seen in neuroblastomas. An excellent correlation of these cells with cells present in histologic material on the surface of the neural defect was illustrated (Blenkinsopp et al., 1984). The method may still prove to be of diagnostic value in the absence of suitable ultrasound equipment.

Molecular Biologic Techniques

At the time of this writing (1991) gene identification in several congenital disorders is within reach. Thus genes of mucoviscidosis (cystic fibrosis), Huntington's disease, and several other heritable abnormalities have been identified and may soon allow prenatal screening.

Amniotic Fluid Embolism

Amniotic fluid embolism is an often fatal complication of childbirth, caused by the transfer of amniotic fluid to maternal circulation, with resulting occlusion of the alveoli by fetal squamous cells. Botero and Holmquist (1979) were the first to describe the finding of anucleated squamous cells in a blood sample obtained from the right heart through a Swan–Ganz catheter.

Several similar case reports have appeared in the literature (summary in Lee et al., 1986). Of note was the use of an antiserum to human keratin that facilitated the recognition of squamous cells (Garland and Thompson, 1983). Clearly, the use of monoclonal antibodies to intermediate keratin filaments would be equally useful.

Other Fluids

From time to time other body fluids are examined cytologically. As an example, Tanaka et al. (1985) reported on washings of a maxillary sinus in a case of carcinoma associated with aspergillosis.

EXFOLIATIVE CYTOLOGY OF THE EYE AND THE ORBIT

During the 1980s, the cytologic methods of diagnosis of diseases of the eye and the orbit have made great strides because of the developments of new targeting techniques, mainly CT, combined with the thin-needle aspiration biopsy. The approaches to this technology and the results of thin-needle aspiration biopsy, which require specialized equipment and skilled operators, will be summarized in Chapter 29.

The external aspects of the eye, the eyelids, and the orbit are accessible, however, to simple cytologic procedures, within the reach of any ophthalmologist and any laboratory of cytology. The technique is based on scraping the visible lesion and preparing fixed or air-dried smears for the diagnosis of inflammatory disorders and some superficial malignant lesions, such as carcinoma in situ of the cornea (DeAzavedo, 1962; Naib et al., 1967; Dykstra and Dykstra, 1969; Naib 1970; Naib, 1981).

Normal Population of Cells in Conjunctival and Corneal Scrape Smears

Scrape smears may be obtained under local anesthesia. The normal cell population consists of squamous cells of corneal origin and cuboidal to columnar epithelial cells of conjunctival origin. Goblet cells may be present.

Inflammatory Lesions

Viral Infections

Viral infections are very common and cause painful inflammation of the conjunctiva and the cornea. Their identification may be of substantial assistance in clinical handling of the patient.

Naib et al. (1967, 1972, 1981) have given excellent descriptions of cytologic findings in eye disorders caused by viruses. These are summarized in Table 27–2. Olding-Stenkvist and Brege applied immunofluorescent techniques for the diagnosis of herpetic conjunctivitis.

Other Inflammatory Processes

Allergic conjunctivitis, a common disorder, is characterized in smears by a large number of eosinophils, mixed with other inflammatory cells.

Bacterial infections result in acute conjunctivitis characterized by a dominance of neutrophils in smears. Gonorrheal conjunctivitis in infected newborn infants is largely a preventable disease. A related organism, *Moraxella* (*Branhamellia*) *catarrhalis*, an encapsulated diplococcus, may also result in a purulent inflammation in an adult. Eyelid infections with staphylococci (sty) rarely require cytologic confirmation. Actinomycosis of the cheek may spread to the orbit.

Chlamydia trachomatis is the cause of a chronic follicular infection (trachoma and inclusion conjunctivitis) that may lead to blindness. The cellular changes were described on p. 342 and illustrated in Fig. 10–35. A number of staining techniques are discussed and illustrated by Duggan et al. (1986).

Mycotic infections are uncommon but may lead to a loss of vision, particularly with Phycomycetes (Zygomycetes). Other fungi, such as *Candida* and *Aspergillus* species, may be observed (Naib, 1981).

Keratitis caused by *Acanthamoeba* species occurs with increasing frequency, mainly in wearers of soft contact lenses. Corneal scrapings may be used for diagnosis (summary in Karayianis et al., 1988). The double-walled cysts of the parasite may be identified by many staining techniques, but also in Papanicolaou stain. An early diagnosis is essential to prevent, by aggressive therapy, a possible loss of vision (Wright et al., 1985; Moore et al., 1985; Jones et al., 1986).

Table 27–2
Cytologic Changes in Viral Infections of the Eye and Adnexa

Disease	Ocular Site	Location of Inclusions	Inclusion Descriptive Features	Remarks
Trachoma	Cornea and conjunctiva	Cytoplasmic in mature cells	Multiple small (0.5 μm), basophilic with halos	Clusters of inclusions from necrotic cells
Inclusion conjunctivitis (frequent in newborn infants)		Cytoplasmic in mature cells	Same as above	Clusters of inclusions
Adenovirus	Conjunctiva	Intranuclear in small cells	Multiple, small eosinophilic, becoming coalescent, basophilic with halos	Few cells involved
Vaccinia	Conjunctiva	Cytoplasmic	Single, large, eosinophilic	
Herpes, simplex and zoster	Conjunctiva and cornea	Intranuclear, often in multinucleated cells with nuclear molding	Enlarged "ground-glass" nuclei becoming eosinophilic, inclusions	In herpes zoster multinucleated cells and eosinophilic inclusions are rare
Measles	Conjunctiva	Multinucleated giant cells	Multiple eosinophilic cytoplasmic inclusions with sharp halos	

(Modified from Naib, Z.M., et al.: Exfoliative cytology as an aid in the diagnosis of ophthalmic lesions. Acta Cytol., *11*:295–303, 1967; Naib, Z.M.: Cytology of ocular lesions. Acta Cytol., *16*:178–185, 1972)

Benign Tumors

Scrapings of benin tumors of the eyelids such as xanthelasma, molluscum contagiosum (a viral disorder), and squamous papillomas may sometimes be of diagnostic advantage (Naib, 1981).

Malignant Tumors of the Conjunctiva

Malignant tumors of the conjunctiva are predominantly squamous carcinomas which, in fortuitous situations, may be diagnosed as carcinomas in situ (Fig. 27–32). Not surprisingly, the clinical presen-

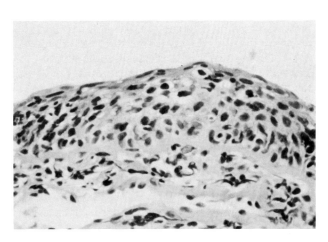

FIGURE 27–32. Epidermoid carcinoma in situ of conjunctiva. (×150)

tation of carcinoma in situ is often misleading, and the lesion is not correctly recognized by ophthalmologists. This was the experience of Dykstra and Dykstra, who used cytologic techniques for the diagnosis of carcinoma of the conjunctiva. In three of their eight cases, the lesion was preinvasive and not suspected clinically.

The presence of human papillomavirus type 16 was reported in a substantial proportion of prema-

lignant and malignant lesions of the conjunctiva and cornea (McDonell et al., 1989). The polymerase chain reaction was used in this study (for further discussion of polymerase chain reaction see Chap. 2; for human papillomavirus, see Chap. 11).

A case of adenocarcinoma of Maibomian glands diagnosed on a scrape of a lesion of the lower eyelid was thought clinically to represent a chalazion (Fig. 27–33).

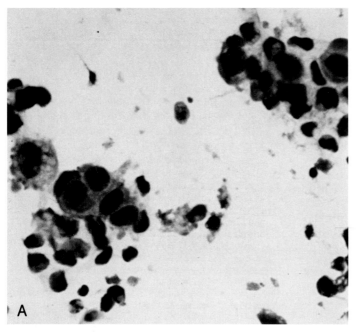

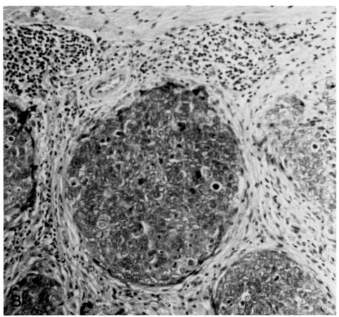

FIGURE 27–33. Adenocarcinoma of the Maibomian glands, originally thought to represent a chalazion. (*A*) Note large cancer cells, singly and in clusters, in the scrape smear of the lesion of the lower eyelid. (*B*) The histologic section shows a carcinoma, reminiscent of a mammary carcinoma. (*A* ×560; *B* ×150. Courtesy of Dr. Clifford Urban, Phoenixville, Pennsylvania)

Malignant Tumors of the Bulbus and the Orbit

Since the diagnosis of these tumors requires, for the most part, an aspiration biopsy, the subject is summarized in Chapter 29.

THE SKIN

Skin lesions are usually amenable to direct surgical biopsies, and the cytologic techniques are rarely used for diagnosis. In some institutions, however, the rapidity of the cytologic diagnosis on scrapes and thin-needle aspirates of skin lesions is appreciated (Graham et al., 1961; Selbach and Heisel, 1962; Conti, 1984). Because the cytologic presentation of skin scrapes and aspirates is quite similar, the topic is summarized in Chapter 29.

It must be noted that some skin lesions have now been shown to be associated with human papillomavirus, as has been discussed in Chapter 11. Therefore, some appreciation of common warts, epidermodysplasia verruciformis and its malignant transformation, and condylomata acuminata is of value in the cytologic assessment of neoplastic lesions of the female genital tract (Jablonska et al., 1983; Jablonska and Orth, 1983; Grüssendorf-Conen, 1987).

BIBLIOGRAPHY

Cerebrospinal fluid
  Books
  Benign disorders
  Lymphomas and related disorders
  Metastatic cancer
  Primary meningeal and brain tumors
Synovial fluids
Miscellaneous fluids
Amniotic fluid and chorionic villus sampling
Eye and eyelids

Cerebrospinal Fluid

Books

Koelmel, H.W.: Atlas of Cerebrospinal Fluid Cells. New York, Springer-Verlag, 1976.
den Hartog Jager, W.A.: Color Atlas of C.S.F. Cytopathology. Philadelphia, JB Lippincott, 1980.
Rosenthal, D.L.: Cytology of the Central Nervous System. Basel, S. Karger, 1984.

Benign Disorders

Benach, J.L., Bosler, E.M., and Hanrahan, J.P.: Spirochetes isolated from the blood of two patients with Lyme disease. N. Engl. J. Med., 308:740–742, 1983.
Bernad, P.G., and Taft, P.D.: Cytologic diagnosis of intraventricular hemorrhage in a neonate. Acta Cytol., 24:4–6, 1980.
Bigner, S.H., Elmore, P.D., Dee, A.L., and Johnston, W.W.: The cytopathology of reactions to ventricular shunts. Acta Cytol., 29:391–396, 1985.
Bigner, S.H., Elmore, P.D., Dee, A.L., Hoffman, M., and Johnston, W.W.: Unusual presentations of inflammatory conditions in cerebrospinal fluid. Acta Cytol., 29:291–296, 1985.
Bigner, S.H., and Johnston, W.W.: The cytopathology of cerebrospinal fluid. I. Nonneoplastic conditions, lymphoma and leukemia. II. Metastatic cancer, meningeal carcinomatosis, and primary central nervous system neoplasms. Acta Cytol., 25:335–353; 461–479, 1981.
Borowitz, M., Bigner, S., and Johnston, W.W.: Diagnostic problems in the cytologic evaluation of cerebrospinal fluid for lymphoma and leukemia. Acta Cytol., 25:665–674, 1981.
Bots, G.T.A.M., Went, L.N., and Schaberg, A.: Results of a sedimentation technique for cytology of cerebrospinal fluid. Acta Cytol., 8:234–241, 1964.
Dalens, B., Bezon, M.-J., Coulet, M., and Raynaud, E.-J.: Cerebrospinal fluid cytomorphology in neonates. Acta Cytol., 26:395–400, 1982.
De la Monte, S., Gupta, P.K., and Hutchins, G.M.: Polymorphous exudates and atypical mononuclear cells in the cerebrospinal fluid of patients with Sjögren's syndrome. Acta Cytol., 29:634–637, 1985.
DeFendini, R., Hunter, S.B., Schlesinger, E.B., Leifer, E., and Roland A.P.: Eosinophilic meningitis in a case of disseminated glioblastoma. Arch. Neurol., 38:52–53, 1981.
Dyken, P.R.: Cerebrospinal fluid cytology: practical clinical usefulness. Neurology, 25:210–217, 1975.
Garcia-Riego, A., Prats, J.M., and Zarranz, J.J.: Sanfilippo disease: Buhot cells in the cerebrospinal fluid. Acta Cytol., 22:282–284, 1978.
Gondos, B., and King, E.B.: Cerebrospinal fluid cytology: diagnostic accuracy and comparison of different techniques. Acta Cytol., 20:542–547, 1976.
Gupta, P.K., Gupta, P.C., Roy, S., and Banerji, A.K.: Herpes simplex encephalitis. Cerebrospinal fluid cytology studies. Acta Cytol., 16:563–565, 1972.
Hansen, H.H., Bender, R.A., and Shelton, B.J.: The cytocentrifuge and cerebrospinal fluid cytology. Acta Cytol., 18:259–262, 1974.
Jaeckle, K.A.: Cerebrospinal fluid morphology in systemic lupus erythematosus with Anton's syndrome. Acta Cytol., 26:532–536, 1982.
Jeren, T., and Beus, I.: Characteristics of cerebrospinal fluid in tuberculous meningitis. Acta Cytol., 26:678–680, 1982.
Kam-Hansen, S.: Reduced number of active T cells in cerebrospinal fluid in multiple sclerosis. Neurology, 29:897–899, 1979.
Kline, T.S.: Cytological examination of the cerebrospinal fluid. Cancer, 15:591–597, 1962.
Kolmel, H.W.: A method for concentrating cerebrospinal fluid cells. Acta Cytol., 21:154–157, 1977.
Lowe, E.: Mollaret's meningitis. A case report. Acta Cytol., 26:338–340, 1982.
Manconi, P.E., Marrosu, M.G., Spissu, A., Todde, P.F., and Ferelli, A.: Plasma cell reaction in cerebrospinal fluid: an additional case report. Neurology, 28:856–857, 1978.

Mathios, A.J., Nielsen, S.L., Barrett, D., and King, E.B.: Cerebrospinal fluid cytomorphology: identification of benign cells originating in the central nervous system. Acta Cytol., *21*:403–412, 1977.

McGarry, P., Holmquist, N.D., and Carmel, Sr. A.: A postmortem study of cerebrospinal fluid with histologic correlation. Acta Cytol., *13*:48–52, 1969.

Nakamura, S., Takase, S., and Itahara, K.: Cytological examination of cerebrospinal fluid in eight patients with neuro-Behcet's disease. Tohoku J. Exp. Med., *132*:421–430, 1980.

Naylor, B.: Cytologic study of intracranial fluids. Acta Cytol., *5*:198–202, 1961.

Naylor, B.: The cytologic diagnosis of cerebrospinal fluid. Acta Cytol., *8*:141–149, 1964.

Nyland, H., and Naess, A.: Lymphocyte subpopulations in blood and cerebrospinal fluid from patients with acute Guillain-Barré syndrome. Eur. Neurol., *17*:247–252, 1978.

Oehmichen, M.: Characterization of mononuclear phagocytes in human CSF using membrane markers. Acta Cytol., *20*:548–552, 1976.

Oehmichen, M., and Huber, H.: Supplementary cytodiagnostic analyses of mononuclear cells of the cerebrospinal fluid using cytological markers. J. Neurol., *218*:187–196, 1978.

Pelc, S., DeMaertelaere, E., and Denolin-Reubens, R.: CSF cytology of acute viral meningitis and meningoencephalitis. Eur. Neurol., *20*:95–102, 1981.

Preissig, S.H., and Buhaug, J.: Corpora amylacea in cerebrospinal fluid. A source of possible diagnostic error. Acta Cytol., *22*:511–514, 1978.

Razavi-Encha, F., Fleury-Feith, J., Gherardi, R., and Bernaudin, J.-F.: Cytologic features of cerebrospinal fluid in Lyme disease. Acta Cytol., *31*:439–440, 1987.

Reinhartz, T., Lijovetzky, G., and Levij, I.S.: Intracellular starch granules in cytologic material. Acta Cytol., *22*:36–37, 1978.

Rozich, J., Holley, H.P., Henderson, F., Gardner, J., and Nelson, F.: Cauda equina syndrome secondary to disseminated zygomycosis. JAMA, *260*:3638–3640, 1988.

Rubinstein, L.J., Herman, M.M., Long, T.F., and Wilbur, J.R.: Disseminated necrotizing leukoencephalopathy: a complication of treated central nervous system leukemia and lymphoma. Cancer, *35*:291–305, 1975.

Sayk, J.: Cytologie der Cerebrospinalflussigkeit. Jena, Gustav Fischer, 1960.

Steere, A.C., Bartenhagen, N.H., and Craft, J.E.: The early clinical manifestations of Lyme disease. Ann. Intern. Med., *99*:76–82, 1983.

Steere, A.C., Grodzicki, R.L., and Kornblatt, A.N.: The spirochetal etiology of Lyme disease. N. Engl. J Med., *308*:733–740, 1983.

Takeda, M., King, D.E., Choi, H.Y., Gomi, K., and Lang, W.R.: Diagnostic pitfalls in cerebrospinal fluid cytology. Acta Cytol., *25*:245–250, 1981.

Yamamoto, L.J., Tedder, D.G., Ashley, R., and Levin, M.J.: Herpes simplex virus Type 1 DNA in cerebrospinal fluid of a patient with Mollaret's meningitis. N. Engl. J. Med., *325*:1082–1085, 1991.

Zaharopoulos, P.: Hemoglobin crystals in fluid specimens from confined body spaces. Acta Cytol. *31*:777–782, 1987.

Lymphomas and Related Disorders

Aaronson, A.G., Hajdu, S.I., and Melamed, M.R.: Spinal fluid cytology during chemotherapy of leukemia of the central nervous system in children. Am J. Clin. Pathol., *63*:528–537, 1975.

Afifi, A.M.: Myeloma cells in the cerebral spinal fluid in plasma cell neoplasia. J. Neurol. Neurosurg. Psychiatry, *37*:1162–1165, 1974.

Aronson, A., Garwicz, S., and Sornas, R.: Cytology of the cerebrospinal fluid in children with acute lymphoblastic leukemia. J. Pediatr., *85*:221–224, 1974.

Astaldi, A., Pasino, M., Rosanda, C., and Massimo, L.: T and B cells in cerebrospinal fluid in acute lymphocytic leukemias. N. Engl. J. Med., *294*:550–551, 1976.

Bigner, S.H., and Johnston, W.W.: The cytopathology of cerebrospinal fluid. I. Nonneoplastic conditions, lymphoma and leukemia. II. Metastatic cancer, meningeal carcinomatosis, and primary central nervous system neoplasms. Acta Cytol., *25*:335–353; 461–479, 1981.

Bodensteiner, D.C., and Skikne, B.: Central nervous system involvement in mycosis fungoides. Diagnosis, treatment and literature review. Cancer, *50*:1181–1184, 1982.

Bonnin, J.M., and Garcia, J.H.: Primary malignant non-Hodgkin's lymphoma of the central nervous system. Pathol. Annu., *22*:353–375, 1987.

Borowitz, M., Bigner, S., and Johnston, W.W.: Diagnostic problems in the cytologic evaluation of cerebrospinal fluid for lymphoma and leukemia. Acta Cytol., *25*:665–674, 1981.

Carbone, A., and Volpe, R.: Cerebrospinal fluid involvement by malignant histiocytosis. Acta Cytol., *24*:172–173, 1980.

Chang, A.H., and Ng, A.B.P.: The cellular manifestations of mycosis fungoides in cerebrospinal fluid. A case report. Acta Cytol., *19*:148–151, 1975.

Domagala, W., Emeson, E.E., Greenwald, E., and Koss, L.G.: A scanning electron microscopic and immunologic study of B-cell lymphosarcoma cells in cerebrospinal fluid. Cancer, *40*:112–116, 1977.

Drewinko, B., Sullivan, M.P., and Martin, T.: Use of the cytocentrifuge in the diagnosis of meningeal leukemia. Cancer, *31*:1331–1336, 1973.

Getaz, E.P., and Miller, G.J.: Spinal cord involvement in chronic lymphocytic leukemia. Cancer, *43*:1858–1861, 1979.

Gold, J.H., Shelbourne, J.D., and Bossen, E.H.: Meningeal mycosis fungoides: cytologic and ultrastructural aspects. Acta Cytol., *20*:349–355, 1976.

Gregory, M.C., and Hughes, J.T.: Intracranial reticulum cell sarcoma associated with immunoglobulin A deficiency. J. Neurol. Neurosurg. Psychiatry, *36*:769–776, 1973.

Hamilton, S.R., Gupta, P.K., Marshall, M.E., Donovan, P.A., Wingard, J.R., and Zaatari, G.S.: Cerebrospinal fluid cytology in histiocytic proliferative disorders. Acta Cytol., *26*:22–28, 1982.

Hautzer, N.W., Aiyesimoju, A., and Robitaille, Y.: "Primary" spinal intramedullary lymphomas: a review. Ann. Neurol., *14*:62–66, 1983.

Levitt, L.J., Fsedon, D.M., Rosenthal, D.S., and Moloney, W.C.: CNS involvement in the non-Hodgkin's lymphomas. Cancer, *45*:545–552, 1980.

Li, C.Y., Witzig, T.E., Phyliky, R.L., Ziesmer, S.C., and Yam, L.T.: Diagnosis of B-cell non-Hodgkin's lymphoma of the central nervous system by immunocytochemical analysis of cerebrospinal fluid lymphocytes. Cancer, *57*:737–744, 1986.

Ludwig, R.A., and Balachandran, I.: Mycosis fungoides. The importance of pulmonary cytology in the diagnosis of a case with systemic involvement. Acta Cytol., *27*:198–201, 1983.

Meyer, R.J., Ferreira, P.P., Cuttner, J., Greenberg, M.L., Goldberg, J., and Holland, J.F.: Central nervous system involvement at presentation in acute granulocytic leukemia. A prospective cytocentrifuge study. Am. J. Med., *68*:691–694, 1980.

Mitsumoto, H., Breuer, A.C., and Lederman, R.J.: Malignant lymphoma of the central nervous system: a case of primary spinal intramedullary involvement. Cancer, *46*:1258–1262, 1980.

Nies, B.A., Malmgren, R.A., Chu, E.W., Del Vecchio, P.R., Thomas, L.B., and Freireich, E.J.: Cerebrospinal fluid cytology in patients with acute leukemia. Cancer, *18*:1385–1391, 1965.

Nies, B.A., Thomas, L.B., and Freireich, E.J.: Meningeal leukemia. A follow-up study. Cancer, *18*:546–553, 1965.

Spriggs, A.I., and Boddington, M.M.: Leukaemic cells in cerebrospinal fluid. Br. J. Haematol., *5*:83–91, 1959.

Wolfson, W.L.: Cytopathologic presentation of cerebral histiocytosis. Acta Cytol., *23*:392–398, 1979.

Zimmerman, H.M.: Malignant Lymphomas. *In* Minckler, J. (ed.): Pathology of the Nervous System. pp. 2165–2178. New York, McGraw-Hill, 1971.

Zimmerman, H.M.: Malignant lymphomas of the nervous system. Acta Neuropathol., *16*:69–74, 1975.

Metastatic Cancer

Aisner, J., Aisner, S.C., Ostrow, S., Govindan, S., Mummert, K., and Wiernik, P.: Meningeal carcinomatosis from small cell carcinoma of the lung. Consequences of improved survival. Acta Cytol., *23*:292–296, 1979.

Bergdahl, L., Boquist, L., Lillequist, B., Thullin, C.A., and Tovi, D.: Primary malignant melanoma of the central nervous system. Acta Neurochir., *26*:139–149, 1972.

Bigner, S.H., and Johnston, W.W.: The cytopathology of cerebrospinal fluid. I. Nonneoplastic conditions, lymphoma and leukemia. II. Metastatic cancer, meningeal carcinomatosis, and primary central nervous system neoplasms. Acta Cytol., *25*:335–353; 461–479, 1981.

Bots, G.T.A.M., Went, L.N., and Schaberg, A.: Results of a sedimentation technique for cytology of cerebrospinal fluid. Acta Cytol., *8*:234–241, 1964.

Chandrasoma, P.T., and Apuzzo, M.L.J.: Stereotactic Brain Biopsy. New York, Igaku-Shoin, 1989.

Cibas, E.S., Malkin, M.G., Posner, J.B., and Melamed, M.R.: Detection of DNA abnormalities by flow cytometry in cells from cerebrospinal fluid. Am. J. Clin. Pathol., *88*:570–577, 1987.

Conrad, K.A., Gross, J.L., and Trojanowski, J.Q.: Leptomeningeal carcinomatosis presenting as eosinophilic meningitis. Acta Cytol., *30*:29–31, 1986.

Doyle, T.J.: Brain metastasis in the natural history of small-cell lung cancer: 1972–1979. Cancer, *50*:752–754, 1982.

Eyha, H., Hajdu, S.I., and Melamed, M.R.: Cytopathology of nonlymphoreticular neoplasms metastatic to the central nervous system. Acta Cytol., *25*:599–610, 1981.

Geisinger, K.R., Hajdu, S.I., and Helson, L.: Exfoliative cytology of nonlymphoreticular neoplasms in children. Acta Cytol., *28*:16–28, 1984.

Glass, J.P., Melamed, M., Chernik, N.L., and Posner, J.B.: Malignant cells in cerebrospinal fluid (CSF): the meaning of a positive CSF cytology. Neurology *29*:1369–1375, 1979.

Gondos, B., and King, E.B.: Cerebrospinal fluid cytology: diagnostic accuracy and comparison of different techniques. Acta Cytol., *20*:542–547, 1976.

Greenberg, M.L., and Goldberg, L.: The value of cerebrospinal fluid cytology in the early diagnosis of metastatic retinoblastoma. Acta Cytol., *21*:735–738, 1978.

Hansen, H.H., Bender, R.A., and Shelton, B.J.: The cytocentrifuge and cerebrospinal fluid cytology. Acta Cytol., *18*:259–262, 1974.

Hoffman, J.S., and Pena, Y.M.: Central nervous system lesions and advanced ovarian cancer. Gynecol. Oncol., *30*:87–97, 1988.

Hust, M.H., and Pfitzer, P.: Cerebrospinal fluid and metastasis of transitional cell carcinoma of the bladder. Acta Cytol., *26*:217–223, 1982.

Johnston, W.W., Ginn, F.L., and Amatulli, J.M.: Light and electron microscopic observations on malignant cells in cerebrospinal fluid from metastatic alveolar cell carcinoma. Acta Cytol., *15*:365–371, 1971.

Kline, T.S.: Cytological examination of the cerebrospinal fluid. Cancer, *15*:591–597, 1962.

Kolmel, H.W.: A method for concentrating cerebrospinal fluid cells. Acta Cytol., *21*:154–157, 1977.

Larson, C.P., Robson, J.T., and Reberger, C.C.: Cytologic diagnosis of tumor cells in cerebrospinal fluid. J. Neurosurg., *10*:337–341, 1953.

Little, J.R., Dale, A.J., and Okazaki, H.: Meningeal carcinomatosis. Arch. Neurol., *30*:138–143, 1974.

McCormack, L.J., Hazard, J.B., Gardner, W.J., and Klotz, J.G.: Cerebrospinal fluid changes in secondary carcinoma of meninges. Am. J. Clin. Pathol., *23*:470–478, 1953.

McCormack, L.J., Hazard, J.B., Belovich, D., and Gardner, W.J.: Identification of neoplastic cells in cerebrospinal fluid by wet-film method. Cancer, *10*:1293–1299, 1957.

McGarry, P., Holmquist, N.D., and Carmel, Sr. A.: A postmortem study of cerebrospinal fluid with histologic correlation. Acta Cytol., *13*:48–52, 1969.

Moore, T.N., Livingston, R., Heilbrun, L., Eltringham, J., Skinner, O., White, J., and Tesh, D.: The effectiveness of prophylactic brain irradiation in small cell carcinoma of the lung. Cancer, *41*:2149–2153, 1978.

Naylor, B.: Cytologic study of intracranial fluids. Acta Cytol., *5*:198–202, 1961.

Naylor, B.: The cytologic diagnosis of cerebrospinal fluid. Acta Cytol., *8*:141–149, 1964.

Olson, M.E., Chernik, N.L., and Posner, J.B.: Infiltration of the leptomeninges by systemic cancer: a clinical and pathologic study. Arch. Neurol., *30*:122–137, 1974.

Pedersen, A.G., Hansen, M., Hummer, L., and Rogowski, P.: Cerebrospinal fluid ACTH as a marker of central nervous system metastases from small cell carcinoma of the lung. Cancer, *56*:2476–2480, 1985.

Sayk, J.: Cytologie der Cerebrospinalflussigkeit. Jena, Gustav Fischer, 1960.

Schmidt, R.M.: Cytological investigation of the cerebrospinal fluid in secondary brain tumors. Schweiz. Arch. Neurol. Psychiatr. *127*:233–236, 1980.

Spriggs, A.I.: Malignant cells in cerebrospinal fluid. J. Clin. Pathol., *7*:122–130, 1954.

Talekar, S.V.: CSF cytology and microbiology using a new in vivo filter technique. J. Neurosci. Methods, *2*:107–108, 1980.

Theodore, W.H., and Gendelman, S.: Meningeal carcinomatosis. Arch. Neurol., *38*:696–699, 1981.

Vannucci, R.C., and Baten, M.: Cerebral metastatic disease in childhood. Neurology, 24:981–985, 1974.

Wasserstrom, W.R., Glass, J.P., and Posner, J.B.: Diagnosis and treatment of leptomeningeal metastases from solid tumors. Cancer *49*:759–772, 1982.

Wertlake, P.T., Markovits, B.A., and Stellar, S.: Cytologic evaluation of the cerebrospinal fluid with clinical and histological correlation. Acta Cytol., *16*:224–239, 1972.

Primary Meningeal and Brain Tumors

Aichner, F., and Schuler, G.: Primary leptomeningeal melanoma: diagnosis by ultrastructural cytology of cerebrospinal fluid and cranial computed tomography. Cancer, *50*:1751–1756, 1982.

Barnard, R.O.: Smear preparations in the diagnosis of malignant lesions of the central nervous system. In Koss, L.G., and Coleman, D.V. (eds.): Advances in Clinical Cytology, pp. 254–269. vol. 1. London, Butterworths, 1981.

Bondeson, L., and Falt, K.: Primary intracranial epidermoid carcinoma. Acta Cytol., *28*:487–489, 1984.

Chandrasoma, P.T., and Apuzzo, M.L.J.: Stereotactic Brain Biopsy. New York, Igaku-Shoin, 1989.

Crisp, D.E., and Thompson, J.A.: Primary malignant melanomatosis of the meninges: clinical course and computer tomographic findings in a young child. Arch. Neurol., *38*:528–529, 1981.

DeFendini, R., Hunter, S.B., Schlesinger, E.B., Leifer, E., and Roland A.P.: Eosinophilic meningitis in a case of disseminated glioblastoma. Arch. Neurol., *38*:52–53, 1981.

Flodmark, O., Fitz, C.R., Harwood-Nash, D.C., and Chuang, S.H.: Neuroradiologic findings in a child with primary leptomeningeal melanoma. Neuroradiology, *18*:153–156, 1979.

Foot, N.C., and Zeek, P.: Two cases of melanoma of the meninges, with autopsy. Am. J. Pathol., *7*:605–617, 1931.

Gandolfi, A., et al.: The cytology of cerebral neuroblastoma. Acta Cytol., *24*:344–346, 1980.

Garbes, A.D.: Cytologic presentation of primary leptomeningeal sarcomatosis. Acta Cytol., *28*:709–712, 1984.

Ginhart, T.D., and Tsukahara, Y.C.: Cytologic diagnosis of pineal germinoma in cerebrospinal fluid and sputum. Acta Cytol., *23*:341–346, 1979.

Kajikawa, H., Ohta, T., Ohshiro, H., Harada, K., Ishikawa, S., Uozumi, T., Kodama, M., and Okada, T.: Cerebrospinal fluid cytology in patients with brain tumors; a simple method using the cell culture technique. Acta Cytol., *21*:162–167, 1977.

Kim, K., Greenblatt, S.H., and Robinson, M.G.: Choroid plexus carcinoma. Report of case with cytopathologic differential diagnosis. Acta Cytol., *29*:876–849, 1985.

Langheim, W., Kernohan, J.W., and Uihlein, A.: Arachnoidal sarcoma of the cerebellum. Cancer, *15*:705–716, 1962.

Liwnicz, B.H., and Rodriguez, C.A.: The central nervous system. *In* Koss, L.G., Woyke, S., and Olszewski, W.: Aspiration Biopsy. Cytologic Interpretation and Histologic Bases. pp. 457–490. New York, Igaku-Shoin, 1984.

Ludwin, S.K., Rubinstein, L.J., and Russell, D.S.: Papillary meningioma. A malignant variant of meningioma. Cancer, *36*:1363–1373, 1975.

Minauf, M., and Summer, K.: Primare Melanoblastose der Leptomeningen. Wien. Z. Nervenheilkd. *30*:150–157, 1972.

Onofrio, B.M., Kernohan, J.W., and Uihlein, A.: Primary meningeal sarcomatosis. A review of the literature and report of 12 cases. Cancer, *15*:1197–1208, 1962.

Pasquier, B., Pasquier, D., N'golet, A., Panh, M.H., and Couderc, P.: Extraneural metastases of astrocytomas and glioblastomas. Clinicopathological study of two cases and review of literature. Cancer, *45*:112–125, 1980.

Schmidt, P., Neuen-Jacob, E., Blanke, M., Arendt, G., Wechsler, W., and Pfitzer, P.: Primary malignant melanoblastosis of the meninges: clinical, cytologic and neuropathologic findings in a case. Acta Cytol., *32*:713–718, 1988.

Spens, N., Parsons, H., and Begg, C.F.: Primary melanoma of the meninges. N.Y. State J. Med., *62*:3777–3780, 1962.

Watson, C.W., and Hajdu, S.I.: Cytology of primary neoplasms of the central nervous system. Acta Cytol., *21*:40–47, 1977.

Wolfson, W.L.: Cytopathologic presentation of cerebral histiocytosis. Acta Cytol., *24*:392–398, 1980.

Zaharopoulos, P., and Wong, J.Y.: Cytology of common primary midline brain tumors. Acta Cytol., *24*:384–390, 1980.

Zulch, K.J.: Primary melanotic tumors. *In* Brain Tumours: Their Biology and Pathology, 3rd ed. pp. 391–393. Berlin, Springer-Verlag, 1986.

Synovial Fluids

Delbarre, F.: Le ragocyte synovial. Presse Méd., *72*:2129–2132, 1964.

Fallet, G.H.: Diagnostic value and possible role of synovial ragocytes in rheumatology. Rev. Rheumatol., *35*:590–600, 1968.

Hollander, J.L., Reginato, A., and Torralba, T.P.: Examination of synovial fluid as a diagnostic aid in arthritis. Med. Clin. North Am., *50*:1281–1293, 1966.

Meisels, A., and Berebichez, M.: Exfoliative cytology in orthopedics. Can. Med. Assoc. J., *84*:957–959, 1961.

Naib, Z.M.: Cytology of synovial fluids. Acta Cytol., *17*:299–309, 1973.

Rawson, A., Abelson, N.M., and Hollander, J.L.: Studies on the pathogenesis of rheumatoid joint inflammation. Ann. Intern. Med., *62*:281–284, 1965.

Suprun, H., and Mansoor, I.: An aspiration cytodiagnostic test for gouty arthritis. Acta Cytol., *17*:198–199, 1973.

Zaharopoulos, P., and Wong, J.Y.: Identification of crystals in joint fluids. Acta Cytol., *24*:197–202, 1980.

Miscellaneous Fluids

Ehya, H.: Cytology of mesothelioma of the tunica vaginalis metastatic to lung. Acta Cytol., *29*:79–84, 1985.

Japko, L., Horta, A.A., Schreiber, K., Mitsudo, S., Karwa, G.L., Singh. G., and Koss, L.G.: Malignant mesothelioma of the tunica vaginalis testis: report of first case with preoperative diagnosis. Cancer, *49*:119–127, 1982.

Kasdon, E.J.: Malignant mesothelioma of the tunica vaginalis propria testis. Cancer, *23*:1144–1150, 1969.

Piscioli, F., Polla, E., Pusiol, T., Failoni, G., and Luciani, L.: Pseudomalignant cytologic presentation of spermatic hydrocele fluid. Acta Cytol., *27*:666–670, 1983.

Rosai, J., and Dehner, L.P.: Nodular mesothelial hyperplasia in hernia sacs. A benign reactive condition simulating a neoplastic process. Cancer, *35*:165–175, 1975.

Tanaka, T., Nishioka, K., Naito, M., Masuda, Y., and Ogura, Y.: Coexistence of aspergillosis and squamous-cell carcinoma in the maxillary sinus proven by preoperative cytology. Acta Cytol., *29*:73–78, 1985.

Tang, C.K., Gray, G.F., and Keuhnelian, J.G.: Malignant peritoneal mesothelioma of an inguinal hernia sac. Cancer, *37*:1887–1890, 1976.

Vassilakos, P., and Cox, J.N.: Filariasis diagnosed by cytologic examination of hydrocele fluid. Acta Cytol., *18*:62–64, 1974.

Wentworth, P., Wagar, S., and Unitt, M.: Atypical cells in spermatocele fluid [letter]. Acta Cytol., *15*:210–211, 1971.

Amniotic Fluid and Chorionic Villus Sampling

Adams, C., Kilpatrick, B., Kabacy, G., Fialko, G., and Dumars, K.W.: Fetal sex determination. Acta Cytol., *17*:233–236, 1973.

Arendzen, J.H., and Huisjes, H.J.: A simple method for prenatal determination of sex. Acta Cytol., *15*:316–317, 1971.

Audy, S., Ivic, J., Kuvacic, I., and Drazancic, A.: Antenatal sex determination in amniotic fluid samples. Acta Cytol., *21*:330–333, 1977.

Barnett, H.R., and Nevin, M.: The value of the Nile blue test in estimating fetal maturity in normal and complicated pregnancies. J. Obstet. Gynaecol. Br. Commonw., 77:151, 1970.

Blenkinsopp, W.K., Chapman, P.A., and Barnard, R.O.: Amniotic fluid cytology in the antenatal diagnosis of neural tube closure defects. *In* Koss, L.G., and Coleman, D.V. (eds.): Advances in Clinical Cytology, vol. 2, pp. 291–306. New York, Masson Publishing, 1984.

Botero, S.D., and Holmquist, N.D.: Cytologic diagnosis of amniotic fluid embolus. Acta Cytol., 23:465–466, 1979.

Brambati, G., Simoni, O., and Danesino, G.: First trimester fetal diagnosis of genetic disorders. J. Med. Genet., *22*:92–99, 1985.

Casadei, R., D'Ablaing, G.I., Kaplan, B.J., and Schwinn, C.P.: A cytologic study of amniotic fluid. Acta Cytol., *17*:289–298, 1973.

Dolynuck, M., Orfei, E., Vania, H., Karlman, R., and Tomich, P.: Rapid diagnosis of amniotic fluid embolism. Obstet. Gynecol., *61*:285–305, 1983.

Doran, T.A.: Chorionic villus sampling as the primary diagnostic tool in prenatal diagnosis. Should it replace genetic amniocentesis? J. Reprod. Med., *35*:935–940, 1990.

Dougherty, C.M., and McCormick, M.: X-chromosomal anomalies in the newborn. Acta Cytol., *17*:423–424, 1973.

Gariepy, G., and Vauclair, R.: Study of ruptured fetal membranes by Nile blue sulphate staining. Acta Cytol., *13*:154, 1969.

Garland, J.W.C., and Thompson, W.D.: Diagnosis of amniotic fluid embolism using an antiserum to human keratin. J. Clin. Pathol. 36:625–627, 1983.

Horwell, D.H., Loeffler, F.E., and Coleman, D.V.: Assessment of a transcervical aspiration technique for chorionic villus biopsy in the first trimester of pregnancy. Br. J. Obstet. Gynaecol., *90*:196–198, 1983.

Hudson, E.A.: The cytological difference between amniotic fluids of male and female fetuses. Br. J. Obstet. Gynaecol., *82*:523–528, 1975.

Hudson, E.A.: The karyopyknotic index of amniotic fluid cells and its relationship to oestrogen concentration. Br. J. Obstet. Gynaecol., *82*:529–535, 1975.

Huisjes, H.J.: Cytologic features of liquor amnii. Acta Cytol., *12*:42–45, 1968.

Johansen, K.: Gestational age assessed by modified amniotic fluid cytology in normal and small-for-date pregnancies. Acta Cytol., *18*:142–148, 1974.

Kazy, Z., Rozovski, I.S., and Bakharev, V.A.: Chorionic biopsy in early pregnancy: a method of early prenatal diagnosis for inherited disorders. Prenat. Diagn., *2*:39–46, 1982.

Lee, K.R., Catalano, P.M., and Ortiz-Giroux, S.: Cytologic diagnosis of amniotic fluid embolism. Report of a case with a unique cytologic feature and emphasis on the difficulty of eliminating squamous contamination. Acta Cytol., *30*:177–182, 1986.

Lewis, B.V., and Chapman, P.A.: A comparison of techniques for determining prenatal sex from liquor amnii. J. Clin. Pathol., *27*:639, 1974.

Makowski, E.L., Prem, K.A., and Kaiser, I.H.: Detection of sex of fetuses by the incidence of sex chromatin body in nuclei of cells in amniotic fluid. Science, *123*:542, 1956.

Morris, H.H.B., and Bennett, M.J.: The classification and origin of amniotic fluid cells. Acta Cytol., *18*:149–154, 1974.

Multicentre randomized clinical trial of chorionic villus sampling and amniocentesis: first report of the Canadian Collaborative Clinical Trial Group. Lancet, *1*:1–6, 1989.

Natelson, S., Scommegna, A., and Epstein, M.B.: Amniotic Fluid: Physiology, Biochemistry and Clinical Chemistry. New York, John Wiley & Sons, 1974.

Rhoads, C.C., Jackson, L.G., and Schlesselman, S.E., et al.: The safety and efficiency of chorionic villus sampling for early prenatal diagnosis of cytogenetic abnormalities. N. Engl. J. Med., *320*:609–617, 1989.

Schrage, R., Boegelspacher, H.-R., and Wurster, K.-G.: Amniotic fluid in the second trimester of pregnancy. Acta Cytol., *26*:406–416, 1982.

Sharma, S.D., and Trussell, R.: The value of amniotic fluid examination in the assessment of fetal maturity. J. Obstet. Gynecol., 77:215, 1970.

Simoni, O., Brambati, B., and Danesino, C., et al.: Efficient direct chromosome analysis and enzyme determinations from chorionic villi sampling in the first trimester of pregnancy. Hum. Genet., *3*:349–357, 1983.

Stenback, F., and Ojala, A.: Determination of fetal maturity by means of amniotic fluid. Acta Cytol., *14*:439–443, 1970.

Van Leeuwen, L., Jacoby, H., and Charles B.: Exfoliative cytology of amniotic fluid. Acta Cytol., *9*:442–445, 1965.

Wachtel, E.G.: Exfoliative Cytology in Gynaecological Practice, 2nd ed. London, Butterworths & Co., 1969.

Eye and Eyelids

Blank, H., and Rake, G.W.: Viral and Rickettsial Diseases of the Skin, Eye and Mucous Membranes of Man. Boston, Little, Brown & Co., 1955.

Bruckner, R., and Ludin, H.: Zur zytologischen Tumordiagnostik in der Ophthalmologie. Ophthalmologica, *133*:169–175, 1957.

Char, D.H., and Norman, D.: The use of computed tomography and ultrasonography in the evaluation of orbital masses. Surg. Ophthalmol., *27*:49–63, 1982.

Coutifari, N., and Nocolaou, D.: Le cyto-diagnostic en ophthalmologie. Arch. Ophthalmol., *19*:360, 1959.

Cristallini, E.G., Bolis, G.B., and Ottaviano, P.: Fine needle aspiration biopsy of orbital meningioma. Report of a case. Acta Cytol., *34*:236–238, 1990.

Czerniak, B., Woyke, S., Daniel, R., Krzyszotolik, Z., and Koss, L.G.: Diagnosis of orbital tumors by aspiration biopsy guided by computerized tomography. Cancer 54:2385–2389, 1984.

Czerniak, B., Woyke, S., Krzysztolik, Z., and Domagala, W.: Fine needle aspiration biopsy of intraocular melanoma. Acta Cytol., *27*:157–165, 1983.

Das, D.K., Das, J., Chachra, K.L., and Natarajan, R.: Diagnosis of retinoblastoma by fine needle aspiration and aqueous cytology. Diagn. Cytopathol., 5:203–206, 1989.

Dubois, P.J., Kennerdell, J.S., Rosenbaum, A.E., Dekker, A., Johnson, B.R., and Swink, C.A.: Computed tomographic localization of fine needle aspiration biopsy of orbital tumors. Radiology, *131*:149–152, 1979.

Duggan, M.A., Pomponi, C., Kay, D., and Robboy, S.J.: Infantile chlamydial conjunctivitis. A comparison of Papanicolaou, Giemsa and immunoperoxidase staining methods. Acta Cytol., *30*:341–346, 1986.

Dykstra, P.C., and Dykstra, B.A.: The cytologic diagnosis of carcinoma and related lesions of the ocular conjunctiva and cornea. Trans. Am. Acad. Ophthalmol. Otolaryngol., *73*:979–995, 1969.

Engel, H., de la Cruz, Z.C., Jimenez-Abalahin, L.D., Green, W.R., and Michels, R.G.: Cytopreparatory techniques for eye fluid specimens obtained by vitrectomy. Acta Cytol., *26*:551–560, 1982.

Engel, H.M., Green, W.R., Michels, R.G., Rice, T.A., and Erozan, Y.S.: Diagnostic vitrectomy. Retina, *1*:121–149, 1981.

Green, W.R.: Diagnostic cytopathology of ocular fluid specimens. Ophthalmology, *91*:726–749, 1984.

Henkind, P., and Friedman, A.: Cancer of the lids and ocular adnexa. *In* Andrade, R., Gumport, S.L., Popkin, G.L., and Rees, T.D. (eds.): Cancer of the Skin. pp. 1345–1371. Philadelphia, W.B. Saunders, 1976.

Jakobiec, F., and Chattock, A.: The role of cytology and needle biopsies in the diagnosis of ophthalmic tumors and simulating condition. *In* Jakobiec, F. (ed): Ocular and Adnexal Tumors. pp. 341–358, Birmingham, Ala., Aesculapius, 1978.

Jakobiec, F.A., Coleman, D.J., Chattock, A., and Smith, M.: Ultrasonically guided needle biopsy and cytologic diagnosis of solid intraocular tumors. Ophthalmology, *86*:1662–1678, 1979.

Karayianis, S.L., Genack, L.J., Lundergan, M.K., and Schumann, G.B.: Cytologic diagnosis of acanthamoebic keratitis. Acta Cytol., *32*:491–494, 1988.

Kennerdell, J.S., Dekker, A., Johnson, B., and Dubois, P.J.: Fine needle aspiration biopsy. Its use in orbital tumors. Arch. Ophthalmol., *97*:1315–1317, 1979.

Kennerdell, J.S., Dubois, P.J., Dekker, A., and Johnson, B.: CT guided fine needle aspiration biopsy of orbital optic nerve tumors. Ophthalmology, *87*:491–496, 1980.

Kimura, S.J., and Thygeson, P.: The cytology of external ocular disease. Am. J. Ophthalmol., *39*:137–154, 1955.

Kopelman, J.E., and Shorr, N.: A case of prostatic carcinoma metastatic to orbit diagnosed by fine needle aspiration and immunoperoxidase staining for prostatic specific antigen. Ophthal. Surg., *18*:599–603, 1987.

Ljung, B.-M., Char, D., Miller, T.R., and Deschenes, J.: Intraocular lymphoma: cytologic diagnosis and the role of immunologic markers. Acta Cytol., *32*:840–847, 1988.

Mandell, D.B., Levy, J.J., and Rosenthal, D.L.: Preparation and cytologic evaluation of intraocular fluids. Acta Cytol., *31*:150–158, 1987.

McDonnell, J.M., Mayr, A.J., and Martin, W.J.: DNA of human papillomavirus type 16 in dysplastic and malignant lesions of the conjunctiva and cornea. N. Engl. J. Med., *320*:1442–1446, 1989.

Moore, R.B., McCulley, J.P., Luckenbach, M., Gelender, H., Newton C., McDonald M.B., and Visvesvara, G.S.: Acanthamoeba keratitis associated with soft contact lenses. Am. J. Opthalmol., *100*:396–403, 1985.

Naib, Z.M.: Cytology of TRIC agent infection of the eye of newborn infants and their mothers' genital tracts. Acta Cytol., *14*:390–395, 1970.

Naib, Z.M.: Cytology of ocular lesions. Acta Cytol., *16*:178–185, 1972.

Naib, Z.M.: Cytology of ophthalmological diseases. *In* Koss, L.G., and Coleman, D.V. (eds.): Advances in Clinical Cytology, vol. 1. pp. 232–253. London, Butterworths, 1981.

Naib, Z.M., Clepper, A.S., and Elliott, S.R.: Exfoliative cytology as an aid in the diagnosis of ophthalmic lesions. Acta Cytol., *11*:295–303, 1967.

Olding-Stenkvist, E., and Brege, K.G.: Application of immunofluorescent technique in the cytologic diagnosis of human herpes simplex keratitis. Acta Cytol., *19*:411–419, 1975.

Otto, R.A., Templer, J.W., Renner, G., and Hurt, M.: Secondary and metastatic tumors of the orbit. Otolaryngol. Head Neck Surg., *97*:328–334, 1987.

Rodriguez, A.: Diagnosis of retinoblastoma by cytology examination of the aqueous and vitreous. Med. Prob. Ophthalmol., *18*:142–148, 1977.

Sagiroglu, N., Ozgonul, T., and Muderris, S.: Diagnostic intraocular cytology. Acta Cytol., *19*:32–37, 1975.

Sanderson, T.L., Pustai, W., Shelley, L., Gelender, H., and Ng, A.B.: Cytologic evaluation of ocular lesions. Acta Cytol., *24*:391–400, 1980.

Schumann, G.B., O'Dowd, G.J., and Spinnler, P.A.: Eye cytology. Lab. Med., *11*:533–539, 1980.

Spoor, T.C., Kennerdell, J.S., Dekker, A., Johnson, B., and Rehkopf, P.: Orbital fine needle aspiration biopsy with B-scan guidance. Am. J. Ophthalmol., *89*:274–277, 1980.

Takeda, M., Maguire, N.L.C., Augsburger, J.J., and Shields, J.A.: Cytologic diagnosis of ocular malignant melanoma. Acta Cytol., *26*:743–744, 1982.

Thelmo, W., Csordas, J., Davis, P., and Marshall, K.G.: The cytology of acute bacterial and follicular conjunctivitis. Acta Cytol., *16*:172–177, 1972.

Thygeson, P.: The cytology of conjunctival exudates. Am. J. Ophthalmol., *29*:1499–1513, 1946.

Vade, A., and Armstrong, D.: Orbital rhabdomyosarcoma in childhood. Radiol. Clin. North. Am., *25*:701–714, 1987.

Westman-Naeser, S., and Naeser, P.: Tumors of the orbit diagnosed by fine needle biopsy. Acta Ophthalmol., *56*:969–976, 1978.

Wolter, R., and Naylor, B.: A membrane filter method: used to diagnose intraocular tumor. J. Pediatr. Ophthalmol., *5*:36–38, 1968.

28

Nipple Secretions and Breast Cysts

ANATOMIC AND HISTOLOGIC CONSIDERATIONS

The female breast is composed of 15 to 20 modified sweat glands surrounded by fat. In the resting (nonlactating) breast the glandular portion is composed of small lobules that are connected by a series of small ducts, with the main excretory ducts opening into the nipple. During pregnancy the entire glandular system of the breast undergoes a marked hypertrophy.

The excretory ducts are lined by one to two layers of cuboidal cells. Small flat myoepithelial cells support the cuboidal cells. Occasionally, the lining of some of the ducts may change to that seen in the apocrine sweat glands (i.e., it will be composed of tall cuboidal cells with eosinophilic cytoplasm; Fig. 28–1).

NIPPLE SECRETIONS

Nipple secretions may have various appearance: milky, watery (collostrum), serous (yellow, watery, and clear), purulent (thick, yellow), blood-tinged, or frankly bloody. Except during lactation and the immediate postlactation period, any discharge from the nipple is abnormal. The nipple secretions may be due to such benign disorders as duct stasis or papilloma. However, occasionally an important endocrine disturbance or an otherwise asymptomatic cancer of the ducts of the breast may cause secretion. The chief value of cytologic examination of nipple secretions lies in the possible early diagnosis of such cancers. The procedure should be confined to those patients who have no palpable masses in the breast or other evidence of breast cancer. If there is clinical or mammographic suspicion of cancer of the breast, other methods of diagnosis, such as aspiration biopsy (see Chap. 29) or excisional biopsy and frozen section, should be applied.

The remarks pertaining to nipple secretions concern only the nonlactating breast.

Cytology of Nipple Secretions in the Absence of Cancer

Endocrine Disturbances

Nipple secretions, resembling either milk, colostrum, or serous secretions (galactorrhea), may

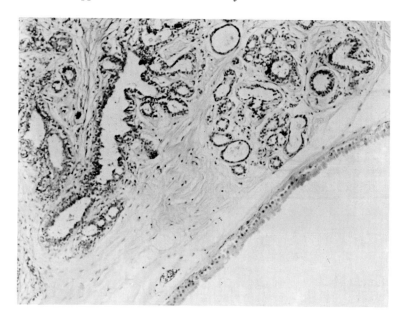

FIGURE 28–1. Cystic disease of the breast. Ducts of various sizes are seen in the field. One large duct (*bottom, right*) is lined by tall, columnar, eosinophilic cells of apocrine type. (×150)

occur in a variety of endocrine disorders affecting the secretion of prolacin or prolactin inhibitor. The most significant of these disorders are pituitary tumors and other diseases of the hypothalamic–pituitary axis. These must be always considered in the differential diagnosis of nipple discharge (see Chap. 9).

Duct Dilatation and Stasis

As a result of inflammatory processes within the breast, or obstruction in the duct system, there may be a partial blockage of the latter with resulting accumulation of greenish-sticky material within the dilated ducts. Such material may escape from the nipple. Cytologically, the predominant component is the "foam cell," a fairly large, markedly vacuolated histiocytelike cell that is of ductal origin and represents a modified duct lining cell (Fig. 28–2A). The ductal origin of such cells may be observed in tissue sections (Fig. 28–2B) and was confirmed by Papanicolaou in tissue culture. The nuclei of the vacuolated cells may contain prominent nucleoli.

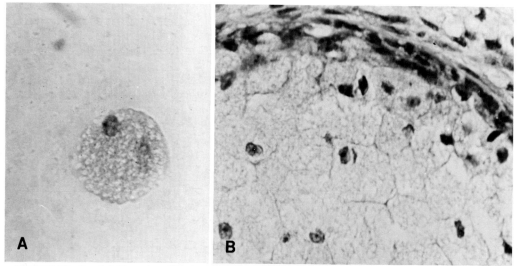

FIGURE 28–2. (*A*) Vacuolated histiocyte or foam cell in nipple secretion. (*B*) Section of breast duct, demonstrating the origin of foam cells from ductal lining. (*A, B* ×560)

In addition to the vacuolated histiocytes, the secretions may contain duct lining cells, singly and in clusters. These cells are small, often oval when single, but somewhat irregular within clusters (Fig. 28–3). An important characteristic of benign duct cells is their good adherence to each other while in clusters. The nuclei are quite large for the small size of cells, but they are even in size and not particularly dark. Larger eosinophilic duct cells with granular cytoplasm, suggesting apocrine metaplasia of duct lining, may be noted in nipple secretions (Fig. 28–4). Such cells have very dark, homogeneous, regularly shaped nuclei, sometimes provided with nucleoli.

Intraductal Papilloma

This common disease of the duct system of the breast may bring about nipple secretions, especially if the lesion is located within the main excretory ducts. Histologically, the papillomas are built around a central core of connective tissue. The lining is that of duct cells, which may vary in size and display nuclear atypia. Apocrine type cells are commonly observed within the papillomas. This histologic picture is reflected in nipple secretions. Clusters of duct cells may be observed. There is often some variation in cell size (Fig. 28–5). In the clusters of large apocrine cells the regular nuclei may appear markedly hyperchromatic.

However, the cells within the clusters display good adherence to each other; the nuclei, although dark, show a homogeneous structure. Even when there is marked nuclear abnormality, as shown in Fig. 28–5B, one should be particularly cautious in making the diagnosis of breast cancer in the presence of papillary clusters and in the absence

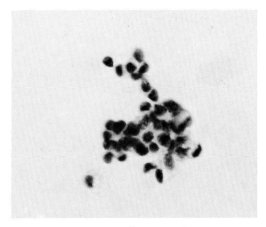

FIGURE 28–3. Duct cells in nipple secretion. Note good adherence of the small cells to each other and small, even nuclei. (×560)

of single cancer cells. The prognosis for many papillary lesions is often very favorable, despite marked cellular abnormalities. Histologic examination of tissues is advisable in questionable cases. It must be pointed out that the association of papillomatous lesions, mainly of the subareolar type, with breast cancer has been repeatedly observed (Bhagavan et al.).

Tuberculosis of the Breast

Nayar and Saxena (1984) reported several cases of tuberculosis of the breast with nipple discharge. In several of these cases epitheloid cells and giant cells of Langhans' type were observed. For cytologic recognition of these cells see pp. 340 and 727.

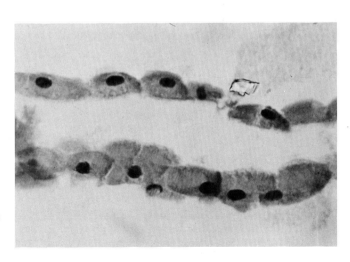

FIGURE 28–4. Apocrine duct cells in nipple secretion. Note the large size of these eosinophilic cells and their dark, even nuclei (cf. Fig. 28–10). (×560)

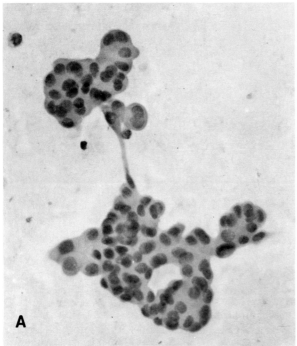

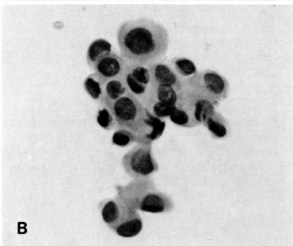

FIGURE 28-5. (*A, B*) Clusters of duct cells originating in an intraductal papilloma. The cells are much larger than those shown in Fig. 28-3, but are well adherent. In (*B*) there is considerable variability in the sizes of the atypical dark nuclei. This degree of abnormality is common in papillomas. In the absence of single abnormal cells, the diagnosis of carcinoma is not warranted; however, a tissue examination should be performed. (*A* ×350; *B* ×560)

Other Rare Findings

Lahiri (1975) observed microfilariae in nipple secretions. Masukawa (1972) observed calcific concretions and fungal organisms in filamentous and yeast forms.

Nipple Secretions in Breast Cancer

Ciatto et al. (1986) studied nipple secretions in 3,687 women to determine the type of fluid that was most likely to harbor mammary carcinoma.

The prevalance of cancer was 3.96% in patients with bloody nipple discharge, followed by purulent discharge (0.83%), serous discharge (0.16%), and milky discharge (0.13%).

Thus, bloody secretions must be examined with particular care, but, unfortunately, other types of secretions cannot be ignored, although the probability of cancer diagnosis is much lower.

Two subtypes of cancer of the breast may manifest themselves in spontaneous nipple secretions: the solid or papillary ductal carcinoma and the duct cell carcinoma associated with Paget's disease of the nipple. Tumors yielding cells of diagnostic value are usually located within the main ducts of the breast.

Duct Carcinoma

In the absence of invasion, the histologic diagnosis of duct cancer is based on the cytologic criteria; the cells forming the tumor are usually significantly larger than normal and display marked nuclear abnormalities. There may also be an alteration in growth pattern, such as abnormal proliferation of papillary processes, often criss-crossing the lumen of the duct (Figs. 28–6E and 28–8D). In the so-called comedocarcinoma, the ducts are lined with cancer cells, but there is necrosis in the center.

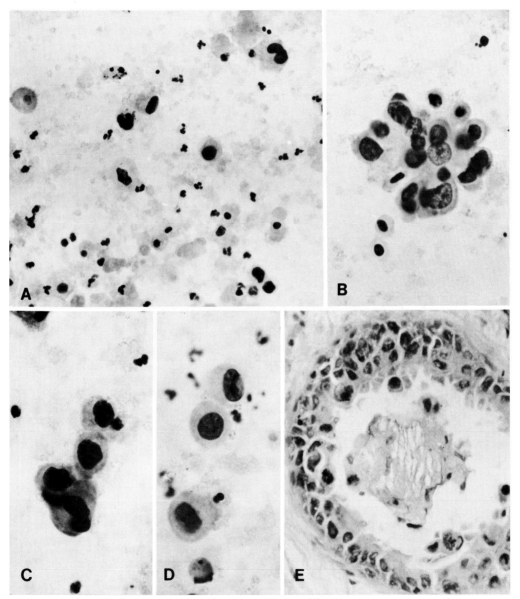

FIGURE 28–6. Intraductal carcinoma of breast in a 54-year-old patient. Diagnosis was made on smear of blood-tinged nipple secretions. (*A*) Overview of smear showing numerous large cancer cells amidst necrotic material and leukocytes. (*B, C, D*) Cancer cells. Note the papillary cluster in (*B*) and single cells and small cell clusters in (*C*) and (*D*). Nuclear enlargement and hyperchromasia and irregular nuclear outline are clearly seen. (*E*) Intraductal carcinoma. The primary tumor was 4 cm distant from the nipple. (*A, E* ×350; *B, C, D* ×560)

In nipple secretions, the cancer cells desquamate singly or in clusters. The tendency of the individual cells to break loose from the cluster is in marked contrast with the compactness of fragments in benign papillomas. The individual cancer cells vary in size and may reach twice or more the size of the benign duct cells. The nuclei of cancer cells are hyperchromatic, irregular, and very large in relation to the cytoplasm (Figs. 28–6 to 28–8). Occasionally, the clusters may show superposition of cells and crowding characteristic of papillary cancers (see Figs. 28–7 and 28–8*A*). Cancer cells may be accompanied by necrotic material and inflammatory cells.

The diagnosis of cancer of the breast in nipple secretions should be made only on irrefutable evidence. If the evidence is questionable, other methods of investigation must be suggested before therapy is instituted.

The diagnosis of a duct carcinoma in nipple secretions of a male patient was reported by Fudji et al. (1986).

Paget's Disease of the Nipple

In a form of duct cancer of the breast, there may be involvement of the nipple that clinically suggests an ulcerating inflammatory lesion. Histologically, the epidermis is permeated with large, clear cancer cells (Paget's cells). Cytologically, in addition to the cells of duct cancer, the nipple secretion contains Paget's cells, which are quite large cancer cells with distinctly abnormal hyperchromatic nuclei and abundant clear cytoplasm (Fig. 28–9). In the absence of spontaneous secretions, direct smear or scraping from the nipple may also be diagnostic of the disease.

Breast Cancer Detection by Cytology of Nipple Secretions

Unfortunately, nipple secretions, whether spontaneous or obtained by a special breast pump, are not a very efficient means of detection of occult carci-

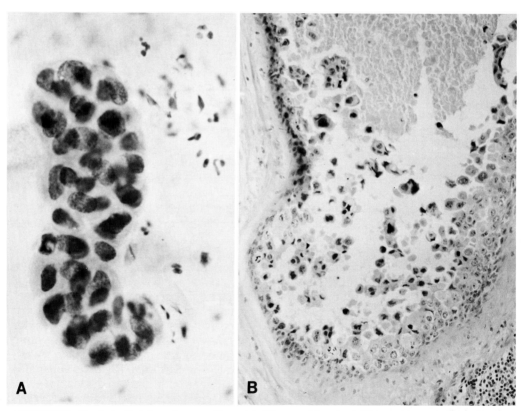

FIGURE 28–7. Intraductal carcinoma of breast in 51-year-old patient. Diagnosis was made on smear of nipple discharge. (*A*) Papillary cluster of cancer cells: Note large size of cells forming the cluster, nuclear enlargement, and hyperchromasia. (*B*) Histologic section of primary tumor 2 cm distant from nipple. (*A* ×560; *B* ×150)

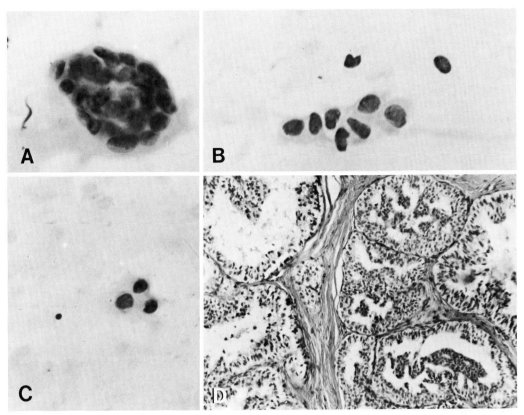

FIGURE 28–8. Duct cell carcinoma. Primary diagnosis by smear. Papillary cluster of crowded cancer cells (*A*) and cancer cells singly and in sheets (*B, C*). The nuclear abnormalities and scanty cytoplasm are readily evident. (*D*) Histologic section of tumor. This cancer occurred in a 36-year-old woman and was completely asymptomatic except for nipple discharge. (*A, B, C* ×560; *D* ×150)

noma of the breast. The results of one breast cancer detection study are shown in Table 28–1, taken from a major paper by Papanicolaou et al. Only 1 case of breast cancer was identified by Papanicolaou among 917 asymptomatic patients. Results reported by other investigators are summarized in Table 28–2. Impressive results were reported by Masukawa, who advocated the use of direct nipple touch preparations using multiple frosted slides.

Sartorius devised a nipple aspiration apparatus with which breast fluid can be obtained by a double vacuum system. The results vary with the age of the population examined. Nipple fluid in amounts sufficient for cytologic examination could be obtained in approximately 55% of all women examined. Fluid could be obtained in only slightly more than 30% of women younger than 20 years of age and older than 60. In a group of women classed as "high-risk group" because of history of breast cancer in a mother or a sister or because of prior breast surgery, the rate of "atypical" cells was higher than in normal women. Malignant cells were observed in 49 patients with documented breast cancer. In 7 of these, all with lesions smaller than 0.8 cm in diameter, the diagnosis was established by nipple cytology alone in the absence of clinical or mammographic evidence of disease. In these patients the localization of the disease was obtained by injecting contrast medium into the ducts (contrast ductography), a procedure which requires less radiation than mammography. Cannulation of individual breast ducts, originally advocated by Sartorius, has been apparently abandoned in favor of contrast ductography. It appears that the nipple aspiration method devised by Sartorius can contribute to the detection of early breast cancer. Similar conclusions were reached by Wunderlich (1977).

The very important diagnostic method of aspi-

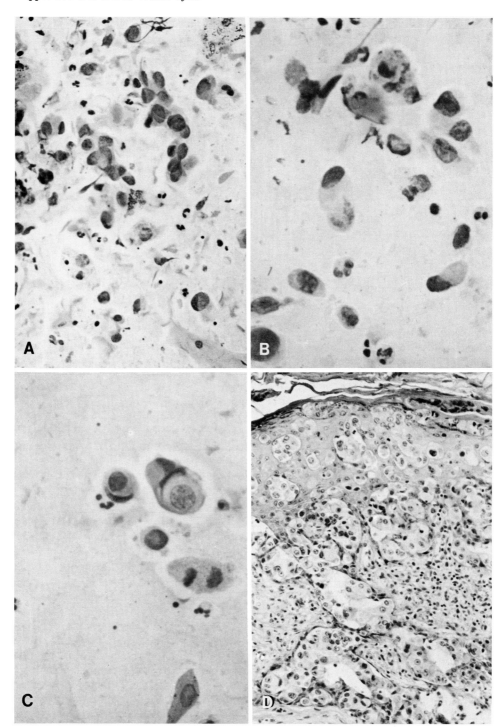

FIGURE 28–9.   Paget's disease of the nipple: smears of nipple discharge. (*A*) Numerous cancer cells singly and in clusters are present in this low-power view. (*B*) Bizarre cancer cells, partly distorted because of poor fixation of material. (*C*) The characteristic cell-in-cell arrangement. Note the clear cytoplasm of the inner cells — a feature likewise observed in tissue sections (*D*) and also reported in extramammary Paget's disease. (*D*) Tissue section, same case. Classic Paget's disease of the nipple with underlying duct carcinoma. (*A, D* ×350; *B, C* ×560)

Table 28–1
Cytology of Nipple Secretions

Asymptomatic patients	Total 917
Secretions obtained (breast pump)	245
Bilateral secretions (mainly premenopausal women)	74
Carcinoma (duct in situ)	1
Symptomatic patients	Total 510
Carcinoma	45
Nipple secretions suspicious or positive	27
Patients with breast cancer	52
Secretions positive	17
Secretions suspicious	10
Carcinoma opposite breast	8
Secretions positive	2

(Papanicolaou G.N., et al.: Exfoliative cytology of human mammary gland and its value in diagnosis of cancer and other diseases of breast. Cancer, *11*:377, 1958)

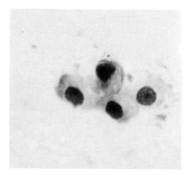

FIGURE 28–10. Apocrine cells in fluid aspirated from breast cyst. Note vacuolated cytoplasm and nuclear degeneration. (×560)

ration biopsy of breast lesions is described in Chapter 29.

Cytology of nipple secretions cannot be considered a replacement for such other methods of breast cancer diagnosis as mammography, but occasionally it contributes in a major way to the salvage of individual patients.

The Cytology of Aspirates from Breast Cysts

Aspiration of breast cysts is a frequent practice, and the fluid thus obtained should be submitted for cytologic investigation. Usually, the fluid from benign breast cysts is fairly rich in vacuolated histiocytes and ductal cells. If there is apocrine metaplasia, cells with granular cytoplasm, prominent nuclei and nucleoli, may be present. Degenerated apocrine cells may display peripherally located, very dark, homogeneous nuclei and prominent nucleoli. However, the cytoplasm is usually abundant and sharply demarcated—an important point in differentiating such cells from cancer (Fig. 28–10). After aspiration, benign breast cysts should no longer be palpable. If there is a residual mass, a reaspiration or tissue biopsy is suggested to rule out the presence of a mammary carcinoma.

Primary carcinoma originating in cyst lining is exceedingly uncommon. The aspiration in such cases contains cancer cells, singly and in clusters. They are in every respect similar to cells of duct carcinoma (Fig. 28–11).

For further comments on cytologic makeup of thin-needle aspirates of the breast, see Chapter 29.

Table 28–2
Cytology of Nipple Secretions in Breast Cancer

Author	Number of Patients With Breast Cancer	Cytologic Classification			
		Cancer	Probable cancer	Papilloma or atypia	Benign
Kjellgren, 1964	25	11	10	3	1
		Positive	Inconclusive		Negative
Masukawa et al., 1966	16	6	8		2
Masukawa, 2nd series, 1972	16	10	5		1

(Data from Kjellgren, O.: The cytologic diagnosis of cancer of the breast. Acta Cytol., *8*:216–222, 1964; Masukawa, T., et al.: The cytologic examination of breast secretions. Acta Cytol., *10*:261–265, 1966; Masukawa, T.: Discovery of psommoma bodies and fungus organisms in nipple secretion with improved breast cytology technique. Acta Cytol., *16*:408–415, 1972)

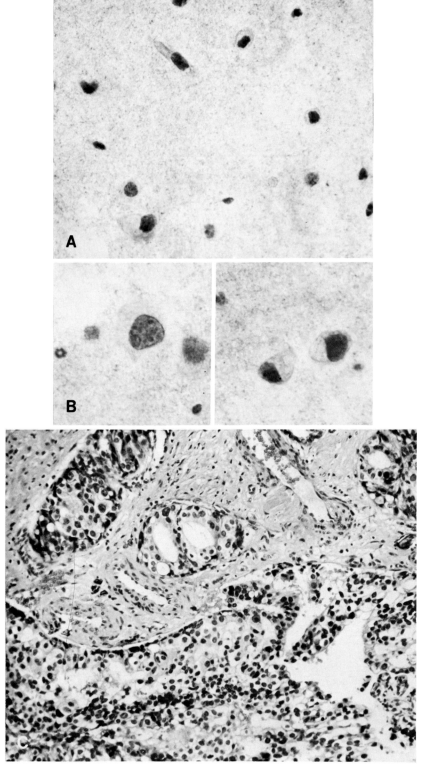

FIGURE 28-11. Mammary carcinoma originating in lining of a breast cyst. Primary diagnosis by aspiration smear. (*A*) Low-power view showing single cancer cells. (*B*) Higherpower view of cancer cells. (*C*) Histologic appearance of cancer, lining the cyst but also showing focal infiltration of the underlying fibrous cyst wall. (*A* ×350; *B* ×560; *C* ×150)

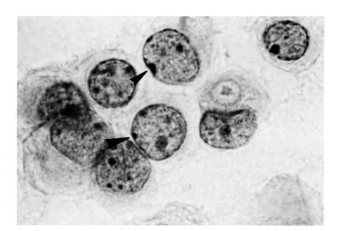

FIGURE 28–12. Sex chromatin bodies (*arrowheads*) in human carcinoma of the breast. Smear preparation; Guard stain. (×560. Savino, A., and Koss, L.G.: The evaluation of sex chromatin as a prognostic factor in carcinoma of the breast. A preliminary report. Acta Cytol., *15*:372–374, 1971)

SEX CHROMATIN AS A PROGNOSTIC FACTOR IN CARCINOMA OF THE BREAST

It has been repeatedly observed that the presence of sex chromatin in breast cancer cells has a favorable prognostic significance (Wacker and Miles; Schiødt; Kallenberger et al.). In a study of 100 consecutive breast cancer patients treated by radical mastectomy, sex chromatin was evaluated on smears obtained by scraping the cut surface of the tumor (Savino and Koss). The presence of 20% or more of cancer cells with identifiable sex chromatin resulted in much more favorable tumor behavior in terms of recurrence (Fig. 28–12). This observation was unrelated to tumor grade or stage at the time of the original surgery and is summarized in Tables 28–3 to 28–5. This simple method of assessment of breast cancer prognosis is probably as accurate as other quantitative methods of DNA measurements or estrogen receptor analysis, discussed on p. 1293. Rosen et al. (1977) found a correlation between the role of sex chromatin bodies and estrogen receptors.

Table 28–3
Distribution of Sex Chromatin Bodies in Breast Cancer

% of Sex Chromatin	No. of Cases	NED*	Recurrence†
1–9	26 } 100%	19 } 82.2%	7 } 17.8%
10–19	47	41	6
20–29	23 } 100%	23 } 100%	0
30 and up	4	4	0
Total	100	87	13

*NED; No evidence of disease from 1 to 5 years.
†Recurrent local or metastatic tumor within 1 to 5 years of follow-up.
(Savino, A., and Koss, L. G.: The evaluation of sex chromatin as a prognostic factor in carcinoma of the breast. A preliminary report. Acta Cytol., *15*:372–374, 1971)

Table 28–4
Correlation Between Sex Chromatin Count and Grade of Tumor

% of Sex Chromatin	Total	Intraductal Carcinoma	Tumor Grade		
			I	II	III Including Infil. Lobular Carcinoma
1–19	73 (100%)	2	1	57* (79%)	13†(17%)
20 and up	27 (100%)	0	0	19 (70%)	8 (30%)

Recurrence: recurrent local or metastatic tumor within 1 to 5 years of follow-up.
*11 Recurrences of tumor.
†2 Recurrences of tumor.
(Savino, A., and Koss, L. G.: The evaluation of sex chromatin as a prognostic factor in carcinoma of the breast. A preliminary report. Acta Cytol., *15*:373–374, 1971)

Table 28–5
Correlation Between Sex Chromatin Counts and Lymph Node Metastases

% of Sex Chromatin	Nodes Positive	Recurrence*	Nodes Negative	Recurrence*
1–19	29–73 (40%)	10	41–73 (60%)	3
20 and up	12–27 (44%)	0	15–27 (56%)	0

*Recurrent local or metastatic tumor within 1 to 5 years of follow-up.
(Savino, A., and Koss, L. G.: The evaluation of sex chromatin as a prognostic factor in carcinoma of the breast. A preliminary report. Acta Cytol., *15*:372–374, 1971)

BIBLIOGRAPHY

(References to Aspiration Biopsy of the Breast are in Chap. 29)

Bhagavan, B.S., Patchevsky, A., and Koss, L.G.: Florid subareolar duct papillomatosis (nipple adenoma) and mammary carcinoma. Report of 3 cases. Hum. Pathol., 4:289–295, 1973.

Ciatto, S., Bravetti, P., and Caraggi, P.: Significance of nipple discharge clinical patterns in the selection of cases for cytologic examination. Acta Cytol., 30:17–20, 1986.

Fudji, M., Ishii, Y., Wakabayashi, T., Itoyanaga, N., Hagiwara, K., Saito, M., and Takahashi, M.: Cytologic diagnosis of male breast cancer with nipple discharge. Acta Cytol., 30:21–24, 1986.

Ghosh, S.N., and Shah, P.N.: Prognosis and incidence of sex chromatin in breast cancer. A preliminary report. Acta Cytol., 19:58–61, 1975.

Groll, M., Takeda, M., and Rakoff, A.: Breast and vaginal hormonal cytology in patients with breast secretions. Acta Cytol., 19:429–430, 1975.

Jenny, J.: Der cytologische Abstrich als Hilfsmittel bei der Diagnose des Mammacarcinomas. Gynaecologia, 152:114–117, 1961.

Kern, W.H., and Dermer, G.B.: The cytopathology of hyperplastic and neoplastic mammary duct epithelium. Cytologic and ultrastructural studies. Acta Cytol., 16:120–129, 1972.

Kjellgren, O.: The cytologic diagnosis of cancer of the breast. Acta Cytol., 8:216–223, 1964.

Lahiri, V.L.: Microfilariae in nipple secretion. Acta Cytol., 19:154, 1975.

Masukawa, T.: Discovery of psammoma bodies and fungus organisms in the nipple secretion with improved breast cytology technique. Acta Cytol., 16:408–415, 1972.

Masukawa, T., Kuzma, J.F., and Straumfjord, J.V.: Cytologic detection of early Paget's disease of breast with improved cellular collection method. Acta Cytol., 19:274–278, 1975.

Masukawa, T., Lewison, E.F., and Frost, J.K.: The cytologic examination of breast secretions. Acta Cytol., 10:261–265, 1966.

Masukawa, T., Wada, Y., Mattingly, R.F., and Kuzma, J.F.: Cytologic detection of minute ovarian, endometrial and breast carcinomas, with emphasis on clinical–pathological approaches. Acta Cytol., 17:316–319, 1973.

McDivitt, R.W., Stewart, F.W., and Berg, J.W.: Tumors of the breast. In Atlas of Tumor Pathology, 2nd Ser., fasc. 2. Washington, D.C., Armed Forces Institute of Pathology, 1968.

Mitsudo, S., Nakanishi, I., and Koss, L.G.: Paget's disease of the penis and adjacent skin. Its association with fatal sweat gland carcinoma. Arch. Pathol. Lab. Med., 105:518–520, 1981.

Murad, T.M., and Synder, M.E.: The diagnosis of breast lesions from cytologic material. Acta Cytol., 17:418–422, 1973.

Nagy, G.K., Jacobs, J.B., Mason-Savas, A., Pomerantz, S.N., and DeCiero, G.J.: Intracytoplasmic eosinophilic inclusion bodies in breast cyst fluids are giant lysosomes. Acta Cytol., 33:99–103, 1989.

Nayar, M., and Saxena, H.M.K.: Tuberculosis of the breast. A cytomorphologic study of needle aspirates and nipple discharges. Acta Cytol., 28:325–328, 1984.

Papanicolaou, G.N., Holmquist, D.G., Bader, B.M., and Falk,

E.A.: Exfoliative cytology of human mammary gland and its value in diagnosis of cancer and other diseases of breast. Cancer, *11*:377–409, 1958.

Rosen, P.P., Savino, A., Menendez-Botet, C., Urban, J.A., Mike, V., Schwartz, M.K., and Melamed, M.R.: Barr body distribution and estrogen receptor protein in mammary carcinoma. Ann. Clin. Lab. Sci., *7*:491–499, 1977.

Sartorius, O.W., and Smith, H.S.: Contrast ductography for the recognition and localization of benign and malignant breast lesions: an improved technique. *In* Logan, W. (ed.): Breast Carcinoma. New York, John Wiley & Sons, 1977.

Sartorius, O.W., Smith, H.S., Morris, P., Benedict, D., and Friesen, L.: Cytologic evaluation of breast fluid in the detection of breast disease. JNCI, *59*:1073–1080, 1977.

Savino, A., and Koss, L.G.: The evaluation of sex chromatin as a prognostic factor in carcinoma of the breast. Acta Cytol., *15*:372–374, 1971.

Vilaplana, E.V., and Jiminez-Ayala, M.: The cytologic diagnosis of breast lesions. Acta Cytol., *19*:519–526, 1975.

Wiman, L.-G., and Skogh, M.: Cytologisk diagnos av Paget's disease of the nipple. Nagra reflexioner kring ett fall med negativ biopsi. Sven. Lakartidn, *57*:3154–3161, 1960.

Wunderlich, M.: Die Exfoliativzytologie der sezernierenden Mamma. Arch. Geschwulstforsch., *47*:627–633, 1977.

29

Aspiration Biopsy

Leopold G. Koss, M.D. and Josef Zajicek, M.D.*

PART I: INTRODUCTION TO TECHNIQUES AND INTERPRETATION

The purpose of aspiration biopsy is to obtain diagnostic material for cytologic study from organs that do not shed cells spontaneously. The bone marrow, spleen, liver, breast, thyroid gland, and lymph nodes were initially the targets of this type of diagnostic procedure. The method now encompasses virtually all organs, as set forth in this chapter and listed in Tables 29–1 and 29–2.

HISTORICAL PERSPECTIVE

Biopsy by aspiration, also known as thin- or fine-needle aspiration biopsy, has become an important diagnostic technique, replacing, to some extent, and complementing tissue pathology in many clinical situations. It is of interest that tissue pathology, which has been the dominant, standard diagnostic technique for the past century, was a relatively late development in the history of human pathology. It became popular only after the introduction of tissue fixatives, cutting instruments, and stains during the 1870s and after the concept of diagnostic biopsy was introduced by the gynecologist Ruge (Ruge, 1890). Before that time, the mi-

*This chapter in the third (1979) edition of this book was Dr. Zajicek's last contribution before his untimely death of prostate cancer in 1979. The chapter required major modifications and restructuring to bring it up to date. Still, an effort was made to preserve as much of Dr. Zajicek's original writing as possible as a tribute to one of the great pioneers of aspiration biopsy.

Special thanks are due to my friends and colleagues, Prof. Stanislaw Woyke, Szczecin, and Prof. Wladyslaw Olszewski, Warsaw, Poland, and to Igaku-Shoin Publishers (New York and Tokyo) for their permission to reproduce in this chapter a number of photographs from the first edition of the book Aspiration Biopsy, Cytologic Interpretation and Histologic Bases (Igaku-Shoin, 1984). Prof. Woyke also provided a number of unpublished photographs, as acknowledged in legends.

Dr. Zajicek's original contribution was aided by a grant from King Gustaf V's Jubilee Foundation. He was assisted by Ingrid Edlund, Lena Warnlöf, and Guy Masson. L.G.K.

Table 29–1
Targets of Transcutaneous Thin-Needle Diagnostic Aspirates: Palpable Lesions

Target Organ	Principal Lesions to Be Identified	Remarks
Salivary glands	*Benign*: mixed tumors (pleomorphic adenomas), Warthin's tumors, cysts *Malignant*: adenoid cystic carcinomas, mucoepidermoid tumors, other rare cancers	Identification of some benign mixed tumors and of adenoid cystic carcinomas may cause difficulties.
Lymph nodes	Metastatic cancers and lymphomas of Hodgkin's and non-Hodgkin's type; inflammatory disorders and AIDS	Precise classification of subtypes of lymphomas often requires tissue evidence.
Thyroid	*Benign*: adenomas, goiters *Malignant*: carcinomas (papillary, follicular, anaplastic, medullary)	Differentiation between follicular adenoma and carcinoma is difficult.
Breast	*Benign*: mastopathy, fibroadenomas *Malignant*: carcinomas: duct type, lobular type; other rare cancers	Scirrhous, colloid (mucus-producing) and papillary carcinomas may be difficult to identfy.
Prostate	*Benign*: prostatic hyperplasia *Malignant*: Prostatic carcinoma	Special instrumentation is required.
Soft-tissue tumors, bone (may require radiologic guidance)	Differentiation of benign lesions from primary and metastatic cancers	Precise classification of spindle cell sarcomas may cause difficulties.

(Modified from Koss, L. G.: Aspiration biopsy—a tool in surgical pathology. Am. J. Surg. Pathol., *12*[Suppl. 1]:43–53, 1988, with permission)

croscopic morphology of disease was studied mainly in cellular preparations that were much easier to secure. Detailed microscopic descriptions of cell aberrations in a broad variety of disease processes, mainly cancer, can be found in many papers and several books on clinical microscopy published before 1860 (Lebert, 1845; Donné, 1845; Beale, 1858).

Ever since syringes or equivalent instruments were introduced into the medical armamentarium, they were used to aspirate collections of fluids that could be examined under the microscope. Some of the earliest descriptions of diagnostic applicability of these instruments go back to the 1830s. The first applications of the aspirated sample pertained to infectious diseases. Perhaps the most notable was the contribution by two British military surgeons, Greig and Gray (1904) who, working in Africa, described in detail the use of aspirates of lymph nodes for the identification of trypanosomes in the diagnosis of sleeping sickness. To the best of my knowledge (LGK) the first diagnosis of a solid tumor based on an aspirated sample, a lymphoma of the

skin, was published by Hirschfeld (1912). Hirschfeld, who used a small-caliber needle, subsequently extended his experience to other tumors, but was prevented by World War I from publishing his results until 1919.

In 1926, a head and neck surgeon and radiotherapist, Hayes Martin, at the Memorial Hospital for Cancer and Allied Diseases in New York City, initiated a system of tumor diagnosis using a syringe with a large-caliber needle. He was assisted in this endeavor by a technician, Edward Ellis, who was Dr. James Ewing's factotum and protegé. In response to a specific query, the reasons for this development were explained many years later in a letter to one of us (LGK), dated June 30, 1980 written by Dr. Fred W. Stewart.

Martin and Ewing were at swords point on the need for biopsy proof prior to aggressive surgery or radiation (in neck nodes since Hayes dealt exclusively in head and neck stuff) and the needle was a sort of compromise. Ewing thought biopsy hazardous—a method of disease spread. The material was seen

Table 29–2
Targets of Thin-Needle Diagnostic Aspirates Requiring Imaging Guidance

Organ System	Methods of Imaging	Principal Lesions to Be Identified	Remarks
Lung and pleura (see Chaps. 19, 20, and 26)	Fluoroscopy or computed tomography (CT)	Lung cancers of various types, carcinoids, metastatic cancers; mesotheliomas.	Chronic pneumonic processes and effects of drugs or radiotherapy may mimic cancer. Pneumothorax is common; 3–4% require treatment.
Mediastinum	Fluoroscopy, CT	Thymomas, lymphomas, thymic germinomas, metastatic cancer	Lymphomas: see lymph nodes, Table 29–1
Liver	Ultrasound, rarely radionuclide uptake, CT for small lesions	Metastatic cancer, primary hepatomas, cystic lesions	Vascular lesions (hemangiomas, angiosarcomas) may prove troublesome because of danger of hemorrhage.
Pancreas	Ultrasound, CT, angiography, retrograde visualization of pancreatic duct system	Carcinoma, islet cell tumors, pseudocysts	Differentiation between well-differentiated carcinoma and chronic pancreatitis may cause difficulties.
Kidney	Ultrasound, CT, intravenous pyelography	Renal carcinomas, Wilms' tumors, oncocytomas, cystic lesions	Solitary cysts may be treated by aspiration.
Adrenals, lymph nodes, retroperitoneal space	CT, ultrasound (for large lesions), lymphangiography (for lymph nodes)	Adrenal tumors and metastatic cancers; retroperitoneal sarcomas; lymphoma.	In reference to sarcomas, see soft-tissue tumors, Table 29–1. In reference to lymphomas, see lymph nodes, Table 29–1.
Brain and spinal cord	CT (stereotactic)	Brain tumors, abscesses, cysts	Special instrumentation and skills required.
Eye and orbit	CT	Primary and metastatic tumors	Special skills required.

(Modified from Koss, L.G.: Aspiration biopsy—a tool in surgical pathology. Am. J. Surg. Pathol., *12*[Suppl. 1]:43–53, 1988, with permission)

mostly by me [FWS]. Ewing at the time was quite inactive. Eddie Ellis merely fixed and stained the slides. He probably looked at them—he was used to looking at stuff with Ewing and really knew more about diagnoses than a lot of pathologists of the period. The needle really spread from neck nodes to the various other regions, especially breast of course. As for publication I don't recall ever being asked if Martin and Ellis could publish it. The drive for paper writing was not so vigorous in the early thirties.

Nonetheless, following the papers published by Martin and Ellis in 1930 and by Coley et al. in 1931, Stewart published in 1933 a classic paper, *The diagnosis of tumors by aspiration,* in which he discussed at length the pros and cons of this method of diagnosis, its achievements, and pitfalls.

The Memorial Hospital system of aspiration of tumors never achieved any significant following in the United States, even though its value was recognized by a few pathologists, and the method was repeatedly described in American publications (Berg, 1961; Godwin, 1956). In Europe, on the other hand, the interest in the method persisted. Thus, in the 1940s two internists, Paul Lopes-Cardozo in Holland and Nils Soderström in Sweden, experimented on a large scale with this system of diagnosis. Both subsequently published books on the subject of thin-needle aspiration with the use of hematologic techniques.

Although both books were published in English, they had virtually no impact on the American diagnostic scene, but were noticed in Europe, particularly in Sweden. Working at the Radiumhemmet, the Stockholm Cancer Center, the radiotherapist–oncologist, Sixten Franzén, and his student and colleague, Josef Zajicek, applied the thin-needle technique first to the prostate and, subsequently, to a broad variety of targets, ranging from lesions of salivary glands to the skeleton. Aided by an imaginative syringe holder designed by Franzén in 1960, the technique soon became an acceptable substitute for tissue biopsies. An extensive bibliography, generated by the Swedish group, supported the value and accuracy of the procedure (Esposti, 1974; Löwhagen and Willems, 1981; Zajicek, 1974, 1979). Although the Swedish authors published in English and also contributed to this book, the impact of thin-needle aspiration technique for many years remained trivial and confined to a few institutions and individuals.

The radical change in attitude and the rapidly growing acceptance of the thin-needle diagnostic aspirates in the United States may be due to several factors. Broad acceptance of cytologic techniques for detection and diagnosis of cancer and other diseases clearly played a major role in these developments. The introduction of new imaging techniques, such as opacification, radionuclide scanning, computed tomography, and ultrasound, not only contributed to improved visualization of organs but also to a roentgenologists's ability to perform a number of procedures, hitherto in the domain of surgeons (Ferucci, 1981; Kamholz, 1982; Zornoza, 1981). After timid beginnings in the early 1970s, documenting that the use of a thin needle was an essentially harmless and beneficial procedure, a new era of diagnosis began. Thus, the morphologic diagnosis of human disease has come full circle. The study of cells that began in the early days of the 19th century and was replaced by the study of tissues for over a century, has been again projective into the forefront of diagnostic endeavors.

At the time of this writing (1991), aspiration biopsy technique is widespread throughout the world. Several textbooks describing the technique and its results in considerable detail have appeared (Frable, 1983; Linsk and Franzén, 1989; Koss et al., 1992; Kline, 1988). The purpose of this chapter is to summarize the essential aspects of aspiration cytology of common entities. The targets of aspiration biopsy are summarized in Tables 29–1 and 29–2.

TECHNIQUE

Introduction

The technique of aspiration biopsy evolved over the years from a very simple procedure, utilizing any type of syringe and needle, to an elaborate, rather complicated system, following a set of fairly rigid rules. The purpose of these rules, developed by trial and error, is to optimize the yield of the sample, thereby making its interpretation easier and more reliable. To follow the procedure accurately requires considerable practice under supervision, followed by clinical experience in obtaining and preparing the sample for microscopic evaluation. Unfortunately, it is not correct that any person capable of handling a syringe and a needle will automatically be qualified to perform aspiration biopsies. It is strongly advised that beginners should practice the technique on surgically removed or autopsy tissues before attempting clinical work. A simple training system is a portion of animal liver wrapped in a surgical glove. The techniques of aspiration and smear preparation can be very effectively practiced on this model.

Instrumentation

Needles

Disposable needles of various lengths and diameters must be available to the operator. The needles should vary in length from 2.5 to 20 cm, and in diameter from 20 to 26 gauge. The selection of the needle depends to a significant extent on clinical experience and the target to be aspirated.

Palpable Lesions. In general, for palpable lesions, needles of small caliber should be used (22 to 26 gauge). Needles with an ordinary, slanted bevel are generally acceptable. For special, very superficial targets, such as the iris of the eye, a shortened bevel may be advantageous (see "The Eye Globe" in Koss et al., 1992).

Nonpalpable Lesions. Such lesions are usually aspirated under the guidance of an imaging modality, such as fluoroscopy (see Chap. 19), computed tomography (CT), ultrasound, and occasionally, other procedures, such as stereotaxic mammography. For virtually all these procedures, except the breast, long needles of 20 or 22 gauge, provided with an obturator, must be used. Such a larger-caliber needle will not bend as easily as the smaller-gauge needles and will be easier to manipulate and guide to the target.

Selection of Needles. The length and the caliber of the needle should fit the size, the location, and the consistency of the target. For small, subcutanous lesions, a 2.5-cm-long small-caliber needle may suffice, whereas for a deeply seated breast lesion, a longer and somewhat larger needle may be required. Another rule has to do with consistency of the lesion: for soft, fleshy lesions (for example, lymph nodes), a larger-caliber needle, such as 22 gauge, can be safely used, as it will help in securing abundant material. For firm lesions, such as subcutaneous nodules likely to be composed mainly of connective tissue, or a very firm mammary mass thought to be a scirrhous carcinoma, a very small-gauge needle (for example, 26 gauge) should be selected, as it will penetrate firm tissue more readily than a larger-caliber needle. Another rule applies to targets that are highly vascular, hence, prone to bleeding, for example, the thyroid. For such organs, small-caliber needles should be used, as they are more likely to prevent significant bleeding that may dilute the sample and render it useless. For cystic lesions, a larger-caliber needle will facilitate removal of the cyst content. The selection of the appropriate needle should occur after a thorough examination of the lesion, its location, size, and depth. For the description of methods and instruments used in aspiration of abdominal organs, see p. 1340 and Figs. 29–98 and 29–99. Aspiration of lung lesions was described in Chapters 19 and 20.

Syringes and Syringe Holders

Disposable plastic syringes, preferably with an off-center tip, are suitable for aspiration biopsy. The off-center tip may provide support for the operator in aspirating small, superficial lesions. The size of the syringe is not critical because *the primary purpose of the syringe is not to become the repository of the aspirated material* (with the exception of cyst contents), *but to serve as a device providing a vacuum.* Smaller syringes, of 5 or 10 ml, are easier to handle than larger syringes. One cardinal rule in selecting a syringe is the tight fit of the needle on the syringe tip. A loosely fitting needle may render the procedure useless and may injure the patient.

A syringe holder, devised by Franzén (Fig. 29–1), permits performance of the aspiration, using the single dominant hand. The advantage of the holder is in letting the operator use his or her other hand to immobilize the target, a very important part of the aspiration procedure. Several syringe holders are commercially available, somewhat differing from each other. The selection depends on the operator's preference, ease of handling and cleaning, and the size and type of the syringe. A syringe holder is not a mandatory instrument. Some operators find it awkward to handle because it in-

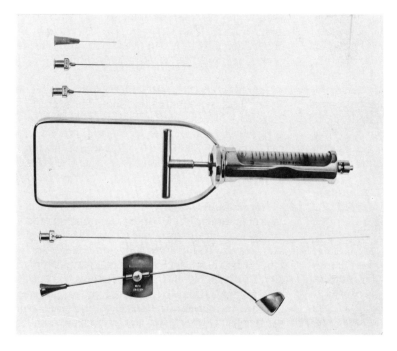

FIGURE 29–1. Apparatus for transcutaneous and transrectal aspiration biopsy: needles of various sizes (*top*), aspiration syringe with a special handle (*center*), needle and needle-guide for transrectal aspiration biopsy (*bottom*). Approximately one-half original size. Although contemporary syringes and syringe holders are somewhat different, this photograph adequately reflects the basic armamentarium necessary for aspiration biopsy.

creases the distance between the dominant hand of the operator and the target and reduces the ability to "feel" the changing consistency of the target. Some operators find that the holder impedes the to-and-fro movements within the target, an important part of the aspiration procedure. Clearly, an adequate aspiration can also be performed without the syringe holder, or, for that matter, even without a syringe (see below).

Other Supplies

A supply of clean transparent glass slides must be readily available during the aspiration procedure. Slides with frosted *ends* are helpful, as the patient's name and other identifying symbols can be inscribed with a pencil. On the other hand, *frosted surface slides are not recommended,* as they tend to tear cells and produce major artifacts during the smearing procedure. If rapid stains are required either to ascertain the quality or quantity of the aspirate, or for a rapid preliminary diagnosis, an appropriate setup must be prepared well in advance of the procedure. If fixation of smears is anticipated for Papanicolaou or hematoxylin–eosin staining, appropriate fixative, such as 70% ethanol, must be at hand. If material is to be secured for paraffin embedding, or if the need for electron microscopy is anticipated, the appropriate fixatives in small glass or plastic containers must be prepared. A small ophthalmic forceps with a sharp tip must be at hand to secure tissue fragments for further processing.

Sterile gloves should be worn by the operator. For patients suspected of having the acquired immunodeficiency syndrome (AIDS), double-gloving may be indicated.

The success or failure of the aspiration procedure depends, to some extent, on the organization of the setup. Some institutions have set aside appropriately equipped areas dedicated to the procedure. Otherwise, the materials can be arranged on movable carts, or even in portable containers.

Aspiration Procedure

With the setup in place, the actual aspiration procedure may be planned. There are several important principles that should be followed.

1. The patient's history, if not already known, must be secured in advance of the procedure.
2. The lesion to be aspirated must be either palpated or visualized and its suitability for aspiration assessed.

3. The procedure is explained to the patient, and an informed consent is secured.
4. The setup is once again checked and the needle, syringe, and other materials selected and *assembled in advance.* The operator should be gloved.

Palpable Lesions

The steps in the actual performance of the aspiration are as follows (Figs. 29–2 and 29–3):

Immobilization of the Lesion. The lesion must be immobilized by the nondominant hand (Fig. 29–2). Failure to immobilize the lesion will often result in an inadequate aspiration. If possible, the skin over the lesion must be stretched with two fingers so that the needle will reach its target by the shortest possible route and not get enmeshed in subcutaneous tissue. Care should be taken to avoid aspirating across large muscles, such as the sternocleidomastoid, as this may be painful to the patient. This may require moving the lesions with the fingers of the nondominant hand before beginning the aspiration. For lesions located near the thoracic cage, care must be taken for the needle not to enter an intercostal space, as this may cause a pneumothorax. Under these circumstances, it is advisable to perform the aspiration procedure with the needle in a plane parallel to the thoracic cage.

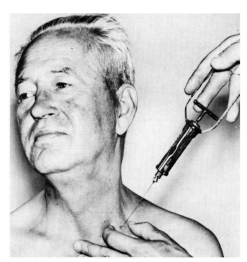

FIGURE 29–2. Transcutaneous aspiration biopsy of a lymph node, showing the position of the left hand fixing the target and the one-hand grip of the apparatus in the right hand of the operator.

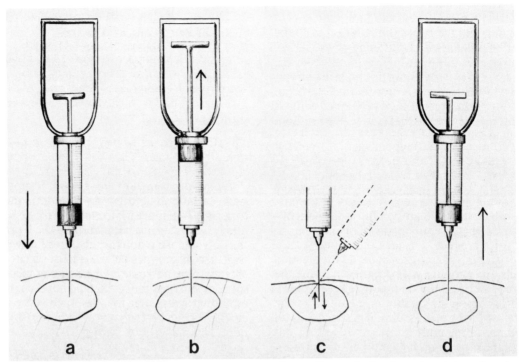

FIGURE 29-3. The technique of aspiration biopsy. The needle attached to the syringe is introduced into the lesion (*a*). The piston is retracted (*b*). The needle is moved back and forth in the lesion and, after partial withdrawal, may be directed into different areas. (*c*). The piston is released before the needle is withdrawn from the lesion (*d*). (Zajicek, J.: Aspiration Biopsy Cytology. Part I. Basel, S. Karger, 1974)

Sterilizing the Field. A simple skin cleansing with an alcohol- or other disinfectant-soaked gauze pad is usually sufficient.

Local anesthesia is not necessary, as a general rule, for palpable lesions. The pain of the anesthesia approximately equals that of the aspiration procedure. Apprehensive patients must be reassured about this.

Penetrating the Lesion. The preassembled aspiration instrument (i.e., the needle attached to the syringe, with or without syringe holder) is firmly grasped by the dominant hand and introduced through the skin into the lesion (Fig. 29-3). The angle and depth of entry should be planned in advance. For small lesions, an aspiration of the central portion of the lesion is indicated. For large lesions that may have a necrotic center, an aspiration of the off-center part of the lesion may be planned.

With experience, a change in tissue consistency will be felt as the needle crosses the subcutaneous tissue and enters the lesion. Care should be taken to place the needle within the center of the lesion or a preselected area of a large lesion. If the needle does not reach the lesion, or if the needle is placed too far beyond the lesion, diagnostic failure will result.

Creation of a Vacuum. The piston of the syringe should be withdrawn; usually 2 to 3 ml of air will create an adequate vacuum.

Obtaining the Material. With the piston of the syringe in the vacuum position, the needle is rapidly moved back and forth *in the same plane,* to loosen up the target and aspirate the tiny tissue fragments dislodged by needle tip *into the lumen of the needle.* Depending on the target, from 3 to 20 movements of the needle are performed. Except for cystic lesions or richly vascularized organs (i.e., the thyroid), nothing should be seen in the barrel of the syringe. *The material in the lumen of the needle is sufficient for diagnostic purposes in most instances.*

Changing the Direction of the Needle. It is often desirable to secure a sample from more than one area of the lesion. For this reason, the direction of the needle must be modified, but this should *never* be done while the needle is still within the lesion, as this will result in hemorrhage. The needle under vacuum *must be withdrawn to the level of the subcutaneous tissue and then redirected.* The aspiration procedure of the new area is repeated, as described above.

Release of the Vacuum and Withdrawal of the Needle. The piston of the syringe *must* be returned to the normal (i.e., nonvacuum) position *before* withdrawal of the needle. Otherwise, the material will be sucked into the barrel of the syringe where, in most instances, it will be irretrievably lost.

Cystic Lesions. The above principles do not necessarily apply to the aspiration of cysts. The cyst content must be aspirated fully, if necessary using another syringe. After aspiration the area must be palpated and, if there is a residual lesion, another aspiration of it should be performed.

Richly Vascularized Targets. Targets known to have an abundant blood supply (i.e., the thyroid) must be sampled rapidly, with only two or three to-and-fro movements of the needle. Otherwise blood will dilute the sample and render it diagnostically useless. The aspiration should be discontinued if blood appears in the barrel of the syringe.

Nonpalpable Lesions

Nearly all nonpalpable lesions are aspirated with the help of roentgenologic imaging devices such as television fluoroscopy (Fig. 29–4), computed tomography (CT), ultrasound, stereotactic mammography, etc. For further discussion of the pertinent techniques see Chapters 19 and 20 (lung), and p. 1340 (abdominal organs). The principles governing the aspiration of palpable lesions are fully applicable, although the aspirations are usually performed by radiologists. Smear preparation and evaluation, however, should remain in the hands of the cytology laboratory.

Aspirations Without a Syringe

As has been pointed out by Zajdela and his group at the Curie Institute in Paris, perfectly adequate samples of palpable lesions may be secured by using a needle not attached to the syringe. The needle is inserted into the lesion, moved back and forth, as described above, and, by capillary suction, sufficient material is obtained to be diagnostically adequate, in most cases. A syringe is attached to the needle to expel the material for preparation of smears or other uses.

Transrectal Aspiration Biopsy

The main use of transrectal aspiration biopsy (Franzén et al., 1960), is in the diagnosis of lesions of the prostate, the ovary, and the parametria. A special needle is used (see Fig. 29–1). It is flexible, about 20-cm long, and 22-gauge except in the proximal 5 cm, where it is slightly thicker and rigid. The transition from the thicker to the thinner part of the needle serves as a marker (see below). A needle guide is required. This is a fine metal tube, curved to fit the line of the palpating finger (see Fig. 29–1, *bottom*). The length of the guide equals that of the thinner part of the needle. To facilitate intro-

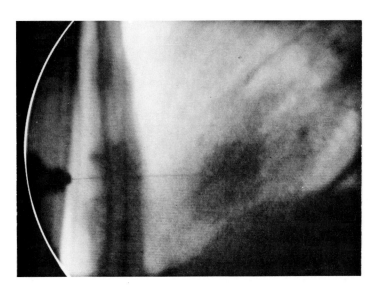

FIGURE 29–4. Transcutaneous aspiration biopsy of a pulmonary lesion. The biopsy is followed on the television screen, which shows the lesion and the needle in position before the aspiration is performed.

duction of the needle into the guide, the latter is enlarged at its proximal end like a funnel. At the distal end of the guide there is a steering ring for the palpating finger. This ring is open on its dorsal aspect and may be adjusted to fit the operator's finger. An adjustable plate midway along the guide serves to support the instrument by resting on the thenar during the operation.

The arrangement of the instrument on the operator's left hand is shown in Fig. 29–5. The index finger of the gloved left hand is passed through the steering ring on the distal part of the finger, leaving the fingertip free. To fix the guide more firmly on the palpating finger and to avoid contamination, a finger-cot is thereafter pulled over the index finger. The support plate is adjusted to rest on the thenar. The best stability of the instrument is obtained if the plate is kept in place by the pressure of the other three fingers of the left hand flexed against the thenar. The needle is introduced through the funnel into the guide until the thicker part of the needle approaches the funnel. At that moment the needle point is nearing the end of the guide immediately below the finger-cot.

The biopsy is made with the patient in lithotomy position. Neither previous preparation of the bowel nor anesthesia is required. Careful digital examination of the lesion to assess its size and consistency is first made. The left index finger, with the instrument arranged as shown in Fig. 29–6, is then inserted into the rectum. The finger must be well lubricated and must be inserted slowly and carefully, as this may be the most uncomfortable moment for the patient, particularly if there is anal spasm. The suspected area is now palpated with the left index finger, after which the needle is advanced into the lesion. Up to this point the plunger of the syringe has been down. When the needle has entered the lesion, the aspiration is performed as described for transcutaneous biopsy.

It must be stressed once again that release of the syringe plunger and *equalization of the pressure before needle withdrawal from the lesion is most important.* Apart from the risk of aspirating tumor cells into the needle track, withdrawal of the needle in vacuum mode may result in the suction of the prostatic material into the barrel of the syringe, where it may be lost, while rectal epithelium and fecal contents enter the needle. These events may render the procedure useless.

When the needle has been pulled back into the guide, the instrument-bearing finger is withdrawn from the rectum.

Special Techniques

Technical pointers in reference to specific organs or organ systems are discussed under the appropriate headings.

The Aspirated Cell Sample

Preparation of Smears

When aspiration biopsy has been completed and after the needle has been withdrawn, the syringe is disconnected from the needle, filled with air, and reconnected. The material in the needle is expelled onto a glass slide, with care being taken to deposit it as a single drop at one end of the slide. The needle tip, therefore, should be brought into light contact with the slide and the aspirate carefully expressed.

The aspirate that has been deposited on the glass slide (Fig. 29–7A) is first inspected visually. It con-

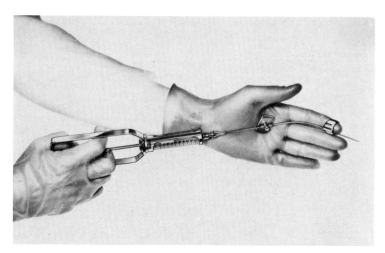

FIGURE 29–5. The instrument for transrectal aspiration biopsy, arranged in the operator's left hand.

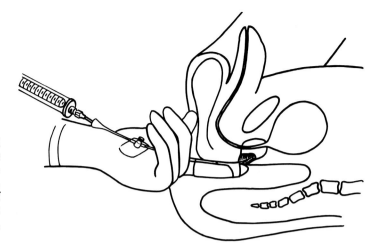

FIGURE 29–6. Position of the left hand during transrectal aspiration biopsy. Prostate in sagittal section showing the needle inserted into the suspected, indurated area. (Franzén, S., et al.: Cytological diagnosis of prostatic tumours by transrectal aspiration biopsy: A preliminary report. Br. J. Urol., *32*:193–196, 1960)

sists of a droplet of fluid, with or without admixture of blood or of semisolid material. Semisolid aspirate is spread along the slide by the use of flat pressure with a thick coverslip (of the type used in a Bürker's blood counting chamber) as shown in Figure 29–7*B*. Another glass slide may also be used in lieu of a coverslip.

An excess of fresh blood or fluid in the aspirate is dealt with as follows: A hematologic type smear is prepared first by touching the droplet with the edge of a thick coverslip. This distributes the fluid evenly along the edge of the coverslip (see Fig. 29–7*C,D*), which is then used to spread the fluid rapidly over the slide (see Fig. 29–7*E*). The large tis-

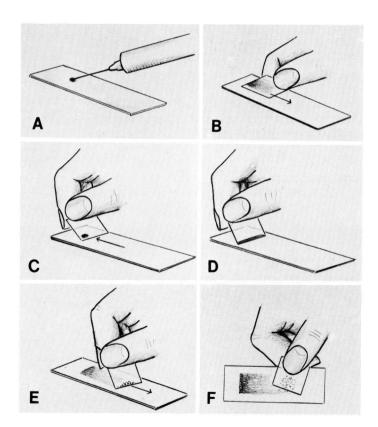

FIGURE 29–7. Preparation of smears. The aspirate is deposited on a glass slide (*A*). Semisolid aspirate is spread by flat pressure with a coverslip (*B*). Aspirate consisting of a droplet of blood or other fluid is evenly distributed along the edge of the coverslip (*C, D*), and spread as for a blood smear (*E*). Tissue fragments that collect at the end of the smear are gently squeezed by firm flat pressure with the coverslip (*F*). (Zajicek, J.: Aspiration Biopsy Cytology. Part I. Basel, S. Karger, 1974)

sue fragments collect at the edge of the smears. They are gently crushed by firm flat pressure with the coverslip (Figs. 29–7*F* and 29–8).

Several other methods of smear preparation have been described (summary in Koss et al., 1992) but they do not necessarily improve the yield of diagnostic material. Three additional techniques must be mentioned:

Cytocentrifuge Preparations. The introduction of immunostaining, used particularly in classification of malignant lymphomas, created the need for multiple samples. This can be achieved either by securing additional material from the lesion or by collecting all materials beyond the primary diagnostic sample (including washings of the syringe and needle with physiologic saline) as a cell suspension, processed by cytocentrifugation (for description of this technique, see Chap. 33). Eight to ten preparations may usually be secured in this fashion.

Cell Block Technique. Larger fragments of tissue may be removed from the aspirated sample for embedding in paraffin and processing as mini-biopsies. The method is often very useful inasmuch as it allows histologic analysis of fragments of tissue and permits the use of multiple sections for special stains.

Receptor and Gene Identification. With the use of specific antibodies, it is now possible to quantitate estrogen and progesterone receptors and other gene products, such as oncoproteins, in mammary carcinoma and other tumors by image analysis (see Chap. 35) and flow cytometry (see Chap. 36). Smears obtained for this purpose must be snap-frozen and kept in deep freeze at −70°C until use. Special processing protocols must be applied to this material (Czerniak et al., 1990; see also Chap. 34).

Fixation and Staining of Smears

There are two fundamental methods of processing smears obtained by aspiration biopsy: fixation and staining with either Papanicolaou or hemotoxylin–eosin, or air-drying of smears followed by hematologic stains. Both methods have their advantages and disadvantages, summarized in Table 29–3.

In general, fixed material allows a better comparison with histology and, therefore, is favored by many pathologists. Air-dried material, stained with Wright's, Wright–Giemsa, or May–Grünwald–Giemsa (MGG) stains requires additional experience and diagnostic adjustment. In air-dried material, the cells are much larger and the nuclei, particularly when somewhat overstained, may mimic cancer when none is present. The benefits of air-dried material is the speed with which it may be stained (particularly with the use of rapid stains such as Diff-Quik or toluidine blue) and the recognition of colloid, mucin, and endocrine cytoplasmic granules.

Rapid stains are particularly useful in preliminary assessment for adequacy of the sample before the patient is released. We use the Diff-Quik stain (Harleco, Gibbstown, New Jersey) for rapid preliminary analysis of the samples. The procedure is as follows:

Diff-Quik Stain. The fixative and the two staining solutions are purchased in gallon containers. The staining procedure is as follows:

1. Fixative   20 sec
2. Staining solution I 20 sec
3. Staining solution II 20 sec
4. Distilled water   10 sec
5. Ethanol 95%   10 sec
6. Absolute ethanol   15 sec
7. Xylene   15–20 sec
8. Mount with a coverslip

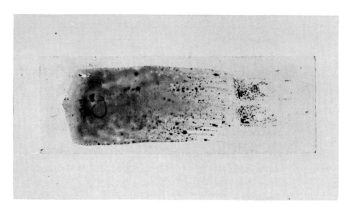

FIGURE 29–8. Slide with stained smear from aspiration biopsy. The solid flattened tissue fragments are seen to the right.

Table 29–3
*Comparison of May–Grüenwald–Giemsa (MGG), Hematoxylin–Eosin, and
Papanicolaou Stains*

Factors	MGG	Hematoxylin–Eosin	Papanicolaou
Preparation of material	Air-drying	Alcohol fixation	Alcohol fixation
Cytoplasmic features	Brings out a variety of cytoplasmic granules and inclusions	Offers little cytoplasmic differentiation	Brings out cytoplasmic keratinization
Nuclear features	Chromatin features difficult to assess; air-drying may induce artifacts	Tends to overstain nuclei unless carefully performed	Excellent identification of nuclear features
Nucleoli	Readily visible as pale intranuclear structures	Adequate, sometimes difficult to see in hyperchromatic nuclei	Adequate, sometimes difficult to see in hyperchromatic nuclei
Mucus and colloid	Well visualized	Require special stains	Require special stains
Familiarity to users	Stain familiar to hematologists	Stain familiar to tissue pathologists	Stain familiar to cytopathologists

The results of Diff-Quik stain are similar to those obtained with the Wright–Giemsa stain. The smears stained with Diff-Quik are readily restained with Papanicolaou stain. No destaining is necessary. The time required for processing the Diff-Quik stained smear is half that required for routine Papanicolaou stain (see Chap. 33).

Nuclear detail is of paramount importance in exfoliative cytology, wherein the recognition of a malignant tumor often depends on scanty cytologic evidence. In aspiration biopsy cytology, using smears that often contain hundreds of unmistakable cancer cells, other problems are encountered. These include precise identification of tumor type, recognition of grade of differentiation, and, when metastases are aspirated, establishing the site of the primary tumor. For such purposes the cytoplasmic details and the staining properties of some cell products, brought out by hematologic stains, are sometimes helpful.

Application of Molecular Biologic and Other Research Techniques to the Aspirated Sample

The sample of cells obtained by the needle aspiration technique is unique, inasmuch as it is a source of viable benign and cancer cells not subjected to prior manipulations. The viability of these cells was investigated by Zajicek (*Diagnostic Cytology,* 3rd ed., 1979) and 80% of them were viable under the conditions prevailing in most aspirations. Consequently, aspirated samples are eminently suitable for further investigations and analysis.

Current applications of the aspirated samples comprise several approaches.

DNA Analysis

DNA analysis of aspirated samples may be performed on fresh aspirates by flow cytometry and, on recent or archival smears, by image analysis. The details of the techniques may be found on pp. 1596 and 1620. The most significant application of these techniques has been for samples of mammary carcinoma, wherein information of potential diagnostic significance has been obtained (see p. 1600). In other cancers, including lymphomas, the value of this type of analysis is insecure.

Immunochemistry

With the development of a broad variety of monoclonal antibodies to various cell components, the aspirated samples have been repeatedly subjected to a broad range of experiments, documenting the presence of a large variety of cell components, such as intermediate filaments. Domagala et al. published extensively on the use of these techniques in accurate classification of various human tumors (see Chap. 34 for details). Of special value is typing of malignant lymphomas. Quantitation of various cell components, including gene products, is discussed in Chapter 35 (image analysis) and 36 (flow cytometry).

Molecular Biology Techniques

Documentation has been provided that gene analysis is possible in the aspirated sample, and it is particularly valuable in the assessment of malignant lymphomas (Lubinski and Huebner, 1989).

Electron Microscopy

The aspirated sample is eminently suitable for transmission and scanning electron microscopy, after appropriate fixation (Domagala and Koss, 1980).

Complications of Aspiration Biopsy

Traumatic complications of fine-needle aspiration biopsy of palpable lesions are infrequent and almost always of a minor degree. A hematoma occasionally forms at the site of aspiration, but causes little or no discomfort. Pneumothorax occurs in about 25% of patients receiving an aspiration biopsy of the lung. As a rule, the lung reexpands spontaneously within a few days, and therapeutic measures are called for in only 1% to 3% of such patients.

Infection, usually with gram-negative organisms, may occur in a very few cases after transrectal aspiration biopsy, mainly in patients with prostatitis. Therefore, needle biopsy of the prostate should be used only in the diagnosis of carcinoma and not to confirm a clinical diagnosis of prostatitis. When this restriction is observed, the frequency of inflammatory complications is negligible. Indeed, the rarity of infection is also surprising in intra-abdominal and transabdominal needle biopsy of organs such as the pancreas or retroabdominal lymph nodes, even when the needle has to pass through hollow viscera, such as the colon, stomach, or gallbladder. The risk of complications does increase, however, if several procedures are performed during the same session.

Dissemination of tumor cells or cell clusters through the needle track or the efferent lymph or blood vessels with resulting spread of the neoplastic growth and impaired prognosis is a risk in aspiration biopsy. This matter is discussed below.

Implantation of Tumor Cells

In experiments on rabbits, aspiration biopsy of lymph nodes metastases from transplantable V_x2 carcinoma was performed with an 18-gauge needle (Engzell et al., 1971). In all cases, carcinoma cells were found outside the capsule of the node at the sites of puncture. Similarly, analysis of blood seeping through the needle track after aspiration biopsy of human mammary carcinoma often shows tumor cells.

These observations suggest that tumor cells may spread along the needle track. Their clinical significance, however, is negligible, even if the needle track is not excised.

Tumor growth along the tracks of needles used for biopsy of palpable tumors has occasionally been reported (summary in Engzell et al., 1971). It must be noted that in such cases the needle used was of a relatively large caliber and the samples were collected for histologic examination. A search of the literature has revealed rare cases of local tumor spread caused by fine-needle aspiration biopsy (summary in Koss et al., 1992).

At Karolinska Hospital, 656 patients in whom cervical lymph node metastases had been diagnosed by aspiration with a 22-gauge needle were followed for up to 5 years. In no case was there any clinical evidence of local tumor growth resulting from the aspiration biopsy.

The question of local tumor dissemination was further studied in patients in whom pleomorphic adenoma (mixed tumor) of the major salivary glands, or carcinoma of the prostate or of the lung had been diagnosed by aspiration biopsy. These tumor types were selected because it was assumed that spread of neoplastic cells resulting in tumor growth along the needle track would be revealed during clinical follow-up.

The incidence of *postoperative* recurrence of pleomorphic adenomas (mixed tumors) of the major salivary glands has been reported as ranging from nil to almost 50%. The high rates of recurrence after excision must be ascribed to incomplete removal of the tumor, leaving small residues.

To study the possibility of local recurrence of pleomorphic adenomas diagnosed by fine-needle aspiration biopsy, 157 patients were followed for up to 10 years. In all cases the affected salivary gland was excised shortly after the aspiration. There were only three recurrences of adenoma. In two of them the primary excision was not complete. In none of the cases was the recurrent growth subcutaneous or cutaneous; accordingly, it could not be attributed to the aspiration biopsy.

Spontaneous extension of prostatic carcinoma through the fascia of Denonvillier and involvement of the rectal mucosa is uncommon and has been recorded in 1.5% of cases (Young, 1945). In our material only one of the 469 patients with prostatic carcinoma, followed for 5 years or more after the cytologic diagnosis, showed evidence of invasion of the rectum by tumor. In necropsy series the frequency of rectal involvement has been reported as 8% to 11%.

In a series of 1,264 malignant pulmonary lesions submitted to aspiration biopsy, neoplastic growth could be demonstrated in the needle track during follow-up in only 1 patient (Sinner and Zajicek, 1976). The diameter of the needles used for the pulmonary lesions was about 0.9 to 1.1 mm, which is greater than that of the needles in aspiration biopsy of palpable lesions (0.6 to 0.7 mm). Additional cases of this type were recorded by Koss et al. (1992).

These clinical studies indicate that local extension of tumor following fine-needle biopsy is a rare occurrence. It may be assumed that, in humans, the number of cancer cells that enter the needle tracks is relatively small and that the cells are destroyed before they can give rise to local tumor growth.

Vascular Dissemination of Tumor Cells

The literature contains numerous reports on the spread of tumor cells through blood vessels in connection with surgery (see Chap. 30). Much less attention has been paid to the possibility of vascular or lymphatic spread in connection with aspiration biopsy. The question, nevertheless, merits serious consideration, since no matter how fine a needle is used, aspiration biopsy inevitably causes microtrauma to the tissues through which the needle passes.

In an experimental approach, efferent lymphatics and veins in rabbits with popliteal lymphnode metastases from V_x2 carcinoma were cannulated (Engzell et al., 1971). Efferent lymph and blood were then sampled and analyzed for tumor cells. After gentle massage of the metastasis-bearing node, carcinoma cells were demonstrated in the lymph in one of seven rabbits and in the blood in one of nine rabbits. Aspiration of the node was thereafter performed. No evidence was obtained that this procedure released V_x2 carcinoma cells into the lymphatic system or bloodstream.

The available data thus indicate that, although it is likely that tumor cells enter the needle tracks in aspiration biopsy, this route of possible dissemination has no practical clinical implication. Distant dissemination of tumor cells through lymphatics or blood vessels following thin-needle biopsy seems to be uncommon. The use of thin-needle aspiration biopsy for the diagnosis of malignant tumors does not appear to have any prognostic significance.

The possible effect of aspiration biopsy on prognosis has been analyzed for carcinoma of the kidney (von Schreeb et al., 1967) and of the breast (Robbins et al., 1954). The 5-year survival rate of 77 patients who were operated on for renal carcinoma following direct injection of contrast medium into the tumor was compared with 73 matched controls without history of injection. There were no significant differences in the respective survival rates. The studies on mammary carcinoma were performed at the Memorial Hospital in New York, where aspiration biopsy has been used for the diagnosis of cancer since the early 1930s. On the basis of a comparative 5-year follow-up, it was concluded that aspiration biopsy had no effect on the survival rates in mammary carcinoma. The 15-year actuarial survival rate among 370 patients who were operated on for mammary carcinoma following aspiration biopsy was later compared with the corresponding rate in 370 matched controls in whom the diagnosis had been made by other means (Berg and Robbins, 1962). The survival rates in the two case series were identical (Fig. 29–9). The writers concluded, "Clinically, no reason can be found not to use aspiration when it is indicated."

INTERPRETATION OF ASPIRATION BIOPSY IN CLINICAL PRACTICE

The primary purpose of the aspiration biopsy is to provide the clinician with a reliable, rapid, and inexpensive method of diagnosis of lesions observed on physical examination or detected by x-ray examination or sonography. The principal advantage of this method of diagnosis is that, in most instances, it requires no hospitalization or anesthesia, as the procedure can be performed on ambulatory patients. The obvious danger of the method is that in the hands of poorly qualified personnel it may lead to major errors of diagnosis with grave harm to the patient. For these reasons, the results of the aspiration biopsy must be rendered *in terms of surgical pathology* and contain a clear and con-

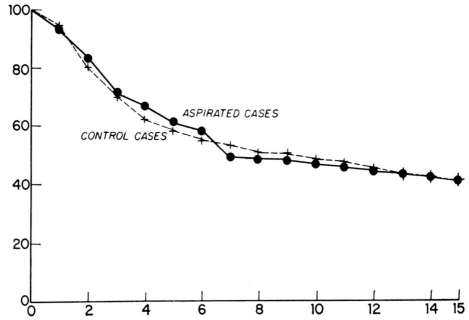

FIGURE 29–9.   Fifteen-year actuarial survival rates for breast cancer patients who had aspiration biopsy (●———●), and their matching controls (+––+). (Berg, J.W., and Robbins, G.F.: A late look at the safety of aspiration biopsy. Cancer, *15*:826–827, 1962)

cise *diagnosis* that will guide the clinician in selecting the optimal therapy. Ancillary terminology, such as Papanicolaou's "classes," if undesirable in exfoliative cytology, is unacceptable for aspiration biopsies.

The interpretation of the cytologic sample obtained by thin-needle aspiration biopsy varies greatly according to the target organ. Cell changes that may be of diagnostic significance in one anatomic setting may be unimportant in another. Thorough knowledge of clinical history and of the spectrum of pathologic changes are essential prerequisites for a successful application of this method of diagnosis to clinical practice.

Translating Cytologic Into Histologic Patterns

A translation of the cytologic into histologic patterns of diseases, mainly tumors, is important in all areas of cytology, but it acquires special significance in aspiration biopsies. There, the pathologist is expected to render a definitive diagnosis, based on combination of the clinical and roentgenologic presentation and the cell sample (Koss et al., 1992). The task is not always easy and sometimes may be compared to an archeologic "dig," wherein an attempt is made to reconstruct edifices and sometimes entire cities from fragments of bricks and walls. Nothing undermines the confidence of clinicians in the value of aspiration biopsy faster than a faulty diagnosis.

There are several fundamental differences between the two diagnostic media. Histologic material represents a two-dimensional cross section of a tissue or organ, wherein the relationship of tissue components to one another is easily recognized. The aspirated material consists of whole cells and tissue fragments, not cut by a knife, but usually in a state of disarray, wherein the relationship of tissue components to one another is jumbled.

The cells and small tissue fragments in the aspirated sample are often sufficient for the accurate diagnosis to be rendered, provided the pathologist is capable of a synthesis of the evidence and is familiar with differences between the histologic section and the smear or cell block. Some of the critical issues are summarized below:

Benign Tissues

Benign Epithelia.   In general, benign lining epithelia and glands appear in the aspirated samples as cohesive sheets of cells, with nuclei of uniform sizes, often showing sharp and distinct cell borders or a honeycomb appearance (see Fig. 29–84 as an example). The epithelial cells are often accompanied by small, spindle-shaped cells with dark nuclei, the myoepithelial cells. It should be noted that the presence of myoepithelial cells is rarely of significance in histologic material, whereas in the aspirated sample, they are synonymous with benign tissues, as they are virtually never seen in cancer. This basic description of benign epithelial structures applies only to some organs, because other configurations of benign epithelia may be observed in various specialized tissues, for example, the salivary glands (see Fig. 29–10), the thyroid (see Fig. 29–25), the liver (see Fig. 29–100), and the mesothelium. The latter is characterized by the presence of multiple, sometimes irregularly shaped nucleoli (see Figs. 25–7 and 29–113*B*). Special forms of benign epithelial cells, such as the oncocytes or Hürthle cells will be described where appropriate.

In general, although benign epithelial cells share some common features, their knowledge for each individual organ is mandatory to avoid mistakes.

Other Benign Structures.   The blood vessels, which in histologic material appear as round or oval cross sections filled with blood, usually appear in the aspirated sample as elongated, sausage-like three-dimensional structures. The blood cells can be seen across the transparent wall.

Connective tissue cells in the aspirated sample often appear as bundles of slender, spindly cells, occasionally provided with visible nucleoli. Fat and cartilage are usually readily identified because of their characteristic morphologic features.

Macrophages, whether mononucleated or multinucleated, are usually readily recognized, as they do not differ in their presentation from that in exfoliated material.

Malignant Tumors

The recognition of malignant cells in adequate samples is usually fairly easy, particularly when a large population of such cells is available for inspection and if they display the classic features of cancer cells, such as large size, variability of shape and configuration, large, hyperchromatic nuclei, and multiple nucleoli (see Fig. 29–66 as an example). A characteristic feature of cancer cells is their poor adhesiveness; hence, as a general rule, *no diagnosis of cancer should be made in the absence of single cancer cells.* Cancer cell clusters often show piling up of cells, lack of the orderly honeycomb relationship, and absence of myoepithelial cells.

Determination of tumor type, on the other hand, may not be easy. Whenever possible, particularly when dealing with metastatic cancers, a review of prior histologic material may be very helpful in determining the identity of the tumor.

Carcinomas.   One common feature of nearly all carcinomas cells is their tendency to form small and large clusters. Clustering is rarely seen in malignant lymphomas and sarcomas. The presence of keratin filaments is also characteristic of nearly all carcinomas. The recognition of specific forms of carcinomas is as follows:

Adenocarcinomas.   In general, adenocarcinomas of various origins tend to form spherical "papillary" clusters or sometimes form glandular structures (examples in Figs. 29–17, 29–67, and 29–87). Single cells may be cuboidal or cylindrical. Such tumors often produce mucin, which can be documented by the simple and inexpensive mucicarmine stain. Specific types of adenocarcinomas with special features, such as hepatocellular carcinoma or carcinomas composed of signet ring cells, will be described in appropriate segments of this chapter.

Squamous Carcinomas.   Keratin-forming tumors have the same appearance in aspiration biopsy material as elsewhere and are generally readily recognized (see Fig. 29–56 as an example). In some tumors, however, the cancer cells may mimic benign squamous cells. Such events occur mainly in aspirations of lymph nodes of the neck, where the cells of the metastatic tumor may be confused with a branchial cyst and vice versa.

Undifferentiated Carcinomas.   Large-cell tumors of this type are usually easy to recognize because the cancer cells in such cases have a classic appearance of cancer (see Fig. 29–68 as an example). Small-cell malignant tumors, on the other hand, may be more difficult to recognize and classify. Oat cell carcinomas often display two populations of nuclei, vesicular and pyknotic, but no nucleoli (see Chap. 20). Other small-cell malignant tumors will be discussed when appropriate.

Malignant Lymphomas.   The many types of malignant lymphomas will be described below (see lymph nodes). In general, the cells of malignant lymphomas tend to be dispersed and rarely form clusters in good preparations (see Figs. 29–48 and

29–50). In thick smears, wherein the material has not been properly dispersed, clustering may be seen. When the lymphomas are of large-cell types, such presentation may be confused with that of a carcinoma (see p. 1286).

Other Tumor Types. There are no general rules in the recognition of the many types of malignant tumors that may be observed in aspirated material. Such tumors will be described wherever appropriate. The reader is referred to highly specialized books listed in the bibliography for description of very uncommon neoplasms.

Cell Products. As described in Chapter 26, various cell products that may be encountered in the cytologic samples are sometimes very helpful in tumor classification. Thus, mucin, melanin, psammoma bodies, and various crystals may be encountered and their presence used to diagnostic advantage. Immunologic techniques that may be applied to the analysis of cytologic samples are described in Chapter 34.

It is quite evident that a thorough knowledge of surgical pathology is an important advantage in the interpretation of aspirated samples. A review of prior histologic material, whenever available, is also extremely helpful in many cases, as is the use of cell blocks. However, even with the help of special stains and a thorough knowledge of patient's history and clinical findings, there will be a residue of aspirated samples wherein the definitive diagnosis may be difficult to achieve. In such cases admitting the limitations of the method and one's knowledge is a better strategy than risking an improper diagnosis.

PART II: ASPIRATION BIOPSY OF PALPABLE LESIONS

The aspirates of palpable lesions (see Table 29–1) will be discussed in anatomic order, beginning with the salivary glands, cysts, and miscellaneous neck structures, the thyroid, the lymph nodes, the breast, skin and soft parts, prostate, and gonads. The data on lymph nodes, although described within the head and neck area, are obviously applicable to all anatomic sites.

THE SALIVARY GLANDS

Normal Structure

The salivary glands are classified as major or minor. The major salivary glands are the parotid, submandibular, and sublingual glands. Minor salivary glands are scattered over the lips, buccal mucosa, palate, larynx, and tongue. The nasopharynx, trachea, and bronchi contain similar small glands. The secretion of the parotid glands is serous, whereas that of the submandibular and sublingual glands is of mixed type, predominantly serous in the submandibular and predominantly mucous in the sublingual glands. The minor salivary glands produce serous, mucous, or mixed secretions.

The major salivary glands are lobulated structures. The secretory units of the lobules—the acini (alveoli)—drain into intralobular ducts. From the lobules, the secretion is conveyed by interlobular ducts to the main secretory duct.

Serous fluid is produced by acinic cells, which have small round nuclei and abundant vacuolated cytoplasm. In smears of aspiration biopsy, the acinic cells usually occur in clusters in which acini are readily recognizable (Fig. 29–10). Dissociated cells are seldom seen. Their presence indicates a breakdown of the acini, usually the result of an inflammatory process. The acini may also contain mucus-secreting cells. These cells resemble the mucous cells of other organs, such as the intestine or the uterine cervix. Although the parotid gland is considered to be serous in type, mucus-secreting cells are sometimes irregularly distributed in the intralobular and interlobular ducts. This explains why mucus-producing tumors may occur in the parotid gland.

The ductal epithelial cells of the salivary glands show small round nuclei and scanty cytoplasm, resembling the lining epithelium of the other glandular organs, such as the breast. Single cells are rarely found in smears of an aspirate.

The salivary glands also contain large oncocytic cells with granular, markedly eosinophilic cytoplasm and round nuclei. The oncocytes are found in the acini and the ducts, and their numbers increase with age. Electron microscopy and histochemical studies of oncocytes have indicated an

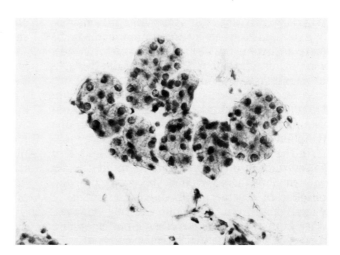

FIGURE 29–10. Aspirate smear from parotid gland. A cluster of normal acini is seen. (Papanicolaou stain ×230)

abundance of mitochondria and a high level of enzymic activity. Similar cells occur in the thyroid gland, where they are called Hürthle or Askanazy cells and where their frequency likewise increases with age. Cells with similar morphologic characteristics in the breast are usually described as sudoriparous or apocrine cells.

Between the basement membrane and the epithelial cells, regardless of configuration, there is a layer of flat myoepithelial cells with elongated nuclei. The myoepithelial cells appear to be involved in the histogenesis of pleomorphic adenoma (mixed tumor).

Lesions of the Salivary Glands

Palpable lesions of salivary glands can be classed as follows:

Classification of Palpable Lesions of the Salivary Glands

Inflammatory lesions and cysts
Benign neoplasms
   Pleomorphic adenoma (mixed tumor)
   Basal cell adenoma
   Adenolymphoma (Warthin's tumor)
   Oncocytoma
Malignant neoplasms
   Acinic cell carcinoma
   Adenoid cystic carcinoma
   Mucoepidermoid carcinoma
   Squamous cell carcinoma
   Undifferentiated carcinoma
   Carcinoma in pleomorphic adenoma (malignant mixed tumor)

Inflammatory Lesions and Cysts

Lymphadenitis. The parotid gland often contains enlarged, hyperplastic lymph nodes that cannot be reliably differentiated by clinical examination from a cyst or a neoplasm. Aspiration biopsy of such a node yields a grayish substance, and microscopy shows lymphoid cells, occasionally mixed with acinic cells and duct epithelium. The presence of salivary gland cells is most often due to inadvertent aspiration of peripheral salivary gland tissue. On rare occasions, however, an intraparotid lymph node may contain a salivary gland component, which may be aspirated together with lymphoid tissue. The cytology of intraparotid lymph nodes otherwise does not differ from that of lymph node aspirates in other anatomic locations (cf. p. 1279).

Sialadenitis. In acute sialadenitis the aspirate from the affected glands contains numerous neutrophilic granulocytes and phagocytes, in addition to gland epithelium. In the early phase of the inflammation many acinic cells may also be aspirated. Later on, the ductal epithelial cells predominate due to widespread destruction of acini.

Lymphoepithelial Lesions and Related Conditions—Mikulicz's and Sjögren's Syndromes. Partial or complete, often bilateral enlargement of the salivary glands occurs in these conditions. Parotid glands are most commonly affected. When the salivary gland lesion is associated with a similar enlargement of lacrimal glands, it is known as Mikulicz's syndrome or disease. When the salivary gland lesion is associated with keratoconjunctivitis, laryngitis, and rhinitis sicca and other generalized manifestations of autoimmune disorders (such as rheumatoid arthritis), it is known as Sjörgen's syndrome. The relationship of the two syndromes is not well understood. Both, however, may lead to, or be associated with, a malignant lymphoma. The purpose of the salivary gland aspiration in such cases is to rule out the presence of a lymphoma.

In the absence of a lymphoma the aspiration smears show a predominantly lymphoid picture, with small and large lymphocytes, stem cells, and phagocytes, together with variable amounts of ductal epithelium. Difficulties arise, however, when immature lymphoid cells, lymphoblasts, and stem cells predominate in the smears. Primary malignant lymphoma in the salivary gland must then be excluded.

Because, under these circumstances, the diagnosis of a malignant lymphoma in the aspirate may be very difficult, a formal surgical biopsy, with the use of lymphocyte markers, is recommended. It must be noted that several years may elapse from the time of first salivary gland enlargement until the development of a malignant lymphoma, which may occur at this or at another anatomic site.

Cysts. Any salivary gland, major or minor, may be the site of a cyst. The cysts are lined by epithelium of ductal, oncocytic, mucus-secreting, or mixed cell type. Transitional forms of epithelium may also occur. Aspirated cystic fluid may be clear and somewhat viscid, resembling saliva, or it may have a more-or-less turbid appearance.

When clear saliva-like fluid has been aspirated, the swelling may disappear. The lesion then is probably a retention cyst, and cytologic analysis of the aspirate may reveal only a few phagocytes. In such cases a clinical checkup after 2 to 4 weeks generally suffices. Cloudy fluid, as a rule, contains inflammatory cells, and after the aspiration a mass often remains palpable at the periphery of the cyst. Residual masses should always be reaspirated and reevaluated according to cytologic findings. It must be noted, however, that Warthin's tumor (see below) and, rarely, malignant tumors may mimic cysts. For these reasons a surgical excision of residual masses may be indicated if the cytologic findings are not conclusively benign.

Benign Neoplasms

Pleomorphic Adenoma (Mixed Tumor). This tumor contains both epithelial and mesenchymal stromal structures (Plate 29–1). It is the most common of all salivary gland neoplasms, constituting about 70% of all tumors.

Cytologic recognition of pleomorphic adenoma is based on the presence of both stromal and epithelial elements in the smears (see Plate 29–1). The stromal structures are most easily recognized in MGG-stained smears (see Plate 29–1*A, E, F*). The intercellular substance in these smears stains predominantly red in myxomatous areas and purplish in areas suggestive of cartilaginous transformation. The stromal cells display oval, elongated nuclei surrounded by gray cytoplasm. The nuclei of the epithelial cells are round, sometimes eccentric, and are surrounded by pale blue cytoplasm. In wet-fixed Papanicolaou-stained smears (see Plate 29–1*C, D*), the mesenchymal structures are characterized by fibers embedded in the matrix, which stains gray, sometimes with a touch of pink. The fibers are very delicate and scarcely visible in some areas, but may be coarse in others.

The epithelial elements usually consist of cohesive sheets of small epithelial cells, which may show a transition to the stromal cells (Fig. 29–11). Occasionally, however, the epithelial cells may be larger and may mimic squamous cells (see Plate 29–1*E*). Such cases may be quite perplexing and difficult to interpret. It is very rare, however, not to be able to differentiate a pleomorphic adenoma from a malignant tumor (see below). Perhaps the most significant difficulty in this regard is the rare, cellular pleomorphic adenoma that may yield epithelial cell clusters arranged in tight "balls," reminiscent of an adenoid cystic carcinoma. On close inspection, the presence of stromal elements and the absence of dispersed cancer cells favor the benign lesion. Because the benign pleomorphic adenomas require a careful and wide excision to prevent recurrence, the diagnostic dilemma is rarely of clinical significance.

Some pleomorphic adenomas may produce specific crystalline proteins. Thus, tyrosine or hippurate crystals, when present in smears, are invariably associated with these lesions, even if the cytologic evidence is scanty (see Fig. 29–11*D*).

Basal Cell Adenoma. Neoplasms of this type are rare and account for only about 2% of all primary tumors of the salivary glands. They are encapsulated and consist of isomorphic cells resembling cutaneous basal cells. The cells are arranged in ductal, trabecular, and solid structures. The stroma is mostly loose (Fig. 29–12*A*). Stromal elements of the types seen in pleomorphic adenomas do not occur in these tumors.

Aspiration biopsy smears contain numerous,

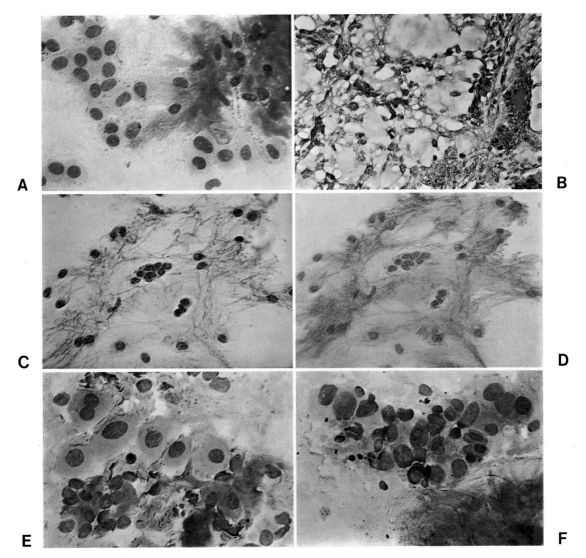

Plate 29–1. Aspiration biopsy smears and a tissue section from mixed tumors of the salivary gland. (*A*) Aspirate from a benign mixed tumor containing on the *right* red-stained myxoid material with embedded cells. On the *left* is a plug of epithelial cells with minimal amounts of intercellular mucus (May–Grünwald–Giemsa stain). (*B*) Tissue section from a benign mixed tumor (combined alcian blue–PAS stain). The epithelial mucus in a duct (on the *right*) and the stellate cells of the myxoid areas are PAS-positive. The ground substance of the myxoid areas stains with alcian blue. (*C*) Aspirate from a benign mixed tumor showing a plug of the epithelial cells and myxoid material consisting of coarse fibrils with embedded stroma cells (Papanicolaou stain). (*D*) The slide in (*C*) after decolorization and restaining with alcian blue–PAS. The cytoplasm of the stromal cells is PAS-positive, but the intercellular substance reacts with alcian blue. (*E*) Aspiration biopsy smear from a benign mixed tumor. The lower part of the slide shows myxoid material with embedded cells. In the upper part are cells showing differentiation toward squamous epithelium. (May–Grünwald–Giemsa stain). (*F*) Aspiration biopsy smear from a malignant mixed tumor. A plug of carcinoma cells is seen adjacent to a fragment of myxoid tissue (May–Grünwald–Giemsa stain). (*A*, *C*–*F* ×320; *B* ×200. Eneroth, C.-M., and Zajicek, J.: Aspiration biopsy of salivary gland tumors: III. Morphologic studies on smears and histologic sections from 368 mixed tumors. Acta Cytol., *10*:440–454)

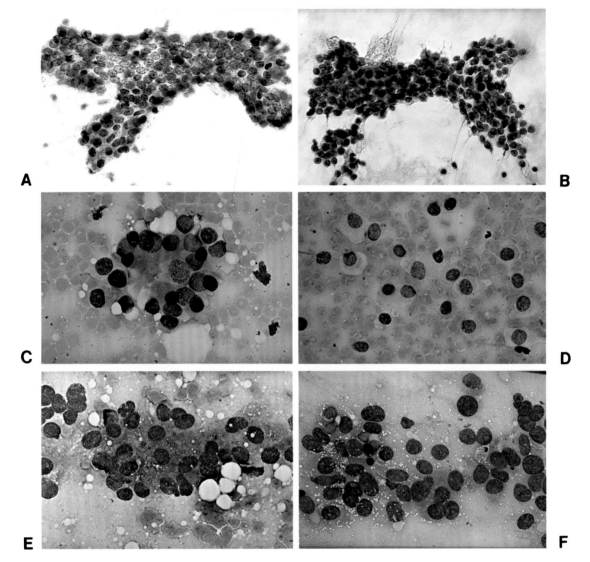

Plate 29 – 2. Aspiration biopsy smears from benign breast conditions and breast carcinomas. (*A*) Aspirate showing a cluster of benign cells imitating ductal structures. (*B*) Aspirate showing a cluster of well-differentiated breast carcinoma, tubular type. The cell size corresponds to the benign epithelium shown in (*A*). The irregular arrangement of the cells, together with slight nuclear hyperchromasia and eosinophilia of the cytoplasm, is helpful in differential diagnosis with duct adenosis and fibroadenoma. (*C*) Aspirate from a well-differentiated breast carcinoma, of ductal type. A glandular structure is shown. In glandular structures the cytoplasm is crowded into a central mass and the nuclei are at the periphery. Unstained round globules adjacent to the acinus are droplets of fat probably aspirated from fatty tissue. Air-dried smear. (*D*) Aspirate from breast carcinoma. The cancer cells are dispersed. When fibrosis is present the cell yield is often scanty and the presence of carcinoma may be overlooked. Air-dried smear. (*E*) Needle aspirate from a lactating breast showing a cluster of acinic cells. These cells have a finely granulated cytoplasm that is very fragile. Air-dried smear. (*F*) Needle aspirate from breast carcinoma. Round carcinoma cell nuclei are surrounded by fragile cytoplasm with poorly delineated cell borders, and containing numerous transparent droplets resembling fat. Histologically this case was classified as a medullary carcinoma. Air-dried smear. (*A, B* Papanicolaou stain, ×250; *C – F* MGG stain, ×400)

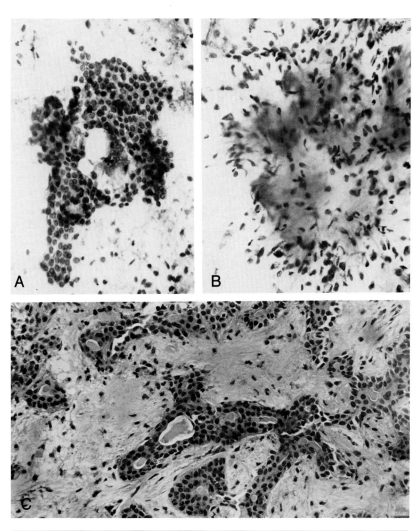

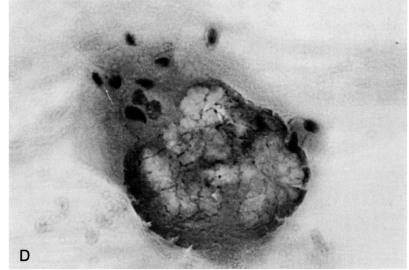

FIGURE 29-11. Pleomorphic adenoma. (*A, B*) Fixed aspiration smears stained with Papanicolaou stain. (*A*) shows a cohesive sheet of small epithelial cells forming a lumen; (*B*) shows an area of myxoid stroma with spindly cells and ground substance staining gray (compare with air-dried, MGG stained smears in Plate 29-1, *A* and *E*). (*C*) Histologic section of the tumor. (*D*) Aspirate from another pleomorphic adenoma containing the characteristic brown, leaf-shaped tyrosine crystals, surrounded by a few benign stromal cells. (*A* and *B* ×400; *C* ×200; *D* ×560. *A*–*C* from Koss, L.G., et al.: Aspiration Biopsy. Cytologic Interpretation and Histologic Bases. New York and Tokyo, Igaku-Shoin, 1984, with permission)

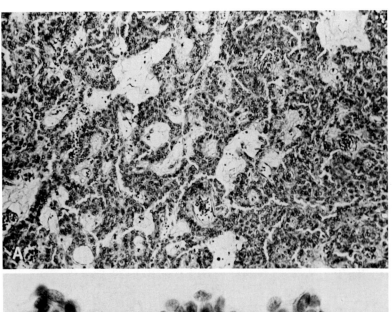

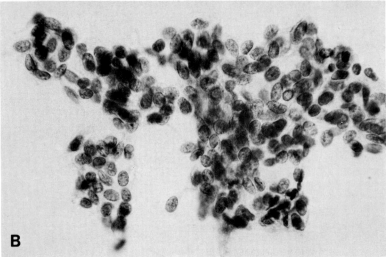

FIGURE 29–12. Basal cell adenoma of parotid. (*A*) Tissue section. (*B*) Needle aspirate showing tightly packed, ovoid neoplastic cells. (*A* ×120; *B*, Papanicolaou stain ×480)

tightly knit cell clusters and a few fragments of stroma. The epithelial cells have a round or ovoid nucleus with a rim of pale cytoplasm (see Fig. 29–12*B*). Dissociated, single cells are rarely seen.

The stromal fragments consist of amorphous matrix in which are embedded cells with elongated nuclei. The matrix stains bright red in MGG smears and is almost translucent in Papanicolaou smears. It appears homogeneous, in contrast with the stromal fragments in pleomorphic adenomas which contain fibrillar elements.

Adenolymphoma (Warthin's Tumor). These benign, slowly growing, and frequently cystic tumors have an epithelial and a lymphoid component. The former consists of cuboidal or polygonal oncocytes (Fig. 29–13*A*), which often form papillary projections. Necrotic material is often present in the lumina of the cysts. The lymphoid and epi-

thelial components are separated from each other by a thin basal membrane.

The aspirates of adenolymphomas often yield only turbid fluid, representing cyst content. Therein one finds occasional oncocytic cells, scattered lymphocytes, and cell debris. If the tumor itself is aspirated, sheets of oncocytic cells and scattered lymphocytes are observed (see Fig. 29–13*B,C*).

The oncocytes aspirated from adenolymphomas show abundant cytoplasm and round, usually central nuclei (see Fig. 29–13*B,C*). In Papanicolaou-stained smears, oxyphilic granulation is seen in the cytoplasm. In air-dried MGG smears the cytoplasm stains slate gray. Very fine granulation of the cytoplasm is seen in some cells. The cytoplasmic outlines are distinct. The oncocytes usually appear in solid aggregates. Single cells are rare, and when present, they usually show signs of cyto-

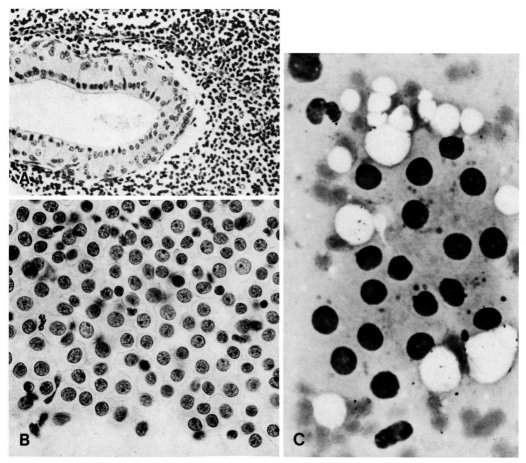

FIGURE 29–13. Adenolymphoma (Warthin's tumor). (*A*) Tissue section showing typical arrangement of oncocytes in two rows, forming a tubular structure that contains some amorphous material. The surrounding stroma contains abundant lymphoid tissue. (*B*) Needle aspirate showing a cluster of oncocytes (fixed smear, Papanicolaou stain). Note the abundant eosinophilic cytoplasm and the honeycomb pattern. (*C*) A cluster of oncocytes in an air-dried smear. Some cytoplasmic granulation is seen. (*A* ×120; *B* ×380; *C*, MGG ×600. *A*: Eneroth, C.-M., and Zajicek, J.: Aspiration biopsy of salivary gland tumors: II. Morphologic studies on smears and histologic sections from oncocytic tumors [45 cases of papillary cystadenoma lymphomatosum and 4 cases of oncocytoma]. Acta Cytol., 9:355–361, 1965)

plasmic degeneration. The morphologic characteristics of oncocytes make them distinguishable from other cells in neoplastic and nonneoplastic lesions of the salivary glands.

Because the oncocytes may undergo squamous metaplasia (Hamperl, 1936), occasional aspirates may contain squamous cells and be mistaken for squamous or mucoepidermoid carcinomas. Two such cases were reported by Zajicek and Eneroth (1970).

Oncocytoma. Oncocytoma is a rare benign tumor made up of large eosinophilic cells (oncocytes) with comparatively small, round nuclei (Fig. 29–14*A*).

Aspiration biopsy yields solid plugs of polygonal cells with abundant granular cytoplasm, resembling the oncocytes of adenolymphoma (see Fig. 29–14*B*).

The oncocytes in adenolymphoma and in oncocytoma are morphologically very similar. The diagnosis of adenolymphoma is supported by the presence of cyst fluid, amorphous material, lymphocytes, and cell debris in the background of the smear. Moreover, pure oncocytomas are very uncommon tumors.

Malignant Neoplasms

Acinic Cell Carcinoma. These slow-growing and deceptively benign-appearing tumors are composed of sheets of small to medium-sized cells with

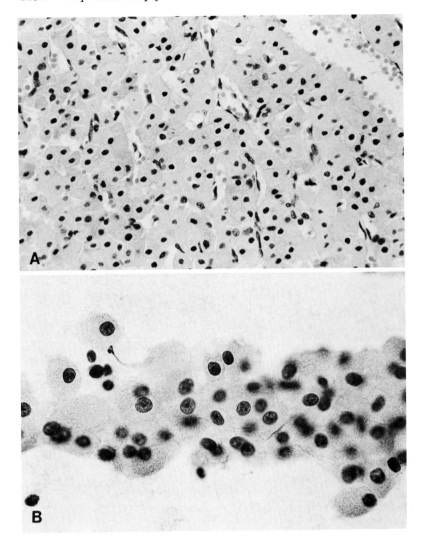

FIGURE 29–14. Oncocytoma: (*A*) Tissue section. (*B*) Needle aspirate showing finely granulated cytoplasm of the large, eosinophilic cells composing the tumor. (*A* ×120; *B*, Papanicolaou stain ×480. *A*: Zajicek, J.: Aspiration Biopsy Cytology. Part I. Basel, S. Karger, 1974)

clear cytoplasm and uniform small nuclei. Occasionally, gland formation may be observed (Fig. 29–15*B*). Metastases may occur late in the course of the disease.

Needle aspirates usually contain acinar, medium-sized cells without nuclear polymorphism or nuclear atypia. In such cases, the cytologist must differentiate between acinic cell tumor and a nonneoplastic enlargement of a salivary gland. With some experience this is not difficult. Aspirate from nonneoplastic lesions of salivary glands contains fragments in which the compact acinic structures are well delineated, and their cells have round, basally located nuclei (see Fig. 29–10). Intact, free acinic cells are rarely seen, although naked nuclei the size of small lymphocytes are frequently scattered throughout the smears. Fragments of ductal epithelium are also usually present.

The yield of cells in acinic cell tumors usually is more abundant than in the nonneoplastic lesions. Ductal epithelium is absent. Acinic structures are discernible, but are not clearly delineated (see Fig. 29–15*A*). Naked, lymphocyte-sized nuclei of acinic tumor cells are numerous, and a lower-power view may give the impression that lymphocytes have been aspirated in addition to tumor cells.

In some cases, the nuclei of aspirated cells are polymorphic and hyperchromatic and contain large nucleoli. Recognition of a malignant tumor is not difficult in such cases, but the recognition of the carcinomas as acinic cell may be cytologically

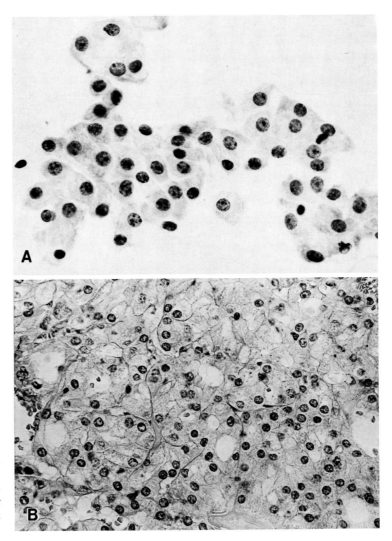

FIGURE 29–15. (*A*) Acinic cell carcinoma: smear, Papanicolaou stain. (*B*) Tissue section from an acinic cell carcinoma. Note the homogeneous tumor structure with cells with clear cytoplasm and small dark nuclei. (×270)

difficult. In poorly differentiated tumors with increased nucleocytoplasmic ratios, the cytologist can only state that a carcinoma is present and that the determination of tumor type must await histologic examination of the tumor.

Adenoid Cystic Carcinoma. Adenoid cystic carcinoma is a highly malignant tumor of salivary glands, often with a slow evolution that may stretch over a period of many years. The histologic appearance of the tumor is very characteristic. The tumor consists of sheets and strands of small cells surrounding cystic spaces of various sizes, each containing a deposit of hyaline amorphous material (Figs. 29–16*A* and 29–17*E*). The hyaline material is an accumulation of fibrillar basement membrane proteins. Elsewhere in the tumor, small

mucus-containing glandular spaces may be observed. Similar tumors may occasionally occur in the major bronchi, the uterine cervix, the breast, and in other organs (see pp. 528 and 831). Occasionally, particularly in recurrent tumors, the characteristic structure may be partially lost, and the tumor may be composed predominantly of sheets of uniform, small malignant cells, with only an occasional cystic space formation.

The cytologic presentation of these tumors in aspirates is usually equally characteristic. The small tumor cells form round aggregates or "balls," wherein, upon focusing up and down, one can discern the presence of the hyaline material (see Figs. 29–16*B* and 29–17*A–D*). With MGG, the hyaline material stains red. Occasionally, isolated hya-

(text continues on page 1260)

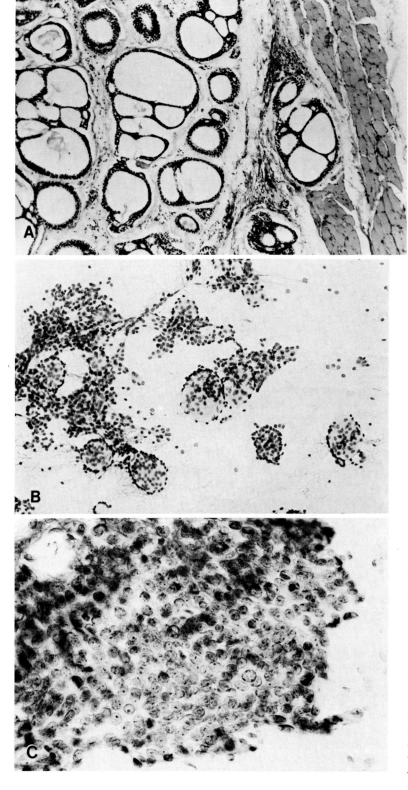

FIGURE 29–16. Adenoid cystic carcinoma. (*A*) Tissue section from an adenoid cystic carcinoma showing acellular cystic spaces containing hyaline material, surrounded by small tumor cells. Intramuscular invasion has taken place. (*B*) Smear of biopsy aspirate from the adenoid cystic carcinoma shown in (*A*). The hyaline material is seen as transparent globules surrounded by carcinoma cells. (*C*) Aspiration biopsy smear from a predominantly solid adenoid cystic carcinoma. (*A*, Van Gieson stain 120; *B*, Papanicolaou stain ×120; *C*, Papanicolaou stain ×360. *A*: Eneroth, C.-M., and Zajicek, J.: Aspiration biopsy of salivary tumors IV. Morphologic studies on smears and histologic sections from 45 cases of salivary tumors IV. Morphologic studies on smears and histologic sections from 45 cases of adenoid cystic carcinoma. Acta Cytol., *13*:59–63, 1969)

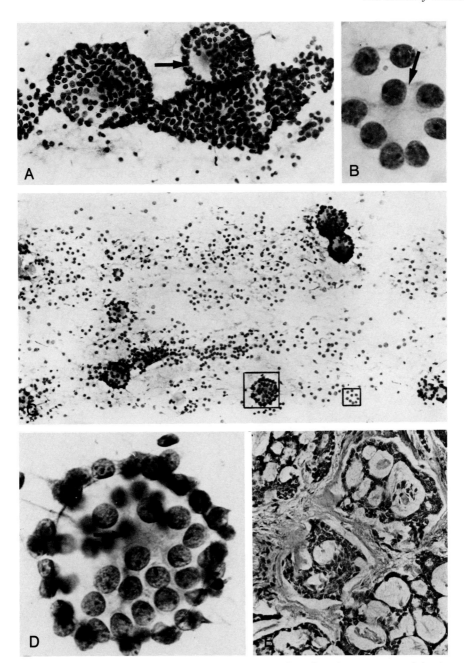

FIGURE 29–17. Adenoid cystic carcinoma: aspirate (*A–D*) and tissue section (*E*). The central panel (*C*) shows a low-power view of the aspirate: spherical clusters (balls) of tumor cells are seen against the background of dispersed cells. Panel (*A*) shows a higher-power view of another field of the aspirate. Hyaline material (*arrow*) may be seen within the spherical cell cluster. (*B–D*) High-power view of the clusters, corresponding to the two *marked* areas in (*C*). The small, monotonous tumor cells with round nuclei and single nucleoli are shown. The hyaline material in the center of the cluster is marked by the *arrow.* (*E*) The characteristic histologic presentation of the tumor with cystic spaces filled with hyaline material (*A* ×200; *B, E* ×800; *C* ×100; *E* ×200. Koss, L.G., et al.: Aspiration Biopsy. Cytologic Interpretation and Histologic Bases. New York, Igaku-Shoin, 1984, with permission)

line cylinders or spheres may also occur. Elsewhere in the smears, dispersed small tumor cells form the background (see Fig. 29–17*C*). It is of note that the cancer cells show very monotonous small, round nuclei, each usually provided with a single small nucleolus. In the poorly differentiated variety, sheets of small, fairly monotonous malignant cells, with somewhat larger and more conspicuous nucleoli (see Fig. 29–16*C*), are seen. Here, the identification of tumor type may be difficult in the absence of prior material. A search for hyaline globules, if successful, ensures the diagnosis.

Mucoepidermoid Carcinoma. This neoplasm is of ductal origin. It contains mucus-secreting, epidermoid and undifferentiated, so-called intermediate cells in various proportions. It is customary to distinguish between well-differentiated (low-grade malignant) and poorly differentiated (high-grade malignant) tumor types.

In smears of aspirates from the well-differentiated, predominantly cystic tumors, mucoid material and mucus-producing cells predominate, but are usually accompanied by scattered, somewhat atypical squamous cells (Fig. 29–18*A,B*). Neither cell type shows conspicuous nuclear abnormalities

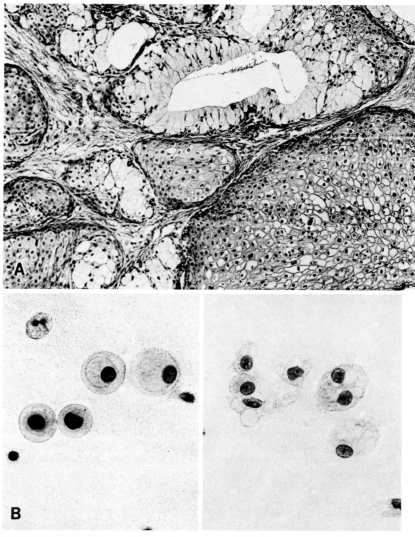

FIGURE 29–18. Mucoepidermoid carcinoma. (*A*) Tissue section showing mucus-producing and epidermoid part of the tumor. (*B*) Needle aspirate containing atypical squamous cells (*left*) and mucus-producing cells with eccentrically located nuclei and foamy cytoplasm (*right*). Nuclear atypia is almost absent. Same case as in (*A*).

(continued)

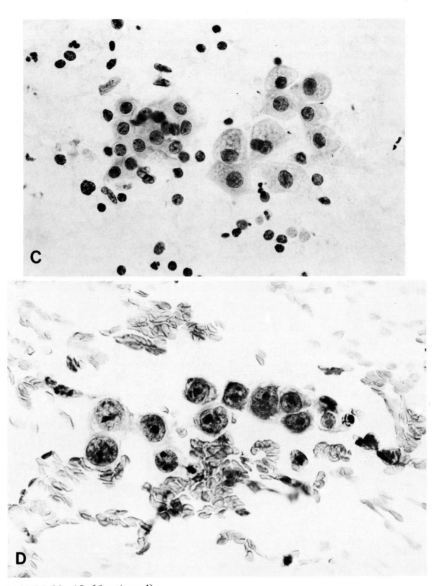

FIGURE 29–18 *(Continued).*
(*C*) Needle aspirate from a moderately differentiated mucoepidermoid carcinoma showing a cluster of mucus-producing cells (*right*) and of intermediate cells (*left*) surrounded by lymphocytic cells. (*D*) Needle aspirate from a poorly differentiated mucoepidermoid carcinoma showing polymorphic undifferentiated carcinoma cells. (*A* ×120; *B, C, D*, Papanicolaou stain ×480. *A:* Zajicek, J., et al.: Aspiration biopsy of salivary gland tumors VI. Morphologic studies on smears and histologic sections from mucoepidermoid carcinoma. Acta Cytol., *20*:35–41, 1976)

of a malignant tumor, but their synchronous presence in a cystic salivary gland lesion is strongly suggestive of a low-grade mucoepidermoid tumor. Mucin can usually be demonstrated in the cytoplasm of the *squamous cells,* a characteristic finding in this group of tumors.

In moderately differentiated, predominantly solid tumors, the smears show mucus-producing, intermediate, and squamous cells (see Fig. 29-18C). Atypia may be seen in all the cell types, but, as a rule, it is most prominent in the squamous cells. In aspirate from poorly differentiated tumors, squamous or undifferentiated carcinoma cells are the dominant cell types (see Fig. 29-18D).

In the previous edition of this book, Dr. Zajicek defined a category of poorly differentiated salivary gland tumors containing conspicuous, single, mucus-rich signet ring cells. He considered this to be a special category of tumors and classified them as *mucous cell* or *adenopapillary carcinomas.* There is no further justification for this classification because these tumors are mere variants of poorly differentiated mucoepidermoid carcinomas (Fig. 29-19).

Squamous Cell Carcinoma.   The well-known potential of the ductal epithelium to undergo squamous metaplasia explains the origin of squamous cell carcinoma in ducts of salivary glands. Squamous cell carcinoma accounts for about 4% of all tumors of the major salivary glands. Whether squamous carcinomas are always derived from foci of squamous cell metaplasia or whether they may

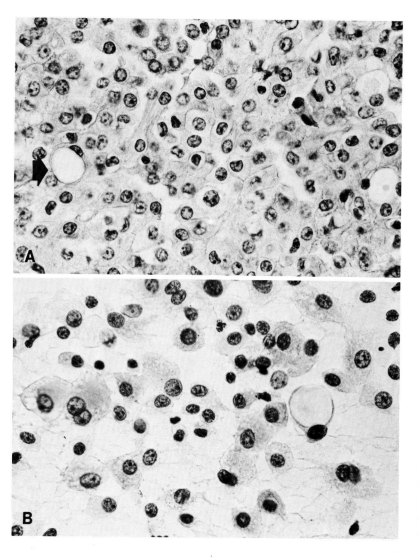

FIGURE 29–19.   Poorly differentiated mucoepidermoid carcinoma with scattered mucus-containing signet ring cells, previously classified as mucous cell adenocarcinoma (adenopapillary carcinoma). (*A*) Tissue section showing a signet ring cell (*arrow*). (*B*) Needle aspirate from the same case. Carcinoma cells have round nuclei surrounded by abundant cytoplasm. One cell exhibits signet-ring form. (*A* ×480; *B*, Papanicolaou stain ×480)

also arise from squamous cell overgrowth of mucoepidermoid tumors is unknown.

When aspirates from different areas of a salivary gland tumor contain only squamous carcinoma cells without admixture of mucus, three possibilities must be considered: *(1)* a primary squamous cell carcinoma, *(2)* a mucoepidermoid carcinoma growing chiefly as a squamous carcinoma, and *(3)* a metastasis from a squamous cell carcinoma elsewhere in the body. The decision cannot be made from the study of an aspirate. The cytologist, while reporting the presence of a squamous carcinoma, must clearly state that the derivation of the tumor can be determined only from the clinical evidence or from histologic study of the excised lesion.

Undifferentiated Carcinoma. When smears of biopsy aspirate from salivary glands contain cancer cells without any of the distinct morphologic characteristics described above, the possibility of an undifferentiated carcinoma must be considered. The cytologic picture in most such cases shows clear-cut cancer cells, and the diagnosis of a malignant tumor is not in doubt. However, the question of primary versus metastatic cancer cannot be answered in this type of material.

Carcinoma in Pleomorphic Adenoma (Malignant Mixed Tumor). Cancer can occasionally occur in pleomorphic adenoma. If the malignant component extends beyond the boundaries of the pleomorphic adenoma into the surrounding tissue, the prognosis becomes unfavorable.

Some risk of cytologic "overdiagnosis" of cancer may occasionally arise from small foci of abnormal cells observed in benign pleomorphic adenomas. The finding of such cells in smears of aspirate may sometimes lead to a discrepancy between the cytologic and the histologic diagnosis.

The risk of diagnostic "overcall" in pleomorphic as well as in monomorphic adenomas can be avoided if, in debatable cases, a histologic study of the tumor is recommended (Fig. 29–20). If, however, the aspirate from several different areas of the tumor contain only cancer cells without evidence of benign adenoma, the lesion is obviously malignant and should be so reported.

Malignant Lymphomas. Primary malignant lymphomas may occur in the salivary glands and mimic other forms of swelling. The aspiration biopsy diagnosis may be very difficult at times because of the synchronous presence of epithelial cells. Furthermore, in some of the cases, the smear and cell patterns may mimic small-cell carcinomas. Because of major therapeutic and prognostic differences between small-cell carcinomas and malignant lymphomas, a surgical biopsy should be recommended for all patients with a cytologic suspicion of a lymphoma. Immunologic workup may still be required to reach the final diagnosis (see Chap. 34).

Metastatic Tumors. Although rare, the involvement of the salivary glands by metastatic tumors is known to occur. Besides lymphomas and leukemias, breast cancer in women and malignant melanomas have been observed from time to time. Metastatic cancers of other types and primary origins may also occur.

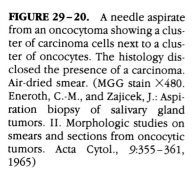

FIGURE 29–20. A needle aspirate from an oncocytoma showing a cluster of carcinoma cells next to a cluster of oncocytes. The histology disclosed the presence of a carcinoma. Air-dried smear. (MGG stain ×480. Eneroth, C.-M., and Zajicek, J.: Aspiration biopsy of salivary gland tumors. II. Morphologic studies on smears and sections from oncocytic tumors. Acta Cytol., 9:355–361, 1965)

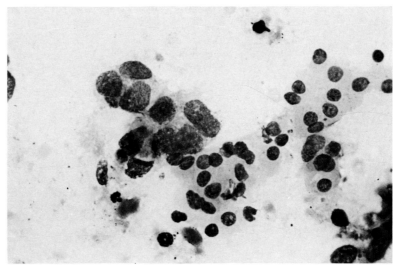

CYSTS OF THE NECK

Cysts of the neck are usually congenital and are generally classified as medial or thyroglossal and lateral or branchiogenic.

Medial Cysts (Thyroglossal Cysts)

Medial cysts, as their name implies, as a rule, arise in the midline of the neck close to the hyoid bone, to which they usually are attached. These cysts are generally considered to be derived from a remnant of the thyroglossal duct, which normally disappears between the sixth to eighth week of intrauterine life.

Clinical examination reveals a doughy swelling in close proximity to the hyoid bone. The swelling must be differentiated from other tumors that can arise in the same region, such as thyroid neoplasms, dermoid or sebaceous cysts, and various lesions of the lymph nodes.

Medial cysts are lined with squamous or columnar epithelium (Fig. 29–21*A*). Aspiration biopsy yields cell-free fluid or semisolid mucoid matter in about 25% of the cases. The nature of the aspirate and the palpatory findings are then helpful in distinguishing the lesion from an enlarged lymph node or a sebaceous cyst. However, the possibility of a thyroid lesion cannot be ruled out, since cystic fluid can often be aspirated from the latter (cf. p. 1271). Cellular aspirates, most often inflammatory cells with admixture of squamous cells and occasionally also with columnar epithelial cells, can be obtained from about 75% of the medial cysts of the

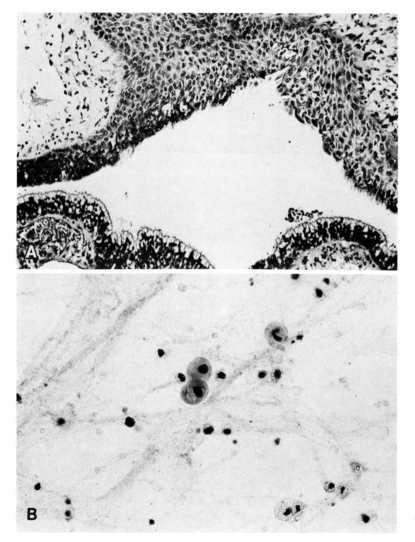

FIGURE 29–21. (*A*) Medial congenital cyst lined with mucus-producing epithelium (*bottom*) and with metaplastic squamous epithelia (*top*). (*B*) Needle aspirate from medial congenital cyst. Two metaplastic squamous epithelial cells are surrounded by inflammatory cells and mucous material. (*A* ×300; *B*, Papanicolaou stain ×300. Zajicek, J.: Aspiration Biopsy Cytology. Part I. Basel, S. Karger, 1974)

neck (see Fig. 29–21*B*). In these cases, cytologic recognition of the palpable swelling as a medial cyst should pose no problems.

Lateral Cysts (Branchial Cleft Cysts)

Lateral cysts of the neck generally appear at the level of the hyoid bone in a lateral position. As a rule, they are more or less covered by the anterior border of the sternomastoid muscle, but they can also occur above and below this position. The histogenesis of lateral cysts has been much discussed. The most widely accepted theory is that they are derived from the second branchial cleft.

The clinical diagnosis of lateral or branchiogenic cyst may be more difficult than that of medial cyst. Numerous other lesions of the same region (below the anterior border of the sternomastoid muscle) have to be taken into account. They include lymph node enlargement, carotid body tumors, lymphangiomas, salivary gland tumors, and lipomas.

The lining of lateral cysts usually consists of squamous epithelium, surrounded, in most cases, by lymphoid tissue. Needle aspirate consists of cell-free fluid in about 10% of the cases. In the other cases the aspirated fluid contains squamous cells (Fig. 29–22). The cell-free fluid is not diagnostic, as it may be also derived from a salivary gland tumor such as cystic pleomorphic adenomas, papillary cystadenolymphomas, mucoepidermoid carcinomas, lymphangiomas, and lymph node metastases of squamous cell or thyroid carcinomas. Consequently, the lesion should be reexamined after the fluid has been aspirated. If any palpable mass remains, it should be aspirated again. An aspiration of the periphery of the cystic mass is sometimes helpful. If there is any uncertainty at all, the lesion should be excised for histologic examination.

The aspirate is indicative of a branchial cyst only in the absence of atypia of squamous cells. *Even the slightest degree of nuclear atypia must trigger the possibility of a metastasis from a well-differentiated squamous cell carcinoma,* especially of the tonsil, floor of the mouth, tongue, or lip origin. Aspirates from lymph node metastases of these tumors occasionally contain squamous carcinoma cells with only trivial morphologic evidence of cancer (see also p. 1293).

It is not always possible, therefore, to distinguish on aspiration biopsy smears between squamous carcinoma cells and squamous cells from a branchiogenic cyst. In doubtful cases, a thorough clinical search must be made for a possible primary

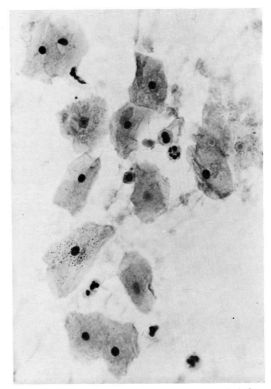

FIGURE 29–22. Smear of fluid from a brachial cleft cyst containing squamous epithelium without nuclear atypia. (Papanicolaou stain ×480)

squamous cell carcinoma before the neck lesion is removed for histologic examination.

THE CAROTID BODY

Tumors may develop from the carotid body (glomus caroticum), a chemoreceptor organ that is most often located on the median aspect of the internal carotid artery close to the carotid bifurcation. Because of the intimate relation of carotid body tumor to the carotid arteries, the arterial pulsations are sometimes transmitted through it and may be felt on palpation of the tumor. The tumor is mobile in the horizontal, but not in vertical, direction. It grows slowly, and the patient may have observed a lump in the neck for many years before seeking medical advice. Carotid body tumors, as a rule, are clinically benign. However, metastases to

(text continues on page 1268)

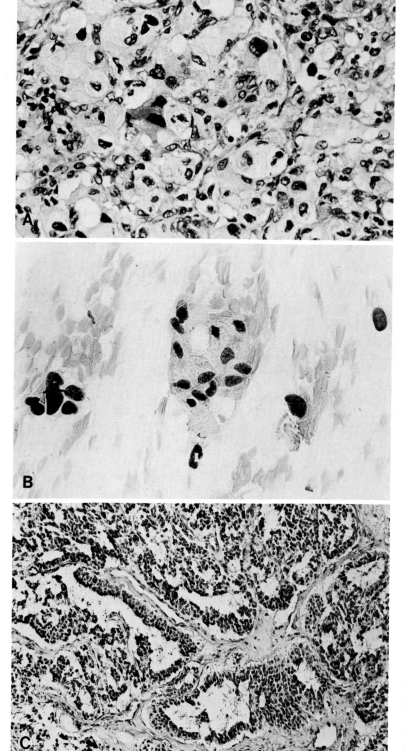

FIGURE 29–23. Carotid body tumors. (*A*) Carotid body, "usual type." Tissue section from an area with pronounced cellular polymorphism. (*B*) Needle aspirate from the same tumor as in (*A*), showing a "syncytium" and scattered cells with a pronounced nuclear polymorphism. (*C*) Carotid body, "adenoma-like" type. The general pattern and cellular morphology strikingly resemble epithelium. Tissue section.

(continued)

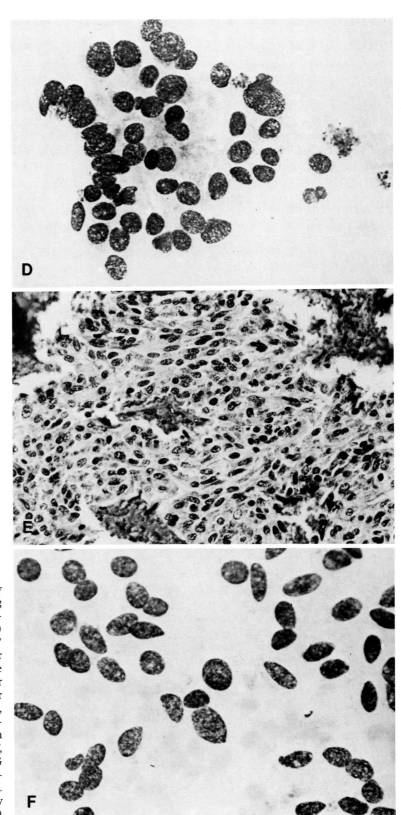

FIGURE 29–23 *(Continued).*
(*D*) Needle aspirate from carotid body tumor with a cell cluster mimicking acinar or follicular structures. Air-dried smear; same case as in (*C*). (*E*) Carotid body tumor, "angioma-like" type. Tissue section showing oval or spindle-shaped cells. (*F*) Needle aspirate from carotid body tumor shown in (*E*). The nuclei are oval or spindle-shaped. Air-dried smear. (*A*, Van Gieson stain ×300; *B*, Papanicolaou stain ×480; *C*, Van Gieson stain ×120; *D*, MGG stain ×600; *E*, Van Gieson stain ×300; *F*, MGG stain ×600. Engzell, U., et al.: Aspiration biopsy of tumours of the neck II. Findings in 13 cases of carotid body tumour. Acta Cytol., *15*:25–30, 1971)

regional lymph nodes and to distant organs may occur.

The aspiration of a carotid body tumor is not without dangers of syncope, paroxysmal hypertension, and bleeding from the richly vascularized tumor or from an inadvertently perforated carotid artery. Hence, if the diagnosis can be established clinically, a surgical removal, rather than an aspiration, should be planned.

Carotid body tumors mimic to a variable extent the histologic structure of the carotid body and can be classified histologically into three groups (LeCompte, 1948): *(1)* the common type, reproducing the normal structure (Fig. 29–23*A*); *(2)* the adenomalike type, with cells resembling epithelium (Fig. 29–23*C*); and *(3)* the angioma-like type, with spindle- or crescent-shaped cells mimicking endothelial cells (Fig. 29–23*E*).

Aspiration biopsy yields in some cases a drop of blood mixed with grossly detectable tissue fragments. In other cases, the aspirates yield mostly blood, with a few scattered small clusters of epithelial cells. The tumor cells have abundant cytoplasm and indistinct cellular borders. The cytoplasm often contains variable amounts of granules that take on a reddish tinge with MGG stain. Pronounced anisonucleosis is present and, in some cases, there are huge nuclei mimicking a highly malignant tumor (see Fig. 29–23*B*). The nuclei are usually round or ovoid, but may be of spindle or crescent shape. In about half of the cases the smears contain areas where the cells are arranged in acinic or follicular structures.

The presence of ovoid or spindle-shaped nuclei (see Fig. 29–23*F*) may result in an erroneous cytologic report of a medullary carcinoma of thyroid, a neurofibroma, or a neurofibrosarcoma. When this picture is seen in aspirate from a tumor of the carotid region, angiography should be performed. Carotid body tumor then characteristically appears as a richly vascularized tumor between the internal and the external carotid arteries.

If the smeared aspirate contains cells in acinic or follicular formations (see Fig. 29–23*D*), the cytologic picture may be mistaken for a metastasis from follicular carcinoma of the thyroid. In follicular carcinoma, however, the cells are more densely packed and the nuclei more uniform, polymorphism being absent as a rule. If the origin of the cells remains in doubt, a careful examination of the thyroid, including a scintiscan, should be performed. As mentioned above, carotid angiography or a CT scan is helpful in debatable situations.

THE THYROID

Normal Structure

The thyroid gland consists of two conical lobes connected anteriorly by the isthmus. A third, smaller central lobe, the pyramidal lobe, is frequently found. The gland is enclosed in a true capsule, which may adhere to the trachea and larynx. The thyroid is richly vascularized and has a high rate of blood flow, which may interfere with surgical biopsy.

The structural unit of the thyroid gland is the follicle, a closed, approximately spherical space lined with epithelial cells. These vary in size from low cuboidal or flat to high columnar. The height and the configuration of the thyroid follicular cells reflect, to some extent, the functional activity. The follicles are filled with colloid, a homogenous eosinophilic substance. Variations in the density and staining properties of the colloid can also be ascribed some functional significance; thin eosinophilic colloid appears to be associated with functional activity, whereas inactive follicles often contain thick eosinophilic colloid.

A number of biochemical tests and radioactive isotope-uptake studies are commonly used to determine the function of the gland. The most important indication for an aspiration biopsy is the so-called cold nodule (i.e., an area of the thyroid without uptake of the isotope).

Aspiration Biopsy Technique

Conventional excisional biopsy has never achieved significant popularity in the diagnosis of thyroid disorders. The essentially nontraumatic nature of thin-needle aspiration biopsy, therefore, has made it an attractive procedure for routine use. In more than 10,000 aspiration biopsies of the thyroid at Radiumhemmet, no untoward complications have arisen, apart from occasional hematomas, which caused no major discomfort (Löwhagen, 1974).

The aspiration is performed with the patient supine. To avoid inadvertent displacement of the gland during the biopsy, the patient is instructed to refrain from swallowing and speaking. Aspirate is always collected from different parts of the palpable gland. Since the thyroid is richly vascularized, the actual aspiration is performed as quickly as possible, in about 1 to 2 seconds, to avoid flooding the syringe with blood.

Because of the safety of aspiration biopsy of the thyroid, the maximum range of indicates becomes evident when the method has been adopted in clinics dealing with thyroid disorders. Virtually all nodular or enlarged thyroids will thus be referred for aspiration biopsy. When the diagnostic program also includes scintigraphic determination of radioactive iodine or other isotope uptake, the aspiration biopsy is usually performed after scintiscan. Immediate aspiration is also advocated by some observers. The cytologic examination helps to disclose the nature of scintigraphically visualized zones with reduced uptake of radioiodine. These "cold" areas are most frequently found to be the site of degenerative cystic changes in a nodular goiter or of carcinoma.

The principal lesions of the thyroid gland that may be identified in aspiration cytology are as follows:

Cysts
Colloid goiters
Thyroiditis
   Acute
   Subacute
   Lymphocytic (Hashimoto's disease)
   "Adenomas"
Carcinomas
   Follicular (see caveats)
   Papillary (and its variants)
   Medullary
   Anaplastic (large and small cell types)
Malignant lymphomas
Metastatic tumors

Cytology of Goiter

The terms *goiter* or *struma* denote any enlargement, which may be diffuse or nodular, of the thyroid gland. The three most common types are the colloid goiter, inflammatory goiter or thyroiditis, and neoplastic goiter caused by benign or malignant tumors.

Colloid Goiter

(Synonyms: *Adenomatous Goiter, Diffuse or Nodular Goiter, Endemic Goiter*)

Colloid goiter is usually due to hyperplasia of the thyroid gland induced by iodine deficiency. Its his-

tologic appearance varies with the developmental stage of the disease. In the early stages, the changes are mainly hyperplastic, with bilateral and diffuse enlargement of the gland made up of small follicles. Later on, some of the follicles may become distended and may coalesce to form nodules, with diameters ranging from less than 1 mm to several centimeters. There are often degenerative changes, such as hemorrhage, necrosis, and scar or cyst formation. Although the process usually involves the entire gland, it may occur focally and produce a solitary nodule. On the scintiscan such a change is often labeled a "cold nodule," which is difficult to distinguish from true neoplasm (Fig. 29–24).

The nature of a needle aspirate from colloid goiter depends on the type of the lesion. The aspirate may be solid, semisolid, or fluid. Solid or semisolid aspirate often consists of amber-colored colloid, which in MGG-stained smears appears bluish-violet and in Papanicolaou smears pink. The cytologic pattern is dominated by follicular cells, sometimes arranged in microfollicles. The follicular cells are small, usually cuboidal, with clear, usually scanty cytoplasm and small, compact, dark spherical nuclei without visible nucleoli. The follicular cells may be dispersed or form spherical clusters or flat sheets wherein the honeycomb-forming cytoplasmic borders may sometimes be recognized (Fig. 29–25). Naked follicular cell nuclei are often seen scattered throughout the smear. In posthemorrhagic nodules or cysts, numerous

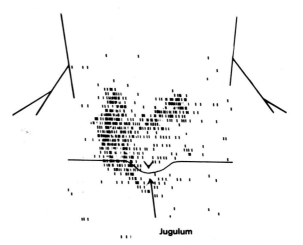

Jugulum

FIGURE 29–24. Scintigram showing areas of reduced radioiodine uptake (cold nodules) in left thyroid and isthmus. At aspiration biopsy 8 ml of cystic fluid was aspirated (cf. Fig. 29–26).

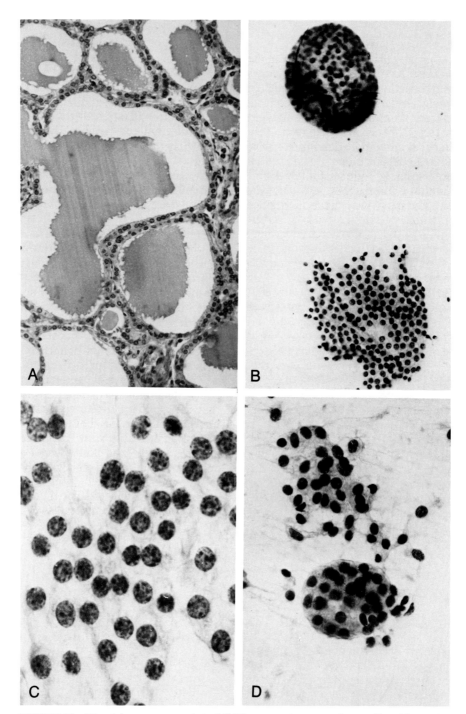

FIGURE 29–25. Adenomatous goiter. (*A*) Tissue section: note the small and large thyroid follicles. (*B–D*) Aspiration smears (fixed material, Papanicolaou stain) showing the characteristic cytologic presentation of benign thyroid disorders. (*B*) A three-dimensional round, sharply outlined cluster of follicular cells representing a whole squashed follicle (*top*) next to a flat sheet of similar cells (*bottom*). Note the monotonous size of the small nuclei. (*C*) High-power view of the sheet of follicular cells shown in (*B*). Although the delicate cytoplasm cannot be clearly seen in this photograph, the nuclei are fairly evenly spaced. Note the even nuclear size, slight granularity of chromatin, and tiny nucleoli or chromocenters. (*D*) A small, round cluster representing a squashed follicle, and a small sheet of follicular cells. Note the delicate cytoplasm and the minimal variability of the nuclei. (*A, B* ×200; *C* ×800; *D* ×400. Koss, L.G., et al.: Aspiration Biopsy. Cytologic Interpretation and Histologic Bases. New York, Igaku-Shoin, 1984, with permission)

macrophages may be observed next to follicular cells (Fig. 29–26).

A fairly high proportion of aspirations in colloid goiter yield cystic fluid. This fluid is sometimes clear and yellow, but most commonly, it is stained brown because of a prior hemorrhage. Such fluid in thyroid aspirates usually indicates degenerative cystic changes in a colloid goiter.

Colloid goiter is the lesion most commonly referred for aspiration biopsy: about 80% of needle aspirates from goiters show features described above.

Thyroiditis

In the *acute* form of thyroiditis, aspiration biopsy yields follicular cells, neutrophilic granulocytes, and macrophages. The clinical picture in these patients is swelling and tenderness of the thyroid gland. In *granulomatous* (subacute, de Quervain's) thyroiditis, the thyroid is slightly to moderately enlarged and there is tenderness on digital examination. The aspirates contain follicular epithelial cells, epithelioid cells, and giant cells of Langhans' type, together with lymphocytes, plasma cells, and some granulocytes (Fig. 29–27).

Lymphocytic thyroiditis or *Hashimoto's disease* is the most frequent form of thyroiditis observed in clinical practice. The disease most often affects women past the age of 40 and is thought to be a form of autoimmune disease. Antithyroid antibodies are often elevated in this condition and the thyroid function may be reduced. Both lobes of the thyroid are usually affected, diffusely enlarged, and firm. In histologic sections, the thyroid is infiltrated with lymphocytes that may also form lymph follicles with germinal centers. The acini are often destroyed or atrophic. A major component of the disease is the transformation of the follicular cells into oncocytes (Hürthle or Askanazy cells). The oncocytes may line glandular structures or form solid sheets of various sizes. The characteristic features of oncocytes, i.e., abundant, eosinophilic, granular cytoplasm and large, often pyknotic nuclei of variable sizes, are usually well seen in Hashimoto's disease.

The various components of the diseased thyroid are usually well represented in aspirated material. In some cases, the aspirates are dominated by lymphocytes of various levels of maturation, and the smear may resemble an aspirate of a hyperplastic lymph node. Further search will usually reveal the presence of oncocytes and scattered follicular cells in clusters (Fig. 29–28). In other cases, the presence of oncocytes is dominant. In aspirates, these large cells form sheets or glandlike structures. The striking, abundant, eosinophilic and granular cytoplasm and the variability in nuclear sizes are usually well seen in smears (Fig. 29–29). Sometimes the nuclei contain fairly large nucleoli. Because of nuclear abnormalities, these cells can be mistaken for malignant cells. On further search lymphocytes and follicular thyroid cells can be observed. On one occasion the follicular cells mimicked a papillary carcinoma (see below).

Thyroid carcinomas and malignant lymphomas may occur in Hashimoto's thyroiditis and their cytologic diagnosis may be exceedingly difficult. If either event is suspected a surgical biopsy should be suggested.

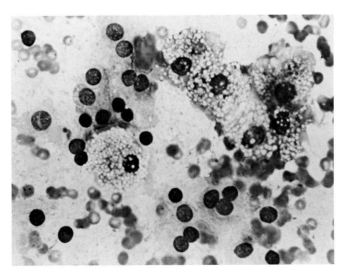

FIGURE 29–26. Benign thyroid cells and foamy macrophages aspirated from a degenerative cystic lesion in a cold nodule (see Fig. 29–24). (MGG stain ×430)

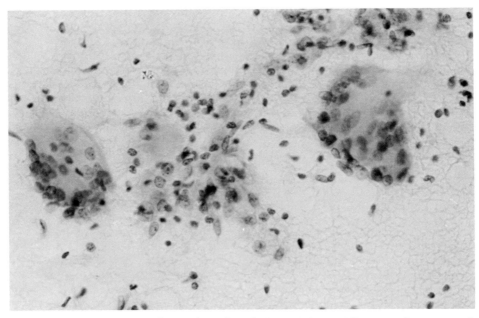

FIGURE 29–27. Aspirate in chronic thyroiditis, de Quervain's type. The smear shows two multinucleated giant cells and, in the *center*, a cluster of spindly, epithelioid cells. Scattered lymphocytes form the background of the smear. (×400. Courtesy of Prof. S. Woyke)

Neoplastic Lesions

Most early, nontoxic goiters are symmetric and of soft, somewhat elastic consistency. In their further development, they often become nodular. This sometimes starts with a solitary nodule arising from focal cystic degeneration or focal hyperplasia. Such a nodule, or *adenoma,* as it is still often called, cannot be reliably differentiated on clinical grounds from "true" adenoma or carcinoma.

The most significant contribution of needle aspiration biopsy of thyroid nodules is a *triage of patients,* separating those who require surgical removal from those who may be safely followed by clinical observations. While the cytologic differentiation of many of the benign nodules from carcinomas is feasible with the use of appropriate techniques, there remains a gray zone, particularly in reference to follicular tumors, where the cytologic techniques may fail. In spite of this limitation, data

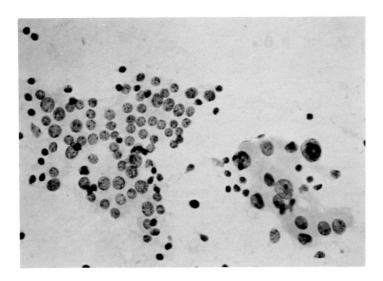

FIGURE 29–28. Smear of aspirate in lymphocytic thyroiditis (Hashimoto's disease). The three components of the smear may be noted: mature lymphocytes in the background and two varieties of epithelial cells: a cluster of normal follicular cells with vesicular nuclei and barely visible, clear cytoplasm (*left*); and a cluster of oncocytes (Hürthle cells; *right*). The latter have abundant, granular, eosinophilic cytoplasm; the nuclei of variable sizes contain visible nucleoli. Nuclear pyknosis is commonly seen in oncocytes (×350. Courtesy of Prof. S. Woyke)

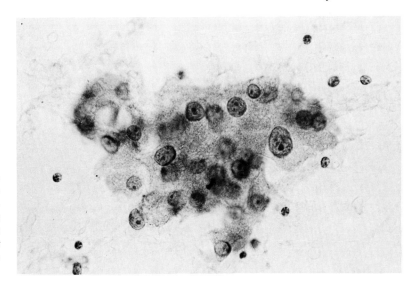

FIGURE 29-29. Chronic lymphocytic thyroiditis (Hashimoto's disease). A few lymphocytes surrounding a group of large oncocytes showing a finely granular cytoplasm and nuclei of variable sizes. Fairly large nucleoli may be noted. (Papanicolaou stain ×480)

accumulated from many institutions, including our own, strongly suggest that the aspiration biopsy technique does contribute in a meaningful way to the preoperative triage. Statistical evidence strongly suggests that by the use of aspiration biopsy the total number of thyroidectomies is significantly reduced, whereas the proportion of carcinomas in the treated population increases significantly (for further discussion of results see below).

As a general rule, smears from nonneoplastic nodules contain much colloid and few cells. In aspirates from neoplastic lesions, by contrast, there is little colloid and the cellularity is high. Still, there are many cases in which this distinction does not apply.

Benign Neoplasms. Follicular adenoma and oncocytic tumors are the most common benign neoplasms of the thyroid gland.

Oncocytic tumors (synonyms: oxyphilic adenoma, Hürthle cell tumor) consist of oncocytes that often show pronounced anisonucleosis with enlarged nucleoli. Their abundant cytoplasm contains eosinophilic granules (Fig. 29-30). These are tumors of uncertain prognosis, which are capable of recurrence and metastases. They should be treated by surgical excision.

In *follicular adenomas* the cells are arranged in follicular structures (Fig. 29-31). Single follicle-lining cells and naked nuclei are also scattered throughout the smear. Anisonucleosis may be

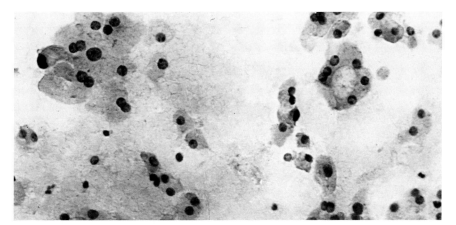

FIGURE 29-30. Aspirate of a Hürthle cell tumor (oncocytic tumor): The smear pattern is dominated by clusters, sheets, and dispersed single oncocytes. The cells are large, with a sharply demarcated, eosinophilic cytoplasm and dark spherical nuclei of uneven sizes. Future behavior cannot be ascertained from the cytologic or histologic appearance of the tumor: some of them will metastasize. (×400)

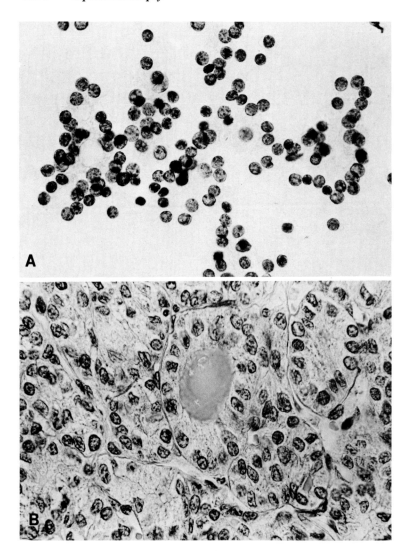

FIGURE 29–31. Follicular adenoma. (*A*) Needle aspirate. Monomorphic neoplastic cells in more-or-less well-preserved follicular formation. (*B*) Tissue-section from the same case. (*A*, Papanicolaou stain ×480; *B* ×480. Zajicek, J.: Aspiration Biopsy Cytology. Part I. Basel, S. Karger, 1974)

present. The nuclear chromatin is uniformly distributed, and the nucleoli are barely visible. It must remembered that a well-differentiated follicular carcinoma may have a very similar cytologic presentation in an aspiration biopsy smear. In such cases, the cytologic diagnosis should, therefore, be "follicular neoplasm or tumor," clearly stating that for a reliable differential diagnosis between follicular adenoma and a low-grade follicular carcinoma, histologic examination is mandatory.

Carcinomas. Thyroid carcinomas are usually classified as follicular, papillary, medullary, anaplastic giant cell (spindle and giant cell), and anaplastic small cell carcinomas.

Follicular Carcinomas. Aspiration biopsy smears from follicular carcinomas are usually highly cellular with little or no colloid. The cells occur singly or in clusters and are often arranged in follicle-like structures. In well-differentiated follicular carcinoma, cellular atypia may be minimal, and the general impression from the smear may suggest a benign event, rather than a carcinoma. In less well-differentiated forms, nuclear atypia is present (Fig. 29–32).

Particularly valuable, in our hands, has been the presence of prominent, large nucleoli within the follicular cells (see Fig. 29–32*B*, *C*). In such cases, the cytologic diagnosis of follicular carcinoma is justified. To be sure, the lesion may be encapsu-

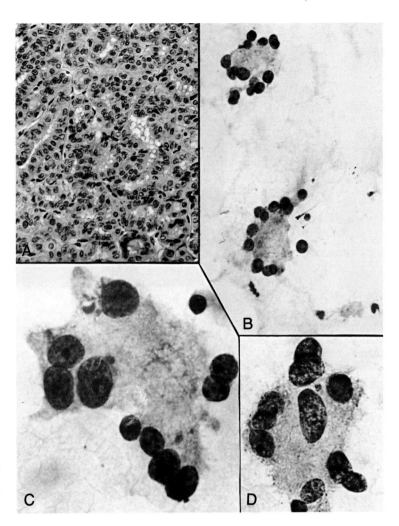

FIGURE 29-32. Poorly differentiated follicular carcinoma of thyroid. (*A*) Histologic appearance of tumor; (*B, C, D*) aspirate. (*B*) The tumor cells form follicle or rosette-like structures around a core of colloid material. Higher magnification of these cells (*C, D*) shows distinctly hyperchromatic, coarsely granular nuclei with visible, large nucleoli. (*A, B* ×200; *C, D* ×800. Koss, L.G., et al.: Aspiration Biopsy. Cytologic Interpretation and Histologic Bases. New York, Igaku-Shoin, 1984, with permission)

lated and the histologic classification may vary between "atypical follicular adenoma" and "follicular carcinoma without invasion," depending on the preference of the pathologist. Still, in at least some of these cases, recurrent or even metastatic tumor may be observed, sometimes many years after the removal of the primary. Because the metastatic lesions may show formation of follicles with colloid, the term *benign metastasizing struma* has been used in the past to describe such events.

Unfortunately, DNA measurements do not provide any diagnostic help. It has been shown that some of the follicular adenomas may be aneuploid and some of the follicular carcinomas diploid (Greenbaum et al., 1985).

Papillary Carcinomas. This group of tumors may have an unusual clinical presentation. Al-

though, in most instances, a primary "cold" nodule is observed in the thyroid (Fig. 29-33), the first clinical manifestation of the tumor may be a metastasis to a lymph node of the neck from a small, occult primary tumor. The faulty term "lateral aberrant thyroid" has been sometimes used in the past to describe these situations.

There are several variants of the papillary carcinoma, including the follicular variant (papillary and follicular carcinoma), which may focally mimic follicular carcinoma, except for the presence of the characteristic "ground-glass," opaque nuclei (see Fig. 26-48). Other interesting features of these tumors include cystic presentation, the presence of psammoma bodies, and the presence of intranuclear cytoplasmic inclusions (nuclear holes) in a variable proportion of the cells. This last feature may also be observed in other types of thy-

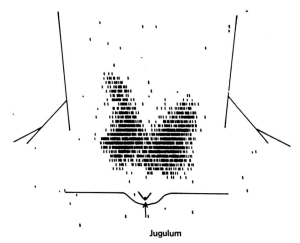

Jugulum

FIGURE 29–33. Scintigram showing area of reduced radioiodine uptake (cold nodule) in right thyroid. Aspiration biopsy revealed a papillary thyroid carcinoma (cf. Fig. 29–34).

roid cancer and in other tumors such as malignant melanomas and bronchioloalveolar carcinomas (see pp. 800 and 1167).

Needles aspirates from papillary carcinomas are usually rich in cells. The cells may be arranged in follicular structures, in papillary fragments, or in monolayered sheets.

In general, the degree of nuclear abnormality in cancer cells is slight. Still, the diagnosis can be made securely on other evidence. The presence of multilayered papillary sheets or clusters is diagnostic of the tumor (Figs. 29–34 and 29–35A). Other characteristic cytologic features of note include nuclear folds or grooves in finely granulated, opaque nuclei of follicular cells (see Fig. 29–35B) and calcified psammoma bodies (see Fig. 29–35C). It must be noted, though, that calcified structures mimicking psammoma bodies may sometimes occur in benign thyroids as well. The in-

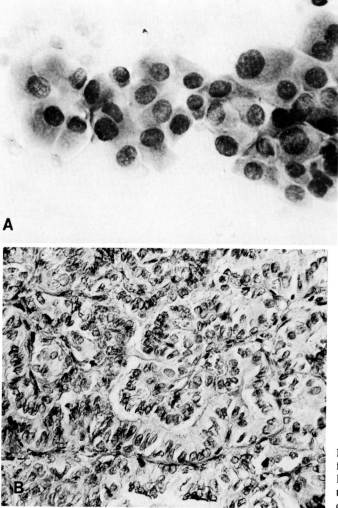

FIGURE 29–34. (*A*) Aspiration biopsy smear from a cold nodule (see Fig. 29–33). Solid papillary plug of thyroid carcinoma. (*B*) Tissue section from a papillary thyroid carcinoma, same case. (*A*, MGG stain ×430; *B* ×300)

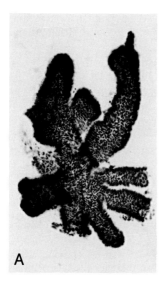

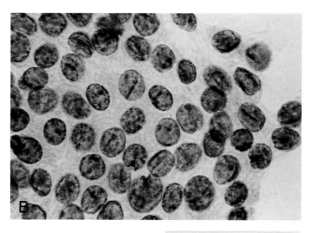

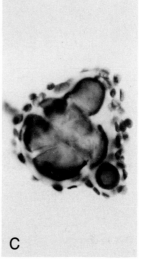

FIGURE 29–35. Various cytologic aspects of papillary carcinomas of the thyroid in aspiration smears. (*A*) A fragment of tumor with papillary configuration, diagnostic of the disease. (*B*) A sheet of follicular cells with opaque nuclei showing nuclear folds or grooves. (*C*) Psammoma bodies with a few follicular cells at the periphery (*A* ×100; *B, C* ×400. Courtesy of Prof. S. Woyke)

tranuclear cytoplasmic inclusions, which are not unique to papillary carcinoma (see above), are often conspicuous (Fig. 29–36) and helpful in the diagnosis when other features are absent or not persuasive. Lymphocytes, foam cells, multinucleated giant cells, and squamous epithelial cells showing degenerative changes are commonly found in aspirates from papillary carcinoma.

On one occasion papillary clusters of follicular cells, suggestive of papillary carcinoma, were observed in an aspirate of chronic lymphocytic thyroiditis (Hashimoto). No evidence of cancer could be found in completely processed thyroid tissue. The source of the papillary clusters was probably atypical follicular cells. Fortunately, such events are very rare.

Medullary Carcinomas. Medullary carcinomas of the thyroid are derived from calcito-nin-secreting C cells and belong to the group of endocrine neoplasms with secretory cytoplasmic granules (see Fig. 1–20). The tumors may occur as a component of a multiple endocrine neoplasia (MEN) syndrome, with synchronous tumors of other endocrine organs, such as pheochromocytomas of adrenal medulla, parathyroid adenomas, etc.

The histologic appearance of the tumor may vary: nests or sheets of polygonal or spindly cells surrounded by a network of capillaries are commonly observed. Formation of amyloid may be conspicuous. The cytologic presentation in aspiration biopsies is fairly characteristic. The smears are cellular, and the large, epithelial cells are usually dispersed. The cytoplasm is abundant, of variable shape, and faintly granular in fixed material, but may show conspicuous red granules in air-dried MGG-stained smears (Fig. 29–37). The nuclei are

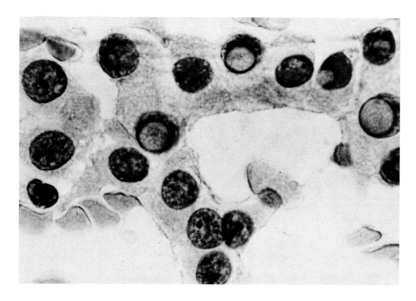

FIGURE 29–36. Needle aspirate from papillary carcinoma. Carcinoma cells exhibiting intranuclear cytoplasmic inclusions (pseudonucleoli). (Papanicolaou stain ×1,200. Zajicek, J.: Aspiration Biopsy Cytology, Part I. Bassel, S. Karger, 1974)

large, atypical, provided with nucleoli, and often eccentric, a feature common to many endocrine tumors. Tumor variants composed wholly or in part of spindly, elongated cells or of small cancer cells must also be recognized. The latter may be mistaken for a malignant lymphoma. An amorphous substance, amyloid, can be observed extracellularly in MGG-stained, air-dried smears.

Anaplastic Carcinomas. These highly malignant, rapidly growing tumors occur in two forms: a spindle and giant cell carcinoma and a small-cell–type carcinoma. The question of appropriate classification of small-cell carcinomas has been repeatedly raised. The possibility that some of these tumors are exceptionally aggressive malignant lymphomas or small-cell medullary carcinomas cannot be ruled out.

Smears of aspirate from anaplastic giant cell carcinoma usually contain necrotic matter, cell debris, inflammatory cells (mainly granulocytes), and large polymorphous, often multinucleated, cells with bizarre nuclei and very prominent nucleoli (Fig. 29–38). These tumors should not be confused with the exceedingly rare carcinomas with giant cells, mimicking the giant cell tumors of bone.

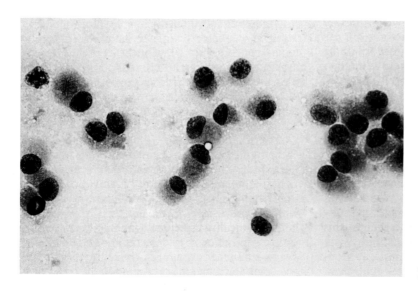

FIGURE 29–37. Needle aspirate from a medullary carcinoma of thyroid. Dissociated cells with moderate variation in the size of eccentric large nuclei. The cytoplasm is granulated. Air-dried smear. (MGG stain ×480)

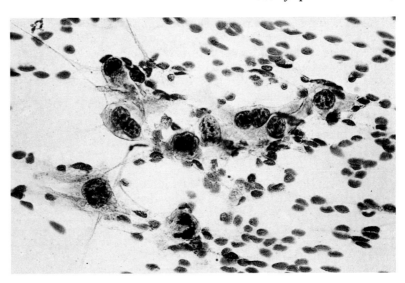

FIGURE 29–38. Needle aspirate from an anaplastic carcinoma of thyroid. Malignant cells with marked variation in size and nuclear abnormalities. (Papanicolaou stain ×480)

In *small-cell anaplastic carcinoma* the aspirate contains malignant cells, with round or oval nuclei and scanty cytoplasm. A point to be noted is that, in tissue sections, small-cell anaplastic carcinoma may be difficult to distinguish from malignant lymphoma. This may give rise to discrepancies between histologic and cytologic reports of this tumor.

Other Malignant Tumors. Malignant lymphomas may be primary in the thyroid, particularly in patients with Hashimoto's thyroiditis. The cytologic presentation of these uncommon tumors is complicated by the synchronous presence of epithelial components. Immune typing of such tumors is diagnostically helpful (Tani et al., 1989).

Metastatic tumors may also involve the thyroid, among them mammary and renal carcinomas. The latter may be composed of elongated, spindly cells and, thus, mimic a sarcoma or a medullary carcinoma.

Efficacy of Thyroid Aspirates

There are few reported series of thyroid aspirates wherein errors of omission or commission have not been made. Thus, the principal role of thyroid aspirates is to triage the common thyroid nodules into those that require surgery and those that may be kept under medical surveillance. In general, this goal has been achieved in most institutions with adequate experience. To give an example, at Montefiore Medical Center, the rate of malignant tumors in thyroid surgery rose from 11% for the years 1974 to 1977 to 31% for the years 1979 to 1981, the latter data reflecting the triage by preoperative aspiration. Similar results were reported from other institutions.

THE LYMPH NODES

Aspiration biopsy of lymph nodes represents perhaps the oldest application of this technique, and there is an extensive literature on this subject. Lymph nodes in every accessible location may be so examined. However, lymph nodes in the head and neck area are, by choice, the most frequent targets of aspiration biopsies.

Since palpable swellings of the neck are readily accessible to surgical exploration, one could assume that there is little need for aspiration biopsy in this region. It is a common experience, however, that once aspiration biopsy becomes a routine diagnostic procedure, the aspirates from lesions of the neck form a significant part of the cytologist's daily work.

The information obtainable from aspiration biopsy of the neck depends on the clinical history. In patients with known primary cancer, the aim is to identify local or distant metastases. In patients with no previously proved cancer, but with enlarged, clinically suspicious lymph nodes, the cytologic examination may determine whether the lesion is a malignant lymphoma or a metastasis from an occult primary tumor. Even when the presumptive clinical impression is lymphadenitis, the clinician may wish to have this diagnosis confirmed.

To obtain an idea of the types of neck lesions studied by aspiration biopsy, 1,245 consecutive cases were reviewed (Zajicek et al., 1967). Thyroid and submandibular gland aspiration biopsies are not included in this figure. In 1,200 cases (96%) the lesion was an enlarged lymph node. The remaining 45 cases included 18 branchial cleft cysts, 2 carotid body tumors, lipomas, and epidermoid inclusion cysts.

The diagnostic results from 1,200 lymph node aspirations are summarized in Fig. 29–39. Benign lymphadenitis was found in about 52% of this series, malignant lymphoma in 10%, and metastatic carcinoma in 38%. The fact that only 305 of the 1,200 patients were subsequently operated on suggests that the aspiration biopsy may have prevented a large number of unnecessary surgical procedures.

Lymph Node Structure

The general structure of lymph node is schematically illustrated in Fig. 29–40. Trabeculae of connective tissue, which extend from the capsule into the substance of the node, provide support and carry blood vessels. In the peripheral (cortical) portions of the nodes there are nodules (follicles) of densely packed lymphocytes (primary nodules or primary follicles). Some of the nodules (Fig. 29–41A) have a pale-stained germinal center.

Between the follicles in the cortical portion and the central (medullary) portion of the lymph node lies diffuse lymphoid tissue—the pulp. In the med-

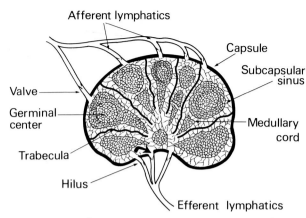

FIGURE 29–40. Diagrammatic representation of the structure of a lymph node.

ullary portion, the pulp is arranged in elongated cords—the medullary cords.

Within recent years much has been learned about the make-up and function of the cells composing the lymph nodes (see Chap. 3). The principal findings pertain to the sequence of events in transformation of lymphocytes and their impact on the understanding of the immune function, and, in the context of this chapter, on classification of malignant lymphomas.

The two principal families of lymphocytes are the B and T cells. Contrary to prior assumptions that the circulating lymphocytes with the well-known compact, spherical nuclei, represent the final step in lymphocyte differentiation, these are, in fact, precursor cells of a series of transformations, many of them taking place in the germinal

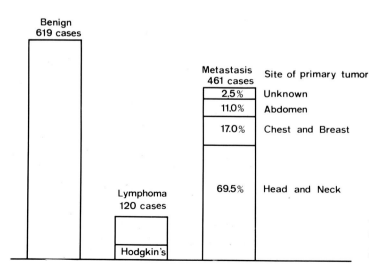

FIGURE 29–39. Cytologic findings in 1,200 consecutive aspiration biopsies of lymph nodes of the neck. (Zajicek, J., et al.: Aspiration biopsy of lymph nodes in diagnosis and research. *In* Rüttimann, A. [ed.]: Progress in Lymphology. Stuttgart, Georg Thieme, 1967)

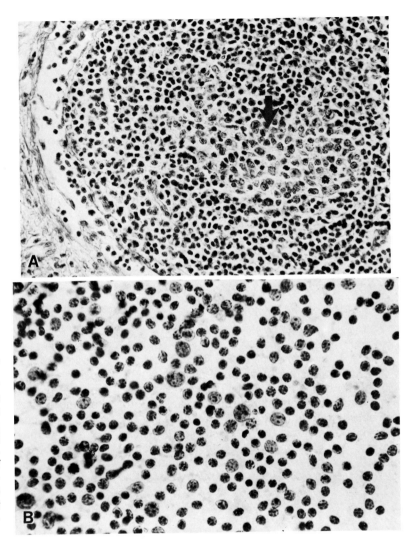

FIGURE 29-41. Lymphadenitis. (*A*) Tissue section from a lymph node with chronic lymphadenitis. The capsule and dilated subcapsular sinuses are seen on the *left*. In the center (*arrow*) is a lymph follicle with a germinal center. The germinal center is surrounded by small- and medium-sized lymphocytes. (*B*) Aspirate smear from a lymph node of the neck with a picture of lymphadenitis. Small lymphocytes, large lymphocytes, and follicle center cells are shown. (*A* ×120; *B*, air-dried smear, MGG stain ×480)

centers of lymph nodes. The sequence, as defined by Lukes and Collins, is as follows:

Small lymphocytes
↓
Small lymphocytes with indented nucleus (small, cleaved cells)
↓
Large lymphocytes with indented nucleus (large, cleaved cells)
↓
Large lymphocytes with noncleaved nucleus
↓
Large cells with prominent nucleoli (immunoblasts)

This sequence of events is the basis of the current classification of malignant lymphomas of non-Hodgkin's type.

It is quite evident from this brief description that the cell population in the lymph follicles is quite variable in reference to cell sizes and configuration. For practical purposes, all the stages of benign lymphocyte transformation may be considered as *follicle center cells.* The lymph nodes also contain cells with phagocytic properties (macrophages) which, when activated and containing fragments of phagocytosed material, are designated as *tingible body macrophages.* Dendritic reticulum cells, nonphagocytic cells of unknown significance, are also observed in lymph nodes.

The following principal lesions of the lymph nodes may be identified in aspiration biopsy:

Hyperplasia (including AIDS-related syndrome)
Granulomatous inflammation
Non-Hodgkin's lymphomas and their subgroups
  (see text)
Hodgkin's disease
Metastatic cancer

Hyperplasia of Lymph Nodes

Hyperplasia is a nonspecific reaction to a broad variety of causative agents, including AIDS-related syndrome, resulting in enlargement of lymph nodes and their lymph follicles. The aspiration smears in this condition are characterized by the presence of lymphocytes and a broad variety of transformed cells, ranging from small, cleaved lymphocytes to a few large immunoblasts. Tingible body macrophages and plasma cells are commonly present. This variegated cytologic picture is characteristic of hyperplastic lymph nodes resulting from inflammation (lymphadenitis) or other causes (Figs. 29–41B, 29–42, and 29–43). In acute lymphadenitis a major component of granulocytes is usually present.

In *infectious mononucleosis* numerous immunoblasts are seen. Immunoblasts are also plentiful in *toxoplasmosis,* wherein epithelioid cells and enlarged macrophages with prominent nucleoli can also be observed. In *tuberculosis* and *sarcoidosis* the dominant features are clusters of epithelioid cells and sometimes multinucleated giant cells. Necrotic material in a smear showing evidence of

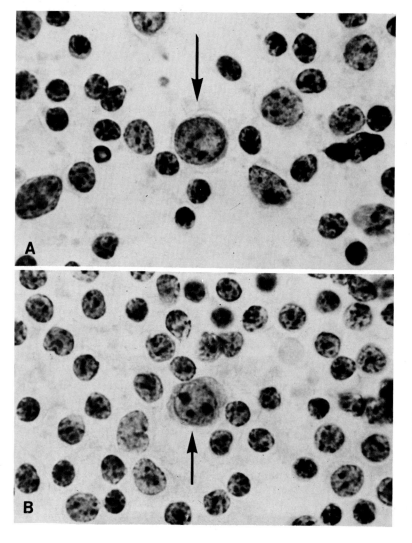

FIGURE 29–42. Needle aspirates from hyperplastic lymph nodes. A large noncleaved cell (*arrow, A*) and an immunoblast (*arrow, B*) are surrounded by lymphocytes in various stages of transformation. (Papanicolaou stain *A, B* ×1,000. Zajicek, J.: Aspiration Biopsy Cytology, Part I. Basel, S. Karger, 1974)

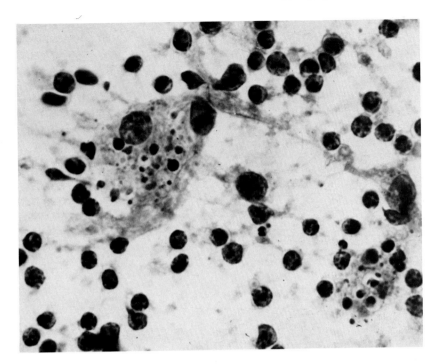

FIGURE 29–43. Hyperplastic lymph node. Large, tingible body macrophages containing phagocytized cell debris are surrounded by lymphocytes in various stages of transformation. (×900. Modified from Koss, L.G., et al.: Aspiration Biopsy. Cytologic Interpretation and Histologic Bases. New York, Igaku-Shoin, 1984, with permission)

granulomatous inflammation is suggestive of tuberculosis (see Fig. 19–56). However, such patterns of smears, with cell detritus, may also be observed in metastatic carcinomas, especially of squamous cell type.

Malignant Lymphomas

This group of diseases has attracted much attention and scientific effort, out of proportion to the frequency of these disorders, which constitute no more than 5% of all human cancers. There are several reasons for this: the malignant lymphomas are treatable, and many are curable; the diseases lend themselves to cytogenetic observations and molecular biologic observations that have enhanced our knowledge of events in human cancer; new classifications of many of these disorders have been proposed in keeping with the current concepts of immunology.

The principal subdivision of malignant lymphomas is into two categories: non-Hodgkin's lymphoma and Hodgkin's disease. In each category, there are several subgroups, with the grouping based in part on immunologic data and in part on morphology. Regardless of classification, all malignant lymphomas have a common denominator: the diseases affect primarily lymph nodes and cause their enlargement. Much less commonly malignant lymphomas occur in lymphoid tissue in other organs. Enlarged lymph nodes lend themselves to an aspiration biopsy; hence, the recognition of this group of diseases in aspirated material is of practical value.

The task is not easy and is complicated by the subdivision of malignant lymphomas into many groupings. It is questionable whether a precise classification of malignant lymphomas can be achieved in the aspirated sample, although, with the addition of the immunologic techniques, at least an attempt in this direction can be made. The important primary question—What is the cause of the lymph node enlargement? Is it a benign process, a metastatic cancer, or is it a primary malignant lymphoma?—can be answered in most instances. The answer can be provided rapidly and therein lies the value of the aspiration biopsy of enlarged lymph nodes.

Non-Hodgkin's Lymphomas

The main subdivision of this group of diseases is based on the recognition of B- and T-type lymphocytes (see Chap. 3). A further subdivision is based on preservation of follicles (follicular lymphoma), or their destruction (diffuse lymphoma). Within each group, there are many variants that have been repeatedly classified over the last 30 years, notably by Rappaport, by Lukes and Collins, and by Lennert (Kiel classification). The new classifications were based on the sequence of events in lymphocyte activation (see p. 1281). The simplest and most practical classification is that provided by a study group sponsored by the National Cancer Institute (United States), which divides non-Hodgkin's lymphomas into three major groups, based on prognosis, as follows:

Low-Grade (Best Prognosis)
Small lymphocytic, plasmacytoid, follicular mixed (small and large cleaved cells)

Intermediate-Grade (Intermediate Prognosis)
Follicular, predominantly large cell
Diffuse, small cleaved cells
Diffuse, small and large cells
Diffuse, large cells (cleaved or noncleaved)

High-Grade (Poor Prognosis)
Large cell, immunoblastic
Lymphoblastic
Small, noncleaved cells
Burkitt's lymphoma

From the point of view of the aspiration biopsy, there are several principles in the recognition of non-Hodgkin's lymphomas:

1. The cell population in the smear can be recognized as being of lymphocytic derivation and is monotonous, or at least significantly less heterogeneous than that derived from hyperplastic lymph nodes.
2. The cells lie singly, or at least do not form conspicuous sheets or groupings, characteristic of epithelial cancers.
3. The cells show features consistent with a malignant lymphoma; these features depend on the degree of maturation and differentiation and differ considerably from one type of lymphoma to another.

If these three features are not observed or cannot be recognized in the cytologic preparation, the diagnosis of a malignant lymphoma, non-Hodgkin's type, cannot be made with any degree of certainty. There are situations in which a large cell type of a malignant lymphoma may mimic a metastatic carcinoma and vice versa. Immunocytochemistry may be helpful in such cases. The presence

of keratin filaments will be in favor of a carcinoma, whereas the expression of the common lymphocyte antigen will favor a lymphoma. For further discussion of immunocytochemistry, see Chapter 34.

Small-Cell Lymphomas. The characteristic features of the small-cell lymphoma in aspirates are as follows:

1. The tumor cells are dispersed, forming very few, if any, small clusters.
2. The cell population is monotonous.
3. The tumor cells resemble lymphocytes by virtue of generally spherical shape and usually scanty rim of basophilic cytoplasm. The size of the tumor cells is from 1½ to twice the size of normal inactive lymphocytes. Hence, the term *small* is used only in relation to other forms of lymphoma.
4. The nuclei also differ from the compact nuclei of normal lymphocytes: they are vesicular and quite often contain coarse clumps of chromatin (see *cellules grumelées*, p. 1160). Small nucleoli are often present.
5. Spontaneous karyorrhexis occurs with a fair frequency in tumors of this type. In the absence of prior treatment or other causes such as a trauma, this phenomenon is strongly suggestive of a lymphoma, even in the absence of classic morphology (see Fig. 26–54).

There are nuclear and cytoplasmic features in the tumor cells that allow further classification of this group of tumors.

Lymphocytic Lymphoma, Diffuse. Tumor cells and their nuclei are approximately spherical with no indentation (Fig. 29–44). Granularity of nuclear chromatin (cellules grumelées or "lumpy cells", see p. 1160) is a common feature. Identical findings may occur in chronic lymphocytic leukemias. The prognosis is good.

Plasmacytoid Lymphoma. The tumor cells are slightly larger. The nucleus is eccentric and the chromatin is arranged in a cartwheel pattern (Fig. 29–45). The prognosis is good.

Cleaved Cells, Diffuse Small-Cell Lymphoma. The tumor cells are usually somewhat larger, and the cell population is less monotonous. The nuclei show a cleavage or a crease, characteristic of this type of lymphoma (Fig. 29–46). The prognosis is fair, but the outcome is guarded.

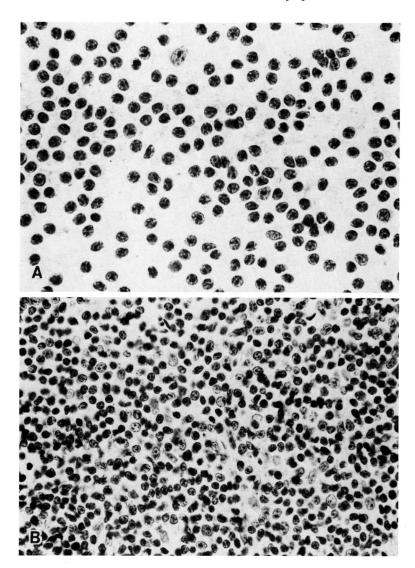

FIGURE 29–44. Small-cell lymphocytic lymphoma: (*A*) Needle aspirate. The smear is composed of monotonous small tumor cells with granular chromatin pattern, but without any obvious malignant features. (*B*) Tissue section. (*A*, Papanicolaou stain ×480; *B* ×480)

FIGURE 29–45. Plasmocytoid small-cell lymphoma, aspiration smear. The small tumor cells have eccentric nuclei with prominent chromatin granules ("lumpy cells"), occasionally symmetrically distributed at the nuclear rim, hence, forming the cartwheel pattern (*arrows*). (×900. Modified from Koss, L.G., et al.: Aspiration Biopsy. Cytologic Interpretation and Histologic Bases. New York, Igaku-Shoin, 1984, with permission)

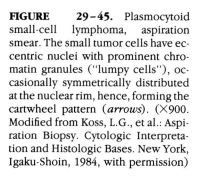

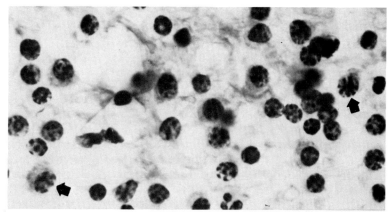

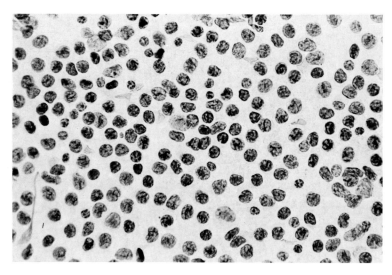

FIGURE 29–46. Needle aspirate from a small-cell, cleaved cell lymphoma. The nuclei show the characteristic creases or cleavage. (Papanicolaou stain ×480)

Large-Cell Lymphomas. The characteristic features of large-cell lymphomas in aspirates are as follows:

1. The tumor cells are dispersed, forming few clusters, although in improperly prepared smears clumping may occur.
2. The cell population is monotonous.
3. The cells are four to ten times larger than normal lymphocytes.
4. The amount of cytoplasm varies. In some cases, the tumor cells show only a narrow rim of basophilic cytoplasm; in other cases, the cytoplasm may be abundant.
5. The nuclei, on the whole, show unmistakable evidence of a malignant tumor: hyperchromasia, and large and multiple nucleoli. Bizarre nuclear shapes are common, with tongues of chromatin protruding from the nuclear contour.

Non–Cleaved-Cell Lymphoma. There is a monotonous population of large tumor cells with a narrow rim of cytoplasm and large hyperchromatic, coarsely granular nuclei provided with single or multiple nucleoli. The latter are not well visualized in air-dried, MGG-stained smears (Fig. 29–47), but are usually prominent in fixed, Papanicolaou-stained smears (Fig. 29–48).

Burkitt's Lymphoma. The smears usually contain an abundant population of noncleaved large lymphoma cells, accompanied by tingible body macrophages (Fig. 29–49*A*), corresponding to the "starry sky" pattern seen in the corresponding tissue sections (see Fig. 29–49*B*).

Large, Cleaved Cell–Type Lymphoma ("Reticulum Cell Sarcoma"). The highly malignant lymphoma is composed of large cells often provided with a significant amount of cytoplasm, and oddly shaped, large nuclei, with large or very large nucleoli (Figs. 29–50 and 29–51). It is not unusual for this type of tumor to be confused with metastatic carcinoma, requiring immunocytologic workup (see Chap. 34).

T-Cell Lymphomas. Most T-cell lymphomas cannot be differentiated morphologically from B-cell lymphomas. Occasionally, however, the T-cell derivation may be suggested in large-cell lymphomas showing a bizarre lobulation of nuclei (Fig. 29–52) or a peculiar cerebriform arrangement of chromatin, best seen in air-dried smears stained with MGG. The latter is characteristically observed in disseminated mycosis fungoides, a T-cell lymphoma of the skin (Fig. 29–53).

Ki-1 Lymphoma. A subgroup of large-cell malignant lymphomas, mostly of T-cell derivation, has been identified within recent years because of their reactivity with Ki-1 antibody. The antibody, originally developed as a marker for Hodgkin's disease, is expressed in large, bizarre, often multinucleated malignant cells with abundant cytoplasm that may mimic to perfection large-cell anaplastic carcinomas (Agnorsson and Kadin, 1988; Tani et al., 1989). The tumor, which is usually but not always keratin negative, can be confidently identified only by its reaction with Ki-1 antibody. The prognosis is poor.

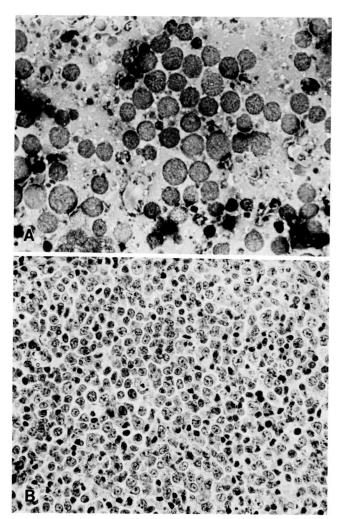

FIGURE 29–47. Noncleaved, lymphoblastic lymphoma: (*A*) Aspirate smear from a malignant lymphoma with monomorphic tumor cell population. Air-dried smear. (*B*) Tissue section of the lymph node with malignant lymphoma shown in (*A*). (*A*, MGG stain ×480; *B* ×300)

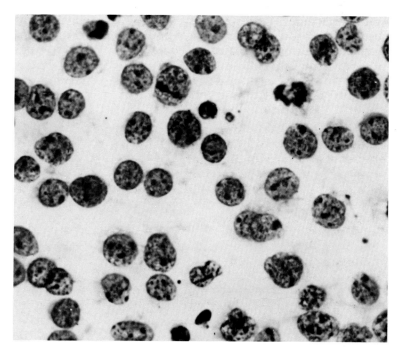

FIGURE 29–48. Aspirate of a noncleaved, large-cell lymphoblastic lymphoma, fixed preparation stained with Papanicolaou stain. Note the coarse granularity of the nuclei and the large, often multiple, and comma-shaped nucleoli. (×900. Modified from Koss, L.G., et al.: Aspiration Biopsy. Cytologic Interpretation and Histologic Bases. New York, Igaku-Shoin, 1984, with permission)

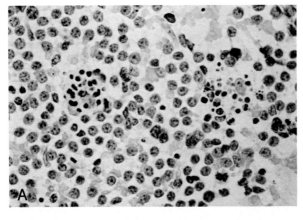

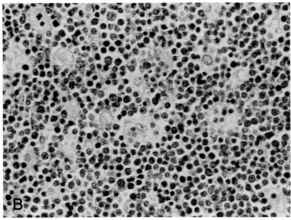

FIGURE 29-49. Burkitt's lymphoma, aspiration smear and tissue section. (*A*) Aspiration smear showing a large-cell noncleaved cell lymphoma and two tingible body macrophages. (*B*) The corresponding tissue section showing the characteristic "starry-sky" patterns in the lymph node. (*A* ×450; *B* ×300. Courtesy of Prof. S. Woyke)

Histiocytic Lymphoma. Until some years ago, many of the large-cell B-cell and T-cell lymphomas were thought to be of histiocytic origin. As a consequence of immunologic studies, these histiocytic lymphomas are now considered to be rare. Their characteristic feature is erythrophagocytosis by large, often bizarre tumor cells with vacuolated abundant cytoplasm. Alpha-1-antitripsin immunostaining may be positive (Tani et al., 1988). For further comments on cytologic presentation of

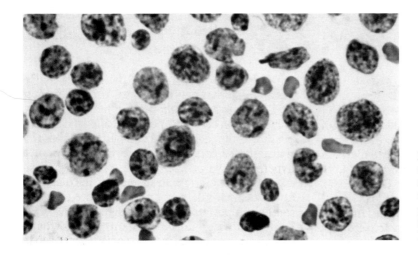

FIGURE 29-50. Large, cleaved cell malignant lymphoma. The nuclei show creases, indentations, and protrusions. (×900. Koss, L.G., et al.: Aspiration Biopsy. Cytologic Interpretation and Histologic Bases. New York, Igaku-Shoin, 1984, with permission)

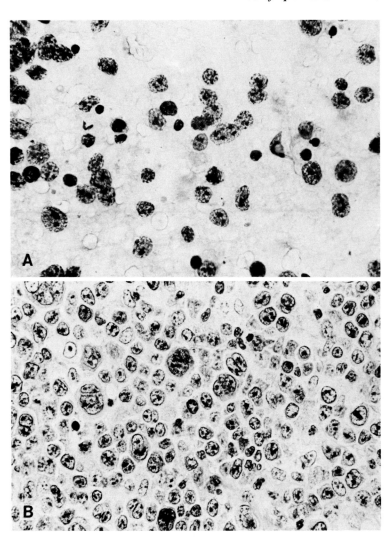

FIGURE 29–51. Immunoblastic (large cell) lymphoma. (*A*) Needle aspirate. The smear consists almost exclusively of polymorphic, irregularly shaped tumor cells with scanty cytoplasm and large, prominent nucleoli. Note the variability in nuclear sizes, also seen in the corresponding tissue section (*B*). Some pyknotic nuclei are also present. (*A*, Papanicolaou stain ×480; *B* ×480. Zajicek, J.: Aspiration Biopsy Cytology, Part I. Basel, S. Karger, 1974)

these rare tumors in cerebrospinal fluid, see Chapter 27.

DIFFERENTIAL DIAGNOSIS OF NON-HODGKIN'S LYMPHOMAS OF LARGE-CELL TYPE

The principal difficulty with this group of tumors is with metastatic carcinomas. In the lymphomas with abundant cytoplasm, particularly in technically poor preparations wherein clustering may occur, an error is easily made. The opposite error (i.e., confusing a metastatic small-cell carcinoma or melanoma with a lymphoma) is less common but also may occur. The knowledge of the clinical data is essential in such cases. Immuno-chemical staining may also assist in establishing the correct diagnosis (see Chap. 34).

Follicular Lymphomas. This group of malignant lymphomas may present substantial diagnostic difficulties because the monotonous population of lymphoma cells may not be seen in smears. Depending on the extent and configuration of the lesions, the smears may mimic the pattern of a hyperplastic lymph node, wherein a mixed population of cells is present. In such cases, the diagnosis of lymphoma must rest on the presence of a substantial proportion of large, malignant cells or, in B-cell tumors, on documentation of monoclonality for immunoglobulins kappa or lambda. Even in

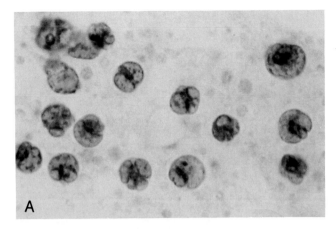

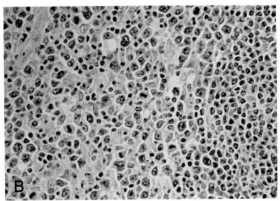

FIGURE 29–52. T-cell lymphoma, aspiration smear and tissue. (*A*) The lymphoma cells are characterized by bizarre convolutions that on superficial scrutiny suggest Reed–Sternberg cells. The nuclei, however, are single. (*B*) Corresponding tissue section showing a large-cell lymphoma (*A* ×900; *B* ×300. Courtesy of Prof. S. Woyke)

these situations, however, removal of the affected lymph node for histologic and immunologic study is a safer way to diagnosis.

Hodgkin's Disease

This malignant disease of the lymphoid tissue, occurring predominantly in young adults, is now usually classified into four histologic types: *(1)* lymphocytic predominance, *(2)* nodular sclerosis, *(3)* mixed cellularity, or *(4)* lymphocytic depletion.

Lymphocytic predominance is usually associated with early stages of the disease. The cases with nodular sclerosis and mixed cellularity are almost equally distributed among the early and advanced stages, whereas lymphocytic depletion is most common in advanced disease.

The unifying feature of all the types of Hodgkin's lymphoma is the presence of Reed–Sternberg cells, which are binucleated, multinucleated, or multilobate large cells with very large nucleoli. The precise derivation of these cells has not as yet been settled. Accompanying the Reed–Sternberg cells are large, mononucleated cells with prominent nucleoli, sometimes referred to as Hodgkin's cells. The background of the smears consists of macrophages, lymphocytes, and polymorphonuclear leukocytes; eosinophils may be present in large numbers. Lacunar cells are variants of Reed–Sternberg cells, characterized by clear cytoplasm and multiple or multilobate nuclei with multiple nucleoli. The lacunar cells are observed mainly in the nodular sclerosis type of Hodgkin's disease.

This histologic grouping tallies to some extent with the findings in smears of aspirates. The smears from the lymphocytic predominance group are dominated by lymphocytes, but they also contain numerous macrophages, some of which are enlarged and have a lobulated nucleus, but lack prominent nucleoli. Large atypical mononucleated cells, resembling basophilic stem cells but provided with large, round, single nucleoli may also be noted (Fig. 29–54*A*).* The finding of such

---

* *Editor's Note: Dr. Fred W. Stewart used to call these cells "one-eyed bandits" and considered them of great diagnostic value in Hodgkin's disease. (LGK)*

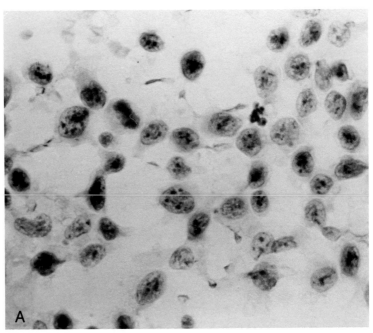

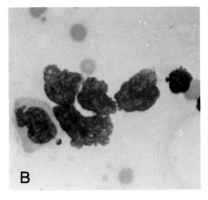

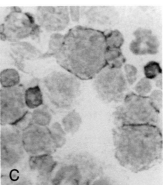

FIGURE 29–53. Aspirate of mycosis fungoides metastatic to a neck node. (*A*) Fixed, Papanicolaou-stained smear showing malignant cells with convoluted, irregularly shaped nuclei, provided with prominent nucleoli. (*B*) Same case, air-dried smear stained with MGG. The bizarre, cerebriform configuration of the chromatin may be noted. (*C*) Positive reaction to staining with an antibody to T-cell epitope. (*A, B, C* ×560. Case courtesy of Dr. Britt-Marie Ljung, University of California, San Francisco)

cells, particularly in association with some eosinophilic granulocytes, should arouse the suspicion of Hodgkin's disease. The definitive diagnosis requires the identification of Reed–Sternberg cells (see Fig. 29–54*B,C*). In smears the Reed–Sternberg cells appear as large, sometimes giant cells, usually with segmented or multiple nuclei similar to those of bone marrow megakaryocytes but containing large nucleoli that may attain the size of erythrocytes.

In the *nodular sclerosing form* of Hodgkin's disease, the aspirates may be selectively taken from cellular areas of the lymph nodes. The smears cannot be distinguished from those in the mixed cellularity type of disease.

In Hodgkin's disease with *mixed cellularity,* aspiration biopsy usually yields abundant material. The cell pattern shows Reed–Sternberg cells in addition to lymphocytes, histiocytes, eosinophils, plasma cells and the abnormal mononucleated Hodgkin's cells.

Lymphocytic depletion is the common feature of several histologic types of Hodgkin's disease. In *diffuse fibrosis,* aspiration biopsy usually yields only a few fibroblast-like cells and giant cells with nucleoli of malignant appearance. This paucity of cells may render the diagnosis of Hodgkin's disease difficult or even impossible. In *Hodgkin's sarcoma,* by contrast, there is usually an abundant yield of polymorphic malignant cells mixed with cells of Reed–Sternberg type.

Histiocytosis is a systemic proliferation of cells

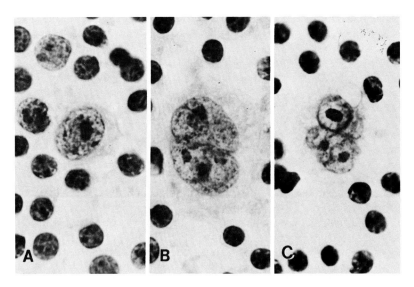

FIGURE 29-54. Needle aspirate from Hodgkin's disease. (*A*) Atypical mononucleated cell with a large nucleolus (a so-called Hodgkin's cell). (*B*) Typical binucleated giant Reed–Sternberg cell. (*C*) Multinucleated giant cell of Reed–Sternberg type. (*A, B, C,* Papanicolaou stain ×1,200)

with features of histiocytes. The several types of histiocytosis are known as Letterer–Siwe disease (malignant form) or eosinophilic granuloma, and Hand–Schüller–Christian disease (benign form, Fig. 29–55). The cytoplasm of the histiocytes is more abundant in the benign than in the malignant form. Numerous eosinophilic granulocytes are seen in smears of some of the benign cases.

Metastatic Carcinomas

Metastatic cancer was found in 461 of 1,200 aspiration biopsy smears from lymph nodes (Zajicek et al., 1967). The distribution according to primary site is shown in Figure 29–39.

The consensus is that aspiration biopsy of lymph nodes in the presence of metastatic cancer is reliable; more than 90% of lymph node metastases are diagnosed from the initial aspiration (Engzell et al., 1971). Berg (1961) listed four circumstances contributing to the diagnostic success in this field: the accessibility of the enlarged lymph nodes to palpation and aspiration; the high cellularity and poor vascularization of the metastases, resulting in a rich yield of tumor cells, with practically no admixed blood; the readiness with which alien epithelial cells can be distinguished from the normal constituents of the node; and that, in most cases, the primary cancer is known and histologically proved.

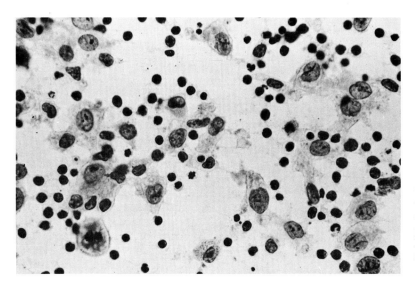

FIGURE 29-55. Needle aspirate from a lymph node in an 8-month-old boy with Hand-Schüller-Christian disease. Large macrophages with vacuolated cytoplasm (histiocytes) are intermingled with lymphocytes. (Papanicolaou stain ×480. Zajicek, J.: Aspiration Biopsy Cytology, Part I. Basel, S. Karger, 1974)

The simplicity of diagnosing metastatic lesions, compared with primary lymphomas, is well exemplified by tumors of the thyroid gland. In direct smears from the thyroid, atypical thyroid cells may be suggestive of adenoma *or* carcinoma. But if thyroid cells are found in smears prepared from a lymph node aspirate, they must be considered malignant unless there is doubt about the origin of the material. In such an event, it must be made clear to all concerned that the diagnosis of metastatic thyroid cancer stands or falls on the clinical judgment.

When the primary cancer is known, the differential cytologic diagnosis of lymph node metastases is simplified by the possibility of comparing the makeup of the aspirated cells with those of the primary tumor. If the primary tumor is unknown, the information contained in the smears may assist in tracing the origin of the metastasis. Metastases of thyroid cancer, as mentioned above, are readily identifiable, especially when they show papillary or follicular structures. Careful palpation of the thyroid may then disclose a firm nodule, which can be shown to have a reduced uptake of radioactive iodine (cf. p. 1269). Aspirate from this nodule may display cells similar to those aspirated from the lymph node.

Pigmented cells from malignant melanoma are easily recognized in smears from lymph nodes. This finding will prompt a search for pigmented skin lesions or for scars of lesions removed for cosmetic reasons. Other features of cells in metastatic melanoma are discussed in Chapter 26.

Even if the specific origin of a metastatic tumor cannot be identified in the aspirate, the identification of tumor type may be quite helpful and narrow the search for a primary site. Thus, the diagnosis of an adenocarcinoma in a Virchow's node will direct the attention to the gastrointestinal tract. The same tumor type in a neck node is more likely to be of breast origin in women or of lung origin in either sex.

A small-cell carcinoma may suggest origin in the lung; when observed in a young patient, particularly in an Asiatic, the possibility of a nasopharyngeal carcinoma must be considered.

The diagnosis of an epidermoid (squamous) carcinoma in a neck node is suggestive of buccal, respiratory tract, or esophagus origin. The same type of cancer observed in a pelvic or retroperitoneal lymph node in a woman is suggestive of cervical or vaginal cancer.

In reference to the keratin-forming cancers observed in a neck node a comment is in order: Metastatic keratinizing squamous cell carcinoma usually undergoes necrosis and even liquefaction. (Fig.

29–56). Aspiration biopsy may fluid, and the smears may be dom erating squamous epithelium, gr gocytes, and foreign body giant c branchial cleft cysts often pres similar picture. Aspiration of the peri, lesion and a careful scrutiny of the slides, however, should reveal unmistakable cancer cells in metastatic carcinoma, whereas the squamous epithelium in smears from branchial cleft cysts usually is monotonous and without nuclear atypia (compare Fig. 29–56*A* with Fig. 29–22).

It is often possible to identify other metastatic tumors, either by morphology (i.e., clear cell carcinoma of the kidney) or by immunochemistry (prostatic carcinoma). The reader is referred to Chapter 34 for further discussion of immunologic markers.

THE BREAST

Aspiration biopsy of mammary lesions has become a quasi-routine clinical procedure in many hospitals and clinics, replacing a preoperative tissue biopsy. There are many notable benefits to this method of diagnosis:

1. Rapidity and, in experienced hands, reliability of the diagnosis of mammary carcinoma
2. The involvement of the cancer patient in choice and planning of treatment
3. The aspiration, under stereotactic control, of mammographically detected lesions as small as 2 to 3 mm in diameter (see p. 1314 for further discussion)
4. The ability to perform quantitation of steroid receptor-binding (estrogen [ER] and progesterone [PR]), proliferation antigen (such as Ki 67), and DNA pattern analysis on smears, thus obviating the need for tissue biopsy (see Chaps. 34 and 35)

Aspiration biopsy is also considered to be the method of choice in the diagnosis of cystic lesions and in distinguishing between diffuse suppurative mastitis and inflammatory carcinoma.

The spectacular development of mammography has given a new impetus to the use of the aspiration biopsy. Excisional biopsy of questionable lesions detected by mammography has certain disadvantages. Should the excised lesion be histologically benign, the scar tissue tends to make subsequent mammographic checks more difficult. In patients for whom the radiologist considers surgi-

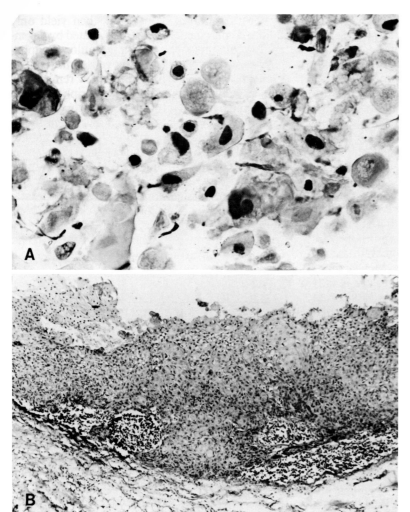

FIGURE 29–56. Lymph node metastasis of a well-differentiated squamous cell carcinoma. (*A*) Smear of fluid aspirated from a cystic lymph node of the neck with metastatic squamous cell carcinoma of the tongue. Note cellular debris and a few obvious squamous cancer cells with large, hyperchromatic nuclei. (*B*) Tissue section from a lymph node with squamous cell carcinoma and remnants of lymphatic tissue close to the capsule (*lower part* of the figure). In the central part of the node, carcinoma has undergone degeneration and liquefaction (*upper part* of the figure). Same case as that in (*A*). (*A*, Papanicolaou stain ×480; *B*, van Gieson stain ×75)

cal intervention unnecessary, aspiration biopsy thus offers a nontraumatic approach to the diagnosis of suspicious or debatable radiologic findings.

There are still some surgeons who resist this method of diagnosis, either for selfish reasons or because they do not trust the laboratory. Breast aspiration is a serious responsibility of the pathologist, and a false-positive diagnosis may result in an unnecessary mutilation of the patient. Whatever caveats have been expressed in this regard in the preceding pages, they must be repeated and reinforced again in reference to the breast: in case of doubt the procedure should be repeated or another opinion sought. A breast once removed cannot be replaced.

The following principal lesions of the female breast can be identified in aspirated samples:

- Mastitis and fat necrosis
- Fibroadenoma
- Lactating adenoma
- Rare benign tumors
- Carcinomas of various types (see text)
- Sarcomas
- Metastatic tumors

Cells of the Normal Breast

The breast is a secretory gland that consists of efferent lactiferous ducts that branch into ductular structures with terminal alveoli or acini. Clusters of

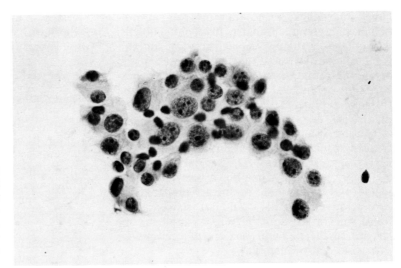

FIGURE 29–57. Needle aspirate from a fibroadenoma, a cluster of duct cells showing some degree of nuclear atypia. The attached oval or comma-shaped cells are myoepithelial cells. Similar cytologic findings may be observed in fibrocystic disease. (Papanicolaou stain, ×480)

terminal alveoli or acini are referred to as lobules (cf. Chap. 28). The epithelial cells lining the ductules and the ducts have scanty cytoplasm and ovoid nuclei. The long nuclear axis is commonly at a right angle to the direction of the duct. There is also an outer layer of myoepithelial cells with nuclei parallel with the ducts.

In smears of needle aspirate, fragments from the efferent ducts (Fig. 29–57) appear as large cohesive clusters showing flat, regularly arranged duct cells. Fragments from ductules or acini are much smaller, and the cells are characteristically arranged in small clusters or sheets.

In pregnancy and lactation, ductular-acinar epithelium differentiates into secretory cells, which show abundant, often vacuolated cytoplasm and round, often dark nuclei with enlarged, round nucleoli (see Fig. 29–69A). Secretory cells can occasionally be seen in aspirates from breasts with fibrocystic disease, but they usually lack the enlarged nucleoli seen in pregnancy.

Myoepithelial cells in smears adhere to the fragments of duct epithelium (see Fig. 29–57) or appear as detached naked, oval or comma–shaped nuclei in the background of the smear (Fig. 29–58). The nuclei of myoepithelial cells have sharp contours and stain darker than do the nuclei of the duct lining cells. They are readily distinguishable from the naked nuclei of carcinoma cells, which usually are round or oddly shaped, and much

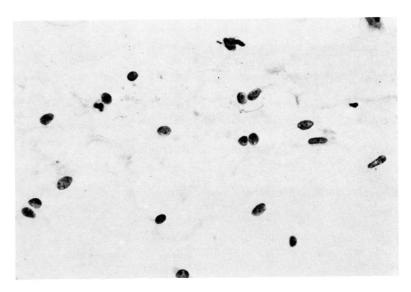

FIGURE 29–58. Needle aspirate from adenosis (fibrocystic disease) of the breast, showing round and oval naked nuclei forming the background of the smear. Some if not all of these naked nuclei are derived from myoepithelium. (Papanicolaou stain, 480)

larger. Nucleoli, as a rule, are much more prominent in carcinoma cells than in myoepithelial cells, wherein they are barely visible. In a smear containing suspicious cells and myoepithelial cell nuclei diagnostic caution is strongly advised. The presence of myoepithelial cell nuclei suggests that the suspicious epithelial cells may be benign, atypical duct cells.

Clusters of apocrine cells of ductal origin are frequently found in breast aspirates (see Fig. 29-71*A*). These cells have round, often dark nuclei and abundant cytoplasm. The cytoplasm is finely granulated and eosinophilic in smears prepared according to Papanicolaou and are slate gray in MGG smears. The apocrine cells resemble the oncocytes in salivary glands and Hürthle cells in the thyroid (see also Chap. 28).

Mucus-producing cells, resembling goblet cells, are occasionally found in breast aspirates, especially in fibrocystic disease. They are the dominant cell type in gelatinous or colloid carcinoma (see p. 1306).

Cytology of Benign Breast Lesions

Mastitis and Abscess

An aspirate from diffuse suppurative mastitis or a breast abscess usually consists of semisolid, purulent material containing numerous inflammatory cells, such as granulocytes, lymphocytes, foam cells, and phagocytes. The diagnosis is usually easy. Sometimes, however, large sheets of foam cells and of macrophages with enlarged nucleoli present problems for the inexperienced examiner. Never-

theless, careful analysis of the general appearance of the smear should clearly reveal the benign nature of such aggregates (Fig. 29-59).

Fat Necrosis

The affected area presents clinically as a firm mass that is partly fixed to the surrounding tissues. When there is no history of trauma, the lesion may be clinically mistaken for carcinoma.

Aspirates from fat necrosis (Fig. 29-60) may contain amorphous material, mainly fat and inflammatory cells: neutrophil granulocytes, lymphocytes, macrophages, epithelioid cells, or foreign body giant cells in varying proportions. Whereas the fat cells in aspirate from the normal breast occur in clusters, in fat necrosis they are enlarged and dissociated. Their cytoplasm is often vacuolated, and it may not always be possible to distinguish these cells from large foamy phagocytes.

Fibrocystic Disease (Benign Mammary Dysplasia)

In the nomenclature proposed by the WHO International Center for the Histologic Definition and Classification of Breast Tumors (1968), the following entities are listed under *benign dysplasia* of the female breast: *(1)* cyst, *(2)* adenosis, *(3)* benign epithelial proliferation in ducts or lobules, *(4)* duct ectasia, and *(5)* sclerosing adenosis. It must be noted that the term *dysplasia* in reference to the breast indicates distinctly benign processes and is therefore at marked variance with the usage of this term as a precancerous lesion (see Chap. 12). For this reason the WHO nomenclature has not gained

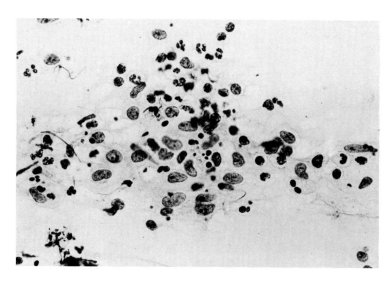

FIGURE 29-59. Needle aspirate from a case of acute mastitis. Macrophages and granulocytes dominate the picture. (Papanicolaou stain ×480)

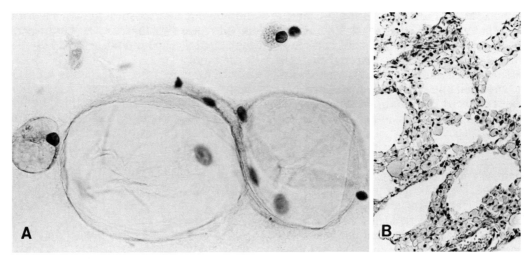

FIGURE 29–60.   Fat necrosis. (*A*) Needle aspirate showing fat cells of various size and a foamy phagocyte (*top*). (*B*) Tissue section showing an area of fat necrosis. (*A*, Papanicolaou stain ×480; *B* ×120. Zajicek, J.: Aspiration Biopsy Cytology. Part I. Basel, S. Karger, 1974)

much acceptance, and the term *fibrocystic disease* is favored in many laboratories, notably in the United States.

In 509 consecutive cases of histologically diagnosed fibrocystic disease, the aspiration biopsy yielded variable amounts of fluid, suggesting that *cysts* occurred in about 40% of the series (Franzén and Zajicek, 1968).

Aspiration of simple cysts yields translucent fluid that may be yellow, brown, green, or blood-stained. Cytologic examination of this fluid usually shows only a few foamy phagocytes (cf. Chap. 28). In cysts lined by papillae-forming epithelium, or in inflamed cysts, the fluid is usually cloudy and richer in cells. Smears from cysts with papillary lining show clusters of apocrine epithelial cells with evidence of degeneration and varying degrees of nuclear atypia (see Fig. 28–4). Carcinomas originating in cyst lining, while rare, do occasionally occur (cf. Chap. 28).

The presence of cysts hampers palpation of the breast. After removal of the cystic fluid, the breast should be palpated again. Palpable lesions remaining after aspiration of a cyst should be reaspirated. Cysts in which *cytologic analysis* of the fluid *suggests papillary proliferation must be excised for histologic study.*

In *adenosis,* smears of needle aspirate contain numerous cell clusters which mimic ductal (duct adenosis) or ductular–acinar structures (lobular adenosis, sclerosing adenosis).

In *benign proliferative processes* affecting *ducts or lobules,* the presence of degenerated epithelial cells and of spindle-shaped myoepithelial cells may be observed (see Figs. 29–57 and 29–58). In air-dried, MGG-stained smears, overstaining of the nuclei and "dirty" appearance of the cytoplasm are additional signs by which cell clusters aspirated from benign intraductal proliferation can be identified. In this respect, air-dried, MGG-stained smears are superior to wet-fixed smears stained with hematoxylin and eosin or according to Papanicolaou.

Table 29–4 summarizes cytologic findings according to predominant type of palpable fibrocystic disease. In 60% of these cases the lesions were solid, and the aspirates showed epithelial cells without noteworthy admixture of fluid. Epithelial

Table 29–4

Aspiration Biopsy Findings, With Approximate Frequency Rates, in Various Types of Fibrocystic Disease of the Breast (Benign Mammary Dysplasia)

Needle Aspirate	Predominant Type of Lesion	% (approx.)
Fluid	Cystic	40
Scanty to moderate cellularity	Fibrotic	58
High cellularity	Adenosis: proliferation in ducts or lobules	2

(Linsk, J., et al.: Cytologic diagnosis of mammary tumors from aspiration smears. II. Studies on 210 fibroadenomas and 210 cases of benign dysplasia. Acta Cytol., *16*:130–138, 1972)

cells were scanty in most of the noncystic abnormalities. They were abundant in only 5.8% of such cases. Comparisons with tissue sections showed that mammary lesions yielding few epithelial cells usually displayed features of extensive fibrosis. When epithelial cells were numerous in needle aspirate, the usual histologic classification was adenosis or benign epithelial proliferation in ducts and lobules.

Benign Neoplasms

Fibroadenoma

Fibroadenomas are encapsulated benign breast tumors characterized by proliferation of connective tissue and of ductal epithelium. Two histologic varieties of mammary fibroadenoma are generally recognized—pericanalicular and intracanalicular —although mixtures of these types are common.

Pericanalicular fibroadenomas (Fig. 29–61*A*) consist of ducts surrounded concentrically by connective tissue. The *intracanalicular type* (Fig. 29–61*B*) results from invagination and distortion of ducts by proliferation of subepithelial connective tissue. The amounts of fibrous and epithelial component vary from case to case. Hyalinization and even calcification of the fibrous component are frequently seen, especially in elderly patients.

The clinical and cytologic presentation of both types of fibroadenoma are identical. Clinical examination characteristically reveals a firm, freely mobile mass, which, however, may be confused with a cyst or a lipoma and, in the elderly, also with a carcinoma.

The aspirates of fibroadenomas are characterized by sheets of benign mammary epithelium. This finding, in combination with a well-circumscribed mass, is strongly suggestive of a fibroadenoma. In about 70% of fibroadenomas, aspiration smears contain numerous sheets of epithelial cells (Fig. 29–62*A*); in about 30% fragments of stroma and myoepithelial cells are also present (Fig. 29–62*B*). By contrast, aspirates from noncystic benign mammary disease generally contain only a few cells; numerous epithelial cells were observed in only 4% of fibrocystic disease and fragments of stroma were present in only 2% (Linsk et al., 1972).

The assessment of epithelial cellularity and the presence of stroma in smears is sufficient for a diagnosis of fibroadenoma in about 70% of cases. In the remaining cases the aspirated material is scanty and mimics fibrocystic disease.

In an occasional fibroadenoma, scattered epithelial cells with markedly enlarged and hyperchromatic nuclei may occur. These, fortunately, very rare cases pose a diagnostic dilemma between a fibroadenoma with atypia and a mammary carcinoma, possibly occurring within the fibroadenoma. In such cases a histologic study of the lesion is mandatory.

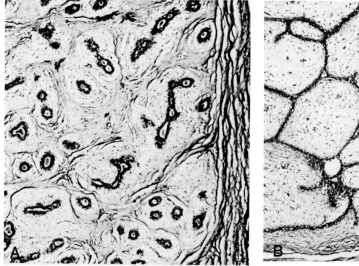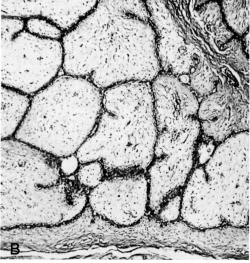

FIGURE 29–61. (*A*) Tissue section from a pericanalicular fibroadenoma. Capsular tissue is seen on the *right.* (*B*) Tissue section from an intracanalicular fibroadenoma: Capsular tissue is seen at *bottom* of photograph. (*A, B* ×120)

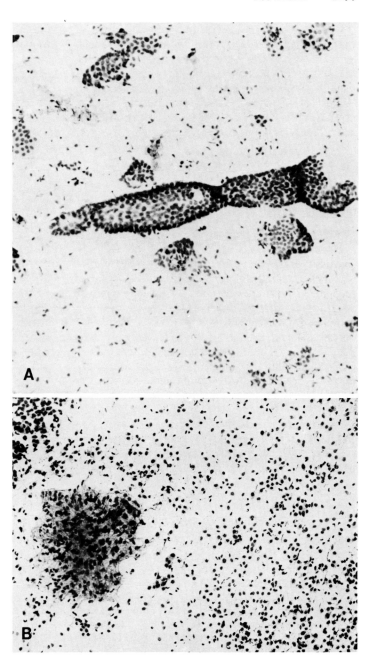

FIGURE 29–62. (*A*) Aspiration smear from a fibroadenoma of the breast. Large sheets of mammary duct cells and dissociated cell elements are seen. The latter comprise stromal and myoepithelial cells. (*B*) Needle aspirate from a fibroadenoma. Cellular smear with a stroma fragment on the *left*. (Papanicolaou stain *A* ×130; *B* ×120)

Lactating Adenoma

Palpable, nodular lesions in breasts of pregnant or lactating women require prompt attention, as they may represent a carcinoma or a benign adenoma. Aspiration biopsy of the breast in lactating adenoma yields numerous, densely packed large lobules, either in large, irregular clusters or as spherical structures, with myoepithelial cells at the periphery. Some of the clusters break up in the process of smear preparation and form flat sheets of cells with cytoplasm studded with large vacuoles and spherical nuclei of equal sizes, each containing one or more prominent, large, sometimes irregular nucleoli (Fig. 29–63). It is the presence of the nucleoli that may mislead an uninformed observer into believing that cancer is present. This error must be avoided at all costs, as it may have tragic consequences.

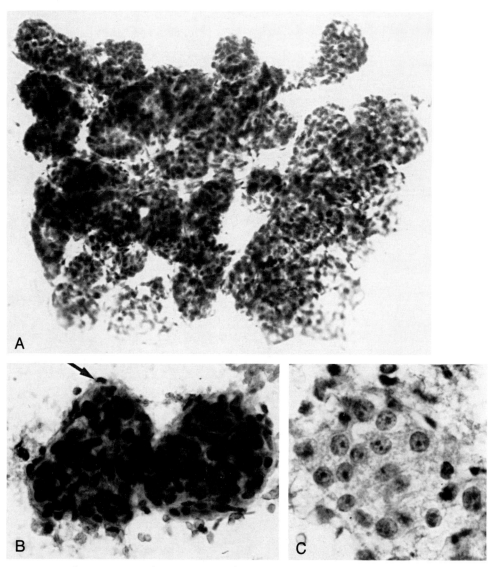

FIGURE 29–63. Lactating adenoma: Smear of an aspirate of a breast nodule in a 28-year-old pregnant woman. (*A*) The aspirate yielded a large number of enlarged mammary lobules, forming thick clusters. (*B*) Two of the lobules under higher magnification. Note the layer of spindly, myoepithelial cells at the periphery (*arrow*). (*C*) A squashed lactating lobule: note the prominent nucleoli and frothy cytoplasm of the lobular cells. (*A* ×60; *B* ×150; *C* ×560)

Duct Papilloma

The main secretory ducts are the most common sites of this neoplasm, which is often associated with hemorrhagic discharge from the nipple. According to the WHO definition, *duct papilloma* is a "regular papillary overgrowth without mitoses or hyperchromatism" (Fig. 29–64C). Most intraductal papillomas are not palpable, but produce nipple discharge, as described and illustrated in Chapter 28. When the lesions are palpable within the breast they can be aspirated.

Aspiration biopsy of duct papilloma usually yields a droplet of clear fluid or blood, containing epithelial fragments. The smears show numerous clusters of columnar ductal epithelial cells, often forming a monolayer. Clusters of apocrine cells may also be observed (see Fig. 29–64A). In the latter, chromatin clumping and pyknotic nuclei are

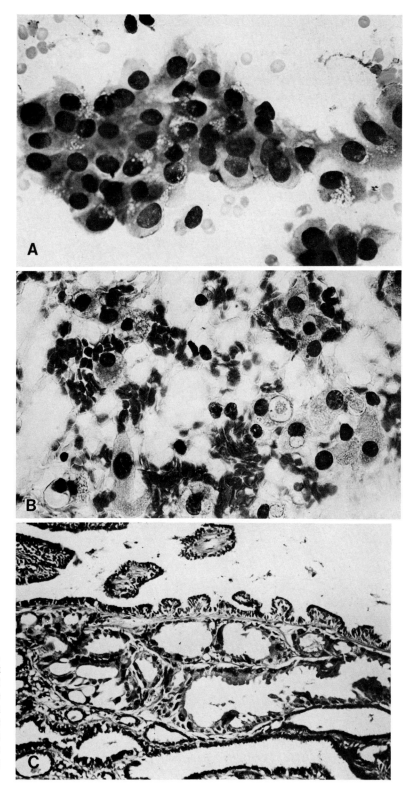

FIGURE 29-64. Duct papilloma. (*A*) Needle aspirate showing a sheet of apocrine cells with large nuclei showing pyknotic degenerative changes. (*B*) Needle aspirate with epithelial cells showing cytoplasmic vacuolization. (*C*) Tissue section from the same case. (*A*, MGG stain ×480; *B*, Papanicolaou stain ×480; *C* ×300)

commonly present. The cytoplasm shows fine vacuoles. Transitional forms between normal epithelial cells and foam cells can be observed. In some cells, the cytoplasm contains a large vacuole, and the cells resemble the signet ring macrophages seen in pleural or ascitic fluid (see Fig. 29–64B; also p. 1092).

The presence of degenerated apocrine cells may also occur in aspirates from breast cysts and from benign intraductal epithelial proliferation (see Fig. 28–4). In cyst aspirates the apocrine cells accompany appreciable volumes of fluid, and in benign intraductal proliferation the apocrine fragments are mixed with normal epithelial clusters.

Nipple Papillomatosis (Florid Papilloma of Nipple)

This entity characteristically involves terminal lactiferous ducts and forms an intricate network of proliferating ducts and tubules that may be mistaken for a carcinoma in a histologic section. The lesion often causes a visible deformity of the nipple.

The cytology of such lesions is usually easily classified as benign, inasmuch as the epithelial cells form cohesive sheets akin to those seen in fibroadenomas, usually accompanied by myoepithelial cells.

Granular Cell Tumor (Myoblastoma)

This uncommon firm tumor of the breast may reach substantial size (2 to 3 cm), and may clinically mimic a carcinoma. It is important to recognize in the aspiration smear (and in the histologic section, for that matter) the characteristic large cells with abundant granular cytoplasm and fairly monotonous, generally spherical nuclei without distinguishing features (Fig. 29–65). The lesion should not be confused with a large-cell duct carcinoma (see below).

Malignant Neoplasms

Carcinoma

Carcinoma of the breast is the most common malignant tumor of the Western woman. The needle

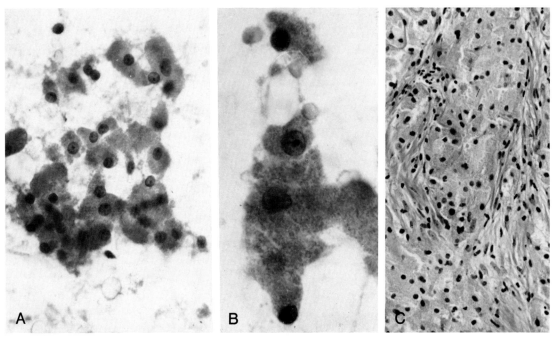

FIGURE 29–65. Granular cell tumor of breast. The aspiration smear (*A*) shows dispersed large cells with abundant, granular cytoplasm and somewhat dark-staining, but otherwise monotonous, nuclei. (*B*) The same cells under higher magnification. (*C*) The histologic section of the same tumor, again showing the granular cytoplasm of the sheet-forming tumor cells. (*A* ×400; *B* ×800; *C* ×200. Koss, L.G., et al.: Aspiration Biopsy. Cytologic Interpretation and Histologic Bases. New York, Igaku-Shoin, 1984, with permission)

aspiration biopsy plays a major role in diagnosis of this group of diseases and, with the availability of new immunologic techniques, also in the estimation of various parameters of possible prognostic value. The role of the needle aspiration biopsy was enhanced still further by acceptance of newer modalities of treatment, i.e., "lumpectomy," followed by radiotherapy, replacing in many instances a mastectomy with equivalent results.

An early and rapid diagnosis of mammary cancer allows the patient's participation in the selection of an optimal therapeutic mode.

With progress in mammography, the needle aspiration biopsy has become important in the diagnosis of occult lesions of the breast. Stereotactic aspiration of small lesions, sometimes measuring only 2 or 3 mm in diameter, is quite effective and accurate in the diagnosis of mammary cancer.

CLASSIFICATION OF MAMMARY CARCINOMA

For the purpose of cytologic diagnosis of clinical value a simple classification of mammary carcinomas is sufficient.*

Carcinomas of Mammary Ducts

Infiltrating duct carcinoma

Solid and gland-forming type
Scirrhous type
Medullary type
Colloid or mucinous type
"Apocrine" type
Tubular type
Papillary type

Intraductal carcinoma (in situ carcinoma of ducts)
Comedo type

Carcinoma of Mammary Lobules

Infiltrating lobular carcinoma
Lobular carcinoma in situ

Rare Types of Mammary Carcinomas

Inflammatory carcinoma
Spindle and giant cell carcinoma
Adenoid cystic carcinoma
Other rare types

Mixed Types of Carcinomas

In the previous editions of this book, Dr. Josef Zajicek presented a complex classification of mammary cancers that was based on cytologic patterns in smears. His classification did not correlate with histologic patterns of disease. This note is therefore of historical interest only.

Not all of these types and subtypes of mammary cancer can be securely identified in aspirates; although some are easy to diagnose, others may present substantial difficulties, as discussed below.

GENERAL CYTOLOGIC PRESENTATION OF MAMMARY CARCINOMA (SEE ALSO COLOR PLATE 29-2)

Aspirates from mammary carcinoma usually yield abundant cancer cells, singly and in clusters (Fig. 29–66A). The only exception is the fibrosing (scirrhous) duct cancer, which may yield only a scanty population of cancer cells. Depending on tumor type, the cancer cells may vary enormously in size, from very large to very small, barely larger than lymphocytes. Customarily, cells of approximately the same type predominate in each individual tumor. The clusters of aspirated cancer cells in breast cancer are often three-dimensional (i.e., composed of several superimposed layers of cells). The clusters are loosely arranged and consequently the cells at the periphery of the cluster tend to become detached. This cell arrangement differs from cell clusters in benign lesions of the breast, which are generally tight and often flat (see Figs. 29–57, 29–62, and 29–66B). The configuration of cell clusters is usually not sufficient for a definitive diagnosis. The presence of single, detached cancer cells is of great diagnostic value. In the absence of single cells, the diagnosis of breast cancer should be made with extreme caution. Isolated cancer cells usually display the customary evidence of cancer, i.e., changed nucleocytoplasmic ratio and such nuclear abnormalities as hyperchromasia and, mainly, large and multiple nucleoli. The significance of sex chromatin bodies in breast cancer cells is discussed on p. 1231.

In about 80% of mammary carcinomas, the diagnosis can be made in a secure fashion, based on the general cell features outlined above. In about 20% of mammary cancers, usually of the well-differentiated types, the cells lack the classic abnormalities, and a confident cytologic diagnosis on needle aspirates may not always be possible, as outlined below. It is particularly advisable not to make the cytologic diagnosis of mammary carcinoma in the presence of inflammation, except on overwhelming evidence.

Infiltrating Duct Cell Carcinoma. This is by far the most common variety of breast cancer.

Solid and Gland-Forming Type of Ductal Carcinoma. The classic cytologic presentation of this tumor is shown in Fig. 29–66A, described above.

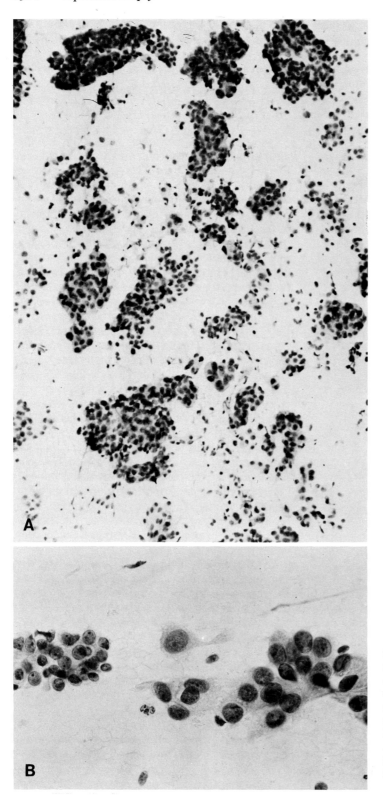

FIGURE 29–66. (*A*) Aspiration smear from a carcinoma of the breast consisting of solid plugs and dissociated carcinoma cells. (*B*) Needle aspirate from a mammary carcinoma. Large carcinoma cells (*right*) compared with benign mammary epithelium (*left*). (Papanicolaou stain, *A* ×130; *B* ×480. *A*, Zajicek, J.: Sampling of cells from human tumours by aspiration biopsy for diagnosis and research. Eur. J. Cancer, *1*:253–258, 1965)

Other variants are shown in Figs. 29–67 and 29–68. Cancer cell arrangement may mimic glandular structures (see Fig. 29–67A). Not uncommonly the cancer cells are dispersed (see Fig. 29–68A). It may be noted that peripheral placement of the nuclei, mimicking giant plasma cells, is common in cells of duct carcinoma.

Scirrhous Carcinoma. Because of marked fibrosis, the aspirate may yield only a few cancer cells, usually with peripheral nuclei. If this cancer cell population is not contaminated by benign cells, the diagnosis may be made with reasonable confidence. If, however, scanty abnormal cells are associated with benign epithelial cells, it is advisable to request a tissue biopsy.

Medullary Carcinoma. These fleshy tumors often mimic grossly a fibroadenoma. A lymphoid component of the periphery, and within the tumor itself, is often present (medullary carcinoma with lymphoid stroma).

The aspirates of the tumor are rich in undifferentiated cancer cells, with irregular nuclei and

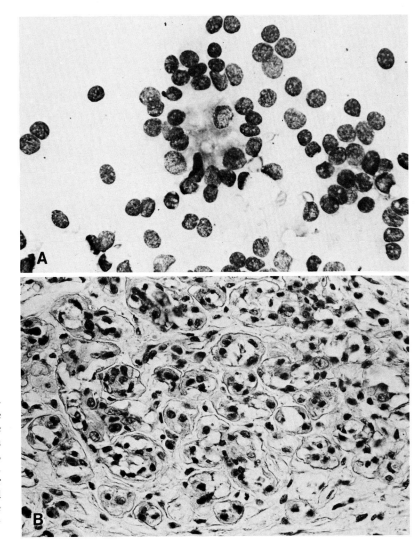

FIGURE 29–67. Mammary carcinoma, ductal type. (A) Needle aspirate. In the center a glandlike structure is shown. The cytoplasm is crowded into a central mass, whereas the nuclei are peripheral. Many large naked nuclei of cancer cells are also present. Air-dried smear. (B) Tissue section of the carcinoma shown in (A). (A, MGG stain ×480; B ×300)

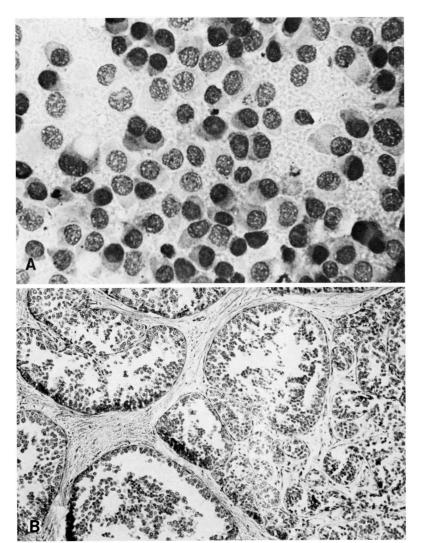

FIGURE 29-68. Infiltrating duct carcinoma. (*A*) Needle aspirate. The cancer cells, spread in a monolayer, appear singly or in small clusters. Note the characteristic peripheral placement of the nuclei in the large cancer cells (air-dried smear). (*B*) Tissue section: enlarged cancerous ducts filled with carcinoma cells exhibiting decreased intracellular cohesiveness. The same case as in (*A*). (*A*, MGG stain ×480; *B* ×120. Wallgren, A., and Zajicek, J.: Cytologic presentation of mammary carcinoma on aspiration biopsy smears. Acta Cytol., *20*:469–478, 1976)

often very large nucleoli (Fig. 29–69). An admixture of lymphocytes is frequently observed. Zajicek pointed out that certain similarities may exist between cells derived from acini of a lactating breast, often provided with nucleoli, and cancer cells in this tumor type. The similarity, illustrated in Fig. 29–69*A,B* is spurious. The degree of cellular and nuclear abnormality in medullary carcinoma is significantly greater than that observed in cells derived from a lactating breast. Still, this example does call attention to the dangers of cytologic diagnosis of mammary carcinoma during pregnancy and lactation.

Colloid (Mucous Cell) Carcinoma. These tumors, often achieving large sizes, are characterized by abundant production of mucus, surrounding clusters of cancer cells (Fig. 29–70). The cancer cells usually form cohesive clusters, with only slight nuclear abnormalities. The diagnosis is based on the presence of mucus bathing the clusters and is easier in air-dried, MGG-stained smears, wherein the mucus stains pink or red. In fixed, Papanicolaou-stained smears, the mucus appears as a gray-staining amorphous substance in the background of the smear. A positive mucicarmine stain of such material will confirm the diag-

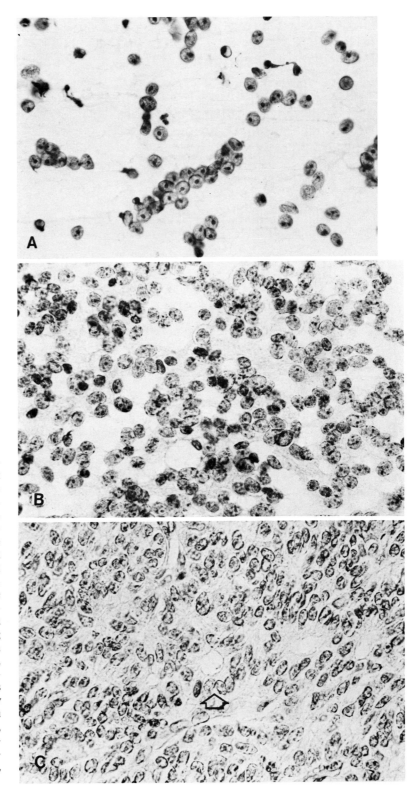

FIGURE 29–69. Comparison of lobular cells from a lactating breast with cells from a medullary carcinoma. (*A*) Needle aspirate of a female breast 7 days after childbirth. Stripped nuclei of secretory (acinic) cells with enlarged nucleoli are shown. (*B*) Needle aspirate from a medullary carcinoma. Naked nuclei of cancer cells dominate the smear. The fragile cytoplasm is seen in the background. The picture vaguely resembles that seen in aspirates from a pregnant breast or a breast during lactation. (*C*) Tissue section from carcinoma shown in (*B*). Glandular, acinus-like structures can be observed (*arrow*). Histologically this case was classified as a medullary carcinoma. (*A, B* Papanicolaou stain ×480; *C* ×480. *B, C*: Wallgren, A., and Zajicek, J.: Cytologic presentation of mammary carcinoma on aspiration biopsy smears. Acta Cytol., *20*:469–478, 1976)

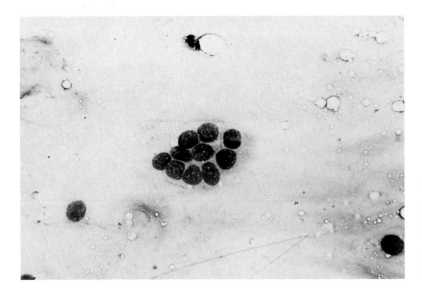

FIGURE 29–70. Mucous cell (colloid) carcinoma. A cluster of carcinoma cells surrounded by mucus. Air-dried smear. (MGG stain ×480. Wallgren, A., and Zajicek, J.: Cytologic presentation of mammary carcinoma on aspiration biopsy smears. Acta Cytol., *20:*469–478, 1976)

nosis. This type of mammary carcinoma may be difficult to diagnose because of the relatively trivial abnormalities in the cohesive clusters of cancer cells. The diagnosis requires a close correlation with clinical findings.

"Apocrine"-Type Carcinoma. There is considerable doubt whether duct cancers of this type are deserving of a separate classification. Still, in practice, one is confronted every once in a while with a mammary carcinoma composed of large cells, with eosinophilic, granular cytoplasm, resembling benign apocrine cells (Fig. 29–71). The differentiation of the benign from the malignant cells is sometimes difficult, inasmuch as the benign apocrine cells may display large nuclei and nucleoli of substantial sizes. The cancer cells are usually dispersed, whereas the apocrine cells usually form cohesive sheets (see Fig. 29–71*A*). As a rule, there is a significant variability in the sizes of the cancer cells, their nuclei, and their nucleoli. Furthermore, the smears from carcinomas usually show at least some cancer cells of the classic type. Still, in case of doubt, a tissue biopsy should be requested for confirmation of the diagnosis.

Tubular Carcinoma. The tumor cells form cohesive, three-dimensional, complex, often branching and angulated epithelial cell clusters and sheets, resembling somewhat the tubular structures seen in fibroadenoma (compare Figs. 29–62*A*, 29–72*A*, and Plate 29–2*A,B*). In carcinoma, however, the tubular structures are surrounded by fat that can be readily recognized in the background of

the smears and corresponds to the tumor tubules infiltrating fat in histologic sections (see Fig. 29–72*C*).

The nuclear abnormalities in tubular carcinoma are relatively trivial: the spherical nuclei are enlarged, but not hyperchromatic and contain tiny nucleoli (see Fig. 29–72*B*). This classic and diagnostic presentation of tubular carcinoma is unfortunately not always seen. In other cases, the tubular structures may be less complex (see Color Plate 29–2*B*) and may mimic to perfection a fibroadenoma. The presence of myoepithelial cells, as observed in one such case, made the diagnosis of carcinoma impossible. Clearly, the clinical and mammographic presentation of the lesion is very important in debatable cases.

Papillary Carcinoma. The cytologic presentation of a papillary carcinoma usually cannot be distinguished from an intraductal papilloma (see Fig. 29–64). It is recommended that all such lesions be surgically excised for histologic examination (see also Chap. 28).

Paget's Disease of the Breast. See Chapter 28.

Intraductal Carcinoma. Depending on size and the number of ducts involved, aspiration biopsy of this tumor type is conducted either in the presence of a palpable tumor or, when incidentally discovered by mammography, under stereotactic conditions (see below). The aspirates do not have any specific cytologic features that would enable

(text continues on page 1131)

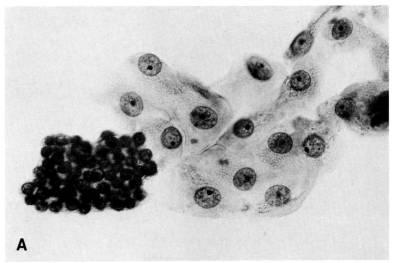

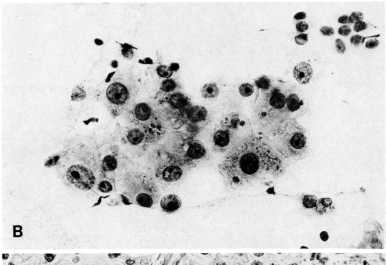

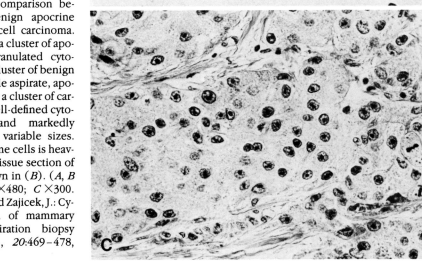

FIGURE 29–71. Comparison between common benign apocrine cells and apocrine cell carcinoma. (*A*) Needle aspirate: a cluster of apocrine cells with granulated cytoplasm adjacent to a cluster of benign duct cells. (*B*) Needle aspirate, apocrine cell carcinoma: a cluster of carcinoma cells with well-defined cytoplasmic borders and markedly abnormal nuclei of variable sizes. The cytoplasm of some cells is heavily granulated. (*C*) Tissue section of duct carcinoma shown in (*B*). (*A, B* Papanicolaou stain ×480; *C* ×300. *B, C:* Wallgren, A., and Zajicek, J.: Cytologic presentation of mammary carcinoma on aspiration biopsy smears. Acta Cytol., *20:*469–478, 1976)

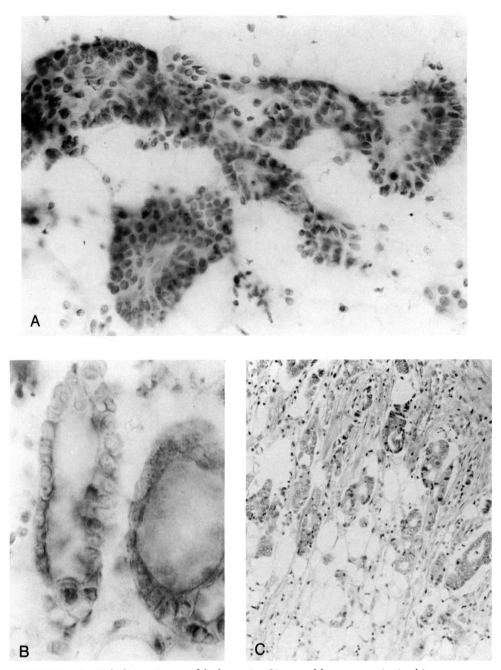

FIGURE 29–72. Tubular carcinoma of the breast in a 51-year-old woman, aspiration biopsy smear and tissue. (*A*) An example of one of the complex, branching, three-dimensional tubular cell clusters infiltrating fat, which is seen in the background. (*B*) High-power view of one of the tubular epithelial clusters to document the minimal cytologic abnormalities, such as nuclear enlargement and barely visible small nucleoli. Note the presence of fat cells surrounding the tubules. (*C*) Tubular carcinoma, infiltrating fat. (*A* ×350; *B* ×560; *C* ×150. Case courtesy of Dr. William J. Frable, Medical College of Virginia, Richmond)

one to diagnose an intraductal lesion. The populations of cancer cells are usually comparable with other solid and gland-forming duct carcinomas (see Figs. 29–66*A*, 29–67, and 29–68).

Lobular Carcinomas. Infiltrating lobular carcinomas, with their characteristic "Indian file" arrangement of cancer cells may be sometimes difficult to aspirate because of considerable fibrosis. The diagnostic problems may be due to scanty evidence of cancer. In most cases, though, a population of small fairly monotonous cancer cells are observed, with many cells showing cytoplasmic vacuoles (Fig. 29–73). The cells are dispersed, but also form clusters and Indian files. A very characteristic feature of lobular carcinomas, primary or metastatic, is the presence of cytoplasmic vacuoles with a central condensation of mucus (Fig. 29–74). In air-dried MGG-stained smears, the mucus stains a violet-reddish color and the term "magenta cells" has been used to describe this phenomenon. The presence of mucus can be readily documented in fixed material with mucicarmine stain.

The diagnosis of *lobular carcinoma in situ* is very rarely made on aspirates. The finding of these small lesions is usually incidental. The cell population, usually very scanty, has the same features as those of infiltrating lobular carcinoma.

Rare Types of Mammary Carcinoma. Mammary carcinomas may occasionally show morpho-

logic features of a squamous carcinoma, giant-cell tumor of bone, chondro-, or osteosarcoma. The cytologic features of such rare tumors have been described elsewhere (Koss et al., 1992) and are being sporadically reported.

Other Forms of Mammary Carcinoma. See Chapter 28 for discussion of Paget's disease of the breast, nipple secretions and mammary lesions associated therewith.

Sarcomas

Cystosarcoma Phyllodes. Clinically, the tumor presents as a large, fairly well-demarcated lesion, sometimes with history of rapid enlargement. Histologically, the tumors resemble a fibroadenoma, with the salient feature of atypia of the periductal stroma. Transitional forms between cellular intracanalicular fibroadenoma and a sarcoma (malignant cystosarcoma phyllodes) may be seen.

Biopsy aspirates characteristically are highly cellular and are dominated by fragments of spindly or polygonal stromal cells, showing nuclear atypia. The degree of nuclear atypia varies from case to case. In some tumors, the nuclei are monomorphic and only slightly larger than the nuclei in ordinary fibroadenoma. In other cases, the nuclei vary considerably in size and shape and may show hyperchromasia, with fairly numerous mitoses, suggesting a malignant neoplasm (Fig. 29–75). The

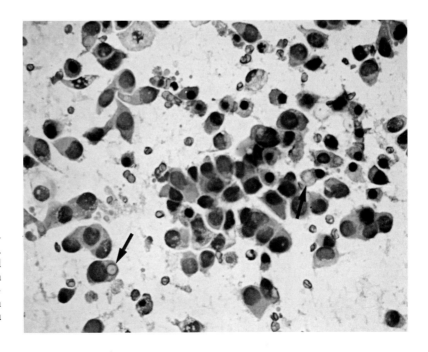

FIGURE 29–73. Infiltrating lobular carcinoma, aspiration smear. The fairly monotonous small cancer cells form clusters, "Indian files" and are dispersed. Cytoplasmic vacuoles (*arrows*) contain mucus, easily documented with a mucicarmin stain. (×560)

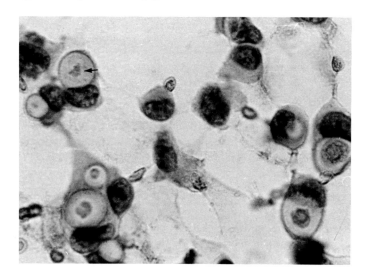

FIGURE 29–74. Infiltrating lobular carcinoma, aspiration smear. Small cancer cells with large, cytoplasmic mucous vacuoles with a central condensation (*arrow*) are characteristic of this tumor (×800. Courtesy of Prof. S. Woyke)

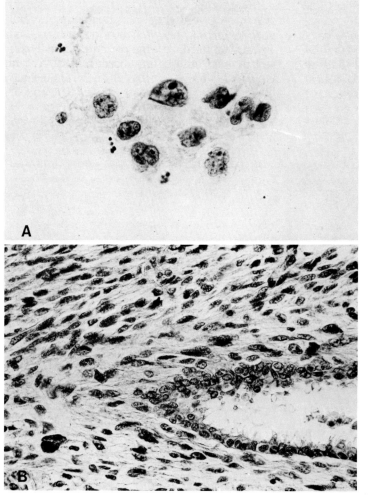

FIGURE 29–75. Cystosarcoma arising in cellular intracanalicular fibroadenoma. (*A*) Aspiration biopsy smear showing cells with polymorphic bizarre nuclei. (*B*) Tissue section from the same case. (*A*, Papanicolaou stain ×480; *B* ×300. Zajicek, J.: Aspiration Biopsy Cytology. Part I. Basel, S. Karger, 1974)

cytologic picture of stromal cells is fairly characteristic and should readily permit differentiation from carcinoma, except in the rare cases of spindle cell carcinoma.

Other Types of Sarcomas. Fibrosarcoma, liposarcoma, stromal sarcoma, angiosarcoma, and malignant lymphoma may, on rare occasions, be primary in the breast. There is very limited information on the cytologic presentation of these uncommon tumors in aspirated material.

Metastatic Tumors. Metastatic carcinomas from various other primary sites may occasionally occur. Metastatic ovarian or renal carcinomas may closely mimic primary mammary cancers.

Accuracy of the Aspiration Biopsy of Palpable Breast Lesions

Aspiration biopsy cytology aims to differentiate benign breast lesions from carcinoma. Table 29–5 shows the cytologic findings in 1,009 histologically diagnosed benign breast lesions studied at the Radiumhemmet in Stockholm between 1955 and 1964. The cytologic report was negative for cancer in more than 97% of the cases. In 2.8% there was a cytologic suspicion of carcinoma. In only one case did the cytologic report state carcinoma. A review of the slides from this case showed that the cell population was unquestionably malignant. The patient died 3 years later of diffuse metastatic carcinoma, and it must be assumed that the negative histologic report reflected incomplete exploration of the breast.

The cytologic findings in 1,068 histologically proved mammary carcinomas from the same period are shown in Table 29–6. Of the total series,

77% were cytologically reported as carcinoma. (In the year 1964, the figure was 83%.) In these cases a radical mastectomy was performed without preoperative histologic confirmation of the cytologic diagnosis. Carcinoma was cytologically suspected in 13% of the total series (11% in 1964). Negative cytologic reports were given in almost 10% of the 1,068 cases (6% in 1964).

Improved diagnostic accuracy was obtained when the aspiration biopsy was repeated in cytologically doubtful or negative, but clinically suspected cases. This was the procedure in 1974 when, as Table 29–6 shows, more than 92% of the breast carcinomas were diagnosed cytologically and 6% were considered cytologically suspect. False-negative cytologic reports were given in about 2% of the cases. But since repeatedly negative needle biopsies do not guarantee that a lesion is benign, surgical biopsy should be done in all clinically doubtful, but cytologically negative, cases.

Some pertinent data from the older literature concerning false-positive and false-negative cytologic reports in carcinoma of the breast are also presented in Table 29–7.

More recent data on sensitivity and specificity

Table 29–5
Cytologic Findings in 1,009 Histologically Verified Benign Lesions Studied 1955–1964

Cytologic Report	Histology: No. of Cases	Benign Lesion (%)
Negative for cancer	980	97.1
Carcinoma suspected	28	2.8
Carcinoma	1	0.1

Table 29–6
Cytologic Findings in 1,068 Histologically Verified Mammary Carcinomas Studied 1955–1964* and in 226 Carcinomas from 1974

Cytologic Report	Histologically Diagnosed Carcinomas			
	1955–1964: 1,068 Cases		1974: 226 Cases	
	Number	%*	Number	%
Negative for cancer	106	9.9 [6.1]	4	1.8
Carcinoma suspected	139	13.0 [11.3]	13	5.7
Carcinoma	823	77.1 [82.6]	209	92.5

*Figures in brackets from 1964.

Table 29–7

Frequencies of False-Positive and False-Negative Reports From Aspiration Biopsy in Cases of Histologically Verified Mammary Gland Carcinoma

Literature	Number of Breasts	Histologically Proved Carcinoma		Aspiration Biopsy			
				False-Positive		False-Negative	
		Number	%	Number	%	Number	%
Cornillot et al. (1974)	2267	1335	58.9	15	1.6	162	12.1
Kreuzer and Boquoi (1976)	602	247	41.0	4	1.1	33	13.4
Rosen et al. (1972)	208	179	86.1	0	0	32	17.9
Shiller-Volkova and Agamova (1960)	263	165	62.7	4	2.4	44	26.7
Smith et al. (1959)	202	80	39.6	3	2.5	19	23.8
Stavric et al. (1973)	250	108	43.2	2	1.4	5	4.6
Zajdela (1975)	2772	1745	62.9	3	0.3	152	8.7
Zajicek (1974)	2077	1068	51.4	1	0.1	106	9.9
TOTAL	8641	4927	57.0	32	0.9	553	11.2

of aspiration biopsies of the breast were provided by Frable (1989), shown in Table 29–8.

These data, taken from several sources, indicate a high level of specificity of the aspiration biopsy, but not at the desirable 100% level that has been achieved in some institutions. The significantly lower level of sensitivity in the American experience, when compared with the European experience, most likely reflects caution because of the legal consequences of a false-positive diagnosis, but it also may reflect inadequate material obtained by untrained medical personnel.

Stereotactic Needle Biopsy of Mammographically Detected Breast Lesions

For study of nonpalpable lesions revealed by mammography, a stereotactic technique of needle biopsy was developed at the Karolinska Hospital (Bolmgren et al., 1977). The patient is placed prone on a special table. The breast is positioned in an aperture in the table top and is held in a stereotactic compression device that allows stereoradiographs to be taken with a superimposed coordinate sys-

Table 29–8

Sensitivity and Specificity of the Thin-Needle Aspiration Biopsy of Mammary Carcinoma

	European Experience 8,434 cases (6 sources)	American Experience 4,763 cases (5 sources)
Sensitivity*	84.5%	70.8%
Specificity†	96.5%	96.7%

$$*Sensitivity = \frac{true\text{-}positive}{true\text{-}positive + suspected + false\text{-}positive}$$

$$†Specificity = \frac{true\ negative}{true\text{-}negative + suspected + false\text{-}positive}$$

(Modified from Frable, W.J.: Needle aspiration biopsy: past, present and future. Hum. Pathol., *20*:504–517, 1989, with permission)

tem. From film projections of the lesion, the true *x, y,* and *z* coordinates can be calculated with the aid of a computer. An instrument holder fitted with a cannula 1-mm thick and an internal stainless steel screw needle is then attached to the device. The cannula is inserted into the mammary tissue, and cellular material is sampled with the screw needle. The sample is deposited on a glass slide and is stained according to conventional cytologic methods.

After the sampling, a small piece of stainless steel suture thread is introduced into the lesion to serve as a marker. Before surgical removal of the lesion, the path between the lesion and the skin is marked by injection of India ink or carbon dust, using a stereotactic device. This has proved to be a very valuable guide for identification of the lesion at surgery, and it simplifies the histopathologic examination of the specimen.

Since these early developments, new machines for stereotactic aspiration of small, mammographically detected breast lesions have been made available, but the fundamental principles, described above, have remained the same. Plain needles have now replaced the screw needle described by Bolmgren et al. in 1977.

With the increasing interest in early detection of mammary cancer, the use of the method is increasing. The efficiency of the procedure must be examined from two points of view:

1. How reliable is the diagnosis of mammary carcinoma established on a small sample of cells aspirated from a lesion barely 2 to 4 mm in diameter?
2. How reliable is the diagnosis of "no cancer cells present" under these circumstances? Is it safe to follow such patients without surgical removal?

Both questions were addressed in a summary of experience with 2,594 nonpalpable breast lesions by Azavedo et al. (1989). Of the 2,005 samples judged to be benign by mammography and cytology, only 1 patient developed carcinoma. Of the 567 samples on which surgical removal of the lesion was recommended either because of mammographic findings or cytologic diagnoses, 451 were diagnosed as mammary carcinoma and the remainder as benign lesions. The conclusions of this paper were that a combination of mammography and stereotactic aspiration of the breast are, in competent hands, a reliable method in the diagnosis "no cancer present". Cytology alone, however, failed in the identification of a substantial proportion of small occult carcinomas.

At the time of this writing (1991), there are no matching data available from any other institution. Clearly, a confirmation of these findings would be highly desirable, as it may lead to avoidance of unnecessary surgery in the majority of patients whose mammographically detected lesions are benign.

THE GONADS

In the previous (1979) edition of this book, Dr. Zajicek described at considerable length the application of aspiration biopsy techniques to the lesions of the ovary and testis.

With the development of new radiologic and clinical techniques, such as computed tomography, ultrasound, and peritoneoscopy, transvaginal or transrectal aspiration of ovarian lesions is rarely, if ever, of clinical value. Furthermore, the danger of rupturing a cystic ovarian carcinoma by the needle tip cannot be ruled out and, consequently, the technique has been abandoned, for all practical intents and purposes. Aspiration biopsy of the testis, on the other hand, is still a clinically valuable technique.

Occasional ovarian aspirates may be obtained at the time of peritoneoscopy. Of special interest are ovarian follicles, aspirated in searching for ova for in vitro fertilization. In the absence of ova, the fluid may be forwarded to the laboratory. Because the interpretation of such samples is sometimes difficult, the original text of the Zajicek contribution is repeated, with minor editorial changes. The segment on testicular lesions has been retained and expanded.

Aspiration biopsy of the gonads is mainly performed in the diagnosis of palpable tumors. The tumor pathology of the ovary and testis is highly complex, owing to the multitude of their cellular constituents. To facilitate understanding of the problems of cytologic diagnosis, a brief survey of the tumor pathology of the male and female gonads is provided.

Classification of Tumors

Tumors of the gonads are classified, on the basis of their origin, into the following main groups: germ cell tumors, sex cord–stromal tumors, and epithelial tumors. The classification of germ cell, sex cord, and epithelial tumors is shown in Table 29–9.

Most of the gonadal tumor types listed are rare

Table 29–9
Tumors of the Ovary and Testis

Nomenclature in Ovary	Cell Origin and Histologic Presentation	Nomenclature in Testis
Germ Cells		
Dysgerminoma	Primordial germ cells	Seminoma
Endodermal sinus tumor (embryonal carcinoma, yolk-sac tumor)	Yolk sac vesicles, endodermal sinuses	Infantile embryonal carcinoma
Choriocarcinoma	Trophoblastic tissue	Choriocarcinoma
Polyembryoma	Multiple embryonic bodies	Polyembryoma
Embryonal carcinoma	Embryonal cells in epithelioid structures	Embryonal carcinoma
Teratomas	Tissues of varying origin and differentiation	Teratomas
1. Immature (embryonal)	Embryonal tissues	1. Immature
2. Mature (adult)*	Mature structures of various embryonic layers	2. Mature*
Dermoid cyst	Cyst containing hair, bone, etc.	Dermoid cyst
3. Monodermal and specialized	Single organ or cell type	3. One-sided development
Struma ovarii	Thyroid tissue	
Carcinoid	Argentaffin cells	Carcinoid
Sex Cord Stromal Cells		
Granulosa-stromal cell tumor	Granulosa cells and theca cells	
Granulosa cell tumor	Granulosa cells	Granulosa cell tumor
Thecoma, fibroma	Theca cells and/or fibroblast-like cells	
Androblastoma	Sertoli cells and Leydig cells	Androblastoma
Sertoli cell tumor (tubular androblastoma)	Sertoli cells	Sertoli cell tumor
Leydig cell tumor (hilus cell tumor)	Leydig cells	Leydig cell tumor
Gynandroblastoma	Granulosa cells and Sertoli cells	Gynandroblastoma
Epithelium		
Serous tumor	Ovarian epithelium	
Mucinous tumor	Endocervical type epithelium	
Endometrioid tumor	Endometrial type epithelium	
Clear cell (mesonephroid tumor)	Unknown	
Brenner tumor	Unknown	Brenner tumor

*The tumor is malignant in the testis, but not in the ovary.
(Modified from Zajicek J.: Aspiration Biopsy Cytology, Part 2. Basel, S. Karger, 1979)

and are mainly of theoretical interest. Carcinomas are by far the most common malignant ovarian tumors. The cytologic presentation of the common tumors of the ovary follows:

Aspiration Biopsy of the Ovary

Clinical interpretation of a palpable enlargement of the ovary is often very difficult. Congestion, fol-licular and other benign cysts, and neoplasm must be considered. Because of the high frequency of minor ovarian enlargement caused by nonneo-plastic conditions, exploratory laparotomy is not always desirable, especially in younger women. Fine-needle aspiration biopsy can provide material for cytologic diagnosis, without excessive discom-fort for the patient and, consequently, this tech-nique has been used in the diagnosis of palpable ovarian enlargement.

The equipment used for ovarian needle aspiration was originally devised for samplings of the tumors of the prostate. The technique is described on page 1241.

The ovary can be aspirated through the vagina or the rectum. The transvaginal approach (Fig. 29–76) is preferable. The vaginal wall can be cleaned before the needle is inserted, whereas the transrectal puncture of a cystic lesion involves some risk of infection.

Non-neoplastic Lesions

The most common palpable non-neoplastic lesions that are investigated by thin-needle aspiration biopsy of the ovary are endometriosis and ovarian cysts, such as follicular and corpus luteum cysts. In endometriosis, the aspirate is composed of old, liquified blood, hemosiderin-containing macrophages, and clusters of poorly preserved epithelial cells. Follicular cysts usually yield clear, cell-free fluid.

In aspirates of *ovarian follicles*, obtained for the purpose of in vitro fertilization, granulosa cells may be present. On microscopic examination, the cells may appear as polygonal, fairly large cells, with granular cytoplasm and spherical nuclei (see Fig. 29–77). The nuclei are sometimes surprisingly large and hyperchromatic. There is usually a background of a few inflammatory cells, small macrophages, and debris. Smears with atypical granulosa cells may sometimes suggest a malignant tumor. This diagnosis should be withheld on the basis of clinical data. In a few such follicles, excised for verification of cytologic findings, only benign ovarian structures were observed (Dr. Ellen Greenebaum, personal communication).

The aspirates from corpus luteum cysts contain old, liquefied blood and foam cells (macrophages) and may be difficult to distinguish from the contents of an endometriotic cyst.

Benign Neoplasms

Benign germ cell tumors, i.e., benign ovarian teratomas (dermoid cysts) and benign epithelial tumors (serous and mucinous cystomas) are the most common benign neoplasms referred for aspiration biopsy.

In dermoid cysts, the aspirates usually contain amorphous matter mixed with sebaceous cells, squamous epithelial cells, and inflammatory cells, including foreign body giant cells. The presence of columnar epithelial cells of respiratory or intestinal type is also indicative of a benign teratoma. The same applies to the presence of hairs, provided that contamination of the smear can be ruled out (Kjellgren and Ångström, 1979).

Benign cystomas, as a rule, yield clear fluid. Sometimes cuboidal, columnar, or mucus-producing epithelial cells can be identified. Otherwise the lesion cannot be distinguished from other cysts.

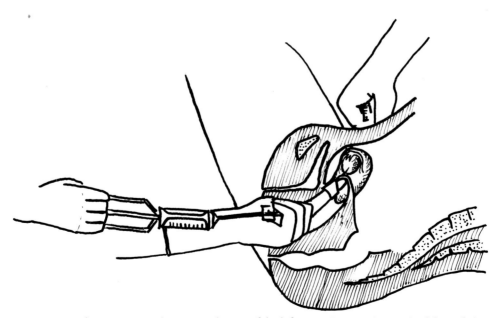

FIGURE 29–76. Transvaginal aspiration biopsy of the left ovary. Pressure is exercised through the abdominal wall to bring the ovary in line with the tip of the needle. (Zajicek, J.: Aspiration Biopsy Cytology. Part II. Basel, S. Karger, 1979)

Granulosa – Theca Cell Tumors.   These tumors are composed of granulosa and theca cells and fibroblast-like stromal cells in varying proportions. Needle biopsy usually yields preponderantly granulosa cells. Granulosa cells appear in smears in variable-sized clusters. The cells have monomorphic, round, oval nuclei, with inconspicuous nucleoli (Fig. 29–77). The presence of nuclear polymorphism and hyperchromasia in association with increased numbers of mitotic figures is suggestive of a malignant variant. Note comments above about the aspirates of ovarian follicles (see also Chap. 16).

Malignant Tumors

Dysgerminoma.   The cells of this tumor are large and round and resemble primordial germ cells. The cytologic presentation in needle aspirates corresponds to that of seminoma in the testis (see Fig. 29–82).

Malignant Teratoma.   Malignant teratomas of the ovary are exceedingly rare. The malignant component may be made up of undifferentiated small malignant cells, resembling neuroblastoma. In a rare case, a carcinoid or a carcinoma, most often of squamous type, may arise in a dermoid cyst.

Carcinomas.   Aspirates from ovarian carcinomas are, as a rule, richer in cells than are aspirates from benign epithelial tumors. The cytologic recognition of a malignant tumor is usually not difficult. Even in well-differentiated types of carci-

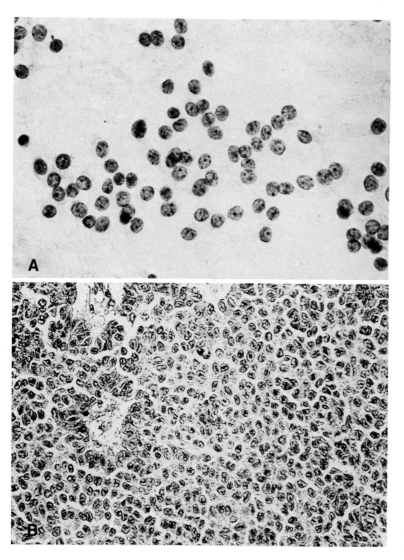

FIGURE 29–77. Granulosa cell tumor, ovary. (*A*) Needle aspirate showing neoplastic cells with monomorphic nuclei exhibiting inconspicuous nucleoli. (*B*) Tissue section of the same tumor. (*A*, Papanicolaou stain ×480; *B* ×120)

noma the smeared aspirate contains groups of cells with characteristic features of an adenocarcinoma, such as nuclear enlargement and hyperchromasia, large nucleoli, and thickening of the nuclear membrane (Figs. 29–78 and 29–79). In serous adenocarcinoma, the cells often appear in monolayer, but such a finding is insufficient for reliable distinction of a serous adenocarcinoma from endometrioid ovarian carcinoma, Mucinous ovarian carcinoma, by contrast, has a distinct cytologic presentation of mucus-producing cells embedded in masses of mucus. It, therefore, is readily distinguishable from other ovarian carcinomas. The same applies to clear cell adenocarcinoma, which resembles clear cell adenocarcinoma of the kidney (p. 1362). In the cystic lesions of "borderline malignancy" the needle aspirates usually are more cellular than in clearly benign cystomas (Fig. 29–80).

The accuracy of aspiration biopsy cytologic diagnosis in ovarian cancer was studied by Kjellgren and Ångström (1971, 1979), and by Geier et al. (1975). In both reports, ovarian cancer was accurately identified in about 92% of cases. The proportion of false-positive cytologic reports in histologically benign lesions was 4% in both studies.

Aspiration Biopsy of the Testis

The usual purpose of testicular needle biopsy is to investigate the nature of a palpable lesion. Aspiration biopsy has also been used to obtain cell samples for the evaluation of spermatogenesis (Persson et al., 1971). Thin needles (external diameter of 0.6 mm) are used, and palpable lesions are aspirated without anesthesia. In the evaluation of fertility, however, local anesthesia is used.

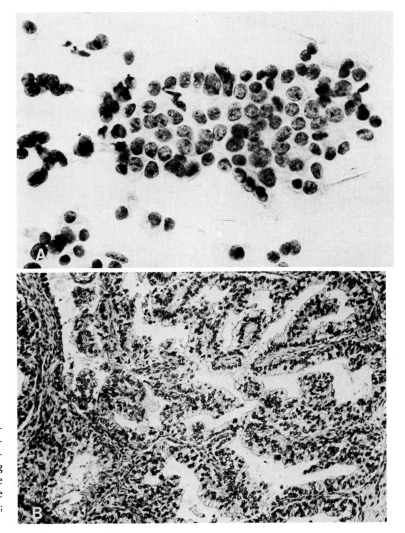

FIGURE 29–78. Serous papillary adenocarcinoma of the ovary. (*A*) Needle aspirate. A cluster of monomorphic malignant cells exhibiting pronounced hyperchromasia of the nuclei. (*B*) Tissue section of the tumor. (*A*, Papanicolaou stain ×480; *B* ×120)

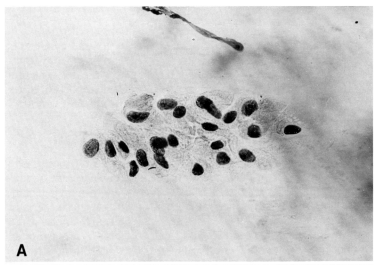

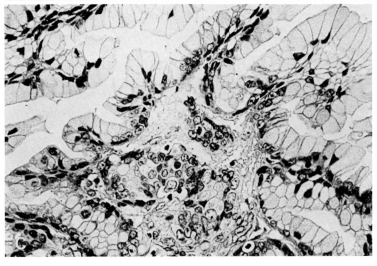

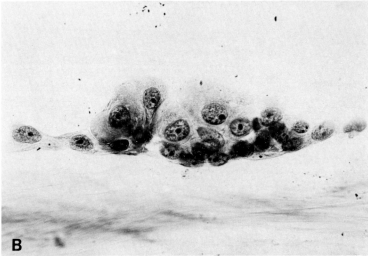

FIGURE 29-79. Mucinous adenocarcinoma of the ovary. (*A*) Needle aspirate. A cluster of mucinous carcinoma cells embedded in mucus. The cells are well differentiated, and nuclear hyperchromasia is the main cytologic sign of malignancy. (*B*) Needle aspirate smear showing a cluster of mucinous carcinoma cells and mucus. Nuclear atypia is more pronounced than in (*A*). (*C*) Tissue section. An area of well-differentiated carcinoma corresponding to the cell type shown in (*A*). (*A*, *B*, Papanicolaou stain ×480; *C* ×300. Zajicek, J.: Aspiration Biopsy Cytology. Part II. Basel, S. Karger, 1979)

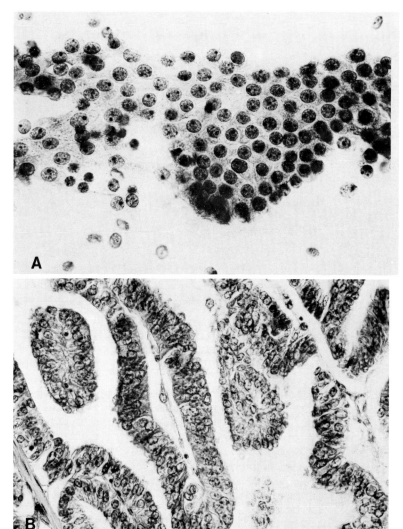

FIGURE 29–80. Serous ovarian cystoma, of borderline malignancy. (*A*) Needle aspirate, a cluster of epithelial cells. Irregular arrangement of the cells, together with some anisonucleosis, suggest the neoplastic nature of the aspirate. (*B*) Tissue section of the same tumor. Stromal invasion could not be ascertained and the neoplasm was classified as a "borderline lesion." (*A*, Papanicolaou stain ×480; *B* ×300)

Normal Cell Populations

Normal cellular constituents of the testis (spermatogonia and other sperm-forming cells, Sertoli and Leydig cells) are observed in aspirates obtained for study of spermatogenesis. They are also observed if the needle is inadvertently introduced into normal parenchyma during the aspiration of a palpable lesion.

Spermatogenic Cells. Aspirates from the normal, sexually mature testis are dominated by spermatogenic cells. Spermatogonia have a round, central nucleus, with an enlarged nucleolus. The cytoplasm is homogenous and has well-defined borders. The most common and readily recogniz-

able are the primary spermatocytes. They have a long prophase, and the nuclei are intensely stained due to reorganization of their chromatin into thick prophase chromosomes (Fig. 29–81). In air-dried, MGG-stained smears the spermatogonia resemble lymphatic blast cells, and an inexperienced observer may suspect the presence of a stem cell lymphoma. A more detailed scrutiny of the smear, however, will reveal numerous transitional cell forms, ranging from spermatogonia to spermatozoa. The secondary spermatozoa and spermatids are characterized by smaller nuclear sizes (these are haploid cells) and condensation of chromatin.

Sertoli Cells. These cells have a round, vesicular nucleus that contains a large nucleolus and is

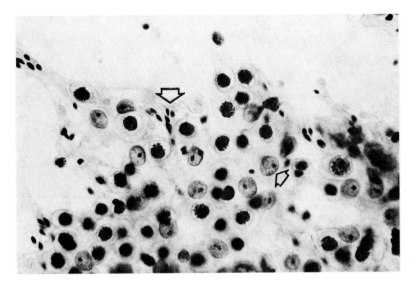

FIGURE 29–81. Needle aspirate of testis, a cell cluster from a seminiferous tubule. Sertoli cells, spermatogenic cells, and spermatozoa (*large arrow*) are recognized. Sertoli cells (*small arrow*) have large vesicle nuclei and indistinct cytoplasmic borders. Spermatogenic cells have distinct cytoplasmic borders. Primary spermotocytes are recognizable by the intensely stained nuclei. (Papanicolaou stain ×480. Zajicek, J.: Aspiration Biopsy Cytology. Part II. Basel, S. Karger, 1979)

surrounded by abundant pale and vacuolated cytoplasm with poorly defined cell borders (see Fig. 29–81). The cytoplasm appears fragile, and naked nuclei are common.

Interstitial or Leydig Cells.   In smeared aspirates, these cells appear singly or in clusters. They are somewhat smaller than Sertoli cells and have a central spherical or oval nucleus. Some Leydig cells are binucleated. The abundant, irregularly delineated cytoplasm is finely granular. As with Sertoli cells, a relative increase of Leydig cells is found in aspirates from juvenile and from atrophic testes.

Inflammatory Lesions

Acute Orchitis.   In acute orchitis, which often complicates other infections (e.g., influenza, mumps, pneumonia, cystitis), the testicles become painful, swollen, and firm. Aspiration biopsy yields abundant material, mainly fibrin, granulocytes, phagocytes, and cell detritus. Such smears should be carefully inspected, since occasionally malignant neoplasms of the testis may be accompanied by acute inflammation. The clinical history is the main guide to correct interpretation of the cytologic findings.

Chronic Orchitis.   Acute orchitis may subside completely or may persist in chronic form. The yield of an aspiration biopsy in chronic orchitis is less than in the acute condition, mainly because of increased fibrosis of the testis. Variable degrees of degeneration and decrease of spermatogenic cells are found, and also relative increase of Sertoli and Leydig cells. Variable numbers of lymphocytes, histiocytes, and plasma cells with scanty admixture of granulocytes are also present in the smears.

Granulomatous Orchitis.   In addition to the cells found in chronic orchitis, aspirates from granulomatous orchitis (usually due to tuberculosis) contain clusters of epithelioid cells and occasional multinucleated giant cells.

Cystic Lesions

Hydrocele (hematocele) and spermatocele are the two most common conditions that can simulate a testicular tumor and from which fluid can be aspirated at needle biopsy.

Aspiration biopsy of *hydrocele* usually yields clear, amber-colored fluid. Centrifugation gives a scanty sediment consisting of mesothelial cells and lymphocytes. Occasionally, the aspirate is hemorrhagic, indicating that bleeding has occurred in the sac of the tunica vaginalis (hematocele). The aspirate in *spermatocele* consists of variable amounts of milky fluid containing spermatozoa (see also Chap. 27).

The removal of fluid from a cystic lesion should be followed by careful examination of the affected testis. If any residual mass is palpable, it should be aspirated again and the material examined cytologically.

For description of mesotheliomas of the tunica vaginalis testis see Chapter 26.

Tumors

Germ cell tumors comprise about 95% of all malignant testicular tumors. Sex cord stromal tumors (Sertoli and Leydig cell tumors) are very rare and are usually benign.

The great majority of germ cell tumors are seminomas, embryonal carcinomas, and teratomas. Contrary to the ovary, where nearly all teratomas are benign, all teratomas of the testis must be considered as malignant. These tumors may occur in pure form or in various combinations. In a series of 834 germ cell tumors. Nefzger and Mostofi (1972) classified 316 (38%) as seminoma, 123 (15%) as embryonal carcinoma, 59 (8%) as teratoma, and 3 (0.4%) as choriocarcinoma. The remaining 333 germ cell tumors were combinations of various types, the most common ones being embryonal carcinoma–teratoma (199 cases; 24% of all the testis tumors), teratoma–embryonal carcinoma–seminoma (6%), embryonal carcinoma–seminoma (5%), and teratoma–serminoma (about 2%). Combinations of various germ cell tumors with choriocarcinoma were found in the residual 3% of the series.

Seminoma. These tumors, derived from seminiferous tubules, are characterized by a homogeneous population of neoplastic cells, usually larger than spermatogonia (Fig. 29–82). The nuclei are round or oval and show evenly distributed chromatin and often have large nucleoli. The cells may appear singly or in loose clusters. They are highly fragile, and spreading of needle aspirate on the slide often results in damage to a substantial part of the

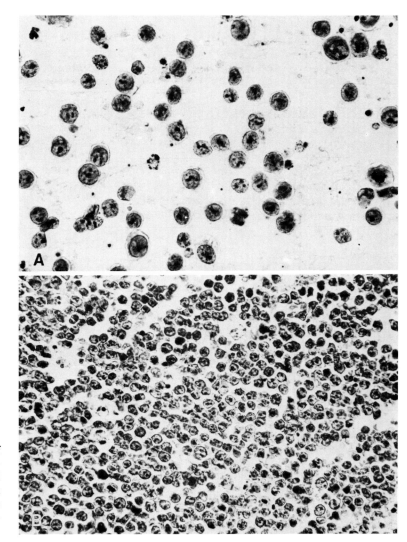

FIGURE 29–82. Seminoma of testis. (*A*) Needle aspirate: monomorphic population of dispersed neoplastic cells resembling blast cells. Note large nucleoli. (*B*) Tissue section of the same tumor. (*A*, Papanicolaou stain ×480; *B* ×300)

neoplastic cell population. In air-dried, MGG-stained smears, the background of the smears, probably composed of cytoplasmic debris, often has a striped, "tigroid" appearance that is quite characteristic of seminoma. The reasons for this peculiar artifact are not clear. Cell degeneration, in particular nuclear pyknosis, is often seen. The lymphocytes and the granulomatous reaction that are histologically observed in a high proportion of seminomas are sometimes observed also in smeared aspirate, although they are usually less impressive than in the tissue sections. In the smears, the lymphocytes are mingled with neoplastic cells, and distinction between lymphocytes and small seminoma cells sometimes may be difficult.

Embryonal Carcinoma. Needle aspirate is usually abundant in pleomorphic cancer cells, which form numerous cohesive clusters arranged in a characteristic epithelial pattern (Fig. 29–83). The nuclei have irregular contours. They contain enlarged nucleoli and show pronounced hyperchromasia and clumping of chromatin. The cytoplasm appears more compact than in seminoma and is usually well preserved.

Teratoma. Several types of tissue, representing two or three embryonal layers, are generally found in these highly malignant testicular tumors. The ectodermal layer, as a rule, is represented by squamous epithelium and neurogenic tissue, the entodermal by gastrointestinal and respiratory tissue,

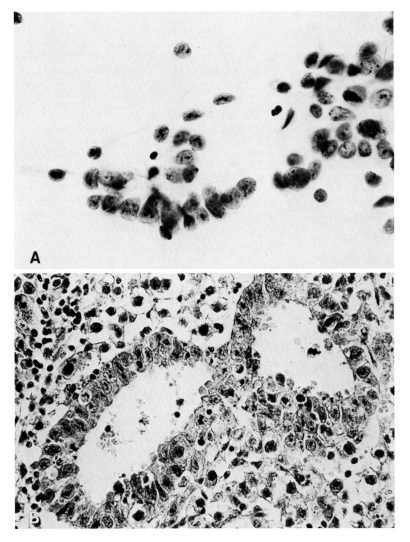

FIGURE 29–83. Embryonal carcinoma of testis. (*A*) Needle aspirate: a cluster of pleomorphic, neoplastic cells, resembling a carcinoma. (*B*) Tissue section from the same case as in (*A*). (*A*, Papanicolaou stain ×480; *B* ×300)

and the mesodermal layer by muscle, cartilage, and bone.

At biopsy, pure teratomas usually are hard on palpation and resist penetration by the needle. The yield of cells is most often scanty. Cytologic diagnosis of tumor may be extremely difficult in such material. Only when a cystic area has been penetrated is abundant fluid obtained. Palpation of the testis after removal of the fluid reveals a hard mass, which on repeated aspiration yields scanty material composed of fragments of epithelial structures, fibroblasts, or fragments of cartilage.

When a teratoma is associated with seminoma, embryonal carcinoma, or choriocarcinoma, as is the case in about 30% to 35% of all such tumors, these associated components predominate in needle aspirates because of their high cellularity and low cohesiveness. The teratoma component, therefore, may be unrecognized. This has some clinical implications, since survival rates are much higher in pure seminoma than in seminoma–teratoma, and are somewhat lower in pure embryonal carcinoma than for the combination of this tumor type with teratoma.

THE PROSTATE

Palpation of the prostate is a routine procedure in the medical examination of men over 40. It is generally accepted that most prostatic carcinomas arise in the posterior lobe of the gland and are detectable by transrectal palpation. The accuracy of digital examination in the diagnostic assessment of prostatic nodules has been estimated to average about 50%.

Newer modes of prostatic examination include ultrasound probes that may reveal small abnormalities not recognizable by palpation.

Most urologists consider histologic examination of prostatic tissue essential for the diagnosis of prostatic carcinoma. Transperineal open biopsy is often said to give the most satisfactory tissue specimen. The less traumatic and technically simpler transrectal punch biopsy with a thick needle has become increasingly popular, and several instruments have been devised for this purpose.

Studies of cell samples obtained by prostatic massage have been discussed in Chapter 23.

Aspiration Technique

The advantages of transrectal aspiration biopsy of the prostate, as used at Radiumhemmet (p. 1241),

are the directness of the approach, the minimal discomfort and trauma from the 22-gauge needle, and the rapidity with which slides can be processed and interpreted. These advantages are illustrated by the following account of 3,002 transrectal aspiration biopsies performed at Radiumhemmet on 2,410 patients during the years 1956 to 1966 (Eposti et al., 1968).

Most of the biopsies were done as office procedures. No anesthesia was used except in a few cases with anal complications, such as inflamed hemorrhoids or fistula. An anesthetic jelly was then applied before the instrument was introduced.

Most of the patients reported no particular pain or discomfort during the puncture and aspiration. Significant discomfort was reported by only a few patients with acute prostatitis and a few with prostatic carcinoma. Repeat biopsies were always readily accepted by the patients.

Complications

In approximately 17,000 transrectal prostatic aspiration biopsies performed at Karolinska Sjukhuset since the method was introduced in 1956, there have been none of the traumatic complications, such as severe bleeding, hematoma, and fistula, that can occur when thick needles are used to obtain specimens for histologic study. A review of 3,002 transrectal aspiration biopsies of the prostate performed between 1956 and 1966 showed complications in 12 cases (0.4%). Two of these patients had slight, transient hematuria (which required no treatment) a few minutes after the aspiration biopsy. In the other 10 cases there were late complications, namely acute epididymitis on the third day after the biopsy in 1 patient and on the tenth day in another, hemospermia a few days after the biopsy in 3 patients, and transient pyrexia in the first 24 hours in 5 patients, all of whom had known prostatovesiculitis and urinary infection.

In the following years, however, when the number of needle biopsies increased sharply, there were four cases of severe, gram-negative septicemia, one with a fatal outcome (Esposti et al., 1975). Further investigations, using a series of 571 aspiration biopsies, showed that among the patients who were referred primarily for cytologic confirmation of prostatitis, febrile reactions were more common than in the patients without clinically suspect prostatitis. In the prostatitis group, the frequency of febrile reactions after needle aspiration was 2.5%. It was 6.3% among prostatitis cases referred from the department of rheumatology and 1.5% in the prostatitis cases from the department of urology.

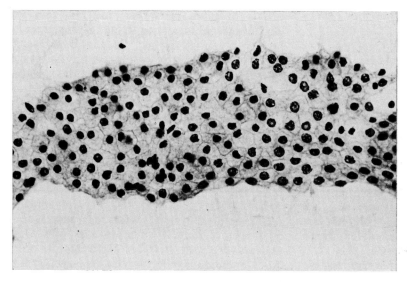

FIGURE 29–84. Aspiration of prostate. A sheet of epithelial cells in needle aspirate from a benign prostatic gland. (Papanicolaou stain ×370)

Of the 246 aspiration biopsies on patients without suspected prostatis, only one was followed by pyrexia (0.4%). The conclusion was that transrectal aspiration biopsy should *not* be undertaken for the diagnosis of prostatitis.

A past history of prostatitis does not in itself contraindicate an aspiration biopsy. When the palpatory findings are equivocal, aspiration biopsy is mandatory. Ten percent of the patients with prostatitis were found by study of needle aspirate to have carcinoma. In the patient with arthritis who is clinically suspected of harboring prostatic cancer, the relatively high risk of a febrile reaction requires that needle biopsy be performed only after the problem has been discussed with the responsible physician and with the patient. Because of the remote possibility of septicemia, every patient undergoing a transrectal aspiration biopsy of the prostate should be advised to contact his own physician or the nearest hospital should a febrile reaction occur. It is still a matter of debate whether prophylactic treatment with antibiotics is effective in preventing septicemia.

Cytology

The microscopy of prostatic smears should begin at low magnification to obtain a general impression of their appearance. In benign hyperplasia one usually sees a thin film of blood or fluid with a few scattered sheets of regularly shaped epithelial cells. If the aspirate has been properly spread on the slide most of the prostatic cell clusters will be found at the end of the slide.

Normal Prostatic Cells and Other Benign Cellular Constituents of Aspirates

Epithelial Cells. Normal prostatic epithelial acinar cells form flat sheets of small cells with clear cytoplasm and small, spherical nuclei of even sizes. The cytoplasmic borders are readily seen as thin lines separating the cells from each other (honeycomb effect) (Figs. 29–84 and 29–85*A,B*). Comma-shaped, dark nuclei of myoepithelial cells may be observed under high power (see Fig. 29–85*B*). Prostatic duct cells are somewhat larger, and

FIGURE 29–85. Aspiration smears of prostate (fixed). Comparison of benign prostatic epithelium (*A, B*) with a low-grade carcinoma (*C, D*). (*A*) Low-power view of a sheet of benign prostatic epithelial cells. Note the flatness of the cluster and the regular spacing of the spherical nuclei of equal size. (*B*) *Framed area* of (*A*) under magnification: The "honeycomb" of cell borders is shown. The nuclei are bland. No nucleoli are seen. The *arrows* point to the dark, comma-shaped nuclei of myoepithelial cells. (*C*) A low-power view of a well-differentiated prostatic adenocarcinoma. Note the piling up of cancer cells in the large cluster and the presence of a "microadenomatous complex" in the *framed* part of the photograph. (*D*) *Framed area* of (*C*) under high magnification. The somewhat enlarged and hyperchromatic nuclei lie at the periphery of the glandular structure, whereas the center thereof is formed by the cytoplasm of the cells. *Small arrows* point to the visible fairly large nucleoli. (*A, C* ×200; *B, D* ×800. Modified from Koss, L.G., et al.: Aspiration Biopsy. Cytologic Interpretation and Histologic Bases. New York, Igaku-Shoin, 1984, with permission)

are usually of cuboidal or columnar shape with one flat surface. Opaque, homogeneous prostatic concretions (corpora amylacea) are not uncommonly seen. Other benign cells, not of prostatic origin, that may be observed in prostatic aspirates and that may be of diagnostic significance are the seminal vesicle cells, urothelial cells, colonic epithelium, and bone marrow cells.

Seminal vesicle cells are often characterized by very large, opaque, dark nuclei and brown, granu-

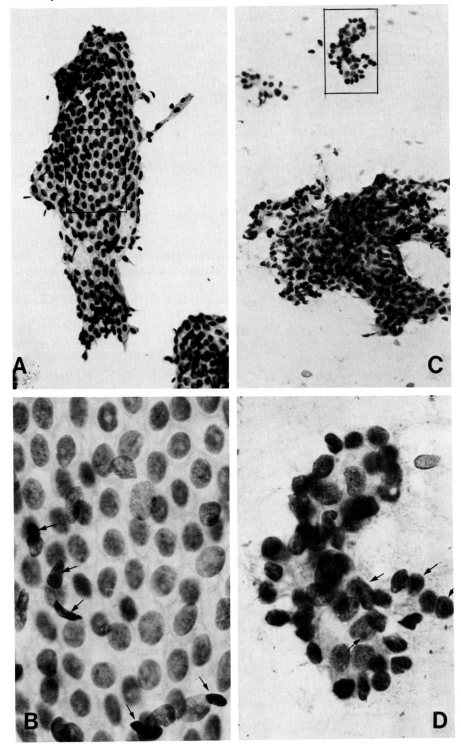

lar deposits of cytoplasmic pigment (Fig. 29–86A,B). These cells may be readily mistaken for cancer cells. Besides the presence of the pigment, another common identifying feature of these cells is the company of spermatozoa and of macrophages with phagocytosed spermatozoa (see Fig. 29–86A).

Urothelial cells are seen in aspirates wherein the needle is too deeply inserted and reaches the trigone of the bladder. Such cells are readily recog-

nized, particularly if the superficial umbrella cells are present in the smear (see Fig. 29–86C).

Colonic epithelium appears in smears if the tip of the needle is withdrawn to the level of the colonic epithelium, before releasing the piston of the syringe to equalize the vacuum. Large, columnar colonic goblet cells, with clear, mucus-containing cytoplasm and peripheral nuclei are usually readily identified (see Fig. 29–86D).

Bone marrow cells, notably megakaryocytes,

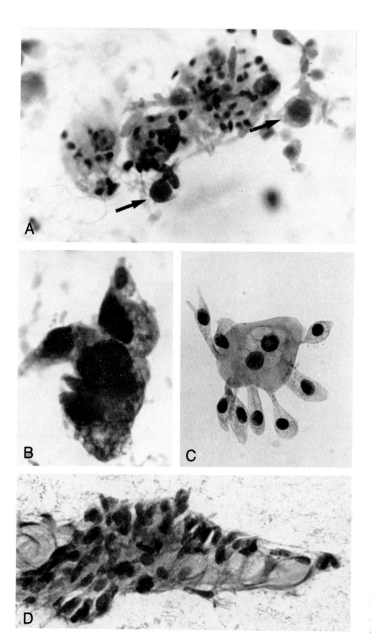

FIGURE 29–86. Benign cells not of prostatic origin observed in aspirations of the prostate. (*A*) Seminal vesicle epithelial cells with large, opaque, hyperchromatic nuclei (*arrows*) and macrophages containing phagocytized spermatozoa. (*B*) Seminal vesicle epithelial cells under high magnification. Note the large, hyperchromatic, yet homogeneous nuclei. Cytoplasmic granules of brown pigment may be noted. (*C*) Urothelial cells from bladder trigone: The center is formed by large binucleated umbrella cell to which several smaller epithelial cells from the adjacent deeper epithelial layer are attached. Note the very sharp cellular borders of the abundant cytoplasm and the spherical nuclei. (*D*) Rectal mucosa. A sheet of goblet cells with clear, mucus-containing cytoplasm and peripheral nuclei. (*A, C, D* ×400; *B* ×800). Modified from Koss, L.G., et al.: Aspiration Biopsy. Cytologic Interpretation and Histologic Bases. New York, Igaku-Shoin, 1984, with permission)

may be observed if the inexperienced operator aspirates the bone marrow from the sacrum (Greenebaum, 1988).

Benign Lesions

In benign prostatic hyperplasia, the typical epithelial cluster is represented by a flat, nonstratified sheet of benign epithelial cells with striking regularity of architecture (see Fig. 29–84). In MGG-stained smears, bluish purple granules of variable size can frequently be seen in the cytoplasm.

Another type of cell grouping in benign prostatic lesions is a multilayered plug of epithelial cells of quasi-papillary appearance and more irregular structure. This may arouse the suspicion of cancer, but higher magnification shows that here, too, the spherical nuclei are of even sizes, and the amount of cytoplasm is constant. The relatively few dissociated cells have the same appearance as the clustered cells.

In prostatitis, the aspiration biopsy smears show variable numbers of inflammatory cells. In acute inflammation, neutrophil granulocytes predominate. In less acute forms, the smears show monocytes, lymphocytes, and neutrophil granulocytes. The prostatic glandular cells often show degenerative changes, such as vacuolization of the cytoplasm, swelling or pyknosis of the nuclei, and cytolysis. Macrophages may be numerous in these smears. The prostatic epithelium sometimes reacts to the inflammation with variation in nuclear size and shape and the presence of small nucleoli. In the presence of nucleoli it is difficult to exclude the possibility of cancer, and we usually recommend repeat biopsy after treatment of the inflammation.

A relatively rare, but distinct, type of inflammatory process is granulomatous eosinophilic prostatis, which is observed in patients with allergic conditions such as bronchial asthma. The inflammatory cell population in aspiration biopsy smears is dominated by plasma cells, multinucleated giant cells, and eosinophilic leukocytes. Despite its comparative rarity, granulomatous eosinophilic prostatitis is clinically important, since it causes induration and partial fixation of the gland and thus may strongly suggest prostatic carcinoma on digitial examination.

Prostatic Carcinoma

The aspirates in prostatic carcinoma usually contain more abundant cells than in benign conditions. Often there is no admixture of blood, which gives a distinctive appearance to the dried, unstained smears.

In smears from well-differentiated cancers the most characteristic feature is the microadenomatous complex. The cytoplasm of the cancer cells is crowded into a central mass, while the enlarged nuclei are arranged at the periphery. When this pattern is repeated throughout the smear without noteworthy nuclear polymorphism, the cytologic picture can be regarded as pathognomonic of well-differentiated prostatic adenocarcinoma (see Figs. 29–85C,D and 29–87).

In moderately well-differentiated adenocarcinoma, this pattern is less evident, and there are more solid groups of malignant cells with pronounced nuclear polymorphism and large, irregularly shaped nuclei.

In smears from poorly differentiated prostatic cancers, the malignant cells are dissociated and may be strikingly polymorphic, with bizarre forms and very large nuclei (Figs. 29–88 and 28–89). In the anaplastic variant, the picture is monotonous, resembling the pattern of leukemia or lymphoma. Clustering and a tendency to form microadenomatous complexes are relatively rare.

On review of the prostatic aspiration biopsies performed at Radiumhemmet in Stockholm during the years 1956 to 1966, the carcinomas were classified as well-differentiated, moderately differentiated, or poorly differentiated tumors (Eposti et al., 1968). In 206 patients with estrogen-treated carcinomas, correlation of cytologic grading and survival rates showed clear prognostic differences. The 3-year survival rate was 80% in the well-differentiated carcinoma, close to 60% when the differentiation was of a moderate degree, but only 20% in poorly differentiated cancer. The same tendency was observed in the 84 patients who could be followed for 5 years (Fig. 29–90).

When the cytologic examination shows poorly differentiated carcinoma, estrogen therapy alone appears inadequate to control the malignant process. At Radiumhemmet such patients are treated by radiotherapy.

These comments on cytologic grading of prostatic carcinoma, written in 1978 by Dr. Zajicek, are still valid today (1991). In the interim, DNA measurements by flow cytometry and image analysis systems have largely confirmed these observations. The well-differentiated carcinomas have, for the most part, a diploid DNA content, whereas the less well-differentiated prostatic cancers, for the most part, are aneuploid. Diploid tumors are often of low stage (confined to the prostate) and offer a better prognosis than aneuploid tumors. Even high-stage diploid tumors have a slower evolution than

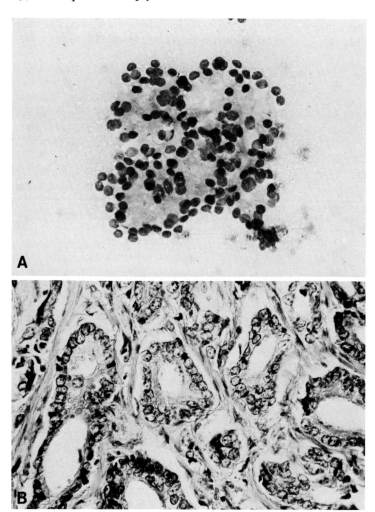

FIGURE 29–87. (*A*) Needle aspirate smear from a well-differentiated prostatic carcinoma. A cell cluster imitating acinar structures (microadenomatous complex) is seen (air-dried smear). (*B*) Tissue section of the tumor shown in (*A*). (*A*, MGG ×270; *B* ×300)

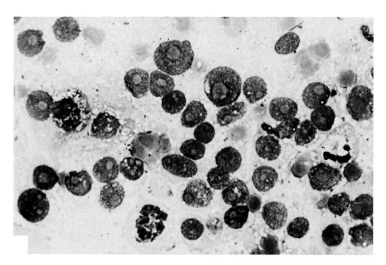

FIGURE 29–88.   Needle aspirate from a poorly differentiated prostatic carcinoma showing polymorphic population of dispersed, single carcinoma cells. (Air-dried smear, MGG ×550)

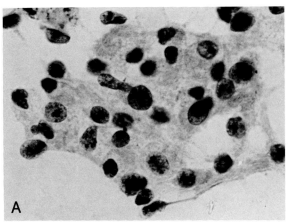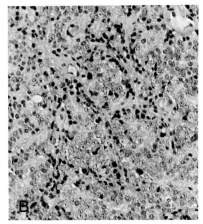

FIGURE 29–89. Aspirate and tissue section of a poorly differentiated prostatic carcinoma. (*A*) Fixed smear; the borders of the cancer cells are not distinct. The nuclei are irregular in shape, hyperchromatic, vary in size, and contain large nucleoli. (*B*) Histologic section of the same tumor. (*A* ×800; *B* ×150)

aneuploid tumors (for further details and references, see Chaps. 34 and 35).

Treatment of prostatic carcinoma by estrogens and synthetic estrogen substitutes can be monitored by prostatic aspirates. A favorable effect of estrogen is reflected in numerical reduction and degenerative changes in the cancer cells, which finally disappear from the aspirate. The prostatic glandular epithelium is transformed into squamous epithelium, and "glycogenic" cells appear (Fig. 29–91). Such changes may be seen in aspiration biopsy smears within a few weeks after the start of treatment (Esposti, 1971). The aspiration should be made from the tumor region that clinically shows least regression.

To ascertain the diagnostic reliability of the aspiration biopsy method in prostatic carcinoma, comparisons were made between the cytologic reports in 162 cases and the histologic findings in the

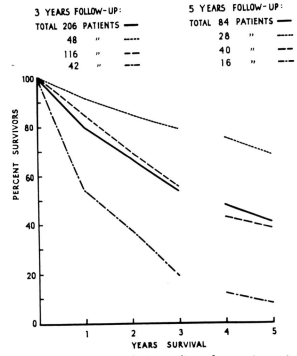

FIGURE 29–90. Cytologic grading of prostatic carcinoma and survival of 206 patients treated with estrogens (January 1956–June 1963).

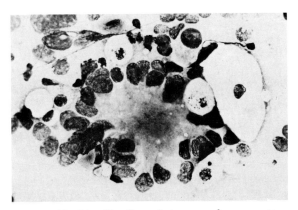

FIGURE 29–91. Needle aspirate smear from an acinar cancer complex after 8 weeks of estrogen treatment. "Glycogenic" squamous cells have appeared. (Air-dried smear, MGG stain ×430)

same cases (Eposti, 1966). There were no erroneous cytologic diagnoses of cancer. Therefore, it was concluded that a report of prostatic carcinoma based on cytologic study of prostatic aspirates can be accepted as reliable. Cancer was diagnosed from the initial aspiration biopsy smears in 90% of the cases of histologically proved carcinoma. By repeating the aspiration biopsy if a clinical suspicion of malignancy persisted after a negative cytologic report, this diagnostic accuracy was increased to 95%. For further discussion of cytology of prostatic carcinoma in urinary sediment see Chapter 23.

THE SKIN

Because of the ease with which punch or excisional biopsies of skin lesions can be obtained, the aspiration biopsy technique has found limited applications in the diagnosis of skin disorders. There are, however, some observers who use aspirations and scrapes of skin lesions when primary or metastatic skin tumors are suspected (Canti, 1984).

Primary Tumors of Skin

Basal Cell Carcinoma and Related Lesions

Tumor scrapes or thin-needle aspirates of this group of tumors yield the characteristic cohesive clusters of epithelial cells. At the periphery of the clusters, palisading of cells may be noted. Very few detached epithelial cells are seen (Fig. 29–92*A*).

Squamous Carcinoma

Fully developed invasive primary squamous carcinomas of the skin are comparatively uncommon. The cytologic features are those of other squamous cancers, including keratin shells ("ghost cells"), as shown in Fig. 29–92*B*.

Malignant Melanoma

Primary malignant melanomas of the skin have some common features that allow the cytologic recognition of the tumor. Chief among the latter is the presence of melanin pigment in the cytoplasm of the tumor cells. Other features include the presence of large, binucleated or multinucleated cells, with nuclei arranged at the periphery, and the frequent presence of intranuclear cytoplasmic inclusions (see Fig. 29–92*C*).

There are several other morphologic variants of malignant melanomas, including the spindle cell type and balloon cell type (discussion in Koss et al., 1992).

Merkel Cell Carcinoma (Primary Neuroendocrine Carcinoma of Skin)

These uncommon, highly malignant tumors, derived from the neuroendocrine cells (Merkel cells), occur in the dermis of elderly patients. The tumors are composed of trabecular sheets or nodules of monotonous, small, tumor cells. The neuroendocrine nature of the tumor was confirmed by ultrastructural studies that revealed numerous membrane-bound, cytoplasmic, dense core granules, and by cytochemistry.

In aspiration smears the tumor cells are either dispersed or form loosely structured clusters. The cytoplasm is very scanty and disintegrates easily with resulting debris and naked nuclei. The nuclei are granular, but the nucleoli are either not visible or very small. The most characteristic feature of these tumors is the presence of spherical, eosinophilic, pink, cytoplasmic inclusions that are located near the nuclei or within nuclear indentations. The inclusions (intermediate filaments or IF buttons) are composed of keratin filaments and are best documented with antikeratin antibodies (Domagala et al., 1987).

The differential diagnosis of Merkel cell carcinomas includes metastatic oat cell carcinoma, metastatic carcinoids, and occasionally other tumors composed of small cancer cells. In none of them are the IF buttons observed; hence, this is a unique morphologic feature of Merkel cell carcinoma in aspirates.

Metastatic Tumors

From time to time, skin and subcutaneous tissue metastases may occur with almost any primary cancer. The most important application of aspiration biopsy, however, is in the diagnosis of recurrent mammary carcinoma in mastectomy scars. An example of such a lesion is shown in Fig. 29–93. An important point of differential diagnosis is subcutaneous endometriosis (discussed below).

SOFT-PART TUMORS

A broad variety of benign and malignant soft-part lesions occasionally may be aspirated. It is not possible within the framework of this summary to discuss all of the entities that may be encountered and that, for the most part, cannot be accurately classified in aspirated material.

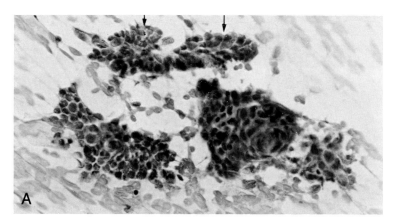

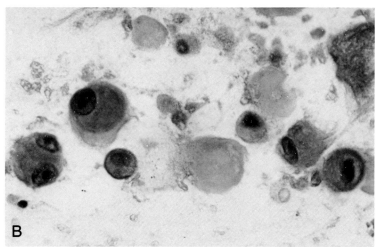

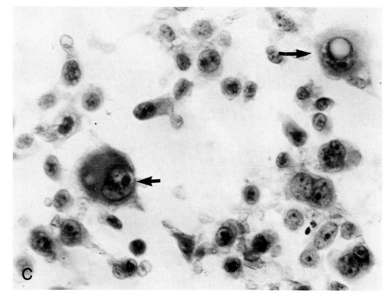

FIGURE 29–92. Aspiration biopsy smears of primary skin tumors. (*A*) Basal cell carcinoma; note the cohesive clusters of small epithelial cells with palisading at the periphery (*arrows*). (*B*) Squamous cell carcinoma; the field contains large cancer cells and keratin shells (ghost cells). (*C*) Malignant melanoma; the field shows cancer cells of variable sizes. One binucleated cancer cell shows a large nucleolus (*small arrow*). One cancer cell contains a large intranuclear cytoplasmic inclusion (*large arrow*). (*A* ×400; *B*, *C* ×800. Modified from Koss, L.G., et al.: Aspiration Biopsy. Cytologic Interpretation and Histologic Bases. New York, Igaku-Shoin, 1984, with permission)

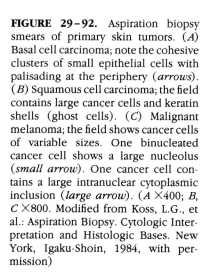

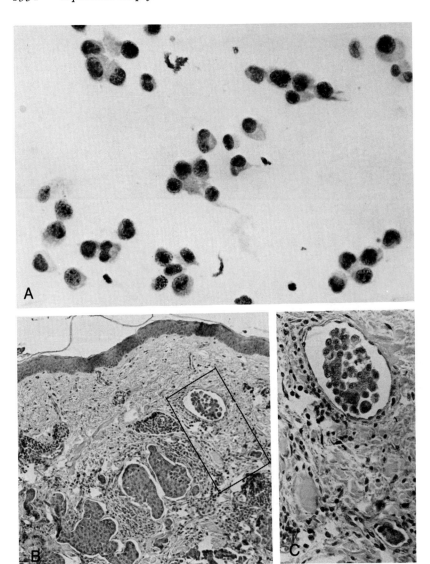

FIGURE 29–93. Metastatic mammary carcinoma to skin. (*A*) Aspiration smear showing dispersed small cancer cells, many with peripheral nuclei. (*B*) Skin biopsy from the same case showing mammary carcinoma in subcutaneous lymphatics. (*C*) An enlargement of the *marked area* in (*B*) to show cancer cells in a subcutaneous lymphatic. (*A* ×400; *B* ×100; *C* ×250. Modified from Koss, L.G., et al.: Aspiration Biopsy. Cytologic Interpretation and Histologic Bases. New York, Igaku-Shoin, 1984, with permission)

Perhaps the most important two questions that can be answered on aspirated material are the following:

1. Is the lesion benign or malignant?
2. Is the malignant lesion a metastatic or a primary tumor, the latter requiring further classification on a tissue biopsy.

There are some important exceptions to these general guidelines. Some soft-part lesions may be accurately recognized in the aspirated material, for example, endometriosis (Fig. 29–94) and neurilemomas (see Fig. 29–97).

Endometriosis in the form of subcutaneous ab-

dominal nodules, often occurring in the area of the umbilicus or in laparotomy scars, is an important source of diagnostic errors. The aspirate usually contains two families of cells: larger cells, representing the lining of the endometrial glands, and smaller, spindly cells of endometrial stroma (see Fig. 29–94). Unless close attention is paid to the differences between these two cell populations, erroneous diagnoses of metastatic adenocarcinoma has been known to occur, sometimes with disastrous results.

The cytologic findings in neurilemoma are described on p. 1339.

Soft-part sarcomas often yield abundant malig-

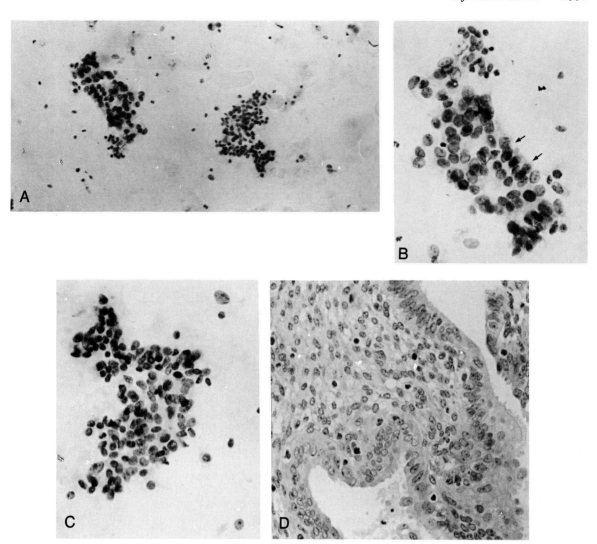

FIGURE 29–94. Endometriosis of abdominal wall. (*A*) A low-power view of the aspiration smear showing two clusters of cells: the endometrial gland cells are somewhat larger cells than the stromal cells. (*B*) Higher magnification of endometrial glandular cells from (*A*). Note the uniform round nuclei and the palisading of the cells on the edge of the cluster (*arrows*), corresponding to the lumen of the gland. (*C*) Higher magnification of the endometrial stromal cells from (*A*). The cells are distinctly smaller than the glandular cells. (*D*) Tissue section of abdominal endometriosis (*A* ×150; *B, C* ×560; *D* ×350. Case courtesy of Dr. James Amberson, Cornell University Medical School, New York, New York)

nant cells. Perhaps the easiest to identify are liposarcomas and chondrosarcomas because of the characteristic features of their cells (see Fig. 29–132). All spindle cell sarcomas are similar in aspirates and, in most instances, require tissue biopsy for further classification. Some of the important points of differential diagnosis include atypical lipomas, pseudosarcomatous fasciitis, and Kaposi's sarcoma in AIDS (see Fig. 29–127 and Koss et al., 1992 for further discussion).

PART III: ASPIRATION BIOPSY REQUIRING IMAGING GUIDANCE

Within the last decades, the introduction of various roentgenologic imaging techniques has facilitated the aspiration biopsy of nonpalpable lesions (see Table 29–2). The oldest of these techniques is fluoroscopy, utilized as early as 1938 for the aspiration of lung tumors (Craver and Binkley, 1938). The results were rather disastrous, because the large-caliber needles used in the aspiration procedure resulted in numerous serious complications, such as pneumothorax, requiring treatment. Several decades later, Dahlgren and Nordenstrøm revived the technique of lung aspiration, with excellent results, when using small-caliber needles and an improved imaging system (see Chaps. 19 and 20, for description of the contemporary technique). Angiography and lymphangiography also provided guidance to aspiration biopsies of abdominal organs and retroperitoneal lymph nodes. However, it is only with the introduction of sophisticated modalities of ultrasound, computed tomography (CT), and stereotactic instruments that interventional radiologists began to aspirate nonpalpable lesions on a large scale, often forcing the practicing surgical pathologists to accept the technique of aspiration biopsy as an important part of the diagnostic armamentarium.

Thin-needle aspiration biopsy can now be applied to the diagnosis of space-occupying lesions anywhere in the human body. Radiologic guidance is particularly useful in the aspiration of thoracic, abdominal, and intracranial lesions, but it is also applicable to other anatomic sites, such as the orbit. There are several important advantages to these techniques: They often spare the patient diagnostic surgical procedures, they can be performed with relatively little discomfort to the patient, and, in experienced hands, they provide a rapid and reliable diagnostic guidance to further treatment.

THORACIC ORGANS

The Lung and the Pleura

The aspiration biopsy of lung lesions was treated in Chapters 19 and 20. Pleural lesions were discussed in Chapter 26.

The Mediastinum

The mediastinal space is the site of space-occupying inflammatory lesions and of primary and metastatic tumors. Among the inflammatory lesions, tuberculosis and histoplasmosis play an important role. The recognition of these processes has been discussed elsewhere in this book (see pp. 727 and 739).

The following principal mediastinal lesions can be recognized in aspirated material.

Anterior Mediastinum
Cysts (including dermoid cysts)
Substernal thyroid
Thymomas
Malignant teratomas
Seminomas
Malignant lymphomas

Central Mediastinum
Metastatic tumors
Malignant lymphomas

Posterior Mediastinum
Schwannomas (neurilemomas)
Other rare tumors

Primary Tumors

A variety of tumors of thymic origin may occur in the anterior mediastinum. Chief among them are the thymomas, benign and malignant teratomas, and malignant lymphomas. Tumors occurring in the posterior mediastinum include neurilemomas and other uncommon soft-part neoplasms.

Thymomas. Thymomas are tumors composed of an epithelial component and T-lymphocytes. The two components may be equally represented or they may be a preponderance of one against the other. The tumors may be associated with myasthenia gravis and hematologic disorders. Most thymomas are asymptomatic and discovered on an incidental chest roentgenogram. The cytologic makeup of the aspiration biopsies of thymomas depends on their composition. In an average tumor, the epithelial and the lymphocytic component will be well represented and are diagnostic of the lesion (Fig. 29–95). In the epithelial variant, the lymphocytic component is poorly represented and the aspirated material is dominated by eosinophilic epithelial cells of variable sizes, which are dispersed but also form sheets and small cell clusters. The cell-in-cell arrangement that is sometimes seen, is reminiscent of Hassal's corpuscles and must be differentiated from "squamous pearls" occurring in metastatic squamous carcinoma. In epithelial thymomas, however, the necrosis, usually seen in metastatic squamous cancer, is not evident (Fig. 29–96). The behavior of thy-

momas cannot be anticipated on the basis of their morphology, although the epithelial spindle cell variant is sometimes considered to have a greater potential for recurrence and metastases.

Benign Teratomas. Benign teratomas of the mediastinum are often cystic and contain elements of the three embryonal layers, dominated by squamous epithelium and skin appendages. There is limited experience with the cytologic presentation of these tumors on aspiration biopsy. Squamous cells and keratinized debris dominate the cytologic picture, but skin appendages (hair shafts, seba-

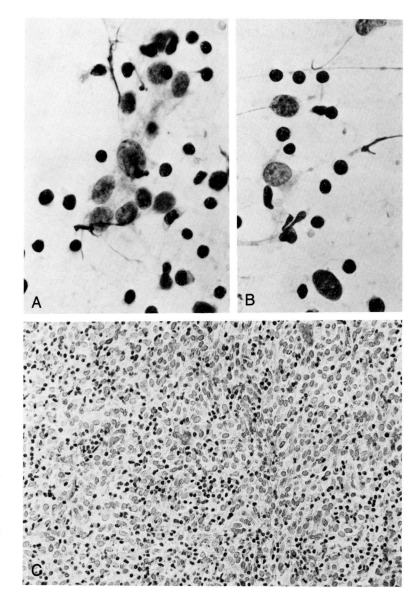

FIGURE 29–95. Thymoma, aspiration biopsy and tissue section. (*A, B*) The smear shows a mixture of epithelial cells and lymphocytes characteristic of this tumor. (*C*) The corresponding tissue section. (*A, B* ×800; *C* ×225. Modified from Koss, L.G., et al.: Aspiration Biopsy. Cytologic Interpretation and Histologic Bases. New York, Igaku-Shoin, 1984, with permission)

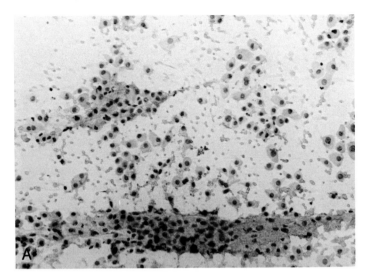

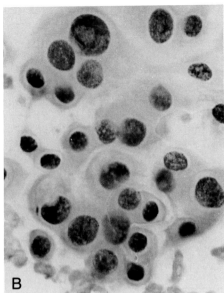

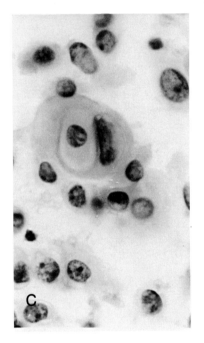

FIGURE 29-96. Epithelial thymoma, an incidental finding in a 74-year-old asymptomatic woman with a sharply demarcated anterior mediastinal mass. (*A*) Overview of the aspiration biopsy smear with dispersed and clustered epithelial cells. There were very few lymphocytes in the smear. (*B, C*) Higher-power view of the epithelial cells. The cells were eosinophilic, sharply demarcated and showing some variability in the sizes of the hyperchromatic nuclei. (*C*) The cell-in-cell arrangement, reminiscent of a Hassal's corpuscle. The patient refused surgery and remained asymptomatic. (*A* ×100; *B, C* ×800. Case Courtesy of Dr. Honig, White Plains Hospital, White Plains, New York)

ceous glands) and other benign epithelial structures may be observed (Koss et al., 1992). A case of a ruptured benign cystic teratoma into the pleural cavity was described by Cobb et al. (1985; see Chap. 25).

Malignant Teratomas. These may contain elements of malignant tumors of several types: embryonal carcinoma, seminoma, or a more mature variant of a carcinoma. An example of a malignant teratoma of the pericardium is shown in Fig. 26-

73. Mediastinal seminomas have the same cytologic presentation as testicular seminomas (see Fig. 29-82).

Malignant Lymphomas. A broad variety of Hodgkin's and non-Hodgkin's lymphomas may occur in the thymus and in the intrathoracic lymph nodes. The non-Hodgkin's lymphomas are usually of T-cell type and often carry an ominous prognosis. The cytologic presentation of these tumors is discussed on p. 1283.

Posterior Mediastinum. An example of the most common primary tumor of the posterior mediastinum, a neurilemoma, is shown in Fig. 29–97. The tumor is readily recognized in an aspirate because the cohesive tumor fragments show palisading of the component cells (Verocay bodies), which is readily visible in the form of dark lines, representing aligned nuclei. A malignant variant of this tumor may also occur. In such cases, dispersed, large, hyperchromatic nuclei may be seen next to spindly cells in cohesive bundles.

Metastatic Tumors

Tumors of lung origin, but also tumors of the larynx, esophagus, and tumors from distant sites, may be observed in the mediastinum. Their cytologic presentation has been repeatedly discussed elsewhere in this book.

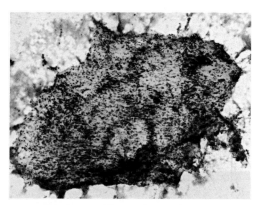

FIGURE 29–97. Mediastinal neurilemoma. A typical low-power view of a cell cluster with dark lines representing nuclear palisading (Verocay bodies), diagnostic of this tumor. (×56. Modified from Koss, L.G., et al.: Aspiration Biopsy. Cytologic Interpretation and Histologic Bases. New York, Igaku-Shoin, 1984, with permission)

ABDOMINAL ORGANS*

The principal purpose of aspiration biopsy of the abdominal organs is the rapid identification of the space-occupying lesions, whether primary tumors or metastases. With experience and skill, this purpose can be achieved in the majority of patients. The benefits of this technique are obvious in several clinical situations:

1. When the patient is thought to have a metastatic or recurrent tumor that cannot be treated by surgery and when a confirmatory aspirate may prevent an unnecessary exploratory laparotomy. Metastases to the liver, adrenal glands, or kidneys, and recurrence of pelvic tumors are the prime examples of this situation.
2. When the patient is thought to have an inoperable primary tumor of unknown type. The aspiration may provide adequate guidance to further clinical steps and to optimal nonsurgical treatment, e.g., in pancreatic cancer and in retroperitoneal lymphoma.
3. When the differential diagnosis between a benign entity and a cancer cannot be made on clinical or roentgenologic evidence and the nature of the lesion can be clarified by aspiration. Examples of this situation include avascular

space-occupying renal lesions and some pancreatic and retroperitoneal lesions.
4. When staging of cancer can be performed by aspiration of pelvic, aortic, or retroperitoneal lymph nodes. Examples include staging of carcinoma of the uterine cervix, endometrium, prostate, and testicular or ovarian tumors.

There are still other clinical situations not specifically listed above when the needle aspiration may prove to be beneficial to the patient, for example, in evacuation of cystic lesions. The principal advantage, however, is in providing a rapid diagnostic decision, thereby minimizing the delay in treatment, while also reducing expenses and operative risk.

Complications

The potential hazards to the patient include perforation of a viscus and dissemination of the tumor along the needle track or through vascular channels. In general, the small perforations of viscera apparently seal rapidly, and peritonitis (except for bile peritonitis; see below) has not, to our knowledge, been recorded. Studies of the safety of the aspiration biopsy of the pancreas in the pig (Coel and Niwagaria, 1978), an animal model chosen because its pancreas is similar histologically and in anatomic location to that of humans, and on mongrel dogs (Goldstein et al., 1977), have shown that

---

*This text, in part, is based on the chapter by Moussouris, H.F., Koss, L.G., Rosenblatt, R., and Kutcher, R.: Thin needle aspiration biopsy of abdominal organs. In Koss, L.G., and Coleman, D.V. (eds): Advances in Clinical Cytology, vol. 2. New York and Paris, Masson Publishing, 1984, with permission.

no significant damage to the abdominal viscera is caused by the thin needle.

Single instances of intrahepatic hemorrhage (Lundquist, 1971) and of intra-abdominal hemorrhage (Zormoza, 1981) have been observed. We observed one case of bile peritonitis after incidental perforation of a Courvoisier gallbladder, not unlike a case described by Schultz (1976). Anecdotal rare cases of pancreatitis have been observed.

The spread of tumor along the needle track is most uncommon, but has been observed occasionally (Ferucci et al., 1979; Gibbons et al., 1977; Smith et al., 1980; Bersenfeld et al., 1988). Although the aspiration biopsy of the breast has been shown to be harmless in reference to patients' survival, similar statistics pertaining to abdominal organs are still scarce. For renal carcinomas, von Schreeb et al. (1967) failed to observe any deleterious effects of diagnostic aspiration on survival. To date, a single death has been reported following a small-caliber-needle aspirate of the liver for a necrotic hepatocellular carcinoma (Riska and Freeman, 1975).

Techniques

Imaging of Abdominal Organs

Within the last 30 years, several roentgenologic techniques have been developed that, combined with the use of small-caliber needles, have completely revolutionized the approach to percutaneous aspiration of space-occupying intra-abdominal lesions. These techniques not only permit precise anatomic imaging and targeting of the lesions, but also allow the planning of a safe access route, thereby reducing the risk of complications. The oldest of these techniques is fluoroscopy combined with opacification studies, followed by radionuclide scanning, computed tomography (CT), and ultrasonography. The choice of the technique depends on the availability of equipment, the training and skill of the person performing the aspiration, and the location and size of the lesion.

Fluoroscopy must be enhanced by opacification studies, i.e., injection of a radiopaque substance that will outline specific targets. Among the opacification techniques are angiography, lymphangiography, intravenous pyelography, and percutaneous transhepatic or endoscopic retrograde cholangiography, each of which serves a different purpose.

Angiography may reveal an abnormal configuration of vessels and of blood supply suggestive of a malignant tumor (tumor blush), or encasement of a vessel by a constricting lesion (see Fig. 29–115B). Lymphangiography may outline the location of pelvic and retroperitoneal lymph nodes and provide data on their size and configuration (see Fig. 29–125.). Intravenous pyelography serves to identify the anatomic outlines of the kidneys and the renal pelves. Transhepatic cholangiography provides information on the distribution of the biliary duct system that may be disturbed by a space-occupying lesion. Endoscopic cholangiography also permits the visualization of the pancreatic ducts.

Each one of these techniques was extensively used for guided aspiration biopsies. Thus, angiography was used by Oscarson et al. (1972) to perform guided aspirations of pancreatic and gastric tumors under fluoroscopic control. Ho et al. (1977) used cholangiopancreatography as a guide to aspiration of the pancreas. Gothlin (1976) and Zornoza et al. (1977) first used lymphangiography as a guide to aspiration of lymph notes. Andersen et al. (1976) and Johansen and Svendsen (1978) used radionuclide scanning as a guide to needle aspirations of the liver. For further accounts of the various techniques, the reader is referred to Zornoza (1981) and to the descriptive parts of this chapter.

Computed tomography, as a guide to fine-needle aspiration of space-occupying lesions, has been successfully used by a number of investigators since the mid-1970s. (Ferucci et al., 1979; Haaga and Alfidi, 1976) This approach offers excellent, reproducible image resolution (see Figs. 29–105 and 29–114A). With the newer instruments, the optimal distance to the lesion and the angle of needle entry may be automatically calculated, displayed on the screen, and recorded for further reference. Verification of the needle tip position prior to tissue sampling is readily accomplished. Computed tomography is particularly useful as a guide to the aspiration biopsy of small, deeply seated lesions; however, it does have some significant disadvantages. The technique is cumbersome and slow; it also involves exposing the patient to a significant amount of radiation. The cost of the use of equipment is also very high.

Ultrasonography also offers a two-dimensional anatomic display (see Figs. 29–108A and 29–115A). When compared with CT, ultrasound has the advantage of greater scanning flexibility and speed, particularly with the use of real-time and operator-controlled hand-held transducers. Electronic calipers, currently available, will automatically calculate the distance to the target; the angle of entry can also be measured. In addition, the absence of radiation exposure and the relatively low cost of the equipment have made ultrasonography the preferred tool for localization of space-occupying lesions in many cases. (Smith et al., 1975; Rasmussen et al., 1972; Rosenblatt et al., 1982). The limiting factor in the use of ultrasound as a guide for thin-needle aspiration is the difficulty in demonstrating the needle tip within solid lesions. Although ultrasonography can demonstrate the tip of the needle within a fluid collection, the acoustical interface between the needle and a solid tumor mass is often not discernible. Therefore, because the precise position of the needle tip, prior to the aspiration, cannot be documented easily, lesions smaller than 3 cm in diameter and situated deeply within an organ may be missed; these should be sampled under CT guidance.

Instrumentation

The needles used for aspiration biopsy at Montefiore Medical Center are stainless steel, 22- or 23-gauge (outer diameter 0.75 mm and 0.64 mm, respectively), and 15 or 20 cm in length. Three types of needles are in use, each with a different tip.* The Chiba needle has a one-sided bevel at a 45° angle. The pencil-point needle is beveled all the way around, and the Greene needle, which was introduced in 1981, has a cutting bevel tip used for acquiring a core of tissue. All needles are introduced into the abdomen with an obturating stylet in place. Disposable 20-ml plastic syringes are used for the aspiration (Fig. 29–98).

Sampling Techniques

Either one of the imaging modalities described above will guide the selection of the entry site for biopsy. Computed tomography and ultrasound will, in addition, provide information on the depth to which the needle will be inserted and the angle of

---

Supplied by Cook Inc., Bloomington, Indiana 47402.

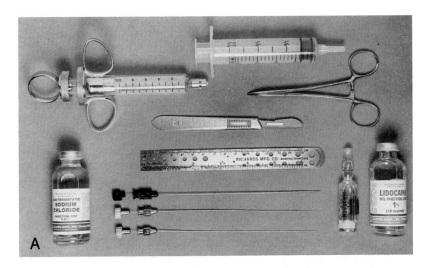

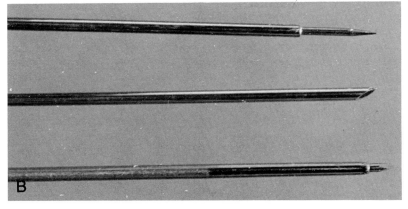

FIGURE 29–98. (*A*) Tray used for abdominal aspiration biopsy. Note the three different needles with stylets. (*B*) Enlargement of the needle tips: *top*, pencil-point needle; *center*, Chiba needle; *bottom*, Greene needle. The caliber of the needles is 22- or 23-gauge and the lengths are from 15 to 20 cm.

approach to the target. The entry site is selected to obtain the shortest distance between the skin and the target lesion. This selection may be influenced by the desire to avoid the costrophrenic angles (and hence pneumothorax) and major vessels, such as the aorta, vena cava, and portal veins.

Following the selection of the entry site, the skin is cleansed and anesthetized. A 2- to 3-mm skin incision facilitates the passage of the biopsy needle. The needle, with the stylet in place, is inserted through the small skin incision, at the previously determined angle and depth. The insertion of the needle is performed during suspended respiration and usually in the same respiratory phase as in the prior localizing study. Special care and experience are required to prevent the deflection of the direction of the thin, flexible needle, particularly in patients with well-developed musculature. This problem can be avoided by initially inserting an 18-gauge needle with a stylet to the depth of subcutaneous fat and muscle. Subsequently, the stylet is removed and replaced by the thin needle, which is then advanced to the target. As the needle reaches the target, the operator is often able to sense a change in the consistency of the tissue. From five to ten rapid (4- to 5-mm) excursions of the needle are performed to loosen the cells. The stylet is then removed and suction applied using a 20-ml disposable syringe. This is followed by a few short excursions through the lesion, using suction. *Suction must be released before the withdrawal of the needle. Except for cysts with a large fluid content, the aspirated material should remain within the needle.* This procedure can be repeated three to four times through the same skin incision, using a different needle and slightly modifying the angle of approach.

Some observers also use a 22-gauge cutting needle, described by Isler et al. (1981) and Wittenberg et al., (1982) that serves to obtain a tissue core biopsy in addition to the cytologic material. The needle is advanced to within a few millimeters of the target. The stylet is then removed, and the cannula, which has a sharp cutting edge, is connected to a 20-ml syringe containing 10 ml of saline. Circular, twisting, downward pressure is then applied to the cannula with one hand, while a maximal negative pressure is created with the syringe in an effort to transfer a small tissue core into the cannula. The ability to obtain histologic and cytologic material from the same lesion is occasionally very helpful.

At Montefiore Medical Center, the procedure currently used for abdominal aspiration is as follows: at least three aspirations, using two different needles, are performed. The first one is performed with a Chiba or, more commonly, with a pencil-point needle. The sample is checked for cell content (see below). If the cellularity of the sample is inadequate, the procedure is repeated once or twice. If no cells are obtained, the procedure is considered unsatisfactory.

If the first or subsequent aspirates are adequate, another pass with the Greene cutting needle is performed to secure, if possible, a small tissue core as a minibiopsy.

In general, the two procedures (i.e., the aspiration of cells and the minibiopsy), when successful, are complementary and increase the probability of an accurate diagnosis. There is yet a further advantage of the use of multiple aspirates. It is not uncommon for the malignant tumors to show multiple patterns of growth that are better represented in multiple aspirates, as will be shown below.

Patient Management Before and After the Aspiration Biopsy

As with most interventional procedures, the patient's consent should be obtained prior to aspiration. Bleeding parameters, such as prothrombin time and platelet count, must be determined. The patient generally has fasted for 4 to 6 hours before the procedure and, at times, mild sedation is given to relieve anxiety. Following the aspiration, vital signs are monitored every 30 minutes for 3 hours. If the procedure is performed on an outpatient basis, the patient is kept under observation by a qualified nurse for a period of 3 to 4 hours.

Collection and Processing of Samples

The quality of the aspirate and the proper handling and preparation of the aspirated sample are crucial to the ultimate success of this diagnostic approach. For this reason, the Swedish cytologists have always advocated that, whenever possible, the same person should perform the aspiration and prepare and interpret the smears. Söderström (1966) has given a fascinating and informative account on the development of the aspiration biopsy in his own clinical practice.

In the United States the aspiration of an abdominal organ is usually performed by roentgenologists. It is mandatory, however, for the material to be processed by a member of the cytology team.

A cart or a portable tray, containing slides, bottles with fixatives, rapid stains, an assortment of necessary instruments, and a microscope, are always ready to use (Fig. 29–99). The cart is manned by a senior cytotechnologist and a pathol-

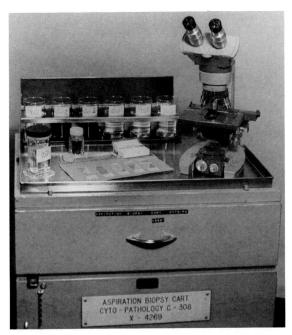

FIGURE 29-99. Aspiration biopsy cart used by cyto-pathology personnel in responding to calls for an aspiration procedure. Note the setup for a Diff-Quik stain in the back and the microscope used to verify the cellularity of the sample.

ogy fellow or resident who are on call from 8:00 AM to 5:00 PM, the customary hours during which the aspirations are performed. It is the duty of the person in charge to obtain the essential clinical and roentgenologic data that may prove important in the interpretation of the material, to pass preliminary judgment on the adequacy of the aspirated sample, and to prepare the material for final processing and interpretation. The procedure is as follows:

1. Upon completion of the aspiration, the syringe, with the needle still attached, is handed to the cytotechnologist. The following sequence of steps is rapidly executed:
2. The syringe is disconnected from the needle, filled with air, and reconnected.
3. A tiny drop of the aspirated material, present in the needle, is carefully expressed onto one end of a clean, glass, microscopic slide. To prevent splattering and loss of material, the needle tip is brought into light contact with the surface of the slide.
   A second slide is placed on top of the first one to obtain an even spread of the material, and the slides are separated. One of the slides is used for a Diff-Quik stain (see p. 1244). The other slide is immediately placed in a jar of 95% alcohol. The procedure is repeated with residual material available within the needle.
4. The first smear is stained with Diff-Quik (HARLECO, Gibbstown, New Jersey) and rapidly examined under the microscope to ensure that the sample contains cells of interest. If only blood or debris is present, the person performing the aspiration is notified and the aspiration procedure may have to be repeated. If the cell content on the slide is adequate, the preparation of material for final interpretation will continue.
5. The number of smears prepared from each aspiration procedure is variable and depends on the amount of material within the needle. Tissue fragments, if identified on the slide before smearing, are gently removed with a small forceps and transferred to buffered formalin or to Bouin's fixative for cell block preparation.
6. Whenever possible, the needle is rinsed with alcohol to secure additional material for a cytocentrifuge preparation. If the aspiration yields a substantial amount of fluid, the material must be centrifuged and smears or cytocentrifuge preparation made from the sediment.
7. We routinely use rapid fixation and Papanicolaou's staining method, except if a lymphoproliferative disorder is suspected. Under the latter circumstance, an air-dried smear or two are also prepared and stained with a hematologic stain. Additional material for immunocytologic studies is also secured.
8. For tissue cores (minibiopsies) obtained with the cutting Greene needle, the core may be expelled directly into the tissue fixative by flushing it out of the needle with the saline already in the syringe. The needle is washed with alcohol, and the residual material saved for cytocentrifuge preparation.
9. Special cytochemical and immunologic stains can be obtained on additional smears, cytocentrifuge preparations, or on cell blocks of aspirates.

Failures of the Aspiration Procedures

A common cause for a false-negative aspirate of cancer is the failure to reach the lesion. The thin needle used for aspiration biopsies is extremely flexible and the needle tip may be easily deflected from its course by the resistance from subcutaneous tissues, by trajectory errors, or by respiratory motion. Thus, when the planned depth has been reached, the needle tip may not be within the target lesion. This happens most often with small lesions (less than 3 cm in diameter) located deeply in the abdomen and when the position of the needle tip cannot be documented before aspiration. Occasionally, because of its firmness and dense consistency, the lesion will offer great resistance to puncture, and the needle tip may buckle, rather than pierce the lesion. This is rather unusual with abdominal lesions. However, the tumor mass may undergo reactive fibrosis, necrosis, hemorrhage, or inflammatory changes that may obscure the malignant nature of the target. Consequently, even an adequate aspiration may not always be of diagnostic value. To some extent, this type of false-negative aspirate may be avoided by multiple aspiration attempts with slight variations in the angle of approach. Faulty laboratory processing techniques may also contribute to false-negative results. The rate of false-negative aspirations may vary, depending on the factors cited.

THE LIVER

Large-core needle biopsy techniques were introduced in Europe in the 1920s for diagnosis of diffuse parenchymal disorders of the liver (Edmondson and Schift, 1975). The current practice is based on the use of relatively short (3.5 to 7 cm in length) cutting needles (Vim-Silverman or Menghini type), varying from 1 to 1.5 mm in diameter, to remove transcutaneously a core of tissue for morphologic study. For malignant tumors, it has been shown by Sherlock *et al.* (1967) that the cytologic evaluation of the residual debris accompanying liver biopsy specimens obtained by the Menghini technique provided additional diagnoses to the histologic evaluation. In a study of 15 patients with confirmed liver involvement by metastatic cancer, in 13 the diagnosis was reached histologically, whereas the cytologic preparations from all 15 patients showed identifiable cancer cells. These observations were confirmed by Grossman et al. (1972) and by Carney (1975).

Lundquist (1972) has attributed the actual introduction of the thin-needle aspiration of the liver to Lucatello in 1895. In our institutions, the liver is the abdominal organ most commonly aspirated, accounting for nearly one-half of abdominal aspirates.

In metastatic cancer, the superiority of the guided thin-needle approach over the Menghini technique has been documented, particularly for lesions in the left lobe of the liver (Rosenblatt et al., 1982). Safety and the acceptance of the nearly painless procedure by the patient are also important. In the absence of hemorrhagic diathesis, few complications of the thin-needle procedure have been observed. A single instance of intrahepatic hemorrhage requiring surgery was reported by Lundquist (1970). Still, in consideration of the large, although unspecified, number of thin-needle aspirations of the liver, the rate of complications appears to be extremely low, probably less than 0.1%.

Indications

Guided, transcutaneous, thin-needle aspiration of the liver is usually performed for sampling of space-occupying lesions suspected of being neoplastic, most commonly a metastatic carcinoma. Hepatocellular carcinoma, which is a common disease in parts of Africa and Asia, is relatively rare in the Western world, where it usually occurs in association with cirrhosis. Cholangiocarcinoma is an even less common primary liver cancer, except in China. Evacuation of a cyst or of a liver abscess is yet another potential benefit of needle aspiration (Haaga et al., 1976).

In the evaluation of diffuse disorders of the liver, such as hepatitis or cirrhosis, the thin-needle approach currently has limited diagnostic usefulness, and histologic investigation is essential for accurate diagnosis.

The following principal lesions of the liver may be recognized in aspirates:

- Cirrhotic liver
- Metabolic disorders
- Cysts and some viral and parasitic disorders
- Hepatomas
- Metastatic tumors

The Cytology of Liver Aspiration in the Absence of Cancer

Normal Liver. Normal liver is never deliberately aspirated. However, on numerous occasions, normal cell components of the liver are incidentally observed. Normal hepatocytes in aspiration smears either form clusters of various sizes or appear singly. The cells are large, polygonal, with distinct or frayed cell borders. The cytoplasm, which stains an orange-brown with the Papanicolaou stain, is granular. Bile canaliculi or small granules of bile may be observed in the cytoplasm of hepatocytes in fresh, well-fixed preparations. The nucleus

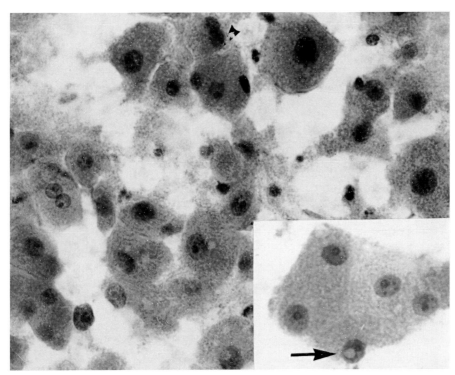

FIGURE 29-100.   Liver aspirate, normal liver cells. Note the polygonal shapes, the granular cytoplasm, and the single or double nuclei of variable sizes. Note also a cluster of liver cells with an intercellular bile canaliculus seen as a focal, oval-shaped separation of the apposed cytoplasmic membranes (*arrowhead*). (*Inset*) A cluster of normal liver cells with large nucleoli and one intranuclear cytoplasmic inclusion (*arrow*). (×700; *inset* ×800)

is round, often dark and homogeneous, and generally contains a central prominent nucleolus. Binucleation is common. In adults, many of the nuclei of normal hepatocytes are tetraploid or even octaploid. Thus, a marked variation in the size of the nuclei is common. Occasionally, intranuclear cytoplasmic inclusions may be present. Narrow, intercellular bile canaliculi can be observed as narrow spaces separating hepatocytes from each other (Fig. 29-100). The canaliculi can be better demonstrated by the use of cytochemical stains (Wasastjerna, 1979).

Cells of bile duct origin appear in smears as flat sheets or tightly knit clusters of cuboidal or columnar cells with even, small, round nuclei (Fig. 29-101). Cells with phagocytic properties, presumably

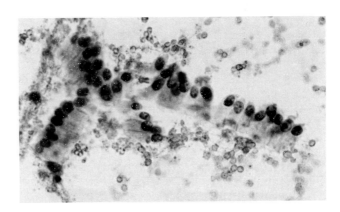

FIGURE 29-101.   Liver aspirate, epithelium of a large bile duct. The columnar configuration of the cells may be noted. In smaller bile ducts the lining cells are cuboidal. (×400)

Kupffer cells derived from the lining of sinusoid capillaries, may be noted occasionally.

Disorders of Metabolism. Liver aspirates often reflect a variety of metabolic disorders. For example, fatty liver due to accumulation of lipids may be observed in the form of large, cytoplasmic vacuoles within the hepatocytes (Fig. 29–102*B*). In obstructive jaundice, crystalline brown-green inclusions of bile may be observed. Dilated bile canaliculi may be demonstrated by means of amino acid naphthylamidase stain (Wasastjerna, 1979). In hemosiderosis, finely granular cytoplasmic deposits of brown pigment may be noted (Fig.

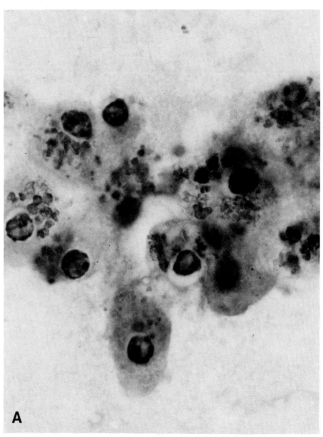

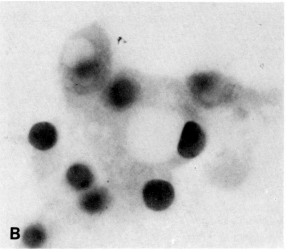

FIGURE 29–102. Abnormalities of liver cells as seen in cytologic material obtained during liver biopsies. (*A*) Hemosiderosis following multiple transfusions. The cytoplasmic granular pigment was shown to contain iron by appropriate stains. (*B*) Fatty metamorphosis: Note cytoplasmic vacuoles. (*A, B* ×1,000. Sherlock, P., et al.: Cytologic diagnosis of cancer from aspirated material obtained with liver biopsies. Am. J. Dig. Dis., *12*: 396–402, 1967)

29–102*A*). The identity of the pigment should be confirmed by a stain for iron to differentiate it not only from bile, but also from lipofuscin. The latter forms small brown granules in the vicinity of the nucleus. Rarely, melanin granules may be observed in benign cells in liver aspirates in disseminated malignant melanoma. Some of the pigment-containing cells are probably the phagocytic Kupffer cells.

Cirrohsis of Liver. Cirrhosis cannot be recognized as such in aspirated material. Rather, the disease is reflected in samples obtained during a search for hepatocellular carcinoma. The characteristic feature of cirrhosis is the presence of benign hepatocytes of variable sizes and configuration. The compact clustering of hepatocytes and other features characteristic of hepatocellular carcinoma (see below) are absent. Bile duct cells, singly and in clusters, may be numerous.

Inflammatory Disorders

Viral Hepatitis. This disorder is not a primary indication for thin-needle aspiration. However, smears have been obtained from contents of Menghini needles after the biopsy core has been removed. The changes of importance included the numerous lymphocytes forming the background of the smear and the great variability in sizes of hepatocytes (Fig. 29–103). Depending on the stage of disease, necrosis of hepatocytes may be observed, affecting a larger proportion of cells in the acute, rather than in the subacute, form of hepatitis.

Cystic Lesions

Abscess of the Liver. The pyogenic abscesses are usually due to ascending bacterial cholangitis or to amebiasis and may be fatal to the patient unless treated.

Thin-needle aspiration under ultrasound or CT guidance may be used to diagnose abscesses that can subsequently be drained with a larger-bore needle, thereby avoiding the necessity for surgical intervention.

Congenital Hepatic Cysts — Solitary Type. Solitary cysts are more frequently observed in women between the ages of 20 and 50 years than in males (Schiff, 1975). If larger than 10 cm in diameter, they may be symptomatic, causing abdominal discomfort. Diagnostic aspiration and therapeutic drainage of these uncommon lesions may be performed. The lining of the cysts is usually composed of a single layer of cuboidal epithelial cells. The smears may also contain a variable amount of benign, hepatic parenchymal epithelium or bile duct epithelial cells.

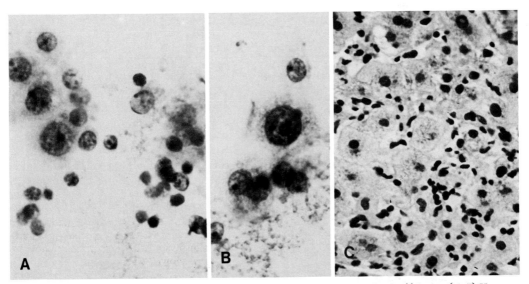

FIGURE 29–103. Acute hepatitis in a 64-year-old woman, aspiration smear and biopsy. (*A, B*) Hepatocytes with frayed cytoplasm showing breakdown of clusters and great variability in nuclear sizes. Note leukocytes in the background. Prominent, large nucleoli may be occasionally observed. (*C*) Hepatic biopsy showing infiltration of hepatic parenchyma by leukocytes. (*A, B* ×560; *C* ×350)

Hydatid Cysts. Worldwide, the echinococcal cyst is the most frequent type of liver cyst. Most cases occur in people from countries where the disease is endemic, such as Greece, Australia, Argentina, and South Africa. In principle, the cysts should not be aspirated because of the danger of anaphylactic shock. Occasionally, however, the nature of the cysts is misjudged, and an aspirate is performed.

The cyst, which is usually unilocular and which may reach 20 cm in diameter, may be, in part, calcified. Roentgenologically, it may be confused with a congenital solitary cyst that similarly may also develop partial calcification of the wall. In aspirates, the identification of the characteristic scolices with hooklets is diagnostic of *Echinococcus granulosus* infestation (Fig. 29 – 104).

Hemangiomas. Cavernous hemangiomas of the liver may reach large size causing pressure symptoms. In ultrasound studies, these congenital lesions appear as echogenic, well-circumscribed, space-occupying masses that may be confused with metastatic tumors. Dynamic radionuclide flow studies and angiography are helpful in the differential diagnosis. Spontaneous rupture, with acute hemoperitoneum, may sometimes occur. The aspiration smears show blood and fragments of fibrovascular connective tissue.

There is limited experience with aspirates of hemangiomas, and the dangers of the procedure have not been fully evaluated, particularly in reference to the rupture of the lesion and intraperitoneal hemorrhage.

Adenomas of the Liver. These lesions occur mainly in young women using contraceptive hormones for an extended period of time. The lesions are usually solitary. Aspiration biopsy usually discloses normal hepatocytes with a marked increase

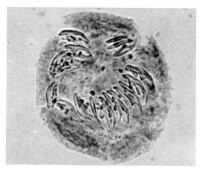

FIGURE 29 – 104. Liver aspirate, echinococcal cyst (*E. granulosus*). Note the scolex with hooklets. (×400)

of cell clusters of ductal origin. The diagnosis must be closely coordinated with clinical and radiologic data.

Malignant Tumors

HEPATOCELLULAR CARCINOMA (HEPATOMAS)

The most frequent type of primary liver cancer is hepatocellular carcinoma. Cholangiocarcinoma is rarely seen. Hepatomas often arise in a background of cirrhosis or viral hepatitis B and have a poor prognosis unless small and treated by surgical removal (Lee et al., 1982). Most of the patients are seen with a right upper quadrant mass, abdominal pain, and weight loss or ascites Alpha-fetoprotein levels are elevated in about 60% of the patients. The tumors vary in the degree of differentiation, from well-differentiated types, resembling normal liver tissue, to anaplastic, small-cell variants. Roentgenologic imaging techniques are often quite helpful in the differential diagnosis of hepatoma from metastatic tumors. Hepatomas usually show a single tumor mass (Fig. 29 – 105); metastatic carcinomas usually form multiple tumor nodules. In the presence of a solitary metastasis or multifocal hepatoma, the differential diagnosis may be very difficult.

Cytology. The cytologic presentation of hepatocellular carcinoma on the aspiration smear reflects the histopathologic pattern. There are several cytologic features that are helpful in the identification of hepatocellular carcinoma:

1. The malignant hepatocytes, presumably because of cytoplasmic fragility, often appear as "naked nuclei." Although this phenomenon may also occur in benign hepatocytes, it is usually confined to a few cells. In hepatomas the presence of naked nuclei is usually very extensive (Fig. 29 – 106*A*).
2. Round or oval clusters of liver cells are often surrounded by a layer of endothelial cells, derived from capillary vessels, corresponding to similar structures occurring in tissue sections (see Fig. 29 – 106*B,C*).
3. Intact malignant hepatocytes show very large nucleoli that may occasionally reach half of the nuclear diameter. Multinucleated tumor cells are common, again characterized by abundant cytoplasm and large nucleoli (Fig. 29 – 107).

Other features of note include the presence of cytoplasmic hyaline inclusions (see Fig. 29 – 107*B*)

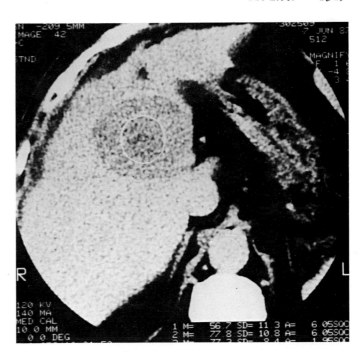

FIGURE 29–105. Hepatocellular carcinoma, typical appearance on a CT scan. A single lesion is present.

and occasionally the presence of intranuclear cytoplasmic inclusions (nuclear holes). This last feature is not unique to hepatoma, as it may also, but rarely, occur in benign hepatocytes (see Fig. 29–100) and in metastatic tumors, mainly melanomas (see Fig. 29–111).

In poorly differentiated hepatocellular carcinomas (hepatoblastomas), the malignant nature of the cells is readily identified, but the tumor type may be difficult to determine.

A characteristic feature of some hepatocellular carcinomas is their ability to produce bile. Bile pigment, in the form of fine, brownish granules, occurs within the cytoplasm of the tumor cells. However, intracellular bile pigment may also occur in necrotic metastatic tumors and in obstructive jaundice. The differential diagnosis of hepatocellular carcinoma comprises metastatic carcinomas and melanomas that may have a similar cytologic presentation. The data on cholangiocarcinoma are scarce. Wasastjerna (1979) described and illustrated a case with cytologic appearance of a duct carcinoma.

Metastatic Tumors

The liver is one of the most frequent sites of metastases. Malignant tumors originating in any site in the body may metastasize to the liver by lymphatic, venous, or arterial routes.

The thin-needle aspiration is the optimal approach to the diagnosis of hepatic metastases.

General Comments

The recognition of metastatic cancer in liver aspirates is usually quite easy. As a rule, the tumor cells show the classic features of cancer: the nuclei are often large, with coarse patterns of chromatin and large and multiple nucleoli. The cytoplasm differs markedly from that of hepatocytes and may display a variety of features that may allow the precise identification of tumor type. The clustering of cells is also fairly characteristic: cells of metastatic carcinoma often form large three-dimensional clusters, unlike any seen in normal liver. The diagnosis is facilitated if the site and the histology of the primary tumor are known. Unfortunately, in about one-third of the cases, the origin of the metastases is obscure.

Metastatic tumors composed of medium-size or small cells are usually readily recognized. The only problem in the differential diagnosis may occasionally occur with metastatic cancers composed of large cells of a size similar to that of hepatocytes. The absence of the characteristic features of hepatocytes described above is a helpful diagnostic clue. Nonetheless, in such cases the differential diagnosis between a metastatic cancer and a poorly differentiated hepatoma may be troublesome at times.

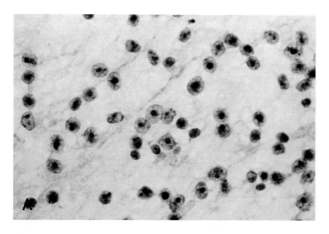

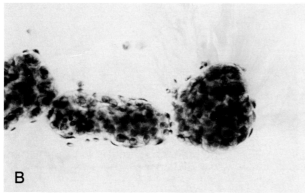

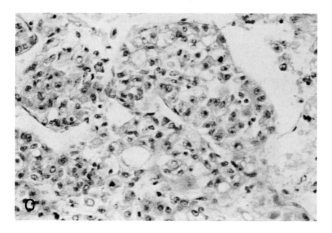

FIGURE 29–106. Hepatocellular carcinoma, aspiration smear and biopsy section. (*A*) Note the numerous "naked nuclei" of hepatocytes in the aspiration smear. (*B*) Typical clusters of hepatocytes encased in peripheral endothelial cells derived from capillaries. (*C*) Needle biopsy showing a trabecular hepatocellular carcinoma. (*A* ×400; *B* ×200; *C* ×250. Courtesy of Prof. S. Woyke)

RECOGNITION OF SPECIFIC TUMOR TYPES

Colon. The characteristic cancer cells are usually large, columnar, and have clear or vacuolated cytoplasm containing mucin (Fig. 29–108). Their nuclei, located at one end of the cell, are usually single, large, with prominent nucleoli and a fine chromatin pattern. The cancer cells are sometimes arranged in a glandular or rosette-like cluster. Unfortunately, this presentation of colon cancer is not always evident. The tumor cells may be smaller and fail to display the cytoplasmic features of diagnostic value (see Fig. 29–108*D*). Under these circumstances the diagnosis of cancer is still readily

(text continues on page 1153)

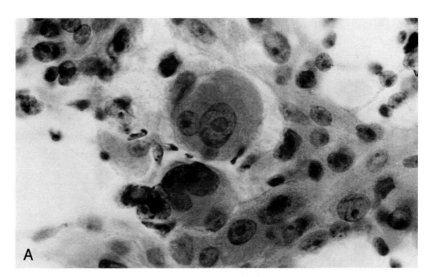

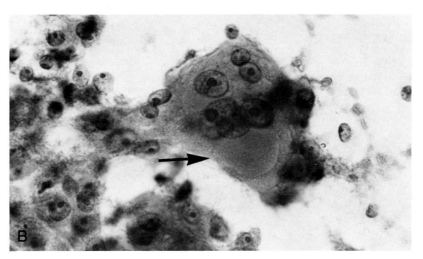

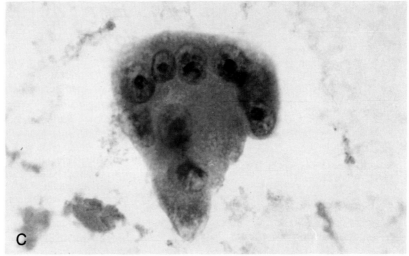

FIGURE 29–107. Hepatocellular carcinomas, liver aspirates. (*A, B*) from a 74-year-old man with a large, single liver mass. The large tumor cells vary in size, and some of them resemble normal hepatocytes. Note the huge nuclei and nucleoli and the intracytoplasmic hyalin inclusion (*arrow*) in one of the giant cells. (*C*) From a 75-year-old man with a large, single liver mass. A single multinucleated tumor giant cell with granular cytoplasm is shown. (*A, B, C* ×600)

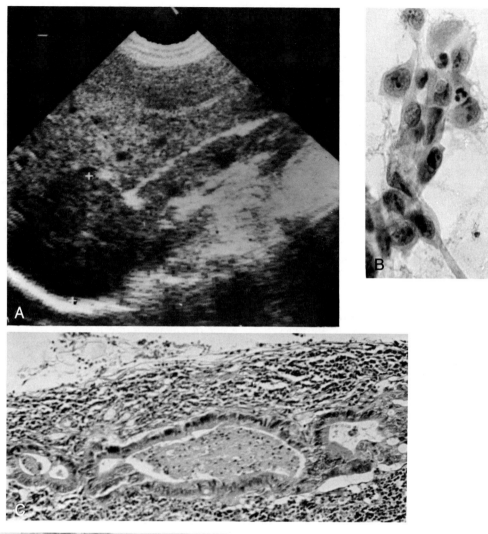

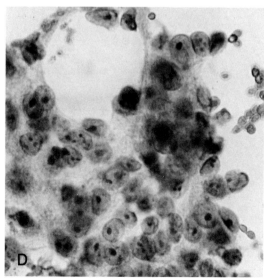

FIGURE 29–108. Metastatic colonic carcinoma in the liver in a 31-year-old man with known colonic carcinoma developing in ulcerative colitis (*A–C*). (*A*) Ultrasound image of a hypoechogenic mass in the posteroinferior aspect of the right liver lobe (*crosses*). (*B*) Cytology of liver aspirate showing the classic, predominantly columnar cancer cells, with large nuclei and nucleoli. (*C*) Section of a lymph node with metastatic colonic carcinoma in prior colectomy specimen. (*D*) Aspirate from a 55-year-old woman with two liver masses. The primary site of tumor cannot be determined in the smear because the small tumor cells show no identifying cytoplasmic features. The diagnosis of cancer is based on nuclear features. (*B, D* ×600; *C* ×150)

established, but the site of origin of the tumor may remain obscure.

Breast. It is uncommon to observe metastatic mammary carcinoma to the liver in the absence of a known primary tumor. The neoplastic cells of ductal carcinoma of the breast are generally round or oval and are seen singly and in clusters (Fig. 29–109). Their nuclei are of moderate size, with nucleoli, and are surrounded by a fair amount of pale cytoplasm. The nucleoli are often multiple and in an eccentric location. The tumor cells may vary from large to quite small. The clusters are of variable sizes, and the cells within them will show nuclear molding. Occasionally, the cancer cells are arranged in Indian file, reflecting lobular or small-cell duct carcinoma. Small signet ring cancer cells, containing mucous cytoplasmic inclusions, are characteristic of lobular carcinomas (see Fig. 29–73 and 29–74).

Squamous Cell (Epidermoid) Carcinoma. The cancer cells are usually large and show marked variability in shape (Fig. 29–110). Round, "tadpole-shaped," oval, spindly, or bizarre cells may occur. The cytoplasm is dense and well demarcated. Keratin-forming cells are common. In general, the nuclear chromatin is deeply hyperchromatic and coarse, and the nuclei are angular in outline. Much necrosis may be seen.

Small-Cell Anaplastic (Oat Cell) Carcinoma. The small neoplastic cells show either dense, hyperchromatic, or vesicular nuclei of a variety of shapes that mold with one another and that exhibit very scanty, if any, cytoplasm. Because of marked nuclear fragility, the smears contain streaks of bluish material representing tumor DNA derived from crushed nuclei. The latter is an important diagnostic feature of these tumors (see Fig. 20–18).

Melanoma. The aspiration smear usually shows large cancer cells with abundant cytoplasm, often containing brown granules of melanin. The amount of melanin is variable. It may be abundant and may even obscure cell structure (Fig. 29–111). The cytoplasm is usually well defined. The nuclei are large, single, or multiple; they may exhibit unusual variability in outline and may have very prominent nucleoli. Intranuclear cytoplasmic inclusions are occasionally seen.

An entity of special clinical interest is the occurrence of metastatic melanoma in patients with a past history of ocular melanoma. The time interval between the surgical removal of the eye and the occurrence of hepatic metastases may be very long, 28 years in a personally observed case. The presence of pigmented malignant melanoma cells in a liver aspirate should always trigger a question: "Does the patient have a glass eye?" The syndrome

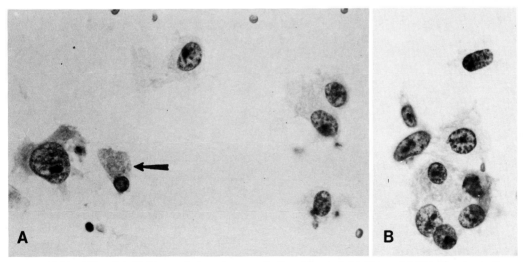

FIGURE 29–109. (*A, B*) Metastatic breast cancer in liver biopsy fluid. The variability of cancer cells and nuclear abnormalities are usually sufficient for diagnosis. In (*A*) a columnar cell with a small nucleus (*arrow*), probably of bile duct origin, serves as a reference point to assess the cell abnormalities. (*A, B* ×560)

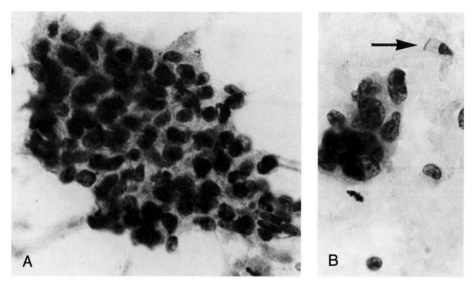

FIGURE 29–110. Metastatic epidermoid bronchogenic carcinoma. (*A*) Liver aspirate; cluster of tumor cells with hyperchromatic nuclei from a 62-year-old man with a lung mass. (*B*) Cluster of similar tumor cells in bronchial washing from the same patient. Note, as a point of reference, a ciliated bronchial epithelial cell (*arrow*). (*B, C* ×600)

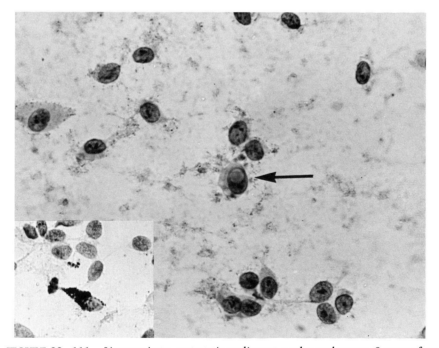

FIGURE 29–111. Liver aspirate, metastatic malignant ocular melanoma, 8 years after enucleation. Note the tumor cells with granular pigment in their cytoplasm, large nuclei, and large nucleoli. One cell shows the classic intranuclear cytoplasmic inclusion (*arrow*). (*Inset*) Masson–Fontana stain of the same preparation to document the presence of numerous granules of melanin. (×600)

of "glass eye and protuberant abdomen" is readily suggested by cytology.

Carcinoid or Islet Cell Tumors. The smears exhibit a population of monotonous, small, round, or polyhedral cells, each with a modest amount of well-defined, delicate basophilic cytoplasm. The nuclei are of even size, small, round, and often peripheral in location. The chomatin is finely granular, and small nucleoli are seen. The neoplastic cells are distributed singly and in sheets, within which small pseudorosette-like clusters can be identified (Fig. 29–112). Argyrophilia may be demonstrated by Grimelius stain. Other immunologic stains may be applied to document the endocrine nature of the tumor (see Chap. 34).

THE SPLEEN

Aspirations of the spleen, although well established among European hematologists, have not found wide acceptance in the United States.

The interested reader is referred to Moeschlin's classic monograph (1947) (in German) and to a brilliant summary by Söderström in Zajicek's book (1979). Söderström described the principal application of splenic puncture in the diagnosis and follow-up of hematologic and lymphoproliferative disorders, such as leukemias and various types of lymphomas. He also described granulomas, storage diseases (Gaucher's and Niemann–Pick), and the rare metastatic cancers. Spleen aspirates may also be used for the diagnosis of parasitic disorders, such as malaria and leishmaniasis. Pasternak (1974) applied the procedure to the diagnosis of amyloidosis.

In the absence of bleeding diathesis, polycythemia, thrombocytosis, or infectious mononucleosis, Söderström (1976) considered the procedure to be safe.

THE PANCREAS

The principal reason for aspiration biopsies of the pancreas is the diagnosis of space-occupying le-

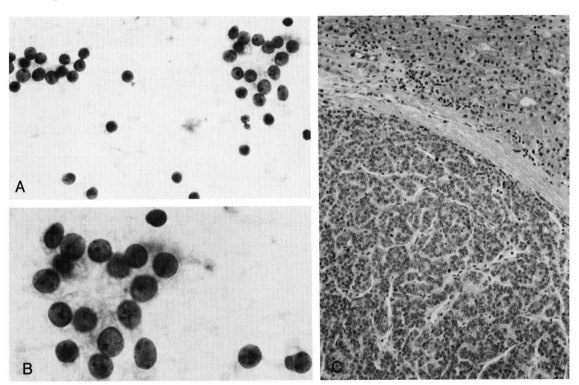

FIGURE 29–112. Metastatic islet cell tumor of pancreas to liver. (*A, B*) Liver aspirate: The smear contained small tumor cells with even spherical nuclei and very small nucleoli. In this example, the rosette-like arrangement of tumor cells was observed, shown under high power in (*B*). (*C*) Confirmatory autopsy evidence showing the islet cell tumor in the liver. (*A* ×400; *B* ×800; *C* ×200. From Koss, L.G., et al.: Aspiration Biopsy. Cytologic Interpretation and Histologic Bases. New York, Igaku-Shoin, 1984 with permission)

sions, mainly pancreatic carcinoma. The differential diagnosis comprises subacute or chronic pancreatis and its sequelae, such as pseudocysts and, rarely, tumors of the islets of Langerhans and other neoplastic lesions.

Before the era of roentgenologic or ultrasound imaging, the diagnostic options were limited to cell collections from the pancreatic ducts obtained by duodenal intubation or direct biopsy of the pancreas secured during exploratory laparotomy. (see Chap. 24). The procedure, designed to obtain the cytologic samples through the duodenum, was extremely complex and time-consuming and had limited success. Direct pancreatic biopsies also presented difficulties in the choice of tissue samples because of the masking of carcinoma by fibrosis and pancreatitis. This surgical approach was not free of subsequent complications, such as fistula formation or acute pancreatitis.

The introduction of fine-needle aspirates represented a major improvement in the diagnostic armamentarium. At first, the aspirates were obtained under direct vision during exploratory laparotomies (Arnesjo et al., 1972). The method made possible the sampling of multiple areas of the pancreas, with improved accuracy, and greatly reduced the risk of complications accompanying open wedge biopsies. With the introduction of precise methods of imaging, a percutaneous approach to cytologic sampling of the pancreas became possible and will be discussed in this section. It must be noted, though, that needle-tract seeding of a pancreatic carcinoma was recorded (Bersenfeld et al., 1988).

Radiologic Aspects

Lesions in the pancreas may be localized and visualized with fluoroscopic techniques by opacifying the pancreatic duct during endoscopic retrograde cholangiography (ERCP) (Goodale et al., 1981). If obstructive jaundice is present, the bile duct system may be opacified by means of percutaneous transhepatic cholangiography. Such studies may demonstrate pressure, obstruction, or encasement of the ducts by tumor. Selective angiography offers visualization of vascular encasement by tumor. In vascular tumors, such as an islet cell tumor, for example, a blush may be seen. The instillation of air into the stomach and duodenum (hypotonic duodenography) may sometimes show pressure effect by a mass located in the head of the pancreas. The latter technique is much less sensitive than the contrast opacification studies. With use of one or more of the opacification studies as a guide to aspi-

ration, Pereiras et al. (1978) achieved an 80% correct diagnosis of cancer of the pancreas in 20 patients. Computed tomography and ultrasound provide direct visualization of the pancreas without the need for opacification studies (see Fig. 29–114*A*). Of the two imaging modalities, CT visualization of the pancreas is more precise. Visualization of the pancreas by CT is enhanced by the administration of oral diatrizoate meglumine (Gastrografin) to outline the gastric antrum and duodenum. Computed tomography is more suitable as a guide to the aspiration of small lesions, when needle-tip placement can be monitored before beginning aspiration. Larger lesions, which at times may be palpable as an area of vague resistance in the epigastrium, can often be demonstrated sonographically, and the relationship to the major prevertebral vessels can be discerned. When regional landmarks, such as the splenic veins, superior mesenteric artery, and major prevertebral vessels, can be identified on sonography, the level of confidence in using this modality as a guide to percutaneous aspiration is enhanced.

Cytology

Cytology of pancreatic aspirates is relatively simple and straightforward. The principal point of differential diagnosis is pancreatitis and pancreatic adenocarcinoma. With reasonable precautions, errors are avoidable.

Normal Pancreas.   It is unusual to see perfectly normal pancreatic cells in aspirates. When they are observed, the cells derived from pancreatic acini form tightly bound flat or spherical clusters of small cuboidal cells, with round nuclei of equal sizes. The chromatin is dispersed, and nucleoli are either not visible or very small. Occasionally, glandlike structures may be observed.

Cells of pancreatic duct lining are generally larger than acinar cells (Fig. 29–113*A*). Depending on the caliber of the duct, the cells are cuboidal or columnar. In flat clusters, the cells are well demarcated and form a honeycomb type of arrangement. Palisade-like arrangement of the ductal cells may also be observed. The cytoplasm of the duct cells is generally clear; and the nuclei are round, of even sizes, and very similar to the nuclei of acinar cells.

An important point of differentiation of ductal epithelium is sheets of mesothelial cells, which are commonly observed in pancreatic aspirates (see Fig. 29–113*B*). The cells are usually separated from each other by clear spaces or "windows." The

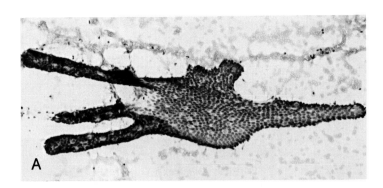

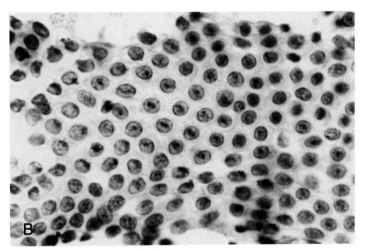

FIGURE 29–113. Pancreatic aspirate. (*A*) Normal ducts: overview to show a portion of a branching duct system. (*B*) A sheet of mesothelial cells with evenly spaced nuclei and prominent nucleoli. (*A* ×120; *B* ×700)

evenly spaced nuclei of these cells often contain nucleoli of substantial sizes that may mislead an uninformed observer. The monotonous size of the cells and their spherical, small nuclei should prevent the erroneous diagnosis of a malignant tumor (for further comments on the cytologic presentation of benign mesothelial cells in aspirates, see Chap. 25).

Occasionally, cells from the islets of Langerhans may be observed as ribbons of small, polyhedral cells, with granular cytoplasm and small, monotonous vesicular nuclei.

Pancreatitis. The cytologic image of pancreatitis is that of an acute or subacute inflammatory process, with numerous leukocytes and necrotic cell debris forming the background. Macrophages with evidence of phagocytic activity are often present, and calcified debris may be encountered. Within this background, clusters of benign, epithelial acinar and ductal cells may be observed. The

epithelial cells often show a degree of atypia in the form of somewhat hyperchromatic dark nuclei. The dark nuclear staining may be enhanced if the smear contains a great deal of blood. Prominent nucleoli are very uncommon and, when they occur, the differential diagnosis with a carcinoma must be considered. Other features of pancreatic cancer, described below and summarized in Table 29–10, are absent.

In general, caution is recommended in the interpretation of aspirates that show evidence of inflammation. The diagnosis of cancer should be made only on irrefutable evidence.

Pancreatic Adenocarcinoma. Carcinoma of pancreatic ducts is the most common type of pancreatic cancer. The neoplastic epithelial cells vary in size and in number. They are usually much larger than benign epithelial cells and occur singly or in small, loosely structured clusters (Fig. 29–114*B*). The cells of ductal carcinoma are character-

Table 29-10
Differentiation of Pancreatic Carcinoma from Benign Pancreatic Cells

Aspiration Smear Features	Benign Pancreatic Epithelium	Pancreatic Duct Adenocarcinoma
Cell cohesiveness in clusters	Excellent	Reduced, loose, or "piled-up" clusters
Single cells	Few	Prominent
Cell size	Uniform	Variable size, depends on tumor type
Nuclear size	Small	Enlarged
Nuclear chromatin configuration	Fine, dispersed	Coarsely granular
Nucleoli	Tiny or absent	Prominent, often multiple

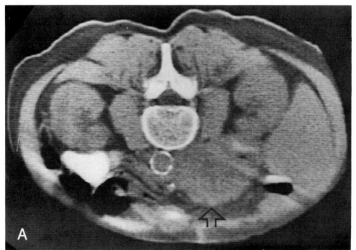

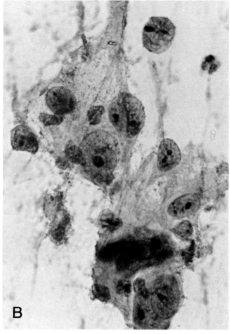

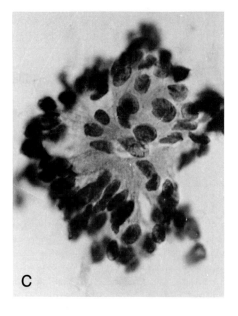

FIGURE 29-114.   Pancreatic carcinoma (*A, B*) from a 66-year-old man with a mass in the head and body of the pancreas. (*A*) CT of pancreas showing a large mass in the head and body of the pancreas (*open arrow*). The cross section of a vertebra is an easily recognized landmark. The aorta appears as a white ring anterior to the vertebral body. (*B*) Aspirate of mass shown in (*A*). Note the huge size of the nuclei and nucleoli in the cancer cells. (*C*) Pancreatic aspirate from a 57-year-old woman with a mass. The columnar cancer cells are arranged in a rosette-like structure, suggestive of gland-forming ductal carcinoma. (*B, C* ×600)

ized by large, coarsely granular, hyperchromatic nuclei, with one or more prominent nucleoli. The cytoplasm is clear or eosinophilic, often poorly preserved. Intracytoplasmic mucin may be demonstrated by histochemical staining. Glandlike clusters of cancer cells, arranged around a central lumen, are not uncommon (see Fig. 29–114C). Such structures are readily differentiated from normal cells by the differences in cell sizes and by the nuclear features.

Acinic cell carcinoma of the pancreas is rather uncommon. The cancer cells are somewhat smaller than the cells of duct cancer but have the same characteristics. Still less common are the highly anaplastic carcinomas that may occur as a large- or a small-cell variant. The malignant nature of such cells is rarely in doubt.

On occasion, pancreatitis may occur in the presence of, or may be associated with, pancreatic adenocarcinoma. The presence of acute or chronic inflammation in the smear should not preclude the search for cancer cells, but diagnostic caution is advised.

In general, the diagnosis of pancreatic carcinoma in an adequate cell sample is not particularly difficult. A summary of the principal points of diagnosis has been provided in Table 29–10.

Aspiration biopsy of the rare mucinous cystic neoplasms of the pancreas has also been reported (Emmert and Bewtra, 1986; Koss et al., 1992). Mucus-producing columnar cells characterize these lesions. Other very rare tumors may also occur (see Bibliography).

Islet Cell Tumors. These tumors are usually located in the body and tail of the pancreas. In some cases, they are multiple. Clinically, the patients may exhibit one or more endocrine abnormalities that reflect the tumor's production of one or more polypeptide hormones. The tumors are composed of nests, sheets, and anastomosing cords of cells, with the characteristic close relationship to capillaries.

The cytology of aspirated islet cell tumors is characterized by a monotonous population of small cells, with pale, delicate, basophilic cytoplasm and small, often eccentric, regular nuclei that have dispersed chromatin and tiny central nucleoli. The tumor cells occur singly or in small clusters that sometimes show a rosette-like arrangement (see Fig. 29–112). As is common in tumors with endocrine features, giant cells with single or multiple large, hyperchromatic nuclei may occur. The presence of such cells has no prognostic value (see also Carotid Body Tumors, p. 1265).

THE KIDNEY AND THE RENAL PELVIS

It is not quite clear who initiated the concept of thin-needle aspiration biopsy of the kidney. As early as 1939, A. L. Dean in New York City aspirated renal cysts with large-caliber needles, using pyelography as the guide to localization. The thin-needle aspirate clearly originated in the Scandinavian countries. Söderström described the method as a long-term user in his book published in 1966. Von Schreeb et al. reported a series of cases in 1967; Kristensen et al. in 1972; and Thommesen and Nielsen, Edgren et al., and Holm et al. each reported a series of cases in 1975.

There is still some controversy over the best use of this technique. In the previous edition of this book (1979), Zajicek stated that the sole purpose of thin-needle aspirates of renal masses was to establish the grade of malignancy in renal carcinomas: for patients with high-grade (poorly differentiated) tumors with poor prognosis, preoperative radiotherapy was advocated; other patients were referred directly for surgical treatment. The grading method is no longer used. However, with growing experience, it has become evident that the scope of the renal aspirates is much broader. The precise preoperative identification of renal tumors includes a wide spectrum of neoplasms, ranging from carcinoma of various types to rare tumors, such as oncocytomas, Wilms' tumors (childhood and adult variants), a variety of cystic neoplasms, tumors of renal pelvic origin, and metastatic tumors.

Ultrasonography (Fig. 29–115A) and CT have been shown to be of major advantage as localization techniques and in separating solid from cystic lesions and cystic neoplasms from benign cysts (Pollack et al., 1982).

Cytology of Normal Kidney

In material aspirated from renal cysts, and sometimes renal tumors, benign renal parenchyma is often observed. The glomeruli appear as sharply circumscribed, round or oval, multilayered structures, sometimes with proximal convoluted tubules still attached. The latter are composed of even, moderately large, cuboidal cells, with granular eosinophilic cytoplasm and even, vesicular, round nuclei (Fig. 29–116A). Isolated cells of proximal tubules may resemble small hepatocytes. Distal convoluted tubules may be removed intact and appear as multilayered tubular structures that must be differentiated from capillary vessels. The latter are recognized by their luminal content of blood cells. Single cells of distal tubule origin ap-

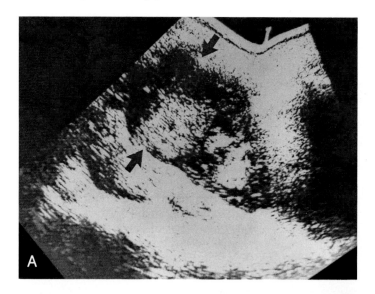

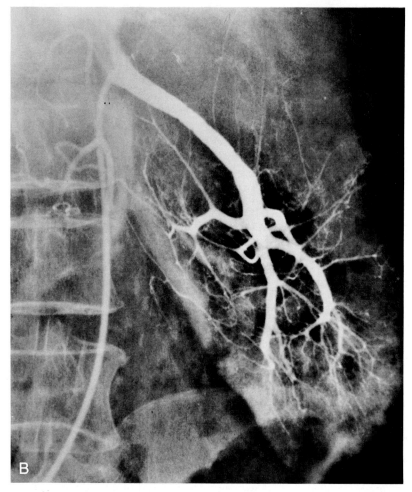

FIGURE 29–115. Examples of ultrasound and angiogram examinations of a patient with a renal cell carcinoma documented by aspiration biopsy and surgery. (*A*) The ultrasound study of the left kidney obtained in the prone position showing an echogenic solid mass in the upper pole (*arrows*). (*B*) An angiogram of the same case displaying an avascular mass with stretching of vessels.

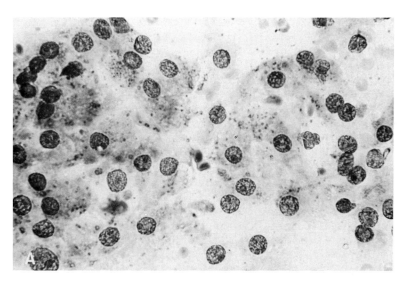

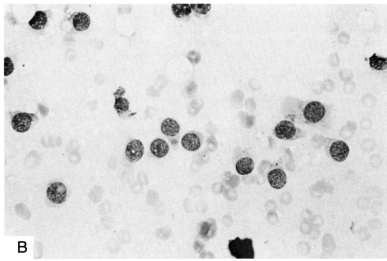

FIGURE 29–116. Normal renal epithelium, needle aspirates. (*A*) Epithelial cells from convoluted tubules. Abundant cytoplasm exhibits fine and coarse granulation. (*B*) Epithelial cells from collecting tubules. The cells have scanty cytoplasm. (*A*, MGG ×480; *B*, MGG ×480. Zajicek, J.: Aspiration Biopsy Cytology. Part II. Basel, S. Karger, 1979)

pear as small, cuboidal cells, with scanty basophilic or eosinophilic cytoplasm and small, round nuclei (see Fig. 29–116*B*).

Benign Lesions

Cysts. Cysts are the renal lesions most commonly aspirated, usually with a large, 18-gauge needle. Renal cysts may be congenital or acquired. The congenital cysts are either single or multiple, as in the polycystic kidney, and may enlarge with age. In the adult form of polycystic kidney, significant enlargement of both kidneys may occur. Acquired cysts are usually due to shrinkage of renal parenchyma secondary to vascular insufficiency and are rarely a cause for alarm. Except for the

adult form of polycystic kidneys, most renal cysts are asymptomatic and are frequently observed as an incidental finding. However, infection or hemorrhage into the lumen of the cyst may cause acute symptoms of pain and sometimes hematuria. Furthermore, renal carcinomas may undergo cystic degeneration, and renal tumors may be associated with renal cysts. Thus, it is common practice today to aspirate single renal cysts of debatable nature for purposes of diagnosis and, in some instances, treatment. A rare large aneurysm of the renal artery may mimic a cyst.

Cytology. The amount of fluid aspirated from renal cysts varies according to cyst size. In exceptional cases, 40 or 50 ml of fluid may be aspirated;

usually, however, only a few milliliters are obtained. In most instances, the fluid is clear, straw-colored, occasionally cloudy or blood-tinged, or, rarely, chocolate brown. It was suggested by Zajicek that clear, straw-colored fluids do not require cytologic study, but cloudy or hemorrhagic fluids, particularly from patients with debatable roentgenologic findings, should be carefully examined. Our experience supports this conclusion.

Fluid sediment from simple cysts contains few small cuboidal epithelial lining cells, with round, even nuclei that cause no problems in interpretation, regardless of whether they occur singly or form small clusters. Mono- and multinucleated macrophages occur in variable numbers and configuration. As a rule, these cells are readily identified because of their small nuclei and abundant cytoplasm with fine vacuoles (Fig. 29–117). However, in one instance seen in consultation, markedly atypical macrophages with large, hyperchromatic nuclei and visible nucleoli were observed; and they caused a significant diagnostic dilemma. As a general rule, the diagnosis of cancer should not be established in cyst fluid except on firm cytologic evidence.

Imaging control of the aspirated kidney is required some days after the aspiration. If there is evidence of a residual lesion, another aspiration may be required.

Renal Abscess. The patients usually experience ipsilateral, severe costovertebral angle pain and tenderness, chills and fever, and often pyuria.

The collection of pus may be limited to the renal pelvis or may involve the entire kidney and perinephric region. The aspiration yields purulent exudate.

Angiomyolipoma. These are benign lesions that are composed of a variable mixture of smooth muscle, adipose tissue, and tortuous thick-walled blood vessels. Although most common in middle-aged and older women, when the lesions are identified in younger persons, there is a high association with tuberous schlerosis (mental retardation, epilepsy, and adenoma sebaceum).

We have observed one such example in a 21-year-old man with tuberous sclerosis, from whom the renal aspirate showed several clusters of small, somewhat elongated cells of benign appearance. The resected kidney contained a 13 × 10 × 10-cm extensively infarcted angiomyolipoma with a predominant smooth-muscle component.

Other Lesions. Benign entities that may present as space-occupying lesions include the fetal hamartoma, cortical adenoma, leiomyoma, and tuberculosis. We have not yet observed any of these entities, and none have been described in available literature.

Malignant Lesions

Renal Carcinoma. Renal carcinomas display a variety of histologic patterns. The most common dominant microscopic feature of the tumors is the

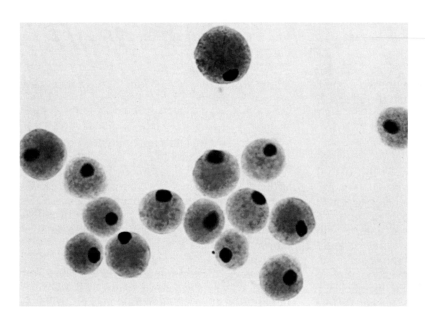

FIGURE 29–117. Aspirate of renal cyst. The sediment was composed of a population of macrophages with finely vacuolated cytoplasm and peripheral small nuclei. (×600)

cell with clear, abundant cytoplasm, filled with delicate vacuoles containing glycogen and lipids, and a central, slightly hyperchromatic nucleus provided with a small, but clearly visible, nucleolus. The clear cells may be arranged in solid sheets, cords, or tubulelike structures. In other tumors, the cytoplasm of the predominant cells is eosinophilic, denser, and more granular, and the nuclear abnormalities may be more conspicuous. The nuclei vary in size, are larger, more hyperchromatic, and contain large nucleoli. Such tumor cells may form solid sheets or have a papillary configuration. In the papillary tumors, the core of the papillae may contain large macrophage-like cells. Also, psammoma bodies may be observed in tumors of this type. There is also a variant of renal carcinomas with highly abnormal spindly tumor cells, imitating sarcomas.

Cytology. Aspirates of renal carcinoma often contain much blood and show considerable necrosis, with cell debris and nuclei stripped of cytoplasm. Within this background, abundant tumor cells are usually seen. Perhaps the most striking feature of renal cancer from which multiple aspirated samples have been obtained is the variability of the cell patterns (Fig. 29–118). Thus, even in the well-differentiated renal cancers that in histologic material may appear quite monotonous, the samples obtained from different parts of the tumor may disclose several coexisting cell patterns. This feature of renal carcinomas has not received any significant emphasis in prior writing on this subject, perhaps because the tumors were studied with only a single aspirate. Thus, the concept of well-differentiated versus poorly differentiated renal carcinomas could not be sustained in our material.

Although the common histologic pattern of orderly clear cell carcinoma of the kidney may appear quasi-benign, the cells aspirated from it are clearly abnormal. The cancer cells are either dispersed or form clusters that are often flat and loosely constructed, but occasionally form gland-like arrangements. The cancer cells are large, much larger than benign tubular cells, and are provided with abundant cytoplasm that is often filled with numerous small vacuoles reflecting lipid droplets (see Fig. 29–118*A,B*). The nuclei vary in size and, although not markedly hyperchromatic, are somewhat larger than the nuclei of normal tubules and have a somewhat coarser granulation of chromatin. The nucleoli, although not very large, are readily seen. Other tumor cells of similar size and configuration have a granular, more opaque, sharply demarcated, eosinophilic cytoplasm. The two cell types, i.e., the cells with vacuolated and those with granular cytoplasm, often occur side by side. Even in the cell samples that appear quite monotonous, it is not uncommon to find single cancer cells or cell clusters containing markedly enlarged, hyperchromatic nuclei. Some of the malignant cells may appear elongated or columnar and may be arranged in clusters, not unlike petals of a flower (see Fig. 29–118*C*). In such cells, the cytoplasm tends to be basophilic and homogeneous and the nuclei show marked enlargement and hyperchromasia. Occasionally, intranuclear cytoplasmic inclusions may occur in renal cancer cells (Fig. 29–119, *inset*). In some tumors, the cancer cells tend to be elongated or spindly and may show a vague similarity to fibroblasts, except for the delicate, vacuolated, abundant, faintly granular cytoplasm and slight enlargement of nuclei (see Fig. 29–119). Such cells correspond to the areas of the primary tumor composed of elongated cells, which may also be seen in metastatic foci.

The cytologic presentation of the predominantly papillary carcinomas is quite characteristic: the tumor cells are large and provided with a delicate, basophilic, slightly granular cytoplasm, and round, large, rather pale nuclei, with finely granular chromatin and large central nucleoli. The cancer cells occur singly or in small, flat clusters and are usually accompanied by numerous macrophages of variable sizes (Fig. 29–120). The latter are characterized by faintly vacuolated, delicate cytoplasm and small, usually single, but sometimes multiple, nuclei. The differential diagnosis between the cancer cells and the macrophages may be rather difficult and must be based on nuclear and nucleolar size, rather than any other features. The macrophages have been traced to the cores of the papillae in the papillary tumors. Their presence in the aspirate must signal the possibility of a papillary carcinoma.

In poorly differentiated tumors, the dominant cancer cells are quite small and occur singly and in small clusters. The cells that have large hyperchromatic nuclei and scanty, clear cytoplasm may resemble those of a large-cell lymphoma, except for the formation of clusters with cell molding. In sections, the tumor is composed of tightly packed, small cancer cells with clear cytoplasm.

In histologic sections of the renal carcinomas, the connective tissue does not appear to be prominent. Yet, in aspirates, it is common to observe fragments of stroma composed of hyaline connective tissue with cancer cells attached (see Fig. 29–118*C*). In still other tumors, the high degree of vascularity will be reflected by the presence of

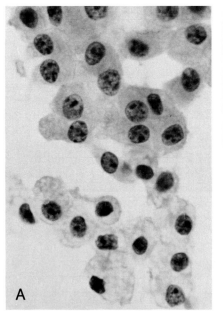

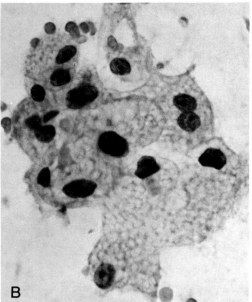

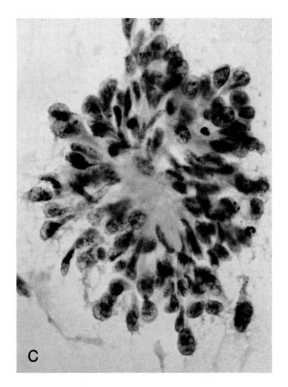

FIGURE 29–118. Renal aspirate, renal cell carcinoma: Different cytologic aspects of the same tumor. (*A*) Clusters of tumor cells with vacuolated clear cytoplasm adjacent to tumor cells with granular cytoplasm. Note the relatively uniform nuclei with granular chromatin and prominent nucleoli. (*B*) Cluster of cells with vacuolated cytoplasm and with marked nuclear abnormalities.(*C*) A papillary fragment of tumor with a central core of homogeneous material. (*A, B* ×700; *C* ×440)

portions of capillary vessels and abundant erythrocytes.

Renal Oncocytoma. Within recent years, a group of solid renal tumors with much better prog-

nosis than the customary renal carcinoma has been identified as tubular adenomas with oncocytic features or renal oncocytomas (Klein and Valensi, 1976). In common with oncocytic tumors of the salivary glands, the thyroid, and the parathyroid,

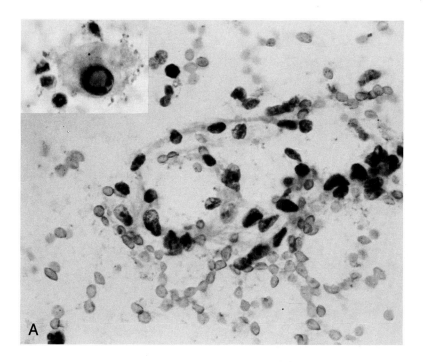

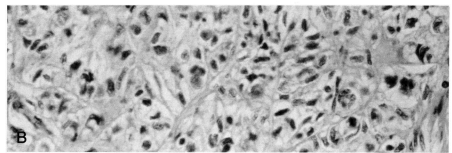

FIGURE 29–119. Renal aspirate, renal cell carcinoma, spindly cell pattern. (*A*) Elongated cancer cells in smear. (*Inset*) A renal carcinoma cell with an intranuclear cytoplasmic inclusion. (*B*) Tissue from the same case. (*A, inset* ×700; *B* ×440)

the tumors are composed of large cells with granular, eosinophilic cytoplasm and large, often multiple, hyperchromatic and pyknotic nuclei. Electron microscopy of the tumor cells discloses a cytoplasm filled with numerous mitochondria. The tumors may reach considerable sizes and may be multiple. Angiography often reveals a space-occupying renal lesion of avascular or hypovascular appearance. Although most oncocytomas appear to behave in a benign fashion, there is evidence that at least some of them may be invasive and perhaps capable of metastasis.

In the case examined and reported by us (Rodriguez et al., 1980), the aspiration smear contained large tumor cells singly and in small clusters. The sharply demarcated cells had abundant, granular cytoplasm and large, spherical or ovoid, smoothly outlined, pyknotic, single or multiple, large nuclei. The cytologic appearance was unlike any other renal neoplasm or normal renal tissue.

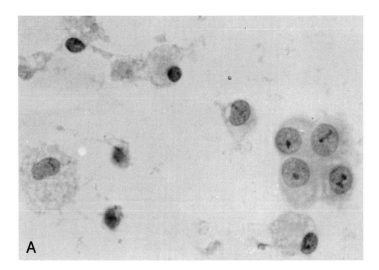

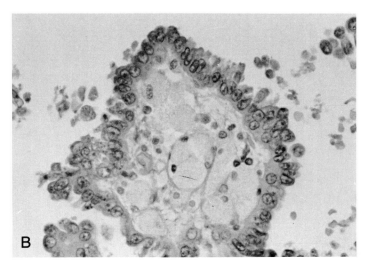

FIGURE 29–120.   Renal aspirate, papillary renal cell carcinoma. (*A*) A small cluster of malignant cells with large, finely granular nuclei and irregular enlarged nucleoli accompanied by several macrophages in the same field. (*B*) Tissue from the same case. Area of papillary carcinoma with macrophages in the stroma. (*A* ×700; *B* ×440)

Nephroblastoma (Wilms' Tumor).   This neoplasm represents approximately 20% of all malignant tumors of childhood. It is seen almost exclusively in young children and rarely in adolescents and adults. Approximately 25% of these patients have metastases to regional lymph nodes, lungs, and liver when first seen. Histologically, this is a mixed malignant neoplasm containing elements of embryonal epithelium mimicking tubules or glomeruli, elements of sarcoma, usually rhabdomyosarcoma, and undifferentiated tumor cells.

Our experience with Wilms' tumor is limited to a few cases in children, provided by Dr. Stanislaw Woyke, and to one case personally observed in an adult. In childhood, the smears are cell rich and are composed predominantly of small cancer cells ar-

ranged in clusters. Single, small, round, or elongated cancer cells can also be seen. Rhabdomyoblasts have not yet been observed. The picture is that of an undifferentiated malignant tumor, and the diagnosis of cancer poses no difficulty.

In a case of a Wilms' tumor occurring in a 54-year-old man, the predominant cell pattern in the aspirate was similar to a small-cell carcinoma, with round and elongated cancer cells that formed occasional clusters, but mainly lay singly (Fig. 29–121). The size of the cancer cells was similar to that of large lymphoblasts. The differential diagnosis comprised a malignant lymphoma or a small cell carcinoma, either primary or metastatic. The biopsy was interpreted as adult Wilms' tumor. In spite of multiple pulmonary metastases, the pa-

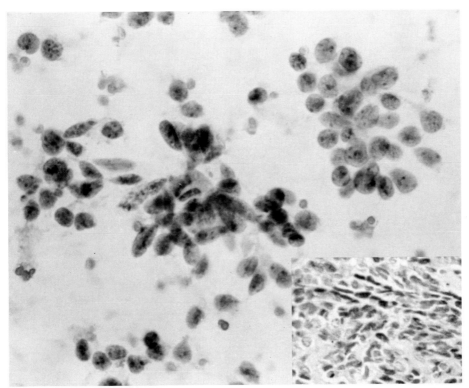

FIGURE 29–121. Renal aspirate, adult Wilms' tumor. Note the monotonous round and elongated, small cancer cells in clusters. (*Inset*) Area of tumor biopsy showing a similar cell pattern. (×700; *inset* ×440)

tient responded dramatically, although temporarily, to a chemotherapeutic regimen suitable for Wilms' tumors.

Renal Pelvic Carcinoma. Carcinoma of this region will frequently present with hematuria and ipsilateral pain. Nearly all the tumors are of urothelial type, and the remainder are either squamous or adenocarcinomas. Our experience is limited to urothelial carcinomas.

In aspiration smears, the neoplastic cells appear singly or in multilayered clusters. The sharply demarcated cells are of moderate size and have a variable amount of cytoplasm that is often eosinophilic. The nuclei are large, obviously malignant, and sometimes pyknotic (Fig. 29–122). For further comments on cytologic diagnosis of renal pelvic tumors, see Chapter 23.

Metastatic Carcinoma to the Kidney. The kidney is occasionally the site of metastases from cancers primary in other organs, such as lung,

breast, colon, thyroid, malignant melanomas, and lymphomas. The kidneys may also be involved in contiguity by cancer from adjacent organs, such as the adrenals and retroperitoneum, including lymphomas (see the section on retroperitoneum). The aspiration biopsy cytology of these lesions is the same as that of the primary neoplasms.

Sarcomas. Approximately 2% to 3% of malignant neoplasms of the kidney are sarcomas and include leiomyosarcoma (the most common type), liposarcoma, rhabdomyosarcoma, and hemangiopericytoma.

We have not seen these tumors in our laboratory.

Complications

In addressing the issue of safety of aspiration for renal tumors, von Schreeb et al. (1969) found no differences in survival of patients with and without aspiration. Yet there is on record a documented

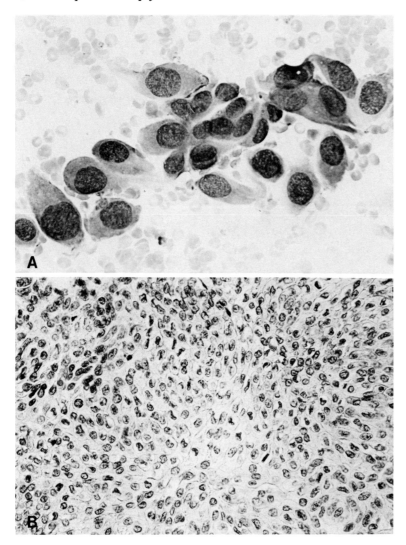

FIGURE 29–122. Urothelial carcinoma of the renal pelvis. (*A*) Needle aspirate: a cluster of cells from a well-differentiated urothelial carcinoma. The cell borders are distinct. Some cells have characteristically elongated cytoplasm (air-dried smear). (*B*) Tissue section of the same tumor. (*A*, MGG stain ×480; *B* ×300)

case of seeding of tumor cells along the needle tract, which was reported by Gibbons et al. (1977). Occasional hematuria was reported by Söderström (1966). We have not observed any complications in our patients.

THE ADRENAL GLANDS

The adrenal glands can be visualized by computed tomography.

The most common tumor of the adrenal is adrenal cortical adenoma, which is usually an incidental finding of no clinical significance. Occasionally, the cortical adenomas (or hyperplasias) have an intense hormonal activity and cause hyperaldosteronism (Conn's syndrome) (White et al., 1980).

Other extremely rare benign lesions are adrenal cysts. Primary malignant tumors of the adrenal glands are uncommon.

Cortical Adenoma

We have observed several cases of large cortical adenomas. In the aspirate, obtained under CT guidance, the cortical cells occurred singly and in flat clusters. The cells had a polyhedral configuration, faintly granular, but clear, cytoplasm, and small nuclei (Fig. 29–123).

Adrenal cortical cells and hepatocytes may be remarkably similar. There are occasional situations wherein the anatomic derivation of the aspirate (liver vs. adrenal) cannot be determined with accuracy. The larger size of the liver cells and the

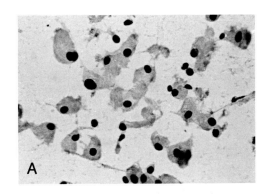

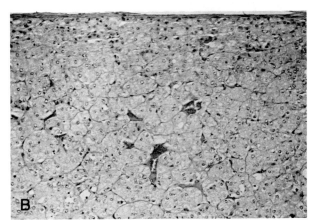

FIGURE 29–123. Aspiration biopsy of a large adrenal cortical adenoma. (*A*) The polyhedral cortical cells vary in size, have a sharply demarcated granular cytoplasm and dark, spherical nuclei with some variability in sizes. (*B*) Histologic section of the surgically removed adenoma. (*A* ×400; *B* ×100)

presence of bile usually allow for an easy differentiation between the cells of the two organs.

Cortical Carcinoma

A case of adrenal cortical carcinoma was illustrated by Zajicek (1974), who emphasized the similarity of this tumor to renal carcinoma. Another case, identified on aspiration, was reported by Levin (1981), who described large, often multinucleated tumor cells, with very large hyperchromatic nuclei and large nucleoli. A word of caution is in order: nuclear hyperchromasia and enlargement may also occur in cells of the normal adrenal cortex and in benign adenomas (see Fig. 29–123). Thus, the diagnosis of adrenal cortical carcinoma may prove to be difficult.

Pheochromocytoma

Pheochromocytoma or paraganglioma is a malignant tumor of the adrenal medulla, or originating in the retroperitoneal space, that may be associated with paroxysmal or sustained hypertension. In its familiar form, the tumor may be associated with

multiple neoplasms of endocrine type, such as medullary carcinoma of the thyroid and parathyroid adenomas (e.g., multiple endocrinopathies, Sipple's syndrome). The behavior of pheochromocytoma cannot be determined on morphologic grounds, and the diagnosis is usually supported by the biochemical demonstration of increased serum and urine levels of catecholamines and their metabolites (Wilson and Ibanez, 1978).

We observed several cases of pheochromocytoma of the adrenal medulla or retroperitoneum in aspirated material. The cell content was modest. The tumor cells, forming small clusters, had fairly monotonous, large, round, hyperchromatic, dark nuclei; nucleoli could not be seen. The cytoplasm was poorly preserved, wispy, and rather scanty; yet in some of the cells, cytoplasmic granularity could be observed (Fig. 29–124*A*). The surgically removed tumor had the classical features of a pheochromocytoma. Formation of rosette-like structures was observed in an adrenal pheochromocytoma (see Fig. 29–124*B*). There are several other reports of pheochromocytoma in aspirates with essentially similar findings.

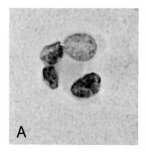
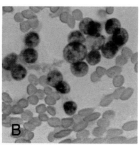
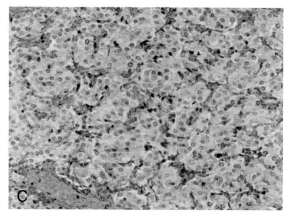

FIGURE 29–124. Retroperitoneal paraganglioma (*A*, *C*) and an adrenal pheochromocytoma (*B*). The aspirate (*A*) contained a few clusters of cells with wispy granular cytoplasm and moderately dark, fairly even nuclei. No nucleoli were seen. (*B*) The aspirate of the adrenal tumor in a 53-year-old woman showed several rosette-forming clusters of similar cells. The center of the clusters was formed by eosinophilic granular material of unknown derivation. (*C*) The tissue corresponding to (*A*) was obtained at surgery. (*A* ×700; *B* ×560; *C* ×175)

Neuroblastoma

We have studied several aspirates from cases of neuroblastoma in children. In most instances, the tumors were metastatic to various sites.

Histologically, the tumor is composed of undifferentiated small cells, often forming small rosettes with delicate neurofibrils filling the lumen. In aspiration smears, the small cancer cells resembled those of an oat cell carcinoma or a highly malignant lymphoma. The nuclei were coarsely granulated and the cytoplasm scanty. Delicate neurofibrils could be observed among the tumor cells. Unlike the cells of a malignant lymphoma, the cells of neuroblastoma formed clusters and rosette-like structures (see Fig. 29–133*B*).

Metastatic Tumors

The adrenal glands are a common site of metastases, most often of lung and mammary origin.

The metastases are often bilateral. Thin-needle aspiration under CT guidance is the ideal technique of diagnosis. The recognition of cells of metastatic carcinoma is usually quite easy as they differ significantly from benign adrenal cells. The primary site of cancer is usually known or suspected, and this facilitates the diagnosis still further. Morphologically, the cells of a neuroblastoma or a Wilms' tumor may resemble those of an oat cell carcinoma, but the age distribution and clinical data usually settle the issue convincingly.

RETROPERITONEAL SPACE

The retroperitoneal space is the site of numerous pathologic processes often requiring morphologic diagnosis as a guide to treatment. Chief among them are primary retroperitoneal sarcomas, malignant lymphomas, and metastatic cancer. One of the important diagnostic targets is the evaluation of the status of lymph nodes for staging of lymphomas, and testicular or pelvic cancers.

This anatomic region was, until recently, explored only by laparotomy. In fact, staging laparotomy for a variety of malignant diseases, such as Hodgkin's or non-Hodgkin's lymphomas, testicular tumors, etc., is still considered by many to be the classic clinical procedure.

The introduction of thin-needle aspiration of retroperitoneal lymph nodes opacified by lymphangiography by Göthlin in 1976 signaled a revolution in the evaluation of patients with retroperitoneal tumors. Computed tomography offers yet another tool to guide thin-needle aspirations of retroperitoneal masses. The aspiration biopsy offers the benefit of speed, good tolerance by patients, low cost, and diagnostic accuracy in experienced hands. The value of this procedure in the precise diagnosis of types of spindle cell sarcomas and typing of non–Hodgkin's lymphomas must yet be established.

Space-occupying lesions of the retroperitoneum that are located above the pelvic brim are approached posteriorly with the patient in either the prone or decubitus position. For lymph nodes and space-occupying lesions of the lower abdomen and pelvis, the patient is supine and the lesion is aspirated transperitoneally. Specific problems pertaining to lymph node aspirates will be discussed below. Care must be exercised to avoid piercing the large vessels. Our experience has shown that incidental penetration of the aorta is not harmful to the patient.

Disorders of Retroperitoneal Lymph Nodes

The first radiologic method that served to elucidate the status of retroperitoneal lymph nodes was lymphangiography. The principle of opacification of lymph nodes by subcutaneous injection of a radiopaque medium into the dorsum of the foot was introduced in 1952 by Kinmoth. It has been repeatedly shown that lymph node abnormalities shown by lymphangiography, such as enlargement or filling defects, did not always correspond to the presence of cancer. The accuracy of the procedure was variously reported between 80% and 90% for metastatic diseases, non-Hodgkin's lymphomas, and Hodgkin's disease. In an important summary based on a large biopsy-controlled experience, Wallace et al. (1977) pointed out the existence of false-positive and false-negative results of lymphangiography. In reviewing the results for Hodgkin's disease, Glatstein et al. (1969) pointed out the difficulty in the interpretation of abdominal lymphangiograms: of 10 equivocal readings in 37 patients, there were 7 negative and 3 positive biopsies

of lymph nodes. Goffinet et al. (1973) also pointed out the existence of false-positive readings due to nonmalignant space-occupying lesions of lymph nodes, such as nonspecific hyperplasia, fibrosis, and granulomas of various kinds.

Göthlin's (1976) introduction of the thin-needle aspiration technique to the sampling of lymph nodes was an important landmark in the assessment of retroperitoneal disease, as confirmed by Wallace et al. (1977). Since then the experience of several investigators has supported the significance and the value of the procedure.

For aspirates performed under fluoroscopic guidance after lymphangiography, the patient is placed in the supine position. The placement of the needle within the lymph node must be verified by slight rotation of the patient to both sides (Fig. 29–125). The appearance of oil droplets in the aspirate indicates the aspiration of the opacifying medium, hence the correct placement of the needle. Pain has been noted by some patients undergoing aspirations of the para-aortic region. This rather tedious technique of lymph node aspiration has been largely replaced by CT. High resolution CT is now extensively used in aspiration of retroperitoneal lesions.

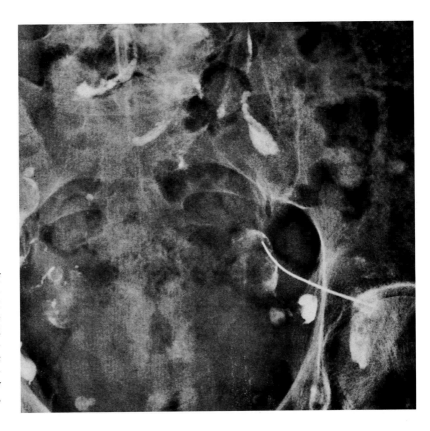

FIGURE 29–125. Cone view of the pelvis following a lymphangiogram in a patient with stage C carcinoma of the prostate. Note the Chiba needle positioned within a filling defect of an abnormal lymph node. The aspirate showed metastatic adenocarcinoma. (Courtesy of Drs. H. Mitty and S. Dan, Mt. Siani Hospital, New York, New York)

Lymphomas and Related Disorders. Hodgkin's and non-Hodgkin's lymphomas, as a group, constitute the most common malignant disease observed in the retroperitoneal space. The lymphomas may occur as a primary event in the retroperitoneum or as a retroperitoneal manifestation of a generalized disorder. The involved lymph nodes may either remain as discrete lesions or there may be matting of adjacent lymph nodes, which, combined with infiltration of adjacent soft tissues, accounts for the formation of a tumor mass.

Cytology. The cytologic manifestations of malignant lymphomas were discussed on pp. 1283–1292.

The same principles are applicable to the retroperitoneal space. The most important point of differential diagnosis of malignant lymphomas is the nonspecific hyperplasia of lymph nodes that may mimic lymphoma. Although this is a relatively uncommon event in the retroperitoneal space, it has occurred in our experience.

Metastatic Disease in Lymph Nodes. Precise staging and therapy of many tumors, mainly of the genitourinary origin, requires the identification of lymph node metastases. Metastases from distant sites may also occur, usually in the presence of known primary tumors (Fig. 29–126).

Cancers of the Female Genital Tract. Thin-needle aspirates of pelvic and retroperitoneal lymph nodes after lymphangiography have been studied in cancer of the uterine cervix and in various malignant tumors originating in the uterus and ovary.

Epidermoid and adenocarcinomas of various types are easy to identify. In Zornoza's summary (1981), the overall efficiency of the aspirates was rated at 70% because of a large proportion of inconclusive or false-negative findings. The importance of an adequate sample obtained by a competent radiologist was stressed.

Cancers of the Male Genital Tract. The results of lymph node aspirates in prostatic cancer and testicular tumors are quite similar to those described for the female genital tract.

Primary Retroperitoneal Tumors

We have had a modest experience in the aspiration diagnosis of primary retroperitoneal tumors, such as leiomyosarcoma and liposarcoma. We have also identified a retroperitoneal neurilemoma (see Fig. 29–97).

The sarcomas were readily recognized as malignant tumors, usually composed of bizarre cancer cells, although their specific classification in aspirates was difficult. In a case of leiomyosarcoma, the cancer cells were spindly and had moderate nuclear abnormalities (Fig. 29–127).

Several other types of sarcomas have been identified in aspirates of the retroperitoneum and were the subject of case reports. Except for well-differentiated liposarcomas, the precise identity of most other tumors cannot be established in aspirates and, in my judgment, this requires tissue evidence for a definitive diagnosis (see also p. 1332). Needle-tract seeding of a retroperitoneal liposarcoma was reported by Hidai et al. (1983).

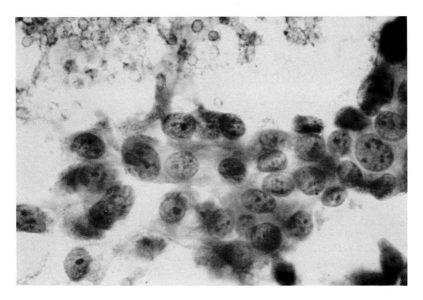

FIGURE 29–126. Retroperitoneal aspirate: cluster of cells of a metastatic carcinoma from the urinary bladder. Note the large cancer cells with large, coarsely granulated nuclei and large nucleoli. (×700)

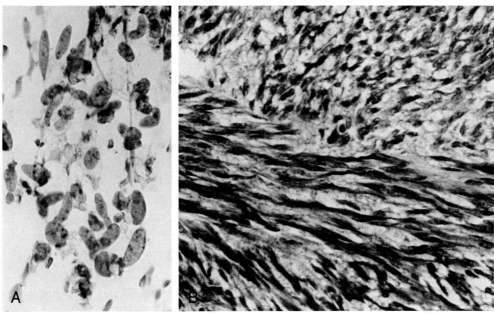

FIGURE 29–127. Aspirate of a retroperitoneal leiomyosarcoma. (*A*) The smear shows numerous scattered, predominantly elongated tumor cells with poorly preserved cytoplasm and nuclei of variable sizes. The nuclear chromatin is finely granular, and nucleoli are visible, although not prominent. (*B*) Tissue section obtained at surgery. (*A, B* ×600)

BONE

Aspiration biopsy of bone marrow, which has been routinely used in hematology for decades, is probably the most widely known application of aspiration biopsy. The method was first applied to bone tumors by Coley et al. (1931).

Aspiration biopsy of space-occupying lesions of bone requires a thorough knowledge of bone pathology and a close correlation with roentgenologic findings. Although some primary cellular bone tumors may be successfully aspirated, sclerosing lesions or roentgenologically debatable lesions should be sampled by open biopsy. The question of reliability of aspiration biopsy of bone as a guide to definitive treatment has not been adequately tested, although the very large experience reported by Schajowicz and Derqui (1968) from Argentina is most impressive.

Perhaps the most valuable application of needle aspiration biopsy to skeletal lesion is metastatic tumors. The procedure, usually successful, often spares the patient open surgery. Still, there are several primary bone lesions that may be recognized with certainty, such as multiple myeloma, giant cell tumor, or chordoma.

Methods

For the aspiration of bony lesions, deep local anesthesia is required, as the penetration of the periosteum is usually very painful. A thick, rigid needle with a stylet or a trocar is introduced into the lesion. After removal of the trocar, a thin needle is placed within the thick needle and the aspiration is performed in the customary fashion. The material is processed as smears or, if tissue fragments are obtained, as a cell block.

Benign Lesions

An important application of aspiration biopsy of skeletal lesions is *osteomyelitis.* The presence of pus, debris, and bony fragments characterize the disorder. In tuberculosis, necrotic caseous material, epithelioid cells, and Langhans'-type giant cells may be present (see Fig. 19–55). Considerable caution is required in the interpretation of giant cells, as these may represent osteoclasts, as in a callus or a reparative granuloma (Fig. 29–128), or may be associated with the presence of an underlying tumor. Other benign lesions of bone that may

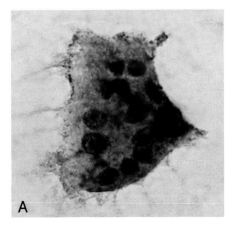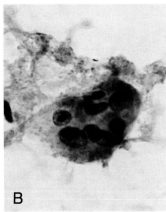

FIGURE 29–128. Osteoclasts in an aspirate of a rib lesion, thought to be a metastatic tumor, but proved to be a callus from an occult fracture. Note the small nuclei of monotonous sizes dispersed throughout the cytoplasm of the giant cells. (*A, B* ×560)

be occasionally sampled are eosinophilic granulomas (Fig. 29–129). The mixed population of small macrophages and eosinophils is quite characteristic of the lesion (cf. Fig. 29–55).

Primary Malignant Tumors

As was noted above, the diagnosis of primary malignant tumors of the skeleton requires close correlation with radiologic findings. The best applications of the aspiration technique are in confirming clinical and radiologic impressions of a known disorder (such as a multiple myeloma or a giant cell tumor) or saving the patient from a technically difficult surgical diagnostic procedure in lesions in some anatomic locations, such as a chordoma of the base of the skull.

Multiple Myeloma

The diagnosis of multiple myeloma is usually established on clinical and biochemical grounds and confirmed by a bone marrow study. Rarely, a localized lesion of bone may require diagnostic clarification in the absence of persuasive clinical data. The customary population of plasma cells is observed in such smears (cf. Fig. 26–58).

Giant Cell Tumor

The classic cytologic presentation is that of a large number of multinucleated giant cells (osteoclasts), accompanied by smaller stromal cells (see Fig. 27–29). The diagnosis must be correlated with clinical and roentgenologic findings because of the ubiquitous presence of osteoclasts in a broad variety of other skeletal disorders (see above and Fig. 29–128).

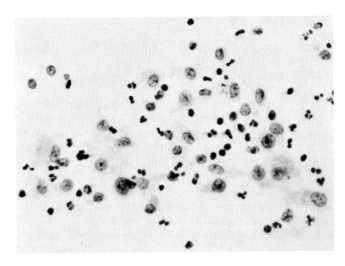

FIGURE 29–129. Eosinophilic granuloma of skull, aspirate. The smear shows a mixture of small macrohages, eosinophils, and lymphocytes. (×400. Courtesy Prof. S. Woyke)

Chordoma

These rare tumors, derived from the remnants of the notochord, occur at the cranial and sacral ends of the spine. The surgical biopsy of the tumors may be sometimes technically difficult, and an aspiration biopsy may confirm a clinical and roentgenologic suspicion. The tumors have a characteristic cytologic presentation: the smear contains clusters of large cells with abundant cytoplasm, studded with small vacuoles, known as physaliferous cells (Fig. 29–130). The nuclei are spherical or oval, somewhat hyperchromatic, with slight variability in sizes. The background of the smears may show fragments of acellular stroma.

One important point of differentiation is a well-differentiated chondrosarcoma, wherein the aspirates may show somewhat similar large cells which, however, usually show only a single cytoplasmic vacuole and which are embedded in cartilaginous stroma (see below and Fig. 29–132).

Osteosarcoma

There is usually a very limited need for an aspiration biopsy of the common juvenile form of this highly malignant tumor because the diagnosis is usually firmly established on clinical and radiologic grounds. There are, however, some exceptions to this rule. On the other hand, aspiration biopsy of the rare adult form of this tumor is sometimes very helpful, particularly in patients with Paget's disease of the skeleton and in bone lesions observed after radiotherapy for another tumor (postradiation osteosarcoma).

Except in the sclerosing type of this tumor, wherein it may be difficult to secure an adequate cytologic sample, the aspirates of other forms of osteosarcoma are rich in bizarre cancer cells (Fig. 29–131). Osteoclasts are often present in such smears and should not lead to an erroneous diagnosis of a giant cell tumor. In view of therapeutic progress, an early diagnosis of an osteosarcoma may be life-saving, and in debatable situations the aspiration biopsy is usually sufficient for the diagnosis of a malignant tumor and sometimes of tumor type.

Chondrosarcoma

On rare occasions aspiration biopsy may be helpful in the diagnosis of a chondrosarcoma, particularly if a recurrence is suspected after treatment of the

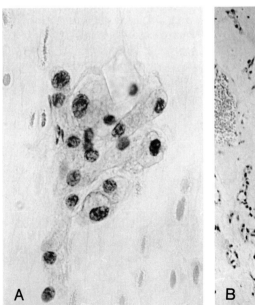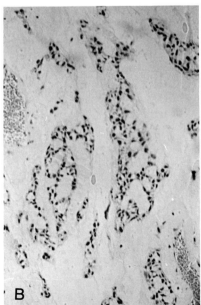

FIGURE 29–130. Chordoma of base of skull. The aspiration smear (*A*) shows a cluster of the large physaliferous cells, with finely vacuolated cytoplasm and oval or spherical nuclei with slight variation in size. The tumor (*B*) was composed of sheets and strands of physaliferous cells embedded in an acellular stroma. (*A* ×400; *B* ×125. Courtesy of Prof. S. Woyke)

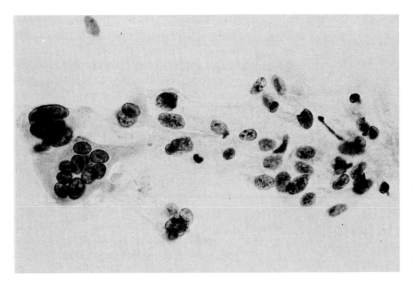

FIGURE 29–131. Needle aspirate from an osteogenic sarcoma. A benign multinucleated cell (osteoclast, *bottom, left*) is seen next to a malignant giant cell and numerous malignant mononucleated cells. (Papanicolaou stain ×480)

primary tumor. The better-differentiated varieties of this tumor may be difficult to sample and usually yield fragments of cartilage matrix with embedded tumor cells (Fig. 29–132). The differentiation between an atypical, but benign, tumor of cartilage and a low-grade chondrosarcoma is based on the degree of nuclear variability and atypia that is usually more pronounced in the malignant variant. The aspirates of a poorly differentiated chondrosarcoma yield cancer cells that are readily recognized as such. The tumor type may be difficult to identify in the cytology sample without the knowledge of clinical and roentgenologic data.

Small-Cell Tumors of Bone

A group of tumors of bone composed of small cells comprises primary malignant lymphomas, Ewing's tumors of childhood, and metastatic tumors, mainly neuroblastoma in children and small-cell carcinomas in adults. The differentiation of these tumors on cytologic grounds is not easy. Similar difficulties may occur in tissue biopsies.

A few diagnostic guidelines may be offered:

In *malignant lymphomas* the cells are generally monotonous and dispersed and show the features described in aspirates of lymph nodes (see p. 1283).

In *Ewing's tumor* and in *neuroblastomas* the cells are arranged in rosettes (Fig. 29–133). The neuroblastoma cells are usually much smaller. The center of the rosettes in Ewing's tumors is composed of homogeneous material, whereas in neuroblastoma it contains neurofibrils that can be demonstrated by special stains.

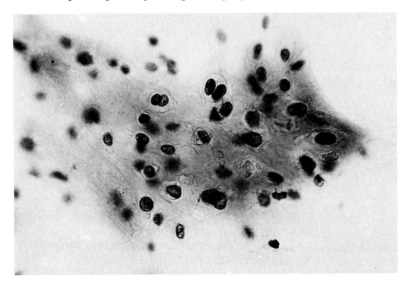

FIGURE 29–132. Needle aspirate from a chondrosarcoma. A fragment of the tumor showing moderate cellular atypia and the characteristic matrix. (Papanicolaou stain ×480)

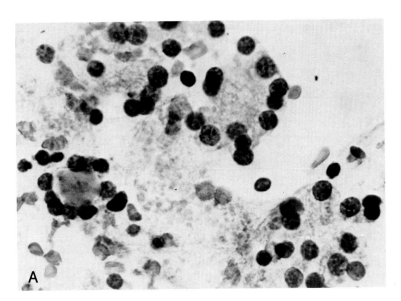

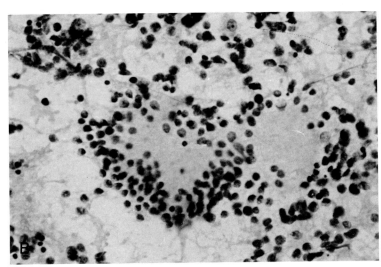

FIGURE 29–133. Ewing's sarcoma and neuroblastoma (*A*) Aspirate of Ewing's sarcoma in a 13-year-old girl. The tumor cells form rosettes with central deposits of homogeneous material. The tumor cells are relatively small, have scanty cytoplasm, and show very little variability in nuclear configuration and sizes.(*B*) Aspirate of a metastatic neuroblastoma. The much smaller, monotonous tumor cells form rosettes with centers filled with thin delicate neurofibrils. Additional fine neurofibrils may be observed in the background of the smear. (*A, B* ×400. *A*: Modified from Koss, L.G., et al.: Aspiration Biopsy. Cytologic Interpretation and Histologic Bases. New York, Igaku-Shoin, 1984, with permission. *B*: Courtesy of Prof. S. Woyke)

Small-cell metastatic tumors occur mainly in adults and are, in nearly all cases, carcinomas. The clustering of cells, combined with a stain for keratin, facilitates the correct identification. The knowledge of clinical history and of radiologic presentation are the essential prerequisites of diagnostic success.

Metastatic Tumors

For all intents and purposes, the aspiration biopsy of metastases is probably the most important application of this technique to skeletal lesions. The value of the method is in rapid recognition of important abnormalities without a formal surgical biopsy that may require considerable delay, may be technically difficult (for example, in the spine), and is nearly always painful.

The technique is applicable to lesions without a known primary site as the first diagnostic procedure. In most such instances the diagnosis of a malignant tumor can be established with ease and the essential characterization of the tumor established (i.e., adenocarcinoma, squamous carcinoma, small-cell carcinoma, etc.). In some instances, specific origin of the tumor may be suggested. For an extensive discussion of metastatic carcinoma see p. 1292.

Mammary Carcinomas

In women, metastatic mammary carcinoma in the presence of an occult primary is not uncommon. The features of mammary carcinoma in aspirated samples were described on pp. 1303–1308. Of special interest is the recognition of lobular carcinoma with its characteristic features documented in Figs. 29–73, 29–74, and 29–135.

Renal Carcinoma

Renal carcinoma of clear cell type may be suspected if the aspirate is composed of fairly monotonous, large cancer cells, with faintly vacuolated and granular cytoplasm (see Fig. 29–118*A*).

Thyroid Cancer

Metastatic thyroid carcinoma may be recognized if the tumor cells form follicles with central colloid. Intranuclear cytoplasmic inclusions are *not*, however, uniquely characteristic of this group of tumors, as they may also occur in metastatic melanomas (see Fig. 29–92*C*), adenocarcinomas of bronchogenic origin, and occasionally in other tumors.

Other tumors may be occasionally recognized as to origin. The reader is referred to the description of specific tumor types for further guidance.

THE ORBIT AND THE EYE GLOBE

Tumors of the eye adnexa were discussed in Chapter 27. With the advent of computed tomography it became possible to obtain aspirated material from space-occupying lesions of the orbit. For summary of techniques and results see Czerniak et al., 1984 and Chapter 18 in Koss et al., 1992.

The Orbit

Benign Lesions

Among the benign orbital lesions of note are cysts, benign tumors of lacrimal glands, and the so-called pseudotumors that may be lymphoid or fibrous. Rarely, meningiomas or benign gliomas of optic nerve may occur.

The aspirates of benign lesions are usually very scanty and great care is required to preserve the material. Only benign mixed tumors of the lacri-mal glands may yield cell-rich aspirates. The cytologic presentation of these tumors is identical with similar tumors occurring in salivary glands (see p. 1252).

The lesion that may cause significant diagnostic difficulties is the benign lymphoid pseudotumor. The aspirate usually does not permit a secure differentiation between a benign, follicle-forming lymphoid lesion and a malignant lymphoma. In any event, even the fate and the significance of the lymphoid pseudotumor is not secure and, in at least some cases, a malignant lymphoma develops with the passage of time (Jakobiec, 1978; Brady and Shields, 1982).

Malignant Lesions

Primary malignant tumors of the orbit are exceedingly rare. Sarcomas of connective tissue, muscle, or malignant lymphomas may be observed. The experience with aspiration biopsy of these tumors is very limited.

Metastatic tumors, on the other hand, are not uncommon, usually in the presence of a known primary, but sometimes as the first manifestation of disease.

A smear from a metastatic prostatic carcinoma is shown in Fig. 29–134. The precise diagnosis could be established by a positive immunostain for specific prostatic antigen. A metastatic mammary carcinoma is shown in Fig. 29–135. The characteristic cytoplasmic vacuoles with central condensation were diagnostic of a metastatic lobular carcinoma (cf. Figs. 29–73 and 29–74). Metastatic cancers from other sites may occur as well. The orbital involvement in malignant lymphoma is known to occur.

In children, orbital manifestations of a neuroblastoma may be the first evidence of disease. The characteristic rosettes formed by the small tumor cells usually permit a rapid recognition of tumor type (see Fig. 29–133). The differentiation from a retinoblastoma of the eye globe is based on examination of the fundus of the eye.

The Eye Globe

Aspiration biopsy of the eye globe is a technically difficult procedure that belongs into the hands of qualified ophthalmologists. Usually, on clinical grounds, the preliminary diagnosis of the space-occupying lesion is suggested, and the aspiration biopsy serves to confirm the clinical impression.

The repertoire of primary eye globe tumors is fairly limited.

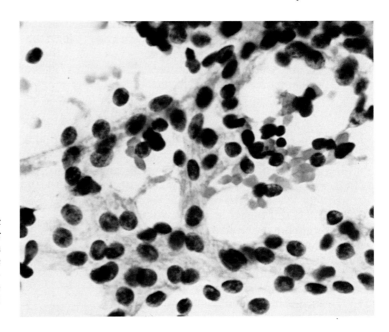

FIGURE 29–134. Metastatic prostatic carcinoma to orbit. The aspiration smear contained medium-sized cancer cells with a tendency to gland formation. The nature of the tumor was confirmed by the presence of specific prostatic antigen. Case from the University of Pittsburgh Medical School. (×560)

In children, the most common malignant tumor is a retinoblastoma that can be unilateral or bilateral. The tumor has very interesting implications in molecular biology of cancer. For a discussion of the retinoblastoma gene (*Rb* gene) see Chap. 2. Aspiration biopsy of a retinoblastoma yields cells that cannot be distinguished on morphologic grounds from cells of related tumors, neuroblastomas (cf. Fig. 29–133) or a medulloblastoma (cf. Figs. 27–2 and 27–13).

In adults, the most common primary tumor is a malignant melanoma that may occur in the iris or anywhere along the retina. Nearly all of these

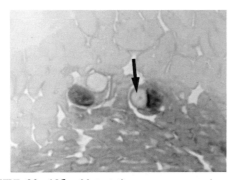

FIGURE 29–135. Metastatic mammary carcinoma to orbit. The cancer cells were few, but had morphologic features diagnostic of a lobular mammary carcinoma: small cancer cells with peripheral nuclei and large cytoplasmic vacuoles, with a central condensation of mucus (*arrow*). (×560)

tumors contain heavily pigmented tumor cells, but they also display other morphologic features of melanoma: cells with marked nuclear abnormalities, multinucleated cells, and intranuclear cytoplasmic inclusions. Pigmented cells resembling dendrites with multiple cytoplasmic extensions may be seen in ocular melanomas (Koss et al., 1992). Perhaps the most difficult to identify is the spindle cell variant of malignant melanoma. The aspirates may contain a fairly monotonous population of elongated cells, with slender cytoplasmic extensions. The nuclei of such cells, however, are hyperchromatic and contain large nucleoli, features that help in the assessment of the malignant nature of the tumor. An interesting feature of malignant ocular melanoma is the propensity of these tumors to form delayed liver metastases, sometimes 20 or more years after the removal of the primary tumor. This writer (LGK) even called this the "syndrome of a glass eye and protuberant abdomen" (see also p. 1353).

Metastatic tumors to the eye globe are rare and are similar to metastatic tumors to the orbit (see above).

THE CENTRAL NERVOUS SYSTEM

The use of cytologic touch preparations of brain biopsies for the rapid diagnosis of tumors was first described by Eisenhardt and Cushing in 1930. The method has had many followers, mainly in the

United Kingdom, and the accuracy of the procedure was considered to be very high (summarized in Barnard, 1981; Liwnicz and Rodriguez, 1984).

With the introduction of computed tomography (CT), the option of precise localization and sizing of space-occupying lesions became available. Furthermore, with growing experience, the benign or malignant nature of these lesions could be determined in most cases. A further refinement of preoperative diagnosis became available with the introduction of magnetic resonance imaging (MRI), which provides visual information on the nature of the lesions of the central nervous system (CNS) with a still higher level of accuracy. This progress in noninvasive diagnostic modalities has not been matched so far by a major progress in therapy of malignant tumors of the central nervous system. Thus, the therapeutic options today remain pretty much the same as they were in the 1930s when Cushing and other pioneers first documented that neurosurgery was possible and was sometimes curative of CNS tumors.

Virtually all patients who are referred for a diagnostic workup are symptomatic. The fundamental questions that must be answered are:

1. Is the lesion benign or malignant?

2. If the lesion is benign, can it be treated?
3. If the lesion is malignant, is it a primary tumor or a metastasis?
4. Is the malignant lesion amenable to treatment?

The introduction of stereotactic CT machines allowed a very accurate placement of thin needles in the space-occupying lesions and led to the development of aspiration techniques. The material could be processed as smears or small tissue fragments (minibiopsies). At the time of this writing (1991), most neurosurgeons and neuropathologists prefer to process the aspirated material as histologic sections. Whether this reflects a lack of training in cytologic techniques or a greater diagnostic accuracy is not clear. In any event, the future of the aspiration biopsy smear as a primary diagnostic modality is unclear.

Principles of Cytologic Diagnosis

The central nervous system is a very complex structure containing a variety of normal cell types (see also Chap. 27). A broad variety of primary tumors may also occur, summarized in Table 29–11.

Table 29–11
A Simplified Classification of CNS Tumors

	Location of Tumor and Prevalence in Population	Subtype	Grade
Neuroepithelial tumors			
Astrocytoma	Cerebrum and cerebellum	Protoplasmic	I
	Any age: pilocytic astrocytoma usually 1st and 2nd decades	Fibrillary	I or II
		Gemistocytic	II
		Pilocytic	I
		Malignant (anaplastic)	III
Glioblastoma (including giant-cell)	Cerebral hemispheres, stem, cord		IV
	45–55 age group		
	More common in men.		
Oligodendroglioma	Mostly frontal/parietal.	Typical	II
	40–55 aged group	Malignant (anaplastic)	III
Ependymoma	Ventricles (particularly the fourth), spinal cord, cerebrum		I–II
	Children and adults	Myxopapillary (sacral)	I–II
		Malignant	III–IV
		Ependymoblastoma	IV
		Subependymoma	I
Choroid plexus papilloma	Fourth ventricle and lateral ventricles		I
Choroid plexus carcinoma	First decade up to adult		III–IV

(continued)

Table 29–11 (continued)

	Location of Tumor and Prevalence in Population	Subtype	Grade
Medulloblastoma	Cerebellum First decade common, young adults rare		IV
Pineal cell tumors	At site of pineal Rare at any age		I–IV
Nerve sheath cells			
Neurofibroma	Cranial nerve root; in association with von Recklinghausen's neurofibromatosis		I
Schwannoma (neurilemmoma)	Intraspinal and intracranial (acoustic neuroma) Adults		I
Meningeal tumors			
Meningioma	Intracranial and intraspinal; more common in females (4:1) Peak incidence 45	Various Malignant	I III
Melanoma (primary)	Rare at any age		IV
Lymphomas			
	Cerebrum (any site); meninges and nerve roots Mostly adults	Primary, "microglioma," "reticulum cell sarcoma"	III–IV
Blood vessel tumors			
Hemangioblastoma	Cerebellum, brain stem, cord Adults 25–45; male preponderance		I
Angioma (+ malformations)	Any site Any age		
Malformations and teratomas			
Germinoma/teratoma	Pineal and suprasellar regions. Age 10–30; male preponderance		III–IV
Craniopharyngioma			
	Suprasellar. Any age but peak 5–25		I
Dermoid/epidermoid cyst	Rare at any age		I
Local (regional) tumors extending to CNS			
Anterior pituitary adenoma	In pituitary fossa, may extend to suprasellar region Adults		I
Chordoma	Base of skull and sacrum Adults		II–III
Cystic adenoid carcinoma	Nasopharynx; sinuses Adults		III

(Modified from Liwnicz, B., and Rodriguez, C.A.: The central nervous system. *In* Koss, L.G., Woyke, S., and Olszewski, W. [eds.]: Aspiration Biopsy. Cytologic Interpretation and Histologic Bases. New York, Igaku-Shoin, 1984, with permission)

The task of the cytopathologist is to differentiate between reactive events in the CNS and tumors. The task is comparatively easy if the makeup of the smear is clearly that of a malignant tumor of high grade. The difficulties occur with low-grade astrocytomas that may mimic reactive gliosis and vice versa.

The recognition of metastatic tumors is comparatively easy, particularly if supported by clinical and imaging data.

Normal and Reactive Cells

Neurons (Ganglion Cells).   Neurons are very large cells, with cytoplasmic processes showing an enormous diversity of morphologic configurations (Liwnicz and Rodriguez, 1984). All neurons have very large nuclei and frequently prominent, large nucleoli. An example is shown in Fig. 29–136.

Glial Cells.   The neurons are surrounded by a supporting apparatus, the glial cells. These may also assume a variety of configurations and are provided with cytoplasmic processes.

In **reactive gliosis** there is often a marked proliferation of glial cells, known as *astrocytes* (Fig. 29–137).

Ependymal and Choroid Plexus Cells.   These epithelial cells with spherical small nuclei generally form flat sheets, wherein the cell borders can be readily identified (Fig. 29–138).

Other Benign Cells.   Cells of meningeal and blood vessel origin may be observed in aspirates.

Benign Space-Occupying Lesions of the Brain

A number of benign disorders may be diagnosed by aspiration biopsy of the brain. The lesions may be cystic or solid, and their accurate diagnosis may be of therapeutic value. Perhaps the most common cystic lesion is cysticercosis, caused by the larval form of the pork tapeworm *Taenia solium*, recognizable by its hooklets similar to hooklets observed in echinococcosis (see Figs. 25–42 and 29–104). Other cystic lesions include abscesses and simple cysts derived from various epithelial components of the CNS, such as the ependyma or the pineal. It must be stressed that some brain tumors may also be cystic, and that the aspiration biopsy may help in distinguishing the benign from the neoplastic cyst. In benign cysts the contents are essentially acellular, whereas abscesses yield pus. In tumors the cysts contain necrotic debris and sometimes necrotic tumor cells.

Among the non-cystic lesions one should consider herpetic encephalitis, progressive multifocal leukoencephalopathy, tuberculosis or syphilitic gumma, and a variety of fungal and parasitic infections, seen with increasing frequency in patients with AIDS. The cytologic presentations of several of these entities are discussed elsewhere in this book (progressive multifocal encephalopathy and

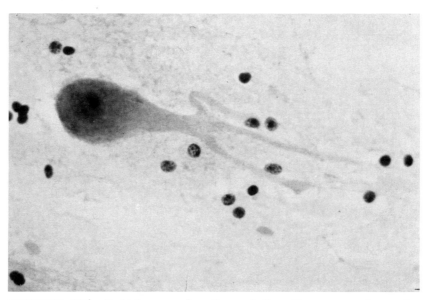

FIGURE 29–136.   Purkinje neuron from the cerebellum. These neurons have a distinctive shape, often resembling an octopus. The surrounding nuclei are mostly those of Bergmann glia. (Smear preparation, Papanicolaou stain ×560. Courtesy of Drs. B. Liwnicz and C. Rodriguez)

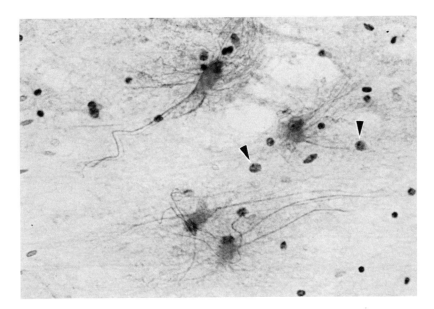

FIGURE 29–137. Reactive gliosis surrounding an infarcted area (not shown in the picture). Reactive astrocytes have multiple processes. For comparison, note the nonreactive astrocytes with only the nuclei visible (*arrowheads*). (Smear preparation, Papanicolaou stain ×560. Courtesy of Drs. B. Liwnicz and C. Rodriguez)

its relationship to the JC strain of polyomavirus, p. 910; cytologic presentations of tuberculosis, p. 727; herpesvirus encephalitis, p. 1188; various parasites, p. 348; and toxoplasmosis of the brain, p. 1193).

Common Primary Brain Tumors (see Table 29–11)

Astrocytomas. These are the most common primary tumors of the CNS, which range in configuration, hence, in grade, from well-differentiated tumors (grade I) to highly malignant, poorly differentiated (grade IV) tumors, the latter is also known as a glioblastoma multiforme.

The *low-grade astrocytomas* are characterized by uniform cells with small nuclei. The presence of capillary vessels in the smears is suggestive of the presence of a tumor, rather than a reactive giosis (Fig. 29–139).

The *high-grade astrocytomas* (glioblastoma multiforme) are readily recognized as malignant (Fig. 29–140). The precise nature of the tumor may require support of clinical and imaging data. The differentiation from metastatic carcinoma may cause diagnostic problems.

Ependymomas. These tumors are characterized by perivascular arrangement of uniform columnar cells (pseudorosettes). In touch prepara-

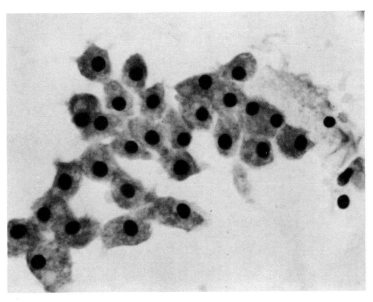

FIGURE 29–138. Sheath of ependymal cells. The cells have uniform round nuclei surrounded by basophilic cytoplasm with well-defined cellular margins. (Smear preparation, Papanicolaou stain ×896. Courtesy of Drs. B. Liwnicz and C. Rodriguez)

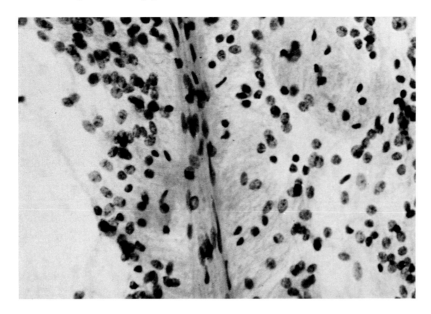

FIGURE 29–139. Papillary structure in astrocytoma. The astrocytes are attached to the capillary blood vessel by thin processes. (Smear preparation, Papanicolaou stain ×560. Courtesy of Drs. B. Liwnicz and C. Rodriguez)

tions, the pseudorosettes may be evident, but in aspirates, this landmark structure may be lost. The presence of uniform columnar cells in smears may permit recognition of the tumor.

Medulloblastoma. This common, highly malignant tumor of childhood and its cytologic presentation were discussed and illustrated in Chapter 27.

Midline Tumors. This term covers a variety of tumors affecting the pineal, the pituitary, and the base of the skull (craniopharyngioma), as they all occur in the midline of the skull. The tumors are not related to one another and, therefore, represent a broad variety of patterns.

Pineal Tumors. These vary from benign teratomas to highly malignant germinomas that resemble testicular seminomas. The classification and cytologic representation of these tumors is similar to testicular tumors and tumors of the anterior mediastinum (see p. 1323).

Pituitary Adenomas. The diagnosis of a pituitary adenoma is usually rendered on clinical and endocrine grounds. The precise classification of these tumors is based on immunohistologic analysis of cell types and their function.

Craniopharyngioma. These uncommon cystic tumors of the base of the skull are very rarely aspirated.

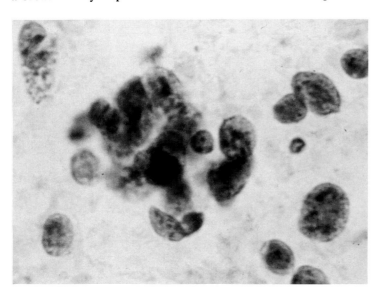

FIGURE 29–140. Glioblastoma. Large, hyperchromatic nuclei showing molding. (Smear preparation, Papanicolaou stain, ×1,020. Courtesy of Drs. B. Liwnicz and C. Rodriguez)

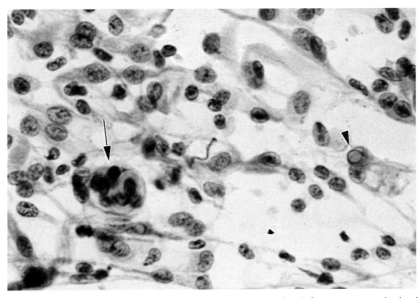

FIGURE 29–141.   Meningioma, aspiration smear. On the *left* is a meningeal whorl (*arrow*). Some of the nuclei contain intranuclear cytoplasmic inclusions (*arrowhead*). (Papanicolaou stain, ×560. Courtesy of Drs. B. Liwnicz and C. Rodriguez)

Other Primary Tumors

Meningiomas.   The aspirates of meningiomas are characterized by sheets of epithelial cells, sometimes forming whorls (Fig. 29–141). The presence of intranuclear cytoplasmic inclusions is common in these tumors.

Nerve Sheet Tumors.   The classic appearance of a neurilemoma (schwannoma) in aspirated material is shown in Fig. 29–97.

Metastatic Tumors

A broad variety of metastatic tumors may affect the CNS. Chief among them are bronchogenic carcinoma, malignant melanoma, and mammary carcinoma. The cytologic presentation of these tumors in aspirates follows the same principles as in cerebrospinal fluid (CSF), described in Chapter 27.

BIBLIOGRAPHY

History and general references
Salivary glands
Lymph nodes and neck organs (other than thyroid gland)
Thyroid
Breast
Testis and ovary
Prostate

Skin and soft part tumors
Mediastinum (for Lung see Chaps. 20 and 21; for Pleura see Chap. 26)
Liver
Pancreas
Spleen
Kidney
Adrenal glands
Retroperitoneum
Bone
Eye and orbit
Central nervous system

History and General References

Beale, L.S.: The Microscope and Its Application to Practical Medicine, 2nd ed. London, John Churchill, 1858.

Berg, J.W.: The aspiration biopsy smear. *In* Koss, L.G.: Diagnostic Cytology and Its Histopathologic Bases, 1st ed. Philadelphia, J.B. Lippincott, 1961.

Coley, B.L., Sharp, G.S., and Ellis, E.B.: Diagnosis of bone tumors by aspiration. Am. J. Surg., *13*:215–224, 1931.

Criborn, C.O., Franzén, S., Unsgaard, B., and Zaijcek, J.: Studies on the effect of aspiration biopsy on the variability of aspirated cells: I. Registration of pressure differences during aspiration. Scand. J. Haematol., *1*:272–279, 1964.

Domagala, W., and Koss, L.G.: Surface configuration of human tumor cells obtained in fine needle aspiration biopsy. Scan. Electr. Micr., *3*:101–108, 1980.

Donné, A.F.: Cours de Microscopie Complémentaires des Etudes Medicales. Atlas execute d'après Nature au Microscope-Daguerreotype. Paris, Balliere, 1845.

Engzell, U., Esposti, P.L., Rubio, C., Sigurdson, A., and Zajicek, J.: Investigation on tumour spread in connection with aspiration biopsy. Acta Radiol., *10*:385–398, 1971.

Eposti, P.L.: Aspiration Biopsy Cytology in the Diagnosis and Management of Prostatic Carcinoma. Stockholm, Stahl and Accidenstryck, 1974.

Eposti, P.-L., Franzén, S., and Zajicek, J.: The aspiration biopsy smear. *In* Koss, L.G.: Diagnostic Cytology and Its Histopathologic Bases, 2nd ed. pp. 565–596. Philadelphia, J.B. Lippincott, 1968.

Ferucci, J.T., and Wittenberg, J.: Interventional Radiology of the Abdomen. Baltimore, Williams & Wilkins, 1981.

Frable, W.J.: Thin Needle Aspiration Biopsy. Philadelphia, W.B. Saunders, 1983.

Franzén, S., Giertz, G., and Zajicek, J.: Cytologic diagnosis of prostatic tumours by transrectal aspiration biopsy. A preliminary report. Br. J. Urol., *32*:193–196, 1960.

Godwin, J.T.: Aspiration biopsy: technique and application. Ann. N.Y. Acad. Sci., *63*:1348–1373, 1956.

Greig, E.D.W., and Gray, A.C.H.: Note on the lymphatic glands in sleeping sickness. Lancet, *1*:1570, 1904.

Hajdu, S.I., and Hajdu, E.O.: Cytopathology of Sarcomas and Other Nonepithelial Malignant Tumors. Philadelphia, W.B. Saunders, 1976.

Hamperl, H.: Ueber das Vorkommen von Onkozyten in verschiedenen Organen und ihren Geschwülsten. Virchows Arch. [A], *298*:327–375, 1936.

Hirschfeld, H.: Bericht ueber einige histologischmikroskopische und experimentelle Arbeiten bei den boesartigen Geschwuelsten. Z. Krebsforsch., *16*:33–39, 1919.

Hirschfeld, H.: Ueber isolierte aleukaemische Lymphadenose der Haut. Z. Krebsforsch., *11*:397–407, 1912.

Johansson, B., and Zajicek, J.: Sampling of cell material from human tumors by aspiration biopsy. Nature, *200*:1333–1334, 1963.

Kamholz, S.L., Pinsker, K.L., Johnson, J., and Schreiber, K.: Fine needle aspiration biopsy of intrathoracic lesions. N.Y. State J. Med., *82*:736–739, 1982.

Kline, T.S.: Aspiration Biopsy Cytology, 2nd ed. New York, Churchhill-Livingstone, 1988.

Koss, L.G., Woyke, S., and Olszewski, W.: Aspiration Biopsy. Cytologic Interpretation and Histologic Bases. New York, Igaku-Shoin, 1984, Ed. 2, 1992.

Lebert, H.: Physologie pathologique ou recherches cliniques experimentales et microscopiques. Paris, Balliere, 1845.

Linsk, J.A., and Franzén, S.: Clinical Aspiration Cytology. 2nd ed. Philadelphia, J.B. Lippincott, 1989.

Lopes Cardozo, P.: Atlas of Clinical Cytology. Hertogenbosch, Targa, 1976.

Lopes-Cardozo, P.: Clinical cytology using the May–Grünwald–Giemsa Stained Smear. Leyden, L. Staflen, 1954.

Löwhagen, T.: Thyroid. *In* Zajicek, J. (ed.): Aspiration Biopsy Cytology, part I. Basel, S. Karger, 1974.

Löwhagen, T., and Willems, J.-S.: Aspiration biopsy cytology in diseases of the thyroid. *In* Koss L.G., and Coleman, D.V. (eds.): Advances in Clinical Cytology. pp. 201–231. London, Butterworth, 1981.

Ludin, H.: Die Organpunktion in der Klinischen Diagnostik. Basel, S. Karger, 1955.

Martin, H.E., and Ellis, E.B.: Aspiration biopsy. Surg. Gynecol. Obstet., *59*:578–589, 1934.

Martin, H.E., and Ellis, E.B.: Biopsy by needle puncture and aspiration. Ann. Surg., *92*:169–181, 1930.

Papanicolaou, G.N., and Traut, H.F.: Diagnosis of Uterine Cancer by the Vaginal Smear. New York, Commonwealth Fund, 1943.

Plesnicar, S., Rubio, C., Sigurdson, A., and Zajicek, J.: Studies on the effect of aspiration biopsy on aspirated cells. Determination of cell viability by dye permeability and trypsin digestion tests on aspirates from lymph nodes, spleen and bone marrow and by lymph node cell cultures with phytohemaglutinin. Acta Cytol., *12*:454–461, 1968.

Rosenblatt, R., Kutcher, R., Moussouris, H.F., Schreiber, K., and Koss, L.G.: Sonographically guided fine needle aspiration of liver lesions. JAMA, *248*:1639–1641, 1982.

Ruge, C.L.: Das Mikroskop in der Gynakologie und der Diagnostik. Z. Geburtshilfe, *20*, 1890.

Sinner, W.N.: Complications of percutaneous transthoracic needle aspiration biopsy. Acta Radiol. [Diagn.] (Stockh.), *17*:813–828, 1976.

Sinner, W.N., and Zajicek, J.: Implantation of metastasis after percutaneous transthoracic needle aspiration biopsy. Acta Radiol. [Diagn.] (Stockh.), *17*:473–480, 1976.

Smetana, H.F.: The needle biopsy in diagnosis. Am. J. Clin. Pathol., *24*:395–405, 1954.

Smith, I.H., Fisher, J.H., Lott, J.S., and Thomson, D.H.: The cytological diagnosis of solid tumors by small needle aspiration and its influence on cancer clinic practice. Can. Med. Assoc. J., *80*:855–860, 1959.

Söderström, N.: Fine-needle Aspiration Biopsy: Used as a Direct Adjunct in Clinical Diagnostic Work. Stockholm, Almqvist & Wiksell, 1966.

Stewart F.W.: The diagnosis of tumors by aspiration. Am. J. Pathol., *9*:801–812, 1933.

Takahashi, M.: Color Atlas of Cancer Cytology. Tokyo, Igaku-Shoin, 1978.

Zajicek, J.: Aspiration Biopsy Cytology. Part 1: Cytology of Supradiaphragmatic Organs. Basel, S. Karger, 1974.

Zajicek, J.: The aspiration biopsy smear. *In* Koss, L.G. (ed.): Diagnostic Cytology and Its Histopathologic Bases, 3rd ed. pp. 1001–1104. Philadelphia, J.B. Lippincott, 1979.

Zajicek, J.: Aspiration Biopsy Cytology. Part 2. Cytology of Infradiaphragmatic Organs. Basel, S. Karger, 1979.

Zajicek, J.: Sampling of cells from human tumours by aspiration biopsy for diagnosis and research. Eur. J. Cancer, *1*:253–258, 1965.

Zornoza, J.: Percutaneous Needle Biopsy. Baltimore, Williams & Wilkins, 1981.

Salivary Glands

Balogh, K., and Roth, S.I.: Histochemical and electronmicroscopic studies of eosinophilic granular cells (oncocytes) in tumours of the parotid gland. Lab. Invest., *14*:310–320, 1965.

Batsakis, J.G.: Tumors of the Head and Neck. Clinical and Pathological Consideration, 2nd ed. Baltimore, Williams & Wilkins, 1979.

Behbehani, A., Dashti, H., Al-Shahawi, M., Awadi, A., Woyke, S., Olszewski, W., Christenson, J.T., and Al-Naqeeb, N.: The value of pre-operative fine-needle aspiration biopsy in planning the management of parotid gland tumours. Med. Principles Pract., *2*:27–34, 1990.

Bondeson, L., Lindholm, K., and Thorstenson, S.: Benign dermal eccrine cylindroma: a pitfall in the cytologic diagnosis of adenoid cystic carcinoma. Acta Cytol., *27*:326–328, 1983.

Bono, A., Chiesa, F., Sala, L., Azzarrelli, A., Pilotti, S., and DiPietro, S.: Fine-needle aspiration biopsy in parotid masses. Tumori, *69*:417–421, 1983.

Bottles, K.T., Ferrell, L.D., and Miller, T.R.: Tyrosine crystals in fine needle aspirates of a pleomorphic adenoma of the parotid gland. Acta Cytol., *28*:490–492, 1984.

Cohen, M.B., Fisher, P.E., Holly, E.A., Ljung, B.M., Lowhagen, T., and Bottles, K.: Fine needle aspiration biopsy diagnosis of mucoepidermoid carcinoma: statistical analysis. Acta Cytol., *34*:43–49, 1990.

Eneroth, C.M., Franzen, S., and Zajicek, J.: Cytologic diagnosis in aspirates from 1000 salivary gland tumours. Acta Otolaryngol. [Suppl.] (Stockh.) *24*:168–171, 1967.

Eneroth, C.-M.: Histological and clinical aspects of parotid tumors. Acta Otolaryngol., *191*:5–99, 1964.

Eneroth, C.-M., Jakobsson, P., and Zajicek, J.: Aspiration biopsy of salivary gland tumors. V. Morphologic investigation on smears and histologic section of acinic cell carcinoma. Acta Radiol., *310*(Suppl.):85–93, 1971.

Eneroth, C.-M., and Zajicek, J.: Aspiration biopsy of salivary gland tumors: II. Morphologic studies on smears and histologic sections from oncocytic tumors (45 cases of papillary cystadenoma lymphomatosum and 4 cases of oncocytoma). Acta Cytol., *9*:355–361, 1965.

Eneroth, C.-M., and Zajicek, J.: Aspiration biopsy of salivary gland tumors: III. Morphologic studies on smears and histologic sections from 368 mixed tumors. Acta Cytol., *10*:440–454, 1966.

Eneroth, C.-M., and Zajicek, J.: Aspiration biopsy of salivary gland tumors. IV. Morphologic studies on smears and histologic sections from 45 cases of adenoid cystic carcinoma. Acta Cytol., *13*:59–63, 1969.

Eusebi, V., Piberi, S., and Usellini, L., et al.: Primary endocrine carcinomas of the salivary gland associated with a lung carcinoid: a possible new association. J. Clin. Pathol., *35*:611–616, 1982.

Foote, F.W., Jr., and Frazell, E.L.: Tumors of the major salivary glands. *In* Atlas of Tumor Pathology, sect. 4, fasc. 11. Washington, D.C., Armed Forces Institute of Pathology, 1963.

Frable, W.J., and Frable, M.A.: Thin needle aspiration biopsy in the diagnosis of head and neck tumors. Laryngoscope, *84*:1069–1074, 1974.

Geisinger, K.R., Reynolds, G.D., Vance, R.P., and McGuirt, W.F.: Adenoid cystic carcinoma arising in a pleomorphic adenoma of the parotid gland: an aspiration cytology and ultrastructural study. Acta Cytol., *29*:522–526, 1985.

Harris, B.R., and Shipkey, F.: Tyrosine-rich crystalloids in neoplasm and tissues of the head and neck. Arch. Pathol. Lab. Med., *110*:709–712, 1986.

Hilborne, L.H., Glasgow, B.J., and Layfield, L.J.: Fine needle aspiration cytology of juvenile hemangioma of the parotid gland. A case report. Diagn. Cytopathol., *3*:152–155, 1987.

Hood, I.C., Qizilbash, A.H., Salama, S.S., and Alexopoulou, I.: Basal-cell adenoma of parotid: difficulty of differentiation from adenoid cystic carcinoma on aspiration biopsy. Acta Cytol., *27*:515–520, 1983.

Humphrey, P.A., Ingram, P., Tucker, A., and Shelburne, J.D.: Crystalloids in salivary gland pleomorphic adenomas. Arch. Pathol. Lab. Med., *113*:390–393, 1989.

Hyman, G.A., and Wolff, M.: Malignant lymphomas of the salivary glands. Review of the literature and report of 33 new cases including four cases associated with the lymphoepithelial lesions. Am. J. Clin. Pathol., *65*:421–438, 1976.

Kline, T.S.: Handbook of Fine Needle Aspiration Biopsy Cytology, 2nd ed. New York, Churchill-Livingstone, 1988.

Kline, T.S., Merriam, J.M., and Shapshay, S.M.: Aspiration biopsy cytology of the salivary gland. Am. J. Clin. Pathol., *76*:263–269, 1981.

Koss, L.G., Spiro, R.H., and Hajdu, S.: Small cell (oat cell) carcinoma of minor salivary gland origin. Cancer, *30*:737–741, 1972.

Koss, L.G., Woyke, S., and Olszewski, W.: Aspiration Biopsy. Cytologic Interpretation and Histologic Bases. New York, Igaku-Shoin, 1984, 2nd Ed., 1992.

Lininger, J.R., Covell, J.L., and Feldman, P.S.: The diagnosis of mucoepidermoid carcinoma of the salivary glands by fine needle aspiration. Acta Cytol., *25*:720, 1981.

Lomax-Smith, J.D., and Azzopardi, J.G.: The hyaline cell: a distinctive feature of "mixed" salivary tumours. Histopathology, *2*:77–92, 1978.

O'Dwyer, P., Farrar, W.B., James, A.G., Finkelmeier, W., and McCabe, D.P.: Needle aspiration biopsy of major salivary gland tumors: its value. Cancer, *57*:554–557, 1986.

Qizilbash, A.H., Sianos, J., Young, J.E.M., and Archibald, S.D.: Fine needle aspiration biopsy cytology of major salivary glands. Acta Cytol., *29*:503–512, 1985.

Schmid, U., Helbron, D., and Lennert, K.: Primary malignant lymphomas localized in salivary glands. Histopathology, *6*:673–687, 1982.

Schultenover, S.J., McDonald, E.C., and Ramzy, I.: Hyaline-cell pleomorphic adenoma. Diagnosis by fine needle aspiration biopsy. Acta Cytol., *28*:593–597, 1984.

Spiro, R.H., Koss, L.G., Hajdu, S.J., and Strong, E.W.: Tumors of minor salivary gland origin. A clinicopathologic study of 492 cases. Cancer, *31*:117–129, 1973.

Whitlach, S.: Psammoma bodies in fine-needle aspiration biopsies of acinic cell tumor. Diagn. Cytopathol., *2*:268–269, 1986.

Young, J.E., Archibald, S.D., and Shier, K.J.: Needle aspiration cytologic biopsy in head and neck masses. Am. J. Surg., *142*:484–489, 1981.

Zajicek, J., Eneroth, C.-M., and Jakobsson, P.: Aspiration biopsy of salivary gland tumors. VI. Morphologic studies on smears and histologic sections from mucoepidermoid carcinoma. Acta Cytol., *20*:35–41, 1976.

Zajicek, J., and Eneroth, C.-M.: Cytological diagnosis of salivary gland carcinomas from aspiration biopsy smears. Acta Otolaryngol. (Stockh.), *263*:183–185, 1970.

Lymph Nodes and Neck Organs (Other than Thyroid Gland)

Agnarsson, B.A., and Kadin, M.E.: Ki-1 positive large cell lymphoma. A morphologic and immunologic study of 19 cases. Am. J. Surg. Pathol., *12*:264–274, 1988.

Bailey, T.M., Akhtar, M., and Ali, M.A.: Fine needle aspiration biopsy in the diagnosis of tuberculosis. Acta Cytol., *29*:732–736, 1985.

Betsill, W.L., and Hajdu, S.I.: Percutaneous aspiration biopsy of lymph nodes. Am. J. Clin. Pathol., *73*:471–479, 1980.

Bottles, K., Cohen, M.B., Brodie, H., Jaffrey, R.B., Nyberg, D.A., and Abrams, D.I.: Fine needle aspiration cytology of lymphadenopathy in homosexual males. Diagn. Cytopathol., *2*:31–35, 1986.

Cardozo, P.L.: The cytologic diagnosis of lymph node punctures. Acta Cytol., *8*:194–204, 1964.

Chan, M.K.M., McGuire, L.J., and Lee, J.C.K.: Fine needle aspiration cytodiagnosis of nasopharyngeal carcinoma in cervical lymph nodes. A study of 40 cases. Acta Cytol., *33*:344–350, 1989.

Chott, A., Augustin, I., Wrba, F., Hanak, H., Öhlinger, W., and Radaszkiewicz, T.: Peripheral T-cell lymphoma. A clinicopathologic study of 75 cases. Hum. Pathol., *21*:1117–1125, 1990.

Christ, M.L., and Feltes-Kennedy, M.: Fine needle aspiration cytology of toxoplasmic lymphadenitis. Acta Cytol., *26*:425–428, 1982.

Engzell, U., Jakobsson, P.A., Sigurdson, A., and Zajicek, J.: Aspiration biopsy of metastatic carcinoma in lymph nodes of the neck. Acta Otolaryngol. (Stockh.), *72*:138–147, 1971.

Engzell, U., and Zajicek, J.: Aspiration biopsy of tumors of the neck. I. Aspiration biopsy and cytologic findings in 100 cases of congenital cysts. Acta Cytol., *14*:51–57, 1970.

Frable, M.A., and Frable, W.J.: Fine needle aspiration biopsy revisited. Laryngoscope, *92*:1414–1418, 1982.

Frable, M.A., and Frable, W.J.: Fine needle aspiration biopsy in the diagnosis of sarcoid of the head and neck. Acta Cytol., *28*:175–177, 1984.

Gertner, R., Podoshin, L., and Fradis, M.: Accuracy of fine needle aspiration biopsy in neck masses. Laryngoscope, *94*:1370–1371, 1984.

Gothlin, J.-H., Rupp, N., Rothenberger, K.H., and MacIntosh, P.K.: Percutaneous biopsy of retroperitoneal lymph nodes. A multicentric study. Eur. J. Radiol., *1*:46–50, 1981.

Hood, I.C., Qizilbash, A.H., Young, J.E.M., and Archibald, S.D.: Fine needle aspiration biopsy cytology of paragangliomas. Cytologic light microscopic and ultrastructural studies of three cases. Acta Cytol., *27*:651–657, 1983.

Joachim, H.L.: Lymph Node Biopsy. Philadelphia, J.B. Lippincott, 1982.

Kardos, T.F., Vinson, J.H., Behm, F.G., Frable, W.J., and O'Dowd, G.J.: Hodgkin's disease: diagnosis by fine needle aspiration biopsy. Analysis of cytologic criteria from a selected series. Am. J. Clin. Pathol., *86*:286–291, 1986.

Katz, R.L., Gritsman, A., Cabanillas, F., Fanning, C.V., Dekmezian, R., Ordonez, N.G., Barlogie, B., and Butler, J.J.: Fine-needle aspiration cytology of peripheral T-cell lymphoma. A cytologic, immunologic and cytometric study. Am. J. Clin. Pathol., *91*:120–131, 1989.

Kim, H., Dorfman, R.F., and Rappaport, H.: Signet ring cell lymphoma. Am. J. Surg. Pathol., *2*:119–132, 1978.

Kline, T.S., Kannan, V., and Kline, I.K.: Lymphadenopathy and aspiration biopsy cytology. Review of 376 superficial nodes. Cancer, *54*:1076–1081, 1984.

Kline, T.S., and Neal, H.S.: Needle aspiration biopsy: diagnosis of subcutaneous nodules and lymph nodes. JAMA, *235*:2848–2850, 1976.

Koo, C.H., Rappaport, H., Sheibari, K., Gerassimos, A.P., Nathwani, B.N., and Winberg, C.D.: Imprint cytology of non-Hodgkin's lymphomas. Based on a study of 212 immunologically characterized cases. Hum. Pathol., *20*(suppl. 1):1–137, 1989.

Koss, L.G., Woyke, S., and Olszewski, W.: Aspiration Biopsy. Cytologic Interpretation and Histologic Bases. New York, Igaku-Shoin, 1984; 2nd ed, 1992.

Layfield, L.J., Glasgow, B.J., and DuPuis, M.H.: Fine-needle aspiration of lymphadenopathy of suspected infectious etiology. Arch. Pathol. Lab. Med., *109*:810–812, 1985.

Le Compte, P.M.: Tumors of the carotid body. Am. J. Pathol., *24*:305–321, 1948.

Lennert, K.: Classification on malignant lymphomas (European concept). *In* Ruttimann, A. (ed.): Progress in Lymphology. pp. 103–109. Stuttgart, George Thieme, 1967.

Lennert, K.: Lymphknoten. Bandteil A: Zytologie und Lymphadenitis. *In* Handbuch der Speziellen Pathologischen Anatomie und Histologie. Berlin, Springer-Verlag, 1961.

Lennert, K.: Malignant Lymphomas Other Than Hodgkin's Disease: Histology, Cytology, Ultrastructure, Immunology. New York, Springer-Verlag, 1978.

Levitt, S., Cheng, L., DuPuis, M.H., and Layfield, L.J.: Fine needle aspiration diagnosis of malignant lymphoma with

confirmation by immunoperoxidase staining. Acta Cytol., *29*:895–902, 1985.

Loseke, L., and Craver, L.F.: The diagnosis of Hodgkin's disease by aspiration biopsy. Blood, *1*:76–82, 1946.

Lubinski, J., Chosia, M., and Huebner, K.: Molecular genetic analysis in the diagnosis of lymphoma in fine needle aspiration biopsies: I. Lymphoma versus benign lymphoproliferation disorders. Anal. Quant. Cytol. Histol., *10*:391–398, 1988.

Lukes, R.J.: A review of the American concept of malignant lymphoma. The evolution of a modern classification. *In* Ruttimann, A. (ed.): Progress in Lymphology. pp. 109–119. Stuttgart, Georg Thieme, 1967.

Lukes, R.J., and Butler, J.J.: The pathology and nomenclature of Hodgkin's disease. Cancer Res., *26*:1063–1081, 1966.

National Cancer Institute sponsored study of classifications of non-Hodgkin's lymphomas: Summary and description of working formulation for clinical usage. The non-Hodgkin's lymphoma pathologic classification project. Cancer *49*: 2112–2135, 1982.

O'Dowd, G.J., Frable, W.J., and Behm, F.G.: Fine needle aspiration cytology of benign lymph node hyperplasias: diagnostic significance of lymphohistiocytic aggregates. Acta Cytol., *29*:554–558, 1985.

Orell, S.R., and Skinner, J.M.: The typing of non-Hodgkin's lymphomas using fine needle aspiration cytology. Pathology, *14*:389–394, 1982.

Pavlovsky, A.: La punction ganglionar: su contribucion al diagnostico clinico-quirurgico de las afecciones ganglionares. Buenos Aires, Aniceto Lopez, 1934.

Pitts, W.C., and Weiss, L.M.: Fine needle aspiration biopsy of lymph nodes. Pathol. Annu., *23*(part 2):329–360, 1988.

Pontifex, A.H., and Klimo, P.: Application of aspiration biopsy cytology to lymphomas. Cancer, *53*:553–556, 1984.

Qizilbash, A.H., Elavathil, L.J., Chen, V., Young, J.E.M., and Archibald, S.D.: Aspiration biopsy cytology of lymph nodes in malignant lymphoma. Diagn. Cytopathol., *1*:18–22, 1985.

Rajwanshi, A., Bhambhani, S., and Das, D.K.: Fine needle aspiration cytology diagnosis of tuberculosis. Diagn. Cytopathol., *3*:13–16, 1987.

Ramzy, I., Rone, R., Schultenover, S.J., and Buhaug, J.: Lymph node aspiration biopsy: diagnostic reliability and limitations—an analysis of 350 cases. Diagn. Cytopathol., *1*:39–45, 1985.

Rappaport, H.: Tumors of the hematopoietic system. *In* Atlas of Tumor Pathology, sect. 3, fasc. 8. Washington, D.C., Armed Forces Institute of Pathology, 1966.

Rosai, J., and Dorfman, R.F.: Sinus histiocytosis with massive lymphadenopathy. Arch. Pathol. Lab. Med., *87*:63–70, 1969.

Silverman, J.F.: Fine needle aspiration cytology of cat scratch disease. Acta Cytol., *29*:542–547, 1985.

Solares, J., and Lacruz, C.: Fine needle aspiration cytology diagnosis of an extracranial meningioma presenting as a cervical mass. Acta Cytol., *31*:502–504, 1987.

Sneige, N., Dekmezian, R.H., Katz, R.L., Fanning, T.V., Lukeman, J.L., Ordořez, N.F., and Cabanillas, F.F.: Morphologic and immunocytochemical evaluation of 220 fine needle aspirates of malignant lymphoma and lymphoid hyperplasia. Acta Cytol., *34*:311–322, 1990.

Spriggs, A.I., and Vanhegan, R.I.: Cytologic diagnosis of lymphoma in serous effusions. J. Clin. Pathol., *34*:1311–1325, 1981.

Stahel, R.: Diagnostische Drusenpunktion. Leipzig, Georg Thieme, 1939.

Strunge, T.: La Ponction des Ganglions Lymphatiques: Une

Description Cytologique Controlee par la Clinique. Copenhagen, Einar Munksgaard, 1944.

Tani, E., Christensson, B., Porwit, A., and Skoog, L.: Immunocytochemical analysis and cytomorphologic diagnosis of fine needle aspirates of lymphoproliferative disease. Acta Cytol., *32*:209–215, 1988.

Tani, E., Löwhagen, T., Nasiell, K., Ost, A., and Skoog, L.: Fine needle aspiration cytology and immunocytochemistry of large cell lymphomas expressing the Ki-1 antigen. Acta Cytol., *33*:359–362, 1989.

Zajdela, A., Ennuyer, A., Bataini, P., and Poncet, P.: Valeur du diagnostic cytologique des adenopathies par ponction aspiration; confrontation cyto-histologique de 1,756 cas. Bull. Cancer (Paris), *63*:327–340, 1976.

Zajdela, A., and Rousseau, J.: Diagnostic cytologique des metastases ganglionnaires. Sa valeur, son interet. Arch. Pathol., *11*:18–23, 1963.

Zajicek, J.: Aspiration Biopsy Cytology. Part I: Cytology of Supradiaphragmatic Organs. Monographs in Clinical Cytology. Basel, S. Karger, 1974.

Zajicek, J., Engzell, U., and Franzen, S.: Aspiration biopsy of lymph nodes in diagnosis and research. *In* Ruttimann, A. (ed.): Progress in Lymphology. George Thieme, Stuttgart, 1967.

Thyroid

Allevato, P.A., Kini, S.R., Rebuck, J.W., Miller, J.M., and Hamburger, J.I.: Signet ring cell lymphoma of the thyroid: a case report. Hum. Pathol., *16*:1066–1068, 1985.

Asp. A.A., Georgitis, W., Waldron, E.J., Sims, J.E., and Kidd, G.S.: Fine needle aspiration of the thyroid. Use in an average health care facility. Am. J. Med., *83*:489–493, 1987.

Baskin, H.J., and Guarda, L.A.: Influence of needle biopsy on management of thyroid nodules: reasons to expand its use. South. Med. J., *80*:702–705, 1987.

Berry, B., MacFarlane, J., and Chan, N.: Osteoclastomalike anaplastic carcinoma of the thyroid: diagnosed by fine needle aspiration cytology. Acta Cytol., *34*:248–250, 1990.

Bodo, M., Dobrossy, L., Sinkovics, J., Tajan, G., and Daubner, K.: Fine needle biopsy of the thyroid gland. J. Surg. Oncol., *12*:289–297, 1979.

Catz, B., Perzik, S.L., Friedman, N.B., and Sacks, H.: Association of lymphocytic thyroiditis with other lesions of the thyroid. Surg. Gynecol., *136*:47–48, 1973.

Chacho, M.S., Greenebaum, E., Moussouris, H.F., Schreiber, K., and Koss, L.G.: Value of aspiration cytology of thyroid in metastatic disease. Acta Cytol., *31*:705–712, 1987.

Chem, K.T., and Rosai, J.: Follicular variant of thyroid papillary carcinoma: a clinicopathologic study of six cases. Am. J. Surg. Pathol., *1*:123–130, 1977.

Chu, E.W., Hanson, T.A., Goldman, J.M., and Robbins, J.: Study of cells in fine needle aspirations of thyroid gland. Acta Cytol., *23*:309–314, 1979.

Cohen, J.P., and Cho, H.T.: The role of needle aspiration biopsy in the selection of patients for thyroidectomy. Laryngoscope, *98*:35–39, 1988.

Deligeorgi-Politi, H.: Nuclear crease as a cytodiagnostic feature of papillary thyroid carcinoma in fine-needle aspiration biopsies. Diagn. Cytopathol., *3*:307–310, 1987.

Droese, M.: Cytological Aspiration Biopsy of the Thyroid Gland. Stuttgart, F.K. Schattauer Verlag, 1980.

Dugan, J.M., Atkinson, B.F., Avitabile, A., Schimmel, M., and Livolsi, V.A.: Psammoma bodies in fine needle aspirate of the thyroid in lymphocytic thyroiditis. Acta Cytol., *31*:330–334, 1987.

Dwarakanathan, A.A., Ryan, W.G., Staren, E.D., Martirano, M.S., and Economou, S.G.: Fine needle aspiration biopsy of the thyroid. Diagnostic accuracy when performing a moderate number of such procedures. Arch. Intern. Med., *149*:2007–2009, 1989.

Einhorn, J., and Franzen, S.: Thin-needle biopsy in the diagnosis of thyroid disease. Acta Radiol., *58*:321–336, 1962.

Gagneten, C.B., Roccatagliata, G., Lowenstein, A., Soto, F., and Soto, R.: The role of fine needle aspiration biopsy cytology in the evaluation of the clinically solitary thyroid nodule. Acta Cytol., *31*:595–598, 1987.

Gardiner, G.W., de Souza, F.M., Carydis, B., and Seeman, C.: Fine needle aspiration biopsy of the thyroid gland: results of a five year experience and a discussion of its clinical limitations. J. Otolaryngol., *15*:161–165, 1986.

Glant, M.D., Berger, E.K., and Davey, D.D.: Intranuclear cytoplasmic inclusions in aspirates of follicular neoplasms of the thyroid. A report of two cases. Acta Cytol., *28*:576–580, 1984.

Goellner, J.R., and Johnson, D.A.: Cytology of cystic papillary carcinoma of the thyroid. Acta Cytol., *26*:797–799, 1982.

Hall, T.L., Layfiled, L.J., Philippe, A., and Rosenthal, D.L.: Sources of diagnostic error in fine needle aspiration of the thyroid. Cancer, *63*:718–725, 1989.

Hamburger, J.I., Husain, M., Nishiyama, R., Nunez, C., and Solomon, D.: Increasing the accuracy of fine-needle biopsy of thyroid nodules. Arch. Pathol. Lab. Med., *113*:1035–1041, 1989.

Hamburger, J.I., and Husain, M.: Semiquantitative criteria for fine needle biopsy diagnosis: reduced false-negative diagnosis. Diagn. Cytopathol., *4*:14–17, 1988.

Hawkins, F., Bellido, D., Bernal, C., Rigopoulou, D., Valdepenas, M.P.R., Lazaro, E., Perez-Barrios, A., and DeAgustin, P.: Fine needle aspiration biopsy in diagnosis of thyroid cancer and thyroid disease. Cancer, *59*:1206–1209, 1987.

Hugh, J.C., Duggan, M.A., and Chang-Poon, V.: The fine-needle aspiration appearance of the follicular variant of thyroid papillary carcinoma: a report of three cases. Diagn. Cytopathol., *4*:196–201, 1988.

Jayaram, G.: Fine needle aspiration cytologic study of the solitary thyroid nodule: profile of 308 cases with histologic correlation. Acta Cytol., *29*:967–973, 1985.

Keiser, H.R., Beaven, M.A., Doppmann, J., Wells, S., and Buja, L.M.: Sipple's syndrome: medullary thyroid carcinoma, pheochromocytoma and parathyroid disease studies in a large family. Ann. Intern. Med., *78*:561–579, 1973.

Keller, M.P., Crabbe, M.M., and Norwood, S.H.: Accuracy and significance of fine needle aspiration and frozen section in determining the extent of thyroid resection. Surgery, *101*:632–635, 1987.

Kini, S.R., Miller, J.M., and Hamburger, J.I.: Cytopathology of papillary carcinoma of the thyroid by fine needle aspiration. Acta Cytol., *24*:511–521, 1980.

Kini, S.R., Miller, J.M. and Hamburger, J.I.: Problems in the cytologic diagnosis of the "cold" thyroid nodule in patients with lymphocytic thyroiditis. Acta Cytol., *25*:506–512, 1981.

Kini, S.R., Miller, J.M., and Hamburger, J.I.: Cytopathology of Hurthle cell lesions of the thyroid gland by fine needle aspiration. Acta Cytol., *25*:647–652, 1981.

Kini, S.R., Miller, J.M., Hamburger, J.I., and Smith, M.J.: Cytopathologic features of medullary carcinoma of the thyroid. Arch. Pathol. Lab. Med., *108*:156–159, 1984.

Kini, S.R., Miller, J.M., Hamburger, J.I., and Smith-Purslow,

M.J.: Cytopathology of follicular lesions of the thyroid gland. Diagn. Cytopathol., *1*:123–132, 1985.

Koss, L.G., Woyke, S., and Olszewski, W.: Aspiration Biopsy. Cytologic Interpretation and Histologic Bases. New York, Igaku-Shoin, 1984, 2nd Ed. 1992.

Lipton, R.F., and Abel, M.S.: Aspiration biopsy of the thyroid in the evaluation of thyroid dysfunction. Am. J. Med. Sci., *208*:736–742, 1944.

Ljungberg, O.: Cytologic diagnosis of medullary carcinoma of the thyroid gland with special regard to the demonstration of amyloid in smears of fine needle aspirates. Acta Cytol., *16*:253–255, 1972.

Löwhagen, T., and Sprenger, E.: Cytologic presentation of thyroid tumors in aspiration biopsy smear. A review of 60 cases. Acta Cytol., *18*:192–197, 1974.

Löwhagen, T., and Willems, J.-S.: Aspiration biopsy cytology in diseases of the thyroid. *In* Koss, L.G., and Coleman, D.V. (eds): Advances in Clinical Cytology. vol. 1. pp. 201–227, London, Butterworths, 1981.

Luck, J.B., Mumaw, V.R., and Frable, W.J.: Fine needle aspiration biopsy of the thyroid: differential diagnosis by videoplan image analysis. Acta Cytol., *26*:793–796, 1982.

Matsuda, M., Sone, H., Koyama, H., and Ishiguro, S.: Fine-needle aspiration cytology of malignant lymphoma of the thyroid. Diagn. Cytopathol., *3*:244–249, 1987.

McCabe, D.P., Farrar, W.B., Petkov, T.M., Finkelmeier, W., O'Dwyer, P., and James, A.: Clinical and pathologic correlations in disease metastatic to the thyroid gland. Am. J. Surg., *150*:519–523, 1985.

Miller, J.M., Kini, S.R., and Hamburger, J.T.: Needle Biopsy of the Thyroid. New York, Praeger Publishers, 1983.

Myren, J., and Sivertssen, E.: Thin-needle biopsy of the thyroid gland in the diagnosis of thyrotoxicosis. Acta Endocrinol., *39*:431–438, 1962.

Nilsson, L.R., and Persson, P.S.: Cytological aspiration biopsy in adolescent goiter. Acta Paediatr., *53*:333–338, 1964.

Pedio, G., Hidinger, C., and Zobeli, L.: Ground-glass nuclei in papillary carcinoma. Acta Cytol., *25*:728, 1981.

Persson, P.S.: Cytodiagnosis of thyroiditis. Acta Med. Scand. [Suppl.], *483*:8–100, 1968.

Ravinsky, E., and Safneck, J.R.: Differentiation of Hashimoto's thyroiditis from thyroid neoplasms in fine needle aspirates. Acta Cytol., *32*:854–861, 1988.

Rudowski, W.: Critical evaluation of aspiration biopsy in the diagnosis of tumors of the thyroid. Am. J. Surg., *95*:40–44, 1958.

Schaffer, R., Miller, H.A., Pfeifer, U., and Ormanns, W.: Cytological findings in medullary carcinoma of the thyroid. Pathol. Res. Pract., *178*:461–466, 1984.

Silverman, J.F., West, R.L., Larkin, E.W., Park, K., Finley, J.L., Swanson, M.S., and Fore, W.W.: The role of fine-needle aspiration biopsy in the rapid diagnosis and management of thyroid neoplasm. Cancer, *57*:1164–1170, 1986.

Söderström, N.: Puncture of goiters for aspiration biopsy. A preliminary report. Acta Med. Scand., *144*:235–244, 1952.

Söderström, N., and Biorklund, A.: Intranuclear cytoplasmic inclusions in some types of thyroid cancer. Acta Cytol., *17*:191–197, 1973.

Sodhani, P., and Nayar, M.: Microfilariae in a thyroid aspirate smear: an incidental findings [Letter]. Acta Cytol., *33*:942–943, 1989.

Sutton, R.T., Reading, C.C., Charboneau, J.W., James E.M., Grant, C.S., and Hay, I.D.: US-guided biopsy of neck masses in postoperative management of patients with thyroid cancer. Radiology, *168*:769–772, 1988.

Tani, E. and Skoog, L.: Fine needle aspiration cytology and immunocytochemistry in the diagnosis of lymphoid lesions of the thyroid gland. Acta Cytol., *33*:48–52, 1989.

Wang, C.A.: Management of thyroid disease based on needle biopsy pathology. Clin. Endocrinol. Metab., *10*:293–298, 1981.

Williams, J.S., Lowhagen, T., and Palombini, L.: The cytology of a giant cell osteoclastoma-like malignant thyroid neoplasm. A case report. Acta Cytol., *23*:214–216, 1979.

Zirkin, H.J., Hertzanu, Y., and Gal, R.: Fine needle aspiration cytology and immunocytochemistry in a case of intrathoracic thyroid goiter. Acta Cytol., *31*:694–698, 1987.

Breast

Abele, J., and Miller, T.: Cytology of well-differentiated and poorly differentiated hemangiosarcoma in fine needle aspirates. Acta Cytol., *26*:341–348, 1982.

Azavedo, E., Svane, G., and Auer, G.: Stereotactic fine-needle biopsy in 2594 mammographically detected non-palpable lesions. Lancet, *1*:1033–1036, 1989.

Bacus, S.S., Bacus, J.W., Slamon, D.J., and Press, M.F.: *HER-2/Neu* oncogene expression and DNA ploidy analysis in breast cancer. Arch. Pathol. Lab. Med., *114*:164–169, 1990.

Bacus, S., Flowers, J.L., Press, M.F., Bacos, J.W., and McCarty, K.S.: The evaluation of estrogen receptor in primary breast carcinoma by computer assisted image analysis. Am. J. Clin. Pathol., *90*:1988.

Bacus, S.S., Goldschmidt, R., Chin, D., Moran, G., Wienberg, D., and Bacus, J.W.: Biologic grading of breast cancer using antibodies to proliferating cells and other markers. Am. J. Pathol., *135*:783–792, 1989.

Berg, J.W., and Robbins, G.F.: A late look at the safety of aspiration biopsy. Cancer, *15*:826–827, 1962.

Boccato, P., Briani, G., d'Atri, C., Pasini, L., Blandamura, S., and Bizzaro, N.: Spindle cell and cartilaginous metaplasia in a breast carcinoma with osteoclastlike stroma cells; a difficult fine needle aspiration diagnosis. Act Cytol., *32*:75–78, 1988.

Bolmgren, J., Jacobson, B., and Norderstrom, B.: Stereotaxic instrument for needle biopsy of the mamma. Am. J. Roentgenol. Radium. Ther. Nucl. Med., *129*:121–125, 1977.

Bondenson, L., and Lindholm, K.: Aspiration cytology of tubular breast carcinoma. Acta Cytol., *34*:15–20, 1990.

Bonneau, H., Sommer, D., and de The, G.: Etude critique de la cytologie tumorale par ponction a l'aiguille fine; à propos de 905 observations. Presse Méd., *68*:909–912, 1960.

Bottles, K., Chan, J.S., Holly, E.A., Chiu, S.-H., and Miller, T.R.: Cytologic criteria for fibroadenoma. Am. J. Clin. Pathol., *89*:707–713, 1988.

Bottles, K., and Taylor, R.N.: Diagnosis of breast masses in pregnant and lactating women by aspiration cytology. Obstet. Gynecol., *66*:76S–78S, 1985.

Clark, G.M., Dressler, L.G., and Owens, M.A.: Prediction of relapse or survival in patients with node-negative breast cancer by flow cytometry. N. Engl. J. Med. *320*:627–633, 1989.

Cornillot, M., and Verhaeghe, M.: Données cytologiques dans les ponctions de tumeurs du sein. Pathol. Biol., *7*:793–802, 1959.

Cornillot, M., Verhaeghe, M., Cappelaere, P., and Clay, A.: Place de la cytologie par ponction dans le diagnostic des tumeurs du sein. Lille Med., *16*:1027, 1971.

d'Amore, E.S.G., Maisto, L., Gatteschi, M.B., Toma, S., and Canavese, G.: Secretory carcinoma of the breast; report of a case with fine needle aspiration biopsy. Acta Cytol., *30*:309–312, 1986.

Doria, M.I., Tani, E.M., and Skoog, L.: Sarcoidosis presenting initially as a breast mass: detection by fine needle aspiration biopsy. Acta Cytol., *31*:378–379, 1987.

Dowlatshahi, K.: Stereotaxic fine needle aspiration cytology of clinically occult malignant and premalignant lesions. Acta Cytol., *32*:193–201, 1988.

Duggan, M.A., Young, G.K., and Hwang, W.S.: Fine-needle aspiration of an apocrine breast carcinoma with multivacuolated, lipid-rich, giant cells. Diagn. Cytopathol., *4*:62–66, 1988.

Duquid, H.L., Wood, R.A., Irving, A.D., Preece, P.E., and Cuschieri, A.: Needle aspiration of the breast with immediate reporting of material. Br. Med. J., *2*:185–187, 1979.

Eisenberg, A.J., Hajdu, S.I., Wilhelmus, J., Melamed, M.R., and Kinne, D.: Preoperative aspiration cytology of breast tumors. Acta Cytol., *30*:135–146, 1986.

Fallenious, A.G., Auer, G.U., and Carstensen, J.M.: Prognostic significance of DNA measurements in 409 consecutive breast cancer patients. Cancer, *62*:331–341, 1988.

Finley, J.L., Silverman, J.F., and Lannim, D.R.: Fine needle aspiration cytology of lactating adenoma. Acta Cytol., *31*:666, 1987.

Fornage, B.D., Faroux, M.J., and Simatos, A.: Breast masses: US-guided fine-needle aspiration biopsy. Radiology, *162*:409–414, 1987.

Frable, W.J.: Needle aspiration biopsy: past, present and future. Hum. Pathol., *20*:504–517, 1989.

Franzén, S., and Zajicek, J.: Aspiration biopsy in diagnosis of palpable lesions of the breast. Acta Radiol., *7*:241–262, 1968.

Gardecki, T.J., Hogbin, B.M., Melcher, D.H., and Smith, R.S.: Aspiration cytology in the preoperative management of breast cancer. Lancet, *2*:790–792, 1980.

Gerdes, J., Lelle, R.J., Pickartz, H., Heidenreich, W., Schwarting, R., Kurtsiefer, L., Stauch, G., and Stein, H.: Growth fractions in breast cancers determined in site with monoclonal antibody Ki-67. J. Clin. Pathol., *39*:977–980, 1986.

Gibson, A., and Smith, G.: Aspiration biopsy of breast tumours. Br. J. Surg., *45*:236–239, 1957.

Glassman, J.A.: Aspiration biopsy for detection of carcinoma of the breast: a critique. J. Int. Coll. Surg., *36*:195–202, 1961.

Grenko, R.T., Lee, K.P., and Lee, K.R.: Fine needle aspiration cytology of lactating adenoma of the breast. A comparative light microscopic and morphometric study. Acta Cytol., *34*:21–26, 1990.

Howell, L.P., and Lindfors, K.K.: Image-directed NAB for occult mammary lesions. *In* Kline T.S., and Kline, I.K. (eds.): Guides to Clinical Aspiration Biopsy. Breast, pp. 197–214. New York, Igaku-Shoin, 1989.

Hsui, J.-G., Hawkins, A.G., d'Amato, N.A., and Mullen, J.T.: A case of pure primary squamous carcinoma of the breast diagnosed by fine needle aspiration biopsy. Acta Cytol., *29*:650–651, 1985.

Jayaram, G.: Cytomorphology of tuberculous mastitis: a report of nine cases with fine needle aspiration biopsy. Acta Cytol., *29*:974–978, 1985.

Kline, T.S., and Kannan, V.: Papillary carcinoma of the breast; a cytomorphologic analysis. Arch. Pathol. Lab. Med., *110*:189–191, 1986.

Kline, T.S., and Kline, J.K.: Guides to Clinical Aspiration Biopsy. Breast. New York, Igaku-Shoin, 1989.

Koss, L.G.: Precancerous lesions of the breast: theoretical and practical considerations. *In* Hollmann, K.H., and Verley, J.M. (eds): New Frontiers of Mammary Pathology. pp. 105–125. New York, Plenum Press, 1983.

Koss, L.G., Woyke, S., and Olszewski, W.: Aspiration Biopsy. Cytologic Interpretation and Histologic Bases. New York, Igaku-Shoin, 1984, 2nd Ed., 1992.

Kreuzer, G., and Boquoi, E.: Aspiration biopsy cytology, mam-

mography and clinical exploration: a modern set up in diagnosis of tumors of the breast. Acta Cytol., *20*:319–323, 1976.

Kreuzer, G., and Zajicek, J.: Cytologic diagnosis of mammary tumors from aspiration biopsy smears. III. Studies on 200 carcinomas with false negative or doubtful cytologic reports. Acta Cytol., *16*:249–252, 1972.

Layfield, L.J., Glasgow, B.J., and Cramer, H.: Fine-needle aspiration in the management of breast masses. Pathol. Annu., 24 (part 2):23–62, 1989.

Linsk, J., Kreuzer, G., and Zajicek, J.: Cytologic diagnosis of mammary tumors from aspiration biopsy smears. II. Studies on 210 fibroadenomas and 210 cases of benign dysplasia. Acta Cytol., *16*:130–138, 1972.

Löwhagen, T., and Rubio, C.A.: The cytology of the granular cell myoblastoma of the breast. Report of a case. Acta Cytol., *2*:314–315, 1970.

Lozowski, M.S., Mishriki, Y., Chao, S., Grimson, R., Pai, P., Harris, M.A., and Lundy, J.: Estrogen receptor determination in fine needle aspirates of the breast. Acta Cytol., *31*:557–562, 1987.

Mahsood, S., Frykberg, E.R., and McLella, G.: Potential value of mammographically guided fine-needle aspiration biopsy in assessment of non-palpable lesions. Am. J. Clin. Pathol., *89*:437, 1988.

Marchetti, E., Bagni, A., Querzoli, P., Durante, E., Marzola, A., Fabris, G., and Nenci, I.: Immunocytochemical detection of estrogen receptors by staining with monoclonal antibodies on cytologic specimens of human breast cancer. Acta Cytol., *32*:829–834, 1988.

Mayer, J.S., and Coplin, M.D.: Thymidine labelling index, flow cytometric S-phase measurements, and DNA index in human tumors. Am. J. Clin. Pathol., *89*:586–599, 1988.

McCarty, K.D., Jr., Miller, L.S., Cox, E.B., Konrath, J., and McCarty, K.S., Sr.: Estrogen receptor analyses: correlation of biochemical and immunohistological methods using monoclonal antireceptor antibodies. Arch. Pathol. Lab. Med., *109*:716–721, 1985.

Murad, T.M., and Scarpelli, D.G.: The ultrastructure of medullary and scirrhous mammary duct carcinoma. Am. J. Pathol., *50*:355–360, 1967.

Naran, S., Simpson, J., and Gupta, R.K.: Cytologic diagnosis of papillary carcinoma of the breast in needle aspiration. Diagn. Cytopathol., *4*:33–37, 1988.

Nicholson, S., Sainsbury, J., and Halcrow, P., et al: Expression of epidermal growth factor receptors associated with lack of response to endocrine therapy in recurrent breast cancer. Lancet, *1*:182–184, 1989.

Nordenstrom, B.: New instruments for biopsy. Radiology, *117*:474–475, 1975.

Nordenskjold, B., Löwhagen, T., Westerberg, H., and Zajicek, J.: ^{3}H-Thymidine incorporation into mammary carcinoma cells obtained by needle aspiration before and during endocrine therapy. Acta Cytol., *20*:137–143, 1976.

Nordenstrom, B., and Zajicek, J.: Stereotaxic breast needle biopsy and preoperative indication of non-palpable mammary lesions detected by mammography. Acta Cytol., *21*:350–351, 1977.

Oertel, Y.C.: Fine Needle Aspiration of the Breast. Stoneham, Mass., Butterworth, 1987.

Paik, S., Hazan, H., Fisher, E.R., Sass, R.E., Fisher, B., Redmond, C., Schlessinger, J., Lippman, M.E., and King, C.R.: Pathologic findings from the National Surgical Adjuvant Breast and Bowel Project: prognostic significance of *erb*B-2 protein overexpression in primary breast cancer. Am. J. Clin. Oncol., *8*:103–112, 1990.

Palombini, L., Fulciniti, F., Vetrani, A., De Rosa, G., Di Benedetto, G., Zeppa, P., and Froncone, G.: Fine-needle aspiration biopsies of breast masses. A critical analysis of 1956 cases in 8 years (1976–1984). Cancer, *61*:2273–2277, 1988.

Perrot-Applanant, M.G., T., Lorenze, F., Jolivet, A., Hai, V., Pallud, C., Spyratos, F., and Milgrom, F.: Immunocytochemical study with monoclonal antibodies to progesterone receptor in human breast tumors. Cancer Res., *47*:2652–2661, 1987.

Pettinato, G., de Chiara, A., Insabato, L., and De Renzo, A.: Fine needle aspiration biopsy of a granulocytic sarcoma (chloroma) of the breast. Acta Cytol., *32*:67–73, 1988.

Rajcic, V.: Cytologic studies of aspiration biopsy of the breast. Critical review of 2890 consecutive biopsies. Minerva Ginecol., *23*:417–419, 1971.

Robbins, G.F., Brothers, J.H. III, Eberhart, W.F., and Quan, S.: Is aspiration biopsy of breast cancer dangerous to the patient? Cancer, *7*:774–778, 1954.

Rosemond, G.P.: Differentiation between the cystic and solid breast mass by needle aspiration. Surg. Clin. North Am., *43*:1433–1437, 1963.

Rosemond, G.P., Burnett, W.E., Caswell, H.T., and McAleer, D.J.: Aspiration of breast cysts as a diagnostic and therapeutic measure. Arch. Surg., *71*:223–229, 1955.

Rosen, P., Hajdu, S.I., Robbins, G., and Foote, F.W.: Diagnosis of carcinoma of the breast by aspiration biopsy. Surg. Gynecol. Obstet., *134*:837–838, 1972.

Rupp, M., Hafiz, M.A., Khalluf, E., and Sutula, M.: Fine needle aspiration in stromal sarcoma of the breast; light and electron microscopic findings with histologic correlation. Acta Cytol., *32*:72–74, 1988.

Sainsbury, J.R.C., Needam, G.K., Malcolm, A., Farndon, J.R., and Harris, A.L.: Epidermal growth factor receptor status as a predictor of early recurrence of and death from breast cancer. Lancet, *11*:1398–1402, 1987.

Salhany, K.E., and Page, D.L.: Fine-needle aspiration of mammary lobular carcinoma in situ and atypical lobulary hyperplasia. Am. J. Clin. Pathol., *92*:22–26, 1989.

Salter, D.R., and Bassett, A.A.: Role of needle aspiration in reducing the number of unnecessary breast biopsies. Can. J. Surg., *24*:311–313, 1981.

Savino, A., and Koss, L.G.: Evaluation of sex chromatin as a prognostic factor in carcinoma of the breast. A preliminary report. Acta Cytol., *15*:372–374, 1971.

Scarff, R.W., and Torloni, H.: Histological Typing of Breast Tumors. Geneva, World Health Organization, 1968.

Sheikh, F.A., Tinkoff, G.H., Kline, T.S., and Neal, H.S.: Final diagnosis by fine-needle aspiration biopsy for definitive operation in breast cancer. Am. J. Surg., *154*:470–475, 1987.

Shiller-Volkova, N.N., and Agamova, K.A.: Cytological examination of punctates as a method of a breast tumor diagnosis. Vopr. Onkol., *6*:54–59, 1960.

Silverman, J.F., Feldman, P.S., Covel, J.L., and Frable, W.J.: Fine needle aspiration cytology of neoplasms metastatic to the breast. Acta Cytol., *31*:291–300, 1987.

Silverman, J.F., Geisinger, K.R., and Frable, W.J.: Fine-needle aspiration cytology of mesenchymal tumors of the breast. Diagn. Cytopathol., *4*:50–58, 1988.

Simi, U., Moretti, D., Iacconi, P., Arganini, M., Roncella, M., Miccoli, P., and Giacomini, G.: Fine needle aspiration cytopathology of phyllodes tumor; differential diagnosis with fibroadenoma. Acta Cytol., *32*:63–66, 1988.

Slamon, D.J., Godolphin, W., and Jones, L.A., et al.: Studies of the *HER-2/neu* proto-oncogene in human breast cancer. Science, *244*:707–712, 1989.

Sneige, N., Zachariah, S., Fanning, T.V., Dekmezian, R.N., and Ordonez, N.G.: Fine-needle aspiration cytology of metastatic neoplasms in the breast. Am. J. Clin. Pathol., *92*:27–35, 1989.

Squires, J.E., and Betsill, W.L.: Intracystic carcinoma of the breast. A correlation of cytomorphology, gross pathology, microscopic pathology and clinical data. Acta Cytol., *25*:267–271, 1981.

Stanley, M.W., Tani, E.M., Horowitz, C.A., Tulman, S., and Skoog, L.: Primary spindle-cell sarcomas of the breast: diagnosis by fine-needle aspiration. Diagn. Cytopathol., *4*:244–249, 1988.

Stavric, G.D., Tevcev, D.T., Kaftandjiev, D.R., and Novak, J.J.: Aspiration biopsy cytologic method in diagnosis of breast lesions. A critical view of 250 cases. Acta Cytol., *17*:188–190, 1973.

Stawicki, M., and Hsiu, J.-G.: Malignant cystosarcoma phyllodes. A case report with cytologic presentation. Acta Cytol., *23*:61–64, 1979.

Steinbrecher, J.S., and Silverberg, S.G.: Signet-ring cell carcinoma of the breast. The mucinous variant of infiltrating lobular carcinoma. Cancer, *37*:829–840, 1976.

Stormby, N., and Bondenson, L.: Adenoma of the nipple; an unusual diagnosis in aspiration cytology. Acta Cytol., *28*:729–732, 1984.

Strobel, S.L., Shah, N.T., Lukas, J.G., and Tuttle, S.E.: Granular-cell tumor of the breast; a cytologic immunohistochemical and ultrastructural study of two cases. Acta Cytol., *29*:598–601, 1985.

Tallent, D.D., and Halter, S.A.: Cytological examination of the breast; a safe, simple and accurate technique. Postgrad. Med. J., *69*:91–94, 1981.

Tani, E.M., and Skoog, L.: Immunocytochemical detection of estrogen receptors in mammary Paget cells. Acta Cytol., *32*:825–828, 1989.

Torres, V., and Ferrer, R.: Cytology of fine needle aspiration biopsy of primary breast rhabdomyosarcoma in an adolescent girl. Acta Cytol., *29*:430–434, 1985.

Volpe, R., Carbone, A., Nicolo, G., and Santi, L.: Cytology of a breast carcinoma with osteoclastlike giant cells. Acta Cytol., *27*:184–187, 1983.

Wallgren, A., Silfversward, C., and Zajicek, J.: Evaluation of needle aspirates and tissue sections as prognostic factors in mammary carcinoma. Acta Cytol., *20*:313–318, 1976.

Wallgren, A., and Zajicek, J.: Cytologic presentation of mammary carcinoma on aspiration biopsy smears. Acta Cytol., *20*:469–478, 1976.

Wallgren, A., and Zajicek, J.: The prognostic value of the aspiration biopsy smear in mammary carcinoma. Acta Cytol., *20*:479–485, 1976.

Wiesman, C., and Liao, K.T.: Primary lymphoma of the breast. Cancer, *29*:1705–1712, 1972.

Woyke, S., Domagala, W., and Gniewosz, Z.: Tuberculosis of the breast clinically mimicking carcinoma, and diagnosed by thin needle aspiration biopsy. Pathol. Res. Pract., *168*:256–261, 1980.

Zajdela, A.: Valeur et interêt du diagnostic cytologique dans les tumeurs du sein par ponction. Etude de 600 cas confrontes cytologiquement et histologiquement. Arch. Anat. Pathol., *11*:85–87, 1963.

Zajdela, A., Ghossein, N.A., Pilleron, J.P., and Ennuyer, A.: The value of aspiration cytology in the diagnosis of breast cancer: Experience at the Fondation Curie. Cancer, *35*:499–506, 1975.

Zajdela, A., Zillhard, P., and Voillemot, N.: Cytological diagnosis by fine needle sampling without aspiration. Cancer, *59*:1201–1205, 1987.

Zajicek, J.: Aspiration biopsy cytology of breast carcinoma. *In* Grundmann, E. (ed.): Early diagnosis of Breast Cancer—Methods and Results. Stuttgart, G. Fischer, 1977.

Zajicek, J.: Breast. *In* Aspiration Biopsy Cytology. Part 1: Cytology of Supradiaphragmatic Organs. Basel, S. Karger, 1973.

Zajicek, J., Caspersson, T., Jakobsson, P., Kudynowski, J., Linsk, J., and Us-Krasovec, M.: Cytologic diagnosis of mammary tumors from aspiration biopsy smears. Comparison of cytologic and histologic findings in 2,111 lesions and diagnostic use of cytophotometry. Acta Cytol., *14*:370–376, 1970.

Zajicek, J., Franzén, S., Jakobsson, P., Rubio, C., and Unsgaard, B.: Aspiration biopsy of mammary tumors in diagnosis and research. Acta Cytol., *11*:169–175, 1967.

Zaloudek, C., Oertel, Y.C., and Orenstein, J.M.: Adenoid cystic carcinoma of the breast. Am. J. Clin. Pathol., *81*:297–307, 1984.

Testis and Ovary

Angström, T., Kjellgren, O., and Bergman, F.: The cytologic diagnosis of ovarian tumors by means of aspiration biopsy. Acta Cytol., *16*:336–341, 1972.

Bjersing, L., Frankendal, B., and Angström, T.: Studies on feminizing ovarian mesenchymoma (granulosa cell tumor). I. Aspiration biopsy, cytology, histology, and ultrastructure. Cancer, *32*:1360–1369, 1973.

Cruciolo, V., and Fulciniti, F.: Fine needle aspiration of the interstitial cell tumor of the testis [Letter]. Acta Cytol., *31*:199, 1987.

Geier, G., Kraus, H., and Schuhmann, R.: Die Punktionszytologie in der Diagnostik von Ovarialtumoren. Geburtshilfe Frauenheilkd., *35*:48–54, 1975.

Geier, G., Kraus, H., and Schuhmann, R.: Fine needle aspiration biopsy in ovarian tumors. *In* DeWatteville, H., et al. (eds.): Diagnosis and Treatment of Ovarian Neoplastic Alterations. pp. 73–76. Amsterdam, Excerpta Medica, 1975.

Gonzalez-Crussi, F.: Testicular and paratesticular neoplasm. *In* Steveberg, S.S. (ed.): Diagnostic Surgical Pathology. pp. 1455–1486. New York, Raven Press, 1989.

Highman, W.J., and Oliver, R.T.D.: Diagnosis of metastases from testicular germ cell tumors using fine needle aspiration cytology. J. Clin. Pathol., *40*:1324–1333, 1987.

Hill, G.S., and Billey-Kijner, C.: Paratesticular structures: nontumorous conditions. *In* Hill, G.S. (ed.): Uropathology. pp. 1101–1134. New York: churchill-Livingston, 1989.

Jayaram, G.: Microfilariae in fine needle aspirates from epididymal lesions. Acta Cytol., *31*:59–62, 1987.

Kjellgren, O., and Angström, T.: Transvaginal and transrectal aspiration biopsy in diagnosis and classification of ovarian tumors. *In* Zajicek, J. (ed.): Aspiration Biopsy Cytology, Part 2: Cytology of Infradiaphragmatic Organs. pp. 80–103. Basel, S. Karger, 1979.

Kjellgren, O., Angstrom, T., Bergman, F., and Wiklund, D.-E.: Fine-needle aspiration biopsy in diagnosis and classification of ovarian carcinoma. Cancer, *28*:967–976, 1971.

Layfield, L.J., Hilborne, L.H., Ljung, B.M., Feig, S., and Ehrlich, R.M.: Use of fine needle aspiration cytology for the diagnosis of testicular relapse in patients with acute lymphoblastic leukemia. J. Urol., *139*:1020–1022, 1988.

Linsk, J.A., and Franzén, S.: Clinical Aspiration Cytology, 2nd ed. pp. 305–318, Philadelphia, J.B. Lippincott, 1989.

Lopez, J., and Aranda, F.I.: Fine needle aspiration cytology of spermatocytic seminoma. Report of a case. Acta Cytol., *33*:627–630, 1989.

Mostofi, F.K., and Price, E.B.: Tumors of the male genital system. *In* Atlas of Tumor Pathology. 2d Series, Fasc. 8. Washington, D.C., Armed forces Institute of Pathology.

Mostofi, F.K., and Sobin, L.H.: Histological Typing of Testis Tumors. Geneva, World Health Organization, 1977.

Papic, Z., Katona, G., and Skrabalo, Z.: The cytologic identifi-

cation and quantification of testicular cell subtypes. Reproducibility and relation to histologic findings in the diagnosis of male infertility. Acta Cytol., *32*:697–706, 1988.

Perez-Guillermo, M., Thor, A., and Löwhagen, T.: Paratesticular adenomatoid tumors. The cytologic presentation in fine needle aspiration biopsies. Acta Cytol., *33*:6–10, 1989.

Perez-Guillermo, M., Thor, A., and Löwhagen, T.: Spermatic granuloma. Diagnosis by fine needle aspiration cytology. Acta Cytol., *33*:1–5, 1989.

Persson, P.S., Ahren, C., and Obrant, K.O.: Aspiration biopsy smears of testis in azoospermia. Scand. J. Urol. Nephrol., *5*:22–27, 1971.

Pettinato, G., Insabato, L., DeChiara, A., and Latella, R.: Fine needle aspiration cytology of a large cell calcifying Sertoli cell tumor of the testis. Acta Cytol., *31*:578–582, 1987.

Piscioli, F., Polla, E., Pusiol, T., Failoni, G., and Luciani, L.: Pseudomalignant cytologic presentation of spermatic hydrocele fluid. Acta Cytol., *27*:666–670, 1983.

Proppe, K.H., and Scully, R.E.: Large cell calcifying Sertoli cell tumor of the testis. Am. J. Clin. Pathol., *74*:607–619, 1980.

Pugh, R.C.B. (ed.): Pathology of the Testis. Oxford, Blackwell Scientific Publications, 1976.

Rupp, M., Hafiz, M.A., Hoover, L., and Sun, C.C.: Fine needle aspiration in the evaluation of testicular leukemic infiltration. Acta Cytol., *31*:57–58, 1987.

Schenck, U., and Schill, W.B.: Cytology of the human seminiferous epithelium. Acta Cytol., *32*:689–696, 1988.

Tao, L.-C., Negin, M.L., and Donat, E.E.: Primary retroperitoneal seminoma diagnosed by fine needle aspiration biopsy: a case report. Acta Cytol., *28*:598–600, 1984.

Teilum, G.: Special Tumors of Ovary and Testis and Related Extragonadal Lesions. Copenhagen, Einar Munksgaard, 1971.

Trainer, T.O.: Histology of the normal testis. Am. J. Surg. Pathol., *11*:797–809, 1987.

Verma, K., Ram, T.R., and Kapila, K.: Value of fine needle aspiration cytology in the diagnosis of testicular neoplasms. Acta Cytol., *33*:631–634, 1989.

Wentworth, P., Wagar, S., and Unitt, M.: Atypical cells in spermatocele fluid. Acta Cytol., *15*:210–211, 1971.

Wheeler, J.E.: Testicular tumors. *In* Hill, G.S. (ed.): Uropathology. pp. 1047–1100. Churchill Livingstone, New York, 1989.

Zajicek, J.: Aspiration biopsy cytology. II. Cytology of infradiaphragmatic organs. Monographs in Clinical Cytology. pp. 104–128. Basel, S. Karger, 1979.

Prostate

Bichel, P., Frederiksen, P., Kjaer, T., Thomessen, P., and Vindeløv, L.L.: Flow microfluorometry and transrectal fine needle biopsy in the classification of human prostatic carcinoma. Cancer, *40*:1206–1211, 1977.

DeGaetani, C.F., and Treutini, G.P.: Atypical hyperplasia of the prostate. A pitfall in the cytologic diagnosis of carcinoma. Acta Cytol., *22*:483–486, 1978.

Droese, M., and Voeth, C.: Cytologic features of seminal vesicle epithelium in aspiration biopsy smears of the prostate. Acta Cytol., *20*:120–125, 1976.

Epstein, N.A.: Prostatic carcinoma: correlation of histologic features of prognostic value with cytomorphology. Cancer, *38*:2071–2077, 1976.

Epstein, N.A.: Prostatic biopsy. A morphologic correlation of aspiration cytology with needle biopsy histology. Cancer, *38*:2078–2087, 1976.

Esposti, P.L.: Aspiration Biopsy Cytology in the Diagnosis and

Management of Prostatic Carcinoma. Stockholm, Stahl and Accidenstryct, 1974.

Esposti, P.-L.: Cytologic diagnosis of prostatic tumors with the aid of transrectal aspiration biopsy: a critical review of 1,110 cases and a report of morphologic and cytochemical studies. Acta Cytol., *10*:182–186, 1966.

Esposti, P.-L.: Cytologic malignancy grading of prostatic carcinoma. Scand. J. Urol. Nephrol., *5*:199–209, 1971.

Esposti, P.-L, Elman, A., and Norlen, H.: Complications of transrectal aspiration biopsy of the prostate. Scand. J. Urol. Nephrol., *9*:208–213, 1975.

Esposti, P.-L., Estborn, B., and Zajicek, J.: Determination of acid phosphatase activity in cells of prostatic tumours. Nature, *188*:663–664, 1960.

Faul, P.: Prostata-Zytologie. Darmstadt, Dr. Dietrich Steinkopff Verlag, 1975.

Ferguson, R.S.: Prostatic neoplasms: Their diagnosis by needle puncture and aspiration. Am. J. Surg., *9*:507–511, 1930.

Franzèn, S., Giertz, G., and Zajicek, J.: Cytological diagnosis of prostatic tumors by transrectal aspiration biopsy: a preliminary report. Br. J. Urol., *32*:193–196, 1960.

Greenebaum, E.: Megakaryocytes and ganglion cells mimicking cancer in fine needle aspiration of the prostate. Acta Cytol., *32*:504–508, 1988.

Helpap, B.: Cell kinetics and cytological grading of prostatic carcinoma. Virchows Arch. [A], *393*:205–214, 1981.

Kaufman, J.J., Rosenthal, M., and Goodwin, W.E.: Methods of diagnosis of carcinoma of the prostate: a comparison of clinical impression, prostatic smear, needle biopsy, open perineal biopsy and transurethral biopsy. J. Urol., *72*:450–465, 1954.

Kline, T.S., Kohler, F.P., and Kesley, D.M.: Aspiration biopsy cytology. Its use in diagnosis of lesions of prostate gland. Arch. Pathol. Lab Med., *106*:136–139, 1982.

Koivuniemi, A., and Tyrkko, J.: Seminal vesicle epithelium in fine-needle aspiration biopsies of the prostate as a pitfall in the cytologic diagnosis of carcinoma. Acta Cytol., *20*:116–119, 1976.

Koss, L.G., Woyke, S., and Olszewski, W.: Aspiration Biopsy. Cytologic Interpretation and Histologic Bases, 2nd ed. New York, Igaku-Shoin, 1992.

Koss, L.G., Woyke, S., Schreiber, K., Kohlberg, W., and Freed, S.Z.: Thin-needle aspiration of the prostate. Urol. Clin. North Am., *11*:237–251, 1984.

Kuo, T., and Gomez, L.G.: Monstrous epithelial cells in human epididymis and seminal vesicles. A pseudomalignant change. Am J. Surg. Pathol., *5*:483–490, 1981.

Leistenschneider, W., and Nagel, R.: Atlas of Prostatic Cytology. Berlin, Springer-Verlag, 1984.

Linsk, J.A., Axelrod, H.D., Solyn, R., and Delaverdac, C.: Transrectal cytologic aspiration in the diagnosis of prostatic carcinoma. J. Urol., *108*:455–459, 1972.

Mulholland, S.W.: A study of prostatic secretion and its relation to malignancy. Proc. Mayo Clin., *6*:733–735, 1931.

Ronstrom, L., Tribukait, B., and Esposti, P.-L.: DNA pattern and cytological findings in fine-needle aspirates of untreated prostatic tumors. A flow-cytofluorometric study. Prostate, *2*:79–88, 1981.

Spieler, P., Gloor, F., Egle, N., and Bandhauer, K.: Cytologic findings in transrectal aspiration biopsy on hormone and radiotreated carcinoma of the prostate. Virchows Arch. [A], *372*:149–159, 1976.

Staehler, W., Ziegler, H., and Volter, D.: Zytodiagnostik der Prostata. Grundriss und Atlas. Stuttgart, F. K. Schattauer Verlag, 1975.

Suhrland, M.J., Deitch, D., Schreiber, K., Freed, S., and Koss, L.G.: Assessment of fine needle aspiration as a screening test for occult prostatic carcinoma. Acta Cytol., *32*:495–498, 1988.

Tanner, F.H., and McDonald, J.R.: Granulomatous prostatitis: histologic study of a group of granulomatous lesions collected from prostate glands. Arch. Pathol., *36*:358–370, 1943.

Zetterberg, A., and Esposti, P.-L.: Cytophotometric DNA-analysis of aspirated cells from prostatic carinoma. Acta Cytol., *20*:46–57, 1976.

Skin and Soft Tissues

Abele, J.S., and Miller, T.: Cytology of well-differentiated hemangiosarcoma in fine needle aspirates. Acta Cytol., *26*:341–348, 1982.

Ahmed, M.N., Feldman, M., and Seemayer, T.A.: Cytology of epithelioid sarcoma. Acta Cytol., *18*:459–461, 1974.

Åkerman, M., Idvall, J., and Rydholm, A.: Cytodiagnosis of soft tissue tumors and tumor-like conditions by means of fine needle aspiration biopsy. Arch. Orthop. Trauma Surg., *96*:61–67, 1980.

Åkerman, M., and Rydholm, A.: Aspiration cytology of intramuscular myxoma: a comparative clinical, cytologic and histologic study of ten cases. Acta Cytol., *27*:505–510, 1983.

Åkerman, M., and Rydholm, A.: Aspiration cytology of lipomatous tumors. A 10 year experience at an orthopedic oncology center. Diagn. Cytolpathol., *3*:295–302, 1987.

Akhtar, M., Ali, M.A., Sabbah, R., Bakry, M., and Nash, J.E.: Fine needle aspiration biopsy diagnosis of round cell malignant tumors of childhood: a combined light and electron microscopic approach. Cancer, *55*:1805–1817, 1985.

Angervall, L., Hagmar, B., Kindblom, L.-G., and Merck, C.: Malignant giant cell tumor of soft tissues. A clinicopathologic, cytologic, ultrastructural, angiographic and microangiographic study. Cancer, *47*:736–747, 1981.

Arora, R., Rewari, R., and Betheria, S.M.: Fine needle aspiration cytology of eyelid tumors. Acta Cytol., *34*:227–232, 1990.

Baez-Giangreco, A., Afzal, M., Mattew, M., and Afaf, A.: Fine needle aspiration in diagnosis of cutaneous leishmaniasis. Ann. Saudi Med., *9*:452–454, 1989.

Bondeson, L., and Andreasson, L.: Aspiration cytology of adult rhabdomyoma. Acta Cytol., *30*:679–682, 1986.

Brown, C.L., Klager, M.R., and Robertson, M.G.: Rapid cytological diagnosis of basal cell carcinoma of the skin. J. Clin. Pathol., *32*:361–367, 1979.

Canti, G.: Skin cytology and its value for rapid diagnosis. Acta Cytol., *23*:516–517, 1979.

Canti, G.: Rapid cytological diagnosis of skin lesions. *In* Koss, L.G., and Coleman, D.V. (eds.): Advances in Clinical Cytology, vol. 2. pp. 243–266. New York, Masson Publishing, 1984.

Dahl, I., and Åkerman, M.: Nodular fasciitis. A cytological and histological study of 13 cases. Acta Cytol., *25*:215–223, 1981.

Domogala, W., Lubinski, J., Lasota, J., Giryn, I., Weber, K., and Osborn, M.: Neuroendocrine (Merkel-cell) skin carcinoma: Cytology, intermediate filament typing and ultrastructure of tumor cells in fine needle aspirates. Acta Cytol., *31*:267–275, 1987.

Hajdu, S.J., and Hajdu, E.O.: Cytopathology of Sarcomas and Other Non-epithelial Malignant Tumors. Philadelphia, W.B. Saunders, 1976.

Hajdu, S.J., and Koss, L.G.: Cytologic diagnosis of metastatic myosarcomas. Acta Cytol., *13*:545–551, 1969.

Hales, M., Bottles, K., Miller, T., Donegan, E., and Ljung, B.M.: Diagnosis of Kaposi's sarcoma by fine needle aspiration biopsy. Am. J. Clin. Pathol., *88*:20–25, 1987.

Hashimoto, C.H., and Cobb, C.J.: Cytodiagnosis of hibernoma: A case report. Cytopathology, *3*:326–329, 1987.

Jayaram, G.: Microfilariae in fine needle aspirates from epididymal lesions. Acta Cytol., *31*:59–62, 1987.

Kapila, K., and Vezma, K.: Gravid adult female worms of *Wuchereria bancrofti* in fine needle aspirates of soft tissue swellings. Report of three cases. Acta Cytol., *33*:390–392, 1989.

Kindblom, L.G., Walaas, L., and Widehn, S.: Ultrastructural studies in the preoperative cytologic diagnosis of soft tissue tumors. Semin. Diagn. Pathol., *3*:317–344, 1986.

Kline, T.S.: Handbook of Fine Needle Aspiration biopsy Cytology. 2nd ed. New York, Churchill Livingstone, 1988.

Koivuniemi, A., and Nickels, J.: Synovial sarcoma diagnosed by fine needle aspiration biopsy. A case report. Acta Cytol., *22*:515–518, 1978.

Layfield, L.J., Anders, K.H., Glasgow, B.J., and Mirra, J.M.: Fine-needle aspiration of primary soft-tissue lesions. Arch. Pathol. Lab. Med., *110*:420–424, 1986.

Leiman, G., Markowitz, S., Veiga-Ferreira, M.M., and Margolius, K.A.: Endometriosis of rectovaginal septum: diagnosis by fine needle aspiration cytology. Acta Cytol., *30*:313–316, 1986.

Linsk, J.A., and Franzén, S.: Melanomas and skin nodules. *In* Linsk, J.A., and Franzén, S. (eds.): Clinical Aspiration Cytology, 2nd ed. pp. 319–336. Philadelphia, J.B. Lippincott, 1989.

Mellblom, L., Akerman, M., and Carlen, B.: Aspiration cytology of neuroendocrine (Merkel-cell) carcinoma of the skin. Report of a case. Acta Cytol., *28*:297–300, 1984.

Merck, C., and Hagmar, b.: Myxofibrosarcoma. A correlative cytologic and histologic study of 13 cases examined by fine needle aspiration cytology. Acta Cytol., *24*:137–144, 1980.

Neifer, R., and Nguyen, G.-K.: Aspiration cytology of solitary schwannoma. Acta Cytol., *29*:12–14, 1985.

Nieberg, R.K.: Fine needle aspiration cytology of alveolar soft-part sarcoma; a case report. Acta Cytol., *28*:198–202, 1984.

Pontiflex, A.H., and Roberts, F.J.: Fine needle aspiration biopsy cytology in the diagnosis of inflammatory lesions. Acta Cytol., *29*:979–982, 1985.

Ramzy, I.: Benign schwannoma. Demonstration of Verocay bodies using fine needle aspiration. Acta Cytol., *21*:316–319, 1977.

Szpak, C.A., Bossen, E.H., Linder, J., and Johnston, W.W.: Cytomorphology of primary small-cell (Merkel-cell) carcinoma of the skin in fine needle aspirates. Acta Cytol., *28*:290–296, 1984.

Walaas, L., Angervall, L., Hagmar, B., and Save-Soderbergh, J.: A correlative cytologic and histologic study of malignant fibrous histiocytoma: an analysis of 40 cases examined by fine-needle aspiration cytology. Diagn. Cytopathol., *2*:46–54, 1986.

Walaas, L., and Kindblom, L.-G.: Lipomatous tumors: a correlative cytologic and histologic study of 27 tumors examined by fine needle aspiration cytology. Hum. Pathol., *16*:6–18, 1985.

Woyke, S., and Czerniak, B.: Fine needle aspiration cytology of metastatic myxopapillary ependymoma. Acta Cytol., *22*:312–315, 1978.

Woyke, S., Domagala, W., Czerniak, B., and Strokowska, M.: Fine needle aspiration cytology of malignant melanoma of the skin. Acta Cytol., *24*:529–538, 1980.

Woyke, S., Olszewski, W., and Eichelkraut, A.: Pilomatrixoma.

A pitfall in the aspiration cytology of skin tumors. Acta Cytol., *26*:189–194, 1982.

Mediastinum

Adler, O., and Rosenberger, A.: Invasive radiology in the diagnosis of mediastinal masses. Radiology, *19*:169–172, 1979.

Dahgren, S.E., and Nordenström, B.: Transthoracic Needle Biopsy. Stockholm, Almqvist & Wiksell, 1966.

Dahlgren, S.E., and Ovenfors, C.O.: Aspiration biopsy diagnosis of neurogenous mediastinal tumours. Acta Radiol. (Stockh.), *10*:289–298, 1970.

Dahlgren, S., Sandstedt, B., and Sundstrom, C.: Fine needle aspiration cytology of thymic tumors. Acta Cytol., *27*:1–6, 1983.

Dyer, N.H.: Cystic thymomas and thymic cysts. Thorax, *22*:408–421, 1967.

Gonzalez-Crussi, F.: Extragonadal teratomas. *In* Atlas of Tumor Pathology, Ser., fasc. 18. Washington, D.C., Armed Forces Institute of Pathology, 1982.

Hurley, M.F.: Cervico-mediastinal thymic cyst: cyst puncture and contrast radiographic demonstration. Br. J. Radiol., *50*:676–678, 1977.

Jareb, M., and Us-Krasovec, M.: Transthoracic needle biopsy of mediastinal and hilar lesions. Cancer, *40*:1356–1357, 1977.

Klatte, E.G., and Yune, H.Y.: Diagnosis and treatment of pericardial cysts. Radiology, *104*:541–543, 1973.

Lalli, A.F., Naylor, B., and Whitehouse, W.M.: Aspiration biopsy of thoracic lesions. Thorax, *22*:404–407, 1967.

Linsk, J.A., and Salzman, A.J.: Diagnosis of intrathoracic tumors by thin needle cytology aspiration. Am. J. Med. Sci., *263*:181–195, 1972.

Nichols, C.R., Roth, B.J., Heerema, N., Griep, J., and Tricot, G.: Hematologic neoplasia associated with primary mediastinal germ-cell tumors. N. Engl. J. Med., *322*:1425–1429, 1990.

Pak, H.Y., Yokota, S.B., and Friedberg, H.A.: Thymoma diagnosed by transthoracic fine needle aspiration. Acta Cytol., *26*:210–216, 1982.

Palombini, L., and Vetrani, A.: Cytologic diagnosis of ganglioneuroblastoma. Acta Cytol., *20*:286–287, 1976.

Palombini, L., Vetrani, A., Vecchione, R., DelBasso, D., and Caro, M.L.: The cytology of ganglioneuroma on fine needle aspiration smear. Acta Cytol., *27*:259–260, 1983.

Ramzy, J.: Benign schwannoma: demonstration of Verocay bodies using fine needle aspiration. Acta Cytol., *21*:316–319, 1977.

Rosai, J., and Levine, G.D.: Tumors of the thymus. *In* Atlas of Tumor Pathology, ser. 2, fasc. 13. Washington, D.C., Armed Forces Institute of Pathology, 1976.

Rosenberger, A., and Adler, O.: Fine needle aspiration biopsy in the diagnosis of mediastinal lesions. AJR, *131*:239–242, 1978.

Sajjad, S.M., Lukeman, J.M., Llamas, L., and Fernandez, T.: Needle biopsy diagnosis of thymoma. A case report. Acta Cytol., *26*:503–506, 1982.

Shimosato, Y., Kameya, T., Nagai, K., and Suemasu, K.: Squamous cell carcinoma of the thymus. An analysis of eight cases. Am. J. Surg. Pathol., *1*:109–121, 1977.

Sterrett, G., Whitabker, D., Shilkin, K.B., and Walters, M.-I.: The fine needle aspiration cytology of mediastinal lesions. Cancer, *51*:127–135, 1983.

Suen, K.C., and Quenville, N.F.: Fine needle aspiration cytology of uncommon thoracic lesions. Am. J. Clin. Pathol., 75:803–809, 1981.

Tao, L.C.: Guides to Clinical Aspiration Biopsy. Lung, Pleura and Mediastinum. New York, Igaku-Shoin, 1988.

Tao, L.C., Pearson, F.G., Delarue, N.C., Cooper, J.D., Sanders, D.E., Weisbroad, G., and Donat, E.E.: Thymoma: a cytomorphologic study and cytologic grading [abstr.]. Acta Cytol., 25:453, 1981.

Wick, M.R., Carney, J.A., Pernatz, P.E., and Brown, L.R.: Primary mediastinal carcinoid tumors. Am. J. Surg. Pathol., 6:195–205, 1982.

Wick, M.R., and Scheithauer, B.W.: Oat-cell carcinoma of the thymus. Cancer, 49:1652–1657, 1982.

Liver

Ajdukiewicz, A., Crowden, A., Hudson, E., and Pyne, C.K.: Liver aspiration in the diagnosis of hepatocellular carcinoma in the Gambia. J. Clin. Pathol., 38:185–192, 1985.

Ali, M.A., Akhtar, M., and Mattingly, R.C.: Morphologic spectrum of hepatocellular carcinoma in fine needle aspiration biopsies. Acta Cytol., 30:294–302, 1986.

Bell, D.A., Carr, C.P., and Szyfelbein, W.M.: Fine needle aspiration cytology of focal liver lesions: results obtained with examination of both cytologic and histologic preparations. Acta Cytol., 30:397–402, 1986.

Bermen, J.J., and McNeill, R.E.: Cirrhosis with atypia: a potential pitfall in the interpretation of liver aspirates. Acta Cytol., 32:11–14, 1988.

Bhatia, A., and Mehrotra, P.: Fine needle aspiration cytology in a case of hepatoblastoma. Acta Cytol., 30:439–441, 1986.

Bizjak-Schwarzbartl, M.: Fine needle aspiration biopsy in the diagnosis of metastases in the liver. Diagn. Cytopathol., 3:278–283, 1987.

Bognel, C., Rougier, P., Leclere, J., Duvillard, P., Charpentier, P., and Prade, M.: Fine needle aspiration of the liver and pancreas with ultrasound guidance. Acta Cytol., 32:22–26, 1988.

Carney, C.N.: Clinical cytology of the liver. Acta Cytol., 19:244–250, 1975.

Dekmezian, R., Sneige, N., Popok, S., and Ordonez, N.G.: A comparative study of two hepatoblastomas and a liver-cell carcinoma. Diagn. Cytopathol., 4:162–168, 1988.

Domagala, W., Lasota, J., Weber, K., and Osborn, M.: Endothelial cells help in the diagnosis of primary versus metastatic carcinoma of the liver fine needle aspirates: an immunofluorescence study with vimentin and endothelial cell-specific antibodies. Anal. Quant. Cytol. Histol., 11:8–14, 1989.

Edmondson, H.A., and Schiff, L.: Needle biopsy of the liver. In Schiff, L. (ed.): Diseases of the Liver, 4th ed. Chap. 9. Philadelphia, J.B. Lippincott, 1975.

Ferucci, J.T., and Wittenberg, J.: CT biopsy of abdominal tumors: aids for lesion localization. Radiology, 129:739–744, 1978.

Ferrucci, J.T., Wittenberg, J., Margolies, M.N., and Carey, R.W.: Malignant seeding of the tract after thin needle aspiration biopsy. Radiology, 130:345–346, 1979.

Ferrucci, J.T., Wittenberg, J., Mueller, P.R., Simeone, J.F., Harbin, W.P., Kirkpatrick, R.H., and Taft, P.D.: diagnosis of abdominal malignancy by radiologic fine needle aspiration biopsy. AJR 134:323–330, 1980.

Frias-Hidvegi, P.: Guides to Clinical Aspiration Biopsy. Liver and Pancreas. New York, Igaku-Shoin, 1988.

Grossman, E., Goldstein, M.J., Koss, L.G., Winawer, S.J., and

Sherlock, P.: Cytological examination as an adjunct to liver biopsy in the diagnosis of hepatic metastases. Gastroenterology, 62:56–60, 1972.

Gupta, S.K., Das, D.K., and Rajwanshi, A.: Cytology of hepatocellular carcinoma. Diagn. Cytopathol., 2:290–294, 1986.

Haaga, J.R., and Alfidi, R.J.: Precise biopsy localization by computed tomography. Radiology, 118:603–607, 1976.

Holm, H.H., Pederson, J.F., Kirstensen, J.K., Rasmussen, S.N., Hancke, S., and Jensen, F.: Ultrasonically guided percutaneous puncture. Radiol. Clin. North Am., 13:493–503, 1975.

Isler, R.J., Ferrucci, J.T., Jr., Wittenberg, J., Mueller, P.R., Simeone, J.F., vanSonnenberg, E., and Hall, D.A.: Tissue core biopsy of abdominal tumors with a 22-gauge cutting needle. AJR, 136:725–728, 1981.

Johansen, P., and Svendsen, K.N.: Scan guided fine needle aspiration biopsy in malignant hepatic disease. Acta Cytol., 22:292–296, 1978.

Johansen, S., and Myren, J.: Fine needle aspiration biopsy smears in the diagnosis of liver diseases. Scand. J. Gastroenterol., 6:583–588, 1971.

Kaminsky, D.B.: Aspiration Biopsy for the Community Hospital. New York, Masson Publishing, 1981.

Kline, T.S.: Handbook of Fine Needle Aspiration Biopsy Cytology, 2nd ed. St. Louis, C.V. Mosby, 1989.

Koss, L.G.: Cytology of liver aspirates. In Koss, L.G.: Diagnostic Cytology and Its Histopathologic Bases, 3rd ed. pp. 863–867. Philadelphia, J.B. Lippincott, 1979.

Koss, L.G.: Cytology of pancreas and bile. In Koss, L.G.: Diagnostic Cytology and its Histopathologic Bases, 3rd ed. pp. 855–858; 868–871. Philadelphia, J.B. Lippincott, 1979.

Koss, L.G., Woyke, S., and Olszewski, W.: Aspiration Biopsy. Cytologic Interpretation and Histologic Bases. New York, Igaku-Shoin, 1984, 2nd Ed., 1992.

Lee, N.W., Wong, J., and Ong, G.B.: The surgical management of primary carcinoma of the liver. World J. Surg., 6:66–75, 1982.

Linsk, J.A., and Franzén, S.: Clinical Aspiration Cytology. Philadelphia, J.B. Lippincott, 1989.

Lundquist, A.: Fine needle aspiration biopsy of the liver. Application in clinical diagnosis and investigation. Acta Med. Scand. [Suppl.], 520:1–28, 1971.

Menghini, G.: One second biopsy of the liver. N. Engl. J. Med., 283:582–585, 1970.

Moussouris, H.F., Koss, L.G., Rosenblatt, R., and Kutcher, R.: Thin needle aspiration biopsy of abdominal organs. In Koss, L.G., and Coleman, D.V. (eds.): Advances in Clinical Cytology, vol. 2. pp. 191–241. New York, Masson Publishing, 1984.

Nguyen, G.K.: Fine needle aspiration biopsy cytology of hepatic tumors in adults. Pathol. Annu., 21(Part 1):321–349, 1986.

Noguchi, S., Yamamoto, R., Tatsuta, M., Kasugai, M., Okuda, S., Wada, A., and Tamura, H.: Cell features and patterns in fine needle aspirates of hepatocellular carcinoma. Cancer, 58:321–328, 1986.

Ong, G.B., and Chan, P.K.W.: Primary carcinoma of the liver. Surg. Gynecol. Obstet., 143:31–38, 1976.

Pedio, G., Landolt, U., Zobeli, L., and Gut, D.: Fine needle aspiration of the liver: significance of hepatocytic naked nuclei in the diagnosis of hepatocellular carinoma. Acta Cytol., 32:437–442, 1988.

Perrault, J., McGill, D.B., Ott, B.J., and Taylor, W.F.: Liver biopsy: complications in 1000 patients. Gastroenterology, 74:103–106, 1978.

Perry, M.D., and Johnston, W.W.: Needle biopsy of the liver for the diagnosis of nonneoplastic liver diseases. Acta Cytol., *29*:385–390, 1985.

Pilotti, S., Rilke, F., Claren, R., Milella, M., and Lombardii, L.: Conclusive diagnosis of hepatic and pancreatic malignancies by fine needle aspiration. Acta Cytol., *32*:27–38, 1988.

Riska, H., and Freeman, C.: Fatality after fine needle aspiration biopsy of liver. Br. Med. J., *1*:517, 1975.

Rosenblatt, R., Kutcher, R., Moussouris, H.F., Schreiber, K., and Koss, L.G.: Sonographically guided fine needle aspiration of liver lesions. JAMA, *248*:1639–1641, 1982.

Schultz, T.B.: Fine needle aspiration biopsy of the liver complicated with bile peritonitis. Acta Med. Scand., *199*:141–142, 1976.

Sherlock, P., Kim, Y.S., and Koss, L.G.: Cytologic diagnosis of cancer from aspirated material obtained at liver biopsy. Am. J. Dig. Dis. *12*:396–402, 1967.

Söderström, N.: Fine Needle Aspiration Biopsy Used as a Direct Adjunct in Clinical Diagnostic Work. New York, Grune Stratton, 1966.

Solbiati, L., Livraghi, T., DePra, L., Ierace, T., Masciadri, N., and Ravetto, C.: Fine needle biopsy of hepatic hemangioma with sonographic guidance. AJR, *144*: 471–474, 1985.

Suen, K.C.: Diagnosis of primary hepatic neoplasms by fine needle aspiration cytology. Diagn. Cytopathol., *2*:99–109, 1986.

Tao, L.C.: Transabdominal Fine Needle Aspiration Biopsy. New York, Igaku-Shoin, 1990.

Wasastjerna, C.: Liver. *In* Zajicek, J. (ed.): Aspiration Biopsy Cytology. Part 2: Cytology of Infradiaphragmatic Organs. Chap. 6. Basel, S. Karger, 1979.

Wittenberg, J., Mueller, P.R., Ferucci, J.T., Jr., Simeone, J.F., van Sonnenberg, E., Neff, C.C., Palermo, R.A., and Isler, R.J.: Percutaneous core biopsy of abdominal tumors using 22-gauge needle. Further observations. AJR, *139*:75–80, 1982.

Zajicek, J.: Aspiration Biopsy Cytology. Part I: Cytology of Supradiaphragmatic Organs. Part II: Cytology of Infradiaphramatic Organs. Basel, S. Karger, Part I, 1974; Part II, 1979.

Zornoza, J.: Abdomen. *In* Zornoza, J. (ed.): Percutaneous Needle Biopsy. Chap. 8. Baltimore, Williams & Wilkins, 1981.

Zornoza, J., Wallace, S., Ordonez, N., and Lukeman, J.: Fine needle aspiration biopsy of the liver. AJR, *134*:331–334, 1980.

Pancreas

Al-Kaisi, N., and Siegler, E.E.: Fine needle aspiration cytology of the pancreas. Acta Cytol., *33*:145–152, 1989.

Banner, B.F., Myrent, K.L., Memoli, V.A., and Gould, V.E.: Neuroendocrine carcinoma of the pancreas diagnosed by aspiration cytology. A case report. Acta Cytol., *29*:442–448, 1985.

Bell, D.A.: Cytologic features of islet cell tumors. Acta Cytol., *31*:485–492, 1987.

Bersenfeldt, M., Genell, S., Lindholm, K., and Ekbers, O.A.P.: Needle-tract seeding after percutaneous fine-needle biopsy of pancreatic carcinoma. Acta Chir. Scand., *154*:77–79, 1988.

Bognel, C., Rougier, P., Leclere, J., Duvillard, P., Charpentier, P., and Prade, M.: Fine needle aspiration of the liver and pancreas with ultrasound guidance. Acta Cytol., *32*:22–26, 1988.

Bondeson, L., Bondeson, A.G., Genell, S., Lindholm, K., and Thorstenson, S.: Aspiration cytology of a rare solid and pap-

illary epithelial neoplasm of the pancreas. Light and electron microscopic study of a case. Acta Cytol., *28*:605–609, 1984.

Bret, P.M., Nicolet, V., and Labadie, M.: Percutaneous fine-needle aspiration biopsy of the pancreas. Diagn. Cytopathol., *2*:221–227, 1986.

Dickey, J.E., Haaga, J.R., Stellato, T.A., Schultz, C.L., and Hau, T.: Evaluation of computed tomography guided percutaneous biopsy of the pancreas. Surg. Gynecol., *163*:497–503, 1986.

Emmert, G.M., and Bewtra, C.: Fine-needle aspiration biopsy of mucinous cystic neoplasm of the pancreas: a case study. Diagn. Cytopathol., *2*:69–71, 1986.

Evander, A., Ishe, I., Sunderquist, A., Tylen, V., and Akerman, H.: Percutaneous cytodiagnosis of carcinoma of the pancreas and bile duct. Ann. Surg., *188*:90–92, 1987.

Fekete, P.S., Nunex, C., and Pitlik, D.A.: Fine needle aspiration biopsy of the pancreas: a study of 61 cases. Diagn. Cytopathol., *2*:301–306, 1986.

Frias-Hidvegi, P.: Guides to Clinical Aspiration Biopsy. Liver and Pancreas. New York, Igaku-Shoin, 1988.

Gupta, P.K., Wakefield, S.J., Fauck, R., and Stewart, R.J.: Immunocytochemical and ultrastructural findings in a case of rare carcinoma of the pancreas with predominance of malignant squamous cells in an intraoperative needle aspirate. Acta Cytol., *33*:153–156, 1989.

Ishihara, A., Sanda, T., Takanari, H., Yatani, R., and Liu, P.I.: Elastase-1-secreting acinar cell carcinoma of the pancreas. A cytologic, electron microscopic and histochemical study. Acta Cytol., *33*:157–163, 1989.

Jones, E.C., Kenneth, C.S., Grant, D.R., and Chan, N.H.: Fine-needle aspiration cytology in neoplastic cysts of the pancreas. Diagn. Cytopathol., *3*:283–243, 1987.

Kline, T.S.: Handbook of Fine Needle Aspiration Biopsy Cytology. 2nd ed. pp. 317–342. New York, Churchill Livingstone, 1988.

Kocjan, G., Rode, J., and Lees, W.R.: Percutaneous fine needle aspiration cytology of the pancreas. Advantages and pitfalls. J. Clin. Pathol., *42*:341–347, 1989.

Koss, L.G., Woyke, S., and Olszewski, W.: Aspiration Biopsy. Cytologic Interpretation and Histologic Bases. New York, Igaku-Shoin, 1984, 2nd Ed., 1992.

Linsk, J.A., and Franzen, S.: Clinical Aspiration Cytology. 2nd ed. pp. 231–234, Philadelphia, J.B. Lippincott, 1989.

Manci, E.A., Gardner, L.L., and Pollock, W.J.: Osteoclastic giant cell tumor of the pancreas. Aspiration cytology, light microscopy and ultrastructure with review of the literature. Diagn. Cytopathol., *1*:105–110, 1985.

Moussouris, H.F., Koss, L.G., Rosenblatt, R., and Kutcher, R.: Thin needle aspiration biopsy of abdominal organs. *In* Koss, L.G., and Coleman, D.V. (eds.): Advances in Clinical Cytology, vol. 2, pp. 191–241. New York, Masson Publishing, 1984.

Mueller, P.R., Miketic, L.M., Simeone, J.F., Silverman, S.G., Saini, S., Wittenberg, J., Hahn, P.F., Steiner, E., and Forman, B.H.: Severe acute pancreatitis after percutaneous biopsy of the pancreas. AJR, *151*:493–494, 1988.

Parsons, L.J., and Palmer, C.H.: How accurate is fine-needle biopsy in malignant neoplasia of the pancreas? Arch. Surg., *124*:681–683, 1989.

Sneige, N., Ordonez, N.G., Veanattukalathil, S., and Samaan, N. A.: Fine needle aspiration cytology in pancreatic endocrine tumors. Diagn. Cytopathol., *3*:35–40, 1987.

Soreide, O., Skoarland, E., and Pederson, O.M., et al.: Fine needle biopsy of the pancreas: results of 204 routinely performed biopsies in 190 patients. World J. Surg., *9*:960–965, 1985.

Tao, L.C.: Transabdominal Fine-Needle Aspiration Biopsy. New York, Igaku-Shoin, 1990.

Trepeta, R.W., Mathur, B., Lagin, S., and LiVolsi, V.A.: Giant cell tumor ("osteoclastoma") of the pancreas: a tumor of epithelial origin. Cancer, *48*:2022–2028, 1981.

Vellet, D., Leiman, G., Mair, S., and Bilchik, A.: Fine needle aspiration cytology of mucinous cystadenocarcinoma of the pancreas. Further observations. Acta Cytol., *32*:43–48, 1988.

Walts, A.E.: Osteoclast-type giant cell tumor of the pancreas. Acta Cytol., *27*:500–504, 1983.

Wilczynski, S.P., Valente, P.T., and Atkinson, B.F.: Cytodiagnosis of adenosquamous carcinoma of the pancreas. Use of intraoperative fine needle aspiration. Acta Cytol., *28*:733–736, 1984.

Spleen

Moeschlin, S.: Die Milzpunktion. Basel, Schwabe, 1947.

Pasternack, A.: Fine needle aspiration biopsy of spleen in diagnosis of generalized amyloidosis. Br. Med. J., *2*:20–22, 1974.

Soderström, N.: How to use cytodiagnostic spleen puncture. Acta Med. Scand., *199*:1–5, 1976.

Soderström, N.: Spleen. *In* Zajicek, J. (ed.): Aspiration Biopsy Cytology. Part 2: Cytology of Infradiaphragmatic Organs. Chap. 9. Basel, S. Karger, 1979.

Kidney

Alanen, K.A., Tyrkko, J.E.S., and Nurmi, M.J.: Aspiration biopsy cytology of renal oncocytoma. Acta Cytol., *29*:859–862, 1985.

Arner, O., Blanck, D., and von Schreeb, T.: Renal adenocarcinoma. Morphology-grading of malignancy-prognosis. Acta Chir. Scand., *346*:11–51, 1965.

Baum, S., Rabinowitz, P., and Malloy, W.A.: The renal scan as an aid in percutaneous renal biopsy. JAMA, *195*:913–915, 1966.

Bennington, J.L., and Beckwith, J.B.: Tumors of the kidney, renal pelvis and ureter. *In* Atlas of Tumor Pathology, ser. 2, fasc. 12. Washington, D.C., Armed Forces Institute of Pathology, 1975.

Bolton, W.K., and Vaughan, E.D., Jr.: A comparative study of open surgical and percutaneous renal biopsies. J. Urol., *117*:696–698, 1977.

Cohen, A.J., Li, F.P., Berg, S., Marchetto, D.J., Tsai, S., Jacobs, S.C., and Brown, R.S.: Hereditary renal-cell carcinoma associated with a chromosomal translocation. N. Engl. J. Med., *301*:592–595, 1979.

Conrad, M.R., Sanders, R.C., and Mascardo, A.D.: Perinephric abscess aspiration using ultrasound guidance. AJR, *128*:459–464, 1977.

Dean, A.L.: Treatment of solitary cyst of kidney by aspiration. Trans. Am. Assoc. Genitourin. Surg., *32*:91–95, 1939.

Domagala, W., Lasota, J., Wolska, H., Lubinski, J., Weber, K., and Osborn, H.: Diagnosis of metastatic renal cell and thyroid carcinomas by intermediate filament typing and cytology of tumor cell in fine needle aspirates. Acta Cytol., *32*:415–421, 1988.

Drut, R., and Pollono, D.: Anaplastic Wilms tumor. Initial diagnosis by fine needle aspiration. Acta Cytol., *32*:774–776, 1987.

Farrow, G.M., Harrison, E.G., Jr., and Utz, D.C.: Sarcomas and sarcomatoid and mixed malignant tumors of the kidney in adults. Cancer, *22*:556–563, 1968.

Flint, A., and Cookingham, C.: Cytologic diagnosis of the papillary variant of renal cell carcinoma. Acta Cytol., *31*:325–329, 1987.

Gibbons, R.P., Bush, W.H., and Burnett, L.L.: Needle tract seeding following aspiration of renal cell carcinoma. J. Urol., *118*:865–867, 1977.

Hamperl, H.: Benign and malignant oncocytoma. Cancer, *15*:1019–1027, 1962.

Hantman, S.S., Barie, J.J., Glendening, T.B., Eisenberg, M.N., and Rapoport, K.D.: Giant renal artery aneurysm mimicking a simple cyst on ultrasound. J. Clin. Ultrasound, *10*:136–139, 1982.

Helm, C.W., Burwood, R.J., Harrison, N.W., and Melcher, D.H.: Aspiration cytology of solid renal tumors. Br. J. Urol., *55*:249–253, 1983.

Iversen, P., and Brun, C.: Aspiration biopsy of the kidney. Am. J. Med., *11*:324–330, 1951.

Kline, T.S.: Handbook of Fine Needle Aspiration Biopsy Cytology, 2nd ed. pp. 433–443. New York, Churchill Livingstone, 1988.

Koss, L.G., Woyke, S., and Olszewski, W.: Aspiration Biopsy. Cytologic Interpretation and Histologic Bases, 2nd ed. New York, Igaku-Shoin, 1992.

Kristensen, J.K., Bartels, E., and Jorgensen, H.E.: Percutaneous renal biopsy under the guidance of ultrasound. Scand. J. Urol. Nephrol., *8*:223–226, 1974.

Kristensen, J.K., Holm, H.H., Rasmussen, S.N., and Barlebo, H.: Ultrasonically guided percutaneous puncture of renal masses. Scand. J. Urol. Nephrol. [Suppl.], *6*:49–56, 1972.

Lang, E.K.: Renal cyst puncture and aspiration: a survey of complications. AJR, *128*:723–727, 1977.

Levine, S.R., Emmett, J.L., and Woolner, L.B.: Cyst and tumor occurring in the same kidney. J. Urol., *91*:1964, 1964.

Linsk, J.A., and Franzen, S.: Clinical Aspiration Cytology, 2nd ed. Philadelphia, J.B. Lippincott, 1989.

Meier, W.L., Willscher, M.K., Novicki, D.E., and Pischinger, R.J.: Evaluation of perihilar and central renal masses using the Chiba needle. J. Urol., *121*:414–416, 1979.

Murphy, W.M., Zambroni, B.R., Emerson, L.D., Moinuddin, S.M., and Lee, L.H.: Aspiration biopsy of the kidney in 152 cases: The value of simultaneously collected cytologic and histologic material in renal cancers. Acta Cytol., *28*:625, 1984.

Nguyen, G.K.: Aspiration biopsy cytology of renal angiomyolipoma. Acta Cytol., *28*:261–264, 1984.

Nguyen, G.K.: Percutaneous fine needle biopsy cytology of the kidney and adrenal. Pathol. Annu., *22*:163–191, 1987.

Orell, S.R., Langlois, S.L., and Marshall, V.R.: Fine needle aspiration cytology in the diagnosis of solid renal and adrenal masses. Scand. J. Urol.. Nephrol., *19*:211–216, 1985.

Pilotti, S., Rilke, F., Alasio, L., and Garbagnati, F.: The role of fine needle aspiration in the assessment of renal masses. Acta Cytol., *32*:1–10, 1988.

Quijano, G., and Drut, R.: Cytologic characteristics of Wilms' tumors in fine needle aspirates. A study of ten cases. Acta Cytol., *33*:263–266, 1989.

Rodriguez, C.A., Buskop, A., Johnson, J., Fromowitz, F., and

Koss, L.G.: Renal oncocytoma. Preoperative diagnosis by aspiration biopsy. Acta Cytol., *24*:355–359, 1980.

Suen, K.C.: Guides to Clinical Aspiration Biopsy: Retroperitoneum and Intestine. Igaku-Shoin, New York, 1987.

von Schreeb, T., Abner, O., Skovsted, G., and Wikstad, N.: Renal adenocarcinoma: is there a risk of spreading tumour cells in diagnostic puncture? Scand. J. Urol. Nephrol., *1*:270–276, 1967.

von Schreeb, T., Franzen, S., and Ljungqvist, A.: Renal adenocarcinoma. Scand. J. Urol. Nephrol., *1*:265–269, 1967.

Von Willebrand, E.: Fine needle aspiration cytology of renal transplants: background and present applications. Transplant. Proc., *17*:2071–2074, 1985.

Zornoza, J., Handel, P., Lukeman, J.M., Jing, B.S., and Wallace, S.: Percutaneous transperitoneal biopsy in urologic malignancies. Urology, *9*:395–398, 1977.

Adrenal Glands

Abrams, H.L., Siegelman, S.S., Adams, D.F., Sanders, R., Finberg, H.J., Hessel, S.J., and McNeil, B.J.: Computed tomography versus ultrasound of the adrenal gland: a prospective study. Radiology, *143*:121–128, 1982.

Heaton, D.K., Handel, D.B., and Ashton, P.R.: Narrow gauge needle aspiration of solid adrenal masses. AJR, *138*:1143–1148, 1982.

Katz, R.L., Patel, S., Mackay, B., and Zornoza, J.: Fine needle aspiration cytology of the adrenal gland. Acta Cytol., *28*;269–282, 1984.

Levin, N.P.: Fine needle aspiration and histology of adrenal cortical carcinoma. A case report. Acta Cytol., *25*:421–424, 1981.

Min, K.-W., Song, J., Boesenberg, M., and Acebey, J.: Adrenal cortical nodule mimicking small round cell malignancy on fine needle aspiration. Acta Cytol., *32*:543–546, 1988.

Mitchell, M.L., Ryan, F.P., and Shermen, R.W.: Pulmonary adenocarcinoma metastatic to the adrenal gland mimicking normal adrenal cortical epithelium on fine needle aspiration. Acta Cytol., *29*:994–998, 1985.

Moussouris, H.F., Koss, L.G., Rosenblatt, R., and Kutcher, R.: Thin needle aspiration biopsy of abdominal organs. *In* Koss, L.G., and Coleman, D.V. (eds.): Advances in Clinical Cytology, vol. 2. pp. 191–241. New York, Masson Publishing, 1984.

Nguyen, G.-K.: Percutaneous fine needle biopsy cytology of the kidney and adrenal. Pathol. Annu., *22*:163–191, 1987.

Nguyen, G.-K.: Cytopathologic aspects of adrenal pheochromocytoma in a fine needle aspiration biopsy. Acta Cytol., *26*:354–358, 1982.

Pinto, M.M.: Fine needle aspiration of myelolipoma of the adrenal gland. Report of a case with computed tomography. Acta Cytol., *29*:863–866, 1985.

Scheible, W., Coel, M., Siemers, P.T., and Siegel, H.: Percutaneous aspiration of adrenal cysts. AJR, *128*:1013–1016, 1977.

White, E.A., Schambelan, M., Rost, C.R., Biglieri, E.G., Moss, A.A., and Korobkin, M.: Use of computed tomography in diagnosing the cause of primary aldosteronism. N. Engl. J. Med., *303*:1503–1507, 1980.

Wilson, R.A., and Ibanez, M.L.: A comparative study of 14 cases of familial and nonfamilial pheochromocytoma. Hum. Pathol., *9*:181–188, 1978.

Yeh, H.C.: Sonography of the adrenal glands: normal glands and small masses. AJR, *135*:1167–1177, 1980.

Retroperitoneum

Bonfiglio, T.A., MacIntosh, P.K., Patten, S.F., Jr., Cafer, D.J., Woodworth, F.E., and Kim, C.W.: Fine needle aspiration cytopathology of retroperitoneal lymph nodes in the evaluation of metastatic disease. Acta Cytol., *23*:126–130, 1979.

Brascho, D.J., Durant, J.R., and Green, L.E.: The accuracy of retroperitoneal ultrasonography in Hodgkin's disease and non-Hodgkin's lymphoma. Radiology, *125*:485–487, 1977.

Cochand-Priollet, B., Roger, B., Boccon-Gibod, J., Ferrand, J., Faure, B., and Blery, M.: Retroperitoneal lymph node aspiration biopsy in staging of pelvic cancer: a cytological study of 228 consecutive cases. Diagn. Cytopathol., *3*:102–107, 1987.

Droese, M., Altmannsberger, M., Kehl, A., Lankisch, P.G., Weiss, R., Weber, K., and Osborn, M.: Ultrasound-guided percutaneous fine needle aspiration biopsy of abdominal and retroperitoneal masses. Accuracy of cytology in the diagnosis of malignancy, cytologic tumor typing and use of antibodies to intermediate filaments in selected cases. Acta Cytol., *28*:368–384, 1984.

Dunnick, N.R., Fischer, R.I., and Chu, E.W.: Percutaneous aspiration of retroperitoneal lymph nodes in ovarian cancer. AJR, *135*:109–113, 1980.

Edeiken-Monroe, B.S.E., and Zornoza, J.: Carcinoma of the cervix: percutaneous lymph node aspiration biopsy. AJR, *138*:655-657, 1982.

Efremides, S.C., Dan, S., Nieburgs, H., and Mitty, H.A.: Carcinoma of the prostate: lymph node aspiration for staging. AJR, *136*:489–492, 1981.

Ennis, M.G., and MacErlean, D.P.: Percutaneous aspiration biopsy of abdomen and retroperitoneum. Clin. Radiol., *31*:611–616, 1980.

Glatstein, E., Guernsey, J.M., Rosenberg, S.A., and Kaplan, H.S.: The value of laparotomy and splenectomy in the staging of Hodgkin's disease. Cancer, *24*:709–718, 1969.

Gothlin, J.H.: Percutaneous transperitoneal fluoroscopy. Guided fine needle biopsy of lymph nodes. Acta Radiol. (Diagn.), *20*:660–664, 1979.

Gothlin, J.H.: Post-lymphographic percutaneous fine needle biopsy of lymph nodes guided by fluoroscopy. Radiology, *120*:205–207, 1976.

Gothlin, J.H., and Hoiem, L.: Percutaneous fine needle biopsy of radiographically normal lymph nodes in the staging of prostatic carcinoma. Radiology, *141*:351–354, 1981.

Hidai, H., Sakuramoto, T., Miura, T., Nakahashi, M., and Kikyo, S.: Needle tract seeding following puncture of retroperitoneal liposarcoma. Eur. Urol., *9*:368–369, 1983.

Kinmoth, J.B.: Lymphography in man. Clin. Sci., *11*:13–20, 1952.

Knelson, M., Haaga, J., Lazarus, H., Ghosh, C., Abdul-Karim, F., and Sorenson, K.: Computed tomography-guided retroperitoneal biopsies. J. Clin. Oncol., *7*:1169–1173, 1989.

Koss, L.G., Woyke, S., and Olszewski, W.: Aspiration Biopsy. Cytologic Interpretation and Histologic Bases. New York, Igaku-Shoin, 1984, 2nd Ed., 1992.

Lagergren, C., and Friberg, S.: Aspiration biopsy of lymph nodes after lymphography. Proc. Swed. Soc. Med. Radiol., *5*:14–15, 1976.

MacIntosh, P.K., Thompson, K.R., and Barbaric, Z.L.: Percutaneous transperitoneal lymph node biopsy as a means of improving lymphographic diagnosis. Radiology, *131*:647–649, 1979.

Mugharbil Z.H., Tannenbaum, M., and Schapira, H.: Retroperitoneal malignant fibrous histiocytoma: case report and literature review. Mt. Sinai J. Med., *54*:158–161, 1987.

Otal-Salaverri, C., Gonzalez-Campora, R., Hevia-Vazquez, A., Lerma-Puertas, E., and Galera-Davidson, H.: Retroperitoneal ganglioneuroblastoma. Report of a case diagnosed by fine needle aspiration cytology and electron microscopy. Acta Cytol., *33*:80–84, 1989.

Pereiras, R.V., Meirers, W., Kunhardt, B., Troner, M., Hutson, D., Barkin, J.S., and Viamonte, M.: Fluoroscopically guided thin needle aspiration biopsy of the abdomen and retroperitoneum. AJR, *131*:197–202, 1978.

Tao, L.C., Negin, M.L., and Donat, E.E.: Primary retroperitoneal seminoma diagnosed by fine needle aspiration biopsy. A case report. Acta Cytol., *28*:598–600, 1984.

Thomson, K.R., House, A.J.S., Gothlin, J.H., and Dolan, T.E.: Percutaneous lymph node aspiration biopsy: experience with a new technique. Clin. Radiol., *28*:329–332, 1977.

Valkov, I., and Bojikin, B.: Fine needle aspiration biopsy of abdominal and retroperitoneal tumors in infants and children. Diagn. Cytopathol., *3*:129–133, 1987.

Zornoza, J., Cabanillas, F.F., Altoff, T.M., Ordonez, N., and Cohen, M.A.: Percutaneous needle biopsy in abdominal lymphoma. AJR, *136*:97–103, 1981.

Zornoza, J., Lukeman, J.M., Jing, B.S., Wharton, J.T., and Wallace, S.: Percutaneous retroperitoneal lymph node biopsy in carcinoma of the cervix. Gynecol. Oncol., *5*:43–51, 1977.

Zornoza, J., Wallace, S., Goldstein, M., Lukeman, J.M., and Jing, B.: Transperitoneal percutaneous retroperitoneal lymph node aspiration biopsy. Radiology, *122*:111–115, 1977.

Bone

Adler, O., and Rosenberger, A.: Fine needle aspiration biopsy of osteolytic metastatic lesions. AJR, *133*:15–18, 1979.

Agarwal, P.K., and Wahal, K.M.: Cytopathologic study of primary tumors of bones and joints. Acta Cytol., *27*:23–27, 1983.

Akerman, M., Berg, N.O., and Persson, B.M.: Fine needle aspiration biopsy in the evaluation of tumor-like lesions of bone. Acta Orthop. Scand., *47*:129–136, 1976.

Ayala, A.G., Raymond, A.K., Ro, J.Y., Carrasco, C.H., Fanning, C.V., and Murray, J.A.: Needle biopsy of primary bone lesions. M.D. Anderson experience. Pathol. Annu., *24*:219–251, 1989.

Coley, B.L., Sharp, G.S., and Ellis, E.B.: Diagnosis of bone tumors by aspiration. Am. J. Surg., *13*:215–224, 1931.

Dahl, I., Akerman, M., and Angervall, L.: Ewing's sarcoma of bone. A correlative cytological and histological study of 14 cases. Acta Pathol. Microbiol. Immunol. Scand., *94*:363–369, 1986.

Dollahite, H.A., Tatum, L., Moinuddin, S.M., and Carnesale, P.G.: Aspiration biopsy of primary neoplasms of bone. J. Bone Joint Surg., *71*:1166–1169, 1989.

Elliot, E.C., McKinney, S., Banks, H., and Fulks, R.M.: Aspiration cytology of metastatic chordoma: a case report. Acta Cytol., *27*:658–662, 1983.

Eneroth, C.-M.: Histological aspects of parapharyngeal tumors. *In* Hamberger, C.A., and Wersall, J. (eds.): Disorders of the Skull Base Region. Nobel Symp., *10*:309–312, 1968.

Franzén, S., and Stenkvist, B.: Cytologic diagnosis of eosino-
philic granuloma-reticulo-endotheliosis. Acta Pathol. Microbiol., *72*:385–390, 1968.

Hajdu, S.I.: Aspiration biopsy of primary malignant bone tumors. Radiat. Ther. Oncol., *10*:73–81, 1975.

Hajdu, S.I., and Melamed, M.R.: Needle biopsy of primary malignant bone tumors. Surg. Gynecol. Obstet., *133*:829–832, 1971.

Kannon, V., and Von-Rudden, D.: Malignant fibrous histiocytoma of bone: initial diagnosis by aspiration biopsy cytology. Diagn. Cytopathol., *4*:262–264, 1988.

Kontozoglou, T., Krakauer, K., and Qizilbash, A.H.: Ewing's sarcoma. Cytologic features in fine needle aspirates in two cases. Acta Cytol., *30*:513–518, 1986.

Kontozoglou, T., Qizilbash, A.H., Sianos, J., and Stead, R.: Chordoma: cytologic and immunocytochemical study of four cases. Diagn. Cytopathol., *2*:55–61, 1986.

Koss, L.G., Woyke, S., and Olszewski, W. Aspiration Biopsy. Cytologic Interpretation and Histologic Bases. New York, Igaku-Shoin, 1984; 2nd ed, 1992.

Layfield, L.J., and Bhuta, S.: Fine-needle aspiration cytology of histiocytosis X: a case report. Diagn. Cytopathol., *4*:140–143, 1988.

Layfield, L.J., Glasgow, B.J., Anders, K.H., and Mirra, J.M.: Fine-needle aspiration cytology of primary bone lesions. Acta Cytol., *31*:177–184, 1987.

Lefer, L.G., and Rosier, P.R.: The cytology of chordoma. Acta Cytol., *22*:51–53, 1978.

Olszewski, W., Woyke, S., and Musiatowicz, B.: Fine needle aspiration biopsy cytology of chondrosarcoma. Acta Cytol., *27*:345–349, 1983.

Ottolenghi, C.E.: Diagnosis of orthopaedic lesions by aspiration biopsy. Results of 1,061 punctures. J. Bone Joint Surg., *37A*:443–464, 1955.

Reif, R.M.: Ewing's sarcoma; cytology of large cell type. Acta Cytol., *24*:175–176, 1980.

Sanerkin, N.G., and Jaffree, G.M.: Cytology of Bone Tumours, A Colour Atlas with Text. Philadelphia, J.B. Lippincott, 1980.

Schajowicz, F., and Derqui, J.C.: Puncture biopsy in lesions of the locomotor system; review of results in 4050 cases, including 941 vertebral punctures. Cancer, *21*:531–548, 1968.

Schajowicz, F., and Hokama, J.: Aspiration (puncture or needle) biopsy in bone lesions. Recent results. Cancer Res., *54*:139–144, 1976.

Silverman, J.F., Larkin, E.W., Carney, M., Weaver, M.D., and Norris, H.T.: Fine needle aspiration cytology of tuberculosis of the lumbar vertebrae (Pott's disease). Acta Cytol., *30*:538–542, 1986.

Sneige, N., Ayala, A.G., Corrasco, C.H., Murray, J., and Raymond, A.K.: Giant cell tumor of bone: a cytologic study of 24 cases. Diagn. Cytopathol., *1*:111–117, 1985.

Snyder, R.E., and Coley, B.L.: Further studies on the diagnosis of bone tumors by aspiration biopsy. Surg. Gynecol. Obstet., *80*:517–522, 1945.

Stormby, N., and Akerman, M.: Cytodiagnosis of bone lesions by means of fine needle aspiration biopsy. Acta Cytol., *17*:166–172, 1973.

Szyfelbein, W.M., and Schiller, A.L.: Cytologic diagnosis of giant cell tumor of bone metastatic to lung. A case report. Acta Cytol., *23*:460–464, 1979.

Thommesen, P., and Frederiksen, P.: Fine needle aspiration biopsy of bone lesions. Clinical value. Acta Orthop. Scand., *47*:137–143, 1976.

Thommesen, P., Frederiksen, P., Lowhagen, T., and Willems, J.-S.: Needle aspiration biopsy in the diagnosis of lytic bone lesions in histiocytosis X, Ewing's sarcoma and neuroblastoma. Acta Radiol. Oncol. Radiat. Ther. Phys. Biol., *17*:145–149, 1978.

Thompson, S.K., and Callery, R.T.: Cytologic diagnosis of a chordoma without physaliforous cells. Diagn. Cytopathol., *4*:144–147, 1988.

Valls, J., Ottolenghi, C.E., and Schajowicz, F.: Aspiration biopsy in diagnosis of lesions of vertebral bodies. JAMA, *136*:376–382, 1948.

Watson, C.W., Unger, P., Kaneko, M., and Gabrilove, J.L.: Fine needle aspiration of osteitis fibrosa cystica. Diagn. Cytopathol., *1*:157–160, 1985.

White, V.A., Fanning, C.V., Ayala, A.G., Raymond, A.K., Carrasco, C.H., and Murray, J.A.: Osteosarcoma and the role of fine needle aspiration. A study of 51 cases. Cancer, *62*:1238–1246, 1988.

Willems, J.-S.: Aspiration biopsy cytology of tumors and tumor-suspect lesions of bone. *In* Linsk, J.A., Franzen, S. (eds.): Clinical Aspiration Cytology, 2nd ed. pp. 349–359. Philadelphia, J.B. Lippincott, 1989.

Eye and Orbit

Char, D.H., and Norman, D.: The use of computed tomography and ultrasonography in the evaluation of orbital masses. Surg. Ophthalmol., *27*:49–63, 1982.

Cristallini, E.G., Bolis, G.B., and Ottaviano, P.: Fine needle aspiration biopsy of orbital meningioma. Report of a case. Acta Cytol., *34*:236–238, 1990.

Czerniak, B., Woyke, S., Daniel, R., Krzysztolik, Z., and Koss, L.G.: Diagnosis of orbital tumors by aspiration biopsy guided by computerized tomography. Cancer, *54*:2385–2388, 1985.

Czerniak, B., Woyke, S., Krzysztolik, Z., and Domagala, W.: Fine needle aspiration biopsy of intraocular melanoma. Acta Cytol., *27*:157–165, 1983.

Das, D.K., Das, J., Chachra, K.L., and Natarajan, R.: Diagnosis of retinoblastoma by fine needle aspiration and aqueous cytology. Diagn. Cytopathol., *5*:203–206, 1989.

Dubois, P.J., Kennerdell, J.S., Rosenbaum, A.E., Dekker, A., Johnson, B.R., and Swink, C.A.: Computed tomographic localization of fine needle aspiration biopsy of orbital tumors. Radiology, *131*:149–152, 1979.

Jakobiec, F., and Chattock, A.: The role of cytology and needle biopsies in the diagnosis of ophthalmic tumors and simulating condition. *In* Jakobiec, F. (ed.): Ocular and Adnexal Tumors. pp. 341–358. Birmingham, Ala., Aesculapius, 1978.

Jakobiec, F.A., Coleman, D.J., Chattock, A., and Smith, M.: Ultrasonically guided needle biopsy and cytologic diagnosis of solid intraocular tumors. Ophthalmology, *86*:1662–1678, 1979.

Kennerdell, J.S., Dekker, A., Johnson, B., and Dubois, P.J.: Fine needle aspiration biopsy. Its use in orbital tumors. Arch. Ophthalmol., *97*:1315–1317, 1979.

Kennerdell, J.S., Dubois, P.J., Dekker, A., and Johnson, B.: CT guided fine needle aspiration biopsy of orbital optic nerve tumors. Ophthalmology, *87*:491–496, 1980.

Kopelman, J.E., and Shorr, N.: A case of prostatic carcinoma metastatic to orbit diagnosed by fine needle aspiration and immunoperoxidase staining for prostatic specific antigen. Ophthal. Surg., *18*:599–603, 1987.

Koss, L.G., Woyke, S., and Olszewski, W. Aspiration Biopsy.

Cytologic Interpretation and Histologic Bases. New York, Igaku-Shoin, 1984; 2nd ed, 1992.

Naib, Z.M.: Cytology of ocular lesions. Acta Cytol., *16*:178–185, 1972.

Naib, Z.M.: Cytology of ophthalmological disease. *In* Koss, L.G., and Coleman, D.W. (eds.): Advances in Clinical Cytology. pp. 232–253, London, Butterworths, 1981.

Naib, Z.M., Clepper, A.S., and Elliot, S.R.: Exfoliative cytology as an aid in the diagnosis of ophthalmic lesions. Acta Cytol., *11*:295–303, 1967.

Otto, R.A., Templer, J.W., Renner, G., and Hurt, M.: Secondary and metastatic tumors of the orbit. Otolaryngol. Head Neck Surg., *97*:328–334, 1987.

Rodriguez, A.: Diagnosis of retinoblastoma by cytology examination of the aqueous and vitreous. Med. Probl. Ophthalmol., *18*:142–148, 1977.

Sagiroglu, N., Ozgonul, T., and Muderris, S.: Diagnostic intraocular cytology. Acta Cytol., *19*:32–37, 1975.

Sanderson, T.L., Pustai, W., Shelly, L., Gelender, H., and Ng, A.B.P.: Cytologic evaluation of ocular lesions. Acta Cytol., *24*:391–400, 1980.

Schumann, G.B., O'Dowd, G.J., and Spinnler, P.A.: Eye cytology. Lab. Med., *11*:533–540, 1980.

Schyberg, E.: Fine needle biopsy of orbital tumors [abstr.]. Acta Ophthalmol. [Suppl.], *53*:11, 1975.

Spoor, T.C., Kennerdell, J.S., Dekker, A., Johnson, B., and Rehkopf, P.: Orbital fine needle aspiration biopsy with B-scan guidance. Am. J. Ophthalmol., *89*:274–277, 1980.

Takeda, M., Maguire, N.L.C., Augsburger, J.J., and Shields, J.A.: Cytologic diagnosis of ocular malignant melanoma. Acta Cytol., *26*:743–744, 1982.

Vade, A., and Armstrong, D.: Orbital rhabdomyosarcoma in childhood. Radiol. Clin. North Am., *25*:701–714, 1987.

Westman-Naeser, S., and Naeser, P.: Tumors of the orbit diagnosed by fine needle biopsy. Acta Ophthalmol., *56*:969–976, 1974.

Wolter, R., and Naylor, B.: A membrane filter method: used to diagnose intraocular tumor. J. Pediatr. Ophthalmol., *5*:36–38, 1968.

Central Nervous System

Adams, J.H., Graham, D.I., and Doyle, D.: Brain Biopsy. The Smear Technique for Neurosurgical Biopsies. Philadelphia, J.B. Lippincott, 1981.

Backlund, E.O.: A new instrument for stereotaxic brain tumor biopsy. Acta Chir. Scand., *137*:825–827, 1971.

Barnard, R.O.: Smear preparations in the diagnosis of malignant lesions of the central nervous system. *In* Koss, L.G., and Coleman, D.V. (eds.): Advances in Clinical Cytology. pp. 254–269, London, Butterworth, 1981.

Boethius, J., Collins, V.P., Edner, G., Lewander, R., and Zajicek, J.: Stereotaxic biopsies and computer tomography in gliomas. Acta Neurochir., *40*:223–232, 1978.

Burger, P.C., and Kleihues, P.: Cytologic composition of the untreated glioblastoma with implications for evaluation of needle biopsies. Cancer, *63*:2014–2023, 1989.

Crain, B.J., Bigner, S.H., and Johnston, W.W.: Fine needle aspiration biopsy of deep cerebrum. A comparison of normal and neoplastic morphology. Acta Cytol., *26*:772–778, 1982.

DelBrutto, O.H., and Sotelo, J.: Neurocysticercosis: an update. Rev. Infect. Dis., *10*:1075–1087, 1988.

Eisenhardt, L., and Cushing, H.: Diagnosis of intracranial tumors by supravital technique. Am. J. Pathol., 6:541–552, 1930.

Grisolia, J.S., and Wiederholt, W.C.: CNS cysticercosis. Arch. Neurol., *39*:540–544, 1982.

Jane, J.A., and Bertrand, G.: A cytological method for the diagnosis of tumors affecting the central nervous system. J. Neuropathol. Exp. Neurol., *21*:400–409, 1962.

Jane, J.A., and Yashon, D.: Cytology of Tumors Affecting the Nervous System. Springfield, Ill., Charles C Thomas, 1969.

Liwnicz, B.H., Henderson, K.S., Masukawa, T., and Smith, R.D.: Needle aspiration cytology of intracranial lesions. A review of 84 cases. Acta Cytol., *26*:779–896, 1982.

McLeod, R., Berry, P.F., Marshall, W.H., Hunt, S.A., Ryning, F.W., and Remington, J.S.: Toxoplasmosis presenting as brain abscess. Diagnosis by computerized tomography and cytology of aspirated purulent material. Am. J. Med., *67*:711–714, 1979.

McMenemey, W.H.: An appraisal of smear-diagnosis in neurosurgery. Am. J. Clin. Pathol., *33*:471–479, 1960.

Rubinstein, L.J.: Tumors of the central nervous system. *In* Atlas of Tumor Pathology, ser. 2, fasc. 6, Washington, D.C., Armed Forces Institute of Pathology, 1972.

Zaharopoulos, P., and Wong, J.Y.: Cytology of common primary midline brain tumors. Acta Cytol., *24*:384–390, 1980.

30

Circulating Cancer Cells

Myron R. Melamed, M.D.

There is no doubt that cancer cells from almost any kind of malignant tumor can and often do enter into the blood circulation and are thereby transported to distant sites, where they may lodge and grow. In fact, this is the only reasonable mechanism to explain discrete metastases in distant organs that are unrelated by lymphatics.[7] Further, it has been shown that visceral metastases are common and survival is shortened when venous invasion by malignant tumor is demonstrated.[8,17,43,51,129]

The original concepts of tumor cell embolization as a mechanism for dissemination of cancer were developed during the 19th century, in parallel with other basic advances in pathology that followed improved microscopy, and the reader may find key references in the historical reviews by Ewing,[35] Willis,[140] and others[50,136,138]

The frequency with which veins are invaded by malignant neoplasms was stressed long ago by Goldmann,[47] who reported grossly visible venous invasion in about 20% of 500 necropsies and microscopic invasion of veins in nearly 10% more (Fig. 30–1). Yet the number of cancer cells that may be found within the bloodstream (excluding the leukemias, of course) is infinitesimal when compared with the number of normal blood cellular elements. In fact, it is extraordinary to find cancer cells in routine blood smears,[11,22,31,38,44,48,61,81,96] and the task of separating or concentrating these cells and giving them their proper identification has proved to be a major technical problem that is still not satisfactorily solved.

HISTORICAL DEVELOPMENT OF STUDIES

The earliest recorded description of free-floating cancer cells in a specimen of blood was that by Ashworth in 1869. He reported finding tumor cells in direct smears of postmortem saphenous venous blood from a 38-year-old man who died with disseminated subcutaneous malignant tumors.[4] Isolated observations of a similar nature were subsequently reported by Schleip[117] and Ward[133] in cases of gastric carcinoma, by Marcus in finger blood from a patient with lung cancer,[75] by Loeper and Loeste in two patients with sarcoma,[66] and by Quensel in the hearts' blood from six of 50 cadavers with various malignant tumors.[94]

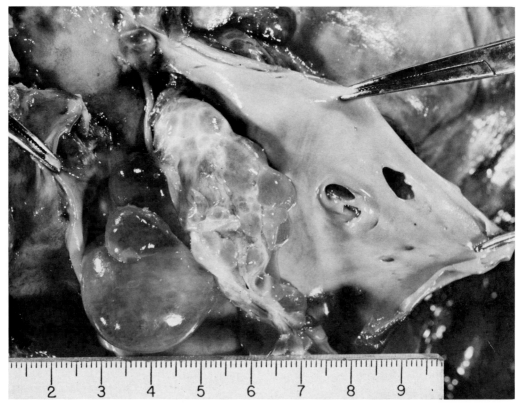

FIGURE 30–1.   Venous invasion by cancer is common, and occasionally there is massive intravascular growth. A testicular teratoma is illustrated here, growing upward within the inferior vena cava. Billroth reported just such a case in 1855 as one of the first examples of venous invasion by cancer (cited by Willis).

In 1934 Pool and Dunlop carried out the first deliberate search for cancer cells in the blood from a series of living patients.[89] Their technique was crude: 5 ml of oxalated blood was hemolyzed with 15% acetic acid and the centrifuged sediment fixed with 10% formalin in alcohol, then embedded in paraffin and step-sectioned. They found what were apparently significant large spherical cells with hyperchromatic nuclei in 17 of 40 cancer cases, but also in one patient with a benign gastric ulcer.

In 1954 Cole, Packard, and Southwick demonstrated cancer cells in the perfusate from the mesenteric vessels of a resected segment of colon with carcinoma.[15] In the following year Fisher and Turnbull studied 25 consecutive patients with colorectal carcinoma undergoing surgical resection and found tumor cells in the blood and perfusate from mesenteric veins of eight (32%).[42] They suggested that tumor cells were dislodged by operative manipulation, and Turnbull et al. subsequently reported that ligation and division of the

lymphovascular pedicle before manipulation of the tumor increased five-year survival.[132]

A study of major importance among the early publications was the work of Engell in 1955, who reported in great detail on the incidence of cancer cells in regional venous and peripheral blood.[32] He used 2 to 5 ml of heparinized blood in most cases, lysed the red cells with 1% saponin, and embedded the remaining cellular sediment in paraffin for serial sections and hematoxylin-eosin stain. Engell found cancer cells in blood draining the tumor area of 63 of 107 colorectal carcinomas (59%), 6 of 8 cases of gastric carcinoma, 3 of 4 cases of lung cancer, and 3 of 6 cases of breast cancer. Peripheral blood from the cubital vein of 14 patients with advanced, inoperable carcinoma was examined, and cancer cells were found in seven; whereas in the peripheral blood from the cubital vein or brachial artery of 79 patients with operable carcinoma, he noted cancer cells in ten. He found cancer cells in the blood more often in patients with the more anaplastic tumors but was unable to demonstrate any relationship to the local extent of the tumor or to operative manipulation. Interestingly, in a follow-up publication 4 years later, he was unable to correlate the presence or absence of cancer cells in the blood with the length of survival.[33]

Engell's work marked the beginning of an extraordinary interest in cancer cells in the blood. During little more than a decade after his second report, there were many other publications concerned with both the technical problems of preparation and cytologic interpretation as well as the actual results and their clinical correlation. Because the accuracy of the examination depends greatly on the quality of the preparation, a brief review of preparatory methods is necessary.

TECHNICAL METHODS

The great variety of techniques that has been proposed for processing specimens is probably a reflection of dissatisfaction with any one of them. Those that are most widely used are based on the methods of Seal,[119-121] Roberts et al.,[103] and Malmgren et al.[73] Their common purpose is the selection or concentration of any cancer cells that may be present, and in general they share certain immediate aims. The most important of these are removal of the red blood cell mass, removal of as many normal leukocytes as possible, maximum preservation of cell morphology, and quantitative reproducibility.

Separation of the red cell mass has been accomplished either by *hemolysis*, initially with water[94] and later with acetic acid,[42,89,107] saponin,[32,34,85] or such enzymes as streptolysin-O[91]; or by *sedimentation*, usually with an accelerating factor such as fibrinogen,[9,103,110] dextran,[2,25,26] phytohemagglutinin,[65] or hemolymph heteroagglutinin.[135]

Sedimentation and separation of cell types may be facilitated by differential centrifugation after suspending the blood in a solution of albumen,[36,70,103] gum acacia,[126] or silicone[120] of specific gravity adjusted between that of the heavier red cells (1.092–1.097) and the lighter cancer cells and lymphocytes (1.056–1.065). Polyvinylpyrrolidone and a detergent "wetting" agent are often added to prevent cell clumping and to keep platelets and cellular debris in suspension during centrifugation. Danielsson[21] suggested using a spiral centrifuge for continuous separation of the lighter cellular elements, but this offers little practical advantage for the relatively small volumes of blood usually examined. Many of the polymorphonuclear leukocytes are also removed by lysis with streptolysin-O or by differential centrifugation since they are heavier than lymphocytes and most cancer cells.

Another rather novel technique for removing phagocytic cells, such as polymorphonuclear leukocytes, involves adding carbonyl iron of 3-μm particle size to heparinized blood and, after 30 minutes of incubation at 37°C, removing the iron-containing cells by stirring the solution with a magnet.[62]

After the blood has been prepared by one or several of these techniques, the final cell suspension is transferred to membrane filters,[119] or centrifuged onto glass slides,[34] or smeared on glass slides, and stained. Much better cell detail is obtained by any of these methods than by the older technique of step-sections of the cell sediment after paraffin embedding.

The best preparations for cytologic detail have been obtained by Roberts et al.,[99,103] using fibrinogen sedimentation to remove most of the red blood cells, and then concentrating any cancer cells in the supernatant plasma by overlaying it on an albumen solution of specific gravity 1.065, followed by centrifugation. Most cancer cells are relatively light and will collect at the plasma-albumen interface, whereas the heavier leukocytes and remaining red blood cells are carried through the interface and collect at the bottom of the tube. The cells are aspirated from the interface, washed, streaked directly on glass slides, and stained with the Papanicolaou stain (Fig. 30–2).

The membrane filters have proved more convenient and more popular and have the advantage of possibly better quantitation (Fig. 30–3).

The choice of stain is a matter of personal preference. Hematoxylin and eosin or the Papanicolaou stain is commonly used with all types of preparations; Wright-Giemsa stains or acridine orange[26] is generally restricted to smears on glass slides.

Direct separation of cells by size alone has been attempted by using either a 10-μm pore membrane filter[138] or a 4.5- to 5-μm pore perforated plastic membrane as a sieve.[121] The latter method gives technically good preparations in addition to its great simplicity. A sample of blood, properly anticoagulated, is simply poured through the perforated plastic membrane. The red blood cells and most of the smaller leukocytes readily pass through. The larger cells, including the cancer cells, are retained and adhere to the plastic membrane. The membrane remains clear and transparent dur-

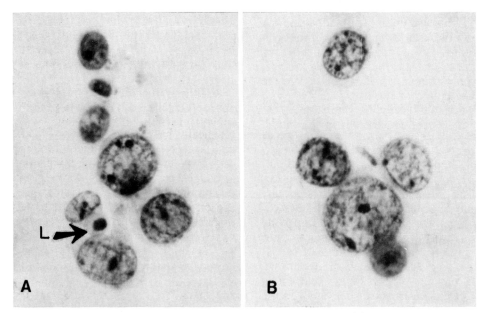

FIGURE 30–2.   Cells of carcinoma of the breast in peripheral blood. (*A*) Group of cancer cells isolated from the antecubital vein during skin preparation prior to surgery. L = lymphocyte. Prepared by fibrinogen sedimentation, differential centrifugation over albumen and smearing directly on a glass slide. (*B*) Direct smear of resected tumor from the same patient. (*A, B,* Papanicolaou stain ×1,000. Dr. E. McGrew, University of Illinois, from Cole, W. H., et al.: The dissemination of cancer cells. Bull. N.Y. Acad. Med., *34*:163–183)

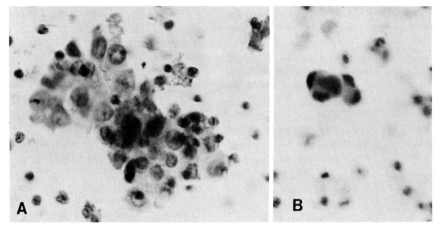

FIGURE 30–3.   (*A, B*) Clumps of cancer cells in venous blood of patients with bronchogenic carcinoma. Specimens on Millipore filters prepared by silicone flotation method of Seal. (*A, B* ×560. Dr. S. H. Seal)

ing staining and can be mounted for screening on a glass slide (see Figs. 30–4 to 30–8).

OBSERVATIONS

The likelihood of finding cancer cells in the blood of patients known to have cancer has been variously reported from less than 1% to as much as 96.5%. There are many reviews of these published figures, and they emphasize the extraordinary differences in results from different laboratories.[12,46,50,83] It is pertinent to note that in later years a growing body of experienced workers in the field have emphasized the danger of misinterpreting certain benign cells in the blood as cancer cells. Probably many of the reported counts of cancer cells in the blood are erroneously high. In our own experience, principally with patients having lung and breast cancer, cancer cells were found in the peripheral venous blood of 1% of the patients or less.

Some of the variation in published reports is due to technical differences in the method of processing, the use of peripheral versus regional venous blood, differences in the number and volume of samples examined, and differences in the type of cancer and the stage of the disease. It seems clear that the likelihood of finding cancer cells is greater in regional venous blood draining the cancer site than in peripheral venous or arterial blood, greater when more specimens or larger volumes of blood are examined,[53] greater late in the course of the disease when cancer is disseminated, and probably greater when tumor masses are disturbed mechanically by manipulation during surgery or physical examination.[7a,60,106,132] It is also worth noting that specimens of blood and perfusate from surgical specimens (or those taken at autopsy) are not to be compared with blood samples drawn by venipuncture from the living patient.

The major source of discrepancies, however, is undoubtedly due to differences in interpretation and classification of certain cells that are rarely found in ordinary blood smears.[30] Megakaryocytes, endothelial cells, and immature hematopoietic cells are not normally expected in peripheral blood smears from individuals without hematologic disorders, but they are found with surprising regularity in the concentrates prepared for cancer cell studies.

Criteria for differential diagnosis of cells likely to be confused with cancer cells in processed specimens of blood have been described in detail by McGrew and associates,[69,71,72] Alexander and Spriggs,[2] Scheinin and Koivuniemi,[114] Griffiths and Salsbury,[50] and the Circulating Cancer Cell Cooperative.[82] Megakaryocytes and immature myeloid cells appear to be the most common of such cells.

Mature megakaryocytes may be very large, commonly measuring as much as 50 to 100 μm or more. In prepulmonic venous blood they characteristically have abundant, finely granular cytoplasm and a cytoplasmic membrane that is either sharply defined or ragged with adherent platelets, although a certain number of the cells are partially or completely stripped of cytoplasm. The nuclei are large and lobulated or multiple, with well-defined chromatin structure. They contain multiple nucleoli, usually at least one in each lobe, but these are sometimes poorly defined with the Papanicolaou stain. Within the nuclei also there are multiple small areas of nuclear clearing about a central chromatin mass, emphasized as characteristic by McGrew (Fig. 30–4). In postpulmonic peripheral blood, megakaryocytes are typically stripped of cytoplasm, and their nuclei are contracted or fragmented and usually dark-staining but still lobulated. Nuclear chromatin detail is often obscured (Fig. 30–5).

Megakaryoblasts are somewhat smaller than mature megakaryocytes and have much less cytoplasm, a large round or bilobed nucleus with more delicate chromatin, and one or several nucleoli.

Some immature myeloid and lymphoid cells are likely to be mistaken for epithelial cancer cells because of their similar size. Cytoplasmic granules are indistinct with the Papanicolaou stain. Nuclei are rounded, reniform, or lobulated. Nucleoli may be multiple and prominent, though they are rarely as large as those in many epithelial cancer cells. Plasma cells and their precursors may be recognized by the peripheral clumping of nuclear chromatin, often asymmetric positioning of the nucleus, and dark cytoplasmic staining with a paranuclear "hof" or clearing.

Large lymphocytes, monocytes, and mononuclear macrophages may measure as much as 20 μm in diameter. Usually, these cells have bland-appearing nuclei and, occasionally, small nucleoli. Poorly preserved cells of this type or cells without specific characteristics may be difficult to identify (Fig. 30–6). They can be mistaken for small cancer cells, particularly if they are degenerating and hyperchromatic. Probably it is this group that accounts for most of what are reported as "atypical" cells.[78]

Endothelial cells can be dislodged by the needle as a specimen of blood is obtained. They may be

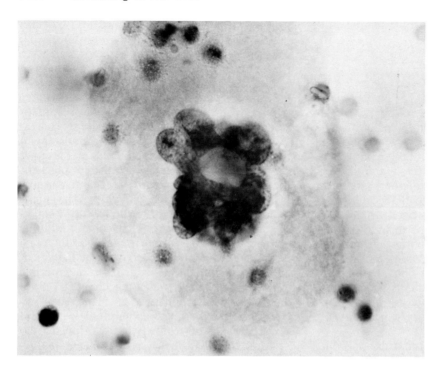

FIGURE 30–4. Megakaryocyte from the prepulmonic (azygos vein) blood. The cell is large with abundant granular cytoplasm and has a well-preserved, multilobulated nucleus with areas of clearing about many chromatin granules. (Seal's Nuclepore sieve method: hematoxylin and eosin. ×1,000. Melamed, M. R., et al.: The megakaryocyte blood count. Am. J. Med. Sci., *252*:301–309, 1966)

present singly, in small sheets, or even as syncytia. They have oval, regular nuclei of 10 to 15 μm in diameter with very delicate or finely punctate chromatin and at least one nucleolus. It is worth deliberately preparing a few specimens that contain endothelial cells, because their appearance is ordinarily quite characteristic, though like all other cells there are circumstances in which they can become quite atypical (Fig. 30–7).

Epithelial (squamous) cells from the skin have been identified in blood specimens obtained by percutaneous venipuncture. Similarly, mesothelial cells have been found in blood samples obtained by transpericardial needle aspiration of the heart.

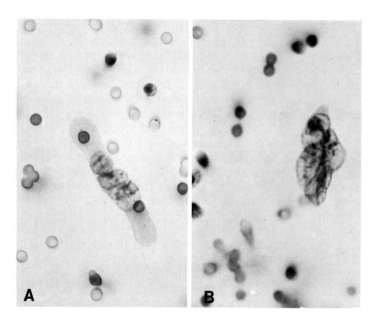

FIGURE 30–5. Megakaryocytes from postpulmonic (antecubital vein) blood. The nuclei are contracted (or fragmented) and have lost most of their cytoplasm. The cell in (*A*) is elongated as if distorted by passage through a narrow capillary. (Seal's Nuclepore sieve method; hematoxylin and eosin, ×800. Melamed, M. R., et al.: The megakaryocyte blood count. Am. J. Med. Sci., *252*:301–309, 1966)

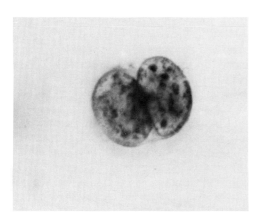

FIGURE 30–6. A binucleated cell from antecubital venous blood of a patient following mastectomy for breast carcinoma. Classification is uncertain. (Seal's Nuclepore sieve technique; hematoxylin and eosin, approx. ×1,000)

These cells appear just as they do in other kinds of cytologic preparations.

A variety of other kinds of cells, including trophoblasts,[28] osteoclasts,[54] Gaucher's cells, and mast cells,[2] have been described, but rarely.

INTERPRETATION

The clinical significance of a finding of cancer cells in the blood is still unknown. Certainly there is no prospect of cancer detection value in this examination. The clinical follow-up studies by Engell[33] failed to demonstrate a convincing relationship between the presence or absence of circulating cancer cells and survival. Early work by Potter and Malmgren also indicated that the presence of cancer cells in the blood was not necessarily followed by metastatic growth.[91] Song et al. reported that patients with localized breast and colon carcinomas had cancer cells in antecubital venous blood more frequently than patients with these same carcinomas that had metastasized to regional lymph nodes.[125] On the other hand, Watne and associates[136] did find a somewhat higher proportion of potentially curable patients among those who had no circulating cancer cells identified; and Drye and coworkers[29] reported that the likelihood of tumor recurrence was greater in patients who had cancer cells in peripheral blood, whereas they found no clinical recurrences in those who did not.

The most impressive clinical association with identifiable cancer cells in the blood has been that of Roberts,[99-103] and Jonasson[60] and their coworkers. They described showers of tumor cells in the blood of patients immediately following tumor trauma or manipulation of surgery and reported that those patients had a 2- to 5-year survival rate that was half of that observed in patients without such tumor cell showers during surgery.

A subsequent report of Roberts and associates[104] five to ten years later reaffirms that survival was unrelated to the finding of cancer cells in the blood except when the cells were found in

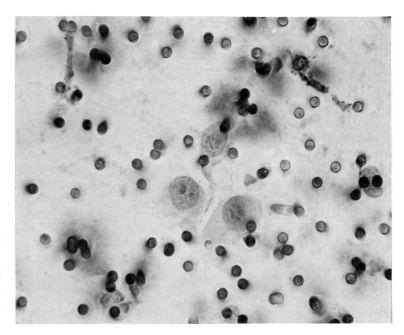

FIGURE 30–7. Endothelial cells from peripheral venous blood of a patient with malignant melanoma. There is an unusual angular irregularity of nucleoli in these cells. (Seal's Nuclepore sieve technique; hematoxylin and eosin, ×560)

showers during or after operation. McDonald and Cole[68] have shown that at least some cancer cells in the regional venous blood of patients with colonic and rectal cancer are viable and can be grown in tissue culture. Moore and coworkers, using a feeder layer of HeLa cells,[79] also reported growth from samples of blood in tissue culture. Roger et al. found tumor cells in mitosis in regional venous blood of two patients given colcemid.[106]

Some of the most rewarding work with cancer cells in the blood has been the study of factors influencing metastases in experimental tumors of animals (Fig. 30–8). With an experimental carcinoma of the cecum in rats,[1] for example, the appearance of cancer cells in the blood can be related to the development of metastases.[13] The circulation and distribution of injected cancer cells can be followed.[49,56] Viability of circulating cancer cells can be demonstrated by injection of blood samples into other susceptible animals.[59] In the case of a transplanted Walker 256 carcinosarcoma within the rat thigh, manipulation of the tumor has been shown to cause showers of tumor cells in the blood.[107]

Not all cancer cells survive in the blood circulation. Many are obviously degenerating and nonviable when they are recovered; others must be incapable of surviving, even though they appear well preserved. Even in dealing with known viable cancer cells, relatively large numbers must be introduced into the blood circulation before survival and growth are assured. The probability of tumor "take" and growth in the experimental animal is directly related to the number of cells inoculated.[6,41,87] Yet, the finding of tumor cells in the blood of patients with cancer, and the fact that some cells may pass through an autotransfusor unit, is a possible contraindication to intraoperative autotransfusion in cancer patients[143] and perhaps to their use as elective blood donors.

Factors affecting survival and distribution of cancer cells in the blood and their potential ability to proliferate are of great interest in understanding the mechanism of blood-borne metastases. The early descriptions of the fate of tumor emboli by Takahashi,[130] Warren and Gates,[134] and later by Saphir[112] and Baserga and Saffiotti,[6] were further clarified by Wood[141] and Zeidman,[146] who have carried out direct observations of the circulation by phase microscopy and microcinematography in living animals. They have demonstrated that intra-arterially injected tumor cells may lodge promptly in the arteriolocapillary bed and become adherent to endothelium but that many surprisingly large tumor cells become greatly elongated or otherwise distorted and pass through the capillary bed. Physical factors, such as capillary diameter, cell size, and flow rate, appear of little importance in determining whether the cancer cells will lodge. Rather it is thought that inherent characteristics of the cell itself,[37] derived by clonal evolution of tumor cell subpopulations,[86] enable the successive steps of invasion, detachment and embolization, lodging, and growth at selected sites that constitute the development of metastasis. The invading tumor cell has lost intercellular (desmosome) and cell substrate junctions and exhibits increased enzymatic activity at its interface with the extracellular matrix.[88] Within minutes after the tumor cell lodges and adheres to capillary endothelium it is enmeshed in a thrombus. This is followed by evidence of endothelial injury. Leukocytes accumulate and then penetrate the endothelium, leaving defects. These defects are subsequently utilized for the migration of other leukocytes as well as the cancer cells. Tumor cells were seen to reach the perivascular connective tissue within three hours.

Blood coagulation appears to play an essential role in the very early development of metastases. Cancer cells are thought to be rich in thromboplastin,[63] promoting thrombus formation and endothelial adhesion. Heparin and fibrinolysin, which interfere with thrombus formation, are known to decrease the incidence of metastases in experimental animals.[13,14,39,40,52,142]

CIRCULATION OF MEGAKARYOCYTES

A fascinating by-product of the studies of cancer cells in blood has been the observations regarding megakaryocytes, which appear to be normally present in the blood circulation. Until recently, platelet production from megakaryocytes was assumed to take place in the marrow, and except in certain disease states, megakaryocytes were thought to remain behind when platelets entered the circulation. Now it can be shown that intact megakaryocytes regularly enter the circulating blood. Because of their large size they are quickly filtered out in the pulmonary and systemic capillaries, and unlike the smaller formed elements of the blood, few megakaryocytes make more than one circuit—hence the relatively small number of these cells in the peripheral venous blood. After passage through the pulmonary capillary bed there is not only a decrease in the number of megakaryocytes in the blood but also a striking change in their morphology. Those present in azygos or vena caval

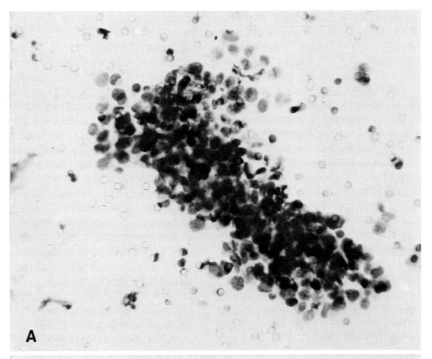

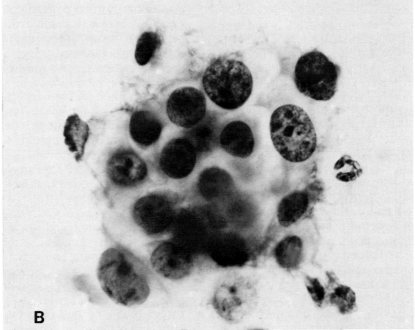

FIGURE 30–8. Cancer cells from aortic blood of rats with experimental cecal tumors produced by implantation of Walker 256 carcinosarcoma.[1] Aliquot portions of the blood produced subcutaneous tumor growth when injected in other animals. (Seal's Nuclepore sieve technique; hematoxylin and eosin.) (*A*) From an animal with widespread metastases. (*B*) From an animal with gross tumor only in cecum and regional lymph nodes. (*A* × approx. 400, *B* ×1,000)

blood draining the marrow-rich ribs or vertebrae are large cells with abundant cytoplasm (see Fig. 30–4). During passage through the lungs their cytoplasm is fragmented and stripped from the nuclei, and platelet production apparently takes place. During passage through peripheral capillaries further distortion occurs, and usually only a few contracted or fragmented, stripped megakaryocytic nuclei remain to be found in peripheral venous blood (see Fig. 30–5). A megakaryocyte blood count is now possible, and preliminary counts on normal individuals have been made.[77] These show marked individual variation, but it can be anticipated that some hematologic abnormalities, including abnormalities of platelet production and function, will be reflected in abnormalities of megakaryocyte number and form in the blood circulation.

The continuing study of cancer cells in the blood is certain to encompass problems in hematology aside from oncology. Whether there will be direct clinical value to individual patients in these examinations is difficult to predict, but their importance in cancer research is already well established.

BONE MARROW

Cancer cells that detach from solid tumors and enter the blood circulation are quickly trapped in capillaries of organs such as lung and liver and removed. Many of these cells lodge and remain in the bone marrow, where they can accumulate in numbers far greater than the cells *in transit* in the blood. Marrow is relatively accessible for study, but by conventional cytologic techniques it has been exceedingly difficult to identify single cancer cells among the great many immature marrow cells.

With recent improvements in immunocytochemical technology and the advent of new polyclonal and monoclonal antibodies, a powerful new tool has become available for the classification of cells not easily identified by cytologic morphology alone. Dearnaley[23,24] and Redding[97] and their associates were the first to use immunocytochemistry to distinguish micrometastatic single cells or small cell clusters within aspirates of bone marrow. They concentrated mononuclear cells of the marrow on a Ficoll gradient and identified isolated cells of breast carcinoma by staining with alkaline phosphatase–labeled antibody to epithelial membrane antigen (EMA). This antigen is expressed on many epithelial cells in addition to breast carcinoma but not on hematopoietic or stromal cells.

Redding et al.[97] found EMA-positive (cancer) cells in the marrow of 31 of 110 patients with breast cancer and in the peripheral blood of only 3 patients. No EMA-positive cells were found in the marrow of 36 control patients without cancer. Further, the probability of finding cancer cells in marrow was greater in patients with larger tumors (39% for tumors larger than 4 cm; 22% for tumors smaller than 4 cm); greater when intramammary vascular invasion was demonstrated in histologic sections (53%) than when no invasion was demonstrated (17%); somewhat greater in lymph-node-positive (32%) compared with lymph-node-negative (24%) patients; and greater in the estrogen-receptor-negative patients with poor prognosis (48%) compared with estrogen-receptor-positive patients (21%). Although long-term follow-up is not available at this writing, the indirect evidence strongly suggests that immunocytologic screening of bone marrow will help in identifying patients at increased risk of metastasis who may profit from more intensive therapy.

Others have since confirmed these early reports and extended them. Schlimok et al.[118] used an anticytokeratin antibody and demonstrated cytokeratin-positive cells in the marrow of 28 of 155 patients with breast cancer and also in 12 of 57 patients with colorectal cancer. Since bone metastases of colorectal cancer are not common, it is presumed that some tumor cells in marrow remain latent. Schlimok et al. also reported staining cancer cells in the marrow in vivo by an anti-EMA monoclonal antibody given intravenously. If confirmed, this may prove of great importance in the design of immunotherapy.

Cote et al.[20] combined three epithelial-specific monoclonal antibodies to achieve higher sensitivity; two were against epithelial membrane antigen and the third against cytokeratin. They found antibody-positive (cancer) cells in the marrow of 35% of patients with operable breast cancer; like Redding et al., they found antibody-positive cells more frequently in the marrow of patients with more advanced disease (Fig. 30–9), and the presence of these cells was predictive of early recurrence.[20a]

Cote et al. also have undertaken a study of patients with prostatic carcinoma, and preliminary results are similar to those of the patients with breast carcinoma (Fig. 30–10). Mansi et al.[74] compared density gradient–enriched marrow aspirates of patients with local versus metastatic prostatic carcinoma, using a mixture of antisera to prostate-specific acid phosphatase, prostate-specific antigen, epithelial membrane antigen, and cytokeratin. They found tumor cells in 11 of 15 patients

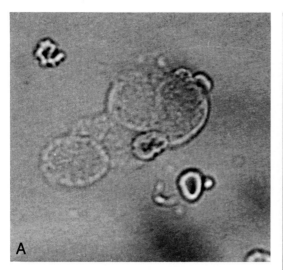
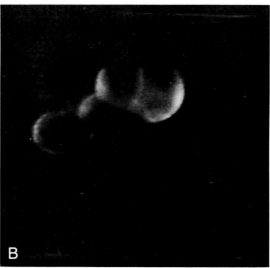
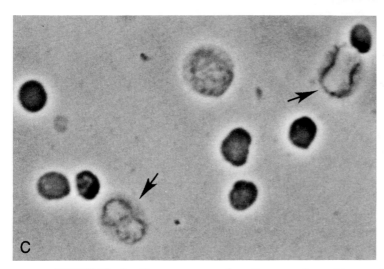
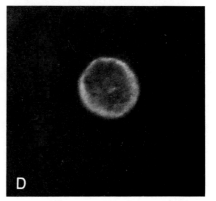

FIGURE 30-9.   Bone marrow aspirate from a patient with stage I breast carcinoma, demonstrating cells recovered from the interface layer of a Ficoll-Hypaque density gradient and reactive with fluoresceinated antibody to epithelial cytokeratins and cell membrane antigen. A cluster of four cells of breast cancer photographed by phase microscopy (*A*), and the same field photographed by fluorescence microscopy (*B*). Another field showing three nucleated single cells by phase microscopy (*C*), and one of those cells (a breast cancer cell) exhibiting fluorescence by fluorescence microscopy (*D*). The *arrows* (*C*) point to two nucleated hemopoietic cells that do not fluoresce. (Reprinted with permission from Cote et al.[20])

with known metastatic carcinoma and 2 of 15 patients with apparently local disease. No patients with benign prostatic hypertrophy had immunoreactive cells in the marrow.

Stahel et al.[127] studied patients with small cell lung cancer and found tumor cells present in the marrow of 69% of 33 patients. Although it is too early to predict whether this new screening technique will revive the hunt for "circulating" cancer cells, it certainly aids in their identification and has reopened the question of clinical significance for the few single malignant cells that are found in this way. Preliminary reports suggest that the finding of cancer cells in marrow does have prognostic value, at least for mammary carcinoma and particularly in predicting bone metastases.[73a] Studies over the

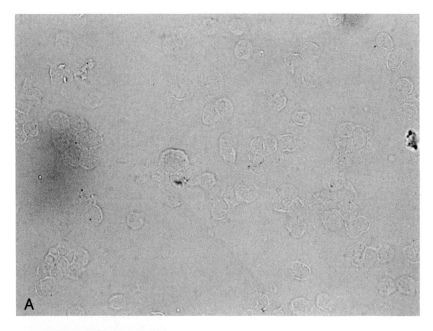

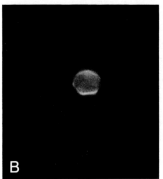

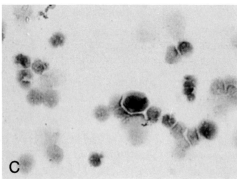

FIGURE 30-10. Bone marrow aspirate from a patient with Stage B prostatic carcinoma, processed as in Fig. 30–9. (*A*) Phase photograph showing many cells present in this field. (*B*) Fluorescence photograph of the same field as in (*A*) showing a single fluorescent cell (of prostatic carcinoma). (*C*) Papanicolaou-stained preparation of the same field showing the inconspicuous nature of the prostatic cancer cell identified by immunofluorescence. (Courtesy of Dr. Richard Cote)

next few years should be extremely important in establishing the possible clinical and research applications of this new methodology.

WOUND WASHINGS

It has been assumed that local recurrence of carcinoma after potentially curative resection may be due to contamination of the operative wound by cancer cells. This type of recurrence is more common with certain kinds of cancer, such as mammary carcinoma or epidermoid cancer of the mouth or pharynx. In an effort to predict which patients would suffer local recurrence, examinations were carried out by Smith and associates on irrigation specimens from the surgical wound taken prior to closure.[123] They reported cancer cells present in 26% of the cases, but subsequent clinical follow-up showed no correlation at all with local or distant metastases or survival.[3]

An alternative explanation for postoperative local recurrence of tumor was proposed by Nash et al.,[84] who suggested that cancer cell seeding in some wounds occurred after closure. They found support for this in the observation that cancer cells were sometimes present in the postoperative drainage of fluid from wounds that had yielded no such cells in previous irrigation specimens at surgery, but their work still lacks clinical substantiation.

The problem of differential diagnosis of tumor cells from actively proliferating connective tissue cells, endothelial and benign epithelial cells, and

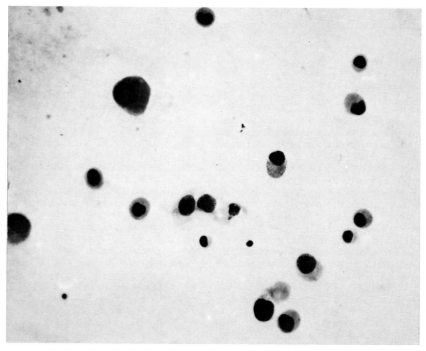

FIGURE 30–11. Cancer cells in thoracic duct lymph from a patient with disseminated malignant melanoma. Many of these huge cancer cells had cytoplasmic melanin. They were viable and grew in tissue culture, where they continued to produce melanin. (Papanicolaou stain ×350).

hematopoietic cells is not to be underestimated. One must have considerable experience with this type of material and maintain good clinicopathologic correlation, if meaningful diagnoses are expected.

THORACIC DUCT LYMPH

Tumor cells have been identified in thoracic duct lymph from approximately 16% of patients with advanced cancers[10] (Fig. 30–11). Technical problems of preparation and interpretation appear to be somewhat simpler than for blood or wound washings.

In a remarkable study of the entire thoracic duct, its tributaries, and draining nodes, Young found involvement by carcinoma in 37% and by lymphoma in 71% of 150 patients with malignant neoplasms at autopsy.[144] Experience with the cytology of thoracic duct lymph is still too limited to suggest what clinical correlations may be possible, but it is an intriguing subject that will surely see more study in the coming years.

BIBLIOGRAPHY

1. Agostino, D., Seal, S.H., and Nickson, J.J.: Capsule implantation: Method for establishing simulated colon carcinoma in rats. Proc. Soc. Exp. Biol. Med., *100*:717–718, 1959.
2. Alexander, R.F., and Spriggs, A.I.: The differential diagnosis of tumour cells in circulating blood. J. Clin. Pathol., *13*:414–424, 1960.
3. Arons, M.S., Smith, R.R., and Myers, M.H.: Significance of cancer cells in operative wounds. Cancer, *14*:1041–1044, 1961.
4. Ashworth, T.R.: Hospital reports. A case of cancer in which the cells similar to those in the tumours were seen in the blood after death. Aust. Med. J., *14*:146–147, 1869.
5. Baserga, R., Putong, P.B., Tyler, S., and Wartman, W.B.: The dose-response relationship between the number of embolic tumor cells and the incidence of blood-borne metastases. Br. J. Cancer, *14*:173–185, 1960.
6. Baserga, R., and Saffiotti, U.: Experimental studies on histogenesis of blood-borne metastases. Arch. Pathol., *59*:26–34, 1955.
7. Batson, O.V.: The function of the vertebral veins and their role in the spread of metastases. Ann Surg., *112*:138–149, 1940.
7a. Breslow, A., Kaufman, R.M., and Lansky, A.R.: The effect of surgery on the concentration of circulating megakaryocytes and platelets. Blood, *32*:393–401, 1968.

8. Brown, C.E., and Warren, S.: Visceral metastases from rectal carcinoma. Surg. Gynecol. Obstet., *66*:611–621, 1938.

9. Buckley, E.S. Jr., Powell, M.J., and Gibson, J.G., II: Separation of formed elements of whole blood by means of Fraction I. J. Lab. Clin. Med., *36*:29–39, 1950.

10. Burn, J.I., Watne, A.L., and Moore, G.E.: The role of the thoracic duct lymph in cancer dissemination. Br. J. Cancer, *16*:608–615, 1962.

11. Carey, R.W., Taft, P.D., Bennett, J.M., and Kaufman, S.: Carcinocythemia (carcinoma cell leukemia). An acute leukemia-like picture due to metastatic carcinoma cells. Am. J. Med., *60*:273–278, 1976.

12. Christopherson, W.M.: Cancer cells in the peripheral blood: A second look. Acta Cytol., *9*:169–172, 1965.

13. Cliffton, E.E., and Agostino, D.: Cancer cells in the blood in simulated colon cancer, resectable and unresectable: Effect of fibrinolysin and heparin on growth potential. Surgery, *50*:395–401, 1961.

14. Cliffton, E.E., and Grossi, C.E.: Effect of human plasmin on the toxic effects and growth of blood-borne metastasis of the Brown-Pearce carcinoma and the V2 carcinoma of rabbit. Cancer, *9*:1147–1152, 1956.

15. Cole, W.H., Packard D., and Southwick, H.W.: Carcinoma of the colon with special reference to prevention of recurrence. J.A.M.A., *155*:1549–1553, 1954.

16. Cole, W.H., Roberts, S., Watne, A., McDonald, G., and McGrew, E.: The dissemination of cancer cells. Bull. N.Y. Acad. Med., *34*:163–183, 1958.

17. Collier, F.C., Enterline, H.T., Kyle, R.H., Tristan, T.T., and Greening, R.: The prognostic implications of vascular invasion in primary carcinomas of the lung: A clinicopathologic correlation of two hundred twenty-five cases with one hundred per cent follow-up. Arch. Pathol., *66*:594–603, 1958.

18. Coman, D.R.: Mechanisms responsible for origin and distribution of blood-borne tumor metastases: A review. Cancer Res., *13*:397–404, 1953.

19. Coombes, R.C., Berger, U., Mansi, J., Redding, H., Powles, T.J., Neville, A.M., McKenna, A., Nash, A.G., Gazet, J.-C., Ford, H.T., Ormerod, M., and McDonnell, T.: Prognostic significance of micrometastases in bone marrow in patients with primary breast cancer. Natl. Cancer Inst. Monogr., *1*:51–53, 1986.

20. Cote, R.J., Rosen, P.P., Hakes, T.B., Sedira, M., Bazinet, M., Kinne, D.W., Old, L.J., and Osborne, M.P.: Monoclonal antibodies detect occult breast carcinoma metastases in the bone marrow of patients with early stage disease. Am. J. Surg. Pathol., *12*:333–340, 1988.

20a. Cote, R.J., Rosen, P.P., Old, L.J., and Osborne, M.P.: Detection of bone marrow micrometastases in patients with early-stage breast cancer. Diagn. Oncol., *1*:37–42, 1991.

20b. Cote. R.J., Rosen P.P., Lesser, M., Old, L.J., and Osborne, M.P.: Prediction of early relapse in patients with operable breast cancer by detection of occult bone marrow micrometastases. J. Clin. Oncol., *9*:1749–1756, 1991.

21. Danielsson, H.: Demonstration of tumour cells in circulating blood with a spiral centrifuge. Svensk. Lakartidn., *58*:140–141, 1961.

22. Dannaker, C.L., Yam, L.T., and McKeown, J.M.: Metastatic carcinoma with carcinocythemia mimicking leukemia. South. Med. J., *72*:622–624, 1979.

23. Dearnaley, D.P., Ormerod, M.G., Sloane, J.P., Lumley, H., Imrie, S., Jones, M., Coombes, R.C., and Neville, A.M.: Detection of isolated mammary carcinoma cells in marrow of patients with primary breast cancer. J. R. Soc. Med., *76*:359–364, 1983.

24. Dearnaley, D.P., Sloane, J.P., Omerod, M.G., Steele, K., Coombes, R.C., Clink, H.M.D., Powles, T.J., Ford, H.T., Gazet, J.-C., and Neville, A.M.: Increased detection of mammary carcinoma cells in marrow smears using antisera to epithelial membrane antigen. Br. J. Cancer, *44*:85–90, 1981.

25. de Carvalho, S.: Detection of nonhemopoietic cells in the circulation on collodion films. J. Lab. Clin. Med., *55*:322–324, 1960.

26. de Mello, R.P.: A new method for detection of cancer cells in peripheral blood using the Bertalanffy fluorochrome method. Acta Cytol., *7*:62–65, 1963.

27. Diddle, E.E., Sholes, D.M. Jr., Hollingsworth, J., and Kinlaw, S.: Cervical carcinoma: Cancer cells in circulating blood. Am. J. Obstet. Gynecol., *78*:582–585, 1959.

28. Douglas, G.W., Thomas, L., Carr, M., Cullen, N.M., and Morris, R.: Trophoblast in circulating blood during pregnancy. Am. J. Obstet. Gynecol., *78*:960–973, 1959.

29. Drye, J.C., Runage, W.T., Jr., and Anderson, A.: Prognostic import of circulating cancer cells after curative surgery. Ann. Surg., *155*:733–740, 1962.

30. Ederer, F., Goldblatt, S.A., and Nadel, E.M.: Analysis of the color micrograph study of the circulating cancer cell cooperative. Acta. Cytol., *9*:50–57, 1965.

31. Ejheckam, G. C., Sogbein, S.K., and McLeish, W.A.: Carcinocythemia due to metastatic oat-cell carcinoma of the lung. Can. Med. Assoc. J., *120*:336–338, 1979.

32. Engell, H.C.: Cancer cells in circulating blood: Clinical study on occurrence of cancer cells in peripheral blood and in venous blood draining tumour area at operation. Acta Chir. Scand. [Suppl. 201]:1–70, 1955.

33. ———: Cancer cells in blood: 5 to 9 year follow-up study. Ann. Surg., *149*:457–461, 1959.

34. Ericksson, O.: Method for cytological detection of cancer cells in blood. Cancer, *15*:171–175, 1962.

35. Ewing, J.: Neoplastic Diseases. 4th ed. Philadelphia, W.B. Saunders, 1940.

36. Fawcett, D.W., Vallee, B.L., and Soule, M.H.: A method for concentration and segregation of malignant cells from bloody, pleural, and peritoneal fluids. Science, *111*:34–36, 1950.

37. Fidler, I.J., and Kripke, M.L.: Metastasis results from pre-existing variant cells within a malignant tumor. Science, *197*:893–895, 1977.

38. Finkel, G.C., and Tishkoff, G.H.: Malignant cells in a peripheral blood smear. Report of a case. N. Engl. J. Med., *262*:187–188, 1960.

39. Fisher, B., and Fisher, E.R.: Experimental studies of factors which influence hepatic metastases. VIII. Effect of anticoagulants. Surgery, *50*:240–247, 1961.

40. ———: Biologic aspects of cancer-cell spread. Fifth National Cancer Conference Proceedings. pp. 105–122, Philadelphia, J.B. Lippincott, 1964.

41. Fisher, E.R., and Fisher, B.: Experimental studies of factors influencing hepatic metastases. I. Effect of number of tumor cells injected and time of growth. Cancer, *12*:926–928, 1959.

42. Fisher, E.R., and Turnbull, R.B.: The cytologic demonstration and significance of tumor cells in the mesenteric venous blood in patients with colorectal carcinoma. Surg. Gynecol. Obstet., *100*:102–108, 1955.

43. Friedell, G.H., and Parsons, L.: Blood vessel invasion in cancer of the cervix. Cancer, *15*:1269–1274, 1962.

44. Gallivan, M.V.E., and Lokich, J.J.: Carcinocythemia

(carcinoma cell leukemia). Report of two cases with English literature review. Cancer, *53*:1100–1102, 1984.

45. Gazet, J.-C.: The detection of viable circulating cancer cells. Acta Cytol., *10*:119–125, 1966.

46. Goldblatt, S.A., and Nadel, E.M.: Cancer cells in the circulating blood: A critical review II. Acta Cytol., *9*:6–20, 1965.

47. Goldmann, E.: Relation of cancer cells to blood vessels and ducts. Lancet, *1*:23–24, 1906.

48. Goodall, P., Spriggs, A.I., and Wells, F.R.: Malignant melanoma with melanosis and melanuria, and with pigmented monocytes and tumour cells in the blood. Br. J. Surg., *48*:549–555, 1961.

49. Griffiths, J.P., and Salsbury, A.J.: The fate of circulating Walker 256 tumor cells. Cells injected intravenously in rats. Br. J. Cancer, *17*:546–557, 1963.

50. ———: Circulating Cancer Cells. American Lecture Series. Springfield, Ill., Charles C Thomas, 1965.

51. Grinnell, R.S.: Spread of carcinoma of the colon and rectum. Cancer, *3*:641–656, 1950.

52. Grossi, C.E., Agostino, D., and Cliffton, E.E.: The effect of human fibrinolysis on pulmonary metastases of Walker 256 carcinosarcoma. Cancer Res., *20*:605–608, 1960.

53. Gurian, J.M., and West, J.T.: Relationship of size of blood sample to yield of "positive" patients in studies of circulating tumor cells. J.N.C.I., *31*:1431–1443, 1963.

54. Haemmerli, G., and Straeuli, P.: Osteoclasten im peripheren Blut: ein Beitrag zur Differentialdiagnose von Tumorzellen im Blut. Klin. Wochenschr., *41*:396–398, 1963.

55. Hansen, M., and Pedersen, N.T.: Circulating megakaryocytes in blood from the antecubital vein in healthy, adult humans. Scand. J. Haematol., *20*:371–376, 1978.

56. Hengesh, J.W., McGrew, E.A., and Nanos, S.: Malignant cells in the peripheral blood of experimental animals. Acta Cytol., *6*:143–147, 1962.

57. Herbeuval, R., Duheille, J., and Goedert-Herbeuval, C.: Diagnosis of unusual blood cells by immunofluorescence. Acta Cytol., *9*:73–82, 1965.

58. Jackson, J.F.: Histochemical identification of megakaryocytes from peripheral blood examined for tumor cells. Cancer, *15*:259–262, 1962.

59. Jonasson, O.: The viability of circulating cancer cells in experimental cancer. Surg. Forum, *9*:577–580, 1958.

60. Jonasson, O., Long, L., Roberts, S., McGrew, E., and McDonald, J.: Cancer cells in the circulating blood during operative management of genitourinary tumors. J. Urol., *85*:1–12, 1961.

61. Krause, J.R.: Rhabdomyosarcoma presenting as carcinocythemia. South. Med. J., *72*:1007–1008, 1979.

62. Kuper, S.W.A., Bignall, J.R., and Luckcock, E.D.: A quantitative method for studying tumour cells in blood. Lancet., *1*:852–853, 1961.

63. Lawrence, E.A., Bowman, D., Moore, D.B., and Bernstein, G.I.: A thromboplastic property of neoplasms. Surg. Forum, *3*:694–698, 1952.

64. Lee, V.W., Chiang, T., and Deodhar, S.D.: Bioassay for quantitating circulating tumor cells in a syngeneic mouse tumor system. Cancer Res. *36*:2053–2058, 1976.

65. Li, J.G., and Osgood, E.E.: A method for the rapid separation of leukocytes and nucleated erythrocytes from blood or marrow with a phytohemagglutinin from red beans (phaseolus vulgaris). Blood, *4*:670–675, 1949.

66. Loeper and Loeste, cited by Ewing, J.: Neoplastic Diseases. 4th ed. p. 55. Philadelphia, W.B. Saunders, 1940.

67. Lugassy, G., Vorst, E.J., Varon, D., Sigler, E., Shani, A., Bassous-Guedj, L., Hurwitz, N., and Berrebi, A: Carcinocythemia: Report of two cases, one simulating a Burkitt lymphoma. Acta Cytol., *34*:265–268, 1990.

68. McDonald, G.O., and Cole, W.H.: Tissue culture of cells recovered from the blood of patients with colonic and rectal cancer. Am. J. Surg., *101*:11–15, 1961.

69. McGrew, E.A.: Criteria for the recognition of malignant cells in circulating blood. Acta Cytol., *9*:58–60, 1965.

70. ———: Concentration of cells from body fluids for cytologic study. Am. J. Clin. Pathol., *24*:1025–1029, 1954.

71. McGrew, E.A., Roberts, S., Watne, A., Jonasson, O., and Cole, W.H.: Circulating blood. *In* Papanicolaou, G.N.: Atlas of Exfoliative Cytology, Suppl. II, Chap. 10. Cambridge, Mass., Harvard University Press, 1960.

72. McGrew, E.A., Romsdahl, M.M., and Valaitas, J.: Differentiation of hematopoietic elements from tumor cells in blood. Acta Cytol., *6*:551–553, 1962.

73. Malmgren, R.A., Pruitt, J.C., Del Vecchio, P.R., and Potter, J.F.: Method for cytologic detection of tumor cells in whole blood. J. Natl. Cancer Inst., *20*:1203–1213, 1958.

73a. Mansi, J.L., Berger, U., Easton, D., McDonnell, T., Redding, W.H., Gazet, J.-C., McKinna, A., Powles, T.J., and Coombes, R.C.: Micrometastasis in bone marrow in patients with primary breast cancer: Evaluation as an early predictor of bone metastases. Br. Med. J., *295*:1093–1096, 1987.

74. Mansi, J.L., Berger, U., Wilson, P., Shearer, R., and Coombes, R.C.: Detection of tumor cells in bone marrow of patients with prostate carcinoma by immunocytochemical techniques. J. Urol., *139*:545–548, 1988.

75. Marcus, H.: Krebsellen im strömenden Blut? Z. Krebsforsch., *16*:217–230, 1917.

76. Mehta, R.D., and Riddell, A.G.: Cancer cells in blood of patients with malignant melanoma treated by regional perfusion. Cancer, *18*:671–673, 1965.

77. Melamed, M.R., Cliffton, E.E., Mercer, C., and Koss, L.G.: The megakaryocyte blood count. Am. J. Med. Sci., *252*:301–309, 1966.

78. Melamed, M.R., Cliffton, E.E., and Seal, S.H.: Cancer cells in the peripheral venous blood. A quantitative study of cells of problematic origin. Am. J. Pathol., *37*:381–388, 1962.

79. Moore, G.E., Mount, D.T., and Wendt, A.C.: The growth of human tumor cells in tissue culture. Surg. Forum, *9*:572–576, 1958.

80. Moore, G.E., Sandberg, A.A., and Schubarg, J.R.: Clinical and experimental observations of occurrence and fate of tumor cells in blood stream. Ann. Surg., *146*:580–587, 1957.

81. Myerowitz, R.L., Edwards, P.A., and Sartiano, G.P.: Carcinocythemia (carcinoma cell leukemia) due to metastatic carcinoma of the breast. Cancer, *40*:3107–3111, 1977.

82. Nadel, E.M., and Goldblatt, S.A. (eds.): The Circulating Cancer Cell Cooperative (CCCC) slide seminar. Acta Cytol., *9*:21–49, 1965.

83. Nagy, K.P.: A study of normal, atypical and neoplastic cells in the white cell concentrate of the peripheral blood. Acta Cytol., *9*:61–67, 1965.

84. Nash, S.C., Malmgren, R.A., Hume, R., and Smith, R.R.: Tumor cells in postoperative wound drainage. Cancer, *15*:221–226, 1962.

85. Nedelkoff, B., Christopherson, W.M., and Harter, J.S.: A method for demonstrating malignant cells in the blood. Acta Cytol., *5*:203–205, 1961.

86. Nowell, P.S.: The clonal evolution of tumor cell subpopulations. Science, *194*:23–28, 1976.

87. Overstreet, R.J., and McDonald, G.O.: The role of cellular dosage on "takes" following inoculation of Walker-256 tumor cells in the rat. Surg. Forum, *8*:161–164, 1957.

88. Pauli, B.U., Schwartz, D.E., Thonar, E.J.-M., and Kuettner, K.E.: Tumor invasion and host extracellular matrix. Cancer Metastasis Rev., *2*:129–152, 1983.

89. Pool, E.H., and Dunlop, G.R.: Cancer cells in blood stream. Am. J. Cancer, *21*:99–102, 1934.

90. Potter, J.F., Longenbaugh, G., Chu, E., Dillon, J., Romsdahl, M., and Malmgren, R.A.: The relationship of tumor type and resectability to the incidence of cancer cells in blood. Surg. Gynecol. Obstet., *110*:734–738, 1960.

91. Potter, J.F., and Malmgren, R.A.: A new technique for the detection of tumor cells in the blood stream and its application to the study of dissemination of cancer. Surg. Forum, *9*:580–593, 1958.

92. Pruitt, J.C., Hiberg, W., and Kaiser, R.F.: Malignant cells in peripheral blood. N. Engl. J. Med., *259*:1161–1164, 1958.

93. Pruitt, J.C., Mengoli, H.F., and Morehead, R.P.: A quantitative clinical and pathologic study of malignant cells in circulating blood. Am. Surg., *29*:383–384, 1963.

94. Quensel, U.: Zur Kenntnis des Vorkommens von Geschwulstzellen im zirkulierenden Blute. Upsala Läkaref. Förh., *26*:1–10, 1921.

95. Raker, J.W., Taft, P.D., and Edmonds, E.E.: Significance of megakaryocytes in search for tumor cells in peripheral blood. N. Engl. J. Med., *263*:993–996, 1960.

96. Rappaport, H.: Tumors of the Hematopoietic System. Plate X D, E. p. 418. Washington, D.C., AFIP, 1966.

97. Redding, W.H., Coombes, R.C., Monaghen, P., Clink, H.M., Imrie, S.F., Dearnaley, D.P., Ormerod, M.G., Sloane, J.P., Gazet, J.-C., Powles, T.J., and Neville, A.M.: Detection of micrometastases in patients with primary breast cancer. Lancet, *2*:1271–1274, 1983.

98. Reiss, R.: Demonstration of carcinoma cells in the blood stream. J. Mount Sinai Hosp. N. Y.: *26*:171–176, 1959.

99. Roberts, S.: Spread by the vascular system. *In* Cole, W.H., McDonald, G.O., Roberts, S., and Southwick, H.W. (eds.): Dissemination of Cancer—Prevention and Therapy. pp. 61–222, New York, Appleton-Century-Crofts, 1961.

100. Roberts, S., Jonasson, O., Long, L., McGrath, R., McGrew, E.A., and Cole, W.H.: Clinical significance of cancer cells in the circulating blood: Two to five year survival. Ann Surg., *154*:362–371, 1961.

101. Roberts, S., Jonasson, O., Long, L., McGrew, E.A., McGrath, R., and Cole, W.H.: Relationship of cancer cells in the circulating blood to operation. Cancer, *15*:232–440, 1962.

102. Roberts, S., Long, L., Jonasson, O., McGrath, R., McGrew, E.A., and Cole, W.H.: The isolation of cancer cells from the blood stream during uterine curettage. Surg. Gynecol. Obstet., *111*:3–11, 1960.

103. Roberts, S., Watne, A., McGrath, R., McGrew, E., and Cole, W.H.: Technique and results of isolation of cancer cells from circulating blood. Arch. Surg., *76*:334–346, 1958.

104. Roberts, S., Hengesh, J.W., McGrath, R.G., Valaitis, J., McGrew, E.A., and Cole, W.H.: Prognostic significance of cancer cells in the circulating blood. Am. J. Surg., *113*:757–762, 1967.

105. Robinson, K.P., McGrath, R., and McGrew, E.: Circulating cancer cells in patients with lung tumors. Surgery, *53*:630–636, 1963.

106. Roger, V., Brennhovd, I., Høeg, K.: Tumor cells in blood: The prognostic significance of tumor cells in blood during palpation and biopsy. Acta Cytol., *16*:557–560, 1972.

107. Romsdahl, M.M., McGrath, R.G., Hoppe, E., and McGrew, E.A.: Experimental model for the study of tumor cells in the blood. Acta Cytol., *9*:141–145, 1965.

108. Romsdahl, M.M., Valaitis, J., McGrath, R.G., and McGrew, E.A.: Circulating tumor cells in patients with carcinoma. J.A.M.A., *193*:1087–1090, 1965.

109. Sakurai, M., Klassen, K.P., and Selbach, G.J.: The presence of malignant cells in the blood of patients with carcinoma of the lung. Acta Cytol., *6*:314–318, 1962.

110. Sandberg, A.A., and Moore, G.E.: Examination of blood for tumor cells. J.N.C.I., *19*:1–11, 1957.

111. Sandberg, A.A., Moore, G.E., and Schulbarg, J.R.: "Atypical" cells in the blood of cancer patients—differentiation from tumor cells. J.N.C.I., *22*:555–559, 1959.

112. Saphir, O.: The fate of carcinoma emboli in the lung. Am. J. Pathol., *23*:245–249, 1947.

113. Scheinin, T.M., and Koivuniemi, A.P.: The occurrence of cancer cells in blood. Surgery, *51*:652–657, 1962.

114. ———: Large benign cells in circulating blood and their significance in the identification of cancer cells. Cancer, *15*:972–977, 1962.

115. ———: Factors influencing the occurrence of circulating malignant cells in lung cancer. Cancer, *16*:639–645, 1963.

116. ———: Megakaryocytes in the pulmonary circulation. Blood, *22*:82–87, 1963.

117. Schleip, K.: Zur Diagnose von Knockenmarkstumoren aus dem Blutbefunde. Z. Klin. Med., *59*:261–282, 1906.

118. Schlimok, G., Funke, I., Holzmann, B., Gottlinger, G., Schmidt, G., Hauser, H., Swierkot, S., Warmecke, H.H., Schneider, B., Koprowski, H., and Riethmuller, G.: Micrometastatic cancer cells in bone marrow: In vitro detection with anticytokeratin and in vivo labeling with anti-17-1A monoclonal antibodies. P.N.A.S. (U.S.A.), *84*:8672–8676, 1987.

119. Seal, S.H.: A method for concentrating cancer cells suspended in large quantities of fluid. Cancer, *9*:866–868, 1956.

120. ———: Silicone flotation; simple quantitative method for isolation of free-floating cancer cells from blood. Cancer, *12*:590–595, 1959.

121. ———: A sieve for the isolation of cancer cells and other large cells from the blood. Cancer, *17*:637–642, 1964.

122. Selbach, G., Sakurai, M., and Bordar, M.: The presence of malignant cells in cadaver blood. Acta Cytol., *7*:159–163, 1963.

123. Smith, R.R., Thomas, L.B., and Hilberg, A.W.: Cancer cell contamination of operative wounds. Cancer, *11*:53–62, 1958.

124. Solanki, D.L., and McCurdy, P.R.: Oat cell carcinoma mimicking leukemia. Postgrad. Med., *68*:213–216, 1980.

125. Song, J., From, P., Morrissey, W.J., and Sams, J.: Circulating cancer cells: Pre- and post-chemotherapy observations. Cancer, *28*:553–561, 1971.

126. Spear, F.: Separation of leukocytes from whole blood by flotation on gum acacia. Blood, *3*:1055–1056, 1948.

127. Stahel, R.A., Mabry, M., Skarin, A.T., Speak, J., and

Bernal, S.D.: Detection of bone marrow metastasis in small-cell lung cancer by monoclonal antibody. J. Clin. Oncol., *3*:455–461, 1985.

128. Stevenson, T.D., and von Haam, E.: A study of factors affecting circulating tumor cells in experimental animals. Acta Cytol., *10*:383–386, 1966.

129. Sunderland, D.A.: The significance of vein invasion by cancer of the rectum and sigmoid: A microscopic study of 210 cases. Cancer, *2*:429–437, 1949.

130. Takahashi, M.: An experimental study of metastases. J. Pathol. Bact., *20*:1–13, 1915.

131. Taylor, F.W., and Vellios, F.: Failure to prove identity of tumor cells in the peripheral blood. Surgery, *44*:453–456, 1958.

132. Turnbull, R.B., Kyle, K., Watson, F.R., and Spratt, J.: Cancer of the colon: The influence of the no-touch isolation technic on survival rates. Ann. Surg., *166*:420–425, 1965.

133. Ward, G.R.: The blood in cancer with bone metastases. Lancet, *1*:676–677, 1913.

134. Warren, S., and Gates, O.: The fate of intravenously injected tumor cells. Am. J. Cancer, *27*:485–492, 1936.

135. Watne, A.L., Cohen, E., Migaiolo, J.A., and Lyon, V.E.: Tumor cell and leukocyte recovery from human blood utilizing *Limulus* heteroagglutinins. Acta Cytol., *10*:255–260, 1966.

136. Watne, A.L., Roberts, S.S., McGrew, E.A., and Cole, W.H.: The occurrence of cancer cells in the circulating blood and their response to surgery and chemotherapy. Acta Un. Int. Cancer, *16*:790–799, 1960.

137. Watne, A.L., Sandberg, A.A., and Moore, G.E.: The vascular dissemination of cancer. Q. Rev. Surg. Obstet., *17*:203–218, 1960.

138. West, J.T., Hume, R., and Kindurys, A.: A one-step filtration technic for recovery of tumor cells from blood. Am. J. Clin. Pathol., *41*:27–32, 1964.

139. Wilder, R.J.: The historical development of the concept of the metastasis. J. Mount Sinai Hosp. N.Y., *23*:728–734, 1956.

140. Willis, R.A.: The Spread of Tumors in the Human Body. St. Louis, C.V. Mosby, 1952.

141. Wood, S., Jr.: Pathogenesis of metastasis formation observed in vivo in the rabbit ear chamber. Arch. Pathol., *66*:550–568, 1958.

142. Wood, S., Jr., Yardley, J.H., and Holyoke, E.D.: The relationship between intravascular coagulation and the formation of pulmonary metastases in mice injected intravenously with tumor suspension. Proc. Am. Assoc. Cancer Res., *2*:260, 1957.

143. Yaw, P.B., Sentany, M., Link, W.J., Wahle, W.M., and Glover, J.L.: Tumor cells carried through autotransfusion. J.A.M.A., *231*:490–491, 1975.

144. Young, J.M.: The thoracic duct in malignant disease. Am. J. Pathol., *32*:253–261, 1956.

145. Zeidman, I.: Experimental studies on the spread of cancer in the lymphatic system. III. Tumor emboli in thoracic duct. The pathogenesis of Virchow's node. Cancer Res., *15*:719–721, 1955.

146. ———: The fate of circulating tumor cells. I. Passage of cells through capillaries. Cancer Res., *21*:38–39, 1961.

147. Zeidman, I., McCutcheon, M., and Coman, D.R.: Factors affecting the number of tumor metastases. Experiments with a transplantable mouse tumor. Cancer Res., *10*:357–359, 1950.

31

Cytologic Techniques in Acquired Immunodeficiency Syndrome (AIDS): A Summary

Acquired immunodeficiency syndrome (AIDS) has been recognized as the end stage of infection with an RNA virus, now known as the human immunodeficiency virus (HIV). The infection is transmitted mainly by sexual intercourse between homosexual males and heterosexual couples and by exchange of blood and blood products, including transfusions. Transplacental infection of infants is well documented. There is some evidence that the infection may also be transmitted by means of accidental skin puncture by needle or other forms of contact with infected blood.

The acute infection results in a brief episode of febrile illness usually lasting a few days. After recovery, patients may remain asymptomatic for periods ranging from a few months to several years, possibly a function of the number of virions transmitted and individual resistance to infection. The final stages of the disease are known as HIV-related syndrome and as AIDS.

Within the few years since the identification of this disease much has been learned about the virus causing it and the range of symptoms. In the Western world the disease is caused by HIV type I, whereas HIV type II has been so far rarely observed outside of Africa. The virus infects and kills a variety of cells, most importantly perhaps a group of T lymphocytes known as helper cells and identified immunologically as CD4+ (positive) cells. There is extensive evidence that macrophages, cells in the gastrointestinal tract, the brain, and other organs, may be directly infected by the virus (review in Levy, 1989).

In HIV-related syndrome and in AIDS the immune response in the affected individuals are profoundly modified. Consequently, a broad range of common and uncommon bacterial, fungal, and viral agents may thrive in immunosuppressed patients. An important example is oral or vaginal candidiasis (*Monilia* infection), which is often the first clinical manifestation of AIDS-related syndrome and of AIDS.

Besides infections, affected individuals may develop a number of other disorders pertinent to the subject matter of this book. These are mainly reactive lymphadenopathies, malignant lymphomas, Kaposi's sarcoma, and squamous carcinomas.

Cytologic techniques are extensively used in the diagnosis of infections and malignant disorders in AIDS.

Since at the time of this writing (1991) AIDS is not curable, the identification of the infectious organisms and neoplastic states is merely a guide to therapy that may prolong the life of the patient.

Nearly all applications of cytology have been discussed under appropriate headings elsewhere in this book. Hence this chapter is merely a summary of applications with references to the appropriate chapters.

BACTERIAL INFECTIONS

Many secondary bacterial infections in AIDS patients can be identified by cytologic techniques.

Tuberculosis. Pulmonary tuberculosis is common in patients with AIDS, particularly in Africa (Goodgame, 1990). Infection with the avian type of *Mycobacterium*, which is extremely uncommon in immunologically normal people, may produce a massive abdominal infection with major lymphadenopathy in patients with AIDS. Except for a possible aspiration biopsy of infected lymph nodes, the disease is not diagnosable by cytologic techniques. For a summary of cytologic findings in bacterial infections, see Table 31–1.

VIRAL INFECTIONS

Every conceivable form of viral infection can occur in patients with AIDS, often in unusual locations.

Thus massive herpetic ulcerations have been described in the perianal region. Asymptomatic or symptomatic cytomegalovirus infection may be observed in the respiratory, urinary, and gastrointestinal tracts. Infection of other organs is rarely recognized prior to autopsy.

Human papillomavirus (HPV) infection in the form of vulvar and anal warts is commonly associated with HIV infection. There is evidence that female patients with HIV infection or AIDS have a higher rate of HPV-associated disorders of the uterine cervix than non-AIDS controls (Schrager et al., 1989; Feingold et al., 1990).

Human polyomavirus type JC has been identified as the cause of progressive multifocal leukoencephaly, a disease identified in brain aspiration biopsies in AIDS patients by Suhrland et al. (1987). Viral inclusions, identical to those observed in the urinary sediments of patients with BK type of infections (see p. 910), have been observed in brain aspirates. For a summary of cytologic findings in viral infections, see Table 31–2.

FUNGAL ORGANISMS

As is the case with viral infections, virtually every known fungal organism can be found in AIDS patients. Cryptosporidiosis, an otherwise rare form of fungal infection, is a common cause of gastrointestinal disease in AIDS resulting in severe diarrhea. This disease is not diagnosable by cytologic techniques. For a summary of cytologic findings in fungal infections, see Table 31–3.

PARASITIC INFECTIONS

One of the most feared complications of AIDS is *Pneumocystis carinii* pneumonia. The disorder is diagnosable by cytologic examination of sputum, bronchial washing, or bronchoalveolar lavage. Other parasitic infections such as *Toxoplasma*

Table 31–1
Bacterial Infections in AIDS

Organism	Organ Site	Medium of Diagnosis	Reference Chapter	Page
Tuberculosis	Lung	Sputum	19	727
		Aspiration biopsy		729
	Lymph nodes and other organs	Aspiration biopsy	29	1282

Table 31–2
Viral Infections in AIDS

Organism	Organ Site	Medium of Diagnosis	Chapter	Page
Cytomegalovirus	Lung	Sputum	19	734
	Urinary tract	Urine	22	907
Herpesvirus	Female and male genital tract	Direct smears	10	351
	Oral cavity	Direct smears	21	869
	Esophagus	Direct smears or balloon	24	1120
	Urinary tract	Urine	22	908
	Central nervous system	Cerebrospinal fluid	27	1188
		Aspiration biopsy	29	1382
Human polyomavirus	Urinary tract	Urine	22	909
	Brain (progressive multifocal leukoencephalopathy)	Aspiration biopsy	29	1382

gondii and superinfection with *Strongyloides stercoralis* have been observed. For a summary of cytologic findings in parasitic infections, see Table 31–4.

NEOPLASTIC DISORDERS

One of the curious aspects of AIDS is the occurrence of a sarcoma of skin of vascular origin known as Kaposi's sarcoma. The disease, usually confined to the skin and subcutis in non-AIDS patients, is aggressive and fully capable of metastases to regional lymph nodes and other organs in AIDS patients. Diagnosis of metastatic Kaposi's sarcoma in pleural fluid and in aspirates of pulmonary and lymph node metastases has been reported.

However, the most common malignant disorder in AIDS is malignant lymphoma. The disease may be nodal and thus diagnosable by needle aspiration biopsy. The central nervous system is commonly affected, and the disease may also be diagnosed by cytologic examinations of the cerebrospinal fluid.

Table 31–3
Fungal Infections in AIDS

Organism	Organ Site	Medium of Diagnosis	Chapter	Page
Candida albicans (monilia)	Oral cavity	Direct smear	21	869
	Vagina & vulva	Direct smear	10	344
	Esophagus	Direct smear or balloon	24	1120
Cryptococcus neoformans	Lung	Sputum	19	736
	Central nervous system	Cerebrospinal fluid	27	1190
Other fungi	Lung	Sputum	19	738
	Female genital tract	Direct smear	10	344
	Miscellaneous sites	See organ systems		

Table 31–4
Protozoan Infections in AIDS

Organism	Organ Site	Medium of Diagnosis	Chapter	Page
			Reference	
Pneumocystis carinii	Lung	Sputum	19	741
		Bronchoalveolar lavage		742
Toxoplasma gondii	Central nervous system	Aspiration biopsy	29	1382
Strongyloides stercoralis	Lung	Sputum	19	743
Miscellaneous organisms	Diverse sites		See organ systems	

Table 31–5
Neoplastic Disorders in AIDS

Type of Disease	Organ Site	Medium of Diagnosis	Chapter	Page
			Reference	
Malignant lymphoma	Effusions	Smears and Cell blocks	26	1153
	Central nervous system	Cerebrospinal fluid	27	1201
	Gastrointestinal tract	Direct smears	24	1058
	Lymph nodes	Aspiration biopsy	29	1283
Kaposi's sarcoma	Skin and lymph nodes	Aspiration biopsy	29	1334
	Effusions	Smears and cell blocks	26	1164
Miscellaneous types	Miscellaneous organs		See organ systems	

Anal carcinomas of the squamous cell type occur in homosexual males and other AIDS victims with a history of anal intercourse. For a summary of cytologic findings in neoplastic disorders, see Table 31–5.

BIBLIOGRAPHY

Pathogenesis
Infections
Neoplastic disorders

Pathogenesis (Summary articles)

Daling, J.R., Weiss, N.S., et al.: Sexual practices, sexually transmitted diseases, and the incidence of anal cancer. N. Engl. J. Med., *317*:973–977, 1987.

Goodgame, R.W.: Aids in Uganda—clinical and social features. N. Engl. J. Med., *323*:383–388, 1990.

Levy, J.A.: Human immunodeficiency viruses and the pathogenesis of AIDS. J.A.M.A., *261*:2997–3006, 1989.

Quinn, T.C., Glasser, D., and Cannon, R.O.: Human immunodeficiency virus infection among patients attending clinics for sexually transmitted diseases. N. Engl. J. Med., *318*:198–203, 1988.

Waisman, J., Rotterdam, H., Niedt, G.N., et al.: AIDS: An overview of the pathology. Pathol. Res. Pract., *182*:729–754, 1987.

Infections (See also specific organs)

Bottles, K., McPhaul, L.W., and Volberdins, P.: Fine needle aspiration biopsy of patients with acquired immunodeficiency syndrome (AIDS): Experience in an outpatient clinic. Ann. Intern. Med., *108*:42–45, 1988.

Broaddus, C., Dake, M.D., Stulbarg, M.S., et al.: Bronchoalveolar lavage and transbronchial biopsy for the diagnosis of pulmonary infections in the acquired immunodeficiency syndrome. Ann. Intern. Med., *102*:747–752, 1988.

Brown, S., Senekjian, E.K., and Montag, A.G.: Cytomegalovirus infection of the uterine cervix in a patient with acquired immunodeficiency syndrome. Obstet. Gynecol., *71*:489–491, 1988.

Chandra, P., Delaney, M.D., and Tuazon, C.U.: Role of special stains in the diagnosis of *Pneumocystis carinii* infection from bronchial washing specimens in patients with the acquired immune deficiency syndrome. Acta Cytol., *32*:105–108, 1988.

Cuarde, L.A., Stein, S.A., Cleary, K.A., et al.: Human cryptosporidiosis in the acquired immunodeficiency syndrome. Arch. Pathol. Lab. Med., *107*:562–566, 1983.

De Fine, L.A., Saleba, K.P., Gobson, B.B., Wesseler, T.A., and Baughman, R.: Cytologic evaluation of bronchoalveolar lavage specimens in immunosuppressed patients with suspected opportunistic infections. Acta Cytol., *31*:235–242, 1987.

Fahey, J.L., Taylor, J.M.G., Detels, R., et al.: The prognostic value of cellular and serologic markers in infection with human immunodeficiency virus type 1. N. Engl. J. Med., *322*:166–172, 1990.

Feingold, A.R., Vermund, S.H., Burk, R.D., Kelley, K.F., Schrager, L.K., Schreiber, K., Munk, G., Friedland, G.H., and Klein, R.S.: Cervical cytologic abnormalities and papillomavirus in women infected with human immunodeficiency virus. Journal of Acquired Immune Deficiency Syndromes, *3*:896–903, 1990.

Gottlieb, M.S., Schroff, R., Schanker, H.M., Weisman, J.D., Fan, P.T., Wolf, R.A., and Saxon, A.: *Pneumocystis carinii* pneumonia and mucosal candidiasis in previously healthy homosexual men: Evidence of a new acquired cellular immunodeficiency. N. Engl. J. Med., *305*:1425–1431, 1981.

Greaves, T.S., and Strigle, S.M.: The recognition of *Pneumocystis carinii* in routine Papanicolaou-stained smears. Acta Cytol., *29*:714–720, 1985.

Grimes, M.M., La Pook J.D., Bar, M.H., et al.: Disseminated *Pneumocystis carinii* infection in a patient with acquired immune deficiency syndrome. Hum. Pathol., *18*:307–308, 1987.

Hildreth, J.E.K., and Orentas, R.J.: Involvement of a leukocyte adhesion receptor (LFA-1) in HIV-induced syncytium formation. Science, *244*:1075–1078, 1989.

Hinnant, K.L., Rotterdam, H.Z., Bell, E.T., et al.: Cytomegalovirus infection of the alimentary tract: A clinicopathological correlation. Am. J. Gastroenterol., *81*:944–950, 1986.

Katz, R.L., Alappatu, C., Glass, J.P., and Bruner, J.M.: Cerebrospinal fluid manifestation of the neurologic complications of human immunodeficiency virus infection. Acta Cytol., *33*:233–244, 1989.

Klatt, E.C., Jensen, D.F., and Meyer, P.R.: Pathology of mycobacterium-avium-intracellulare infection in acquired immunodeficiency syndrome. Hum. Pathol., *18*:709–714, 1987.

Knowles, D.M., Chamulak, G.A., Subar, M., et al.: Lymphoid neoplasia associated with the acquired immunodeficiency syndrome (AIDS): The New York University Medical Center experience with 105 patients (1981–1986). Ann. Intern. Med., *108*:744–753, 1988.

Lebenthal, S.W., Hajdu, S.I., and Urmacher, C.: Cytologic findings in homosexual males with acquired immunodeficiency. Acta Cytol. *27*:597–604, 1983.

Levine, A.M., Meyer, P.R., Begandy, M.M., et al.: Development of B-cell lymphoma in homosexual men: Clinical and immunologic findings. Ann. Intern. Med., *100*:7–13, 1984.

Masur, H., Michelis, M.A., Greene, J.B., Onorato, I., Vande Stouwe, R.A., Holzman, R.S., Wormser, G., Brettman, L., Lange, M., Murray, H.W., and Cunninghan-Rundles, S.: An outbreak of community-acquired *Pneumocystis carinii* pneumonia: Initial manifestation of cellular immune dysfunction. N. Engl. J. Med., *305*:1431–1438, 1981.

Miles, P.R., Baushman, R.P., and Linnemann, C.C., Jr.: Cytomegalovirus in the bronchoalveolar lavage fluid of patients with AIDS. Chest, *97*:1072–1076, 1990.

Mizusawa, H., Hirano, A., Llena, J.F., and Kato, T.: Nuclear bridges in multinucleated giant cells associated with primary lymphoma of the brain in acquired immune deficiency syndrome (AIDS). Acta Neuropathol., *75*:23–26, 1987.

Ognibene, F.P., Shelhamer, J., Gill, V., Macher, A.V., Loew, D., Parker, M.M., Gelmann, E., Fauci, A.S., Parillo, J.E., and Masur, H.: The diagnosis of *Pneumocystis carinii* pneumonia in patients with the acquired immunodeficiency syndrome using segmental bronchoalveolar lavage. Am. Rev. Respir. Dis., *129*:929–932, 1984.

Orenstein, M., Webber, C.A., and Heurich, A.E.: Cytologic diagnosis of *Pneumocystis carinii* infection by brochoalveolar lavage in acquired immune deficiency syndrome. Acta Cytol., *29*:727–731, 1985.

Phair, J., Munoz, A., and Detels, R.: The risk of *Pneumocystis carinii* pneumonia among men infected with human immunodeficiency virus type 1. N. Engl. J. Med., *322*:161–165, 1990.

Rhoads, J.L., Wright, C., Redfield, R.R., and Burke, D.S.: Chronic vaginal candidiasis in women with human immunodeficiency virus infection. J.A.M.A., *257*:3015–3107, 1987.

Schrager, L.K., Friedland, G.H., Maude, D., Schreiber, K., Adachi, A., Pizzuti, D.J., Koss, L.G., and Klein, R.S.: Cervical and vaginal squamous cell abnormalities in women infected with human immunodeficiency virus. Journal of Acquired Immune Deficiency Syndromes, *2*:570–575, 1989.

Siegal, F.P., Lopez, C., Hammer, G.S., et al.: Severe acquired immunodeficiency in male homosexuals, manifested by chronic perianal ulcerative herpes simplex lesions. N. Engl. J. Med., *305*:1439–1444, 1981.

Stover, D.E., Zaman, M.B., Hajdu, S.I., Lange, M., Gold, J., and Armstrong, D.: Bronchoalveolar lavage in the diagnosis of diffuse pulmonary infiltrates in the immunosuppressed host. Ann. Intern. Med., *101*:1–7, 1984.

Striale, S.M., and Gal, A.A.: A review of pulmonary cytopathology in the acquired immunodeficiency syndrome. Diagn. Cytopathol., *5*:44–54, 1989.

Suhrland, M.J., Koslow, M., Perchick, A., Weiner, S., Alba Greco, M., Colquhoun, F., Muller, W.D., and Burstein, D.: Cytologic findings in progressive multifocal leukoencephalopathy. Report of two cases. Acta Cytol., *31*:505–511, 1987.

Weldon-Linne, C.M., Rhone, D.P., and Bourassa, R.: Bronchoscopy specimens in adults with AIDS. Comparative yields of cytology, histology and culture for diagnosis of infectious agents. Chest, *98*:24–28, 1990.

Whiteside, M.E., Barkin, J.S., May, R.G., et al.: Enteric coccidiosis among patients with the acquired immunodeficiency syndrome. Am. J. Trop. Med. Hyg., *33*:1065–1072, 1984.

Zaharopoulos, P., Schnadig, V.J., Davie, K.D., Boudreau, R.E., and Weedn, V.W.: Multiseptate bodies in systemic phaeohyphomycosis diagnosed by fine needle aspiration cytology. Acta Cytol., *32*:885–891, 1988.

Neoplastic Disorders (See also specific organs)

Birx, D.L., Redfield, R.R., and Tosato, G.: Defective regulation of Epstein-Barr virus infection in patients with acquired immunodeficiency syndrome (AIDS) or AIDS-related disorders. N. Engl. J. Med., *314*:874–879, 1986.

Butler, J.J., and Osborne, B.M.: Lymph node enlargement in patients with unsuspected human immunodeficiency virus infections. Hum. Pathol., *19*:849–854, 1988.

Daling, J.R., Weiss, N.S., Hislop, T.G., Maden, C., Coates, R.J., Sherman, K.J., Ashley, R.L., Beagrie, M., Ryan, J.A., and Corey, M.D.: Sexual practices, sexually transmitted diseases, and the incidence of anal cancer. N. Engl. J. Med., *317*:933–937, 1987.

Greenspan, J., Greenspan, D., and Lannette, E.T.: Replication of Epstein-Barr virus within the epithelial cells of oral 'hairy' leukoplakia, and AIDS-associated lesion. N. Engl. J. Med., *313*:1456–1471, 1986.

Ioachim, H.L., Lerner, C.W., and Tapper, M.L.: The lymphoid lesions associated with the acquired immunodeficiency syndrome. Am. J. Surg. Pathol., *7*:543–553, 1983.

Knowles, D.M.: Malignant lymphomas occurring in association with acquired immunodeficiency syndrome. Lab. Med., *17*:674–678, 1986.

Knowles, D.M., Chamulak, G.A., Subar, M., et al.: Lymphoid neoplasia associated with the acquired immunodeficiency syndrome (AIDS): The New York University Medical Center experience with 105 patients (1981–1986). Ann. Intern. Med., *108*:744–753, 1988.

Lebenthal, S.W., Hajdu, S.I., and Urmacher, C.: Cytologic findings in homosexual males with acquired immunodeficiency. Acta Cytol., *27*:597–604, 1983.

Levine, A.M., Meyer, P.R., Begandy, M.M., et al.: Development of B-cell lymphoma in homosexual men: Clinical and immunologic findings. Ann. Intern. Med., *100*:7–13, 1984.

Lind, P., Syrjänen, S., Syrjänen, K., Koppang, H.S., and Aas, E.: Immunoreactivity and human papillomarvirus (HPV) on oral precancer and cancer lesions. Scand. J. Dent. Res., *94*:419–426, 1986.

Lowenthal, D.A., Straus, D.J., and Campbell, S.W.: AIDS-related lymphoid neoplasia. The Memorial experience. Cancer, *61*:2325–2337, 1988.

Lustbader, I., and Sherman, A.: Primary gastrointestinal Kaposi's sarcoma in a patient with acquired immuno-deficiency syndrome. Am. J. Gastroenterol., *82*:894–895, 1987.

Meyer, P.R., Yanagihara, E.T., Parker, J.W., and Lukes, R.J.: A distinct follicular hyperplasia in the acquired immune deficiency syndrome (AIDS) and the AIDS related complex: A pre-lymphomatous state for B cell lymphoma? Hematol. Oncol., *2*:319–347, 1984.

O'Murchadha, M.T., Wolf, B.C., and Neiman, R.S.: The histologic features of hyperplastic lymphadenopathy in AIDS-related complex are nonspecific. Am. J. Surg. Pathol., *11*:94–99, 1987.

Poelzleitner, D., Huebsch, P., Mayerhofer, S., Chott, A., and Zielinski, C.: Primary pulmonary lymphoma in a patient with acquired immune deficiency syndrome. Thorax, *44*:438–439, 1989.

Stanley, M.W., and Frizzera, G.: Diagnostic specificity of histologic features in lymph node biopsy specimens from patients at risk for the acquired immunodeficiency syndrome. Hum. Pathol., *17*:1231–1239, 1986.

Ziegler, J.L., Beckstead, J.A., Volberding, P.A., Abrams, D.I., Levine, A.M., Lukes, R.J., Gill, P.S., Burkes, R.L., Meyer, P.R., Metroka, C.E., Mouradian, J., Moore, A., Riggs, S.A., Butler, J.J., Cabanillas, F.C., Hersh, E., Newell, G.R., Laubenstein, L.J., Knowles, D., Odajnyk, C., Rahael, B., Koziner, B., Urmacher, C., and Clarkson, B.D.: Non-Hodgkin's lymphoma in 90 homosexual men. N. Engl. J. Med., *311*:565–570, 1984.

Part 3

Techniques in Diagnostic Cytology

32

Clinical Procedures in Diagnostic Cytology*

PREPARATION AND FIXATION OF SMEARS AND FLUID SPECIMENS

The quality of the cytologic diagnosis depends in equal measure on the excellence of the clinical procedure used to secure the sample and on laboratory procedures used to process the sample. In this chapter the clinical procedures used to secure cytologic samples from various body sites will be described in detail. Aspiration biopsy procedures, described in Chapters 19, 20, and 29, will not be repeated here. The laboratory procedures are discussed in Chapters 33 and 34.

In general, material for cytologic examination is obtained either in the form of smears prepared by the examining physician, gynecologist, surgeon, or his or her assistant, at the time of the clinical examination, or in the form of brushes or fluid specimens that are forwarded to the laboratory for further processing.

Smears

Prior to the preparation of smears it is important to secure the necessary materials and lay them out on a suitable, conveniently located surface within the reach of the operator:

1. Instrument(s) used to obtain smears.
2. Clean microscopic glass slides of good quality, preferably with frosted ends (0.96–1.06 mm in thickness).
3. Suitable pencil or, if plain slides are used, a diamond marker for identification of slides. Each slide should be identified with patient's name or identifying number. If several body sites are to be studied, the slides must be appropriately identified by symbols. The following symbols may be used: V = vagina, C = cervix, E = endocervix, EN = endometrium, LB = left bronchus, RB = right bronchus, and so on. The precise origin of each smear with the accompanying symbol must be noted on the laboratory form.
4. Paper clips used to separate the slides from each other if liquid fixative is used.
5. Fixative (see p. 1452).

Carol Bales, CT (ASCP), made several useful suggestions during the preparation of this chapter. L. G. K.

6. Laboratory form with clear identification of the patient and appropriate *history*. The minimum data required on each patient comprise:

Date of procedure.
Name of physician or health facility submitting the sample.
Patient's name and address.
Sex.
Age.
Source and site of origin of the specimen with identifying symbols (see above).
Method of collection.
Presumed clinical diagnosis.
Summary of prevailing symptoms.
Prior treatment, if any.
Prior cytology or histology.
For routine gynecologic specimens add:
    Date of last menstrual period.
    Contraceptive history.
    Obstetric history.

Preparation of Smears

For most diagnostic purposes, well-prepared and well-fixed smears are required. Air drying of smears should be avoided, unless specifically desired as in some forms of aspiration biopsy (see p. 1244).

Every effort should be made to place as much as possible of the material obtained on the slide and to prepare a thin, uniform smear. Thick smears with overlapping cell layers are difficult or impossible to interpret. Considerable skill and practice are required to prepare excellent smears by a single, swift motion without loss of material or air drying. Excessive crushing of material, particularly common with brush preparations, must be avoided. The practice of relegating the smear preparations to unskilled personnel is not fair to the patient. If the person obtaining diagnostic material is not familiar with the technical requirements of smear preparation, competent help must be secured in advance.

Fixation

Except in special situations in which the preparation of air-dried material is required or desirable (see Aspiration Biopsy, Chapter 29), immediate fixation of smears is essential for correct interpretations.

Two types of fixatives are commonly used: fluid fixatives and spray fixatives. Both are described in detail in Chapter 33, and hence only a brief summary is required here.

Fluid Fixatives. These are prepared in bottles of suitable sizes, provided with caps, or in Coplin jars with covers. Commonly used fixatives are 95% ethanol, 70% ethanol, or their substitutes, discussed on p. 1452. For all practical purposes, 95% ethyl alcohol is a suitable universal fixative for smears. The bottle or the Coplin jar must carry a label with suitable identification of the patient. If more than one glass slide is placed in the same fixative bottle, it is essential that each slide be correctly identified. A paper clip placed on the frosted or marked end of every other slide will prevent adherence of slides to each other. It is unwise to use a single specimen bottle or Coplin jar for more than one patient. Errors of identification and occurrence of "floaters," or free-floating cells, may cause serious diagnostic mishaps.

The smears must be placed in the container with fluid fixative while still wet, making sure that there is sufficient fixative to cover the smeared area. The container must be immediately closed with cap or cover and forwarded to the laboratory together with the laboratory form. Alternatively, the smears can be removed from the fixative after 15 to 30 minutes and placed in an appropriate container for shipment to the laboratory. The liquid fixative should be filtered before it is used again to avoid contamination with floaters.

Spray Fixatives. These contain water-soluble polymers or plastics and are described in detail in Chapter 33. When correctly used, spray fixatives protect the smears from drying by forming an invisible film on the surface of the slides. Spray fixatives may be used in lieu of fluid fixatives, that is, *immediately* after the process of smear preparation has been completed. Correct use of the spray fixatives calls for several precautions:

1. The spray must be smooth and steady, and the operation of the nozzle must be checked before the smear is obtained.

2. The distance between the nozzle of the spray and the smear to be sprayed must be about 10 to 12 inches (25 to 30 cm), as shown in Figure 32–1. If the spray is held too close to the smear, several mishaps commonly occur: the cells may be dislodged by the force of the spray, or the evaporation of the spray vehicle may freeze and irreversibly damage the cells. An artifact may also occur, inasmuch as normal squamous cells may acquire a perinuclear halo, rendering them similar to koilocytes. If the nozzle is too far from the target, insufficient fixative will reach the surface. Although there is no evi-

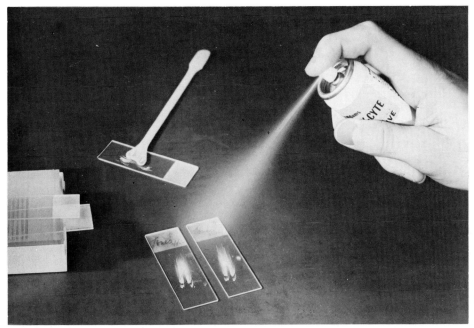

FIGURE 32–1. Use of coating fixatives for smears of uterine cervix obtained with a wooden spatula. Immediate application of fixative is essential. (Clay-Adams Inc., New York, N.Y.)

dence at this time that the materials contained in the various spray preparations are harmful, it is advisable to protect the patient and the medical personnel from inhalation of the spray by using a face mask or by performing the procedure, under a protective glass plate or a hood.

Smears coated with spray fixative are *air dried* and placed in cardboard slide containers and forwarded to the laboratory in this fashion.

Other Fixatives for Smears. Inexpensive liquid-coating fixatives may be prepared in the laboratory and used in lieu of spray fixatives. Carbowax fixative, described on p. 1453, is an example. A few drops of this fixative may be placed on the surface of the smear. After drying (5 to 10 minutes) the slides may be placed in slide containers for shipment.

Fluid Specimens

Fluid specimens may be obtained from a variety of body sites, such as the respiratory tract, gastrointestinal tract, urinary tract, or effusions, and the clini-cal procedures used in their collection are described below. As is discussed in detail on p. 1457 in Chapter 33, unless the laboratory has the facilities for immediate processing of fluid specimens, it is advisable either to collect such specimens in bottles with fixative prepared in advance or to add the fixative shortly after collection. The common fixative of nearly universal applicability to fluids is 50% ethanol. *Ether-containing fixatives should never be added to fluids.* Generally the volume of the fixative should be the same or slightly in excess of the volume of the fluid to be studied.

The volume of the fluid rarely need be larger than 100 ml. Screw cap bottles of 250-ml content, containing 50 ml of 50% ethanol, are suitable for most specimens. Special fixation is required for gastric material (see p. 1465), and it is sometimes advisable to collect effusion fluids in anticoagulants (see p. 1463).

The fluids, particularly sputum and urine, can also be collected in fixatives containing 2% carbowax in 50% or 70% ethanol. For further discussion of these fixatives and processing of specimens by Saccomanno's method for sputum and Bales's method for urine, see pp. 1460 and 1465.

CLINICAL PROCEDURES FOR CYTOLOGIC STUDY OF VARIOUS BODY SITES

The Female Genital Tract

Cytologic Techniques in Gynecologic Practice*

The successful practice of diagnostic cytology depends to a large extent on good fixation of smears. The often scanty cytologic evidence must be technically satisfactory. Therefore, it is recommended that a fixative of the clinician's choice be kept near at hand before smears are obtained.

The patient should not douche for 24 hours before the genital smears are obtained.

Preferably, smears should not be taken during menstrual bleeding because of contamination with blood, endometrium, debris, and histiocytes.

Vaginal Smear. This smear is best obtained as the fist step in the gynecologic examination, prior to introduction of the speculum. The patient is placed in lithotomy position. The posterior fornix of the vagina is aspirated with the blunt end of a slightly curved glass pipette fitted with a rubber bulb. During aspiration the end of the pipette should be gently moved from side to side to ensure a good sampling of cells. The aspirate is spread rapidly on a clean glass slide, which is fixed without delay.

The late Dr. Genevieve M. Bader graciously reviewed this part of the manuscript and made several useful suggestions.

Advantages and Disadvantages. The advantage of the vaginal smear lies chiefly in the ease with which it is obtained, even in the presence of an intact hymen. The vaginal smear is efficient in the detection and the diagnosis of endometrial cancer, but it will *fail* to nearly 50% of all precancerous lesions of the cervix (Table 32–1). No gynecologic examination can be considered complete unless a vaginal smear is accompanied by a cervical smear.

Comment. Within recent years, the vaginal pool smear obtained by aspiration of the contents of the vaginal fornix has fallen into disuse. This unjustified neglect occurred for two reasons: one was the reduction of cost and labor in cervical cancer screening that could be obtained by securing a single cervical smear; the other was the time and skill involved in the screening of the vaginal sample, which is often very rich in cells and difficult to interpret. Yet the vaginal smear complements the cervical sample and offers several major advantages, particularly in women past the age of 40.

Cells from the endometrium, the fallopian tube, the ovary, and occasionally from other, more distant sites are found in the vaginal pool smear and usually not in the direct smear of the uterine cervix. The endocervical aspiration, which sometimes replaces the vaginal pool smear, is not widely used and is technically more difficult. The vaginal smear may be used for a rough estimation of the hormonal status. For these reasons, the vaginal smear should be maintained in the armamentarium of cancer detection.

A satisfactory vaginal smear should contain a good sample of cells of squamous epithelial origin.

Table 32–1
*Comparison of the Respective Usefulness of Cervical and Vaginal Smears — Cytologic Findings in 77 Cases of Carcinoma In Situ of the Cervix**

	Cervical Swab		Vaginal Smear	
	No.	*%*	*No.*	*%*
Positive	56	72.7	16	20.8
Suspicious	19	24.7	18	23.4
Atypia	1	1.3	28	36.3
Negative	0	0	14	18.2
Quantity not sufficient	1	1.3	1	1.3
Total	77	100.0	77	100.0

*Simon, T.R., Durfee, G.R., and Ricci, A.: The value of the vaginal aspiration smear as compared with the cervical swab smear in the detection of in situ carcinoma of the cervix and adenocarcinoma of the fundus. Transactions of the Third Annual Meeting of the Inter-Society Cytology Council, pp. 75-85, November 1955.

The background should be free of foreign material, such as medical jellies. Air drying of smears should be avoided (see above). Mucus, leukocytes, *Trichomonas vaginalis*, fungi, or spermatozoa, either intact or degenerated, do not disqualify a smear. The presence of endocervical cells is exceptional in vaginal smears.

The **vaginal smear for hormonal studies** should be obtained by scraping the lateral wall of the vagina at some distance from the cervix. These smears are reliable only in the evaluation of the hormonal status of the female, provided that other complicating factors, such as inflammation and medication, have been ruled out, as discussed in Chap. 9. The fixation is the same as described on p. 1430.

Cervical Smear. This smear is a reliable means for the diagnosis of cervix cancer, but it fails to provide much information about the status of the endometrium (Table 32–2).

The cervical smear must be obtained under direct vision after introduction of the speculum. However, under no circumstances should the speculum be lubricated with medical jellies, since the foreign material may readily contaminate the smear. If there are difficulties in introducing the speculum, a few drops of normal saline solution may be used to moisten it. Several methods of obtaining cytologic material from the uterine cervix are available.

Cotton Swab Smear. The entire portio of the cervix is swabbed under pressure with an applicator tipped with nonabsorbent cotton, which is introduced into the external os as far as possible. The cervical mucus and the cellular material are spread rapidly by rolling the applicator on a slide. Immediate fixation is mandatory.

Advantages and Disadvantages. The method is easily performed and nontraumatic. If the smear is obtained carefully and the material adequately spread on the slide, sufficient diagnostic evidence is usually obtained. The disadvantage is the scarcity of material obtained by clinicians who are not thoroughly familiar with the method.

Cervical Scraper or Spatula (Ayre). A wooden tongue depressor, cut with scissors to fit the contour of the cervix, may be used. Commercially prepared plastic and wooden scrapers are currently widely available. One end of the scraper is somewhat longer than the other so that it fits the external os and reaches the endocervical canal. The scraper is rotated under pressure, the longer end being used as a pivot within the external os (see Fig. 3, p. 6). The material is spread on a slide and fixed immediately.

Advantages and Disadvantages. Abundant and diagnostically valuable material is obtained by this method. The disadvantages are that the method may occasionally be traumatic to the patient, and the tip of a scraper that does not fit the external ox may fail to remove some of the valuable material from the squamocolumnar junction. The use of a scraper as opposed to the cotton-tipped applicator is a matter of individual preference. Still, smears obtained with scrapers are often easier to screen.

Endocervical Aspiration. By means of a small cannula attached to a syringe or, preferably, to a

Table 32–2
Comparison of the Respective Usefulness of Cervical and Vaginal Smears —
Cytologic Findings in 29 Cases of Adenocarcinoma of Endometrium *

	Cervical Swab		Vaginal Smear	
	No.	*%*	*No.*	*%*
Positive	5	17.2	16	55.1
Suspicious	7	24.2	6	20.7
Atypia	5	17.2	0	0
Negative	12	41.4	7	24.2
Total	29	100.0	29	100.0

*Simon, T.R., Durfee, G.R., and Ricci, A.: The value of the vaginal aspiration smear as compared with the cervical swab smear in the detection of in situ carcinoma of the cervix and adenocarcinoma of the fundus. Transactions of the Third Annual Meeting of the Inter-Society Cytology Council, pp. 75–88, November 1955.

large rubber bulb, the contents of the endocervical canal are aspirated, subsequently expelled on a slide, smeared, and fixed in the usual fashion.

Advantages and Disadvantages. The method provides valuable information about the status of the endocervical canal and the endometrium and may be helpful in localizing an endocervical lesion. The method fails to provide information about the status of the vaginal portio of the cervix and therefore should not be used alone.

In our hands, with the use of a commercially available instrument, endocervical canal aspiration failed to provide useful information about the status of the endocervical canal or the endometrium in asymptomatic women (Koss et al., 1984; see also Chap. 14).

Endocervical Brushing Instruments. Several types of small brushes for sampling of the endocervical canal have been introduced within recent years (Fig. 32–2). The popularity of these instruments is based, to a significant extent, on the concept that an adequate cervical smear must contain endocervical cells (see below, p. 1438). This writer does not necessarily subscribe to this notion because he believes that the plug of endocervical mucus, occluding the external os, is the most important source of abnormal cells. For some of the brushes to be used, the mucus plug must be removed, and this important evidence is lost.

Advantages and Disadvantages. The endocervical brush yields endocervical cells in virtually all the smears, thus increasing the proportion of adequate cervical smears. The performance of the brush in some hands has apparently increased the diagnosis of precancerous cervical lesions and endocervical adenocarcinomas, particularly when combined with a cervical scraper (Boon et al., 1986).

Among the disadvantages, the loss of the cervical mucus plug is poorly compensated by the brush, and the evidence presented in favor of a better yield of malignant or premalignant lesions has not been adequately documented.

Other disadvantages of the brush include the difficulty in the interpretation of thick clusters of endocervical cells scraped from the endocervical surface. There is also evidence that many patients experience bleeding or spotting after the use of this instrument.

Because the brush, at best, samples the endocervical canal and the transformation zone and provides no information on the status of the squamous epithelium of the exocervix, the brush *must* be used in association with another instrument, such as a cervical scraper, to secure a sample from the entire endocervix.

An interesting instrument, the Cervex brush, was introduced some years ago. The brush-like instrument consists of a flat array of flexible plastic strips. The central strips are longer and thus enter the endocervical canal (Fig. 32–3). Several rotations of the instrument ensure sampling of the entire cervical epithelium with adequate representation of endocervical cells.

Mixed Smears from Cervix and Vagina (Fast Smear). Frost advocates the use of a combined smear from both these sites on a single slide. The efficiency of this sample is probably somewhat below that of the direct cervical smears in the detection of abnormalities of the cervical epithelium. The mixed smear offers limited information pertaining to the hormonal status.

Triple Smear Method (V.C.E. Smear). Wied and Bahr advocate placing material from three sources (vagina, portio, endocervix) on a single specially prepared and etched glass slide. This offers the advantage of rapid screening of material. The method requires considerable dexterity on the part of the clinician to obtain material rapidly in order to avoid drying of smears. The procedure is as follows:

1. Obtain a vaginal smear with a wooden tongue depressor. *Do not smear* but hand the tongue depressor to an assistant.
2. Obtain routine cervical scrape smear—*do not smear* but hand the scraper to an assistant.
3. Obtain an endocervical specimen with either a premoistened cotton swab or an endocervical aspirator.
4. Smear all three specimens beginning with the endocervical material on the V.C.E. slide in appropriate slots.
5. Fix slide immediately.

Vaginal Tampon Smear. A tampon, usually produced from a nonabsorbent material such as nylon mesh, is introduced into the vagina by the patient, subsequently removed, and "stamped" on a slide. The usual method of fixation is used.

Advantages and Disadvantages. The advantages of this method are the ease of application and the facility of investigating a large number of women by a small number of medical personnel.

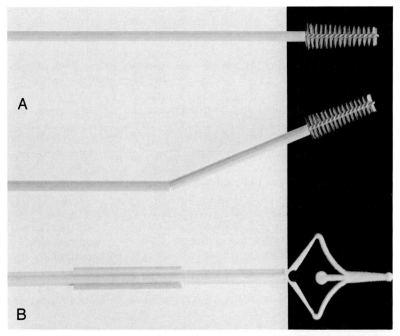

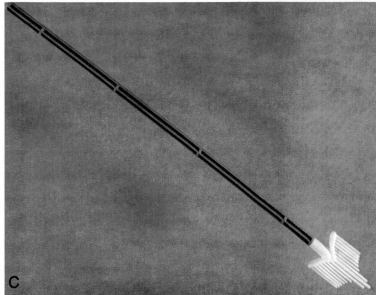

FIGURE 32–2. Newer instruments for sampling of the cervix. (*A*) Cytobrush Plus (Medscand, Malmö, Sweden). The shaft of the instrument is breakable, and the brush can be used for microbiologic culture. (*B*) Accelon (Medscand, Malmö, Sweden). An instrument for synchronous sampling of the endocervical canal and exocervix. (*C*) Cervex brush (Rovers, B.V. and Unimar, Inc., Wilton, Conn.). (*A* and *B* courtesy of Dr. Nils Stormby, Malmö, Sweden; (*C*) courtesy of Mr. W.P.G. Rovers, Oss, Holland.)

The major disadvantages are the relatively poor quality of cellular material obtained by this method and the marked distortion of the component cells, which may render the interpretation quite difficult. The method is not reliable in detecting early cancerous changes of the cervical mucosa. Also, the patient is deprived of the benefits of a clinical examination. The method is recommended only if facilities for a complete gyneco-logic examination, including standard cervical and vaginal smears, are not available.

Irrigation Smear. Koch and Stakemann and Davis introduced a self-administered pipette for collection of cytologic material for purposes of cancer detection. The device, which is disposable, is made up of a fixative-filled plastic bulb attached to a pipette. The device may be mailed to the patient, accompanied by a set of simple instructions. The patient inserts the pipette into the vagina and by compressing the elastic bulb expresses the fixative. The bulb is then released, and the pipette is slowly withdrawn from the vagina. The fixative plus the cells is aspirated back into the pipette. The pipette is sealed and mailed back to the laboratory.

The fluid is spun down in a centrifuge and the sediment smeared on two, three, or more slides. Residual material may be kept indefinitely. Davis considers 50 to 100 cells per low-power field as an adequate smear.

The screening of this material requires a great deal of attention to detail, since abnormal cells may be few and far apart. In many ways the material obtained by irrigation resembles a diluted vaginal smear. Accurate evaluation of this type of material is of necessity time-consuming.

Following very encouraging reports on the use of the pipette by Davis and by Koch and Stakemann, Richart (1965) pointed out that irrigation smears failed to reveal 40% to 50% of early neoplastic lesions of the cervix. A similar result was reported by Muskett et al. (1966) on a smaller group of carefully controlled patients.

In following years a number of additional reports on this subject appeared. Reagan and Lin (1967), Mattingly et al. (1967), Anderson and Gunn (1967), Carrow et al. (1967), and Husain (1970) rendered reports ranging from highly skeptical to enthusiastic. It is generally considered that self-administered smears should not be recommended, unless the patient has no access to a more direct method of cytologic sampling.

Endometrial Aspiration.   Several instruments have been designed to facilitate collection of material from the endometrial cavity. Some of the methods are in all respects similar to that of the endometrial biopsy and fail to show any distinct advantage as a sampling procedure. The ideal method of aspirating the endometrial cavity—one that would provide an adequate sampling of the entire endometrium and that would be painless, nontraumatic, and easy to perform in asymptomatic patients—has yet to be developed.

However, very adequate material may be obtained with the help of the endometrial cannula of Jordan (Fig. 32–3). This cannula may be introduced into the endometrial cavity without preliminary dilatation of the endocervical canal. A 20-ml syringe provides the negative pressure necessary for aspiration of material.

Several variants of the simple instrument devised by Jordan have been produced and are marketed under a variety of trade names. For ex-

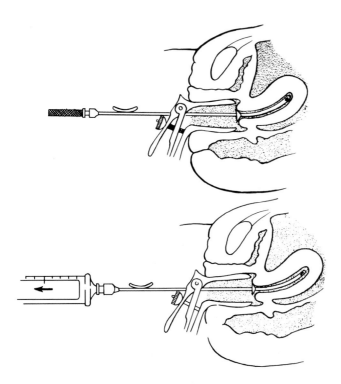

FIGURE 32–3. Technique of endometrial aspiration using Jordan's Aspiration Cannula (United Surgical Supplies Co., Inc., Mamaronek, N.Y.) In the upper drawing the cannula with its obturator in place is located within the endometrial cavity. In the lower drawing the obturator is removed, and suction is exercised by means of a syringe. (Drs. M. J. Jordan and G. M. Bader)

ample, a disposable syringe-cannula combination* (Isaacs's) and a cannula associated with a small portable vacuum bottle replacing the syringe (Vakutage)† have been suggested for endometrial aspirations. Similarly, many instruments for direct endometrial sampling have been devised, such as a brush originally suggested by Ayre, a variant thereof devised by Matsubuchi in Japan, or a plastic applicator devised for this purpose (MiMark).‡

All of the commercial instruments have some features in common: they are relatively costly to use and cause varying degrees of discomfort, particularly to the asymptomatic postmenopausal patient who should be the principal target of endometrial cancer detection. The performance of these devices, often enthusiastically endorsed in the initial stages, is usually excellent in the symptomatic or hospital populations. Their performance as tools of endometrial cancer detection has been tested and resulted in the detection of a substantial number of occult endometrial carcinomas (Koss et al., 1984). See Chapter 14 for further details.

Regardless of the instrument used, there are two ways of examining endometrial material. Smears can be prepared from aspirated samples and handled as any other smear from the genital tract. Alternatively, the material may be placed in fixative (such as 50% alcohol), spun down, embedded in paraffin, and examined as microbiopsies. The advantages and disadvantages of both methods of procedure are discussed at some length in Chapter 14. In general, it may be stated that the histologic sections are easier to interpret, except in cases of advanced endometrial carcinoma where both diagnostic media are equally efficient.

The indications for endometrial aspiration were outlined on p. 571. The method should be used generously in menopausal patients, since it provides a reliable means for the diagnosis of early endometrial carcinoma.

Other Methods of Endometrial Sampling. For description and discussion of several other instruments used in the cytologic diagnosis of endometrial lesions, see Chapter 14, p. 571.

Kendall Co., Boston, Massachusetts 02101.

†Warner-Lambert Co., Morris Plains, New Jersey 07950.

‡Simpson/Basye, Inc., Wilmington, Delaware 19804.

Use of Special Procedures to Increase the Accuracy of Biopsies of the Cervix

SCHILLER'S IODINE TEST

In the absence of a grossly visible lesion, painting the cervix (or the vagina) with a solution of iodine (Schiller's test) may assist in localizing epithelial abnormalities. Normal epithelium is rich in glycogen, which combines with iodine to form a mahogany-brown stain.

Actively proliferating epithelium, such as in situ carcinoma, fails to take iodine stain and remains unstained or poorly stained. Schiller's iodine test provides only a very general guidance in the search for areas to be biopsied. Certain keratinizing cancers of the portio may contain glycogen and stain with iodine. On the other hand, benign abnormalities, such as eversion of the endocervical mucosa or leukoplakia, may fail to stain with iodine. Schiller's test gives no information on the status of the endocervix (see Color Plate 12–2).

Richart carefully evaluated the Schiller test by means of a colpomicroscope and found that about one quarter of the patients with known carcinoma in situ and nearly one half of the patients with known cervical intraepithelial neoplasia failed to display a significant abnormality with this test.

Rubio and Thomassen confirmed Richart's observations in a study of 87 patients with precancerous intraepithelial lesions and 100 normal women serving as controls. The study, which was controlled by histologic examination of each of four quadrants of the cone specimens in the 87 patients, revealed a high percentage of false-positive and false-negative areas. Most important, Schiller's test proved unreliable in detecting or rejecting areas of precancerous abnormalities at the surgical margin of the conization specimen. There were numerous Schiller-positive (unstained) areas on the surfaces of the normal cervices.

Thus, Schiller's test can only be considered as a poor substitute for colposcopy in the detection of precancerous lesions and should be used as a guide to biopsies only if colposcopy is not available.

TOLUIDINE BLUE STAIN

Richart (1963) advocated the use of 1% aqueous solution of toluidine blue for delineation of precancerous lesions and carcinoma in situ in vivo.

The method is as follows: The cervix is cleaned with a mucolytic solution, prepared as follows: to a 1-oz. (30-ml) cup, the bottom of which has been covered by Caroid powder, 1% solution of acetic acid is added. Following cleansing the cervix is dried with cotton balls. The solution of toluidine is then applied with a cotton-tipped applicator. After several minutes the excess stain is blotted with cotton. The cervix is then washed again with the 1% acetic acid solution, and the areas retaining stain are noted. After the second washing with acetic acid the nonneoplastic epithelium of the cervix becomes decolorized or contains only a faint residuum of stain, whereas the areas of neoplasia retain a royal-blue stain. Inflammatory areas and endocervical columnar epithelium (such as that in eversions) may retain the stain but stain blue-black.

The staining reaction correlated with nuclear density, since toluidine blue is a nuclear stain. Accordingly, the intensity of the positive (royal-blue) stain reflected to some degree the nuclear density of the underlying lesion and was less intense in low-grade lesions (dysplasia) than in fully developed carcinoma in situ.

Richart indicated that the toluidine blue stain is much more sensitive than the Schiller test, particularly in low-grade lesions (dysplasia), many of which are Schiller-negative. This was the case in 10 of 18 such lesions discussed in detail in this contribution.

COLPOSCOPY

The colposcope is an instrument that allows a visual examination of the epithelium of the portio under a magnification of up to 20 times (see p. 476). This method may reveal lesions not visible to the naked eye. The colposcope provides excellent guidance in obtaining cervical biopsies; its drawback is its inability to provide information on the status of the endocervical canal.

The principles of colposcopy are based on the identification of abnormal vascular patterns and abnormalities of epithelial configuration. A skilled colposcopist will recognize the abnormalities of the transformation zone and adjacent surface of the cervix. For further details the reader is referred to the extensive bibliography cited.

The colposcope has proved an indispensable tool in the handling of patients suspected of harboring precancerous intraepithelial lesions of the cervix. Its use, which was described in detail on p. 477, is essential and must be encouraged.

Management of Patients with Abnormal Cytology

Uterine Cervix. The suggested handling of such patients is summarized in Fig. 12–54. The diagram emphasizes the need for colposcopic examination of all patients showing evidence of cervical intraepithelial neoplasia or repeatedly atypical smears. It suggests the sequence of clinical procedures in the presence and in the absence of colposcopic abnormalities. In the latter case a review of cytologic evidence is essential before any other diagnostic procedures are contemplated (for further discussion see p. 478, Chap. 12).

Endometrium. If cytologic suspicion or diagnosis of endometrial carcinoma is expressed, an endometrial biopsy or a diagnostic curettage is mandatory.

Ovary and Tube. An ultrasound examination, sometimes followed by laparoscopy or an exploratory laparotomy may be necessary in some cases, as outlined in Chapter 16.

Standards of Adequacy of Cytologic Examination of the Female Genital Tract

The primary purpose of cytologic examination of the female genital tract is the detection of cancer and precancerous states. The following represents a *modified* summary of the conclusions of a Study Group that was convened at the Center for Disease Control in Atlanta, Georgia, in 1973 for the purpose of establishing standards of adequacy of the cytologic examination of the female genital tract.

The value of the cytologic examination in the detection of epithelial abnormalities of the female genital tract depends critically on the quality of the specimen received in the laboratory. A poorly obtained or poorly fixed cellular sample may be interpreted incorrectly by the cytopathologist.

UTERINE CERVIX

An adequate cervical cytologic sample (Papanicolaou smear) should be obtained *under direct visualization* and contain an adequate number of well-preserved epithelial cells.

In an ideal screening situation, a sampling of the endocervix is desirable. This may be achieved by means of an endocervical aspiration, by sampling with a premoistened, nonabsorbent cotton swab applicator, or by using other effective collection devices such as endocervical brush instruments (see above).

The cell population may vary in numbers according to the patient's age and hormonal status. Samples with sparse cellularity, with poor preservation, or exhibiting other factors interfering with diagnostic interpretation (e.g., excessive blood, inflammatory cells) should be considered inadequate.

The presence or absence of identifiable endocervical cells does not appear to have a major bearing on the adequacy or inadequacy of the cervical or endocervical cytologic sample, especially in postmenopausal women with atrophy of the uterine cervix. The presence of endocervical cells in an otherwise adequate negative sample does not rule out the possibility of an epithelial abnormality. Conversely, abnormal cells may occur in the absence of endocervical cells. Cytologic identification of squamous metaplasia is not always possible and is not an adequate criterion of a satisfactory smear. The presence of endocervical mucus, containing leukocytes, suggests that the endocervical canal has been sampled and the endocervical mucus plug dislodged.

The diagnostic accuracy of routine cervical smears, regardless of technique, is not absolute. Therefore, *a minimum of three consecutive cervical smears, at intervals of 6 to 12 months, should be obtained* before the patient is considered free of disease. Subsequent screening may take place at longer intervals every other or third year. Because of low sensitivity, the use of self-administered devices for screening for carcinoma of the cervix is not recommended. The average cytopathology laboratory is not proficient in processing and interpreting this type of material.

Additional Comments on Cervical Smear Adequacy. The issue of smear adequacy has become more acute with the introduction of the Bethesda system (see Chapter 12, p. 486), which places upon the pathologist the responsibility of identifying inadequate specimens. The potential legal consequences of failing to identify a cervical smear as "inadequate" in a woman in whom invasive cancer subsequently develops can be catastrophic. On the other hand, the rejection of too many smears as inadequate results in significant fiscal and emotional burdens on women and society (Koss, 1990).

With the introduction of endocervical brushes a number of papers suggested that the presence of endocervical cells in the smear was an important landmark of cervical smear adequacy (Trimbos and Arenz, 1986) Boon et al. (1986) also suggested that the combination of the endocervical brush and Ayre's cervical spatula resulted in an increased detection rate of precancerous lesions. Other observers, including this writer, are not persuaded that this is the case but that it may merely reflect more careful screening of material known to be the target of a research project. Further, in women approaching or reaching menopause, there is often a retraction of the "transformation zone," placing the endocervical epithelium out of reach of the brush. The issue is still further complicated because there is no evident agreement whether the "adequate" smear should contain endocervical columnar cells or squamous "metaplastic" cells as evidence of proper sampling. Thus the issue of what constitutes an adequate cervical smear has not been settled at this time (1991) and probably never will achieve consensus. Although the presence of endocervical cells is desirable, their absence need not disqualify the smear as inadequate. For further comments see also Chapter 12, p. 474.

ENDOMETRIUM

Increasing attention must be given to the use of cytologic and histopathologic techniques in the detection of precancerous and cancerous endometrial lesions, because of evidence of increasing incidence of malignant diseases at this site. Such efforts should be directed primarily at women past the age of 40 and at women with evidence of menstrual abnormalities.

To improve the detection of cancer of the endometrium and its precursors, *a vaginal pool smear should be included in the examination of all women at risk.* This sampling method has a lower sensitivity and specificity than comparable methods used for the detection of cervical abnormalities. The problem is compounded by difficulties in the morphologic recognition of the cellular patterns of endometrial abnormalities. A major educational effort, directed at clinicians, pathologists, and cytotechnologists, appears desirable.

Where practical, cytologic or microbiopsy techniques that directly sample the endometrium should be used to improve the detection or diagnosis of early endometrial cancer. Such methods also have been shown to be effective screening tools when properly used. For further comments on endometrial cancer detection, see Chapter 14.

Adnexa

Cancer of the ovaries and fallopian tubes remains a major cause of mortality. The state of the art pertaining to the detection and early diagnosis of this group of diseases is unsatisfactory.

Cytologic sampling of the cul-de-sac or direct needle aspirations of adnexal masses may be helpful. Vaginal pool smears, and occasionally endocervical aspirates, have been shown to contain cancer cells of ovarian and tubal origin; unfortunately, most of the lesions so diagnosed were advanced. There is a distinct need for developing better methods of detection of cancer of the ovaries and fallopian tubes.

The Respiratory Tract

The cellular material from the respiratory tract either may be the result of a spontaneous expectoration or may be obtained artificially. The *sputum* is the result of a spontaneous "deep" cough bringing up material from the small bronchi and the alveoli. The cough reflex may be simulated artificially by means of inhalation of cough-stimulating substances. Spontaneous expectorations must be collected in fixative (50% to 70% alcohol). The fixed specimens may be processed at leisure. If adequate laboratory facilities are available for immediate processing, fresh specimens of sputum may be submitted.

Collection of Sputum

One third of a wide-mouth glass bottle is filled with fixative, and the patient is instructed to expectorate the following morning directly into the container. Morning specimens resulting from overnight accumulation of secreta yield the best diagnostic results. Three specimens on three successive days should be collected to ensure a maximum of diagnostic accuracy. The patient must be carefully instructed not to spit into the fixative without a deep cough, since *saliva is of no diagnostic value.*

Sputum Pool. If Saccomanno's fixative and method are used (see p. 1460), a single sample containing three morning sputum specimens may be collected (*3-day sputum pool*). This is particularly helpful in lung cancer detection programs.

Aerosol Method of Sputum Induction. The method of inducing deep-cough sputum by aerosol inhalation outlined here is based on techniques developed by Dr. H. A. Bickerman and his associates at Columbia-Presbyterian Medical Center, New York City.*

A hypertonic saline solution with propylene glycol is placed in a heated nebulizer and vaporized by means of an air pump or an oxygen cylinder. Several types of nebulizers are available at present, and instructions for use accompany each† (Fig. 32–4).

Fifteen percent saline and 20% propylene glycol‡ may be used for asymptomatic patients; 10% saline solution and 20% propylene glycol for pa-

---

Bickerman, H.A., Sproul, E.E., and Barach, A.L.: An aerosol method of producing bronchial secretions in human subjects: A clinical technique for the detection of lung cancer. Dis. Chest., 33:347–362, 1958.

†*Manufacturers: Inhalation Equipment Company, 1686 Second Avenue, New York, N.Y.; The de Vilbiss Company, Somerset, Pa.; Schoeffel Instrument Company, Westwood, N.J.*

‡*NaCl 150 g, propylene glycol 200 ml, aqua dist. q.s. ad. 1,000 ml. Filter before using.*

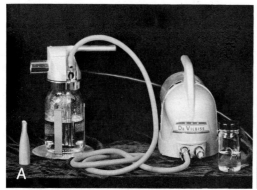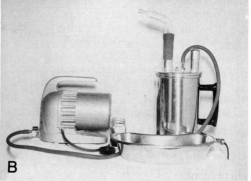

FIGURE 32–4. Nebulizers for stimulation of cough reflex; OEM Company (*A*) and Inhalation Equipment Company (*B*). In this set-up the solution is vaporized by means of an air pump (the de Vilbiss Company, Somerset, Pa., Air Compressor No. 501). The mouthpiece is shown standing on left in (*A*). The bottle contains fixative (50% alcohol).

tients with evidence of heavy bronchial irritation or pulmonary emphysema.

Vapors from these solutions are nontoxic. The only known after-effect may be bronchospasm in persons with asthma or severe emphysema. A solution of 5% propylene glycol in normal saline solution is advised for such cases. The patient should use a bronchodilator a few minutes before inhalation and after, if necessary.

The solution should be allowed to heat until vapors at the mouthpiece register at least 110°F (43°C). The patient should be seated approximately ½ inch (1.25 cm) from the mouthpiece and instructed to breathe in and out through the mouth at as normal a rate as possible. Persons with chronic postnasal discharge should clear the nasopharyngeal passage before inhalation.

Patient cooperation is important in obtaining good material. In most cases the vapors are tolerated easily; those few patients who complain of dizziness or slight nausea may be given a rest period. A deep cough occurs usually within 5 to 15 minutes. The resulting sputum should be preserved in 50% ethyl alcohol. Fresh sputum may be distinguished from saliva in the alcohol by its appearance in clusters of small globules—usually green or yellow in color but occasionally whitish. Saliva is loose and transparent before the alcohol shrinks it into white strands or balls. It is advisable to obtain two plugs of sputum so that the material is adequate for cytologic study.

Fresh sputum may also be collected for prompt processing.

Patients who give no evidence of response after 5 minutes of inhalation may be asked to take a deep breath and to hold it a few seconds, once every minute only (breathing too deeply or too rapidly may cause dizziness and/or bronchospasm). If there is no spontaneous cough at the end of the second 5-minute period, the patient may be asked to induce a deep cough (without overstrain), which in most cases will produce sputum. This procedure may be repeated once or twice if necessary so long as the patient is not under strain. Patients who have not been able to bring up material at the end of a 20-minute period should be released. Occasionally, sputum can be brought up any time from several minutes to several hours after the inhalation period. If not, the procedure can be repeated.

A small percentage of persons are unable to produce sputum by this method: those with diminished cough reflex or unusually dry tracheobronchial mucosa and patients with mental or emotional disorders.

Applications. Satisfactory sputum specimens may be produced by this method in 80% to 85% of all cooperative patients. Therefore, the method is eminently suitable for cancer detection in asymptomatic persons or patients who are not capable of producing a good specimen of sputum. Several surveys of asymptomatic patients have been undertaken by this method throughout the United States.* The results of these surveys, including the National Lung Cancer Detection Program, are cited on p. 818. A further application of induced sputum is in the diagnosis of *P. carinni* infections in patients with AIDS (see p. 741).

Precautions. Explosive cough causes aerosols that may contain pathogenic organisms. Therefore, appropriate measures should be taken to minimize hazard to employees and other patients.

OTHER METHODS OF ARTIFICIAL PRODUCTION OF SPUTUM

A variety of inhalants and procedures have been suggested to induce sputum. We have no personal experience with them.

Advantages and Disadvantages. Sputum may be obtained readily and painlessly and gives a very good representative sample of the mucosa of the entire respiratory tract. Three satisfactory specimens of sputum or a 3-day pooled sample will result in diagnosis of over 80% of lung cancer.

Its disadvantages are (*1*) the very large number of cells that have to be inspected, a task that for an inexperienced observer may be time-consuming; (*2*) the failure to provide any information pertaining to the localization of the lesion within the respiratory tract.

BRONCHIAL ASPIRATES AND WASHINGS

Bronchial aspirates are obtained by suction during bronchoscopic procedures.

Bronchial washings† are obtained in the following manner. With the bronchoscope in position, the patient is placed on the table in such a manner that the suspicious lung is dependent. The tip of the bronchoscope is placed as close as possible to the

---

Smokers Survey, supported by an American Cancer Society Grant, No. 22960 ACS. Participating services: The Thoracic Service (W.G. Cahan, M.D.), the Department of Preventive Medicine (E. Day, M.D.), and the Cytology Service (L.G. Koss, M.D.).

†*The procedure was kindly outlined by Dr. William G. Cahan.*

area to be investigated. About 10 ml of normal saline solution is instilled in small portions of 2 to 3 ml at a time and reaspirated while the patient is asked to cough. The flexible tip of the aspirator may be placed also in the opening of some of the smaller bronchi and the procedure repeated. All of the cellular material is collected in a Clerf's cell collector. *It is mandatory that all of the material collected be placed in alcohol fixative (see p. 1460) without delay unless immediate processing is available.* Additional material may be obtained by rinsing the bronchoscope after withdrawal. The procedure has to be performed very carefully if good results are to be achieved.

To localize the tumor to a lung or a specific lobe, separate bronchoscopes should be used for each area of investigation; otherwise, contamination of the specimens will occur.

Advantages and Disadvantages. The procedure allows for localization of a cancer to a specific lung or a portion thereof. The specimens are easier to screen because of lesser cellularity than that in sputum.

The disadvantages of aspirates and washings are twofold: (*1*) the procedure is highly unpleasant to the patient; (*2*) it has to be performed by a highly skilled physician; otherwise, the sample obtained may be unsatisfactory. In a teaching hospital where the procedure is often done by physicians in training, poor samples are frequently seen. At Memorial Hospital the diagnostic reliability of aspirates and washings was only on the order of 40% of all lung cancers. It is most uncommon to obtain positive evidence of cancer from aspirates and not to see any cancer cells in a satisfactory specimen of sputum from the same patient. However, the contrary occurs quite often. Therefore, for the general purpose of diagnosis of lung cancer, sputum is preferred, whereas the localization of the tumor must be accomplished with the help of the flexible bronchoscope and brushing.

TRACHEAL ASPIRATION*

This method may be used to perform washings of the trachea and the main bronchi without bronchoscopy. After careful local anesthesia of the nares, the larynx, and the pharynx, the patient is placed in sitting position on the examining table. A French catheter (no. 14 or 16, depending on the pa-

Cahan, W.G., and Farr, H.W.: The tracheal aspiration—an additional method for the early diagnosis of carcinoma of the lung. Cancer, 3:475–480, 1950.

tient) is moistened in saline solution and introduced through a naris. The catheter is introduced into the larynx while the examiner exercises traction on the tongue. Saline solution with tetracaine (Pontocaine) is instilled into the trachea, and the catheter is advanced to the carina. If the patient's head is rotated sharply, the catheter may be introduced into the contralateral main bronchus. A total of 18 ml of Pontocaine and saline solution in 2-ml portions is instilled and reaspirated with the catheter in various positions. Upon withdrawal the catheter is flushed with saline solution, and the entire collected material is placed in fixative. The same procedure may be applied to laryngectomized patients (see Fig. 20–57).

Advantages and Disadvantages. The procedure is performed relatively easily in ambulatory patients. Its usefulness is limited to patients who are not able to bring up sputum or to cases in which the sputum has failed consistently to reveal cancer cells. No information pertaining to the location of the tumor can be obtained by tracheal aspiration. Occasionally, the method may yield cancer cells when everything else has failed.

BRONCHIAL BRUSHING

In 1964 Hattori et al. reported remarkable diagnostic results by the application of a brushing technique under fluoroscopic guidance to obtain cytologic specimens from selected peripheral bronchi. This technique was made possible by the use of x-ray television, a set of specially designed small brushes, and perhaps also the great skills and patience of the investigators. When the customary methods of diagnosis failed, Hattori's method yielded diagnostic material in over 50% of small cancers. Tumors less than 3 cm in diameter are accessible to this diagnostic procedure.

The diagnostic evaluation of the bronchial tree has been revolutionized with the use of radiopaque catheters. These can be used to guide a brush or a biopsy forceps to the lesion under fluoroscopic control. Flexible fiberoptic instruments also allow bronchial brushings or biopsy under visual control. The diagnostic yield of bronchial brushing has been discussed on p. 852. The fiberoptic brush specimens, if properly obtained and fixed, offer the advantage of evaluation of multiple areas of the bronchial tree without resorting to biopsies, a procedure particularly helpful in the evaluation of patients suspected of harboring occult bronchogenic carcinoma. The method is equally helpful in the diagnosis of peripheral lung lesions. *Great care and skill are required in the preparation of smears from brush specimens.* The brush must be gently yet rapidly rotated *on a small area* of the surface of the slide and the smear fixed immediately. If the bronchoscopist or assisting nurse does not have experience with smear preparation, it is better to cut off the brush, place it in a bottle of 50% ethanol, and send it to the laboratory where smears can be prepared. Other methods of retrieval of material include ultrasound or Vortex mixer treatment of the brush in a balanced salt solution. This treatment, of short duration, detaches the cells from the brush. The salt solution with cells is forwarded to the laboratory. Most unfortunately, the diagnostic value of bronchial brushing is often significantly reduced by the bronchoscopist's inability to prepare adequate smears. Crushed or air-dried bronchial smears are of limited diagnostic value.

The limitation of the method is the time required for the procedure, especially in the absence of localizing lesions. Hence, the method can only be applied to patients whose evaluation is mandatory. The method cannot replace sputum for occult cancer detection.

Bronchoalveolar Lavage. The technique and applications of this procedure are discussed in Chapter 19.

RECOVERY OF MALIGNANT CELLS OF PULMONARY ORIGIN IN GASTRIC WASHINGS

Reports, notably by Bernhardt et al. and by Bangle et al., pointed out that swallowed sputum recovered from the stomach may occasionally contribute to the diagnosis of lung cancer. The methods of recovery are essentially similar to those used for the diagnosis of gastric cancer (see p. 1445). Recovery of malignant cells from gastric washings calls for a careful assessment of their origin (e.g., lung, esophagus, stomach) before treatment.

ASPIRATION BIOPSY OF LUNG LESIONS

This is discussed in Chapters 19 and 20. Laboratory methods of preparation of smears are discussed in Chapter 29.

Oral Cavity and Adjacent Sites

ORAL LESIONS

A vigorous scrape of the lesion with either a tongue depressor or its metal-made equivalent suffices usually to obtain adequate cytologic material. Rapid spread of the material on a clean glass slide and immediate fixation in 95% alcohol are mandatory to prevent drying effect. Hutter and Gerold used an ordinary endometrial curet to good advantage (see Chapter 21). There does not appear to be a great need for fancy instrumentation.

In Vivo Staining of Oral Lesions. Applying Richart's method of staining the uterine cervix (see p. 1437) with 1% solution of toluidine blue (following cleansing with 1% acetic acid). Niebel and Chomet as well as Shed et al. (see Chap. 21) were able to demonstrate oral carcinoma in the absence of conventional mucosal changes. The clinically inconspicuous areas of carcinoma in situ stained deeply with the dye and could not be decolorized with acetic acid. Shedd et al. also reported successes with recurrent carcinoma. The method proved particularly successful with preinvasive or small invasive carcinomas. In the latter setting the method helped to outline the surface occupied by the marginal areas of carcinoma in situ, thus assisting in the planning of surgical therapy.

The method is not infallible and not diagnostic per se of cancer. It merely indicates an increase in the number of nuclei with affinity for toluidine blue; thus the reaction may be positive in nonspecific ulcerations and in the presence of granulation tissue. The diagnosis of cancer must still rest on microscopic identification of cancer cells and on confirmatory biopsy.

NASOPHARYNX

Ali suggested the use of a cotton-tipped applicator to obtain material for cytologic investigation. Possibly the use of a scraping instrument of some kind may result in improved results (see Chap. 21).

LARYNX

A cotton-swab smear of larynx may be a useful adjunct to clinical diagnosis if biopsy is not contemplated. The use of more elaborate techniques, such as brushing, does not appear to offer any substantial advantage in the collection of material. A surprisingly large number of occult laryngeal carcinomas was diagnosed on sputum cytology during search for occult lung cancer (see p. 881).

PARANASAL SINUSES

Washing of paranasal sinuses with saline solution and the immediate addition of an equal amount of 50% alcohol offers the means of an occasional cytologic diagnosis of cancer in a debatable clinical situation. The method probably should enjoy greater popularity than is the case today, and it may lead to improved and earlier diagnosis of admittedly uncommon cancers that are difficult to treat.

Urinary Tract

Urine. Multiple voided urine specimens are invaluable in assessing the status of the lower urinary tract. Catheterized urine is acceptable. For cytologic evaluation of the bladder, three morning samples of urine, each of about 50 to 100 ml, obtained on consecutive days are recommended. Hydration of patients by forced intake of fluids (1 glass of water every 30 minutes for a 3-hour period) is advocated by some observers (Naib, 1976). Unless the urine can be processed immediately, it is advisable to collect it in an equal amount of fixative, such as a solution of 2% Carbowax in 70% ethanol. For this purpose 250-ml glass containers partly filled with fixative should be prepared in advance. For other methods of processing urinary sediment, see Chapter 33, p. 1465.

Bladder Irrigation (Washings). Washings of the bladder with physiologic saline solution or Ringer's solution, obtained at the time of cystoscopy, have been advocated by some observers as a diagnostic method. The specimen is collected in fixative and processed in the form of either smears or filters.

Beautiful cytologic preparations may be obtained by this method. The disadvantage of the method is its limited use, confined to symptomatic patients. In special situations when cytologic evaluation of the bladder epithelium is required, the method offers distinct diagnostic advantages. The method is not suitable for routine screening but has been used for flow cytometric measurements of DNA content in monitoring patients with bladder tumors (see Chapter 23, p. 988).

Renal Pelvis and Ureters. For suspected lesions of the renal pelvis or the ureter, examination of voided urine is often satisfactory. Special procedures, such as retrograde catheterization or direct brushing, may assist in the localization of the lesions of the upper urinary tract, although the material is often difficult to interpret (see Chapters 22 and 23).

Each specimen must be mixed with an equal amount of 50% ethyl alcohol, unless processed without delay. Specimens must be labeled as to type (voided or catheterized) and, for ureteral specimens and brushings, as to origin (right or left).

Rapid Screening of Urinary Sediment. DeVoogt et al. advocate the use of phase contrast microscopy for rapid study of the urinary sediment at the bedside. Sternheimer suggested the use of a simple supravital stain for the same purpose. Toluidine blue or methylene blue may also be used. Such methods are applicable for cancer detection in routine urinalysis (for technical details see Chapter 33).

Prostatic Secretion. Prostatic secretion should be obtained by prostatic massage and collected directly on a clean glass slide that has been coated with a small drop of Mayer's albumin. The fluid must be spread with a second clean glass slide. The smear must be allowed to dry slightly around the edges of the slide and placed in fixative.

Collection of Urine After Prostatic Massage. A voided urine specimen should be collected before massage and again after massage. An equal amount of 2% Carbowax in 70% ethyl alcohol should be added to each specimen and labeled, indicating whether it was obtained before or after massage.

Gastrointestinal Tract

General Description of Procedures

Fiberoptic Instruments. The introduction of flexible fiberglass optics has not only revolutionized the endoscopy of the gastrointestinal tract (and other organs, such as the respiratory tract) but also allowed direct sampling by cytology or by biopsy of any visible lesion. A variety of instruments specially adapted to the inspection of the esophagus, stomach, duodenum, and colon are in existence. The principles of collection of material for cytologic sampling are the same for all organs.

Fiberoptic Procedures. This procedure may now be performed on any patients with radiographic abnormalities or clinical symptomatology pointing to a lesion. The flexible instruments are provided with an accessory channel through which a brush, a plastic tube, or a small biopsy forceps may be passed. This arrangement permits brushing, lavage, or a biopsy of any area in the upper gastrointestinal tract under direct visual control. The patients generally tolerate the procedure much better than similar procedures with rigid instruments. *Cytologic sampling must be performed prior to biopsy.*

Brushing. Preparation of slides and fixative for cytologic sampling must precede the clinical procedure. Clean glass slides with identifying marks engraved with diamond pencil should be placed in readiness within the reach of the physician or the assistant. *Paper clips must be placed on every other slide to prevent sticking.* A bottle with fixative (50% to 95% ethyl alcohol) should be held *open.* The bottle should have a sufficiently wide opening so that the glass slides fit without contact with glass.

Upon completion of brushing, the brush must be carefully, yet rapidly, withdrawn from the instrument and the smears prepared without delay either by the physician or by a trained assistant. *The cytologic material should not be crushed. The brush should be gently rotated* on a limited area of the surface of the clean slide and, to prevent drying, *the slide must be immediately placed* in the fixative. Usually a brush yields two to four smears. If suitable expertise in preparation of brush smears is not available, is is best to cut off the whole brush and place it in fixative. The smears may then be prepared in the laboratory. Other methods for submitting a brush sample are discussed on p. 1442 in reference to bronchial brushing.

Lavage.   Lavage is limited to the esophagus and stomach. A syringe with 50 to 100 ml of saline solution or Ringer's solution is attached to the plastic tube and a jet of fluid directed at a lesion or an area chosen by the endoscopist. The fluid must be *collected by a second intubation* with a Levin tube after withdrawal of the endoscope. *Immediately after aspiration of the fluid an equal volume of 95% alcohol* must be added and the fluid forwarded to the laboratory for further processing.

Brushing vs. Lavage.   In skilled hands and in the presence of a visible lesion brushing offers certain advantages to the patient, since it does not require a second intubation. However, many physicians not particularly skilled in brushing techniques often send to the laboratory material of such poor technical quality that no diagnosis is possible. In such instances, lavage is definitely the favored method of specimen collection. Lavage also offers the advantage of sampling a larger area and is definitely indicated if no localizing lesion is present.

Cytologic Sampling of Component Organs

Esophagus.   Washings of the esophagus are best obtained during direct esophagoscopy. Small amounts of physiologic saline solution or Ringer's solution (10 to 20 ml) are injected through the esophagoscope and aspirated. It is imperative to place all material in fixative (50% alcohol) without delay. *The washings should be obtained prior to biopsy.*

A Levin tube may be used in ambulatory patients. It may be passed to the cardia or to the level of obstruction. Raskin et al. advocate an "esophageal swallow." With a Levin tube in place and a 100-ml syringe attached to it, the patient is instructed to swallow 100 ml of saline solution. Gentle aspiration is maintained, and the aspirate is placed in fixative. Additional washings of segments of the esophagus may be obtained subsequently by withdrawing the Levin tube a few centimeters at a time.

Brushing of the esophagus may be performed at the time of esophagoscopy with fiberoptic instruments. The method of smear preparation is described above. The sampling of the esophagus by the balloon technique was discussed in Chapter 24, p. 1025.

Stomach.   Numerous "blind" abrasive methods for obtaining cytologic material from the stomach have been advocated prior to the advances in fiberoptic gastroscopy. However, Schade's experience and our own indicate that these methods were mainly of assistance in obtaining samples from advanced tumors with necrotic surfaces. Early gastric cancers readily yield diagnostic material when the stomach is washed with a solution of physiologic saline solution or Ringer's solution. Chymotrypsin,* a mucus-dissolving enzyme, may be added to the saline solution.

Preparation of the Patient.   In patients with pyloric obstruction, several lavages should be performed until the returns are clear. In other patients simple withdrawal of food and drink for 8 hours is sufficient preparation. Gastric washings should precede the barium swallow.

Lavage.   The Levin tube is passed to the 70-cm mark. *No lubricants other than glycerin should be used.* Five hundred ml of Ringer's solution is instilled in small portions, aspirated, and discarded. Subsequently, 500 ml of fresh Ringer's solution (or acetate buffer solution at pH 5.6 if chymotrypsin is used) is instilled and reaspirated several times while the patient is rotated from side to side for 10 minutes. If chymotrypsin is used, the specimen should be placed on ice immediately to stop the action of the enzyme. Rapid centrifugation is also required. If plain saline solution or Ringer's solution is used, the addition of an equal amount of 95% al-

---

Armour Pharmaceutical Company, P.O. Box 511, Kankakee, Ill., 60901.

cohol will allow good preservation of the cells. The specimen may be processed at leisure.

Numerous variants of the above techniques have been suggested, but they do not appear to offer tangible advantages. The secret of an adequate gastric sample is not the type of liquid used to wash the stomach but the preparation of the patient and the skill and patience of the person in charge of the procedure.

Fiberoptic Procedures. In patients suspected of harboring a gastric lesion fiberoptic examination of the stomach with biopsies, brushings, or both is preferable to blind lavage.

Duodenum. The preparation of the patient is the same as that for gastric lavage. Sedation may be required. Raskin et al.* advocate the following intubation procedure.

The patient sits on a cot, elevated 16 inches at one end. A double-lumen gastroduodenal radiopaque tube (Diamond tube), with a 3- to 5-g. weight at the tip, is passed through the mouth to a position just below the cardioesophageal junction (45 cm.). The patient is placed on his left side, with head elevated, and fed an additional 15 cm. of tubing so that the tip of the tube will be lying just proximal to the antrum along the greater curvature. The patient then sits up and bends forward, taking a few deep breaths. The tip of the tube slips into the antrum as the anterior wall of the stomach falls away from the posterior wall. Next the patient is placed on his right side (feet elevated), and 10 more cm. of tubing is slowly introduced, which should send the tube into the first part of the duodenum. Finally, the patient lies on his back for 2 minutes and swallows an additional 15 cm. of tube. A check of the tube's position fluoroscopically will reveal the tip of the tube between the second and third portions of the duodenum. The complete intubation usually requires about 15 minutes.

Duodenal Drainage: Tape the tube to the side of the patient's face. Before the actual collection is started, the stomach is aspirated to remove the residuum. Connect the gastric and duodenal segments to a Gomco vacuum pump (120 mm. Hg pressure). The gastric secretion is drained directly into a large collecting jar; the duodenal aspirate is trapped in 50-ml. plastic tubes immersed in an ice-water bath. Secretin may be injected intravenously after a 20-minute control period has shown duodenal juice to be consistently alkaline to litmus paper and the gastric juice to be acid.

---

*Raskin, H.F., Kirsner, J.B., and Palmer, W.L.: Gastrointestinal Cancer: Definitive Diagnosis by Exfoliative Cytology. Monograph from the Department of Medicine, University of Chicago.

Three 10-minute samples are collected, and the gastric and duodenal secretions are checked frequently with litmus paper in order to ensure independent collection.

Record the volume of the 30-minute postsecretin pancreatic secretion and then centrifuge the fluid for 5 minutes. Decant the supernatant, which is saved for bicarbonate determination, and smear the sediment on glass slides for cytology study.

Colon
Lavage. The preparation of a patient is the same as that for a barium enema. A cathartic by mouth, 2 oz. of mineral or castor oil, taken 12 hours prior to collection of the material, is necessary. On the morning of the procedure, cleansing enemas must be administered until the returns are clear. Actual collection of the cytologic material may take place 1 to 2 hours later. From 500 to 1,000 ml of warm Ringer's solution is instilled with the patient in the left decubitus position. Massage of the colon and rotation of the patient are very helpful in obtaining better cytologic material. The fluid is collected after 3 to 5 minutes. The addition of alcohol to the sample is optional. If none is added, immediate centrifugation is advised. The processing of the sediment is outlined in the section on techniques (Chapter 33).

Other Methods of Cell Collection. Spjut et al. suggested a silicone-foam enema for cytologic examination of the colon. The material solidifies shortly after injection and is expelled by the patient in the form of a cast, faithfully reproducing the contours of the colon. The cast may be washed off, the fluid is spun down, and the sediment is examined microscopically.

The use of encapsulated polyurethane foam for the diagnosis of colonic carcinoma has been suggested by Cromarty. The foam sponge may be retrieved, fixed, and a cell block prepared from the material adherent to the sponge surface.

Katz et al. advocate the use of a pulsating saline lavage (500 to 1,000 ml) with the help of a dental irrigation unit attached either to a rigid or to a flexible colonoscopic instrument. The saline solution is collected in equal volume of 95% ethyl alcohol and the sediment processed after centrifugation as smears or cell blocks. These authors report substantial diagnostic success not only with the diagnosis of primary colon cancer but also with colon cancer occurring in ulcerative colitis. Other methods of lavage are discussed in Chapter 24.

Cell Collection During Sigmoidoscopy or Colonoscopy. Brushing of mucosal abnormalities at the time of fiberoptic examination of the colon is the generally accepted procedure in patients suspected of harboring a colonic lesion. High-risk patients (patients with multiple polyps, ulcerative colitis of long duration, and past history of colonic cancer) should receive frequent examinations. Brush specimens must be carefully processed and labeled as to the site of origin.

Search for Occult Blood in Stools as a Means of Colon Cancer Detection. The poor outlook of patients with colonic cancer has led within recent years to the development of several simple slide-like devices that, upon contact with a sample of stool, disclose the presence of occult blood. The detection system carries with it a substantial margin of error. In the majority of patients the bleeding is due to causes other than cancer. However, in a number of patients colon cancers in early stages have been documented and successfully treated (Gnauck, 1977). The diagnosis of colon cancer is based primarily on radiographic studies and colonoscopy. Brushing of suspected areas or of colonic polyps discovered by means of such studies may contribute to the identification of malignant disease.

Body Fluids

Pleural, pericardial, or ascitic fluids may be collected in tubes or syringes that may be either plain or heparinized to prevent coagulation. Cells in such fluids do not deteriorate very rapidly.

There are certain advantages in the processing of unfixed fluids: layering of many cancer cells in the buffy coat of the centrifuged sample may be achieved. The cells adhere better to the slides. The unfixed specimens are better suited for filter preparation and for examination with hematologic techniques. Finally, such specimens lend themselves to the determination of specific gravity and protein content.

The common anticoagulants that can be used are heparin, 5 to 10 units per ml of fluid to be placed in the collecting vessel; *or* 3.8% sodium citrate, 1 ml per 10 ml of fluid; *or* EDTA, 1 mg per 1 ml of fluid.

However, if the fluids cannot be processed within 12 hours after collection, the addition of 50% ethyl alcohol as a fixative is beneficial. The size of the sample need not exceed 200 ml of fluid with an equal amount of fixative added. The practice of salvaging large amounts of fluid for cytologic examination is not recommended.

Cerebrospinal Fluid and Other Fluids of Small Volume

The volume of the sample has considerable bearing on diagnostic accuracy: the larger the sample, the better the results. If several samples are obtained, the second or the third should be used for cytology.

The addition of an equal amount of 50% ethyl alcohol to the sample is recommended if a delay in processing is anticipated. If a hematologic examination of the spinal fluid is required (for example, in leukemia), an unfixed sample is preferable, to be processed by cytocentrifugation (see Chapter 33).

Nipple Secretions

These should be collected by applying the slide directly to the nipple, followed by immediate fixation. Breast secretions obtained by breast pump or cannulation of the ducts require that smears be prepared with skill and rapidity and fixed immediately.

BIBLIOGRAPHY

Additional references on technical procedures are appended in Chapter 33.

The female genital tract
The respiratory tract
The urinary tract
The prostate
The gastrointestinal tract
Effusions and other fluids
(See also specific organs.)

The Female Genital Tract

Alons-von Kordelaar, J.J., and Boon, M.E.: Diagnostic accuracy of squamous cervical lesions studied in spatula-cytobrush smears. Acta Cytol., *32*:801–804, 1988.

Anderson, W. Frierson, H., Barber, S., et al.: Sensitivity and specificity of endocervical curettage and the endocervical brush for the evaluation of the endocervical canal. Am. J. Obstet. Gynecol., *159*:702–707, 1988

Anderson, W.A.D., and Gunn, S.A.: Cytologic detection of cancer. Considerations for its future: a comparative examination of the Papanicolaou and acridine orange technics. Acta Cytol., *6*:468–470, 1962.

———: Premalignant and malignant conditions of the cervix uteri. Tissue validity study of the vaginal irrigation smear method. Cancer, *20*:1587–1593, 1967.

Ayre, J.E.: Selective cytology smear for diagnosis of cancer. Am. J. Obstet. Gynecol., *53*:609–617, 1947.

Bader, G.M., Simon, T.R., Koss, L.G., and Day, E: Study of detection-tampon method as screening device for uterine cancer. Cancer, *10*:332–337, 1957.

Boon, M.E., Alons-von Kordelaar, J.J., and Rietveld-Scheffers, P.E.: Consequences of the introduction of combined spatula and cytobrush sampling for cervical cytology. Improvement in smear quality and detection rates. Acta Cytol., *30*:264–270, 1986.

Bredahl, E., Koch, F., and Stakemann, G: Cancer detection by cervical scrapings, vaginal pool smears and irrigation smears. A comparative study. Acta Cytol., *9*:189–193, 1965.

Brunschwig, A.: Method for mass screening for cytological detection of carcinoma of cervix uteri. Cancer, *7*:1182–1184, 1954.

————: Detection of endometrial adenocarcinoma by tampon-smear method. Cancer, *10*:120–123, 1957.

Carrow, L.A., Hilker, R.R.J., Elesh, R.H., and Eggum, P.R.: Evaluation of the vaginal irrigation smear technique. Am. J. Obstet. Gynecol., *97*:821–827, 1967.

Creasman, W.T., and Lukeman, J.: Unreliability of urinary cytology in detecting gynecologic malignancy. Cancer, *30*:148–149, 1972.

Davis, H.J.: The irrigation smear. A cytologic method for mass population screening by mail. am. J. Obstet. Gynecol., *84*:1017–1023, 1962.

————: The irrigation smear: Accuracy in detection of cervical smear. Acta Cytol., *6*:459–467, 1962.

Deckert, J.J., Staten, S.F., and Palermo, V.: Improved endocervical cell yield with cytobrush. J. Fam. Pract., *26*:639–641, 1988.

Frost, J.K.: Gynecologic and obstetric cytopathology. *In* Novak, E.R., and Woodruff, J.F.: Novak's Gynecologic and Obstetric Pathology, ed. 7. Philadelphia, W.B. Saunders, 1974.

Gusberg, S.B.: Relative efficiency of diagnostic techniques in detection of early cervical cancer; comparative study with survey of 1,000 normal women. Am. J. Obstet. Gynecol., *65*:1073–1080, 1953.

Held, E., Schreiner, W.E., and Oehler, I.: Bedeutung der Kolposkopie und Cytologie zur Erfassung des Genitalkarzinoms. Schweiz. Med. Wochenschr., *84*:856–860, 1954.

Hinselmann, H: Einführung in die Kolposkopie. Hamburg, P. Hartung, 1933.

Hinselmann, H.: Die Kolposkopie; eine Einleitung; mit einem Beitrag über die Kolpophotographie von A. Schmitt. Wuppertal-Elberfeld, W. Girardet, 1954.

Husain, O.A.N.: The irrigation smear. Am. J. Obstet. Gynecol., *106*:138–146, 1970.

Jordan, M.J., and Bader, G.: New cannula for obtaining endometrial material for cytologic study. Obstet. Gynecol. *8*:611–612, 1956.

Kiricuta, I., and Munteanu, S.: Patient-obtained cell collection for cytologic examination of vaginal smears. Am. J. Obstet. Gynecol., *105*:286–288, 1969.

Koch, F., and Stakemann, G.: Irrigation smear: Accuracy in gynecologic cancer detection. Dan. Med. Bull., *9*:127–131, 1962.

Kolstad, P., and Stafl, A.: Atlas of Colposcopy. ed. 2. Baltimore, University Park Press, 1977.

Koss, L.G.: Detection of carcinoma of the uterine cervix. J.A.M.A., *222*:699–700, 1972.

Koss, L.G.: Cytologic diagnosis of carcinoma of the uterine cervix. *In* Gray, L.A. (ed): Dysplasia, Carcinoma In Situ and Micro-Invasive Carcinoma of the Cervix Uteri, pp. 190–227. Springfield, Ill., Charles C Thomas, 1966.

Koss, L.G.: The new Bethesda system for reporting results of smears of the uterine cervix. J.N.C.I. *82*:988–991, 1990.

Koss, L.G., and Hicklin, M.D.: Standards of adequacy of cytologic examination of the female genital tract. Conclusions of a study group on cytology. Obstet. Gynecol., *43*:792–793, 1974.

Koss, L.G., Schreiber, K., Oberlander, S.G., Moussouris, H., and Lesser, M.: Detection of endometrial carcinomas and hyperplasia in asymptomatic women. Obstet. Gynecol., *64*:1–11, 1984.

Mattingly, R.F., Boyd, A., and Frable, W.J.: The vaginal irrigation smear: A positive method of cervical cancer control. Obstet. Gynecol., *29*:463–470, 1967.

Maynard, J.M., Tierney, J.T., O'Neill, R., and Deutsch, A.M.: Cervical screening with the Davis pipet on a door-to-door basis. Pub. Health Rep., *84*:553–557, 1969.

McLean, B., Talbot, F.G., and Jend, W., Jr.: Detection of uterine cancer in industry. Arch. Indust. H., *18*:261–267, 1958.

Mestwerdt, G.: Atlas der Kolposkopie. ed. 2. Jena, Gustav Fisher, 1953.

Muskett, J.M., Carter, A.K., and Dodge, O.G.: Detection of cervical cancer by irrigation smear and cervical scrapings. Brit. Med. J. *2*:341–342, 1966.

Navratil, E.: Colposcopy. *In* Gray, L.A. (ed.): Dysplasia, Carcinoma in Situ and Micro-Invasive Carcinoma of the Cervix Uteri. pp. 228–283. Springfield, Ill., Charles C Thomas, 1964.

Nieburgs, H.E.: Comparative study of different techniques for diagnosis of cervical carcinoma. Am. J. Obstet. Gynecol., *72*:511–515, 1956.

Papanicolaou, G.N.: Cytological evaluation of smears prepared by tampon method for detection of carcinoma of uterine cervix. Cancer, *7*:1185–1190, 1954.

Reagan, J.W., and Lin, F.: An evaluation of the vaginal irrigation technique in the detection of uterine cancer. Acta Cytol., *11*:374–382, 1967.

Richart, R.M.: A clinical staining test for the in vivo delineation of dysplasia and carcinoma in situ. Am. J. Obstet. Gynecol., *86*:703–712, 1963.

————: The correlation of Schiller-positive areas on the exposed portion of the cervix with intraepithelial neoplasia. Am. J. Obstet. Gynecol., *90*:697–701, 1964.

————: Evaluation of the true false negative rate in cytology. Am. J. Obstet. Gynecol., *89*:723–726, 1964.

————: Colpomicroscopic studies of the distribution of dysplasia and carcinoma in situ on the exposed portion of the human uterine cervix. Cancer, *18*:950–954, 1965.

Richart, R.M., and Vaillant, H.W.: The irrigation smear. False-negative rates in a population with cervical neoplasia. J.A.M.A., *192*:199–202, 1965.

————: Influence of cell collection techniques upon cytologic diagnosis. Cancer, *18*:1474–1478, 1965.

Rubio, C.A., and Thomassen, P.: A critical evaluation of the Schiller test in patients before conization. Am. J. Obstet. Gynecol., *125*:96–99, 1976.

Shingleton, H.M., and Gore, H., Straughn, J.M., Austin, J.M., Jr., and Littleton, H.J.: The contribution of endocervical smears to cervical cancer detection. Acta Cytol., *19*:261–264, 1975.

Simon, T.R., Durfee, G.R., and Ricci, A.: Value of vaginal aspiration smear as compared with cervical swab smear in detection of in situ carcinoma of cervix and adenocarcinoma of fundus. *In* Transactions of the Third Annual Meeting of the Inter-Society Cytology Council, pp. 77–85, 1955.

Smith, P., and Crozier, E.H.: Cytology of voided urine in the diagnosis of gynecologic malignancy. Obstet. Gynecol., *41*:440–442, 1973.

Song, Y.S., Fanger, H., and Murphy, T.H.: Significance of performing dual smear examinations in mass screening survey for uterine cancer. Am. J. Obstet. Gynecol., *78*:1309–1311, 1959.

Soost, H.J.: Die Bedeutung des Ortes der Entnahme fur die zytologische Krebsfahrtensuche. Krebasarzt, *13*:408–420, 1958.

Trimbos, J.B., and Arenz, N.P.W.: The efficiency of the cytobrush versus cotton swab in the collection of endocervical cells in cervical smears. Acta Cytol., *30*:261–263, 1986.

Wachtel, E.: Exfoliative Cytology in Gynaecological Practice. Washington, D.C., Butterworth, 1964.

Wespi, H.J.: Early Carcinoma of the Uterine Cervix; Pathogenesis and Detection (translated by Marie Schiller.) rev. ed, New York, Grune & Stratton, 1959.

Wied, G.L.: Importance of site from which vaginal cytologic smears are taken. Am. J. Clin. Pathol, 25:742–750, 1955.

Wied, G.L., and Bahr, G.F.: Vaginal, cervical and endocervical cytologic smears on a single slide. Obstet. Gynecol., *14*:362–367, 1959.

Wied, G.L., Messina, A.M., Meier, P., and Blough, R.R.: Fluorospectrophotometric analysis of cervical epithelial cells. Acta Cytol., 8:61–67, 1964.

Wolfe, L.A.: Colpomicroscopy; its value in microscopic examination of uterine cervical epithelium in vivo. Am. J. Obstet. Gynecol., *76*:1163–1171, 1958.

The Respiratory Tract

Bangle, R., Jr., Hohl, E.M., Maple, F., and Hart, S.: Technique of esophageal-gastric aspiration for collecting swallowed sputum in diagnostic pulmonary cytology. Acta Cytol., *9*:362–364, 1965.

Bean, W.J., Graham, W.L., Jordan, R.B., and Eavenson, L.W.: Diagnosis of lung cancer by the transbronchial brush biopsy technique. J.A.M.A., *206*:1070–1072, 1968.

Bernhardt, J., Killian, J.J., and Eastridge, C.: Gastric washings as a source of malignant cells from bronchial secretions. J.A.M.A., *183*:189, 1963.

Bibbo, M., Fennessy, J.J., Lu, C-T., Straus, F.H., Variakojis, D., and Wied, G.L.: Bronchial brushing technique for the cytologic diagnosis of peripheral lung lesions. A review of 693 cases. Acta Cytol., *17*:245–251, 1973.

Dahlgren, S.E., and Lind, B.: Comparison between diagnostic results obtained by transthoracic needle biopsy and by sputum cytology. Acta Cytol., *16*:53–58, 1972.

Ellis, F.H., Jr., Woolner, L.B., and Schmidt, H.W.: Metastatic pulmonary malignancy; study of factors involved in exfoliation of malignant cells. J. Thorac. Surg., *20*:125–135, 1950.

Erozan, Y.S., and Frost, J.K.: Cytopathologic diagnosis of cancer in pulmonary material: A critical histopathologic correlation. Acta Cytol., *14*:560–565, 1970

Grunze, H.: Cytologic diagnosis of tumors of the chest. Acta Cytol., *17*:148–159, 1973.

Hattori, S., Matsuda, M., Sugiyama, T., and Matsuda, H.: Cytologic diagnosis of early lung cancer: Brushing method under x-ray television fluoroscopy. Dis. Chest, *45*:129–142, 1964.

Herbut, P.A., and Clerf, L.H.: Bronchogenic carcinoma; diagnosis by cytologic study of bronchoscopically removed secretions. J.A.M.A., *130*:1006–1012, 1946.

Johnston, W.W., and Frable, W.J.: The cytopathology of the respiratory tract. Am. J. Pathol., *84*:372–414, 1976.

Koss, L. G., Melamed, M.R., and Goodner, J.T.: Pulmonary cytology—a brief survey of diagnostic results from July 1st,

1952, until December 31st, 1960. Acta Cytol., 8:104–113, 1964.

Ozgelen, F.N., Brodsky, S.L., and DeGroat, A.: Examination of merits and intrinsic limitations of exfoliative cytology in 465 cases of lung cancer. J. Thorac. Cardiovasc. Surg., *49*:221–230, 1965.

Russell, W.O., Neidhardt, H.W., Mountain, C.F., Griffith, K.M., and Chang, J.P.: Cytodiagnosis of lung cancer. A report of a four-year laboratory clinical, and statistical study with a review of the literature on lung cancer and pulmonary cytology. Acta Cytol., 7:1–44, 1963.

Wandall, H.H.: Study on neoplastic cells in sputum, as contribution to diagnosis of primary lung cancer. Acta Chir. Scand. [Suppl.], *93*:1–143, 1944.

The Urinary Tract

Crabbe, J.G.S.: Cytology of voided urine and special reference to "benign" papilloma and some of the problems encountered in the preparation of the smears. Acta Cytol., 5:233–240, 1961.

Deden, C.: Cancer cells in urinary sediment. Acta Radiol. [Suppl.], *115*:1–75, 1954.

deVoogt, H.J., Beyer-Boon, M.E., and Brussee, J.M.: The value of phase contrast microscopy for urinary cytology, reliability and pitfalls. Acta Cytol., *19*:542–546, 1975.

deVoogt, H.J., Rathert, P., and Beyer-Boon, M.E.: Urinary Cytology. Berlin, Springer-Verlag, 1977.

Esposti, P.L., and Zajicek, J.: Grading of transitional cell neoplasms of the urinary bladder from smears of bladder washings. A critical review of 326 tumors. Acta Cytol., *16*:529–537, 1972.

Harris, M.J., Schwinn, C.P., Morrow, J.W., Gray, R.L., and Browell, B.M.: Exfoliative cytology of the bladder irrigation specimen. Acta Cytol., *15*:385–399, 1971.

Naib, Z.M.: Exfoliative Cytopathology. ed. 2. Boston, Little, Brown and Company, 1976.

Papanicolaou, G.N., and Marshall, V.F.: Urine sediment smears as diagnostic procedure in cancers of urinary tract. Science, *101*:519–520, 1945.

Sarnacki, C.T., McCormack, L.J., Kiser, W.S., Hazard, J.R., McLaughlin, T.C., and Belovich, D.M.: Urinary cytology and clinical diagnosis of urinary tract malignancy: A clinicopathologic study of 1,400 patients. J. Urol., *106*:761–764, 1971.

Sternheimer, R.: A supravital cytodiagnostic stain for urinary sediments. J.A.M.A., *231*:826–832, 1975.

Trott, P.A., and Edwards, L.: Comparison of bladder washings and urine cytology in the diagnosis of bladder cancer. J. Urol., *110*:664–666, 1973.

Umiker, W.: Accuracy of cytologic diagnosis of cancer of the urinary tract. Acta Cytol., 8:186–193, 1964.

Umiker, W., Lapides, J., and Soureene, R.: Exfoliative cytology of papillomas and intraepithelial carcinomas of the urinary bladder. Acta Cytol., *6*:255–266, 1962.

The Prostate

Clarke, B.G., and Bamford, S.B.: Cytology of prostate gland in diagnosis of cancer. J.A.M.A., *172*:1750–1753, 1960.

Frank, I.N., and Scott, W.W.: Cytodiagnosis of prostatic carcinoma: Follow-up study. J. Urol., *79*:983–988, 1958.

Richardson, H.L., Durfee, G.R., Day, E., and Papanicolaou, G.N.: Role of cytology in detection of early prostatic cancer. *In* Homburger, F., and Fishman, W.H. (eds.): The Laboratory Diagnosis of Cancer of the Prostate. pp. 14–17. Boston, Tufts University School of Medicine, 1954.

The Gastrointestinal Tract

Ayre, J.E., and Oren, B.G.: Colon brush. A new diagnostic procedure for cancer of the lower bowel. Am. J. Dig. Dis., *2*:74–80, 1957.

Bader, G.M., and Papanicolaou, G.N.: Application of cytology in diagnosis of cancer of rectum, sigmoid, and descending colon. Cancer, *5*:307–314, 1952.

Bedine, M.S., and Cocco, A.E.: A comparison of washing and brushing cytology and biopsy in the diagnosis of malignant disease of the esophagus, stomach and colon. Gastrointest. Endosc., *19*:75–78, 1972.

Bemvenuti, G.A., Prolla, J.C., Kirsner, J.B., and Reilly, R.W.: Direct vision brushing cytology in the diagnosis of colorectal malignancy. Acta Cytol., *18*:477–481, 1974.

Bourke, J.B., Brown, C.L., Swann, J.C., and Ritchie, H.D.: Exocrine pancreatic function studies, duodenal cytology, and hypotonic duodenography in the diagnosis of surgical jaundice. Lancet, 1:605–608, 1972.

Brandborg, L.L., Taniguchi, L., and Rubin, C.E.: Is exfoliative cytology practical for more general use in the diagnosis of gastric cancer? A simplified chymotrypsin technique. Cancer, *14*:1074–1080, 1961.

Cabré-Fiol, V.: Cytologic Diagnostic of Esophageal and Gastric Cancer. pp. 219–225. *In* Advances in Gastrointestinal Endoscopy, Proc. 2nd World Congress, July 1–11, 1970.

Cameron, A.B., and Thabet, R.J.: Recovery of malignant cells from enema returns in carcinoma of colon. Surg. Forum, *10*:30–33, 1959.

Cook, G.B.: Silicone foam enema as a diagnostic aid in cancer of the rectum and colon. Dis. Colon Rectum, 7:195–196, 1964.

Cooper, W.A., and Papanicolaou, G.N.: Balloon technique in cytological diagnosis of gastric cancer. J.A.M.A., *151*:10–14, 1953.

Cromarty, R.: Colon cytology simplified using enteric coated encapsulated polyurethane foam as a cellular collecting agent. A preliminary report. Act Cytol., *21*:158–161, 1977.

DeLuca, V.A., Jr., Eisenman, L., Moritz, M., Feldstein, E., Bautista, A., Macionus, R., Carillo, H., and Laborda, O.: A new technique for colonic cytology. Acta Cytol., *18*:421–424, 1974.

Dreiling, D.A., Nieburgs, H.E., and Janowitz, H.D.: The combined secretion and cytology test in the diagnosis of pancreatic and biliary tract cancer. Med. Clin. North Am. *44*:801–815, 1960.

Fukuda, T., Shida, S., Takita, T., and Sawada, Y.: Cytologic diagnosis of early gastric cancer by the endoscope method with gastrofiberscope. Acta Cytol., *11*:456–459, 1967.

Galambos, J.T., and Klayman, M.I.: The clinical value of colonic and exfoliative cytology in the diagnosis of cancer beyond the reach of the proctoscope. Surg. Gynecol. Obstet., *101*:673–679, 1955.

Gibbs, D.D.: Exfoliative cytology of the stomach. New York, Appleton-Century-Crofts, 1972.

Gnauck, R.: Screening for colorectal cancer with haemoccult. Leber Magen Darm., *7*:32–35, 1977.

Henning, N., and Witte, S.: Atlas der Gastroenterologischen Zytodiagnostik. 2nd. ed. Stuttgart, Georg Thieme, 1968.

Johnson, W.D., Koss, L.G., Papanicolaou, G.N., and Seybolt, J.F.: Cytology of esophageal washings; evaluation of 364 cases. Cancer, 8:951–957, 1955.

Katz, S.: Newer diagnostic techniques: Rectocolonic exfoliative cytology—a new approach. Dis. Colon Rectum, *17*:3–5, 1974.

Kline, T.S., and Yum, K.K.: Fiberoptic coloscopy and cytology. Cancer, *37*:2553–2556, 1976.

Kobayashi, S., Prolla, J.C., and Kirsner, J.B. Brushing cytology of the esophagus and stomach under direct vision by fiberscopes. Acta Cytol., *14*:219–223, 1970.

Prolla, J.C., and Kirsner, J.B.: Handbook and Atlas of Gastrointestinal Exfoliative Cytology. Chicago, University of Chicago Press, 1972.

Raskin, H.R., Kirsner, J.B., and Palmer, W.L.: Role of exfoliative cytology in the diagnosis of cancer of the digestive tract. J.A.M.A., *169*:789–791, 1959.

Raskin, H.R., Moseley, R.D., Jr., Kirsner, J.B., and Palmer, W.L.: Cancer of the pancreas, biliary tract and liver. CA, *11*:137–148, 166–181, 1961.

Raskin, H.R., and Pleticka, S.: The cytologic diagnosis of cancer of the colon. Acta Cytol., 8:131–140, 1964.

———: Exfoliative cytology of the colon. Fifteen years of lost opportunity. Cancer, *28*:127–130, 1971.

Schade, R.O.K.: Gastric Cytology, Principles, Methods and Results. London, Edward Arnold, 1960.

Shida, S.: Biopsy smear cytology with the fibergastroscope for direct observation. Gann Monograph #11, Early Gastric Cancer. pp. 223–231. Tokyo, Tokyo Press, 1971.

Smithies, A., Lovell, D., Hishon, S., Pounder, R.E., Newton, C., Kellock, T.D., Misiewica, J.J., and Blerdis, L.M.: Value of brush cytology in diagnosis of gastric cancer. Br. Med. J., *373*:326, 1975.

Spjut, H.J., Margulis, A.R., and Cook, G.B.: The silicone-foam enema: A source for exfoliative cytological specimens. Acta Cytol., 7:79–84, 1963.

Effusions and Other Fluids

Drewinko, B., Sullivan, M.P., and Martin, T.: Use of the cytocentrifuge in the diagnosis of meningeal leukemia. Cancer, *31*:1331–1336, 1973.

Gondos, B., and King, E.B.: Cerebrospinal fluid cytology: Diagnostic accuracy and comparison of different techniques. Acta Cytol., *20*:542–547, 1976.

Grunze, H.: The comparative diagnostic accuracy, efficiency and specificity of cytologic technics used in the diagnosis of malignant neoplasm in serous effusions of the pleural and pericardial cavities. Acta Cytol., 8:150–163, 1964.

Masukawa, T., Kuzma, J.F., and Straumfjord, J.V.: Cytologic detection of early Paget's disease of breast with improved cellular collection method. Acta Cytol., *19*:274–278, 1975.

McGrew, E.A., and Nanos, S.: The cytology of serous effusions. *In* Wied, G.L., Koss, L.G., and Reagan, J.W. (eds.): Compendium on Diagnostic Cytology. ed. 4. Chicago, Tutorials of Cytology, 1976.

Naylor, B.: The cytological diagnosis of cerebrospinal fluid. Acta Cytol., 8:141–149, 1964.

Papanicolaou, G.N., Holmquist, D.G., Bader, G.M., and Falk, E.A.: Exfoliative cytology of human mammary gland and its value in diagnosis of cancer and other diseases of breast. Cancer, *11*:377–409, 1958.

Spriggs, A.I.: The Cytology of Effusions in the Pleural, Pericardial and Peritoneal Cavities. ed. 2. London, William Heinemann, 1972.

Tavel, M.E.: Ascites; etiological considerations with emphasis on value of several laboratory findings in diagnosis. Am. J. Med. Sci., *237*:727–743, 1959.

33

Part I: Cytologic Techniques;* Part II: Principles of Operation of a Laboratory of Cytology

Carol E. Bales, B.A., CT(ASCP), CT(IAC), CFIAC, and Grace R. Durfee, B.S., CT(ASCP)

PART I: CYTOLOGIC TECHNIQUES

Within recent years most cytology laboratories have experienced a dramatic increase in the number and types of specimens submitted for cytologic evaluation. Fiberoptic instruments and thin-needle aspirations have allowed physicians to obtain cells from almost all anatomic sites. Screening programs for the early detection of carcinoma from areas other than the female genital tract have also been implemented in some institutions. This diversity of body sites from which samples are obtained and the many procedures developed to cope with large numbers of specimens have led to the evolution of a subspecialty in cytology, that of cytopreparatory techniques.

In the past, the cytotechnologist-screener frequently was also responsible for collection, preparation, and staining of material. As a result, many of the pitfalls affecting the quality of the micro-

---

Immunocytologic procedures and stains are discussed in Chapter 34.

scopic preparations to be screened were learned firsthand. However, many laboratories now employ personnel whose primary function is cytopreparation, with the cytotechnologist participating solely in a supervisory capacity. A thorough understanding of basic cytopreparatory techniques is required to effectively oversee or modify these procedures according to the needs of a laboratory.

This chapter, therefore, describes the basic techniques involved in cytopreparation, stressing the importance of the nature and type of the specimen rather than the site of origin.

Accurate cytologic interpretation of cellular material is dependent on: (1) methods of specimen collection, (2) fixation and fixatives, (3) preservation of fluid specimens prior to processing, (4) preparation of material for microscopic examination, and (5) staining and mounting of the cell sample. These steps will be considered separately because of the important role each plays in affecting the quality of the microscopic preparation.

A series of films produced by the American Society of Cytology on a grant from the American Cancer Society may be useful for training preparatory personnel. The following films along with supplemental literature can be purchased or rented from Health Education Resources, 4733 Bethesda Avenue, Bethesda, Md. 20014.

Cytopreparation With Micro Slides
Cytopreparation With Membrane Filters
Fixation in Diagnostic Cytology
Papanicolaou Stain: Principles
Papanicolaou Stain: Materials and Methods
Coverslipping in Diagnostic Cytology
Sputum Specimens: Collection and Preparation
Bronchoscopy Specimens: Collection and Preparation

METHODS OF SPECIMEN COLLECTION

A detailed description of the clinical methods involved in the collection of cellular material for cy-

Table 33–1
Equivalent Concentrations of Several Alcohols for Purposes of Cell Fixation

100% Methanol
95% Ethanol
95% Denatured alcohol
80% Propanol
80% Isopropanol

tologic evaluation can be found in Chapter 32, and in chapters dealing with specific organs or organ systems.

FIXATION AND FIXATIVES

Fixation of Smears

Rapid fixation of smears is necessary to preserve cytologic detail of cells spread on a glass slide. If smears are allowed to air-dry prior to fixation, marked distortion of the cells occurs.

For many years the fixative of choice for gynecologic and other smear preparations was the one recommended by Papanicolaou, namely, a solution of equal parts of ether and 95% ethyl alcohol. Subsequently, it has been necessary to abandon this original and excellent fixative because ether presents a fire hazard. Ninety-five percent ethyl alcohol (ethanol) is now employed as a fixative by most laboratories, with excellent results. This method of fixation may be used for all smears prepared at the side of the patient, such as vaginal, cervical, and endometrial aspiration smears; prostatic smears; breast smears; and aspiration biopsy smears. It is also used for the final fixation of all smears prepared in the laboratory from fresh fluids or those initially collected in 50% alcohol or other preservatives.

Smears should remain in the 95% ethyl alcohol fixative for a minimum of 15 minutes prior to staining. However, prolonged fixation of several days or even weeks will not materially alter the appearance of the smear. If there is a necessity for saving smears in 95% ethyl alcohol over a period of time, better cellular preservation and less evaporation are assured by storing the specimens in capped containers in the refrigerator.

To obtain ethanol without federal taxation, a license is required. Laboratories that do not have such a license may use other alcohols. However, to obtain results similar to those seen with 95% ethanol, different concentrations must be used. Table 33–1 shows equivalent concentrations of various alcohol fixatives as suggested and tested by Danos-Holmquist.

These substitutes may also be used with membrane filters, except that 100% methanol cannot be used for Millipore filters.

All alcohol fixatives should be discarded or filtered after each use with a good-grade, medium-speed filter such as Whatman #1, and the concentration should be tested with a hydrometer before reuse.

Wet fixation with alcohol is recommended for all nongynecologic material. For gynecologic material, coating fixatives may be used.

Coating Fixatives

A number of agents* on the market today can be sprayed or applied with a dropper to freshly prepared smears, thus eliminating the use of bottles and fixing solutions. Hairsprays with a high alcohol content that contain a minimum of lanolin or oil are also effective as a fixative. Most of these agents have a dual action in that they fix the cells and, when dry, form a thin, protective coating over the smear. These fixatives have practical value in any situation in which smears must be mailed to a distant cytology laboratory for evaluation. The practice of using coating fixatives has, in fact, spread to many institutions with their own cytology laboratories. The method is *not recommended* for smears prepared from fluids within the laboratory.

Instructions for applying the coating fixative accompany the respective preparation and should be followed carefully. Cans should be shaken well prior to each use to ensure optimal dispersal and adequate fixation. As in any good method of fixation, *the coating fixative should be applied immediately to fresh smears.* The distance from which the slides are sprayed with an aerosol fixative affects the quality of the cytologic detail. The optimal distance differs with the brand of fixative used. Danos-Holmquist tested Aqua Net (Chesebrough-Ponds, Greenwich, Conn. 06830) hairspray and

Richard Allen (Box 351, Richland Mich. 49083) fixative held from 1 to 24 inches from the slide. Increments of 1 to 2 inches were used. Table 33–2 summarizes the results of this study. Ten to 12 inches (25 to 30 cm) is the optimal distance recommended for the aerosol fixatives tested. Each brand of spray fixative should be similarly tested, since there is a widespread tendency to hold the can too close to the slide. Aerosol sprays are not recommended for bloody smears because they cause clumping of erythrocytes. For further comments on the use of coating fixatives, see p. 1482 and Fig. 33–1.

Coating fixatives may also be prepared inexpensively within the laboratory. Two such methods are given below.

Polyethylene Glycol (Carbowax) Fixative (*T. Ehrenreich and S. Kerpe, 1959*)

95% Ethyl alcohol	50 ml
Ether†	50 ml
Polyethylene glycol (Carbowax compound 1540‡)	5 g

Soften the polyethylene glycol in an incubator at 56°C and add the 95% ethyl alcohol or the ether-alcohol mixture. Let stand for several hours at room temperature, or use frequent agitation to hasten the dissolution of the polyethylene-glycol. The solution may be dispensed in small dropper bottles.

Freshly made smears are placed on a flat surface, and the slides are covered immediately by five or six drops of the fixative. Allow the slide to dry for five to seven minutes or until an opaque, waxy film forms over the surface.

Spray-Cyte: Curtin Matheson Scientific, Inc., 357 Hamburg Turnpike, Wayne, N.J. 07470-2185. Pro-Fix: Scientific Products, 1430 Waukegan Rd., McGraw Park, Ill. 60085-6787. Sprayfix: Surgipath Medical Industries, Inc. P.O. Box 769, Grayslake, Ill. 60030.

---

†*Ether may be eliminated and 100 ml of 95% alcohol used.*
‡*VWR Scientific, P.O. Box 13645, Philadelphia, Pa. 19101-9711.*

Table 33–2
Quality of Cytologic Detail With Aerosol Fixation at Various Distances

Fixative	Distance	Cytologic Appearance	Fixation
Aqua Net* Hair Spray	⎰ 8–24 inches	Delicate chromatin detail	Good
	⎱ 1–7 inches	Chromatin: hazy hypochromatic, nuclear shrinkage, cilia lost and cytoplasm distorted	Poor
Richard Allen† Fixative	⎧ 14–24 inches	Loss of chromatin detail; nuclear swelling	Poor
	⎨ 6–13 inches	Delicate chromatin detail	Good
	⎩ 1–5 inches	Loss of chromatin detail; nuclear swelling	Poor

* Aqua Net hairspray, Fabergé Inc., 65 Railroad Avenue, Ridgefield, New Jersey 07657.
† Richard Allen Medical Industries, Inc., 1335 Dodge Avenue, Evanston, Illinois 60204.

Diaphane Fixative
(G. N. Papanicolaou and E. L. Bridges, 1957)

3 parts	95% ethyl alcohol
2 parts	Diaphane*

Mix thoroughly at room temperature.

Fresh wet smears are placed on a flat surface and covered immediately with enough solution to form a thin coating over the slide — approximately 0.25 or 0.5 ml (5 or 6 drops) per slide. Allow the Diaphane coating to dry thoroughly (20 to 30 minutes) to a hard, smooth film that protects the smear. When smears are received in the laboratory, place in 95% ethyl alcohol to remove Diaphane before staining.

SOME POINTERS IN THE PROCESSING OF SMEARS PREPARED WITH COATING FIXATIVES

Unless removed prior to staining, all coating fixatives will contaminate the staining solutions, particularly the hematoxylin. Most of the water-soluble coating fixatives should be removed prior to the regular staining procedure by maintaining two separate dishes of 95% ethyl alcohol and leaving the slides in each solution for 5 or 10 minutes. The 95% ethyl alcohol used for washing out the coating fixative should be filtered or changed at least once each day, the number of times depending on the number of slides that are washed.

Manufacturers of spray fixatives occasionally use in their products concentrations of alcohol greater than those normally used for optimal fixation. This results in increased cellular shrinkage, which may cause loss of nuclear detail because of chromatin condensation. The increased density of the cell wall also can impede the penetration of light green dye, with resulting excessive cytoplasmic eosinophilia. Increasing the staining time in eosin-alcohol (EA) may give better cytoplasmic staining; however, better nuclear detail cannot be achieved. All commercial spray fixatives must be tested before acceptance, and the results compared with smears that have been fixed in 95% ethyl alcohol.

Special-Purpose Fixatives

10% Buffered Formalin

Formaldehyde solution (37–40%)	100 ml
Tap water	900 ml

---

*A synthetic resin made by Will Scientific, Inc., Box 1050, Rochester, N. Y. 14063.

Neutral Buffered Formaldehyde Solution

37–40% Formaldehyde solution	100 ml
Water	900 ml
Acid sodium phosphate, monohydrate	4 g
Anhydrous disodium phosphate	6.5 g

Bouin's Solution

1.2% (saturated) aqueous picric acid	750 ml
37–49% formaldehyde solution	250 ml
Glacial acetic acid	50 ml

Picric Acid Fixative

Picric acid	13 g
70% Ethyl alcohol	1000 ml

Formalin Vapor Fixation

Some staining procedures require formalin vapor fixation. Place 1 to 2 ml of formalin solution of required concentration in a Coplin jar. Immediately after preparation of the smear, drop the slide into the Coplin jar, cell end up (label end down), and tightly cover jar. The length of time required for fixation varies according to procedure.

Carnoy's Fixative

95% Ethanol	60 ml
Chloroform	30 ml
Glacial acetic acid	10 ml

This fixative will hemolyze red blood cells and, therefore, is useful for bloody specimens. However, shrinkage of the epithelial cells is greater than that observed in specimens fixed in 95% ethanol. The staining time in hematoxylin must be reduced to prevent overstaining. Place the bloody smear in Carnoy's fixative for 3 to 5 minutes until the sediment becomes colorless, and then transfer to 95% ethanol or its equivalent. Nuclear chromatin will be lost if the cell sample remains in Carnoy's fixative for longer than 15 minutes.

This fixative must be prepared *fresh* when needed and discarded after each use. Carnoy's fixative loses its effectiveness on standing, and the chloroform can react with acetic acid to form hydrochloric acid. This fixative may be used for Millipore filters but will damage Nuclepore and Gelman filters.

Rehydration of Air-Dried Smears

Some years ago, the use of unfixed, air-dried gynecologic smears was advocated by some workers.

Such smears required rehydration in the laboratory prior to staining. In view of the wide availability of inexpensive fixatives, there is no justification for this procedure because air-dried smears are often difficult to interpret and are fraught with error.

The rehydration procedure described below may be used for inadequately fixed smears. It must be noted that squamous cells may appear restored to a considerable extent after rehydration procedures, whereas cells of secretory type often suffer irreparable damage.

The simplest rehydration technique that seems to work as well as, if not better than, most techniques has been developed by R. G. Bonime, of New York City.* Air-dried cytologic specimens are placed in a 50% aqueous solution of glycerine for 3 minutes followed by two rinses in 95% ethyl alcohol, and then are stained by the routine Papanicolaou method.

Mailing of Unstained Smears

Unstained smears may be mailed to distant cytologic laboratories after the application of coating fixatives previously discussed (see p. 1453). A variety of mailing containers are commercially available, ranging from plastic cylinders to cardboard containers, and if properly used, they will prevent breakage in the mail.

If coating fixative solutions are not available, the following method has been used for many years and gives very good results.

Glycerine Method†

Smears are first fixed in 95% ethyl alcohol for a minimum of 15 minutes. The slides are then removed, and one or two drops of glycerine are placed on the smear and covered with a clean glass slide. The slides may now be wrapped in wax paper and mailed to the laboratory in a suitable container.

PRESERVATION OF FLUID SPECIMENS PRIOR TO PROCESSING

Preservation of cellular morphology until the sample can be processed is essential to accurate cyto-

---

*Obstet. Gynecol., 24:783–790, 1966.

†See Bibliography: Ayre, J.E., and Dakin, E., 1946.

logic interpretation. For the purpose of this discussion, "prefixation" refers to the collection of a fluid specimen in a medium that will preserve morphology up to the time of slide preparation. "Fixation" refers to the final slide preparation. A "fresh sample" is one to which no fixative or preservative has been added.

Fresh Material

Specimens may be submitted to the laboratory without preservative if facilities for immediate processing are available. The length of time between collection and preparation of the sample before cellular damages occur depends on pH, protein content, enzymatic activity, and the presence or absence of bacteria. It is not possible to predict these variables even in specimens from the same anatomic site. However, the following guidelines will usually yield acceptable results.

1. *Specimens with a high mucus content*, such as sputums, bronchial aspirates, or mucocele fluid, may be preserved for 12 to 24 hours if refrigerated. Refrigeration slows the bacterial growth that causes cellular damage and the breakdown of mucus. Mucus apparently coats the cells, protecting them against rapid degeneration. The cells in specimens without thick mucus or specimens diluted with saliva are not as well protected and may deteriorate more rapidly.
2. *Specimens with a high protein content*, such as pleural, peritoneal, or pericardial fluids, may be preserved for 24 to 48 hours with refrigeration. The protein-rich fluid in which the cells are bathed acts as a tissue culture medium in preserving cellular morphology.
3. *Specimens with low mucus or protein content*, such as urine or cerebrospinal fluid, will endure only a 1- to 2-hour delay even if refrigerated. The fluid medium in which these cells are bathed contains enzymatic agents capable of causing cell destruction. Refrigeration may inhibit bacterial growth but does not protect the cells.
4. *Specimens with low pH*, such as gastric material, must be collected on ice and be prepared within minutes of collection to prevent cellular destruction by hydrochloric acid.

Prefixation of Material

Prefixation may preserve some specimens for days without deterioration of cells. Some of the disadvantages of prefixation are precipitation of protein, hardening of cells in spherical shapes, and condensation of chromatin. The most common solutions used for this purpose are discussed below.

1. *Ethyl alcohol (ethanol)* (50% solution) was once considered the best universal fixative for fluid specimens.

   Its effectiveness as a preservative, particularly of urine samples, has come under scrutiny in recent years. In 1980 Crabtree and Murphy found that when it was added to urine samples after arrival in the laboratory, degenerative changes continued to occur with a processing delay of 24 hours; fresh unfixed urine yielded the highest number of well-preserved cells. Pearson et al. (1981) resuspended well-preserved benign and malignant urothelial cells in urine samples at pH 4.5, 6.0, and 8.0. Samples with and without the addition of an equal volume of 50% methanol were processed at ½-, 2-, 24-, and 72-hour intervals. Morphologic features of cells suspended in urine with a pH of 4.5 were better preserved than in other samples regardless of whether alcohol was added. The addition of methanol, however, improved preservation of detail in samples of pH higher than 4.5. This same study also found the pH of the first morning voiding to be lower than that of subsequent voidings and that 1 g of vitamin C taken the night before sample collection significantly reduced the pH. However, if one opts to use it as a preservative, ethanol should be added in equal volume to the fluid. Ethyl alcohol in a concentration higher than 50% should not be used in collecting fluids rich in protein, because the sediment becomes hardened and very difficult to spread on glass slides, particularly if the delay in processing is greater than 1 hour. However, 95% ethyl alcohol may be effectively used in the collection of gastric washings. *Fixative containing ether or acetone should never be used for liquid specimens that cannot be smeared on slides immediately after collection.* Hardening of the sediment makes the subsequent preparation of smears almost impossible.

2. *Saccomanno's fixative* is 50% alcohol, which contains approximately 2% Carbowax 1540.* Carbowax infiltrates and occupies submicroscopic spaces, preventing cell collapse, and thus protects the cells during air drying. Cells adhere well to glass slides as a consequence of air drying. This fixative, a variant of the fixative proposed by Ehrenreich and Kerpe in 1959 (see p. 1453), was first used by Saccomanno for prefixation of sputum but can be used for fluid specimens from other sites. Carbowax 1540 is solid at room temperature, with a melting point of 43° to 46°C. To avoid the necessity of melting it whenever the fixative is made, *a stock solution of Carbowax* can be prepared as follows: pour 500 ml of water or 50% ethyl alcohol into a 1000-ml graduated cylinder. Melt Carbowax in an incubator or hot-air oven at 50° to 100°C. Add 500 ml of the melted Carbowax to the graduated cylinder. This mixture will not solidify and can be stored in a liter screwcap bottle.

   A liter of Saccomanno's fixative can be prepared by mixing 434 ml of water, 526 ml of 95% ethyl alcohol, and 40 ml of the water- or alcohol-based stock solution. The final concentration of alcohol will be slightly different, depending on which stock solution is used; however, this difference is not critical. Never use absolute alcohol for preparation of Saccommano's fixative, since it may contain dehydrating agents that cause mucus to become hard and rubbery and difficult to blend.

3. *Mucolexx*† is a commercial, mucoliquefying preservative designed for use in the collection of mucoid and fluid specimens. Its active ingredients are polyethylene glycol, methanol, buffering agents, and aromatics. An equal volume of undiluted Mucolexx added to the specimen is recommended by the manufacturer.

4. *Many other preservatives have been developed for use with automated cytology systems* that may someday have practical application for routine cytology. The formulas are too numerous to be discussed in this section.

   Table 33–3 summarizes the use of the preservatives described.

Comment

The decision to prepare slides from fresh or prefixed material will be influenced by the volume of specimens processed by the laboratory, the number of trained personnel available to prepare the material, and the cooperation of the physicians and nursing staff involved in collection of the sam-

*VWR Scientific, P.O. Box 13645, Philadelphia, Pa. 19101-9711.

†Scientific Products, 1430 Waukegan Rd., McGraw Park, Ill. 60085-6787, Cat. no. 7745.

Table 33-3
Directions for Use of Several Fixatives

Preservative	Specimen	Instructions
50% ethanol Saccomanno Mucolexx }	All body sites except gastric	Sputums: Have the patient expectorate directly into cups containing 50 ml of preservative and shake well. Other specimens: add an equal volume of preservative and mix well.
70% ethanol	Sputum, bronchial aspirates, and washings	Same as above.
95% ethanol	Gastric, bronchial, and other saline washings	Add an equal volume of preservative and mix well.

ple. We do not recommend one method in preference to another but believe that consistency is important. For example, if sputum or urine samples are routinely collected in 50% ethanol, unfixed samples should be fixed immediately upon arrival in the laboratory to ensure uniformly consistent cytologic artifacts for microscopic evaluation.

PREPARATION OF FLUIDS FOR MICROSCOPIC EXAMINATION

Many papers have been published comparing the diagnostic accuracy of different techniques. Often the results of these studies contradict one another. A detailed discussion of the advantages and disadvantages of each method is not possible in this chapter. As with collection techniques, the methods used for preparing specimens will vary according to the volume of specimens processed, personnel available, and collection techniques. The most commonly used procedures can be divided into the following categories: (1) direct or sediment smears on glass slides, (2) cytocentrifuge preparations, (3) preparation with membrane filters, and (4) preparation of cell blocks.

Materials Required

1. Petri dishes and brown paper toweling.
2. Curets, applicator sticks, forceps, or similar instruments. The nasal curet in Fig. 33-1 is one such instrument that can be easily rinsed in a germicidal solution and flamed after each specimen.
3. *Mayer's albumin* is available commercially or can be prepared in the laboratory as follows:

   Mix by stirring 1 volume of fresh egg whites or reconstituted dried egg albumin (1 g of albumin per 20 ml of distilled water) with an equal volume of pure glycerol. Filter this mixture through damp muslin or coarse filter paper in an oven (55°C to 58°C). Add a few crystals of thymol or camphor to prevent growth of molds. Store this solution in small screw-capped bottles at a temperature of −20°C. The bottle of albumin currently in use must be refrigerated.
4. Copper paper clips for keeping the slides separated in the fixative.
5. Glass slides. Slides should be 0.95 to 1.06 mm in thickness to ensure good microscopic illumination. Slides may be plain, totally frosted (Dakin), albuminized, or coated with another adhesive (see below) and can be labeled perma-

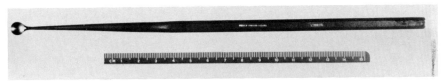

FIGURE 33-1. A small curet-type spoon successfully used in this laboratory for transferring sediment from centrifuge tube or sputum to slide. (United Surgical Supplies Co., Inc., Port Chester, N.Y.)

nently with a diamond-point pencil or black laboratory ink. A lead pencil (no. 3 hardness) can be used for temporary identification of slides with frosted ends. Permanent paper labels can be applied after coverslipping. If totally frosted slides are used, gentle spreading is required to prevent cellular damage, and the use of a mounting medium having a refractive index close to that of glass, such as Fisher Scientific Permount, will help eliminate the granular refractile background of these slides. The choice of plain, frosted, or albuminized slides will depend on the adhesiveness of the material to be smeared. Albuminized slides should be prepared one to several days before use to allow the slides to become tacky.

Preparation of Albuminized Slides. Arrange the slides on a clean tray, and using a dropper, place a drop of Mayer's albumin on each one. With the fingertip covered by a thin rubber cot, spread the albumin thinly and evenly over the entire slide, or lay another slide on top, rubbing the two slides together to obtain uniformly coated slides. Keep the coated slides in a dust-proof area of the laboratory, in a closed slide box, or cover with wax paper.

6. Bottles of 95% ethyl alcohol or equivalent (see p. 1452).

7. Centrifuge tubes, 50-ml capacity, preferably disposable plastic tubes with a screw cap.

8. Centrifuge: 50-ml tube capacity with a horizontal head. Cell fractionation studies have shown that cells sediment best at 600 × gravity in 10 minutes. To determine the centrifuge speed or revolutions per minute (rpm) required to equal 600 × gravity for an individual centrifuge:
   a. Measure the radius of the centrifuge from the center pin of the rotating head to the end of the extended cup (Fig. 33–2).
   b. Place a straight edge on the chart in Fig. 33–3 intersecting the rotating radius and 600 gravities. The point at which the straight edge intersects the speed scale is the recommended rpm.

Other Adhesives

The adhesive *gelatin chrome alum* was found to be superior to albumin for transferring cells from membrane filters to glass slides; it may also be of use for routine slide preparation of poorly adhesive samples. The method described by Adler consists of 1 g of gelatin plus 0.1 g of chrome alum dissolved in 100 ml of distilled water, to which 1 ml of 10% thymol in ethanol has been added. Slides are dipped once, drained, their backs wiped off, and then allowed to dry. Slides are stored as previously

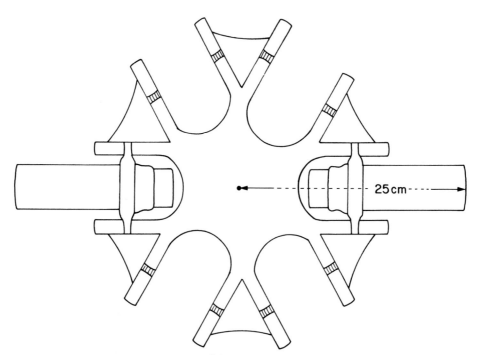

FIGURE 33–2. Determination of the rotating radius of the centrifuge.

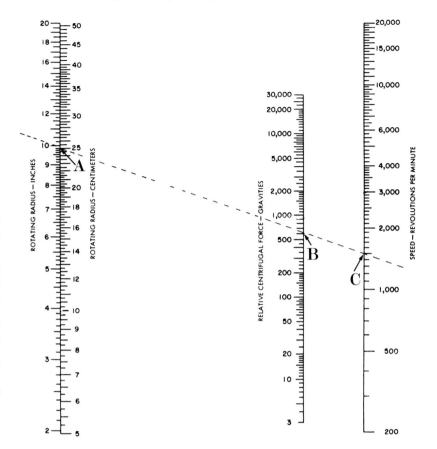

FIGURE 33-3. Chart to be used for the determination of centrifuge speed (revolutions per minute) at gravity 600. The scale on left shows the length of the rotating radius in centimeters or inches. The central scale shows relative centrifugal force or gravities. The right scale shows centrifuge speed expressed as revolutions per minute. In the example given, a straight line intersects the rotating radius at 25 cm, or approximately 10 inches (*A*), and the centrifugal force at 600 gravities (*B*). An extension of this line shows 1,500 as the number of revolutions per minute for optimal centrifugation (*C*).

described for albuminized slides. They may be stored for weeks. However, maximal cell adhesion has been reported when the dipping solution is made up one day prior to use.

Poly-L-lysine is a potent cell adhesive that is particularly useful in experimental work (scanning electron microscopy) and in immunocytochemistry (Haung et al., 1983*).

A 0.1% stock solution of poly-L-lysine in deionized water (molecular weight 380,000) is commercially available from Sigma Diagnostics.† The stock solution is diluted 1 : 10 or 1 : 20 in deionized water. Clean glass slides are placed in the diluted solution at room temperature for five minutes and are oven-dried. Dried slides are ready to use. The

coated slides significantly improve adhesion of cells and tissues.

Another excellent adhesive is *3-aminopropyltriethoxysilane* (3-APTES), also from Sigma Diagnostics. The compound adheres to glass and binds to cell surface. A 2% solution of 3-APTES in acetone is prepared. The solution may be used to coat clean slides, as described above, but may also be used to better attach cells and tissues to slides in archival material.‡ We successfully used this compound in an in situ hybridization procedure of archival cervical smears with DNA biotinylated probes of human papillomavirus.§

Another cell adhesive occasionally used is Elmer's glue.

*Domagala, W., Emeson, E.E., and Koss, L.G.: A simple method of preparation and identification of cells for scanning electron microscopy. Aca Cytol., 23:140–146, 1979.

Huang, W.M., Givson, S.J., Facer, P., Gu, J., Polak, J.M.: Improved section adhesion for immunocytochemistry using high molecular weight polymers of L-lysine as a slide coating. Histochemistry, 77:275, 1983.

†P.O. Box 14508, St. Louis, Mo. 63178, catalog no. P8920.

‡Rule, A.H., Naber, S.P., Perry, C., Waters, G., Coburn, E.W., Moblaker, H., DeLellis, R., and Wolfe, H.: Cells and tissues covalently bound to silinized glass slides. Lab. Invest., 60:81A, 1989.

§Liang, X-M., Wieczorek, R.L., and Koss, L.G.: In situ hybridization with human papillomavirus using biotinylated DNA probes on archival cervical smears. J. Cytochem. Histochem., 39:771–775, 1991.

Preparation of Direct or Sediment Smears on Glass Slides

Specimens consisting of a small amount of material that adheres well to glass slides (e.g., cervical scrapes, brushing, needle aspirates) can be smeared directly on a slide. Details of the clinical handling for each are given in Chapter 32.

Sputum and Bronchial Aspirates

FRESH OR PREFIXED IN 50% ALCOHOL (Fig. 33–4)

Selection of proper particles is critical in correct processing of sputum. To select the bloody, discolored, or solid particles, the sputum must be carefully inspected. This may be done by pouring the specimen into a Petri dish and examining it against a black background. In lieu of Petri dishes, excellent results may be obtained by pouring sputum specimens on two or three thicknesses of brown paper toweling. The paper toweling absorbs most of the fluid portion of the specimen and allows the selection of particles. Sputum is often difficult to transfer to slides in small amounts because of its viscous, ropy consistency. The use of two specially designed curet-type instruments, nasal curets (see Fig. 33–1), or applicator sticks, one in each hand, is required.

Select any bloody, discolored, or solid particles,

if present, and place a small portion of each particle, not larger than the size of a small pea, on each of four plain slides, two of which have paper clips. With a clean glass slide crush the particle of sputum on each of the four slides, using a rotary motion. Then, with overlapping horizontal strokes, spread the material evenly over the slide so that the final preparation is only slightly thicker than a blood smear. *Place the prepared slides immediately in the 95% ethyl alcohol fixative, or its equivalent (see p.1452),* alternating the clipped slide with an unclipped one so that the smeared surfaces remain separated. In the absence of particles, sputum samples from at last four different portions of the specimen must be smeared.

If cell blocks are to be prepared, save the part of the specimen remaining after preparation of smears and proceed as outlined on page 1472.

Specimens fixed in 70% alcohol are prepared as described above; however, *albuminized slides* should be used. If the sample has become hard or rubbery, a drop of water on the slide will soften it.

Saccomanno's Technique (Fig. 33–5)

1. To a specimen received in Saccomanno's fixative, add sufficient 50% ethanol to make a total volume of 50 to 100 ml. If specimen is received in 50% alcohol, add a sufficient amount of Saccommano's stock solution (see p. 1456) to achieve a final concentration of approximately

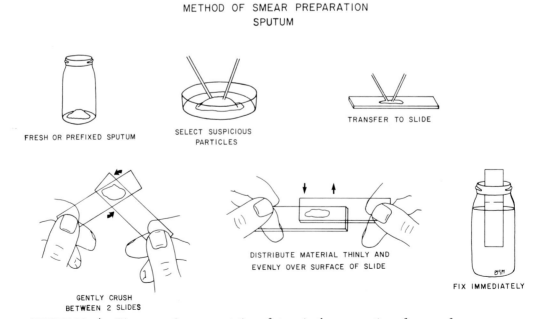

METHOD OF SMEAR PREPARATION
SPUTUM

FRESH OR PREFIXED SPUTUM

SELECT SUSPICIOUS PARTICLES

TRANSFER TO SLIDE

GENTLY CRUSH BETWEEN 2 SLIDES

DISTRIBUTE MATERIAL THINLY AND EVENLY OVER SURFACE OF SLIDE

FIX IMMEDIATELY

FIGURE 33–4.   Diagrammatic representation of steps in the preparation of smears from sputum.

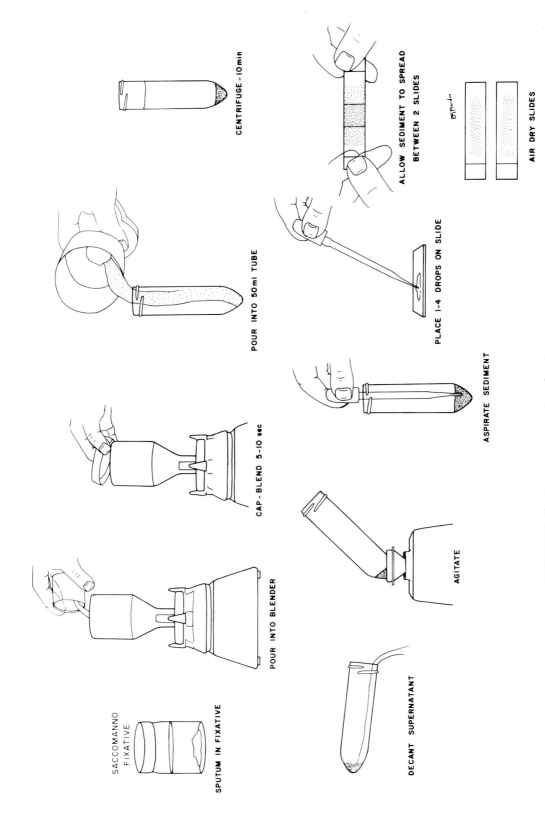

CENTRIFUGE-10min

ALLOW SEDIMENT TO SPREAD
BETWEEN 2 SLIDES

AIR DRY SLIDES

POUR INTO 50ml TUBE

PLACE 1-4 DROPS ON SLIDE

CAP-BLEND 5-10 sec

ASPIRATE SEDIMENT

POUR INTO BLENDER

AGITATE

SACCOMANNO
FIXATIVE

SPUTUM IN FIXATIVE

DECANT SUPERNATANT

FIGURE 33-5. Sputum preparation after Saccomanno.

2% Carbowax. For example, to 45 to 50 ml of specimen, add 4 ml of Saccomanno's stock solution and mix well. Specimen should remain in this fixative approximately 1/2 hour before processing.

2. Pour the specimen into a semimicro container* and blend in a Waring Blendor† at high speed for 5 to 10 seconds. Container should remain capped during blending.

3. Pour blended specimen into a 50-ml test tube. If flecks and fine threads are still visible, return to blender for an additional 5 to 10 seconds. Cells are not damaged unless specimen is blended excessively.

4. Centrifuge specimen for 10 minutes at rpm determined for your centrifuge (see p. 1458).

5. Decant supernatant, leaving a few drops of fluid to mix with the granular, pale sediment. Resuspend sediment by agitating the tube on a vortex mixer.‡

6. Prepare smears by placing a few drops of the resuspended sediment in the center of a clean slide. The number of drops depends on the consistency of the sediment: use only one to two drops if the sediment is thick; use two to four drops if the sediment is thin and watery. Place a second, clean slide over the material and allow it to spread evenly between the two slides. Gently pull the slides apart with an easy sliding motion. Albuminized slides are not necessary, since the preparations are allowed to air-dry.

7. Allow slides to air-dry until ready for staining. Smears may be stored for months in this condition without adverse effects. *As with coating fixatives, the slides should be rinsed in 95% alcohol for at least 10 minutes before staining to remove the Carbowax.* Failure to rinse the slides properly will impede the stain's penetration of the cell, alter the staining results, and contaminate the staining solutions.

8. We have found it useful to use three semimicro containers on rotating bases. After the first specimen is blended and poured into a centrifuge tube, the semimicro container is filled with a 1:10 dilution of household bleach (sodium hypochlorite) for cleaning purposes

and allowed to stand while the second container is being used for the next specimen. The second container is used and then filled with bleach while the first container is emptied of bleach and placed under a faucet of hot running water. The third container is used for the third specimen and filled with bleach while the second container is put under running water and the first container is ready to use again. Many laboratories use only one container and just rinse it well under running water between samples.

Precautions

Harris, in a letter to the editor (Acta Cytol., 21: 493, 1977), quotes a personal communication dated September 28, 1976, from J.E. Forney, Bureau of Laboratories, Center for Disease Control, Atlanta, Georgia:

[T]he household blender has been shown to be one of the most hazardous pieces of equipment used in the laboratory in terms of production of potentially infectious aerosols.

The blending step should be carried out in a safety-type blender which has been properly checked and maintained to prevent any leakage.

Even when using the safety-type blender container, it should not be opened for at least one hour after the blending operation has been completed, because it takes that long for the infectious aerosols to settle in the atmosphere within the blender jar.

The alternative would be to place the blender in a negative pressure cabinet which has an airflow velocity across the face of the cabinet of at least 75 linear feet per minute.

Saccomanno states in a letter to the editor (Acta Cytol., 21: 495, 1977):

[W]e have not experienced any infection in our laboratory utilizing this technique on over 125,000 specimens. We are aware that our area is not endemic for tuberculosis or fungal diseases. Also, that we have added 3 mg. of Rifampin to each fixative bottle with the understanding that this may be helpful, and that a similar amount can be added to the specimen on arrival in the laboratory before preparation. Finally, a negative pressure hood should be used when possible.

Saccomanno (personal communication, August 1990) believes that blending pulmonary secretions poses no undue risk of exposure to the AIDS virus. His laboratory continues to blend samples under a negative-pressure hood, and his technologists wear gloves during the procedure (see p. 1517 for a discussion of universal precautions).

Scientific Products, 1430 Waukegan Rd., McGraw Park, Ill. 60085-6787—Container, Semi-Micro Stainless Steel, Eberbach—catalog no. S8395-1.

†*Scientific Products—Stirrer, Blendor, 2 speed, Waring—catalog no. S8346-1.*

‡*Scientific Products, 1430 Waukegan Rd., Vortex-Genie mixer, catalog no. 12-812. McGraw Park, Ill. 60085-6787.*

Preparation of Rifampin Solution.* Empty the contents of a 300-mg capsule of rifampin† into 100 ml of 50% ethyl alcohol and blend at high speed in Waring Blendor. One ml of rifampin solution should be added to each 50 ml of fixative just before it leaves the laboratory for distribution to patients or hospital wards.

As an added precaution, add another milliliter of rifampin solution to each specimen of sputum returned to the laboratory and let stand for 24 hours before processing.

Pleural, Peritoneal, and Other High-Protein Fluids (Fig. 33–6)

FRESH SPECIMENS

1. Pour specimen into 50-ml centrifuge tubes with screw cap and centrifuge for 10 minutes at recommended rpm (see p. 1458).
2. Pour off the supernatant. If there is only a small cell button, the tube should be inverted on paper toweling or gauze and allowed to stand until the tube is well drained. This prevents dilution of the sediment with the supernatant that runs down the sides of the tube. However, watch closely to prevent loss of the cell button on the paper toweling. Excess protein and blood coating the cells can interfere with the staining reaction. Washing the sediment once or twice with a balanced salt solution at this point will markedly improve the quality of the stain.

   If the sample is very bloody, the centrifugation may produce a buffy coat containing leukocytes and mesothelial and tumor cells, which may be observed above the layer of red blood cells. To not disturb the buffy coat, a Pasteur pipette can be used to remove all the supernatant. Under these circumstances direct smears of the buffy coat may be obtained with excellent concentration of cells.
3. Transfer the sediment or buffy coat to a clean glass slide. Most well-drained sediments adhere well to clean slides; however, albuminized slides may be used. The following three methods are most frequently used for preparation of slides.

A. Place one to two drops of sediment on a slide by means of a disposable glass pipette or an instrument such as a nasal curet (see Fig. 33–1). Place a second clean slide over the sediment and allow it to spread evenly between the two slides. Gently pull slides apart with an easy sliding motion. *Fix immediately* by dropping slides into 95% ethyl alcohol or its equivalent (see p. 1452). Uneven cell distribution ("ribbing effect") will occur if a smooth continuous motion is not used when immersing the slides in alcohol.

B. Dip a thin, tightly wound cotton swab premoistened with supernatant in the sediment. Gently roll the swab in one direction over the surface of the slide. Fix smears immediately as described above.

C. Touch a bacteriology wire loop to the sediment. Move the loop quickly in a longitudinal, then horizontal direction over the surface of the slide. Immediately fix slide as described above.

Clotted Specimens

Fluids high in protein or bloody fluids that were not collected in an anticoagulant may form clots. Clots may be gently twisted or pressed against the side of the container by means of a wooden stick to wring out the fluid and trapped cells. The fluid should be processed as described above and the remaining clot processed as a cell block.

Bloody Fluids

Smears may be prepared as described for fresh specimens. However, erythrocytes may obscure the epithelial cells on smears made from excessively bloody fluids.

Several methods are available for handling bloody samples, such as flotation techniques to separate the erythrocytes from other cellular elements (see p. 1511); hemolyzing the erythrocytes before slide preparation; lysing them after slide preparation with Carnoy's fixative (see p. 1454 for formula and special staining requirements); and lysing them after the slide has been stained.

Method of Erythrocyte Hemolysis Prior to Slide Preparation. Add to 50 ml of sample *one* of the following: 1 ml of glacial acetic acid, *or* a few drops of a special hemolyzing agent such as Zap-Isoton used with the Coulter counter, *or* 0.1 normal HCl until a uniformly brown color appears. Centrifuge the sample and discard the supernatant. Wash the sediment twice in a balanced salt solu-

---

*Personal communication from Dr. Geno Saccomanno, Grand Junction, Colorado.

†Rifadin, Dow Pharmaceuticals. The Dow Chemical Company, P.O. Box 68511 Indianapolis, Ind. 46268.

Rimactane, CIBA Pharmaceutical Company, Division of Ciba–Geigy Corp., Summit, N.J. 07901.

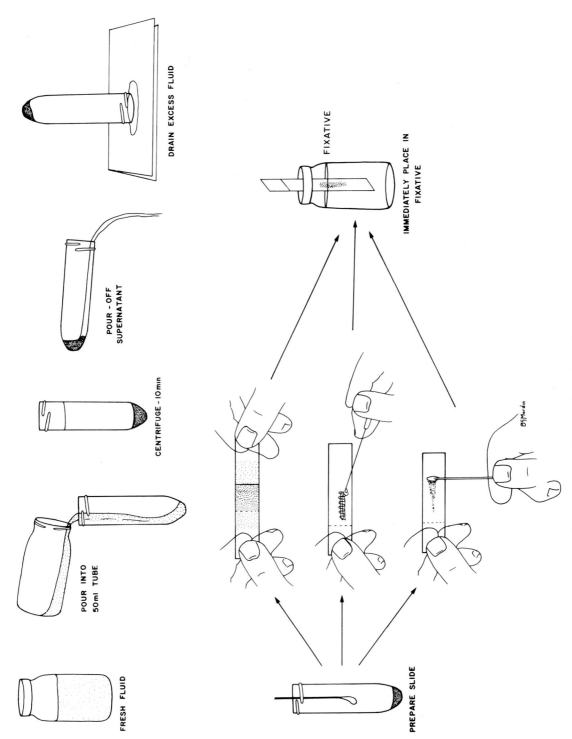

FRESH FLUID

POUR INTO 50ml TUBE

CENTRIFUGE - 10min

POUR-OFF SUPERNATANT

DRAIN EXCESS FLUID

PREPARE SLIDE

FIXATIVE

IMMEDIATELY PLACE IN FIXATIVE

FIGURE 33-6. Preparation of smears from body fluids.

tion. Prepare slides as described for fresh specimens.

Method of Erythrocyte Hemolysis After Slide Preparation. Pieslor et al. recommend the following method, which is suitable for both stained and unstained slides. The hemolyzing agent is a 2M urea solution commercially available as Technicon Platelet Diluent (Technicon Corp., Tarrytown, N.Y.), or it can be prepared by dissolving 120 g of powdered urea (J.T. Baker Chemical Co., Phillipsburg, N.J.) in 1 L of distilled water.

After a minimum of 5 minutes of fixation in 95% ethanol, bloody smears are placed in a Coplin jar containing the urea solution for 20 to 30 seconds, then transferred back to the ethanol fixative and stained routinely.

To lyse cells from stained slides, remove coverslip and take slides back through xylene and alcohol to water. Place slide in urea for 5 to 10 minutes, transfer to 95% alcohol, and then restrain slide with routine stain.

Prefixed Fluids

Prepare slides as described under fresh specimens; however, the use of albuminized or adhesive-coated slides is essential.

Bronchial and Gastric Washings Collected in Normal Saline Solution

1. Pour washings into 50-ml plastic screw-cap centrifuge tubes and centrifuge for 10 minutes at predetermined rpm (see p. 1458).
2. Pour off supernatant. If the sediment is very mucoid, smears may be prepared as described for sputums and bronchial aspirates (see Fig. 33–4). Sediment that contains only a small amount of mucus can be prepared by the two-slide pull method described for pleural, peritoneal, and other high-protein fluids (see Fig. 33–6). If the sediment has no visible mucus, it should be prepared as described for urine sediment (see below). The Saccomanno technique may be used by centrifuging the washing for 10 minutes at the proper rpm, discarding the supernatant, adding 50 ml of Saccomanno's fixative to the sediment, and letting it stand for 2 hours. The slides are then hand-prepared as described in steps 2 through 7 of the Saccomanno technique for sputums (see p. 1460). If the bronchial washing is collected in Saccomanno's fixative, steps 1 through 7 of the same procedure may be used.

Urine, Cerebrospinal Fluid, and Other Watery Fluids

A variety of methods have been developed to deal with the unique characteristics of fluids with low cellularity and low protein content. Cytocentrifuge preparations, membrane filters, Leif buckets, and direct smears from the sediment yield adequate preparations if specimens are handled with care. In our laboratory, a combination of cytocentrifuge and direct smears of the sediment is used. Prevention of cell loss and satisfactory preservation of morphologic detail are the two goals of the procedure. Cell loss may be substantial if slides are wet fixed in alcohol. Beyer-Boon and Voorn-den Hollander (1978) estimated the loss to be from 74% to 98%. With the semiautomated technique developed in this laboratory (Bales, 1981), the cytocentrifuge preparations using Shandon Cytospin* (Fig. 33–7), result in cell-rich monolayer preparations of excellent morphologic quality. The method is applicable to urines, cerebrospinal fluids, and other specimens with a low cell content. Likewise, the smears made directly from the sediment are generally rich in cells and exhibit outstanding cellular detail.

Bales's Method (Acta Cytol., *25*: 895–899, 1981)

Materials Required. The following materials are required for the procedure:

1. Carbowax 1540 (VWR Scientific, P.O. Box 13645, Philadelphia, Pa. 19101-9711.
2. Ethanol (95% solution).
3. Oxford Series P-700 Micro-pipetting system (Fisher Scientific Company, Springfield, N.J. 07081, with one pipette each of capacities 3 μl (Cat. #21-180-23), 50 μl (catalog no. 21-180-38), and 200 μl (catalog no. 21-180-42) and plastic disposable tips (catalog no. 21-240-10).
4. Standard Repipet Dispenser of 1-ml capacity (Fisher Scientific, catalog no. 13-687053).
5. Repipet Jrs. Variable Volume Dispenser of 5-ml capacity (Fisher Scientific, catalog 13-687-59A).
6. Vortex-Genie Mixer (Fisher Scientific, catalog 12-812).
7. Plastic test tubes of 50-ml capacity.
8. Clean glass slides.

Shandon, Inc., 171 Industry Dr. Pittsburgh, Pa. 15275.

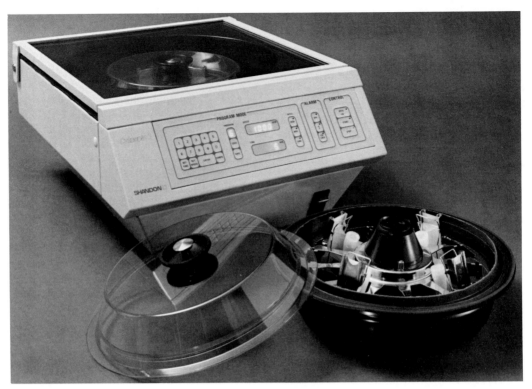

FIGURE 33–7. Shandon's Cytospin II cytocentrifuge. The reader is referred to the manufacturer's manual for technical details of use.

Procedure

Preparation of Carbowax Stock Solution. Carbowax 1540 is solid at room temperature, with a melting point of 43° to 46°C. To avoid the necessity of melting it whenever the fixative is made, a stock solution of Carbowax can be prepared as follows. Pour 500 ml of water into a 1,000-ml graduated cylinder. Melt the Carbowax in an incubator or hot-air oven at 50° to 100°C. Add 500 ml of the melted Carbowax to the graduated cylinder. This mixture will not solidify and can be stored in a liter screw cap bottle.

Preparation of 2% Carbowax Solution in 70% Ethanol. A liter of 2% Carbowax fixative in 70% ethanol is prepared by mixing 223 ml of water, 737 ml of 95% ethyl alcohol, and 40 ml of the water-based stock solution of Carbowax.

Preliminary Preparation of Sample. The preliminary preparation of a sample is carried out in the following steps (Fig. 33–8), using fresh urine or urine prefixed in an equal volume of 50% ethanol:

1. Centrifuge 50 ml of the sample for 10 minutes at 600 g.
2. Pour off the supernatant and invert the centrifuge tube on paper toweling to drain the sediment well.
3. Using a Vortex mixer, briefly agitate the well-drained sediment.
4. Proceed to cytocentrifuge or smear preparations as desired.

Preparation of Cytocentrifuge Slides. To prepare slides by cytocentrifugation, use the following steps (Fig. 33–9):

1. Aspirate *precisely* 3 µl of the sediment obtained in the preliminary preparation of the sample.
2. Expel the sediment into a test tube containing 400 µl of 2% solution of Carbowax into alcohol. (Test tubes can be filled in advance using a repipette set to dispense 400 µl of fixative. These tubes must be stored in the refrigerator until needed.)
3. Briefly agitate the mixture on a Votex mixer to prevent formation of cell aggregates.

PRELIMINARY PREPARATION OF SAMPLE

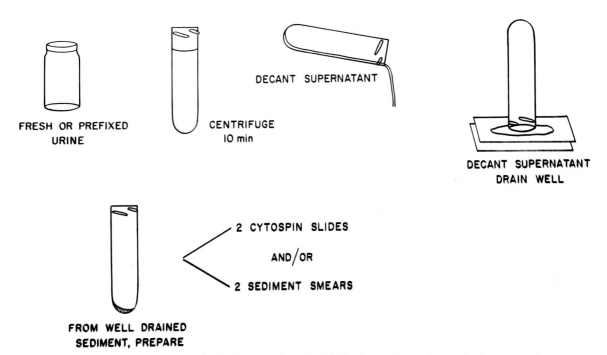

FIGURE 33–8. Bales's method of preparation of voided urine sediment for cytologic examination (see Figs. 33–9 and 33–10).

4. Aspirate 200 μl with an automatic pipette and place in a cytocentrifuge chamber.
5. Repeat step 4 and place the remaining 200 μl in the opposed cytocentrifuge chamber.
6. Spin for 5 minutes, remove slides, and allow them to air-dry for 10 to 30 minutes in a dust-free environment.
7. Rinse slides in 95% alcohol for 10 minutes prior to staining.

Preparation of Smears. Smears may be prepared from the sediment as follows (Fig. 33–10):

1. Add 3 to 5 ml of the 2% Carbowax solution to the sediment obtained in the preliminary preparation of the sample and agitate on a Vortex mixer.
2. Let stand in a vertical position for 10 minutes, and thereafter centrifuge at 600 g for 10 minutes.
3. Pour off the supernatant and drain the sediment as described in step 3 of the preliminary preparation of sample. Agitate the sediment on the Vortex mixer.
4. Aspirate 50 μl of the sediment by means of an

automatic pipette and place on a clean glass slide. Lay second clean slide on top of the sediment and let the sediment spread spontaneously between the two slides. Pull the slides apart with a gentle gliding motion. Place the two slides with the gray sediment face up, and let them air-dry for 10 to 30 minutes in a dust-free location.
5. Rinse the dry slides for 10 minutes in 95% ethanol prior to staining.

Results. Cell-rich, yet flat, monolayer cytocentrifuge preparations of urine and cerebrospinal fluid were routinely obtained by the use of this method. The epithelial cells, whether benign or malignant, were exceptionally well preserved. There was virtually no overlapping of cells. Minimal drying artifacts were occasionally observed in polymorphonuclear leukocytes. The method provided sufficient detail for it to be used routinely in image analysis of sediments of voided urine with excellent results (Koss et al., 1984, 1985, 1987, 1988; Sherman et al., 1986). Examples of the results are shown in Figs. 22–20, 22–30, 22–51, 23–35, and 23–36. Equally good results were ob-

PREPARATION OF CYTOSPIN SLIDES

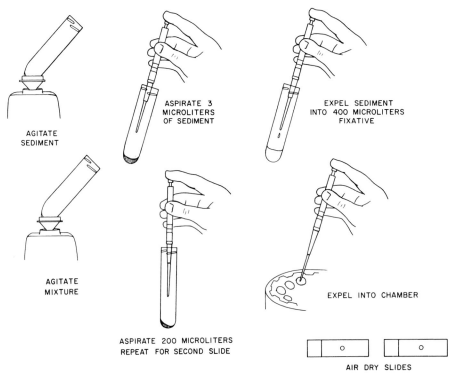

AGITATE
SEDIMENT

ASPIRATE 3
MICROLITERS
OF SEDIMENT

EXPEL SEDIMENT
INTO 400 MICROLITERS
FIXATIVE

AGITATE
MIXTURE

ASPIRATE 200 MICROLITERS
REPEAT FOR SECOND SLIDE

EXPEL INTO CHAMBER

AIR DRY SLIDES

FIGURE 33–9. Bales's method of preparation of voided urine sediment for cytologic examination by cytocentrifugation (see Figs. 33–8 and 33–10).

tained in cerebrospinal fluid. Examples thereof are shown in Figs. 27–2, 27–5, 27–18, 27–33, and 27–34.

The method is highly recommended and can be executed by technical personnel with minimal training and experience.

Comment. Major objections to the use of the cytocentrifuge include distortion of cellular morphology due to air-drying artifact and loss of cells by absorption of fluid into the filter card. Both of these difficulties have been overcome with the technique described. The rare drying artifact of polymorphonuclear leukocytes rarely affects epithelial cells; hence, the diagnostic value of the preparation is not reduced. During the developmental stages of this procedure, the quantification of sediment necessary to achieve a monolayer cytocentrifuge preparation was studied by flow cytometry. The particle counts obtained in this manner proved to be of no assistance in achieving the goal. After considerable trial and error, it was determined that the volume of sediment, rather than the

particle count, was crucial to achieving cytocentrifuge preparations with minimal overlap of cells and satisfactory morphologic characteristics. The precise amount of sediment (3 μl) obtained by means of an automated calibrated pipette has consistently resulted in monolayer cytocentrifuge preparations. Our procedure was developed using the Cytospin I. In 1981 Shandon introduced the Cytospin II with slightly different features, one of which is the automatic formation of an air bubble between the cell suspension and the slide. Boon et al. (1983) compared cell recovery rates between the Cytospin I and II. Recovery rates from the Cytospin II were consistently twice as high as those with the Cytospin I. When, however, the air bubble was deliberately introduced into the chambers of Cytospin I, the recovery rates were similar. Our method, when used with Cytospin II, requires an adjustment of cell concentration in cell-rich samples to prevent overlapping. The volume of sediment used remains the same.

Precaution: After processing of Carbowax-treated samples, the sample chamber should be

PREPARATION OF SEDIMENT SMEAR

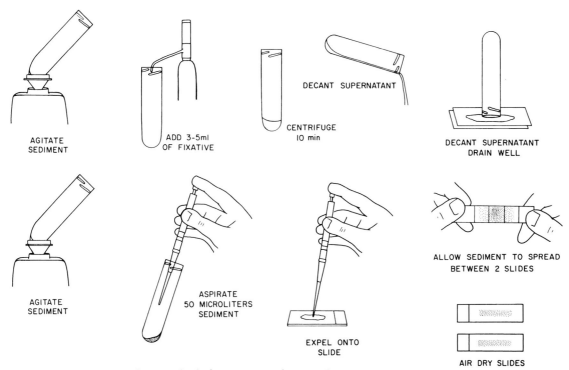

AGITATE SEDIMENT

ADD 3–5ml OF FIXATIVE

DECANT SUPERNATANT

CENTRIFUGE 10 min

DECANT SUPERNATANT DRAIN WELL

AGITATE SEDIMENT

ASPIRATE 50 MICROLITERS SEDIMENT

EXPEL ONTO SLIDE

ALLOW SEDIMENT TO SPREAD BETWEEN 2 SLIDES

AIR DRY SLIDES

FIGURE 33–10. Bales's method of preparation of smear of voided urine sediment for cytologic examination (see Figs. 33–8 and 33–9).

washed thoroughly, not just soaked in a disinfectant. Chambers that are merely rinsed and allowed to dry, even after weeks of disuse, can contaminate other specimens with residual well-preserved cells from previous runs. Washing the chambers with a small brush or soaking them in bleach usually prevents this from occurring. Alternatively, the chambers can be sterilized with boiling water or autoclaved at a maximum temperature of 120°C, or they can be cleaned with a chemical sterilizing agent such as Decon 90*.

Leif's Centrifugal Cytology Buckets

A bucket method whereby cells suspended in small amounts of fluid, for example, in cerebrospinal fluid, can be spun directly onto glass slides was developed by Leif (1971) and is marketed by Coulter Electronics.† The three-chamber bucket,

which can be adapted with almost any laboratory centrifuge, allows simultaneous processing of three samples. The manufacturer provides detailed guidance on the use of the bucket. This author has no personal experience with the method; however, on review, slides prepared in this manner exhibited excellent cytologic detail with uniform cell distribution. The cells are wet-fixed during centrifugation, thereby avoiding air-drying artifacts.

Preparation with Membrane Filters

The use of membrane filters for the concentration of cancer cells suspended in fluid was first introduced by Dr. Sam H. Seal of the Sloan-Kettering Institute. Gelman,‡ Millipore,§ and Nuclepore‖

Markson Scientific, Inc., Box 767, Del Mar, Calif. 92014.

†*Coulter Electronics, Inc., 690 W. 20th St., Hialeah, Fla. 33010.*

‡*Scientific Products, McGraw Park, Ill. 60085-6787.*

§*Millipore Filter Corp., Bedford, Mass. 01730-9903.*

‖*VWR Scientific, P.O. Box 13645, Philadelphia, Pa. 19101-9711.*

are the trade names of the most commonly used filters. Each filter has different physical, chemical, and optical properties and must be handled differently to obtain optimal results.

Gelman and Millipore filters are made of cellulose, are approximately 140 μm thick, and are opaque white in appearance until cleared in xylene and mounted in a mounting medium with a similar refractive index. The Nuclepore is a colorless, transparent membrane 10 μm thick made of polycarbonate. Rectangular sheets (19 $\times$ 42 mm Millipore and Nuclepore, 17 $\times$ 42 mm Gelman), 25-mm disks, and 47-mm disks that can be cut in half to make two slides are available. The pore diameter most frequently used for cytologic preparation is 5 μm.

The materials needed, specimen requirements, and method of filtration are essentially the same for all three types of filters, and the general setup is shown in Fig. 33–11. The major differences are related to staining and the mounting of the filters.

Materials Needed

1. Membrane filters.
2. Filter holder to fit membrane to be used.*
3. Vacuum flask, tubing, and a three-way stopcock.*
4. Vacuum source with regulator and gauge.*
5. Forceps (nonserrated).
6. Balanced salt (electrolyte) solution, such as Hanks' balanced salt solution, Cutter's Polysal, or Abbot's Normosol. Normal saline solution is frequently used but is reported to cause nuclear and cytoplasmic distortion.
7. Petri dishes.
8. 95% Ethyl alcohol.

Millipore Filter Corp., Bedford, Mass. 01730-9903.

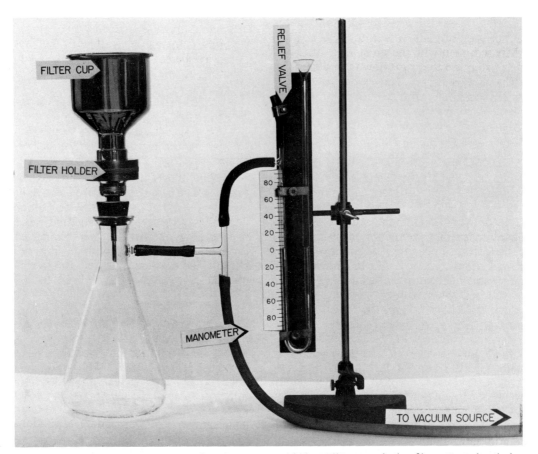

FIGURE 33–11. The apparatus used in conjunction with the Millipore and other filters. For a detailed description, see text. The filtration may be accomplished also in the absence of negative pressure. (Seal, S. H.: Cancer, *12*:590–595, 1959)

9. Ball-point pen with indelible ink.

Specimen Requirements

For best results, the specimens should be collected fresh. Prefixation coagulates proteins that may clog the filters and harden the cells into spherical shapes, preventing flattening of the cells on the membrane's surface.

Small-volume and clear fluids may be filtered directly without prior centrifugation, with the exception of urine specimens. Urine contains salts that are in solution at body temperature but that may precipitate when the urine cools to room temperature. Even though the urine appears grossly clear, these salts may clog the filters. Body cavity fluid specimens also contain debris and protein that may clog the filters. Therefore, urine samples, body cavity fluids, and other voluminous fluid samples should be centrifuged for 10 minutes at the recommended rpm (see p. 1458); the supernatant poured off; and the sediment resuspended in a balanced salt solution. Centrifuge this sample again and *carefully* pour off the supernatant. Once washed, cells do not adhere well to the centrifuge tube. Mix sediment with the small amount of balanced salt solution that runs down the side of the tube. The sample is now ready for filtration.

Mucoid specimens must be liquefied by use of a mucolytic agent, such as Mucolexx (see p. 1456), or by blending as described in the Saccomanno technique. The specimen should then be centrifuged and washed as described above.

Method of Filtration (Fig. 33–12)

1. Label Millipore and Gelman filters with indelible ink to identify patient and the cellular side of the filter. Nuclepore filters may be marked with a hard lean pencil. If a 47-mm filter is used, the left and right sides should be labeled, since the filter will be cut in half.
2. Pre-expand Millipore and Gelman filters in a Petri dish filled with 95% ethyl alcohol for 10 to 15 seconds. This prevents wrinkling of the filter when refixed in alcohol. Moisten Nuclepore filters in a Petri dish filled with a balanced salt solution.
3. Moisten the grid of the filter setup with balanced salt solution. Using nonserrated forceps, lay the pre-expanded or premoistened filter on the grid, label side up.
4. Place the funnel on top of the filter. Do not clamp funnel to base. Add 15 to 20 ml of balanced salt solution to funnel and start the vac-

uum. The filter will be flattened by allowing a portion of the salt solution to pass through the filter. Stop the vacuum at this point and clamp the funnel to the grid.

5. Add 50 to 100 ml of balanced salt solution to the funnel. By means of a disposable pipette, add one to two drops of the sediment to the solution in the funnel.
6. Start vacuum (up to 100 mg of Hg for Millipore and Gelman filters and up to 20 mg of Hg for Nuclepore filters). As the specimen filters, add balanced salt solution from a squeeze bottle to rinse filter well. The stream of the squeeze bottle should be directed against the sides of the funnel to minimize aerosol sprays and to prevent disturbance of the cells on the surface of the filter. Stop the vacuum as soon as the flow of liquid begins to slow down. The filter should appear to be clean. Red blood cells will give the filter a reddish hue. To lyse these red blood cells, add a few milliliters of 50% ethanol. If the filter is not overloaded, it will change from red to white. If the filter appears clean, add more salt solution and restart vacuum until a small amount of solution remains. The surface of the filter should always be covered with fluid, and not merely moist or wet-looking. *Never permit the filter to dry.*
7. Add 20 to 30 ml of 95% ethanol to fix the cells in situ. After 1 minute, carefully restart the vacuum to pull the fixative through the filter. Stop the vacuum when a small amount of alcohol still remains to cover the filter.
8. Unclamp the funnel, remove the wet filter with a nonserrated forceps, and place the filter, cell side up, in a Petri dish with 95% ethanol. The filter is ready for staining after remaining in fixative for one-half hour (see pp. 1484 and 1487 for special staining and mounting requirements).
9. Place funnel, forceps, and grid in disinfectant solution.

Filters are excellent means of recovering cells from sparsely cellular specimens; however, we do *not* recommend their use for effusions. To ensure good cytomorphology the limitations and advantages of the different filters must be understood. Careful attention to the chemical, physical, and optical properties of the filters will maximize their efficiency and minimize their limitations (Table 33–4).

The methods of staining, mounting, and dissolving filters are described on pp. 1484, 1487, and 1488.

METHOD OF FILTER PREPARATION

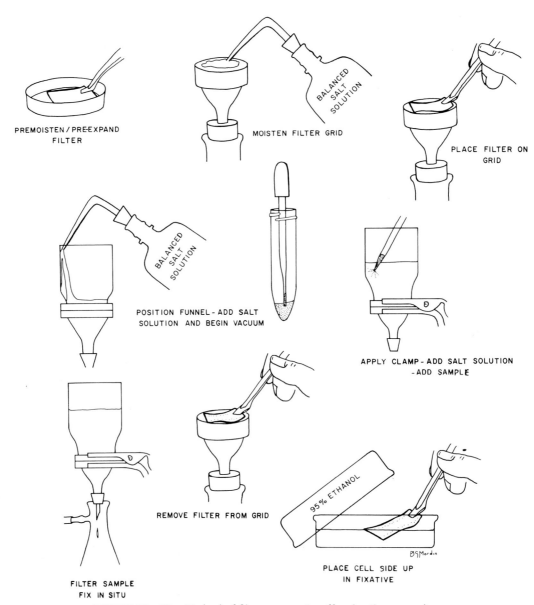

FIGURE 33–12. Method of filter preparation (for details see text).

Preparation of Cell Blocks

Cell block technique or paraffin embedding of sediments of fluids is among the oldest methods of preparing material for microscopic examination. The method uses histologic techniques for processing and thus offers one major advantage: multiple sections of the same material may be processed for routine stains, such as hematoxylin and eosin, and for special stains that may serve for identification of mucin, melanin, or other cell products and for identification of bacteria and fungi.

With the development of excellent cell preparation techniques, described in the foregoing pages, the cell block technique has been abandoned by many laboratories. This neglect is not justified in our opinion. The cell block technique should be used for processing all residual material remaining

Table 33–4
Effects of Various Common Chemicals on Filters

	Little or No Effect	Some Effect	May Dissolve or Deform
Millipore Filter	Chloroform Formalin 100% Isopropanol Xylene 100% 2-Propanol	95% Ethanol: Swells	Acetone Methanol 100% Ethanol
Gelman Filter	Formalin 100% 2-Propanol 100% Isopropanol Xylene 100% Methanol 100% Ethanol	95% Ethanol: Swells	Chloroform Acetone
Nuclepore Filter	Formalin 100% 2-Propanol 100% Isopropanol 100% Methanol 100% Ethanol 95% Ethanol	Xylene: Curls if left longer than 10 to 15 min.	Chloroform

after completion of cytologic preparations. This material often contains valuable diagnostic evidence and tissue fragments that cannot be processed by cytologic techniques. Richardson et al. (1955) have shown that additional diagnoses of cancer can be obtained in 5% of fluid specimens if smear technique is supplemented by cell block sections of residual material. The additional benefit of cell block technique is the recognition of histologic patterns of disease that sometimes cannot be reliably identified in smears or filter preparations.

Sputum, effusions, urine sediment, and material from the gastrointestinal tract are particularly suitable for cell block processing, as are all tissue fragments incidentally obtained during any diagnostic cytologic procedure.

In our experience the best fixatives for cell blocks are Bouin's fixative and picric acid fixative (see p. 1454). Buffered formalin may cause major brown precipitates but preserves DNA for analysis.

Fixed Sediment Method

1. Mix sediment or tissue fragments in one of the fixatives recommended for cell blocks. If the sediment is bloody, the blood may be hemolyzed prior to the addition of fixative by one of the methods described on p. 1452. Fibrin clots can be wrung out as described on p. 1463 and placed in fixative. Steps 2 and 3 are not necessary for fibrin clots.

2. Centrifuge this mixture for 10 minutes at the appropriate rpm (see p. 1458) and let stand from 2 hours to overnight without disturbing the sediment.
3. Pour off supernatant and drain tube well by inverting the tube on a paper towel.
4. Carefully remove the packed sediment or fibrin clot from the test tube by means of a spatula and wrap it in lens paper. Place wrapped sediment in a carefully labeled tissue cassette.
5. Put tissue cassette into a jar of the *same type* of fixative used in step 1. Process as tissue.

Bacterial Agar Method (3% Agar)

Steps 1 through 3 are the same as for the fixed sediment method.

4. If sediment becomes hard and packs well, gently remove it from the test tube with a spatula and place it, conical side up, on a paper towel.
5. Slice the sediment in half from the top to the bottom of the conical portion with a scalpel.
6. Place the cut side of the packed sediment in a small pool of melted agar that has been spread on a glass slide or in a Petri dish. Cover all exposed areas of the sediment with melted agar and let stand a few minutes to harden. *Care must be exercised to avoid bubbles in the agar.*
7. Trim the excess agar from the sediment, and place the agar button in a tissue cassette.
8. Same as step 5 of the fixed sediment method.

If sediment does not pack well or only a small amount is available after completion of steps 1 through 3, a few drops of melted agar should be added to the test tube and mixed thoroughly with sediment. After the agar hardens, gently remove the agar button from the test tube and cut it in half as described in step 5 before placing it into fixative.

Preparation of Agar

The 3% agar is prepared by dissolving 3.0 g of bacterial agar in 100 ml of boiling water. The dissolved agar should be poured into individual sterile glass tubes with a screw cap. Cap the tubes loosely until the agar cools and hardens. When the agar has cooled, tighten the caps and place the tubes in a refrigerator until ready for use. When it is needed, melt the agar in a 60°C water bath. Discard unused agar at the end of the day.*

Plasma-Thrombin Clot Method

1. Thoroughly mix a few drops of outdated blood plasma obtained from blood bank with the fresh unfixed sediment. If the sample was prefixed with alcohol, the sediment must be washed several times with a balanced salt solution, since alcohol inhibits the clotting action of plasma and thrombin.
2. Add the same number of drops of thrombin solution† as of the pooled plasma and mix well.
3. This mixture will form a clot in 1 to 2 minutes if the reagents are fresh and not too cold. Place resulting clot in a cassette that has been lined with lens paper to prevent the clot from oozing through the holes.
4. Same as step 5 of the Fixed Sediment Method. This clot is very soft and a spatula instead of a forceps is recommended for transfer to the embedding mold.*

Regardless of which of the three methods is used, the dehydrated paraffin-infiltrated cell block may be processed just as any other tissue. Histology laboratories usually process the cell blocks. However, if this service is not available, the following *dehydration and embedding procedure* may be used.

The melted agar and plasma may be colored with a small amount of food coloring to ensure contrast with the paraffin.

†*Thrombin, 500 units, topical, 1 vial: Add 10 ml of distilled water. Available from Parke Davis & Co., Rochester, Mich. 48307.*

Dehydration after fixation by placing the cassettes in the following solutions:

A.	70% Alcohol (ethyl)	1 hour
B.	95% Alcohol (ethyl)	1 hour
C.	95% Alcohol (ethyl)	30 minutes
D.	95% Alcohol (ethyl)	30 minutes
E.	Absolute alcohol	1 hour
F.	Absolute alcohol	1 hour
G.	Absolute alcohol	1 hour
H.	Xylol	1 hour
I.	Xylol	1 hour
J.	Paraffin	2 hours
K.	Paraffin	at least 2 hours

Embed in clean paraffin, trim blocks, cut sections at 4 to 6 μm, and mount on slides according to standard histologic techniques.

Simplified Technique

In 1988 Krogerus and Anderson introduced a simple technique for the preparation of cell blocks from material obtained by fine-needle aspiration, brushings, and effusions. The technique is unique in that the procedure is carried out in the sample tube, ensuring minimal cell loss. No transfer of cells to a cassette is necessary, eliminating the need for wrapping paper, agar, or thrombin (see above). The procedure is as follows:

1. In a 50-ml plastic, conical centrifuge tube, fix cell sample with 50% alcohol for 1 hour.
2. Spin sample at 300 g for 7 minutes, and pour off supernatant.
3. Resuspend cell pellet in 3 ml of acetone for 10 minutes.
4. Spin sample at 300 g for 10 minutes. Pour off acetone.
5. Place tubes for 1 hour on a warm plate (not more than 60°C).
6. Add melted paraffin to the dry, warm pellet.
7. After paraffin has solidified, tap the bottom of the tube to remove block.
8. Cut and process the conical end of the paraffin block as you would any tissue section.

THE PAPANICOLAOU STAIN

Innumerable staining techniques are available today, both for routine and for special cytochemical purposes. Consideration of all of them would be out of place in the present volume. Only those techniques that have practical value in diagnostic cytology or that are mentioned in the text are reported here. Numerous special volumes, listed in the appended bibliography, are available and may be consulted if additional staining techniques are desirable.

For routine diagnostic cytology, the Papanicolaou stain is recommended.* The use of the Papanicolaou stain results in well-stained nuclear chromatin, differential cytoplasmic counterstaining, and cytoplasmic transparency. Modifications of the original Papanicolaou stain (1942) were published by Dr. Papanicolaou in 1954 and 1960. A setup for the Papanicolaou stain is shown in Fig. 33–13. Many modifications have been published by others. The intensity of nuclear stain, the depth of cytoplasmic staining, and color of cytoplasm are largely a matter of personal preference. Seven somewhat different modifications are described in

(text continues on page 1478)

Two films are available: The Papanicolaou Stain: Principles and The Papanicolaou Stain: Materials and Methods. See p. 1452 for source, or check with the local chapter of The American Cancer Society.

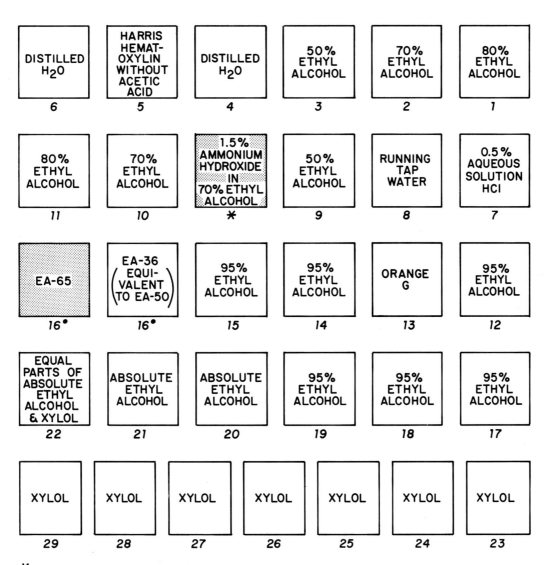

✶ FOR URINES ONLY

**● USE EA 36 FOR GYNECOLOGIC SMEARS
USE EA 65 FOR ALL OTHER SPECIMENS**

FIGURE 33–13. Diagrammatic representation of a set-up for Papanicolaou stain. For modifications see Table 33–5.

Table 33-5
Papanicolaou Stains

	Technique I Regressive (Papanicolaou 1954)	Technique II Progressive (Papanicolaou 1960)	For Slides and Nucleopores (Gill)	For Millipore and Gelman Filters (Gill)	For Carbowax Fixed Smears (Miller)	For Carbowax Fixed Sputums (Saccomanno)	For Urine Sediment Smears (Durfee)
Hydration	80%, 70%, 50% EtOH and water 10 dips each	Same as Tech. I	2 water rinses 10 dips each	2 water rinses 10 dips each	3 rinses water 10–15 dips each†	Tap water† Several changes	80%, 70%, 50% and water 5 dips each
Nuclear Stain	Harris hematoxylin half strength without acetic acid 6 min.	Harris Hematoxylin full strength with 4% acetic acid 45 sec.	Gill hematoxylin 2 min.	Gill hematoxylin 2 min.	Hematoxylin 30–45 sec.	Lillie-Mayer hematoxylin modified‡ 1 min.	Harris hematoxylin without acetic acid 6 min.
Rinse	2 water rinses 10 dips each	2 water + 1 50% EtOH rinses 10 dips each	Same as Tech. I	Same as Tech. I	3 water rinses 10 dips each	Running tap water until clear	Distilled water 5 dips
Differential Extraction	0.25% HCl 6 dips	Not necessary	Not necessary	0.05% HCl up to 30 dips Filter should appear pale yellow	0.25% HCl 1 quick dip	Not necessary	0.5% HCl in 70% alcohol 3–5 dips
Bluing	Running tap water 6 min.	1.5% NH₄OH in 70% EtOH 1 min.	Scott's tap water substitute 1 min.	Scott's tap water substitute 1 min.	3 water rinses and 4 dips in 1.5% NH₄OH in 70% EtOH		Water 5 dips 50% EtOH 5 dips 1.5% NH₄OH in 70% alcohol 1 min.
Rinse and Hydration	50%, 70%, 80%, and 95% EtOH 10 dips each	Same as Tech. I	2 water + 2 95% EtOH rinses 10 dips each	2 water + 2 95% EtOH 10 dips each	3 water + 2 95% EtOH rinses 10–15 dips each	2 rinses 95% EtOH 1 min. each	70%, 80% and 95% EtOH 5 dips each

	OG-6 1½ min.	OG-6 1¼ min.	Modified OG-6 1½ min.	Modified OG-6 2 min.	OG-6 1½ min.	OG-6 2½ min.	OG-6 1½ min.
Cytoplasmic Stain	OG-6 1½ min.	OG-6 1¼ min.	Modified OG-6 1½ min.	Modified OG-6 2 min.	OG-6 1½ min.	OG-6 2½ min.	OG-6 1½ min.
Rinse	3 rinses 95% EtOH 10 dips each	Same as Tech. I	Same as Tech. I	3 rinses 95% EtOH 1 min. each	2 rinses 95% EtOH 10 dips each	3 rinses 95% EtOH 1 min. each (Agitate)	2 rinses 95% EtOH 5 dips each
Cytoplasmic Stain	EA 36, 50, 65 1½ min.	EA-65 3 min.	Modified EA 6–10 min.	Modified EA for filters 8 min.	EA-65 2 min.	EA modified for Carbowax 1½ min.	EA-36 1½ min.
Rinse	3 rinses 95% EtOH 10 dips each	Same as Tech. I	Same as Tech. I	3 rinses 95% EtOH (4, 2, and 1 minute) No dips!	Same as Tech. I	3 rinses 95% EtOH 1 min. each (Agitate)	Same as Tech. I
Dehydration	3 rinses abs. EtOH 10 dips each	Same as Tech. I	Same as Tech. I	3 rinses abs. isopropyl alcohol 1 min. each	3 rinses abs. EtOH and 1 rinse abs. EtOH and xylene 1:1 15–20 dips each	2 rinses abs. EtOH 1 min. each	2 rinses abs. EtOH and 1 rinse abs. EtOH: xylene 1:1 5 dips each
Clearing	3 rinses in xylene 10 dips each until coverslipped	Same as Tech. I	Same as Tech. I Nuclepore limit 1 hour	Same as Tech. I	Same as Tech. I	Same as Tech. I Minimum 5 min.	7 rinses in xylene 5 dips each until coverslipped

* Use all solutions in the order indicated.
† Slide should be rinsed in 95% EtOH prior to hydration for 10–15 min.
‡ See Table 33–8.
COMMENTS: EtOH indicates ethyl alcohol. Substitutions with other alcohols are possible. Concentrations listed in Table 33–1 may be used for guidance, but experimentation is required for optimal results.
Hematoxylins — see Table 33–8 for formulas.
OG stains — see Table 33–10 for formulas.
EA stains — see Table 32–11 for formulas.

Table 33–5. Times may be varied to suit personal preference.

Principal Characteristics of the Various Modifications of the Papanicolaou Stain

Hematoxylin. Papanicolaou Technique I uses Harris hematoxylin regressively. The cells are intentionally overstained and excess hematoxylin is removed by differential extraction in HCl.

Papanicolaou Technique II, originally described for urinary and gastric preparations, uses hematoxylin progressively. Differential extraction in HCl is not necessary, since the reduction in staining time prevents overstaining of the cytoplasm. Mayer hematoxylin and Gill hematoxylin rarely overstain regardless of staining time and are always used progressively. Progressive staining is usually recommended for cell samples that do not adhere well to glass slides, since the running water bath can be eliminated.

Eosin-Alcohol Stain. EA-36 and the commercial preparation, EA-50, have a similar formula. Each contains twice the amount of light green used in EA-65. This increased amount of light green in EA-50 and EA-36 tends to stain the background of thick nongynecologic smears too intensely, and for such smears EA-65 is preferred. EA-65 is also recommended by some authors for gynecologic smears, since the cytoplasmic staining reaction can help differentiate adenocarcinomas of the endocervix (pink) from those of the endometrium (blue). However, all of the EA formulas may be used for every type of sample stained.

Bluing. The substitution of bluing solutions for running water may be used for slides that frequently shed cells. The formulas for several such solutions are given below.

Hydration. The use of a series of graded alcohols (50%, 70%, 80%, and 95%) for hydration and dehydration was thought to minimize cell distortion. Gill replaced this series with one-step hydration and dehydration, which reportedly does not increase cell shrinkage.

Materials Required

Staining Dishes

The type of staining dishes and slide carriers to be used depends on the number of cytologic specimens processed in any given laboratory. If the number of specimens is small, glass staining dishes (250 ml) with removable glass or metal carriers holding 10 slides are adequate. Large numbers of slides are handled more quickly and easily if staining dishes of 1,000-ml capacity, accommodating a carrier for 60 slides, are utilized. Glass dishes* are preferred for the stains and acid and alkaline solutions. Stainless steel dishes† may be used for all other solutions. The stainless steel dishes are more expensive than glass dishes but more practical in the long run.

Stains

The prepared Papanicolaou stains (EA 50, EA 65, and OG 6) may be obtained commercially.‡ Most of the companies making these stains also manufacture hematoxylin.

The commercially prepared stains are time-saving and usually very satisfactory, although it may be necessary to adjust the staining time or alter the dilution to achieve optimum staining results.

The stains may be prepared in the laboratory at a substantial saving. The formulas and methods of preparing stains and solutions used in the Papanicolaou staining method are given below.

Preparation of Stains and Solutions Used in the Papanicolaou Stain

The preparation of the essential solutions used in the Papanicolaou staining method is shown below. The formulas indicated may be used for the variants of Papanicolaou stain as shown in Table 33–5. A detailed discussion of general properties of dyes and chemicals may be found in the section on other stains, p. 1489.

Graded Alcohols. The formulas are listed in Table 33–6.

Solutions of Hydrochloric Acid. The formulas are listed in Table 33–7.

The glass staining dish is 202 mm long, 112 mm wide, and 72 mm deep.

†*The stainless steel staining dish is 205 mm long, 85 mm wide, and 75 mm deep. It may be purchased from Lipshaw Manufacturing Co., 7446 Central, Detroit, Mich. 48210.*

‡*Ortho Pharmaceutical Corporation, Raritan, N.J. 08869; Paragon C & C Co., Inc., 190 Willow Ave., Bronx, N.Y. 10454; Clay-Adams, 141 East 25th Street, New York, N.Y. 10010; Scientific Products, 1430 Waukegan Rd., McGaw Park, Ill. 60085-6787.*

Table 33–6
Preparation of Graded Alcohols (1,000 ml)

Desired Concentration (%)	Volume of Water (ml)	Volume of 95% Alcohol (ml)
50	474	526
70	263	737
80	160	840

Table 33–7
Preparation of Solutions of Hydrochloric Acid (1,000 ml)*

Desired Concentration (%)	1N HCl (ml)		Concentrated HCl (Approx. 12N) (ml)
0.5	60	or	5
0.25	30	or	2.5
0.05	6	or	0.5

* To a 1,000-ml graduated cylinder containing 700 ml water, add the volume of acid required for desired concentration. Let cool and add additional water to bring total volume to 1,000 ml.

Bluing Solutions. There are several formulas for the bluing solutions of approximately equal value.

a. *Ammonium hydroxide in 70% alcohol*
   Add 15 ml of NH_4OH (28% to 30% weight/volume concentration) to 985 ml of 70% ethanol.
b. *Lithium carbonate*
   Stock solution: 1.5 g of $LiCO_3$ in 100 ml of water.
   Working solution: Add 30 drops of stock solution to 1,000 ml of water.
c. *Scott's Tap Water Substitute*
   Dissolve in 1,000 ml of water 2 g of sodium bi-carbonate and *either* 10 g magnesium sulfate, anhydrous ($MgSO_4$), *or* 20 g magnesium sulfate, crystalline (Epsom salt).
d. *Tap water* can be used as a bluing agent if pH is higher than 8.

Alum Hematoxylin. The formulas for several variants are listed in Table 33–8.

Table 33–8
Formulas for Alum Hematoxylin (1 Liter)

Ingredients	Harris	Mayer	Lillie-Mayer	Gill (Half) Oxidized
Hematoxylin C.I. 75290	5 g	1 g	5 g	2 g*
Absolute methanol	50 ml	—	—	—
Water	1,000 ml	1,000 ml	700 ml	730 ml
Glycerol	—	—	300 ml	—
Ethylene glycol	—	—	—	250 ml
Chemical ripening agent	Mercuric oxide (HgO) 2.5 g	Sodium iodate ($NaIO_3$) 0.2 g	Sodium iodate ($NaIO_3$) 0.2–0.4 g	Sodium iodate† ($NaIO_3$) 0.20 g
Aluminum ammonium sulfate (alum)	100 g	50 g	50 g	23.5 g or 17.6 g Aluminum sulfate
Glacial acetic acid	None‡ or 40 ml§	None, 40 ml or 1 g citric acid	20 ml‖	20 ml or 1 g citric acid
Preservative	—	50 g Chloral hydrate	—	—
Stated Life	Months to years	2–3 months	Months to years	Over 1 year

* 2.0 g anhydrous hematoxylin should be used. If the crystalline form is used, 2.36 g is required. Catalogs do not always describe whether anhydrous or the crystalline form is available. The anhydrous form is a fine powder that tends to cake. The crystalline form consists of small crystals that shift readily when the bottle is rotated while tilted.
† The sodium iodate should be weighed accurately to ± 0.01 g.
‡ This formula is diluted with an equal volume of water for the Papanicolaou stain—Technique I.
§ This formula is full strength for Papanicolaou stain—Technique II.
‖ Saccomanno's technique substitutes 20 ml of normal acetic acid (16 ml of glacial acetic acid per 100 ml of water).

Method of Preparation

Harris

1. Dissolve hematoxylin in alcohol.
2. Dissolve alum in water and bring to a boil.
3. Add dissolved hematoxylin to alum and water and bring again to a boil.
4. Remove flask from heat.
5. Immediately add mercuric oxide.
6. Stir this solution until a dark purple color appears.
7. Plunge flask into water bath to cool.
8. Filter and store in a dark bottle.

Mayer, Mayer-Lillie, and Gill (Half Oxidized)

Combine the ingredients in the order listed in Table 33–8 and stir on a magnetic mix for approximately 1 hour at room temperature.

Availability of Commercial Hematoxylin

The hematoxylin shortage in 1973 resulted in the submission of new sources of hematoxylin to the Biological Stain Commission. For details refer to Danos Holmquist, *The Cytotechnologist Bulletin,* *12*:1–4, 1975. Hematoxylin submitted for evaluation after October 1973 is variable in quality. Some batches must be used in amounts of 5 to 6 g to equal the staining intensity of 1 to 2 g of old batches. Some of the new hematoxylin contains an alcohol-insoluble residue, resulting in loss of staining quality. Damien (*The Cytotechnologist Bulletin, 14*:12, 1977) stated that Chromabrand, Catalog no. 5B535. Certification no. ZH4 dated December 1974, is alcohol soluble and requires only the usual 5 g per liter of Harris hematoxylin. A list of hematoxylins certified by the Stain Commission is shown in Table 33–9.

Cytoplasmic Counterstains (Orange G [OG] and Eosin-Alcohol [EA])

The formulas for OG stains are listed in Table 33–10 and for EA stains in Table 33–11. The dyes are listed according to Color Index Number (C.I. No.) for accurate identification (see p. 1489). *The ingredients should be mixed as listed vertically and stored in well-stoppered dark bottles. Filter before using.*

Aqueous Stock Solutions for EA (Called for in Table 33–11)

A: 2% Light green SF yellow, C.I. No. 42095.
B: 10% Bismarck brown, C.I. No. 21000.
C: 3% TDC (total dye content) light green SF yellow, C.I. No. 42095.

Table 33–9
Hematoxylin Certified by the Biologic Stain Commission

Company Code	Prior to 1973 Numbers	Since 1973 Numbers
EH	1 through 30	33 and greater
CH	1 through 43	44 and greater
LH	1 through 38	39 and greater
PH	1 through 3	
NH	1 through 36	
AcH		1 and greater
BaH		1 and greater
BcH		1 and greater
TH		1 and greater
ZH		3 and greater
LeH		1 and greater

D: 20% TDC Eosin Y, C.I. No. 45380.
E: 3% TDC fast green FCF, C.I. No. 42053.

Alcoholic Stock Solutions Made From the Aqueous Stock Solutions

F: 0.1% Light green: 50 ml of solution A + 950 ml of 95% ethyl alcohol.
G: 0.5% Bismarck brown: 5 ml of solution B + 95 ml of 95% ethyl alcohol.
H: 0.5% eosin: 5 g Eosin + 1,000 ml of 95% ethyl alcohol.

PREPARATION OF % SOLUTIONS

Weight per volume solutions are used in making the stock aqueous and alcohol solutions for the counterstains used in the Papanicolaou staining techniques. For example, a 10% aqueous solution of OG would consist of 10 g of OG dye dissolved in 100 ml of water.

Table 33–10
*Preparation of Orange G (OG) Stains**

Ingredients	OG-6	OG Modified
Orange G-C. I. No. 16230	10% Aqueous: 50 ml	10% Aqueous (TDC): 20 ml
95% Ethyl alcohol	950 ml	980 ml
Phosphotunstic acid	0.15 g	0.15 g

* Mix ingredients and store in a well-stoppered, dark bottle. Filter before using.

Table 33-11
Preparation of Eosin-Alcohol (EA) Stains

Ingredients	EA-36	EA-65	EA-Modified for Slides	EA-Modified for Filters*	EA — For Saccomanno Prep.
Light green	Solution F 450 ml	Solution F 225 ml	Solution G 10 ml	Solution C 5 ml	Solution F 325 ml
Fast green	—	—	—	Solution E 5 ml	—
Bismarck brown	Solution G 100 ml	Solution G 100 ml	—	—	Solution G 100 ml
Phosphotungstic acid	2 g	6 g	2 g	2 g	—
Lithium carbonate saturated (see p. 1479)	10 drops	—	—	—	—
Eosin	Solution H 450 ml	Solution H 450 ml	Solution D 20 ml	Solution D 20 ml	Solution H 450 ml
95% Ethyl alcohol	—	225 ml	700 ml	700 ml	125 ml
Absolute methanol	—	—	250 ml	250 ml	—
Glacial acetic acid	—	—	20 ml	20 ml	—

* For Gelman or Millipore only; Nucleopores may be stained with slides.

Modified EA and OG are based on Total Dye Content (TDC). The original formulas for EA and OG did not take into consideration the variability of the percentage of dye content from one batch of dye to another. For this reason the use of TDC has been suggested to standardize the concentration of dyes in the EA and OG staining solution. The percentage dye concentration is printed on the label of certified dyes. To determine the weight of dye needed, divide number of grams of dye required by the percentage dye concentration. For example, if a 10% aqueous solution of OG was required and the dye content of the OG was 80%, 10 g/.80 = 12.5 g of that particular dye batch is needed. Alternately, if a 10% aqueous solution of Bismarck brown Y was needed and the dye content of the batch was 52%, 10 g/.52 = 19.23 g in 100 ml of water is needed to equal a TDC of 10%.

Important Factors Influencing Staining Results

Maintenance of Solutions and Stains

Solutions may be used over a longer period of time if the slide carrier is rested on several thicknesses of paper toweling for a few seconds after removing it from the solutions. The life expectancy of stains may be increased by storing them in dark bottles when not in use and in keeping staining dishes covered.

The frequency of replacement of solutions required to ensure crisp, well-stained slides is dependent on the volume of slides processed daily. Daily microscopic checks are recommended. The following schedule may be adjusted depending on the volume and nature of material processed.

Hematoxylin remains relatively constant in staining characteristics and seldom requires discarding if small amounts of fresh stain are added daily to replace stain loss due to evaporation. However, the use of coating or Carbowax fixatives may result in contamination, making frequent changes necessary.

OG-EA loses strength more rapidly than hematoxylin and should be replaced each week or as soon as the cells appear gray, dull, or without crisp contrasting colors.

Bluing solutions and HCl should be replaced at least once daily.

Water rinses should be changed after each use.

Alcohols used during the rehydrating and dehydrating process prior to the cytoplasmic stains should be checked occasionally with a hydrometer and should be replaced weekly or may be discarded each day to avoid the necessity of filtering these solutions. The alcohol rinses following the cytoplasmic stains are usually changed on a rotating basis after each use. The alcohol rinse immediately following the stain is discarded and the other two rinses are moved into the first and second position, and the fresh, unused dish of alcohol is placed in the third position. This rotation continues after each staining run. The absolute alcohols should be changed weekly and can be kept water-free with the addition of Silica Gel pellets.*

Xylene should be changed as soon as it appears tinted with any of the cytoplasmic stains. Water in the xylene will make the solution appear slightly milky. The clearing process may be disturbed, and tiny drops of water can be seen microscopically on a plane above the cell on a slide. The addition of Silica-Gel pellets to the absolute alcohols will minimize the possibility of water contamination of xylene. Linde Molecular Sieves† can be added to the xylene to absorb any water that may be present.

Dipping Slides

Agitation of the slides by dipping is necessary to remove excess dye. If slides are not rinsed properly, a dull rather than sharp, crisp picture results. Slides should be dipped gently to avoid cell loss, and the slide carrier should not hit the bottom of the staining dish. Each dip should last approximately one second. Dipping too slowly will result in too much decolorization. However, one or two dips more or less will not affect results.

Intensity of Staining Reaction

The desired intensity of nuclear and cytoplasmic stains is one of personal preference and varies with different cell samples. Individual experimentation is necessary. The quality of the stained slides is also dependent on the solubility, percentage of dye concentration, etc., of the dyes used in making EA, OG, and hematoxylin, as discussed in the section of this chapter devoted to stain preparation.

Factors other than timing, however, may influence the nuclear and cytoplasmic staining intensity.

NUCLEAR STAIN TOO PALE

Understaining of the nucleus may occur for one or more of the following reasons:

1. Contamination of hematoxylin with Carbo-

Sigma Chemical Co., P.O. Box 14508, Saint Louis, 63178. Catalog no. S7500 Type II.
†*Union Carbide Corporation, Linde Division, Baltimore, Md. 21207.*

wax or coating fixatives, which reduce its ability to penetrate the nucleus.
2. Time in hematoxylin is not increased for Carbowax-fixed specimens wherein the nuclei tend to resist hematoxylin penetration.
3. Decolorizing action of HCl continues if it is not removed carefully with running tap water.
4. Smears may have been permitted to air-dry prior to fixation.
5. Excessive time in chlorinated tap water will bleach the nuclear stain.
6. Carnoy's fixative results in loss of nuclear material if the smears are left in it for too long a time (see p. 1454).
7. The pH of the tap water or bluing agent is not sufficiently alkaline to blue properly.
8. Single cells may appear understained if thick areas of the smears are correctly stained.
9. Stain may become diluted if water is not drained from racks prior to immersion in hematoxylin.
10. If the timing of staining in hematoxylin is based on material collected in fixatives, unfixed material may have to be stained longer to achieve the same intensity of staining.
11. Concentration of HCl is greater than recommended or there were too many dips in HCl.
12. Expiration date of commercially prepared stain may have been overlooked.
13. Stain may be too old and should be replaced.
14. Inadequate mixing of the contents of aerosol and spray can fixatives can result in poorly distributed fixation. Staining may be uneven and muddy in appearance. Shake all fixatives well prior to use.
15. Slides sprayed with aerosol fixatives at too close or too far a range result in pale, poorly stained slides. See page 1453 for details.
16. Waxes and oils from hairspray fixatives alter staining reactions if not adequately removed. Some brands may require the soaking of slides overnight in 95% alcohol, rather than merely rinsing them in alcohol prior to staining.

NUCLEAR STAIN TOO DARK

Overstaining of the nucleus may occur for one or more of the following reasons:

1. Cells fixed for a few minutes in modified Carnoy's shrink, causing some chromatin condensation. Therefore, staining time in hematoxylin must be decreased.
2. If time is based on staining slides prepared from fresh material, less time must be used for prefixed material.

3. Too few dips in HCl or acid concentration is less than recommended.
4. If single cells are well stained, thick areas of the slide may appear overstained.
5. Nuclepore filters that are dissolved prior to staining sometimes require less staining time in hematoxylin (see p. 1484).
6. The smears may have been prepared directly from very bloody or high-protein fluids. The sediments from these fluids should be washed with a balanced salt solution prior to slide preparation (see p. 1463).
7. Slides were fixed in higher concentration of alcohol than is normally used.

CYTOPLASMIC STAINS UNSATISFACTORY

The cytoplasmic stain may be unsatisfactory for the following reasons:

1. If cytoplasmic stain is too pale, the slides may have been dipped excessively or remained too long in the alcohol rinses, which removes cytoplasmic color.
2. If there is no differential cytoplasmic staining (all cells appear pink), the slide may have been permitted to air-dry prior to fixation, the slide may contain coccoid bacteria that alter staining reaction, or the stain may need replacement. If the slides were fixed with coating fixatives containing concentrations of alcohol greater than normally used, increased shrinking of the cells will occur. Increased timing is required in the EA for the dye to penetrate the dense cell wall.
3. Cytoplasm that appears somewhat gray or purple may result from excessive time in the hematoxylin or failure to remove excess hematoxylin from the cytoplasm with HCl.
4. When there is improper stain distribution, the margins of the cell clusters may stain blue or green, and the central thick portion of the smear may stain red or orange. This is the consequence of insufficient staining time or the lack of agitation during staining and rinsing. The slides should be gently dipped to distribute dye throughout the thick portions of the smear and to remove excess dye trapped in the background.
5. If cytoplasm stains well but the colors appear too blue, green, or pink, the EA formula may have to be changed. EA 50 and 36 contain twice as much light green as EA 65. EA 50, the commercial form of EA 36, varies somewhat from manufacturer to manufacturer. Experimentation with different brands of EA 50 and laboratory EA 36 and 65 is necessary to obtain a cytoplasmic stain that is acceptable.
6. Inadequate mixing of the contents of aerosol and spray can fixatives can result in poorly distributed fixation. Staining may be uneven and muddy in appearance. Shake all fixatives well prior to use.
7. Slides sprayed with aerosol fixatives at too close or too far a range result in pale, poorly stained slides. See page 1430 for details.
8. Waxes and oils from hairspray fixatives alter staining reactions if not adequately removed. Some brands may require the soaking of slides overnight in 95% alcohol rather than merely rinsing them in alcohol prior to staining.
9. Controlling the pH of the EA by the addition of 2 ml of glacial acetic acid per 100 ml of stain may give better and more consistent results.

Contamination Control

Hematoxylin, EA, and OG-6 should be filtered at least once daily and after staining any slides containing known cancer cells. The alcohols used for rehydration and dehydration, the absolute alcohols, and xylenes must also be filtered or replaced daily. To avoid cross-contamination from one slide to another in the same staining rack, it is recommended that those specimens notorious for shedding cells be stained in different staining dishes or at different times. It is generally recommended that gynecologic and nongynecologic material be stained separately. However, no contamination problems have occurred while staining sputums prepared according to Saccomanno or urine and spinal fluid prepared by the method described in this chapter together with the gynecologic slides. Other fluids, particularly those wet fixed in alcohol, must be stained in separate racks and the stains filtered after each run. A good-quality, medium-speed filter paper, such as Whatman #1, removes most cells. In the *Cytotechnologist Bulletin*, vol. *12*, 1975, Gill describes a stain filtration and storage system using a membrane filter to remove all cells. Effusions containing numerous cancer cells most frequently shed tumor cells that may attach to other slides. For this reason, quick preparation using a drop of sediment mixed with toluidine blue and examined immediately can be used to screen out these fluids, which should be stained at the end of the day in a separate rack.

Regardless of the care used in staining, cross-contamination of slides may occur, and it is particularly disturbing if "malignant floaters" occur. If this happens, all solutions and stains should be immediately filtered or discarded. It is also wise to make a microscopic check of the mounting medium at this time to eliminate the possibility of its being a source of contamination.

Important Factors Influencing the Staining Results of Filters

Millipore and Gelman filters should not be attached to a glass slide for staining. Clipping these filters to glass slides traps the stains and results in stain-streaked preparations. Clamp-style paper clips (Fig. 33–14) that allow filters to hang freely during the staining process may be used. Nuclepore filters may be clipped to a glass slide for staining.

Nuclepore filters differ in that prominent outlines of the filter pores remain after staining. Since the filter is birefringent, these pores cannot be made invisible by mounting in a medium of matching refractive index. A number of techniques have been developed to eliminate the pore outline. Cowdrey (St. Luke's Hospital, Cleveland, Ohio) developed a process for dissolving the Nuclepore prior to staining. This method, which has been modified recently, allows the slide to be placed in a staining rack and be stained in the usual manner.

Other methods include dissolving the filter after staining, transferring the cells from the filter to a glass slide, and using a polarized light with a mounting medium with a refractive index that matches one of the two indices of the filter. Details of these procedures are discussed below.

1. During the staining sequence, Nuclepore filters behave similarly to glass slides with the exception of clearing in xylene. The time in xylene should be limited to 10 to 15 minutes to prevent the filters from curling and rolling up tightly.
2. The background of Millipore and Gelman filters will stain with hematoxylin and the cytoplasmic stains. If the background is too heavily stained, cytologic detail and cellular contrast are obscured. For this reason, Gill suggests the use of Mayer's or Gill's hematoxylin over Harris's, which may stain the filter too intensely. After the water rinse following hematoxylin, the filter is slowly dipped approximately 30 times in an 0.025% or 0.05% solution of HCl. The filter should appear pale yellow at this point. Apparently the extremely low concentration of HCl does not decolorize the cells but is sufficient to partially decolorize the background of the filter.
3. As with hematoxylin, the background of the Millipore and Gelman filters is stained by EA and OG. To minimize stain retention, the filters should be rinsed for a longer period. Following OG the slides must remain in three sequential 95% alcohol rinses, 1 minute each, with minimal dipping. The filters are stained for a longer period in EA and are rinsed for 4 minutes, 2 minutes, and 1 minute, respectively, in three sequential 95% alcohol rinses. It is important that no dipping should occur during this sequence. Dipping will cause the stain to be removed from the cells as well as the filter background.
4. Absolute isopropyl alcohol must be substituted for the three final absolute ethanol rinses when staining Millipore filters. Absolute ethyl alcohol can soften and dissolve these filters.

Dissolving Nuclepore Filters Prior to Staining (Fig. 33–15)

1. Place Nuclepore filter, cell side *down, on a clean glass slide. Do not allow filter to dry.*
2. *Quickly* blot the Nuclepore with Whatman No. 1 filter paper folded in half to make a double thickness. Roll a glass rod, print roller, or use finger pressure once over and back the length of the filter.
3. Alcohol should remain under the filter. Quickly flood the filter with chloroform from a Pasteur pipette.
4. Place slide, still covered with chloroform, in a Coplin jar filled with chloroform for 20 to 30 minutes. Transfer slide to 95% alcohol. If a cloudy film appears, return slide to chloroform for 15 to 20 more minutes and then return again to alcohol. The slide may be placed in a rack for routine staining. Never permit the slide to air-dry.

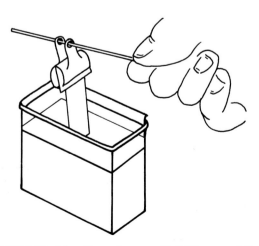

FIGURE 33–14.   Clamp for use with Millipore and Gelman filters.

METHOD OF DISSOLVING NUCLEPORE FILTER
BEFORE STAINING

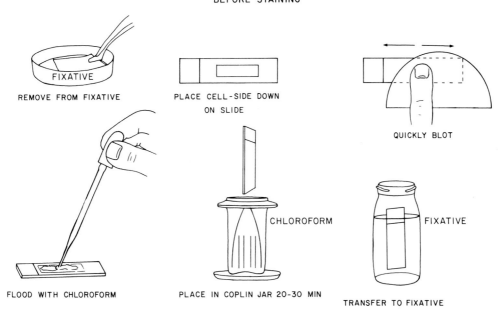

METHOD OF DISSOLVING NUCLEPORE FILTER
AFTER STAINING

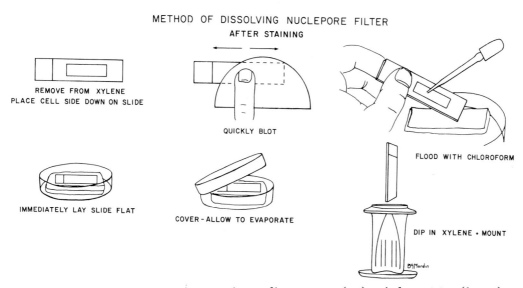

FIGURE 33–15. Dissolving Nuclepore filters prior to (*top*) and after staining (*bottom*).

Dissolving Nuclepore Filter After Staining (see Fig. 33–15)

1. Remove filter from xylene.
2. Place filter cell side down on dry glass slide or coverslip.
3. Blot filter with absorbent towel or filter paper. Roll a glass rod across, or press finger across the surface to flatten filter at the same time.
4. Tilt slide or coverslip over a 4 × 4 gauze pad in a *glass* Petri dish. Start at center, working toward each end, and gently flood the filter with chloroform from a Pasteur pipette.
5. Immediately place the slide or coverslip on the gauze and flood again with chloroform.
6. Place cover on Petri dish and allow chloroform to evaporate. High relative humidity and rapid

evaporation will cause the filter to become cloudy.

7. After evaporation is complete, dip slide or coverslip in xylene and mount with Histoclad.

NOTE: This procedure has been reported to cause some undesirable nuclear distortion.

Transferring Cells from a Membrane Filter to a Glass Slide

A variety of imprint techniques, in which a filter is pressed cell side down against a glass slide to transfer cells, have been reported. In 1983 Nielsen et al. compared cell recovery rates from Millipore filters, using plain glass slides or slides coated with egg albumin-glycerine, Apathy's syrup, and gelatin-chrome alum. Filter preparations were made from urine preserved in Esposti's fixative (50 ml of glacial acetic acid, 225 ml of purified water, and 225 ml of methanol) and pressed against the slides. Egg albumin-glycerine and Apathy's syrup did not increase the transfer of cells when compared with slides without adhesives. The percentage of cells recovered varied from less than 10% to slightly more than 70%. However, gelatin-chrome alum (see p. 1458 for formula) had a pronounced adhesive effect. In every instance, at least 94% and sometimes as many as 99% of the cells were transferred (see reference for details of procedure).

Destaining Slides

Occasionally it is desirable to restain poorly stained slides, slides that have faded because of age, or when special stains are desirable. The following procedure is useful.

1. To remove the coverslip:
   A. Soak in xylene until coverslip falls off, or
   B. Heat slides on a warming plate at 60°C for 3 to 4 hours, or
   C. Place slides in freezer with coverslip down for a few minutes to half an hour (the older the slide, the less time required). The coverslip should separate from the slide around the edges and should appear frosty. A razor blade should be slipped around the edges where the separation exists, and the coverslip will come off easily.
2. Soak slide in xylene to remove old mounting medium.
3. Rinse slides well in two to three rinses each of absolute ethanol, 95% ethanol, and water. One minute in each of the alcohols and water is usually sufficient to remove all counterstains.
4. Place slides in aqueous 0.2% to 0.5% solution of HCl or 1% HCl in 70% alcohol for 5 minutes to 1 hour to remove hematoxylin. Slides should be checked under the microscope to see when decolorization has occurred.
5. Remove acid by rinsing in running tap water for 10 to 15 minutes. To ensure complete removal of the acid, slides should be placed in Scott's tap water substitute with a pH of approximately 8.2 and rinsed again in tap water.
6. Slides are now ready for restaining. If only the removal of cytoplasmic stains is desired, steps 1 through 3 may be used. Slides are then ready for restaining in OG and EA.

MOUNTING THE CELL SAMPLE

Mounting Medium

Mounting medium creates a permanent bond between the slide and the coverslip. This permanent bond protects the cell film from mechanical damage, air-drying effect, and stain fading. Thus, the slides may be stored permanently front to back with no damage to the cell film. To properly visualize cellular morphology, the refractive index of the glass, cellular material, coverslip, and mounting medium should closely match one another. Table 33–12 lists the refractive indices of various material used in cytology.

Regardless of the mounting medium used, it is important to maintain its pH as close to neutral as possible to prevent the fading of stains. One gram of 2, 6-di-tert-butyl-p-cresol* can be added to 100 ml of any mounting medium to inhibit the fading of stains. The mounting medium will thicken as the solvent evaporates. For consistency to be maintained, each new bottle of mounting medium should be checked by counting the number of drops that fall from a pipette filled with the fresh medium for 5 seconds. The number of drops should be noted on the label for future reference. Each week the medium should be checked in a similar manner to determine if the addition of a solvent is necessary.

As can be determined from Table 33–12 Eukitt and Pro-Texx are best suited for Gelman and Millipore filters. Permount and Kleermount can also be used with good results. Histoclad is suitable for Nuclepore filters. However, because of the two refractive indices of this filter, the mounting medium cannot make the pores invisible. Some microsco-

J.T. Baker Chemical Company, Phillipsburg, N.J. 08865

Table 33–12
Refractive Indices of Various Materials Used in Cytology

Slides, Filters, Coverslips	Refractive Index	Mounting Media	Refractive Index
Glass slide	1.515	Eukitt	1.4948
Glass slides, frosted	1.515	Harleco, HSR	1.5202
Coverslip #1 thinness	1.523	Histoclad	1.586
Gelman filter	1.47	Permount	1.5144
Millipore filter	1.495	Pro-Texx	1.495
Nuclepore filter	1.584 and 1.616	Coverbond	1.54

pists find these pores distracting and prefer to dissolve the filter to eliminate the pores. The filters may be dissolved prior to or after staining, as described on pp. 1484 and 1485. Permount or Harleco HSR may be used with plain or frosted glass slides.

Optically Eliminating Pores in Nuclepore Filters

Nuclepore filters have two refractive indices (1.584 and 1.616). It is therefore not possible to eliminate the outline of the pores by using a mounting medium with a similar refractive index. Ocklind, however, developed a method whereby he can visually eliminate the pores by using a specially made mounting medium with an index of 1.584 in combination with polarized light. Details of the method and mounting medium preparation are available in the cited reference.

Coverslips

No. 1 glass coverslips in size 24 × 50 to 60 mm are recommended. The objectives of most microscopes are corrected for use with 0.170- and 0.180-mm coverslips, implying that a No. 1½ coverslip would do well. However, this correction is based on the assumption that tissue sections that are thinner than cytologic preparations are being examined. The thinner No. 1 coverslip will usually compensate for this difference in thickness.

Coverslipping the Cell Sample

Practice is necessary to achieve well-mounted slides, free of air bubbles and artifacts. A minimum of mounting medium should be used. Too much

mounting medium interferes with microscopic detail, making the cell film appear hazy or milky when examined with the high dry objective. If the mounting medium and coverslip are applied too slowly, a common artifact appears as a brown, refractile pigment-like substance on the surface of the cells (Fig. 33–16). This artifact is caused by air trapped on the surface of the cell when xylene is allowed to evaporate. If this artifact occurs, the slide may be soaked in xylene, absolute alcohol, and 95% alcohol, rinsed in running tap water, and restained in OG and EA. In stubborn cases, after the running water rinse, the slide may be placed in glycerine for ½ hour and rinsed well in tap water prior to reapplication of the counterstains.

Method of Coverslipping Glass Slides and Dissolved Nuclepore Filters (Fig. 33–17)

1. Remove slide from xylene.
2. Place one or two drops of mounting medium on the glass slide or coverslip.

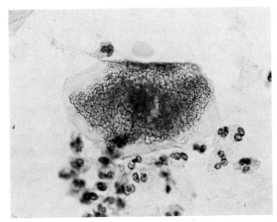

FIGURE 33–16. Common coverslipping artifact—the appearance of a brown pigment-like substance on the surface of squamous cells. (×560)

METHOD OF COVERSLIPPING

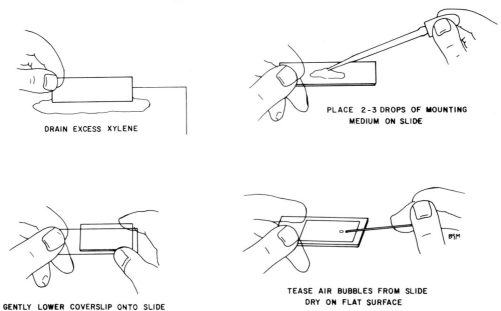

DRAIN EXCESS XYLENE

PLACE 2-3 DROPS OF MOUNTING
MEDIUM ON SLIDE

GENTLY LOWER COVERSLIP ONTO SLIDE

TEASE AIR BUBBLES FROM SLIDE
DRY ON FLAT SURFACE

FIGURE 33–17. Method of coverslipping.

3. Lower the coverslip over the glass slide to which mounting medium has been applied. Bubbles should be avoided at this point. Alternately, if the mounting medium is applied to the coverslip, lower the glass slide over the coverslip and then turn slide right side up. To prevent the possibility of contaminating the dropper and mounting medium with cells, the dropper should never touch the surface of the slide.
4. Gently tease bubbles from under the coverslip with an applicator stick and wipe excess xylene and mounting medium from slide.

Cooking Slides. Graham's method of "cooking" slides allows them to be immediately screened and filed front to back. This procedure is not suitable for Millipore and Gelman filters.

1. Remove slide from xylene.
2. Place three to four drops of mounting medium on glass slide and invert coverslip on top of glass slide.
3. Place slide on an electric hot plate set at the medium temperature and covered with aluminum foil.
4. Leave the slide on the hot plate until the mounting medium bubbles evenly over the entire slide.
5. Remove the slide from the hot plate with for-

ceps and press the surface of the coverslip to expel bubbles and excess mounting medium. Allow the slide to cool for a few minutes.
6. Clean the slide of excess mounting medium by rinsing in xylene or by removal with a razor blade.

Coverslipping Millipore and Gelman Filters. Prior to mounting, 47-mm filters should be cut in half and the excess margin trimmed from all filters. This may be performed with scissors or a scalpel. The filters should be kept wet with xylene during cutting.

1. Dip a clean glass slide in xylene and drain off excess.
2. Place three to four drops of mounting medium on the glass slide and spread over the surface of the slide with the dropper or applicator sticks.
3. Remove filter from xylene and place filter *cell side up* on paper toweling to drain excess xylene. *Do not allow filter to dry.*
4. Place the filter *cell side up* on the glass slide, flatten the filter, and remove air bubbles by rolling an applicator stick or glass rod from the center out to each side of the filter.
5. Place four drops of mounting medium on the filter and gently lower a coverslip over the sur-

face of the slide. *Do not drain excessive mounting medium.*

6. After carefully wiping the excess mounting medium from the bottom of the slide, allow slide to dry on a flat surface.

An alternate method of mounting Millipore and Gelman filters is as follows:

1. Remove filter from xylene.
2. Soak filter in undiluted mounting medium for 5 minutes. A separate dish should be used for each filter to avoid contamination. Miller Plowden suggests the use of disposable 70 × 17 mm aluminum foil dishes* and recycling of the mounting medium by filtering it through a 7-μm pore size Millipore Duralon filter.†
3. Remove the filter from the mounting medium and suspend the filter to allow the excess mounting medium to drain from the filter surface. The drops should stop falling. Excess mounting medium will make focusing difficult, and the cells will appear milky or cloudy.
4. Lay the filter on a clean glass slide, *cell side up,* and gently lower the coverslip. Expel air bubbles that have been trapped by gentle pressure of an applicator stick.
5. Allow slide to dry on a flat surface.

Each of these two method minimizes the risk of xylene evaporation and the drying of the filter, which can produce fernlike opacities.

Filters should be allowed to dry thoroughly on a flat surface before being permanently filed.

OTHER ROUTINE AND SPECIAL STAINS USEFUL IN DIAGNOSTIC CYTOLOGY‡

The use of stains other than the Papanicolaou stain in routine diagnostic cytology has been limited. However, the ease with which cells can be obtained with the aid of a fine needle from organs that are not accessible to exfoliative cytology and advances in the understanding of the histochemical properties of cells may result in the greater application of these stains in the future. The stains listed in this text are routinely performed in most histology laboratories. The principal staining procedures and their purpose are listed in Table 33–13 on pp. 1492 to 1505.

Factors Influencing Staining Results

Timing

All the staining procedures listed in this text may be used for cell blocks or smears unless otherwise indicated. Since there is a marked variation in the thickness of cell block paraffin sections and smears, it will be necessary to vary the times of staining in the different dyes to obtain good results. Individual experimentation is required.

DYES

Dye powders should be obtained from reputable manufacturers§ and certified by the Biologic Stain Commission. Certification ensures that minimum dye content levels are met and that the dye has been tested in staining procedures to see that it produces the classically described results. Dyes should be stored in a cool, dark place.

Color Index Numbers (C.I. No.)

Names of dyes vary from region to region and country to country. For this reason, dyes have been cataloged by a five-digit number that unequivocally identifies the dye. The color index number should be specified when purchasing all dyes. For each dye listed in this text the C.I. No.‖ is provided if available.

Dye Solubility and Impurities

The solvent for most dyes is either alcohol or water, or both. The methods described for preparation of the stains should be carefully adhered to in order to ensure maximum solubility. Most of the dyes currently available are purer than those produced in the past. However, all dyes with a dye content of less than 100% contain impurities that may help or hinder the staining reaction. It is therefore necessary to compare the results obtained from the dyes of different manufacturers and between two batches from the same manufacturer.

(text continues on page 1492)

Arthur H. Thomas — Catalog no. 3844-F20.

†*Millipore Filter Corp., Bedford, Mass., 01730, Catalog no. NSG04700.*

‡ *We gratefully acknowledge the assistance of Ms. Gina Powell, H.T. (ASCP), former Chief Histotechnologist at the Montefiore Hospital and Medical Center, for her guidance and advice on this section.*

§*All dyes used in the procedures listed in this text can be obtained from Bio/Medical Specialists, P.O. Box 1687, Santa Monica, Calif. 90406, and E. Gurr Ltd., 42 Upper Richmond Road, W., London SW 14.*

‖*Source: Lillie and Fullmer, 1976.*

Table 33–13
Stains With Special Purpose

Category	Use	Stain	Fixative
Histologic Sections or Aspiration Smears	Routine stain for paraffin sections and cell blocks	1. Hematoxylin and eosin 2. Hematoxylin—orange eosin	*A. 95% ethyl alcohol or equivalent †B. All fixatives listed on p. 1454
Hormonal Evaluation (Smears Only)	A single stain to differentiate superficial and intermediate cells	Shorr	A. 95% ethyl alcohol or equivalent
	Rapid wet method to differentiate superficial and intermediate cells	Rakoff	None
Barr's Body	Sharply differentiate sex chromatin from nuclear chromatin	1. Biebrich–Scarlet (Guard stain) 2. Acetic–Orcein 3. Cresyl–Violet (Moore and Barr) 4. Feulgen reaction	A. 95% ethyl alcohol or equivalent
Pigments	Bile	Fouchets method	A. 95% ethyl alcohol or equivalent B. All fixatives listed on p. 1454
	Melanin	Ferous ion uptake	Same as above
	Hemosiderin (Iron)	Prussian blue (Peris's)	A. 95% ethyl alcohol or equivalent B. 10% buffered formalin
Microorganisms and Parasites	Sharply delineates fungi and *Pneumocystis carinii*	Grocotts's methenamine silver (Churukian and Schenk)	A. 95% ethyl alcohol or equivalent B. 10% buffered formalin
	Stains fungi and cyst wall of *Pneumocystis carinii*	Gram–Weigert (Krajian)	A. 95% ethyl alcohol or equivalent, or air-dry B. 10% buffered formalin
	Stains most fungi	Periodic acid Schiff	A. 95% *ethyl* alcohol B. 10% buffered formalin
	Capsule of cryptococcus	Mucicarmine (Mayer's)	A. Absolute ethanol or propanol B. 10% buffered formalin
	Stains most microorganisms and parasites	Giemsa Gram	A. 95% ethyl alcohol or equivalent or air-dried smears B. All fixatives listed on p. 1454

* A = Fixative recommended for use with smears.
† B = Fixative recommended for histologic sections.

Table 33–13
Stains With Special Purpose (Continued)

Category	Use	Stain	Fixative
Carbohydrates	Stains all carbohydrates to identify colloid, fungi, glycogen, mucin, and so on	Periodic acid Schiff	A. 95% ethyl alcohol B. 10% buffered formalin
	Same as above except glycogen is eliminated	Periodic acid Schiff with diastase digestion	Same as above
	Specific for epithelial mucins	Mucicarmine (Mayer's)	A. Absolute ethanol or propanol B. 10% buffered formalin
Lipids	Stains all lipids	Sudan Black B	A. 37%–40% formalin vapors B. 10% buffered formalin
	Stains neutral fats to determine if histiocytes have phagocytized fat in lipid pneumonia	Oil Red O	Same as above
	Determination of fetal maturity	Nile blue sulfate	None
Nucleic Acids	Specific for DNA	Feulgen reaction	A. 95% ethyl alcohol or equivalent B. 10% buffered formalin
	Specifically differentiates RNA and DNA	Methyl green-pyronin (Kurnick's variant)	Same as above
Hematologic or Air-Dried Smears	Blood and bone marrow smears. Preferred by some for all cytologic material	1. Wright stain 2. Giemsa stain 3. Wright–Giemsa 4. May–Grünwald Giemsa	A. Air-dried or 95% methyl alcohol
Wet Cell Samples	Determination of fetal maturity	Nile blue sulfate	None
	Hormonal evaluation	Rakoff	None
	Differentiates histiocytes and leukocytes from neoplastic and mesothelial cells	Neutral red–Janus green (Foot and Holmquist)	None
	Rapid method for examining wet sediment	1. Thionine blue 2. Methylene blue 3. Toluidine blue	None
Fluorescence	Differentiation of benign and malignant cells	Acridine orange	A. 95% ethyl alcohol or equivalent

* A = Fixative recommended for use with smears.
† B = Fixative recommended for histologic sections.

Total Dye Content

Dyes certified by the Biologic Stain Commission must meet *minimum* dye content levels. However, there is still a marked variation in percentage dye concentration from one batch of dye to another. For example, the minimum percentage dye concentration of Bismarck Brown Y for certification is 45% and the percentage concentration of a recent batch submitted for certification was 52%. Unfortunately, very few published methods include the percentage dye content of the dye used. Several attempts should be made to adjust the amount of dye used before a new method or stain is condemned. As soon as good results are obtained, greater precision and accuracy will result if the amount of actual dye used is calculated. The percentage dye content of certified dyes is printed on the label. For example, if good results were obtained with 5 g of 93% basic fuchsin, the weight of the actual dye used was 4.65 g (5 g $\times$ 0.93). The amount of basic fuchsin required to yield similar results can then be calculated for different batches of dye. For example, the number of grams of dye needed to yield 4.65 g of actual dye from an 88% dye concentration of basic fuchsin would be:

$$\text{Number of grams of new batch required} = \frac{\text{Total actual dye required}}{\text{Concentration (new batch)}}$$

or

$$xg = 4.65 \text{ g}/.88 = 5.28 \text{ g}$$

In other words, 5.28 g of that particular batch of basic fuchsin is needed to obtain 4.65 g of actual dye.

The percentage dye concentration of the dyes used in the methods described in this text were not available; thus individual experimentation will be required to determine the amount of dye needed to yield good results.

Preparation of Dyes and Solutions

Most staining solutions do not need to be prepared fresh whenever they are used. However, in some cases two or more stock solutions are mixed immediately prior to use. Some of the methods presented in this text will list both stock and working solutions. When this is the case, it is always the working solution that is to be used in the staining procedure itself.

Table 33–13 lists the special stains contained in this text. Under Fixative, *A.* refers to the fixative recommended for smears and *B.* refers to the fixa-

tive recommended for cell blocks. The use of improper fixatives will render staining results invalid in some procedures. Thus, close attention to the recommended fixative is suggested.

Routine Stains for Histologic Sections (Tissue and Cell Blocks)*

Hematoxylin-Eosin

PREPARATION OF STAINS

Modified Harris's Hematoxylin

Hematoxylin, C.I. No. 75290	5	g
Absolute alcohol (ethyl)	50	ml
Alum (ammonium or potassium)	100	g
Distilled water	1,000	ml
Mercuric oxide	2.5 g	

1. Dissolve hematoxylin in alcohol.
2. Dissolve alum in water by aid of heat. Remove from heat and mix the two solutions.
3. Heat mixture to boiling point. Remove from heat and add mercuric oxide.
4. As soon as mixture turns a dark purple, cool quickly by plunging the vessel into cold water.
5. When cool, add 8.0 ml of glacial acetic acid to enhance nuclear stain.

Eosin

Eosin, Y, C.I. No. 45380	16 g
Potassium dichromate	8 g
Picric acid (saturated aqueous)	160 ml
95% Alcohol (ethyl)	160 ml
Distilled water	1,280 ml

Dissolve eosin and potassium dichromate in water; warm slightly if required. Add picric acid and alcohol

STAINING PROCEDURE

Begin with step 1 for paraffin sections and step 8 for smears.

1.	Xylol	5 minutes
2.	Xylol	5 minutes
3.	Absolute ethyl alcohol	15 dips
4.	Absolute ethyl alcohol	25 dips
5.	95% Ethyl alcohol	15 dips
6.	80% Ethyl alcohol	15 dips
7.	70% Ethyl alcohol	15 dips
8.	Wash in distilled water	15 dips

---

*In some laboratories these stains are used for aspiration smears.

9. Harris's hematoxylin (modified — 2 minutes or according to preference).
10. Wash in running tap water until excess stain is removed (approximately 1 minute)
11. Acid alcohol (1.5 ml of concentrated HCl in 650 ml of 70% ethyl alcohol) — two to three dips or until specimen is red in color.
12. Wash in running tap water — 30 seconds
13. Lithium carbonate solution (1.5 ml saturated lithium carbonate solution, 650 ml of 70% ethyl alcohol — 1 minute.
14. Wash in tap water — 15 dips
15. 50% Ethyl alcohol — 15 dips
16. Eosin — approximately 20 seconds
17. Wash in running (tap water until excess stain is removed (approximately 1 minute)
18. 95% Ethyl alcohol — 15 dips
19. 95% Ethyl alcohol — 15 dips
20. Absolute ethyl alcohol — 15 dips
21. Absolute ethyl alcohol — 1 minute
22. Xylol — 15 dips
23. Xylol — 15 dips
24. Xylol — 5 to 10 minutes.
25. Mount

STAINING PROCEDURE

Begin with step 1 for paraffin sections and step 7 for smears.

1. Xylol — 5 minutes
2. Xylol — 5 minutes
3. Absolute ethyl alcohol — 3½ minutes
4. Absolute ethyl alcohol — 3 minutes
5. 95% Ethyl alcohol — 3 minutes
6. 95% Ethyl alcohol — 3 minutes
7. Tap water until clear (5–6 dips)
8. Hematoxylin (Harris's) — 3–7 minutes according to preference
9. Distilled water — 10 dips
10. Aqueous solution of 0.05% HCl — 2–5 dips
11. Wash in running water — 6 minutes
12. Lithium carbonate solution (tap water and two drops of saturated lithium carbonate) — 1 minute
13. 50% Ethyl alcohol — 10 dips
14. 70% Ethyl alcohol — 10 dips
15. 80% Ethyl alcohol — 10 dips
16. 95% Ethyl alcohol — 10 dips
17. Orange and eosin stain — 3 minutes
18. 95% Ethyl alcohol — 10 dips
19. 95% Ethyl alcohol — 10 dips
20. Absolute ethyl alcohol — 10 dips
21. Absolute ethyl alcohol — 10 dips
22. ½ Absolute alcohol and ½ xylol — 10 dips
23. Xylol, 3–5 changes — 10 dips each
24. Mount

Hematoxylin-Orange-Eosin (H.L. Richardson et al., 1949)

PREPARATION OF STAINS

Harris's Hematoxylin Stain

Steps 1 through 4 — proceed as outlined for modified Harris hematoxylin.

Step 5 — add 40 ml of glacial acetic acid to enhance nuclear staining.

Orange and Eosin Stain

Eosin Y, C.I. No. 45380	2.25	g
Orange G, C.I. No. 16230	2.75	g
Distilled water	50	ml
95% Ethyl alcohol	950	ml
Phosphotungstic acid	2	g

1. Dissolve eosin and orange in distilled water.
2. Add 95% alcohol and phosphotungstic acid.

Stains Used in Hormonal Evaluation

Shorr's Stain (1941)

USE

A single differential stain for hormonal evaluation in vaginal smears.

COMPOSITION

For the stain S3, this is as follows:

Ethyl alcohol (50%)	100	ml
Biebrich scarlet, C.I. No., 26905	0.5	g
Orange G, C.I. No. 16230	0.25	g
Fast-green FCF, C.I. No. 42053	0.075	g
Phosphotungstic acid	0.5	g
Phosphomolybdic acid	0.5	g
Glacial acetic acid	1.0	ml

METHOD

The solution should not be used until all the ingredients have dissolved completely.

1. Aspirate the vaginal secretion by means of a dry pipette with rubber bulb attached. Expel and smear on a glass slide.
2. Fix, while wet, in 95% ethyl alcohol. Fixation for 1 or 2 minutes is adequate.
3. Stain for approximately 1 minute in Solution S3.
4. Carry through 70%, 95%, and absolute alcohol, dipping slide 10 times in each solution.
5. Clear in xylol and mount.

RESULTS

The stain provides a sharp differentiation between cornified and noncornified squamous cells. The former stain a brilliant orange-red; the latter take on a green stain that is deeper in the younger cells and paler in the more mature ones. Other constituents, such as leukocytes, erythrocytes, bacteria, and spermatozoa, are differentiated satisfactorily.

Rakoff's Method

PURPOSE

Rapid method of hormonal evaluation using wet smear method.

PREPARATION OF STAIN

Rakoff Stain
Light green, C.I. No. 42095
                    5% Aqueous solution 83 ml
Eosin, E.I. No. 45380
                    1% Aqueous solution 17 ml
Mix these two solutions.

METHOD

1. Moisten cotton-tipped applicator with saline solution and make several vertical strokes along the lateral middle third of the vagina.
2. Drop swab into a test tube containing 1 to 2 ml of saline solution.
3. Place three drops of the Rakoff stain into the test tube and gently stir the solution with swab.
4. Transfer one to two drops of this mixture to a glass slide and coverslip.

RESULTS

Cytoplasm stains brightly eosinophilic and basophilic. Vesicular nuclei are distinctly stained, while pyknotic nuclei have sharply stained margins but are pale.

Stains Used in the Identification of Sex Chromatin

Although vaginal smears may be used for the purpose of sex chromatin identification, buccal smears are preferable. Obtain scrapings of buccal mucosa by drawing edge of metal spatula firmly over an area. Discard the first material and gently scrape the same area a second time to obtain deeper and better preserved cells.

Smears taken from the soft palate also yield an abundance of well-preserved intermediate cells with vesicular nuclei.

Make smear and immediately fix in 95% ethyl alcohol. It is always good procedure to run a control buccal smear along with the test smear.

One hundred single cells are counted. Count only those cells with unwrinkled, well-preserved, vesicular nuclei.

If only unequivocal sex chromatin bodies are counted, the count for males should be 0, and the count for females 20% to 40%.

Bierbrich Scarlet–Fast Green (H.R. Guard, 1959)

PREPARATION OF STAINS

Biebrich Scarlet Stain
Biebrich scarlet-water soluble, C.I.
    No. 26905
    (Harleco)   1.0 g
Phosphotungstic acid   0.3 g
Glacial acetic acid   5.0 ml
50% Ethyl alcohol   100.0 ml

Fast-Green Stain
Fast-green FCF (Harleco), C.I. No.
    42053   0.5 g
Phosphomolybdic acid   0.3 g
Phosphotungstic acid   0.3 g
Glacial acetic acid   5.0 ml
50% Ethyl alcohol   100.0 ml

STAINING PROCEDURE

Our laboratory has found the following procedure to be satisfactory.

1. From fixative transfer smear to 70% alcohol for 2 minutes.
2. Stain in Biebrich scarlet for 5 minutes.
3. Rinse in 50% alcohol.
4. Differentiate in fast-green FCF from 2 to 5 hours.

   During this step, check the differentiation under a microscope at hourly intervals. When all the cells reveal green cytoplasm, and all the

vesicular nuclei are also green, the reaction is complete, which is usually in approximately 4 hours. However, the pyknotic nuclei will not be differentiated and will be bright red.
5. Rinse in 50% alcohol and let remain in the alcohol for 5 minutes.
6. Dehydrate in 70%, 95%, and absolute alcohols for 2 minutes each.
7. Clear in 3 changes of xylol for 2 minutes each.
8. Mount with a permanent mounting medium.

RESULTS

The nuclei stain pale green; the sex chromatin stains pink to red and is seen as a V-shaped or triangular condensation with the base attached to the nuclear membrane. A narrow halo is usually noted around the unattached sides.

A thin single or multiple strand of chromatin material is often observed running from the sex chromatin body toward the center of the nucleus. For further details see Chapter 6.

Acetic Orcein Stain
(After Lillie, 1965, p. 158)

PREPARATION OF STAINS

Acetic Orcein Stain

Orcein (natural)	1 g
Hot glacial acetic acid	45 ml
Distilled water	55 ml

Heat acid to 80° to 85°C in flask placed in beaker containing water. Add orcein while shaking or stirring rapidly. Add distilled water while continuing to stir or shake flask. Stopper flask and place under cold running water. When the stain has cooled, filter and store in a brown bottle. The stain keeps very well.

Fast-Green Stain

Fast green, C.I. No. 42053	0.03 g
95% Ethyl alcohol	100 ml

Add fast green to the alcohol, and stir or shake to dissolve.

STAINING PROCEDURE

1. Fix smears in 95% ethyl alcohol for 30 to 60 minutes.
2. Hydrate slides through 80%, 70%, and 50% ethyl alcohol and distilled water—5 dips each.
3. Stain in acetic orcein stain for 5 minutes (a control slide should be used, as staining time in acetic orcein may vary according to the age of stain).
4. Wash for 10 seconds in distilled water.
5. Dehydrate in 50%, 70%, 80%, 95% ethyl alcohol—5 dips each.

6. Stain in fast green for 1 minute.
7. Wash in 95% ethyl alcohol, absolute ethyl alcohol, absolute ethyl alcohol, and equal parts of xylol—5 dips each. Clear in xylol for 5 minutes.
8. Coverslip preparation, using Permount.

RESULTS

The sex chromatin body stains red, and the cytoplasm stains pale green. This stain also may be used for chromosomal preparations.

Cresyl violet (Moore and Barr)

PREPARATION OF SOLUTIONS

Cresyl violet	1 g
Distilled water	100 ml

STAINING PROCEDURE

1. Water	5 min
2. Cresyl violet	7 min
3. 4. } 95% alcohol	5 min (total)
5. Absolute alcohol	5 min
6. Xylene	15 dips
7. Mount with permanent mounting medium.	

RESULTS

The nuclei stain pale pink, and the sex chromatin stains deep pink to violet.

Stains for Pigments

Fouchet's Method for Bile

PREPARATION OF SOLUTIONS

Fouchet's Stock Solution
A. 25% Aqueous trichloroacetic acid
B. 10% Aqueous ferric chloride

Fouchet's Working Solution

Solution A	100 ml
Solution B	10 ml

Van Gieson's Picro-Fuchsin

1% Aqueous acid fuchsin, C.I. No. 42685	10 ml
Saturated aqueous picric acid	100 ml

STAINING PROCEDURE

Begin with step 1 for paraffin section and step 8 for smears.

1. Xylol	5 minutes
2. Xylol	5 minutes
3. Absolute ethyl alcohol	15 dips
4. Absolute ethyl alcohol	15 dips
5. 95% Ethyl alcohol	15 dips
6. 80% Ethyl alcohol	15 dips

7. 70% Ethyl alcohol	15 dips
8. Wash in distilled water	15 dips
9. Fouchet's working solution	5 minutes
10.⎫ Distilled water	1 minute each
11.⎭	
12. Van Gieson's picro-fuchsin	5 minutes
13.⎫ 95% Alcohol	15 dips each
14.⎭	
15.⎫ Absolute alcohol	15 dips each
16.⎭	
17.⎫ Xylene	15 dips each
18.⎭	

19. Mount with permanent mounting medium.

RESULTS

Bile pigments stain olive green, collagen stains red, and the background stains yellow.

Ferrous Ion Uptake for Melanin

PREPARATION OF SOLUTIONS

1. Prepare a 2.5% aqueous solution of ferrous sulfate.
2. Prepare a 1.0% solution of potassium ferricyanide in 1% acetic acid.
3. Nuclear fast red, C.I. No.60760. (Kernechtrot):

Heat to dissolve 0.1 g of nuclear fast red in a 5% solution of aluminum sulfate. Let cool, filter, and add a grain of thymol.

STAINING PROCEDURE

Begin with step 1 for paraffin sections and step 8 for smears.

1. Xylol	5 minutes
2. Xylol	5 minutes
3. Absolute ethyl alcohol	15 dips
4. Absolute ethyl alcohol	15 dips
5. 95% Ethyl alcohol	15 dips
6. 80% Ethyl alcohol	15 dips
7. 70% Ethyl alcohol	15 dips
8. Wash in distilled water	15 dips
9. Ferrous sulfate solution	1 hour
10.⎫	
11.⎬ Distilled water	1 minute each
12.⎭	
13.	
14. Potassium ferricyanide	30 minutes
15. 1% Acetic acid	15 dips
16. Distilled water	15 dips
17. Nuclear fast red	1–2 minutes
18. Distilled water	15 dips
19. 95% Ethyl alcohol	15 dips
20. Absolute ethyl alcohol	15 dips

21.⎫ Xylol	15 dips
22.⎭	

23. Mount in permanent mounting medium.

RESULTS

Melanin stains dark blue to dark green, and the background stains red to pink.

Prussian Blue Reaction for Hemosiderin (Iron) (Perls's)

PREPARATION OF SOLUTIONS

A. Potassium ferrocyanide	2% aqueous	
B. Hydrochloric acid	2%	
C. Neutral red, C.I. No. 50040	1% aqueous	

STAINING PROCEDURE

Begin with step 1 for paraffin embedded tissue sections and with step 8 for smears.

1. Xylol	5 minutes
2. Xylol	5 minutes
3. Absolute ethyl alcohol	15 dips
4. Absolute ethyl alcohol	15 dips
5. 95% Ethyl alcohol	15 dips
6. 80% Ethyl alcohol	15 dips
7. 70% Ethyl alcohol	15 dips
8. Wash in distilled water	15 dips
9. Equal parts solution A and B	30 minutes
10.⎫	
11.⎬ Distilled water	15 dips each
12.⎭	
13. Neutral red	10 to 15 seconds
14.⎫	
15.⎬ Distilled water	15 dips each
16.⎭	
17.⎫ 95% Alcohol	15 dips each
18.⎭	
19.⎫ Absolute alcohol	15 dips each
20.⎭	
21.⎫ Xylene	15 dips each
22.⎭	

23. Mount

RESULTS

Ferric-iron-containing pigments (hemosiderin) stain blue; the nuclei stain red.

Stains for Microorganisms and Parasites

As a result of the AIDS epidemic, laboratories have been challenged by the dramatic increase of samples submitted for determination of the presence of organisms that cause opportunistic infections. Most notably, an increasing number of patients are presenting with respiratory infection as a complication of AIDS. *Pneumocystis carinii* is high on the list of pathogens responsible for these infections. Gomori's and Grocott's methenamine silver stain have been the traditional methods of choice for demonstrating this organism. The silver stain has a greater individual sensitivity as compared to that of other methods since it gives good contrast between the background of the smear and the organism. An abundance of literature has sprung from modifications of the stain to make it easier and quicker to perform. A number of rapid methods have been reported that use hot plates, water baths, and microwave ovens to speed impregnation of the silver.

With experience gained from seeing numerous positive cases, many have reported success with other rapid stains such as Diff-Quick, cresyl violet, and the routine Papanicolaou smear. In the routine Papanicolaou stain, organisms appear in foamy, honeycombed masses that stain eosinophilic or basophilic and are often two-toned. Ghali et al. reported that *Pneumocystis* emits bright fluorescence when routine Papanicolaou-stained smears are examined under ultraviolet illumination (for further comments see Chapter 19).

Many of these alternatives have been used successfully in our laboratory. The sensitivity of each method in detecting *Pneumocystis carinii* ultimately depends on the experience of the observer rather than the specificity of the stain.

Rapid Methenamine-Silver Stain
Grocott's Method
(Churukian and Schenk)

PURPOSE

Demonstrates *Pneumocystis carinii* and fungi.

PREPARATION OF SOLUTIONS

1. Methenamine silver nitrate

Stock Solution
Mix 100 ml of 3% methenamine (hexamethylenetramine) and 5 ml of 5% silver nitrate. Shake well.

Working Solution
Mix 25 ml of the stock solution with 25 ml of distilled water and 2 ml of 5% borax (sodium borate).

2. Fast Green FCF, C.I. No. 42053

Stock Solution
Dissolve 0.2 g of fast green in 100 ml of 0.2% acetic acid.

Working Solution
Mix 10 ml of stock solution with 40 ml of distilled water.

3. Prepare 5% solution of chromium trioxide.
4. Prepare 1% solution of sodium bisulfite.
5. Prepare 0.2% solution of gold chloride.
6. Prepare 2% solution of sodium thiosulfate.

STAINING PROCEDURE

Start with step 1 for paraffin-embedded histologic sections and with step 8 for smears.

1. Xylol	5 minutes
2. Xylol	5 minutes
3. Absolute ethyl alcohol	15 dips
4. Absolute ethyl alcohol	15 dips
5. 95% Ethyl alcohol	15 dips
6. 80% Ethyl alcohol	15 dips
7. 70% Ethyl alcohol	15 dips
8. Wash in distilled water	15 dips
9. 5% Chromium trioxide (Place Coplin jar with solution and slides in a 43°C water bath.)	2 minutes
10. Transfer Coplin jar to a 58°C water bath	15 minutes
11. Tap water	15 dips
12. 1% Sodium bisulfite	30 seconds
13. Running tap water	15 seconds
14. 15. 16. 17. } Distilled water	15 dips each
18. Methenamine—silver (freshly mixed working solution) Place Coplin jar with solution and slides in 43° water bath.	2 minutes
19. Transfer Coplin jar to a 58°C water bath	23 minutes
20. 21. 22. 23. } Distilled water	15 dips each
24. 0.2% Gold chloride (depends on freshness)	20 to 30 dips
25. 26. } Distilled water	15 dips each
27. 2% Sodium thiosulfate	1 minute
28. Running tap water	15 seconds
29. Fast green (working solution)	30 seconds

30. Running tap water   15 seconds
31.⎫
32.⎬ Distilled water   15 dips each
33.⎫
34.⎬ 95% Ethyl alcohol   15 dips each
35.⎫
36.⎬ Absolute ethyl alcohol   15 dips each
37.⎫
38.⎬ Xylol   15 dips each
39. Mount with permanent mounting medium.

RESULTS

Pneumocystis carinii and fungi stain black, sharply delineated; glycogen and mucin stain rose to gray; and the background stains pale green.

Gram-Weigert Stain
(Krajian Method)

PURPOSE

Demonstration of fungi and cyst wall of *Pneumocystis carinii.*

PREPARATION OF SOLUTIONS

Eosin
Eosin Y, C.I., No 45380   1 g
Distilled water   100 ml

Gentian Violet (Sterling's)
Crystal violet C.I. No. 42555   5 g
95% Ethyl alcohol   10 ml
Aniline oil   2 ml
Distilled water   88 ml

Dissolve the crystal violet in the 95% ethyl alcohol and add this to the mixture of aniline oil and water that has been previously filtered.

Iodine Solution (Gram's)
Iodine   1 g
Potassium iodide   2 g
Distilled water   300 ml

Dissolve the potassium iodide in water and then add the iodine.

STAINING PROCEDURE

Start with step 1 for paraffin sections and with step 8 for smears.

1. Xylol   5 minutes
2. Xylol   5 minutes
3. Absolute ethyl alcohol   15 dips
4. Absolute ethyl alcohol   15 dips
5. 95% Ethyl alcohol   15 dips
6. 80% Ethyl alcohol   15 dips
7. 70% Ethyl alcohol   15 dips
8. Wash in distilled water   15 dips
9. Eosin   5 minutes
10. Water   15 dips
11. Gentian violet   10 minutes
                              (paraffin sections)
                                  5 minutes
                       (smears and frozen sections)
12. Iodine: Flood slides to wash
    off gentian violet and then
    place in iodine   3 minutes
13. Blot with filter paper
14. Aniline oil and xylol 1:1   5 minutes
       (agitate slowly until no color rinses out)
15. Blot with filter paper
16. Xylol—2 changes   15 dips each
17. Mount with permanent mounting medium.

RESULTS

Pneumocytis carinii (cyst wall), gram-positive bacteria and fungi violet, gram-negative organisms are not stained, and fibrin stains blue-black.

Gram's Stain

PURPOSE

Distinguishes gram-negative from gram-positive bacteria.

PREPARATIONS OF SOLUTIONS

Lillie's Crystal Violet
Crystal violet, C.I. No 42555   5 g
95% Alcohol   50 ml
Ammonium oxalate   2 g
Distilled water   200 ml

Dissolve the crystal violet in the alcohol and the ammonium oxalate in water. Combine the two mixtures and filter prior to using.

Lugol's Iodine
Iodine   1 g
Potassium iodide   2 g
Distilled water   100 ml

In a mortar with a small volume of water grind the iodine and potassium iodide. Pour off the supernatant, add another small volume of water, and grind again. Continue these steps until the crystals are completely dissolved. Add remaining water to this solution.

Neutral Red, C.I. No. 50040
Prepare a 1% aqueous solution.

STAINING PROCEDURE

Start with step 1 for paraffin sections, with step 8 for fixed smears, or step 9 for air-dried smears.

1. Xylol — 5 minutes
2. Xylol — 5 minutes
3. Absolute ethyl alcohol — 15 dips
4. Absolute ethyl alcohol — 15 dips
5. 95% Ethyl alcohol — 15 dips
6. 80% Ethyl alcohol — 15 dips
7. 70% Ethyl alcohol — 15 dips
8. Wash in distilled water — 15 dips
9. Crystal violet — 1 to 2 minutes
10. Tap water — 10 dips
11. Lugol's iodine — ½ to 1 minute
12. Tap water — 10 dips
13. Acetone — 10 to 15 dips
14. Running tap water — 5 to 10 minutes
15. Neutral red — ½ to 1 minute
16.–17. } Tap water — 15 dips each
18.–19. } 95% Alcohol — 15 dips each
20.–21. } Absolute alcohol — 15 dips each
22.–23. } Xylene — 15 dips each
24. Mount in permanent mounting medium.

RESULTS

Gram-positive organisms stain blue-black, gram-negative organisms stain red, and the background stains pink.

Stains for Carbohydrates

Periodic Acid Schiff Reaction (PAS)

PREPARATION OF SOLUTIONS

Periodic Acid
Prepare a 1% aqueous solution.

Schiff Reagent

Distilled water	100	ml
Basic fuchsin, C.I. No. 42500	1	g
Sodium or potassium metabisulfite	2	g
1N HCl	20	ml
Activated charcoal	0.3	g

Bring water to a boil and remove from heat. When solution cools to 60°C add the basic fuchsin. Filter and then add the sodium or potassium metabisulfite and HCl. Pour this solution in a stoppered, dark bottle and keep at room temperature for 18 to 24 hours. Add the charcoal and vigorously shake mixture for 1 minute. Filter this solution and store at 0° to 5°C. Discard this reagent when a pink color develops.

Sodium Metabisulfite Solution
(Stock Solution)
Prepare a 10% aqueous solution.

(Working Solution)
5 ml of stock mixed with 100 ml of distilled water.

Pal's Bleach

Oxalic acid	0.5	g
Potassium sulfite	0.5	g
Distilled water	100	ml

Fast Green

Fast green FCF, C.I. No. 42053	1	g
1.0% Acetic acid	100	ml

Weigert's Iron Hematoxylin
(Solution A)

Hematoxylin	1	g
Alcohol 95%	100	ml

(Solutin B)

Ferric chloride 29% aqueous	4	ml
Distilled water	95	ml
HCl, concentrated	1	ml

(Working Solution)
Equal parts of Solutions A and B.

STAINING PROCEDURE

Start with step 1 for paraffin sections and step 8 for smears.

1. Xylol — 5 minutes
2. Xylol — 5 minutes
3. Absolute ethyl alcohol — 15 dips
4. Absolute ethyl alcohol — 15 dips
5. 95% Ethyl alcohol — 15 dips
6. 80% Ethyl alcohol — 15 dips
7. 70% Ethyl alcohol — 15 dips
8. Wash in distilled water — 15 dips
9. Periodic acid — 10 minutes
10. Running tap water — 10 minutes
11. Distilled water — 15 minutes
12. Schiff reagent — 15 minutes
13.–14.–15. } Sodium metabisulfite rinses — 2 minutes each
16. Running tap water — 10 minutes
17. Weigert's hematoxylin — 4 minutes
18. Running tap water — 5 to 10 minutes
19. Pal's bleach — 1 dip

20.	Running tap water	5 minutes
21.	Distilled water	15 dips
22.	Fast green	1 dip
23.	Distilled water	15 dips
24. 25. }	95% Ethyl alcohol	15 dips each
26. 27. }	Absolute ethyl alcohol	15 dips each
28. 29. }	Xylol	15 dips each
30.	Mount with permanent mounting medium.	

RESULTS

All carbohydrates and fungi stain magenta, nuclei stain black, and the background stains green.

Periodic Acid Schiff (PAS) With Diastase Digestion

PREPARATION OF SOLUTION

The same solutions as used for the PAS without diastase digestion with the addition of the following:

Diastase Solution

Diastase of malt, USP	0.5 g
Distilled water	100 ml

STAINING PROCEDURE

The staining procedure is the same as that for PAS except that one of the slides is placed in the diastase solution for 20 minutes prior to step 9.

RESULTS

All carbohydrates, including glycogen and fungi, will be PAS-positive (magenta red) in standard PAS-stained slide. Glycogen will be unstained in the diastase-treated slide.

Mayer's Mucicarmine

PREPARATION OF SOLUTIONS

0.25% Metanil Yellow Solution

Metanil yellow, C.I. No. 13065	0.25 g
Distilled water	100 ml
Glacial acetic acid	0.25 ml

Mucicarmine Solution
(Stock Solution)

Carmine, C.I. No. 75470	1.0 g
Aluminum chloride, anhydrous	0.5 g
Ethyl alcohol (50%)	100 ml
Aluminum hydroxide	1.0 g

Pour the alcohol in a 250-ml flask and add the carmine and aluminum hydroxide. In a mortar, grind the aluminum chloride and add it to the flask. Mix the solution well, rapidly bring it to a boil, and boil for 2½ minutes. Shake the mixture frequently. Place the flask under running tap water to cool it rapidly. Filter and store. Shelf life is approximately 3 months.

(Working Solution)

Mucicarmine stock	25 ml
Tap water	75 ml

Pal's Bleach (see p. 1499)
Weigert's Iron Hematoxylin
(see p. 1499)

STAINING PROCEDURE

Start with step 1 for paraffin sections and with step 8 for smears.

1.	Xylol	5 minutes
2.	Xylol	5 minutes
3.	Absolute ethyl alcohol	15 dips
4.	Absolute ethyl alcohol	15 dips
5.	95% Ethyl alcohol	15 dips
6.	80% Ethyl alcohol	15 dips
7.	70% Ethyl alcohol	15 dips
8.	Wash in distilled water	15 dips
9.	Weigert's hematoxylin	4 minutes
10.	Running tap water	4 minutes
11.	Pal's bleach	1 dip
12.	Running tap water	10 minutes
13.	Mucicarmine	60 minutes
14.	Distilled water	5 dips
15.	Metanil yellow	1 minute
16.	Distilled water	5 dips
17. 18. }	95% Alcohol	15 dips each
19. 20. }	Absolute alcohol	15 dips each
21. 22. }	Xylene	15 dips each
23.	Mount in permanent mounting medium.	

RESULTS

Mucin stains deep rose to red, capsule of *Cryptococcus* stains deep rose to red, nuclei stain black, and other tissue elements stain yellow.

Stains for Lipids

Sudan Black B for Smears

PREPARATION OF SOLUTIONS

Sudan Black B
(Stock Solution)

Sudan Black B, C.I. No. 26150	0.3 g
Absolute ethyl alcohol	100 ml

Shake the mixture vigorously and frequently for 1 or 2 days until the dye is dissolved. Then filter.

Buffer

Phenol crystals	16 g
Absolute ethyl alcohol	30 ml
*Na_2HPO_4	0.119 g in 100 ml of water

Sudan Black B
(Working Solution)

Sudan black B Stock	30 ml
Buffer	20 ml

Filter, using suction through double-thickness #1 filter paper. This solution will keep for 2 to 3 weeks.

*Mayer's Hematoxylin: MHS-1
Eosin Y, C.I. No. 45380: 0.01% Aqueous
Acetic Acid: 0.5% Solution

STAINING PROCEDURE

1.	Fix smear in formalin vapors (see p. 1454)	10 minutes
2.	Air-dry	10 minutes
3.	Sudan black B	30 minutes
4.	70% Ethyl alcohol (2 changes)	2 minutes each
5.	Distilled water	15 dips
6.	Mayer's hematoxylin	5 minutes
7.	Distilled water	10 to 15 minutes
8.	0.01% Eosin Y	1 dip
9.	0.5% Acetic acid	1 dip
10.	Distilled water	15 dips
11.	Blot and air-dry	

RESULTS

Phospholipids and granules of granulocytic series stain black, RBC stain pink, and nuclei stain blue.

Oil Red O Fat Stain

PURPOSE

Occasionally it may be necessary to stain smears for fat. This may be the case with sputum or bronchial washings if there is a suspicion that the patient may have lipoid pneumonia. When fat stain is required, smears should be prepared from fresh, unfixed material and fixed in formalin vapors (see p. 1454).

PREPARATION OF STAINS AND MOUNTING MEDIUM

Oil red, O, C.I. No. 26125	1–2 g

Sigma Chemical Co. P.O. Box 14508, St. Louis, Mo. 63178.

Alcohol, 70%	50 ml
Acetone	50 ml

Harris's hematoxylin is used as a counterstain.

Glycerine Jelly

Gelatin	10 g
Distilled water	60 ml
Heat until gelatin is dissolved. Add:	
Glycerin	70 ml
Phenol	1 ml

STAINING PROCEDURE

1. Dip in 70% alcohol for just a second.
2. Place in a tightly closed container of oil red 0 for 5 minutes or longer (up to 1 hour).
3. Wash very quickly in 70% alcohol.
4. Wash in water.
5. Counterstain in Harris's hematoxylin for a few minutes.
6. Wash in water.
7. Blue in ammonia water. If smears appear too dark when removed from hematoxylin, differentiate in 1% acetic acid in water solution for a few seconds and then blue in ammonia water.
8. Wash in water.
9. Mount in glycerine jelly.

RESULTS

Fat stains orange to bright red, and nuclei stain blue.

Nile Blue Sulfate, C.I. No. 51180
(Brosens and Gordon)

PURPOSE

Estimation of fetal maturity.

METHOD

Directly on a clean glass slide, mix one drop of amniotic fluid (fresh) with 1 drop of 0.1% aqueous solution of Nile Blue A. Apply a coverslip† and examine this preparation under a low-power objective. Count the percentage of orange-stained cells per 500 cells. If clusters are encountered, the number of cells in each cluster can be estimated.

PRINCIPLE

Studies have shown that only cells originating from sebaceous glands stain orange by this method. Therefore, the presence of large numbers of these cells indicates the functional maturity of

---

†*Earlier publications suggested heating the slide prior to coverslipping.*

Table 33–14
Baseline for Fetal Maturity Established by Rosen and Gordon (56 Patients)

Maturity (Weeks)	Orange-Stained Cells (%)
>40	>50
38–40	10–50+
34–38	1–10
<34	<1

sebaceous glands, which is directly related to fetal maturity. Table 33–14 lists some criteria for estimation of fetal maturity by this method.

The method is cited only for its historical value. Obstetric ultrasound has now replaced the need for amniotic fluid study, which is not without danger of infection and induced abortion.

Stains for Nucleic Acids

The Feulgen Stain*

USE

Specific staining of double-stranded deoxyribonucleic acid.

PROCEDURE

1. Bring paraffin sections through xylene and alcohol to water as usual, with the usual iodine thiosulfate sequence for removal of mercurial precipitates if required, or use alcohol-fixed smears.
2. Place in normal hydrochloric acid (preheated) at 60° C for 10 minutes.
3. Immerse in Schiff's reagent (see p. 1499) for 10 minutes.
4. Wash 2 minutes in each of three successive baths of 0.05 M metabisulfite. The sulfite baths should be discarded daily.
5. Wash 5 minutes in running water.
6. Counterstain a few seconds in 0.01% fast-green FCF C.I. No. 42053 in 95% alcohol. The stain does not wash out in alcohol, but if it is too intense, it may be removed promptly in water.
7. Complete the dehydration with 100% alcohol; clear through one change of alcohol and xylene (50:50) and two of xylene. Mount in polysty-

rene, ester gum, Permount, HSR, or other synthetic resin or in balsam.

RESULTS

Nuclear chromatin is a deep red-purple.

Kurnick's Methyl Green–Pyronin Variant†

USE

Demonstration of ribonucleic acid.

PROCEDURE

1. Fix in any one of the following: Carnoy, cold 80% alcohol, cold acetone, neutral formalin; embed and section in paraffin as usual or use frozen dried material embedded in paraffin directly. Alcohol fixed smears may be used.
2. Deparaffinize and hydrate as usual.‡
3. Stain 6 minutes in repurified 0.2% methyl green§ in water or in pH 4.2 M/100 acetate buffer. (The solution should be extracted in a separate funnel by shaking with successive changes of chloroform until no more color is extracted.)
4. Blot dry and dehydrate with two changes of n-butyl alcohol.
5. Stain 30 to 90 seconds in acetone freshly saturated with pyronin.‖ For more delicate staining, dilute one part of the saturated solution with nine parts of acetone and prolong the time somewhat.
6. Clear directly in cedar oil, wash in xylene, and mount in terpene resin (Permount, HSR).

RESULTS

Blue-green chromatin, red nucleoli, pink to red cytoplasm.

Stains for Hematologic Material and Air-Dried Smears

Wright's Stain

USE

Identification of blood cells. Used by some for routine diagnostic purposes.

---

*R.D. Lillie, 1976, p. 171.

†R.D. Lillie, 1965, p. 154.
‡Smears need only to be rinsed in distilled water prior to step 3.
§Methyl green, C.I. No. 42585.
‖Pyronin, C.I. No. 45005.

PREPARATION OF SOLUTIONS

Wright's Stain
(Stock Solution)

Wright's stain	0.5 g
Absolute methyl alcohol	100 ml

Buffer (pH 6.4)

KH_2PO_4	6.63 g
Na_2HPO_4	2.56 g
Distilled water	1,000 ml

Wright's Stain
(Working Solution)

Wright's stain stock	25 ml
Buffer	75 ml

STAINING PROCEDURE

1. Remove slides from 95% methyl alcohol and air-dry.
2. Flood slides with working solution of Wright's stain. Allow to stand until a metallic sheen appears (2–5 minutes).
3. Gently rinse slide with a stream of buffer from wash bottle to remove scum.
4. Rinse the slide under a thin stream of running tap water until thinner parts of smear turn pale purple or pinkish red.
5. Allow slide to dry. Dip dry slide in xylene and mount in gum damar in xylene or other suitable mounting medium.

Giemsa Stain

PREPARATION OF STAIN

Giemsa Stain
(Stock Solution)

Azure II—Eosin	2.0 g
Azure II	1.0 g
Azure B—Eosin	1.0 g
Azure A—Eosin	0.5 g

1. Mix 250 ml of glycerine with 250 ml of methyl alcohol.
2. Dissolve all dyes in this solution.
3. Let stand at room temperature overnight.
4. Shake mixture well for 5 to 10 minutes.
5. Pour, without filtering, into a dark screw cap bottle and store at room temperature.

Giemsa Stain
(Working Solution)

1. Mix 5 ml of Giemsa stock solution and 65 ml of water.

STAINING PROCEDURE

Start with step 1 for paraffin sections and with step 8 for smears.

1. Xylol	5 minutes
2. Xylol	5 minutes
3. Absolute ethyl alcohol	15 dips
4. Absolute ethyl alcohol	15 dips
5. 95% Ethyl alcohol	15 dips
6. 80% Ethyl alcohol	15 dips
7. 70% Ethyl alcohol	15 dips
8. Wash in distilled water	15 dips
9. Giemsa working stain	2 hours
10. 1% Acetic acid	1 quick dip
11. Blot slide with bibulous paper	
12. 100% ethyl alcohol—until there is only a slight bluish tint to the alcohol that runs off the slide	
13. Xylene	10 dips
14. Xylene	10 dips
15. Mount with permanent mounting medium.	

Wright-Giemsa Stain

PREPARATION OF STAINS

Wright's Stain (see above)
Giemsa Stain (see above)

Phosphate Buffer (pH 6.8)

Potassium phosphate monobasic	7.32 g
Sodium phosphate dibasic anhydrous	2.8 g
Distilled water	100 ml

STAINING PROCEDURE

1. Remove slide from methyl alcohol and drain off excess alcohol.
2. Place slide horizontally on rack or flat surface.
3. Flood slide with Wright stain—3 minutes.
4. Flood slide with buffer—4 minutes. Mix the stain and buffer by blowing gently on the slide. A metallic sheen appears.
5. Rinse slide well with tap water and drain off excess water.
6. Mix one drop of Giemsa with 1 ml of buffer. This must be fresh and made daily. Flood slide with this mixture for 20 minutes.
7. Rinse well with tap water.
8. Dehydrate smear with 10 dips in each of two 95% alcohols: one absolute alcohol and two xylenes.
9. Mount in permanent mounting medium.

Modified May-Grünwald–Giemsa (MGG) Stain (Zajicek)

PURPOSE

Routine stains for air-dried cytologic preparations (aspiration biopsy smears).

PREPARATION OF SOLUTIONS

May-Grünwald Reagent
(Stock Solution—Keeps 2 Weeks)

Eosin—methylene blue	1.0 g
Absolute methanol	100 ml

May-Grünwald Reagent
(Working Solution)

May-Grünwald stock	40 ml
Absolute methanol	20 ml

Giemsa Stain
(Stock Solution)

Azure II—Eosin	⎫	0.6 g
Azure II	⎬ Incubate at 37°C, 3h	0.16 g
Glycerin	⎭	50 ml
Absolute methanol		100 ml

Giemsa Stain
(Working Solution)

Giemsa stock	10 ml
Distilled water	90 ml

STAINING PROCEDURE

1.	May-Grünwald solution	5 minutes
2.	Running water	1 minute
3.	Giemsa solution	15 minutes
4.	Running water	1 to 2 minutes
5.	Air-dry. No mounting necessary.	

RESULTS

Nuclei stain blue, cytoplasm stains pink to rose, and bacteria stain blue.

Stock solutions of May-Grünwald and Giemsa reagents are also comercially available from several manufacturers. Follow manufacturers' instructions to prepare working solutions. The staining procedure may vary somewhat, and testing is recommended for optimal results.

For a description of a rapid equivalent of the MGG stain, see Chapter 29, p. 1244.

Stains for Wet Cell Films

Supravital Staining of Sediments of Serous Effusion

(N.C. Foot and N.D. Holmquist, 1958)

USE

Differentiation of macrophages and leukocytes from neoplastic and mesothelial cells in effusions.

PROCEDURE

Saturated solutions of neutral red C.I. No. 50040 and of Janus green C.I. No. 11050 are prepared in separate well-stoppered bottles of absolute alcohol. Dilute solutions are then made from each of these by adding 20 to 50 drops of neutral red stock solution to 10 ml of absolute alcohol and 15 to 30 drops of the saturated solution of Janus green to the same quantity of absolute alcohol. For use, 5 to 10 drops of the dilute Janus green solution are added to 2 ml of the dilute neutral red. One or 2 drops of this mixture are placed on a clean side, another slide is inverted over this, and the two are drawn apart so that an evenly distributed film is left on one side of either slide. Of course, placing sediment on the unprepared surface of the glass will produce totally negative results. The films dry quickly and keep indefinitely. For use: smear sediment on dry film and coverslip.

The neutral red appears to be the more efficacious stain and may be used alone, although Janus green is useful in identifying lymphocytes, which take it up rather diffusely.Neutral red stains the granules (or the vacuoles) of the macrophages a brilliant orange-red within a few seconds after the cover glass has been dropped over the preparation; it also stains polymorphonuclear leukocytes in a very similar manner but acts more slowly. Janus green colors the mitochondria in most of the cells in a specimen and is not particularly specific. Its power to stain lymphocytes diffusely sky blue is very helpful at times. Neoplastic or mesothelial cells, with few exceptions, do not stain at all by this method.

Rapid Stains for Wet Sediment and Preliminary Examination of Aspiration Biopsies

PURPOSE

Harris and Keebler suggest the use of these stains as: (1) a control when setting up new cytopreparatory procedures; (2) a check on the cellular preservation of a sample; (3) a method of identifying highly positive samples so they may be stained separately; (4) a check on existing cytopreparatory methods; and (5) a means of estimating the cellularity of a sample to help achieve a monolayer of cells and to prevent overloading filter preparation.

Other observers recommend the use of these stains as a definitive diagnostic procedure for some fluid specimens, such as urine, effusions and spinal fluid. The stains can also be used in preliminary assessment of aspiration biopsy samples.

Three different stains are listed below. Either one or them can be used, depending on individual preference.

PREPARATION OF SOLUTIONS

Thionin Blue

Thionin blue, C.I. No. 52000	1 g
25% Ethyl alcohol	100 ml
Glacial acetic acid	2 drops

Dissolve, let stand 30 minutes, filter, and store in a dark bottle. Frequent filtration and refrigeration are required.

Methylene Blue

Methylene blue-N.F. C.I.No. 52015	1.5 g	
95% Ethyl alcohol	30	ml
0.1 N Potassium hydroxide	2	ml

Dissolve dye in the alcohol and add the potassium hydroxide. Store in dark bottles and refrigerate.

Toluidine Blue

Toluidine blue, C.I. No. 52040	0.5 g	
95% Ethyl alcohol	20	ml
Distilled water	80	ml

Dissolve dye in alcohol and add water. Filter and store in a dark bottle in the refrigerator.

STAINING PROCEDURE

1. Place a drop of centrifuged sediment on a glass slide.
2. Place a small drop of dye on the slide and mix with an applicator stick.
3. Coverslip and let stand 2 to 5 minutes before examining microscopically.
4. To temporarily preserve this preparation, apply Vaseline or hot wax around the edges of the coverslip.

RESULTS

Methylene blue and toluidine blue stain all cells blue-purple, but distinct differences should be observed in the staining of the cytoplasm and the nucleus. In a well-differentiated preparation the nucleoli are visible as more purple structures within the nucleus. Thionin blue gives similar results except that erythrocytes remain unstained.

FLUORESCENCE TECHNIQUES

The principle of these techniques is the demonstration of certain substances that emit visible light when viewed in ultraviolet light, usually of 350- to 400-nm wavelength. The equipment needed includes:

1. *Microscope.*
2. *Light Source.* A mercury vapor lamp in appropriate housing.
3. *Source Filter.* A Corning glass filter 5113, ½ stock thickness, or similar filter.
4. *Barrier Filter.* Kodak Wratten G (15 G) (or its equivalent) lacquered filter placed above objective lens.

Techniques for Use with Smears

Acridine-Orange (AO) Fluorescence

PURPOSE

Differentiation of malignant cells from benign cells.

AO fluorescence had been at one time advocated as a replacement for Papanicolaou stain in screening of cervical smears. The method did not achieve the claimed success and was largely abandoned. Nonetheless, AO fluorescence is a valuable research technique (see Chap. 36). For this reason, the staining methods and results have been retained.

PRINCIPLE

AO combines with the deoxyribonucleic acid (DNA) and with ribonucleic acid (RNA). When viewed in ultraviolet light, the DNA emits yellowish green fluorescence, whereas the RNA emits red fluorescence. Depending on the pH of the buffer solution used in conjunction with AO, it is possible to emphasize either nuclear or cytoplasmic fluorescence. In cancer cells there is commonly an increase of the nuclear DNA and often an increase in the nucleolar and cytoplasmic RNA associated with increased protein synthesis (see p. 47). By staining of smears at pH 6, the brilliant red cytoplasmic fluorescence will be evident. By staining of smears at pH 3.8, the yellowish green to orange fluorescence of DNA will be emphasized.

Method of Bertalanffy (pH 6) (1960)

PREPARATION OF SOLUTIONS

AO Stock Solution. Prepare 4.1% aqueous stock solution of a good-quality AO (E. Gurr's michrome acridine-orange* or G.T. Gurr's acridine-orange†). Store indefinitely in refrigerator.

---

*Obtainable from K. and K. Laboratories, Inc., 121 Express St, Plainview, N.Y. 11803.

†Obtainable from ESBE Laboratory Supplies, Toronto 4, Ontario, Canada.

Phosphate Buffer—pH 6. The phosphate buffer is a combination of M/15 potassium dihydrophosphate and M/15 sodium phosphate mixed in proportion to pH 6. The solutions are prepared by dissolving 9.072 g of potassium dihydrophosphate (KH_2PO_4) in 1,000 ml of distilled water, and 9.465 g of sodium phosphate (Na_2HPO_4) in 1,000 ml of distilled water. To obtain the buffer, mix 230 ml of potassium dihydrophosphate solution with 40 ml of sodium phosphate solution.

Calcium Chloride. This is used for differentiation in M/10 solution. It is prepared by dissolving 11.099 g of calcium chloride in 1,000 ml of distilled water. All these solutions will keep indefinitely even at room temperature.

PROCEDURE

1. Hydrate rapidly through graded ethyl alcohol solutions—80%, 70%, 50%, to distilled water.
2. Rinse briefly in 1% acetic acid solution.
3. Wash in distilled water.
4. Stain 3 minutes in 0.1% stock AO in phosphate buffer solution (1 part A.O. stock to 9 parts of phosphate buffer).
5. Transfer for at least 1 minute to phosphate buffer to remove excess dye. If batches of slides are processed, they may remain in buffer for several hours while they are examined successively.
6. Differentiate 1 to 2 minutes in M/10 calcium chloride until nuclei (especially of leukocytes) show bright green fluorescence. The time for differentiation can be standardized by trial.
7. Rinse with phosphate buffer by using a polyethylene wash bottle.
8. Mount wet, using a few drops of buffer under coverslip, and examine.

The time of the procedure is approximately 6 to 7 minutes. After microscopic examination, slides can be destained by placing them in 50% ethyl alcohol and then restained by the Papanicolaou technique or other method.

Modification (F.D. Bertalanffy and K.P. Nagy, 1962)

This technique is applicable to frozen and paraffin sections but can serve as a rapid 1-minute procedure for smears. The method uses higher concentrations of the AO staining and $CaCl_2$ differentiating solutions, reducing the time of preparing a smear or specimen to 1 or 2 minutes.

PROCEDURE

1. Same as step 1 above but may be omitted for rapid diagnosis of frozen section.
2. Stain in pH 6 buffered 0.1% solution of AO for 10 seconds.
3. Buffer in pH 6 phosphate buffer as in original technique: 1 minute for sections; a few dips for smears.
4. Differentiate in 1 M solution of calcium chloride 5 to 30 seconds for sections, depending on thickness; 3 to 10 seconds for smears.
5. Same as step 7 above.

NOTE: For paraffin sections continue in 70% alcohol or alcoholic compound fixatives. Avoid fixation in formalin. Sections stained by the fluorescence method may be destained in 50% alcohol and restained for histologic study by routine methods.

RESULTS

Mature superficial squamous cells show fairly green fluorescent cytoplasm; intermediate squamous cells, a brownish cytoplasm. The size and appearance of nuclei further distinguish these two cell forms. Parabasal and basal cells appear brown or reddish brown. Sheets of atrophic squamous cells exhibit brownish orange to red cytoplasmic fluorescence and must be recognized by the normal morphology of nuclei.

Normal endocervical cells are reddish brown. Endocervical cells in inflammatory conditions such as chronic irritation and trichomoniasis appear red (probably from the increased RNA content) and must be distinguished from malignant cells by the normal morphologic characteristics of the nuclei. Malignant cells as a rule show flaming orange to red cytoplasmic fluorescence and greenish yellow fluorescence of the dense hyperchromatic nuclei. Degenerating tumor cells show a progressive loss of RNA, and therefore the cytoplasmic fluorescence is weak.

Trichomonads fluoresce reddish brown with small yellow nuclei. Leukocytes show bright green, fluorescent lobulated nuclei and unstained cytoplasm. Lymphocytes and monocytes usually have dense green nuclei surrounded by a narrow rim of reddish cytoplasm. Hemoglobin prevents fluorescence, and so the erythrocytes are not visible; therefore blood does not interfere with fluorescent microscopy.

Candida albicans (Monilia) mycelia and spores appear brilliant red.

Bacteria fluoresce reddish brown to red. In

smears of nongynecologic material, cells such as respiratory epithelial cells, macrophages and mesothelial cells may show increased cytoplasmic fluorescence requiring evaluation on the basis of morphology.

A Ten-Second Acridine-Orange Staining Technique
(H.L. Riva and T.R. Turner, 1962)

PREPARATION OF SOLUTIONS

Mix 0.25 g of AO* in 1,000 ml of 2.0% acetic acid in distilled water. Add 0.2 ml of Tween 80, a wetting agent (to increase cellular clarity and assist dye in penetrating mucus and debris).

Add 0.1 g of powdered Merthiolate† to prevent growth of fungus and bacteria.

Prepare 2% ethyl alcohol in normal saline solution (for differentiation).

Normal saline solution.

PROCEDURE

Smears may be examined immediately or after fixation.

Specimens of urine, fluids, and sputa are prepared as follows: smears are made on slides without albumin and immediately fixed in 95% alcohol. Gynecologic specimens or all smears made at the side of the patient are immediately fixed in 95% ethyl alcohol.

1. Hold slide with pair of tissue forceps and agitate for 3 seconds in a bottle of AO solution. (Bring AO solution up to volume daily and change weekly.)
2. Agitate for 3 seconds in 2% ethyl alcohol (change daily) in normal saline solution for differentiation.
3. Rinse by agitating in normal saline solution (change daily) for 4 seconds (slides may be left in saline solution indefinitely).

If a smear is not properly differentiated, repeat agitation in 2% ethyl alcohol solution and rinse. Vigorous agitation in all the solutions produces the best results.

Immediately prior to examination of a slide, coverslip using saline solution as a mounting me-

---

National Analine Division, Allied Chemical Corp., Rector St., New York, N.Y. 10006.

†*Thimerosal, Eli Lilly & Co., Box 618, Indianapolis, Ind. 46206.*

dium. Remove excess saline solution by blotting slide gently between layers of paper toweling. If slide dries out during examination, carefully lift coverslip (do not slide) and remount. Remove coverslip, dry, and file after examination. If slides become faded, restain by above method without destaining. Restained smears may require a longer time in the 2% alcohol solution followed by rinsing to obtain optimum differentiation.

RESULTS

In screening slides using the above staining technique, emphasis is placed on the increased fluorescent intensity of the nucleus and not of the cytoplasm. Once attention is drawn to the increased fluorescence in the nucleus, the cell is evaluated according to the standard morphologic criteria. The nuclei of normal cells may fluoresce brightly, but the brilliance is smooth and confined within the nucleus. The nuclei of abnormal cells fluoresce with a glowing brilliance that often seems to be above the nucleus.

Comments

The fluorescent techniques are based on the presence of DNA and RNA and are therefore not specific for cancer cells. The techniques have been advocated for the rapidity of the staining procedure and the alleged ease and speed in screening. Under ideal circumstances it is perhaps easier to spot a brilliantly fluorescent group of cancer cells than to screen for a few clusters or single malignant cells in the routinely prepared Papanicolaou smear.

It is false to assume that screening by the fluorescent methods does not demand conventional basic training and experience in the morphologic aspects of cytology, with a thorough knowledge of the drawbacks and pitfalls of the fluorescence technique. Each slide must be screened with the same thoroughness as the routine Papanicolaou smear, and the ease of screening by the fluorescent method has been disputed by some workers, who have found it not only tedious but very tiring on the eyes.

Although the fluorescence method may be based on morphology, it is attended by certain pitfalls. Bright fluorescence may obscure morphologic detail. Actively growing cells may fluoresce brilliantly and are easily mistaken for cancer cells. Endocervical and endometrial cells often exhibit a bright red fluorescent cytoplasm and increased nuclear fluorescence mimicking poorly differentiated cancer cells. Occasionally, the cytoplasm may glow to such an extent that the fluorescence spills over and obscures the nuclear structure. Histiocytes usually fluoresce a yellowish green, although on occasion the cytoplasm fluoresces a pinkish orange, but an important identifying characteristic, the lacy cytoplasm, is not visible. Degenerating malignant cells from necrotic tumors show very little if any increased fluorescence, and their recognition must depend on morphologic criteria. The intensity of fluorescence in early malignant growths, particularly well-differentiated carcinoma in situ, is not marked, and considerable experience is necessary for diagnosis.

If the screener wishes to mark clusters or single cells for a further check by another cytotechnologist or the pathologist, it is difficult to mark the exact area on the coverslip. The coverslip tends to move when pressure is exerted on it, and the cells often drift away as well. Although the bottom of the slide may be marked with diamond pencil or felt marking pen, the cells have a tendency to drift from the site.

Every smear deemed malignant, suspicious, or questionable by the fluorescence method must be restained and rescreened by the Papanicolaou method. This entails the removal of the coverslip from the specimen and the possibility of losing valuable material.

As there is difficulty in marking a specimen in a liquid mounting medium, there is also difficulty in comparing the two methods on the basis of cellular appearance. The necessity of restaining and rescreening specimens is in itself a time-consuming process. The Papanicolaou method yields a preparation that is easily marked and checked by others and can be used for teaching purposes. The specimen can then be filed for future reference without the necessity of restaining the material.

The fluorescence technique is useful in exceptional cases when it is combined with routinely stained specimens, such as the infrequently encountered effusion containing macrophages or atypical mesothelial cells that may be difficult to distinguish from malignant cells. In our opinion this method is not sufficiently practical or accurate as a routine method for cytologic screening but may be used as an adjunct or research tool.

Fluorescent Stains for Flow Cytometry

As discussed in Chapter 36, fluorescent stains (fluorochromes) have extensive application in flow cytometry. Such techniques may also be used for visual assessment of cells. There are numerous fluorochromes available for such studies. The two common ones are AO and propidium iodide. Only dyes of the highest degree of purity should be used.

Acridine Orange*

A stock solution is prepared by dissolving 50 mg of purified AO* in 50 ml of distilled water and stirring for 8 hours at room temperature in a dark glass flask, to prevent AO degradation by oxidation or light. This stock solution must be kept at 4°C in a tightly stoppered brown bottle, for not longer than 4 months. Prior to use, the stock solution will be diluted ten times and kept cold. It should be used only on the day on which it was prepared. A working solution is made immediately before use by diluting .17 ml of this solution up to 2 ml with TKM.† For AO staining, cells are combined with 1 ml of the final dilution of AO to a suspension of 2×10^5 cells in 1 ml of TKM for an AO concentration of 4.25×10^{-6} g/ml and will be allowed to equilibrate for 5 minutes at 25°C. All fluorescence measurements must be completed within ten minutes after staining. This procedure has been repeatedly tested by constructing concentration curves. We consistently obtained optimal differential staining of green and red fluorescence with the staining procedure described above.

Propidium Iodide (PI)

PI‡ is used for measurement of DNA in flow cytometry. This stain is considered a reliable indicator of DNA concentration and is less sensitive to environmental conditions than AO. A stock solution containing 250 mg of PI in 100 ml of distilled water is prepared. This mixture is stirred at room temperature until dissolved and then stored in a dark brown bottle at 4°C. The unused solution is discarded after 6 months. A working solution is prepared by diluting the stock solution 50 times with 0.1% sodium citrate. The cells are stained with PI by resuspending 1×10^5 cells in 1 ml of PI working solution. The cells are allowed to stand for at least 5 minutes but not more than 15 minutes at 4°C before fluorescence measurements. For further comments, see Appendix to Chap. 36.

Polyscience, Inc., Paul Valley Industrial Park, Warrington, Pennsylvania 18976.

†*TKM solution: 50 mM Tris, pH 7.2; 25 mM KCl; 5 mM MgCl₂.*

‡*Cal-Biochem. 10933 N. Torrey Pines Rd., La Jolla, Calif. 92037.*

SPECIAL TECHNIQUES

Special techniques have been devised for the isolation of cells either from very small samples or from very complex samples.

Sedimentation Technique for Cerebrospinal Fluid
(G. Th. A.M. Bots, L.N. Went and A. Schaberg, 1964)*

PRINCIPLE

This technique is based on the principle of slow absorption of fluid by hard filter paper. If the ab-

---

Acta Cytol., 8:234–241, 1964. A modification of this method was also published by S. Eneström (Acta Neurol. Scand, 41:153–159, 1965).

sorption is very slow, the cells will not be absorbed and will sink to the slide placed beneath. The absorption is slowed down by placing a heavy weight on the filter paper.

APPARATUS (Fig. 33–18)

Slide holder.
Tube holder.
Weights.
Glass tube 15 mm in diameter and 20 mm high.
Filter paper (Green 602 or Schleicher and Schöll 602 hard is acceptable).
The apparatus can be constructed in a machine shop.

PROCEDURE

Approximately 1 ml of fresh cerebrospinal fluid is placed in a small glass tube 15 mm in diameter and 20 mm high. The open end of the tube is placed against a glass slide covered with a piece of filter

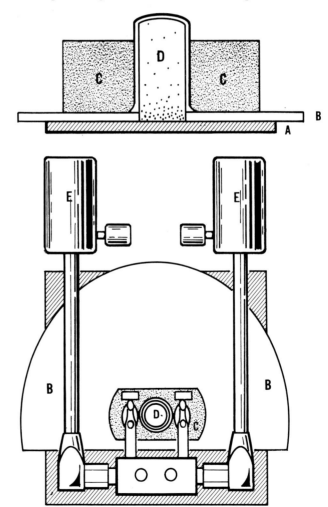

FIGURE 33–18. Apparatus for sedimentation technique for spinal fluid. (*Top*) Cross section of the apparatus. (*A*) Glass slide. (*B*) Filter paper. The rate of fluid absorption is regulated by weights, placed on top of the rubber block C. (*C*) Rubber block with a hole accommodating a glass tube filled with spinal fluid. (*D*) Glass tube with open end resting on glass slide. (*Bottom*) View of the apparatus from above. Parts are as above. (*E*) Adjustable weights. The pressure is transmitted via the rubber block C and regulates the rate of fluid absorption by the filter paper (*B*). (After Bots, G. Th. A. M., et al.: Results of a sedimentation technique for cytology of cerebrospinal fluid. Acta Cytol., 8:234–241, 1964)

paper (Fig. 33–18). The paper is perforated, and the size of the hole corresponds to the internal diameter of the tube. Place tube within the hole. The cells sink to the bottom of the tube and settle on the slide, and the fluid portion of the specimen is slowly removed by the filter paper. A large percentage of the cells is taken up by the paper at the beginning of sedimentation if the filter paper is completely dry. This absorption can be partially prevented by passing 0.5 ml of saline solution through the tube before introducing the cerebrospinal fluid.

To regulate the rate of sedimentation and to limit the loss of cells, the glass tube is placed in a block of rubber in which a hole has been bored. Attachment of adjustable weights to the rubber block allows control of speed of fluid absorption. A weight of 3 kg applied on the correct filter paper results in sedimentation of 1 ml of cerebrospinal fluid with a normal protein content in approximately 25 minutes.

When the protein content of the cerebrospinal fluid is high, the rate of sedimentation is slower. If the quantity of fluid is not appreciably decreased in approximately 30 minutes, the weights on the lever must be adjusted to reduce the pressure. Sedimentation time of less than an hour can be achieved fairly consistently by the use of this procedure. After sedimentation is complete, the preparation is allowed to dry. The cells may be stained by the Giemsa method or other methods.

The disadvantage of this method lies in cell distortion due to dryness. However, if proper adjustment is made to prevent this, excellent diagnostic results can be achieved.

RESULTS

Bots et al. reported that malignant cells were detected cytologically in 16 of 31 cases with histologically conformed tumors or leukemias localized in the central nervous system. Identification of tumor type was possible in 13 of the 16 positive cases.

Excellent results with an essentially similar method were reported by Eneström.

Pasteur Pipette Method (G.R. Durfee, G. Welborne, and L.G. Koss)

PURPOSE

The method can be used advantageously for cerebrospinal fluid and other fluids with sparse cell population.

MATERIALS (Fig. 33–19)

1. Prepare microcentrifuge tubes by cutting off tops of 5¾-inch Pasteur pipettes at indentation, so that final length of the tube is 4¾ inches. Flame tip of tube to close opening.
2. Nine-inch disposable Pasteur pipettes with standard dropper bulb for transfer of fluid specimen or for removal of supernatant fluid.
3. Clinical centrifuge* with 4-place No. 215 horizontal head, trunnion rings, and shields for accommodating 50-ml tubes. Use cylindrical rubber blocks* that fit shields and extend ¹⁄₁₆ inch above lip of shield. The blocks are bored to accommodate five of the above constructed microtubes. Each block is grooved slightly the entire length of one side to facilitate removal if a tube breaks and liquid seeps between shield and block, creating undue suction.
4. Slides covered with Mayer's albumin.

PROCEDURE

Place closed-tip microtube in bored rubber blocks. Mix specimen thoroughly. Transfer fluid into each tube with 9-inch Pasteur pipette with bulb. Place tip of transfer pipette into tube as far as narrowed portion and gently drop specimen while withdrawing pipette slowly. Fill to a half inch from the top of microtube. Balance and centrifuge at approximately 200 rpm for 30 minutes.

After centrifugation gradually remove supernatant fluid with 9-inch pipette by starting from top and using gentle suction as narrow portion of tube is approached. Care must be taken not to suck up specimen button formed at tip. A few drops of liquid will remain in tip over specimen button. Lay tip of microtube on an albuminized slide and cut off tip with a vial file below button. The few drops of liquid left in the tip of microtube are usually sufficient to expel the button onto slide. If the button is not expelled, place dropper bulb on microtube and gently force out. Smear button on albuminized slide with tip of microtube and dry in air for 5 to 10 seconds before placing in fixative (95% ethyl alcohol). Occasionally, spinal fluids are clear and will not yield a visible button after centrifugation. In these instances make smear of the few drops of fluid remaining in the tip of tube. Stain by the routine Papanicolaou method.

———
International Equipment Company, 300 Second Ave., Needham, Mass. 02194.

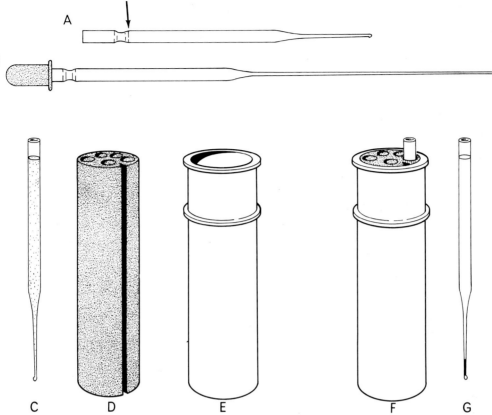

FIGURE 33-19. Pasteur pipette method for small amounts of fluid. (*A*) Pasteur pipette with tip flamed off. The top should be cut at indentation (*arrow*). (*B*) Full-length Pasteur pipette with rubber dropper bulb used for transfer of fluid or for removal of supernatant fluid. (*C*) Pasteur pipette cut to size with tip flamed, filled with fluid to be processed. (*D*) Rubber block accommodating five pipettes and fitting into centrifuge shield (*E*). The groove in the rubber block facilitates removal. (*F*) Pipette with fluid placed in rubber block within the centrifuge shield. (*G*) Pipette after centrifugation. The sediment is shown as a black deposit at bottom of tube.

Flotation Techniques

The principle of separation and enrichment of a specific cell population in a fluid by flotation techniques is based on documented differences in specific gravity (SG). Red blood cells have an SG of 1.092 to 1.097; leukocytes have an average SG of about 1.065, and cancer cells average 1.056 (Seal, 1959). Several flotation techniques using various media of cell separation have been developed and used with varying degrees of success for separation of cancer cells in fluids and the circulating blood. In general, the methods achieve good concentration of cells in fluids, but their preservation is not optimal.

Seal's Method for the Isolation of Free-Floating Cancer Cells from the Blood

PRINCIPLE

This method utilizes the differences in SG to separate cancer cells and lymphocytes from erythrocytes and polymorphonuclear leukocytes. A solution of blended silicone with a specific gravity of 1.075 serves as a separating medium. Ideally, cancer cells and lymphocytes should accumulate on the surface of the silicone, whereas the heavier erythrocytes and polymorphonuclear leukocytes should collect under the silicone.

BLENDING OF SILICONES

Silicone 702 may have the desired specific gravity of 1.075. However, it is safe to obtain also silicones 555 (SG 1.06) and 710 (SG 1.10) for blending purposes. The copper sulfate method (Phillips et al.) is used to determine the accurate specific gravity. *Not all silicones blend.* Consult the manufacturer for further information.

MATERIALS NEEDED

1. Silicones 702, 555, and 710 (2 lb. of each).*
2. Copper sulfate solutions (with an SG of 1.065 to 1.084).†
3. Filter equipment. One needs 200 type SM 47 mm, plain white filters, and a hydrosol simplified filter holder, catalog number XX 20-047-10.‡
4. PVP (polyvinylpyrrolidone, 1 lb.).§ (This product is used to decrease the matting of cells on the surface of the silicone and to keep small particles in suspension.)
5. Oxyethylated tertiary octyl phenol formaldehyde polymer (4 oz.).‖ (This wetting agent is used to prevent agglutination of cells.)
6. EDTA (disodium ethylenediaminetetra-acetate dihydrate, 10 oz.).# (This product is a chelating agent that prevents the formation of fibrin.)
7. General Electric Dri-Film SC 87 (4 oz.).**
8. Saponin (100 g.)†† (It is used to hemolyze erythrocytes remaining after removal of the supernatant.

Available from the Dow Corning Corporation, Midland, Mich. 48640.

†*Available from the Hartmann-Leddon Co., 60th and Woodland Ave., Philadelphia, Pa. 19142.*

‡*All are available from the Millipore Filter Corp., Bedford, Mass. 01730.*

§*Available under the name Plasdone C from the Commercial Development Department of General Aniline and Film Corp., 435 Hudson St., New York, N.Y. 10014.*

‖*Available under the name WR 1339 from the Special Chemical Department of Winthrop Laboratories, 90 Park Ave., New York, N.Y. 10016.*

#*Available under the name Sequestrene NA 2 from Geigy Industrial Chemicals, Division of Geigy Chemical Corp., Ardsley, N.Y. 10502.*

**Available from the Silicone Products Department, Chemical and Metallurgical Division, General Electric Co., 133 Boyd St., Newark, N.J. 07103.*

††*Available under the name Practical Saponin from Eastman Chemical Products, Inc., Subsidiary of Eastman Kodak Co., 343 State St., Rochester, N.Y. 14652.*

9. Microscopic mounting medium, xylene solution (8 oz.).‡‡
10. Two gross of 2 × 3 inch microscope slides, and 10 oz. of 50 mm No. 1 cover glasses.

SOLUTIONS NEEDED

1. Ten percent buffered formalin. Make 18 L (enough to fill a 5-gallon carboy) by dissolving 117 g of dibasic sodium phosphorus and 72 g of monobasic sodium phosphorus in 10.1 L of distilled water. When these chemicals have dissolved, add 1,800 ml of 40% formalin and bring to 18.1 L with distilled water.
2. PVP solution. Make 10 L by dissolving 350 g of PVP in 8.1 L of normal saline solution. When the PVP has dissolved, add 10 ml of WR 1339 and 25 g of EDTA; bring to 10 L with normal saline.
3. Saponin. Use a 2% solution in normal saline solution and make 200 ml at a time.

PROCEDURE

1. In the following order, place 10 ml of silicone, with a specific gravity of 1.075 in the bottom of a 50-ml siliconized centrifuge tube. Carefully overlay the silicone with 20 ml of PVP solution. Add 10 ml of fresh heparinized blood to the PVP solution and centrifuge at 1,500 rpm (500 × g) for 15 minutes, bringing the centrifuge up to speed rapidly. Following centrifugation, one will note the red cell mass under the silicone and, on its surface, little whitish islands (Fig. 33–20). These are the polymorphonuclear neutrophic leukocytes. Between the silicone-supernatant interface is a grayish layer containing lymphocytes, cancer cells, and a few red blood cells.
2. Aspirate the supernatant to about ¼ inch above the silicone and discard. This removes most of the platelets (SG 1.032). Using a bulb pipette, wash the surface of the silicone with 50 ml of PVP solution and place the washings in a 50-ml long conical centrifuge tube. To hemolyze any remaining red blood cells, add three or four drops of 2% saponin to the washings, stopper the tube, and gently invert and right the tube for 1 minute. Centrifuge at 800 rpm (250 × g) for 30 minutes.
3. Again aspirate the supernatant to about ¼ inch above the sediment, discard, and resuspend the sediment in the little PVP solution remaining by tapping the bottom of the tube vigorously in

---

‡‡*Also available from Eastman Chemical Producs.*

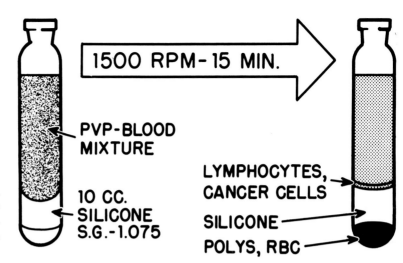

FIGURE 33–20. Appearance of siliconized centrifuge tube before (*left*) and after (*right*) centrifugation. (Seal, S. H.: Cancer, *12*:590–595, 1959)

Figure labels: 1500 RPM – 15 MIN. / PVP-BLOOD MIXTURE / 10 CC. SILICONE S.G.-1.075 / LYMPHOCYTES, CANCER CELLS / SILICONE / POLYS, RBC

the palm of the hand. Fill the tube with 10% buffered formalin and allow to fix overnight.

4. The following day, collect the cells on a type SM Millipore filter (pore size 5 μm) (see p. 1470), rinsing the centrifuge tube thoroughly with buffered formalin. Because the cells are now fixed and thus hardened, pressure regulation during filtration is no longer necessary. Remove the filter from its holder, clamp to a 2 × 3 inch microscope slide with spring hair clips, and stain.

Albumin Technique (McGrew and Nanos)

This method serves to enrich the yield of tumor cells in complex specimens, such as blood or hemorrhagic fluids. The method uses an albumin solution to separate cancer cells from other cells by specific gravity. The results are similar using either Solution A or B.

PREPARATION OF SOLUTIONS

Solution A

Patho-o-cyte 2 (25%)*	4 ml
Physiologic saline solution	1 ml

or

Solution B

Patho-o-cyte 3 (30%)*	3.5 ml
Physiologic saline solution	1.5 ml

1. The specimen must be collected in an anticoagulant and should contain no clots. Centrifuge

sample and prepare sediment smears as described by one of the methods on p. 1463.

2. Resuspend remaining sediment in 5 ml of the original fluid.
3. Place 5 ml of Solution A or B (see above) in a 10-ml plastic tube.
4. Carefully layer 5 ml of the original or resuspended sample over the albumin suspension. Avoid mixing the two solutions.
5. Carefully balance the tube and centrifuge at 2500 rpm for 10 minutes. Allow the centrifuge to come to a complete stop. *Do not use brake.*
6. Aspirate with a syringe and an 18-gauge needle with the bevel filed off and the layer of cells floating at the interphase of the albumin and sample (see Fig. 33–21).
7. Resuspend this layer of cells in a balanced salt solution, centrifuge, and prepare slides by one of the methods described on p. 1463.

Other Flotation Techniques

Besides albumin and silicone gradients, other materials have been recommended for the same purpose. Many of the solutions used were originally developed for other purposes. The solutions are commercially produced and highly standardized.

FICOLL METHOD

The Ficoll-triosil method was initially introduced by Böyum in 1968 for separation of lymphocytes from the blood. Ficoll is a cross-linked polymerized sucrose.

Elequin et al. advocated the use of Ficoll† gra-

Available in 50-ml vials from Miles Laboratories, Inc., Kankakee, Ill. 60901.

†*Pharmacia Fine Chemicals, Division of Pharmacia, Inc., 800 Centennial Ave., Piscataway, N.J. 08854.*

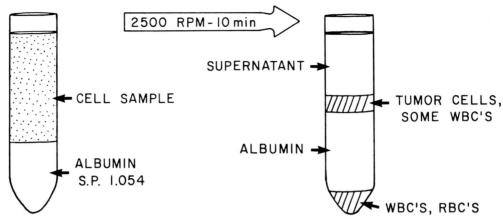

FIGURE 33–21.   Flotation method for separation of cancer cells from body fluids, after McGrew and Nanos.

dient of SG 1.050 to 1.052 for isolation of cancer cells from cell suspensions, followed by the use of a cytocentrifuge for preparation of cell spreads. The centrifuged sample contained a clear band of cancer cells and leukocytes that could be removed by pipette and placed in the cytocentrifuge well. Although good concentration of cancer cells was obtained, the preservation of the cells on the slide was not optimal.

HYPAQUE* (SODIUM DIATRIOZOTE) TECHNIQUE

Spriggs (1975) advocated the use of 25% Hypaque solution, originally used as an intravenous contrast medium in radiography, for separation of erythrocytes from bloody fluids. The fluids are collected with EDTA (2 mg per ml of fluid) to prevent coagulation. After initial centrifugation of fluid to produce a cell button (time and speed are not critical), the gradient is prepared in a round-bottom centrifuge tube by mixing about 4 ml each of Hypaque solution and supernatant fluid. The remaining supernatant is discarded. The cells from the hemorrhagic button from the original fluid are gently mixed and layered on top of the gradient. The mixture is centrifuged for 15 minutes at 3,000 rpm. The erythrocytes are at the bottom of the tube and the white cells above. The white cells are removed with a pipette, and a smear is prepared either directly or after further centrifugation. The method offers good concentration of cancer cells, but their preservation is not optimal.

---

*Sterling Organics, Division of Sterling Drugs, 90 Park Ave., New York, N.Y. 10006.

Digestion of Lung Tissue and Sputum for the Detection of Ferruginous (Asbestos) Bodies (Smith and Naylor, 1972)

MATERIALS

1. Laundry bleach, such as Clorox, which is a 5.25% solution of sodium hypochlorite
2. 300- to 500-ml glass containers
3. Chloroform
4. 50% Ethyl alcohol
5. 50-ml centrifuge tubes
6. 95% Ethyl alcohol
7. Nuclepore filters, 8 to 12 μm pore size, and filtering setup

PROCEDURE

This technique may be used for lung tissue or sputum samples. However, the sputum is digested in a matter of minutes, whereas tissue samples require 24 hours or more.

1. Select approximately 5 g of pulmonary parenchyma from a fresh or fixed lung. Avoid bronchi, bronchioles, large blood vessels, and areas of consolidation.
2. Cut lung tissue into small pieces.
3. Place the pieces of lung or sputum into a glass jar and add approximately 200 ml of bleach. If greater than 5 g of lung is to be digested, increase the amount of bleach proportionately.
4. Let the pieces of lung stay in this solution until the *entire* sample is dissolved. This may require 24 to 72 hours. If the tissue is not completely dissolved in 24 hours, pour off the su-

pernatant and add fresh bleach. This step should be repeated every 24 hours until digestion is complete. Sputum liquefies immediately. However, several hours may be required if one wishes to completely remove all cellular structures.

5. Carefully decant the bleach without disturbing or losing any of the sediment.
6. Add 20 ml of chloroform to the jar. Swirl it around to clean the sides of the jar. Then add 20 ml of 50% ethyl alcohol and shake the jar vigorously to suspend all sediment.
7. Centrifuge this mixture in 50-ml centrifuge tubes for 10 minutes at 600 to 800 rpm. Three visible layers should appear:
   Top layer: alcohol
   Middle layer: Carbonaceous material
   Bottom layer: chloroform
8. Pour off the supernatant. If a visible black, gray, or golden sediment remains in the tip of the tube, repeat steps 6 and 7 until there is no visible sediment.
9. Add 95% ethyl alcohol to the centrifuge tube and mix well.

10. Filter this solution through a Nuclepore filter. Using 95% alcohol, wash the centrifuge tube out several times and wash down the sides of the funnel.
11. After allowing all the fluid to pass through the filter, let the filter dry out for 10 to 15 seconds before turning off the vacuum.
12. Place the completely dry, *unstained filter*, sediment side down, on a coverslip.
13. Place the coverslip on a flat surface, flood it with chloroform, and let the chloroform evaporate completely.
14. Dip the dry coverslip into xylol and mount it on to a glass slide.

QUANTITATION OF ASBESTOS BODIES

The method can be used for quantitation of ferruginous bodies per gram of material. If this is the purpose, several filters may have to be used for each specimen to facilitate counting (see Chap. 19).

For a discussion of immunocytologic techniques, see Chapter 34.

PART II: PRINCIPLES OF OPERATION OF A LABORATORY OF CYTOLOGY

LABORATORY SAFETY

Chemical, electrical, fire, and infectious hazards are of paramount concern for all individuals working in the cytopreparatory laboratory. It is imperative that all personnel thoroughly understand the procedures to follow in case of emergencies and the methods used to minimize the possibility of accidents and infection. State and federal agencies that license or inspect laboratories require that safety standards and regulations be met. Guidelines for the preparation of a detailed safety manual are listed in this section. References listed at the conclusion of the chapter may be consulted for further details.

Every employee should know the location of:

1. Fire extinguishers
2. Fire blankets
3. Fire alarm and emergency exits
4. Eye wash equipment
5. Safety shower

Every employee should know the correct procedures to follow for:

1. Chemical splash to the eye or body
2. Fire, explosion, or electrical shock
3. Storage, handling, disposal, and emergency treatment necessary for all chemicals used in the laboratory
4. Handling and disposal of potentially infectious material

General Guidelines for Storing and Handling Chemicals and Electrical Equipment (Table 33–15)

1. Store chemicals in their original containers, if possible, or in appropriate chemical-resistant plastic containers.
2. A cool, well-ventilated metal cabinet or closed room should be used to store volatile, flammable, and explosive materials.

Table 33–15
Essential Safety-Related Properties of Some Common Chemicals Used in Cytopreparatory Laboratories

Name of Chemical	Properties	Maximum Permissible Atmospheric Concentration	Symptoms of Poisoning
Acetone	* Flash point − 17°C Highly inflammable	1000 ppm†	Inhalation or ingestion: Pulmonary congestion with edema, dyspnea, decreased respirations, and stupor
Concentrate acids or alkali			Corrosive burns
Alcohol			
Ethyl	Flash point 14°C Readily inflammable	1000 ppm	Stupor, flushing, nausea, and vomiting
Isopropyl	Flashpoint 12°C Inflammable	400 ppm	Stupor, coma, hypotension. 8 oz. (240 ml) probably fatal.
Methyl	Flash point 10°C Inflammable	200 ppm	May be fatal, decreased respiration, virtigo, dimness of vision, headache, convulsions; may lead to loss of vision
Ammonium hydroxide (concentrated)	Fumes formed when bottles are near volatile acids. Becomes boiling hot in reaction with H_2SO_4	50 ppm	Corrosive burns from eye and skin contact, inhalation, and ingestion
Chloroform	Nonflammable: Forms toxic gas when in contact with heat	25 ppm	Drowsiness, coma—irritant to skin and mucous membranes
Ether	Flash point—29°C Mixed with air can cause explosions. Store in airtight containers in a cool (8°–15°C) place away from sparking apparatus. Do not refrigerate (<8°C).	400 ppm	Exerts a narcotic action somewhat similar to alcohol. Irritant to skin and mucous membranes
Formalin	Flash point 60°C Should be stored in a well-closed container in a moderately warm place	—	Irritant to skin and mucous membranes, contact dermatitis, bronchitis, and occasionally asthmatic attack
Xylene	Flash point 4°C Flammable	100 ppm	Dizziness, weakness, headache, nausea, vomiting, euphoria, ventricular arrhythmia, convulsions

* Flash point: The lowest temperature at which vapors above a volatile combustible substance ignite in air when exposed to flame.
† Parts per million.

3. Appropriate fire-fighting equipment should be in the immediate area.
4. Do not transfer chemicals with a pipette in the mouth. Use pumps for transferring large volumes and a bulb pipette for small volumes.
5. Volatile, toxic, or irritating chemicals should be transferred under a fume hood.
6. Label all laboratory reagents with date of preparation or delivery and attach poison sticker where indicated.
7. When diluting solutions, always add the concentrated chemical to the water.
8. Never smoke or eat in an area where chemicals are stored or in use.
9. Wear safety glasses when working with caustic chemicals.

10. Wash hands after handling any chemical.
11. Staining and coverslipping should take place in a well-ventilated area or under a fume hood. Avoid inhaling vapors during these procedures.
12. Make certain that all electrical equipment is grounded properly.
13. Never handle electrical switches or controls with wet hands.

Infectious Hazards

With the growing concern of exposure to AIDS in the workplace, it is necessary to emphasize the need to treat blood and body fluids from *all* patients as potentially infective. The Centers for Disease Control estimates that the 1.5 to 2 million individuals seropositive for human immunodeficiency virus (HIV) in the United States in 1991 will quadruple by 1995. All specimens, including the outside of the specimen jar, should be considered contaminated with potentially infectious organisms. Infections may occur from direct contact or from inhaling aerosols created by centrifuging, blending, stirring, and pouring. Written procedures should be a part of the standard operating manual of each laboratory.

The following are excerpts applicable to the laboratory from "Recommendations for Prevention of HIV Transmission in Health-Care Setting," MMWR, *36*(Suppl. 25): 35–185, 1987.

Precautions to Prevent Transmission of HIV

UNIVERSAL PRECAUTIONS

Since medical history and examination cannot reliably identify all patients infected with HIV or other blood-borne pathogens, blood and body-fluid precautions should be consistently used for *all* patients. This approach, previously recommended by CDC, and referred to as "universal blood and body-fluid precautions" or "universal precautions," should be used in the care of *all* patients, especially including those in emergency-care settings in which the risk of blood exposure is increased and the infection status of the patient is usually unknown.

1. All health-care workers should routinely use appropriate barrier precautions to prevent skin and mucous-membrane exposure when contact with blood or other body fluids of any patient is anticipated. Gloves should be worn for touching blood and body fluids, mucous membranes, or non-intact skin of all patients, for handling items or surfaces soiled with blood or body fluids, and for performing venipuncture and other vascular access procedures. Gloves should be changed after contact with each patient. Masks and protective eyewear or face shields should be worn during procedures that are likely to generate droplets of blood or other body fluids to prevent exposure of mucous membranes of the mouth, nose, and eyes. Gowns or aprons should be worn during procedures that are likely to generate splashes of blood or other body fluids.
2. Hands and other skin surfaces should be washed immediately and thoroughly if contaminated with blood or other body fluids. Hands should be washed immediately after gloves are removed.
3. All health-care workers should take precautions to prevent injuries by needles, scalpels, and other sharp instruments or devices during procedures; when cleaning used instruments; during disposal of used needles; and when handling sharp instruments after procedures. To prevent needlestick injuries, needles should not be recapped, purposely bent or broken by hand, removed from disposable syringes, or otherwise manipulated by hand. After they are used, disposable syringes and needles, scalpel blades, and other sharp items should be placed in puncture-resistant containers for disposal; the puncture-resistant containers should be located as close as practical to the use area. Large-bore reusable needles should be placed in a puncture-resistant container for transport to the reprocessing area.
4. Although saliva has not been implicated in HIV transmission, to minimize the need for emergency mouth-to-mouth resuscitation, mouthpieces, resuscitation bags, or other ventilation devices should be available for use in areas in which the need for resuscitation is predictable.
5. Health-care workers who have exudative lesions or weeping dermatitis should refrain from all direct patient care and from handling patient-care equipment until the condition resolves.
6. Pregnant health-care workers are not known to be at greater risk of contracting HIV infection than health-care workers who are not pregnant; however, if a health-care worker develops HIV infection during pregnancy, the infant is at risk of infection resulting from perinatal transmission. Because of this risk, pregnant health-care workers should be especially familiar with and

strictly adhere to precautions to minimize the risk of HIV transmission.

Implementation of universal blood and body-fluid precautions for *all* patients eliminates the need for use of the isolation category of "Blood and Body Fluid Precautions" previously recommended by CDC for patients known or suspected to be infected with blood-borne pathogens. Isolation precautions (e.g., enteric, "AFB" should be used as necessary if associated conditions, such as infectious diarrhea or tuberculosis, are diagnosed or suspected.

PRECAUTIONS FOR LABORATORIES

Blood and other body fluids from *all* patients should be considered infective. To supplement the universal blood and body-fluid precautions listed above, the following precautions are recommended for health-care workers in clinical laboratories.

1. All specimens of blood and body fluids should be put in a well-constructed container with a secure lid to prevent leaking during transport. Care should be taken when collecting each specimen to avoid contaminating the outside of the container and of the laboratory form accompanying the specimen.
2. All persons processing blood and body-fluid specimens (e.g., removing tops from vacuum tubes) should wear gloves. Masks and protective eyewear should be worn if mucous-membrane contact with blood or body fluids is anticipated. Gloves should be changed and hands washed after completion of specimen processing.
3. For routine procedures, such as histologic and pathologic studies or microbiologic culturing, a biological safety cabinet is not necessary. However, biological safety cabinets (Class I or II) should be used whenever procedures are conducted that have a high potential for generating droplets. These include activities such as blending, sonicating, and vigorous mixing.
4. Mechanical pipetting devices should be used for manipulating all liquids in the laboratory. Mouth pipetting must not be done.
5. Use of needles and syringes should be limited to situations in which there is no alternative, and the recommendations for preventing injuries with needles outlined under universal precautions should be followed.
6. Laboratory work surfaces should be decontaminated with an appropriate chemical germicide after a spill of blood or other body fluids and when work activities are completed.
7. Contaminated materials used in laboratory tests should be decontaminated before reprocessing or be placed in bags and disposed of in accordance with institutional policies for disposal of infective waste.
8. Scientific equipment that has been contaminated with blood or other body fluids should be decontaminated and cleaned before being repaired in the laboratory or transported to the manufacturer.
9. All persons should wash their hands after completing laboratory activities and should remove protective clothing before leaving the laboratory.

Implementation of universal blood an body-fluid precautions for *all* patients eliminates the need for warning labels on specimens since blood and other body fluids from all patients should be considered infective.

Environmental Considerations for HIV Transmission

No environmentally mediated mode of HIV transmission has been documented. Nevertheless, the precautions described below should be taken routinely in the care of *all* patients.

STERILIZATION AND DISINFECTION

Standard sterilization and disinfection procedures for patient-care equipment currently recommended for use in a variety of health-care settings —including hospitals, medical and dental clinics and offices, hemodialysis centers, emergency-care facilities, and long-term nursing-care facilities— are adequate to sterilize or disinfect instruments, devices, or other items contaminated with blood or other body fluids from persons infected with blood-borne pathogens including HIV.

Instruments or devices that enter sterile tissue or the vascular system of any patient or through which blood flows should be sterilized before reuse. Devices or items that contact intact mucous membranes should be sterilized or receive high-level disinfection, a procedure that kills vegetative organisms and viruses but not necessarily large numbers of bacterial spores. Chemical germicides that are registered with the U.S. Environmental Protection Agency (EPA) as "sterilants" may be used either for sterilization or for high-level disinfection depending on contact time.

Contact lenses used in trial fittings should be disinfected after each fitting by using a hydrogen peroxide contact lens disinfecting system or, if compatible, with heat (78° C-80° C [172.4° F-176.0° F]) for 10 minutes.

Medical devices or instruments that require sterilization or disinfection should be thoroughly cleaned before being exposed to the germicide, and the manufacturer's instructions for the use of the germicide should be followed. Further, it is important that the manufacturer's specifications for compatibility of the medical device with chemical germicides be closely followed. Information on specific label claims of commercial germicides can be obtained by writing to the Disinfectants Branch, Office of Pesticides, Environmental Protection Agency, 401 M Street, SW, Washington, D.C. 20460.

Studies have shown that HIV is inactivated rapidly after being exposed to commonly used chemical germicides at concentrations that are much lower than used in practice. Embalming fluids are similar to the types of chemical germicides that have been tested and found to completely inactivate HIV. In addition to commercially available chemical germicides, a solution of sodium hypochlorite (household bleach) prepared daily is an inexpensive and effective germicide. Concentrations ranging from approximately 500 ppm (1 : 100 dilution of household bleach) sodium hypochlorite to 5,000 ppm (1 : 10 dilution of household bleach) are effective depending on the amount of organic material (e.g., blood, mucus) present on the surface to be cleaned and disinfected. Commercially available chemical germicides may be more compatible with certain medical devices that might be corroded by repeated exposure to sodium hypochlorite, especially to the 1 : 10 dilution.

SURVIVAL OF HIV IN THE ENVIRONMENT

The most extensive study on the survival of HIV after drying involved greatly concentrated HIV samples, i.e., 10 million tissue-culture infectious doses per milliliter. This concentration is at least 100,000 times greater than that typically found in the blood or serum of patients with HIV infection. HIV was detectable by tissue-culture techniques 1–3 days after drying, but the rate of inactivation was rapid. Studies performed at CDC have also shown that drying HIV causes a rapid (within several hours) 1–2 log (90%–99%) reduction in HIV concentration. In tissue-culture fluid, cell-free HIV could be detected up to 15 days at room temperature, up to 11 days at 37° C (98.6° F), and up to 1 day if the HIV was cell-associated.

When considered in the context of environmental conditions in health-care facilities, these results do not require any changes in currently recommended sterilization, disinfection, or housekeeping strategies. When medical devices are contaminated with blood or other body fluids, existing recommendations include the cleaning of these instruments, followed by disinfection or sterilization, depending on the type of medical device. These protocols assume "worst-case" conditions of extreme virologic and microbiologic contamination, and whether viruses have been inactivated after drying plays no role in formulating these strategies. Consequently, no changes in published procedures for cleaning, disinfecting, or sterilizing need to be made.

HOUSEKEEPING

Environmental surfaces such as walls, floors, and other surfaces are not associated with transmission of infections to patients or health-care workers. Therefore, extraordinary attempts to disinfect or sterilize these environmental surfaces are not necessary. However, cleaning and removal of soil should be done routinely.

Cleaning schedules and methods vary according to the area of the hospital or institution, type of surface to be cleaned, and the amount and type of soil present. Horizontal surfaces (e.g., bedside tables and hard-surface flooring) in patient-care areas are usually cleaned on a regular basis, when soiling or spills occur, and when a patient is discharged. Cleaning of walls, blinds, and curtains is recommended only if they are visibly soiled. Disinfectant fogging is an unsatisfactory method of decontaminating air and surfaces and is not recommended.

Disinfectant-detergent formulations registered by EPA can be used for cleaning environmental surfaces, but the actual physical removal of microorganisms by scrubbing is probably at least as important as any antimicrobial effect of the cleaning agent used. Therefore, cost, safety, and acceptability by housekeepers can be the main criteria for selecting any such registered agent. The manufacturers' instructions for appropriate use should be followed.

CLEANING AND DECONTAMINATING SPILLS OF BLOOD OR OTHER BODY FLUIDS

Chemical germicides that are approved for use as "hospital disinfectants" and are tuberculocidal when used at recommended dilutions can be used to decontaminate spills of blood and other body fluids. Strategies for decontaminating spills of blood and other body fluids in a patient-care setting are different than for spills of cultures or other materials in clinical, public health, or research laboratories. In patient-care areas, visible material should first be removed and then the area should be decontaminated. With large spills of cultured or concentrated infectious agents in the laboratory, the contaminated area should be flooded with a liquid germicide before cleaning, then decontaminated with fresh germicidal chemical. In both settings, gloves should be worn during the cleaning and decontaminating procedures.

LAUNDRY

Although soiled linen has been identified as a source of large numbers of certain pathogenic microorganisms, the risk of actual disease transmission is negligible. Rather than rigid procedures and specifications, hygienic and common-sense storage and processing of clean and soiled linen are recommended. Soiled linen should be handled as little as possible and with minimum agitation to prevent gross microbial contamination of the air and of persons handling the linen. All soiled linen should be bagged at the location where it was used; it should not be sorted or rinsed in patient-care areas. Linen soiled with blood or body fluids should be placed and transported in bags that prevent leakage. If hot water is used, linen should be washed.

Special Precautions for Operation of a Cytopreparatory Laboratory

Notwithstanding the general rules summarized above, certain procedures that are specific for a cytopreparatory laboratory must be observed.

1. Laboratory request slips accompanying specimen should not remain wrapped around the specimen containers. The slips should be removed and placed in an area away from the preparation counter.
2. Prepare specimens in a room or area away from other work areas.
3. Process all specimens under a laminar flow hood. Disposable gloves, gowns, aprons, and face paper masks must be worn, particularly if there is a possibility of a spray of droplets (for example, blending of sputum). Remove such attire before leaving the laboratory and dispose of it in containers for infectious waste. Staining of specimens, however, may be performed in an open, well-ventilated area and does not require a laminar flow hood.
4. Cover the counter of the working area with absorbent paper toweling moistened with a disinfectant.
5. Inspect centrifuge tubes for cracks. Use disposable screw-cap plastic centrifuge tubes. Never

centrifuge or vortex in an open tube. Add a germicidal solution (1:10 dilution of 5.25% sodium hypochlorite [bleach]) between the centrifuge tube and trunnion cup.
6. Cytocentrifuge chambers must be decontaminated with germicidal solution.
7. Never pipette samples by mouth.
8. Develop the habit of keeping your hands away from your mouth, nose, eyes, and face.
9. Wash hands thoroughly after handling any specimen, including the outside of the specimen jar.
10. Discard needles into a special needle disposal container and residual fluids into an autoclaveable, splashproof container containing a small amount of disinfectant. Autoclave the container before disposing of the contents.
11. Contaminated equipment should be autoclaved before washing or disposal. Preferably this should be done in the laboratory area. If this is not possible, the material should be placed in a leakproof plastic bag and sealed. The sealed bag should be placed inside a leakproof autoclaveable pail with a cover.
12. Laboratory benches, work counters, and all surfaces where infectious material is handled should be disinfected after completion of specimen preparation.
13. Equipment used in the cytopreparation laboratory should not be used in other areas of the laboratory.
14. Limit the flow of traffic into and out of the cytopreparation area.
15. Never smoke, eat, or drink in the cytopreparatory laboratory.

SCREENING AND MARKING OF SMEARS

Slides are placed in the mechanical stage holder of the microscope with the label *always* on the same side, either left or right. The slides are best screened vertically, and there should be a slight overlapping of the screened areas so that no cells will be missed (Fig. 33–22). Although some individuals prefer to screen cytologic slides horizontally, this procedure may produce visual fatigue, since any optical aberrations in the glass slide or the cover glass are more noticeable and annoying. For screening, we recommend a 10× objective lens and 15× ocular lenses. This optical system will ensure optimal evaluation of small cells. For detailed examination of cells, a 40× objective lens should be used. Oil immersion is of limited use in diagnostic cytology.

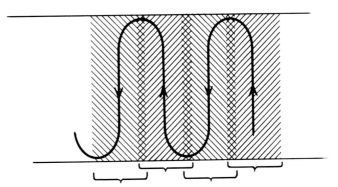

FIGURE 33–22. Diagram of correct screening of smears. A slight overlap of the fields of vision ensures that no important evidence is overlooked.

When marking cells, switch to a scanning lens and, using a pen with a fine point, place an ink dot next to the cell. The position of this mark in relation to the cells in question *should always be the same* (Fig. 33–23). A circle may be placed around the cells in the same way. A short time is required to master the technique of coordinating the hand while looking through the microscope.

The importance of proper screening of slides hardly needs to be emphasized. Marking of slides will facilitate the examination of the same cell or group of cells on numerous occasions or by several observers. Proper screening and marking of slides are indispensable in a well organized cytology laboratory.

ORGANIZATION OF THE CYTOLOGY LABORATORY

Federal and state agencies are in the process of revising and enacting accreditation regulations with which all laboratories will be required to comply. Organization, methods of reporting, quality control, and personnel requirements will no longer be matters of personal choice. The suggestions for the organization of a cytology laboratory, discussed below, should be in compliance with future government guidelines.

Screening of cytology material should be performed by well-trained and certified cytotechnologists. The duties of the cytotechnologists include cytopreparation or supervision of it; screening and marking of material; formulation of a preliminary diagnosis; and formulation of a final diagnosis in certain well-defined circumstances, such as the screening of an asymptomatic population.

The organization of a well-run, large laboratory of cytology is based on a system of checks and cross-checks to minimize errors. Such a system is outlined in Fig. 33–24. This system is based on identification of two major classes of material, one from symptomatic patients and the other from surveys of well population. Symptomatic patients include:

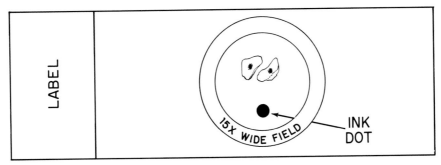

FIGURE 33–23. Diagram suggesting a method of marking slides. The actual marking takes place under direct vision with a low-power scanning lens. In this diagram the dot is placed beneath the cells, as originally suggested by Papanicolaou. However, any other location of marking dots is acceptable, provided that it is constant and observed by all members of the same laboratory.

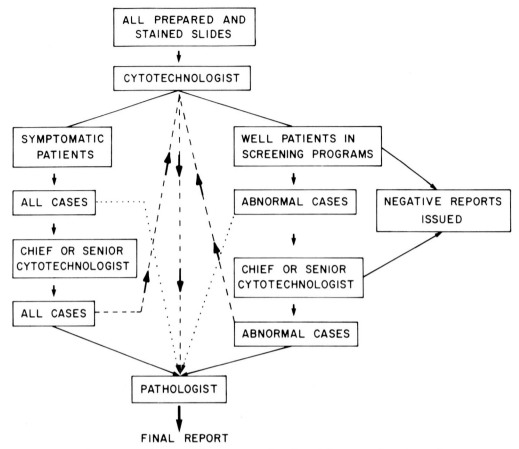

FIGURE 33–24. Suggested system of organization for a large laboratory of cytology offering a number of options (see text).

1. All patients from whom nongynecologic material is collected. Exceptions are special projects, such as screening for early lung cancer in asymptomatic patients, or rapid screening of all urine samples submitted for routine analysis.
2. Patients from whom gynecologic smears are obtained and who have a history of:

   A. Abnormal uterine bleeding
   B. Prior abnormal smears
   C. Cancer or precancerous states
   D. Radiation therapy

The diagram shown in Fig. 33–24 offers a number of options in the handling of material. The first option (*solid lines*) suggests that all cases requiring review by a pathologist should be funneled through a senior or chief cytotechnologist. This system deprives the less experienced cytotechnologists of contact with the pathologist. The second option (*broken lines*) provides for a review of material by a senior cytotechnologist prior to presentation of the

cases by the original screener to the pathologist. The third option (*dotted lines*) offers all cytotechnologists the opportunity to present cases directly to the pathologist. Regardless of the system adopted, channels of consultation at all levels of performance should remain open. It is particularly important for cytotechnologists at all levels of experience to be present when important diagnostic conclusions are reached on material screened by them. Open discussion of problem cases should be encouraged.

Quality Control

Quality control regulations vary, depending on the agency or association responsible for accrediting a laboratory. Each laboratory director must be aware of and strictly adhere to local and federal regulations. We recommend that a quality control program include the following:

1. Correlate cytologic diagnoses with surgical, autopsy, and clinical findings on all patients.
2. Rescreen those cases in which the cytology and histology or clinical history do not correlate.
3. At the time of screening, provide records of prior histologic and cytologic examinations for each patient.
4. Maintain a cross-file or record-keeping system to allow data retrieval for statistical evaluation, such as percentage of positives.
5. Prepare annual statistical correlation reports.
6. Retain reports and slides in a readily accessible area for at least 3 years, and keep cases exhibiting major abnormalities on file as long as the patient is alive but not less than 5 years.
7. Set up internal performance evaluation programs to demonstrate the competency and accuracy of technical personnel.
8. Encourage participation of cytotechnologists in continuing education programs, both internal and external.
9. In our experience the most important aspect of quality control is the constant review and correlation of cytologic findings with surgical and autopsy material. Particularly valuable is rescreening of previous material in patients who subsequently develop important abnormalities. For example, prior "negative" smears in patients with neoplastic lesions of the uterine cervix often will reveal missed evidence of disease. To this effect a constant review of records is mandatory. *A computerized recording system combining cytologic and tissue diagnoses is of great assistance in such efforts.* A satisfactory internal quality control system is difficult to devise. This may, in part, be accomplished by rescreening a certain percentage of negative smears (e.g., 10%, as now required by the Centers for Disease Control) or by inserting material of known diagnostic values into the routine flow and checking the performance of cytotechnologists and pathologists against this standard. The latter system requires destaining, restaining, and renumbering of known cases, a rather formidable procedure.

Reporting of Cytologic Material

A summary of the information that must accompany every cytologic specimen can be found in Chapter 32, p. 1430. The report must include:

1. Name of patient and the laboratory accession number.
2. Name of individual or facility to which the report is addressed.
3. Name and address of the laboratory.
4. The following dates:
   A. Sample collection.
   B. Sample received in the laboratory.
   C. Report issued.
5. Cytologic diagnosis.
6. Identification of cytopathologist and cytotechnologist responsible for the report.

Comment

Throughout this volume it has been pointed out that an accurate cytologic diagnosis of disease is both possible and desirable; therefore, the reports should be expressed in simple language that can be readily understood by the clinician. At one time, Papanicolaou's classification of smears performed a very useful role. However, it was abandoned in this laboratory many years ago in favor of a nomenclature in keeping with the principle of surgical pathology. Thus, the presence of cancer is always reported, and at all times an effort is made to determine — whenever possible — the histologic type, origin, and, occasionally, probable anatomic location of the tumor. In the absence of cancer, a simple diagnosis of "negative for malignant cells" is sufficient. If there is evidence of a noncancerous disease, this fact is also noted. The Bethesda reporting system for cervical smears is summarized on p. 486.

No matter how skillful the pathologist may be, in a certain number of cases it will not be possible to make a definite diagnosis on the strength of the cytologic evidence available. This situation may be due to insufficient sampling of a lesion, to the unfavorable anatomic location of the lesion, or to the nature of a lesion that may be difficult to classify even on the strength of very ample cytologic or histologic material. In such situations a descriptive diagnosis of the findings is, in our experience, more satisfying than any classification and is usually acceptable to the clinician as well. Such descriptive diagnoses should not become the repositories of ignorance but may well express the uncertainty of the observer. The diagnosis of "suspicious" should be made only if a lesion has a definite neoplastic slant, although more evidence is needed for a definitive diagnosis. In such instances it is wise to state, whenever possible, what type of lesion is anticipated. If the evidence is too scanty even for the diagnosis of "suspicious," it is best to withhold any opinion and simply ask for more material, never failing to mention the reason for the request.

If these simple principles of cytologic diagnosis are observed, the mutual respect of the pathologist for the clinician and of the clinician for the pathologist will be maintained in the field of diagnostic cytology.

Several illustrative examples of diagnoses from this laboratory are offered below.

Cervix and vagina—Diagnosis: Negative for malignant cells. Trichomonas infestation.

Cervix and vagina—Diagnosis: Suspicious. Smear pattern suggestive of CIN Gr. I (low-grade lesion, mild dysplasia). Suggest colposcopy.

Cervix and vagina—Diagnosis: Positive for malignant cells. Smear pattern of CIN Gr. III (high-grade lesion, carinoma in situ), keratinizing type. Suggest colposcopy.

Cervix and vagina—Diagnosis: Positive for malignant cells. Endometrial adenocarcinoma.

Sputum—Diagnosis: Negative for malignant cells. Changes suggestive of hyperplasia of bronchial mucosa are noted (bronchiectasis?).

Sputum—Diagnosis: Suspect adenocarcinoma. Additional evidence needed for further evaluation.

Sputum—Diagnosis: Positive for malignant cells. Necrotic squamous carcinoma.

Bronchial brushing—Diagnosis: There is no evidence of cancer, but the degree of atypia of bronchial lining cells calls for further investigation. Please submit more material.

Body fluids—Diagnosis: Positive for malignant cells. The type of tumor cannot be determined from the evidence available.

Urine—Diagnosis: Positive for malignant cells. Urothelial carcinoma.

BIBLIOGRAPHY

Adler, C.: Gelatin-chrome alum: A better section adhesive. Histo-logic, *8*:115–116, 1978.

Affandi, M.Z.: Use of hairspray as a smear fixative. Acta Cytol., *33*:419, 1989.

Anderson, G.H., Flynn, K.J., Hickey, L.A., LeRiche, J.C., Matisic, J.P., and Suen, K.C.: A comprehensive internal quality control system for a large cytology laboratory. Acta Cytol., *31*:895–899, 1987.

Arnold, J.B., Komp, D.M., Peterson, W.H., Johnston, C.L., and dos Santos-Neto, J.G.: The cytocentrifuge, a useful tool in cancer diagnosis. Va. Med., *100*:708–712, 1973.

Ayre, J.E., and Dakin, E.: Cervical cytology tests in cancer diagnosis: Glycerine technique for mailing. Can. Med. Assoc. J., *54*:489–491, 1946.

Bahr, G.F.: Some considerations of basic cell chemistry. *In* Keebler, C.M., Reagan, J.W., and Wied, G.L. (eds.): Compendium in Cytopreparatory Techniques, ed. 4. pp. 1–6. Chicago, Tutorials of Cytology, 1976.

Baker, J.R.: Cytological Technique: The Principles Underlying Routine Methods, ed. 5. London, Chapman and Hall Ltd., 1966.

Bales, C.E.: A semi-automated method for preparation of urine sediment for cytologic examination. Acta Cytol., *25*:323–326, 1981.

Barr, W.T.: Effects of sunlight on stained sections mounted in various media. Stain Technol., *45*:9–14, 1970.

Barr, W.T., Powell, D.E.B., and Raffan, J.B.: Cellular contamination during automatic and manual staining of cytological smears. J. Clin. Pathol., *23*:604–607, 1970.

Barrett, D.L.: Cytocentrifuge technique. *In* Keebler, C.M., Reagan, J.W., and Wied, G.L. (eds.): Compendium on Cytopreparatory Techniques, ed. 4. pp. 80–83. Chicago, Tutorials of Cytology, 1976.

Barrett, D.L., and King, E.B.: Comparison of cellular recovery rates and morphological detail obtained using membrane filter and cytocentrifuge techniques. Acta Cytol., *20*:174–180, 1976.

Barrett, D.L., and King, E.B.: Cytologic preparations from tissue: Cell suspension followed by membrane filtration. Cytotech. Bull., *13*:38–39, 1976.

Battifora, H., and Hidvegi, D.: Improved apparatus for spinal fluid cytomorphology. Acta Cytol., *22*:170–171, 1978.

Benestad, H.B., Rytomaa, T., and Svenson, T.: Some methods of assaying inhibitors of cell proliferation. Exp. Hematol., *8*:961–970, 1980,

Bennet, M.J., Ruberg, J., and Dixon, S.: A new semiautomated method for the concentration of cerebrospinal fluid for cytologic examination. Tech. Bull. Reg. Med. Tech., *38*:247–251, 1978.

Berkhan, E.: Measurement of DNA in cells of vaginal smears. A simple staining procedure for the pulse cytophotometric measurement. Arztl. Lab., *18*:77–79, 1972.

Berkow, R., and Talbott, J.H. (eds.): The Merck Manual of Diagnosis and Therapy. Rahway, N.J., Merck Sharp & Dohme Res. Labs., 1977.

Bertalanffy, F.D.: Fluorescence microscopy of cytodiagnosis of cancer. Postgrad. Med., *28*:627–633, 1960.

——: Evaluation of the acridine-orange microscopic method for cytodiagnosis of cancer. Ann. N.Y. Acad. Sci., *93*:715–750, 1962.

Bertalanffy, L., Masin, M., and Masin, F.: New and rapid method for diagnosis of vaginal and cervical cancer by fluorescence microscopy. Cancer, *11*:873–887, 1958.

Beyer-Boon, M.E., and Voorn-den Hollander, M.J.A.: Cell yield with various cytopreparatory techniques for urinary cytology. Acta Cytol., *22*:589–594, 1978.

Biggs, P.J., and Sarkar, R.K.: Cytologic examination of bronchoscopic biopsy supernates. Acta Cytol., *31*:83, 1987.

Blair, J.E., Lennette, E.H., and Truant, J.P.: Manual of Clinical Microbiology. Baltimore, Williams & Wilkins, 1970.

Boccato, P.: Polyvalent fixative for staining of fine needle aspirates. Acta Cytol., *29*:647–648, 1985.

Boccato, P., and Bovincini, A.: Modification of Fischer's method for urine cytology. Acta Cytol., *25*:5–6, 1981.

Bodily, H.L., Updyke, E.L., and Mason, J.O. (eds.): Diagnostic Procedures for Bacterial, Mycotic and Parasitic Infections. ed. 5. Am. Pub. Health Assoc. Inc., 1970.

Boon, M.E., Wickel, A.F., Ruth, A.M., and Davoren, M.B.: Role of the air bubble in increasing cell recovery using cytospin I and II. Acta Cytol., *27*:699–702, 1983.

Booth, E.: Safety and health in the cytology laboratory. Cytotech. Bull., *13*:66–67, 1976.

Borgstrom, E., Wahren, B., and Gustafson, H.: Fluorescence

methods for measuring the A, B, and H isoantigens on cytological material from bladder carcinoma. Urol. Res., *13*: 43–45, 1985.

Bots, G. Th. A.M., Went, L.N., and Schaberg, A.: Results of a sedimentation technique for cytology of cerebrospinal fluid. Acta Cytol., *8*:234–241, 1964.

Bowling, M.C., Smith, I.M., and Wescott, S.L.: A rapid staining method for *Pneumocystis carinii*. Am. J. Med. Tech., *39*: 267–268, 1973.

Böyum, A.: Separation of leucocytes from blood and bone marrow. Scand. J. Clin. Lab. Invest. [Suppl.], *21*:97, 1968.

Bush, C.L., and Nelson, G.E.: Xylene—dangers of its use in the histology and cytology laboratory. Lab. Med., *8*:16, 1977.

Chalvardjian, A.M., and Grawe, L.A.: A new procedure for the identification of *Pneumocystis carinii* casts in tissue sections and smears. J. Clin. Pathol., *16*:383–384, 1963.

Chamberlain, D.W., Braude, A.C., and Rebuck, A.S.: A critical evaluation of bronchoalveolar lavage: Criteria for identifying unsatisfactory specimens. Acta Cytol., *31*:599–605, 1987.

Chandra, P., Delaney, M.D., and Tuazon, C.: Role of special stains in the diagnosis of *Pneumocystis carinii* infection from bronchial washing specimens in patients with the acquired immune deficiency syndrome. Acta Cytol., *32*:105–108, 1988.

Chang, J.P., Anken, M.A., and Russell, W.O.: Sputum cell concentration by membrane filtration for cancer diagnosis. Acta Cytol., *5*:168–172,1961.

Chang, S.C., and Russell, W.O.: A simplified and rapid filtration technique for concentrating cancer cells in sputum. Acta Cytol., *8*:348–349, 1964.

Chu, E., Malmgren, R.A., DeWitt, S.H., and Ross, G.T.: Millipore technique for nuclear sex chromatin. Acta Cytol., *10*:89–92, 1966.

Churukian, C.J., and Schenk, E.A.: Rapid Grocott's methenamine—silver nitrate method for fungi and *Pneumocystis carinii*. (Letter to the Editor.) Am. J. Clin. Pathol., *68*:427–428, 1977.

Clark, G., ed.: Staining Procedures Used by the Biological Stain Commission. ed. 3. Baltimore, Williams & Wilkins, 1973.

Clark, G.: Comparison of various oxidants for alum hematoxylin. Stain Technol., *49*:225–227, 1974.

Cole, E.C.: Studies on hematoxylin stain. Stain Technol., *18*:125–142, 1943.

Collins, D.N., Kaufmann, W., and Albrecht, R.: New York State computerized proficiency testing program in exfoliative cytology: Evaluation. Acta Cytol., *15*:468–472, 1971.

Collins, D.N., Kaufmann, W., and Clinton, W.: Quality evaluation of cytology laboratories in New York State: (Expanded Program, 1971–73). Acta Cytol., *18*:404–413, 1974.

Coon, J.S., and Weinstein, R.S.: Detection of A,B,H tissue isoantigens by immunoperoxidase methods in normal and neooplastic urothelium. Comparison with the erythorocyte adherence method. Am. J. Clin. Pathol., *76*:163–171,1981.

Couture, M.L., Freund, M., and Katubig, C.P., Jr.: The isolation and identification of exfoliated prostate cells from human semen. Acta Cytol., *24*:262–267, 1980.

Crabtree, W.N., and Murphy, W.M.: The value of ethanol as a fixative in urinary cytology. Acta Cytol., *24*:452–455, 1980.

Cummings, D.: Mayer's mucicarmine stain for mucin. *In* Keebler, C.M., Reagan, J.W., and Wied, G.L. (eds.): Compendium on Cytopreparatory Techniques, ed. 4. p. 111. Chicago, Tutorials of Cytology, 1976.

Curry, H., Thompson, D.W., Dietrich, M., Lipa, M., Massarella, G.R., Taves, I.R., Wood, D.E., and Zuber, E.: Proficiency testing in cytology laboratories in Ontario, Canada: A

decade of experience: I. Introduction and description of the testing model. Acta Cytol., *31*:203–214, 1987.

Curry, H., Thompson, D.W., Dietrich, M., Lipa, M., Massarella, G.R., Taves, I.R., Wood, D.E., and Zuber, E.: Proficiency testing in cytology laboratories in Ontario, Canada: A decade of experience: II. Results of initial surveys. Acta Cytol., *31*:215–219, 1987.

Curry, H., Thompson, D.W., Dietrich, M., Lipa, M., Massarella, G.R., Taves, I.R., Wood, D.E., and Zuber, E.: Proficiency testing in cytology laboratories in Ontartio, Canada: A decade of experience: III. A precision study of consistency and reproducibility in cytology reporting. Acta Cytol., *31*:220–225, 1987.

Dakin, E.S.: Improved adhesion and visibility of cytologic preparations by the use of the frosted glass slide. Science, *124*:474–475, 1955.

Damien, Sister Mary: Tips on Technique. (Letter to Editor.) Cytotech. Bull., *14*:12, 1977.

Danos, M.L.: Fixatives for Cytologic Use. *In* Keebler, C.M., Reagan, J.W., and Wied, G.L., (eds.): Compendium on Cytopreparatory Techniques. pp. 7–9. Chicago, Tutorials of Cytology, 1976.

Danos, M.L.: The Papanicolaou Staining Procedure. *In* Keebler, C.M., Reagan, J.W., and Wied, G.L. (eds.): Compendium on Cytopreparatory Techniques, ed. 4. pp. 10–15. Chicago, Tutorials of Cytology, 1976.

Danos, M.L.: Hematoxylin crisis—what does it mean to you? Cytotech Bull., *12*:1–4, 1975.

Danos, M.L., Holmquist, M.: The effect of distance in aerosol fixation of cytologic specimens. Cytotech. Bull., *15*:25–27, 1978.

Dart, L.H., Jr., and Turner, T.R.: Fluorescence microscopy in exfoliative cytology; report of acridine orange examination of 5491 cases, with comparison by Papanicolaou technic. Lab. Invest. *8*:1513–1522, 1959.

Davis, J.R., Hindman, W.M., Paplanus, S.H., Trego, D.C., Wiens, J.L., and Suciu, T.N.: Value of duplicate smears in cervical cytology. Aca Cytol., *25*:533–538, 1981.

DeFine, L.A., Saleba, K.P., Gibson, B.B., Wesseler, T.A., and Baughman, R.: Cytologic evaluation of bronchoalveolar lavage specimens in immunosuppressed patients with suspected opportunistic infections. Acta Cytol., *31*:235–242, 1987.

Dekker, A., and Bupp, P.A.: Cytology of serous effusions: A comparative study of two slightly different preparative methods. Acta Cytol., *20*:394–399, 1976.

del Vecchio, P.R., DeWitt, S.H., Borelli, J.I., Ward, J.B., Wood, Jr. T.A., and Malmgren, R.A.: Application of Millipore filtration technique to cytologic material. J.N.C.I., *22*:427–431, 1959.

Dempster, W.T.: Rates of penetration of fixing fluids. Am. J. Anat., *107*:59–72, 1960.

DeWitt, S.H., del Veechio, P.R., Borelli, J.I., and Hilberg, A.W.: A method for preparing wound washings and bloody fluids for cytologic evaluation, J.N.C.I., *19*:115–121, 1957.

Disbey, B.D., and Rack, J.H.: Histological Laboratory Methods. Edinburgh, Livingstone, 1970.

Dore, C.F., and Balfour, B.M.: A device for preparing cell spreads. Immunology, *9*:403–405, 1965.

Drewinko, B., Sullivan, M.P., and Martin, T.: Use of the cytocentrifuge in the diagnosis of meningeal leukemia. Cancer, *31*:1331–1336, 1973.

Drijver, J.S., and Boon, M.E.: Manipulating the Papanicolaou staining method: Role of acidity in the EA counterstain. Acta Cytol., *27*:693–698, 1983.

Drijver, J.S., and Boon, M.E.: Tertiary butanol as a substitute for xylene as a clearing agent. Acta Cytol., *27*:210, 1983.

Dubay, E.C., and Grubb, R.D.: Infection Prevention and Control. St. Louis, C.V. Mosby, 1973.

Duggan, M.A., Pomponi, C., Kay, D., and Robboy, S.J.: Infantile chlamydial conjunctivitis. A comparison of Papanicolaou, Giemsa and immunoperoxidase staining methods. Acta Cytol., 30:341–346, 1986.

Dunlap, L.A., Warters, R.L., and Leif, R.C.: Centrifugal cytology. III. The utilization of centrifugal cytology for the preparation of fixed stained dispersions of cells separated by bovine serum albumin buoyant density centrifugation. J. Histochem. Cytochem., 23:369–377, 1975.

Dyken, P.R., Shirley, S., Jill Trefz, B.S., and El Gammal, T.: Comparison of cytocentrifugation and sedimentation techniques for CSF cytomorphology. Acta Cytol., 24:167–170, 1980.

Ehrenreich, T., and Kerpe, S.: New and rapid method of obtaining dry, fixed cytological smeas. J.A.M.A., 170:1176–1177, 1959.

Elefson, D.E.: Infectious hazards in cytology. In Keebler, C.M., Reagan, J.W., and Wied, G.L. (eds.): Compendium on Cytopreparatory Techniques, ed. 4. pp. 91–94. Chicago, Tutorials of Cytology, 1976.

Elequin, F.T., Franco, M.M., Ghossein, N.A., and Schreiber, K.: A quick method for concentrating and pocessing cancer cells from serous fluids and fine needle nodule aspirates. Acta Cytol., 21:596–599, 1977.

Elevitch, F.R., and Brunson, J.G.: Rapid identification of malignant cells in vaginal smears by cytoplasmic fluorescence. Surg. Gynecol. Obstet., 112:3–10, 1961.

Elias, A., Linthorst, G., Bekker, B., and Vooijs, P.G.: The significance of endocervical cells in the diagnosis of cervical epithelial changes. Acta Cytol., 27:225–229, 1983.

Eneström, S.: Some aspects on technique and clinical evaluation of CSF cytology. Acta Neurol. Scand., 41:153–159, 1965.

Engel, H., de la Cruz, Z.C., Jimenez-Albalahin, L.D., Green, W.R., and Michels, R.G.: Cytopreparatory techniques for eye fluid specimens obtained by vitrectomy. Acta Cytol., 26:551–560, 1982.

Fawcett, D.W., and Vallee, B.L.: Studies on the separation of cell types in serosanguinous fluids, blood, and vaginal fluids. J. Lab. Clin. Med., 39:354–364, 1952.

Fawcett, D.W., Valley, B.L., and Soule, M.H.: A method for concentration and segregation of malignant cells from bloody pleural and peritoneal fluids. Science, 111:34, 1950.

Fleischer, R.L., Price, P.B., and Symes, E.M.: Novel filter for biological materials. Science, 143:249–250, 1964.

Fleury, J., Escudier, E., Pocholle, M.-J., Carre, C., and Bernaudin, J.-F.: Cell population obtained by bronchoalveolar lavage in Pneumocystis carinii pneumonitis. Acta Cytol., 29:721–726, 1985.

Fleury-Feith, J., Escudier, E., Pocholle, M.J., Care, C., and Bernaudin, J.F.: The effects of cytocentrifugation on differential cell counts in samples obtained by bronchoalveolar lavage. Acta Cytol., 31:606–610, 1985.

Foot, N.C.: The identification of mesothelial cells in sediments of serous effusions. Cancer, 12:429–437, 1959.

Foot, N.C., and Holmquist, N.D.: Supravital staining of sediments of serous effusions: Simple technique for rapid cytological diagnosis. Cancer, 11:151–157, 1958.

Freeman, J.: Hair spray: An inexpensive aerosol fixative for cytodiagnosis. Acta Cytol., 13:416–419, 1967.

Frost, J.K., Gill, G., Hankins, A.G., LaCorte, F.J., Miller, R.A., and Hollander, D.H.: Cytology filter preparations: Factors affecting their quality for study of circulating cancer cells in the blood. Acta Cytol., 11:363–373, 1967.

Gelman Instrument Company: Gelman Membrane Filtration Products, Ann Arbor, 1973.

General Electric: Nucleopore Membrane Filters—Application Handbook, GEZ-4351. Techniques for Exfoliative Cytology. Phesanton, California, 1967.

Ghali, V.S., Garcia, R.L., and Skolom, J.: Fluorescence of Pneumocystis carinii in Papanicolaou smears. Hum. Pathol., 11:907–909, 1980.

Gigliotti, F., Stokes, D.C., Cheatham, A.B., et al.: Development of murine monoclonal antibodies to Pneumocystis carinii. J. Immunol. Methods, 154:315–322,1986.

Gill, G.W.: Dissolving nucleopore filters on micro slides before staining and without allowing air-drying. The Cytotechnologist Bulletin, 27:1980.

Gill, G.W.: Exfoliative Cytology. Millipore Application Report AR-24, 1969.

———: Principles and Practice of Cytopreparation. In Alman, N.H., and Melby, E.C. (ed.): Handbook of Laboratory Animal Science III. pp. 519–551. Cleveland, C.R.C. Press, 1976.

———: A cross contamination control and stain storage system. Cytotech Bull., 12:12–13, 1975.

———: Comparative filter techniques. Acta Cytol., 19:207–210, 1975.

———: Methods of cell collection on membrane filters. In Keebler, C.M., Reagan, J.W., and Wied, G.L. (eds.): Compendium on Cytopreparatory Techniques. pp. 34–44. Chicago, Tutorials of Cytology, 1976.

———: Cytopreparation of prefixed sputum specimens. In Keebler, C.M., Reagan, J.W., and Wield, G.L. (eds.): Compendium on Cytopreparatory Techniques. ed. 4. Chicago, Tutorials of Cytology, 1976.

Gill, G.W., Frost, J.K., and Miller, K.A.: A new formula for a half-oxidized hematoxylin solution that neither overstains nor requires differentiation. Acta Cytol., 18:300–311, 1974.

Gomori, G.: A new histochemical test for glycogen and mucin. Am. J. Clin. Pathol., 10:177–179, 1946.

Graham, R.M.: The Cytologic Diagnosis of Cancer. ed. 3. Philadelphia, W.B. Saunders, 1972.

Greaves, T.S., and Strigle, S.M.: The recognition of Pneumocystis carinii in routine Papanicolaou-stained smears. Acta Cytol., 29:714–720, 1985.

Green, F.J.: Getting more uniform results from biological stains. Lab. Management, 7:22–23,35–36, 1969.

Grimm, R.: Tips on technique. (Letter to the Editor.) Cytotech Bull., 12:12–13, 1975.

Grocott, R.G.: A stain for fungi in tissue sections and smears using Gomori's methenamine-silver nitrate technic. Am. J. Clin. Pathol., 25:975–979, 1955.

Guard, H.R.: New technic for differential staining of sex chromatin, and determination of its incidence in exfoliated vaginal epithelial cells. Am. J. Clin. Pathol., 32:145–151, 1959.

Gubin, N.: Hematoxylin-and-eosin staining of fine needle aspirate smears. Acta Cytol., 29:648–650, 1985.

Hansen, H.H., Bender, R.A., and Shelton, B.J.: The cytocentrifuge and cerebrospinal fluid cytology. Acta Cytol., 18:259–262, 1974.

Harpst, H.C., Ware, R.E., Eisenberg, R.B., and O'Dell, J.B.: Exfoliative cytology of the urinary tract. Evaluation of the Millipore technic. Acta Cytol., 5:195–197, 1961.

Harris, M.J.: Laboratory safety. In Keebler, C.M., Reagan, J.W., and Wied, G.L. (eds.): Compendium of Cytopreparatory Techniques. ed. 4. pp. 84–90. Chicago, Tutorials of Cytology, 1976.

Harris, M.J.: Cell block preparations. 3% bacterial agar and plasma-thrombin clot methods. Cytotech. Bull., *11*:6–7, 1974.

Harris, M.J., Bibbo, M., Rao, C., and Wied, G.L.: Cytopreparatory techniques for the endometrial jet wash specimen. Acta Cytol., *16*:508–516, 1972.

Harris, M.J., and Keebler, C.M.: Cytopreparatory Techniques. *In* Keebler, C.M., Reagan, J.W., and Wied, G.L. (eds.): Compendium of Cytopreparatory Techniques. ed. 4. pp.45–58. Chicago, Tutorials of Cytology, 1976.

Heinzl, J.: Tips on technique. (Letter to the Editor.) Cytotech. Bull., *13*:30, 1976.

Henry, M.J., Burton, L.G., Stanley, M.W., and Horwitz, C.A.: Application of a modified Diff-Quik stain to fine needle aspiration smears: Rapid staining with improved cytologic detail. Acta Cytol., *31*:954–955, 1987.

Hidvegi, D.F., and Hultgren, S.: Mending broken slides. Acta Cytol., *29*:495–496, 1985.

Hindman, W.M.: A proposal for quality control in gynecologic cytology. Acta Cytol., *31*:384–385, 1987.

Hindman, W.M.: An effective quality control program for the cytology laboratory. Acta Cytol., *20*:233–238, 1976.

Hollander, D.H.: An oil-soluble antitoxidant in resinous mounting media to inhibit fading of Romanowsky stains. Stain Technol., *38*:288–289, 1963.

Hollander, D.H., and Frost, J.K.: Annual bands in synthetic-resin mounted microscopic slides. Acta Cytol., *14*:142–144, 1970.

———: Antioxidant inhibition of stain fading and mounting medium crazing. Acta Cytol., *15*:419, 1971.

Holm, K., Grinsted, P., Poulsen, E.F., and Fenger, C.: Can hairspray be used as a smear fixative?: A comparison between two types of coating fixatives. Acta Cytol., *32*:422–424, 1988.

Holmes, W.C.: The microscopists's need for data on dye solubilites. Stain Technol., *2*:40–43, 1927.

Hopwood, D.: Fixatives and fixation: A review. Histochem. J., *1*:323–360, 1969.

Horai, T., and Ueki, A.: The cell concentration method using acetylcysteine for sputum cytology. Acta Cytol., *22*:580–583, 1978.

Horobin, R.W.: The impurities of biological dyes: Their detection, removal, occurence, and histological significance—a review. Histochem. J., *1*:231–265, 1969.

Horwitz, R.I., and Feinstein, A.R.: Alternative analytic methods for case-control studies of estrogens and endometrial cancer. N. Engl. J. Med., *299*:1089–1094, 1978.

Husain, O.A.N., Butler, E.B., Evans, D.M.D., MacGregor, J.E., and Yule, R.: Quality control in cervical cytology. J. Clin. Pathol., *27*:935–944, 1974.

The International Academy of Cytology's policy statement on the frequency of gynecologic screening. Acta Cytol., *24*:371–372, 1980.

Jampolis, R.W., McDonald, J., and Clagett, O.T.: Mineral oil granuloma of the lungs: An evaluation of methods for identification of mineral oil in tissue. Surg. Gynecol. Obstet., *97*:105–119, 1953.

Jimenez-Joseph, D., and Gangi, M.D.: Application of diatex compound in cytology: Use in preparing multiple slides from a single routine smear. Acta Cytol., *30*:446–447, 1986.

Juniper, K., and Chester, C.L.: A filter membrane technique for cytological study of exfoliated cells in body cavity fluids. Cancer, *12*:278–285, 1959.

Kaltenbach, F.J., Hillemanns, H.G., Fetig, O., and Hilgarth, M.: Thrombin cell block technic in gynecological cytodiagnosis. Acta Cytol., *17*:128–130, 1973.

Kaplow, L.S.: Commercial hair sprays as fixatives for hematological cytochemistry. Stain Technol., *46*:177–182, 1971.

Keebler, C.M., and Reagan, J.W. (eds.): A Manual of Cytotechnology. ed. 4. Chicago, American Soc. Clin. Pathol., 1976 (reprint of 1962 edition).

Keebler, C.M., Reagan, J.W., and Wied, G.L. (eds.): Compendium on Cytopreparatory Techniques, ed. 3. Chicago, Tutorials of Cytology, 1974.

———: Compendium on Cytopreparatory Techniques. ed. 4. Chicago, Tutorials of Cytology, 1976.

Kelly, L.V.: Recovery of diagnostic cells from bloody effusions. cytotech. Bull., *14*:12, 1977.

Kirk, R.S., and Boon, M.E.: A comparison of the efficiency of diagnosis of early cervical carcinoma by general practitioners and cytology screening programs in the Netherlands. Acta Cytol., *25*:259–262, 1981.

Kivlahan, C., and Ingram, E.: Papanicolaou smears without endocervical cells: Are they adequate? Acta Cytol., *30*:258–260, 1986.

Klinkhamer, P.J.J.M., Vooijs, G.P., and de Haan, A.F.J.: Intraobserver and interobserver variability in the quality assessment of cervical smears. Acta Cytol., *33*:215–218, 1989.

Klosevych, S.: Photomicrography-importance of the cover glass thickness. J. Biol. Photogr., *34*:1–6, 1966.

———: Further notes on the importance of cover glass thickness. J. Biol. Photogr., *34*:101, 1966.

Knudtson, K.P.: Mucolytic action of hyaluronidase on sputum for the cytological diagnosis of lung cancer. Acta Cytol., *7*:59–61, 1962.

Kölmel, H.W.: A method for concentrating cerebrospinal fluid cells. Acta Cytol., *21*:154–157, 1977.

Komp, D.M., and Cox, B.J.: Cytocentrifugation in the management of central nervous system leukemia. J. Pediatr., *81*:92–994, 1972.

Koprowska, I.: Early use of the vaginal smear for cervical cancer detection. Acta Cytol., *25*:202, 1981.

Koss, L.G.: The attack on the annual "Pap smear." Acta Cytol., *24*:181–183, 1980.

Koss, L.G., Deitch, D., Ramanthan, R., and Sherman, A.B.: Diagnostic value of cytology of voided urine. Acta Cytol., *29*:810–816, 1985.

Koss, L.G., Eppich, E.M., Medler, K.H., and Wersto, R.P.: DNA cytophotometry of voided urine sediment: Comparison with results of cytologic diagnosis and image analysis. Anal. Quant. Cytol. Hist., *9*:398–404, 1987.

Koss, L.G., Sherman, A.B., and Eppich, E.: Image analysis and DNA content of urothelial cells infected with human polyomavirus. Anal. Quant. Cytol., *6*:89–94, 1984.

Koss, L.G., Sherman, A.B., and Adams, S.E.: The use of hierarchic classification in the image analysis of a complex cell population. Experience with the sediment of voided urine. Anal. Quant. Cytol., *5*:159–166, 1983.

Krogerus, L.A., and Anderson, L.C.: A simple method for the preparation of paraffin—embedded cell blocks from fine needle aspirates, effusions and brushings. Acta Cytol., *32*:585–587, 1988.

Lecioni, L.J., Amezaga, L.A.M., and LoBianco, V.S.: Urocytogram and pregnancy. I. Methods and normal values. Acta Cytol., *13*:279–287, 1969.

Lefer, L.G., Rosier, R.P., and Dornseif, B.E.: Resolution of irregular staining pattern of Pap smears. Acta Cytol., *22*:66, 1978.

Leif, R.C., Bobbit, D., Railey, C., Guarino, V., DerHagopian, R., Ng, A.B.P., and Silverman, M.: Centrifugal cytology of nipple aspirate cells. Acta Cytol., *22*:255–261, 1980.

Lillie, R.D.: Histopathologic Technic and Practical Histochemistry. ed. 3. New York, Blakiston Div., McGraw-Hill, 1965.

Lillie, R.D., and Fullmer, H.: Histopathologic Technic and Practical Histochemistry. ed. 4. New York, McGraw-Hill, 1976.

Lindberg, L.G., and Ohlin, B.: Specimen fixation in urinary cytology. Acta Cytol., 22:142–145, 1978.

Liu, W.: A simplified cytologic staining technique. Am. J. Clin. Pathol., 54:767–768, 1970.

Loughman, N.T.: *Pneumocystis carinii*: Rapid diagnosis with the microwave oven. Acta Cytol., 33:416–417, 1989.

Luna, L.G. (ed.): Manual of Histologic Staining Methods of the Armed Forces Institute of Pathology. ed. 3. New York, McGraw-Hill, 1968.

Luzzato, R., and Teloken, C.: Use of the cytobrush in the diagnosis of male urethral herpesvirus infection. Acta Cytol., 33:417–418, 1989.

McAlpine, L.L., and Ellsworth, B.: A modified membrane filter technique for cytodiagnosis. Techn. Bull. Reg. Med. Techn., 39:154–156, 1969.

McCarty, S.A.: Solving the cytopreparation problem of mucoid specimens with a mucoliquifying agent (MucoLexx) and Nuclepore filters. Acta Cytol., 16:221–223, 1972.

McCarty, K.S., Jr., Miller, L.S., Cox, E.B., Konrath, J., and McCarty, K.S., Sr.: Estrogen receptor analyses: Correlation of biochemical and immunohistological methods using monoclonal antireceptor antibodies. Arch. Pathol. Lab. Med., 109:716–721, 1985.

McGrew, E., and Nanos, S.: The cytology of serious effusions. *In* Wied, G.L., Koss, L.G., and Reagan, J.W.: Compendium on Diagnostic Cytology, ed. 4. pp. 370–379. Chicago, Tutorials of Cytology, 1976.

———: The Cytology of Serous Effusions. *In* Keebler, C.M., Reagan, J.W., and Wied, G.L. (eds.): Compendium on Cytopreparatory Techniques. ed. 4. pp. 75–79. Chicago, Tutorials of Cytology, 1976.

McLennan, B.L., Oertel, Y.C., Malmgren, R.A., and Mendoza, M.: The effect of water soluble contrast material on urine cytology. Acta Cytol., 22:230–233, 1978.

Mallory, F.B.: Pathological Technique. p. 130. New York, Hafner, 1961.

Mandell, D.B., Levy, J.J., and Rosenthal, D.L.: Preparation and cytologic evaluation of intraocular fluids. Acta Cytol., 31:150–158, 1987.

Manual of Histologic and Special Staining Technics. Armed Forces Institute of Pathology. ed. 2. New York, McGraw-Hill, 1960.

Manufacturing Chemists Association. Guide for Safety in the Chemical Laboratory. ed. 2. New York, Van Nostrand Reinhold, 1972.

Markowitz, S., and Leiman, G.: Cytologic detection of *Pneumocystis carinii* by ultraviolet light examination of Papanicolaou-stained sputum specimens. Acta Cytol., 30:79–80, 1986.

Marsan, C., Pasteur, X., Alepee, B., Laurent, J.-L., Accard, J.-L., Cava, E., Eloit, P., and Maoret, J.: Automatic cytopathologic diagnosis of bronchial carcinoma: I. Cytocentrifugation of bronchial brushings for image analysis. Acta Cytol., 26:545–550, 1982.

Marshall, P.N., and Horobin, R.W.: The oxidation products of hematoxylin and their role in biological staining. Histochem. J., 4:493–503, 1972.

Marwah, S., Devlin, D., and Dekker, A.: A comparative cytologic study of 100 urine specimens processed by the slide centrifuge and membrane filter techniques. Acta Cytol., 22:431–434, 1978.

Masin, F., and Masin, M.: Sputum blending. Acta Cytol., 22:442–443, 1978.

Masukawa, T.: Improved cell collection technique in breast cytology. Cytotech. Bull., 7:7, 1970.

Melamed, M.R.: Quality control in the cytology laboratory. Acta Cytol., 20:203–206, 1976.

Melder, K.K., and Koss, L.G.: Automated image analysis in the diagnosis of bladder cancer. Applied Optics, 26:3367–3372, 1987.

Menzies, D.W.: Nucleolar definition in hemalum and eosin staining. Stain Technol., 37:41–42, 1962.

Meyers, D.S., and Gillies, W.F.: Rapid staining technique for fine needle aspiration of the lung. Acta Cytol., 26:265–266, 1982.

Mikel, U.V., and Johnson, F.B.: A simple method for the study of the same cells by light and scanning electron microscopy. Acta Cytol., 24:252–254, 1980.

Miller, F.: Cytopreparatory methods—collection, smearing, staining, screening and reporting. *In* Keebler, C.M., Reagan, J.W., and Wied, G.L. (eds.): Compendium on Cytopreparatory Techniques. ed. 4. pp. 59–69. Chicago, Tutorials of Cytology, 1976.

Millipore Corporation: 1975 Millipore Catalogue and Purchasing Guide, Bedford, Mass. 01730.

Minami, R., Yokota, S., and Teplitz, R.L.: Gradient separation of normal and malignant cells—II. Application to in vivo tumor diagnosis. Acta Cytol., 22:584–588, 1978.

Mitchell, H., Medley, G., and Drake, M.: Quality control measures for cervical cytology laboratories. Acta Cytol., 32:288–292, 1988.

Morris, H.H.B., and Bennett, M.J.: The classification and origin of amniotic fluid cells. Acta Cytol., 18:149–154, 1974.

Mowry, R.W.: Alcian blue and alcian blue-periodic acid Schiff stains for carbohydrates. *In* Manual of Histologic and Special Staining Technics. Armed Forces Institute of Pathology, ed. 2. pp. 142–144. New York, McGraw-Hill, 1960.

Mygind, H., and Bjerregaard, B.: Value of the filter imprint technique in aspiration biopsy cytology. Acta Cytol., 30:75–78, 1986.

Mygind, H., and Lauritzen, A.F.: Influence of prefixation and fixation times on cellular preservation and epithelial cellularity in filter imprints. Acta Cytol., 31:950–953, 1987.

Nagalotimath, S.J., Patil, P.V., and Pai, N.: Cytodiagnosis of smears prepared from sediment of biopsy specimen fixatives. Acta Cytol., 31:531–532, 1987.

Nagasawa, T., and Tatsumi, J.: Cytocentrifugal disc plate for preparation of cytologic samples. Acta Cytol., 30:447–450, 1986.

Naib, Z.M.: Exfoliative Cytopathology, ed. 2. Boston, Little, Brown & Co., 1976.

Naylor, B.: The elimination of a "ribbing" effect observed in cytologic smears. Am. J. Clin. Pathol., 30:143–144, 1958.

Nelson, K.W., Ege, J.F., Jr., Roos, M., Woodman, L.E., and Silverman, L.: Sensory response to certain industrial solvent vapors. J. Industrial Hygiene Toxicology, 25:282–285, 1943.

Nieburgs, H.E.: Cytologic Technics for Office and Clinic. New York, Grune & Stratton, 1956.

Nielsen, M.L., Fischer, S., Hogsborg, E., and Therkelsen, K.: Adhesives for retaining prefixed urothelial cells on slides after imprinting from cellulosic filters. Acta Cytol., 27:371–375, 1983.

Niwayama, G., Walker, B., and Neal, C.: Modified filter preparation for effusion cytology. Cytotech. Bull., 13:10, 1976.

Noble, P.B., Cutts, J.H., and Carroll, K.K.: Ficoll flotation for the separation of blood leukocyte types. Blood, *31*:66–73, 1968.

Nuclepore Corporation: Nucleopore Specifications and Physical Properties, Pleasanton, California 94566, 1973.

———: Diagnostic Cytology. Pleasanton, California, 1975.

Occupational Exposure to Xylene. Washington, D.C.: Education and Welfare, U.S. Dept of Health, 1975.

Ocklind, G.: Optically eliminating the visible outlines of pores in intact polycarbonate (Nuclepore) filters. Acta Cytol., *31*:946–949, 1987.

O'Hara, C.M., and Birmingham, S.P.: Sputum fixatives: How safe is 50 per cent alcohol? Acta Cytol., *20*:400–403, 1976.

Olson, N.J., Gogel, H.K., Williams, W.L., and Mettler, F.A.: Processing of aspiration cytology samples: An alternate method. Acta Cytol., *30*:409–412, 1986.

Orenstein, M., Webber, C.A., and Huerich, A.E.: Cytologic diagnosis of *Pneumocystis carinii* infection by bronchoalveolar lavage in acquired immune deficiency syndrome. Acta Cytol., *29*:727–731, 1985.

Pak, H.Y., Yokota, S., Teplitz, R.L., Shaw, S.L., and Werner, J.L.: Rapid staining techniques employed in fine needle aspirations of the lung. Acta Cytol., *25*:178–184, 1981.

Papanicolaou, G.N.: A new procedure for staining vaginal smears. Science, *95*:438–439, 1942.

———: Atlas of Exfoliative Cytology. Cambridge, Mass., Harvard University Press, 1954.

Papanicolaou, G.N., and Bridges, E.L.: Simple method for protecting fresh smears from drying and deterioration during mailing. J.A.M.A., *164*:1330–1331, 1957.

"The Papanicolaou Stain," supplementary literature to the films "The Papanicolaou Stain: Principles" and "The Papanicolaou Stain: Materials and Methods," 1975. Available from Wexler Film Productions, 801 N. Seward St., Los Angeles, California 90038

Paris, A.L., and Solomon, D.E.: Conference on the state of the art in quality control measures for diagnostic cytology laboratories (Multiple authors). Acta Cytol., *33*:423–490, 1989.

Pearson, J.C., Kromhout, L., and King, E.B.: Evaluation of collection and preservation techniques for urinary cytology. Acta Cytol., *25*:327–333, 1981.

Pedersen, B., Brons, M., Holm, K., Pedersen, D., and Lund, C.: The value of provoked expectoration in obtaining sputum samples for cytologic investigation: A prospective, consecutive and controlled investigation of 134 patients. Acta Cytol., *29*:750–752, 1985.

Pelc, S.: Cytocentrifugation of cerebrospinal fluid with dextran: Improvement of the standard technique using the cytospin apparatus. Acta Cytol., *26*:721–724, 1982.

Periasamy, K.: A technique of staining sections of paraffin-embedded plant materials without employing a graded ethanol series. J. R. Micr. Soc., *87*:109–112, 1967.

Permissible Levels of Toxic Substances in the Working Environment. 6th session of the Joint ILO-WHO Committee on Occupational Health, Geneva, 1968.

Pfitzer, P., Wehle, K., Blanke, M., and Burrig, K.F.: Fluorescence microscopy of Papanicolaou-stained bronchoalveolar lavage specimens in the diagnosis of *Pneumocystis carinii*. Acta Cytol., *33*:557–558, 1989.

Pharr, S.L., and Farber, S.M.: Cellular concentration of sputum and bronchial aspirations by tryptic digestion. Acta Cytol., *6*:447–454, 1962.

Phillips, R.A., Van Slyke, D.D., Dole, V.P., et al.: cited by Seal, S.H. (1959).

Pieslor, P.C., Oertel, Y.C., and Mendoza, M.: The use of 2-molar urea as a hemolyzing solution for cytologic smears. Acta Cytol., *23*:137–139, 1979.

Piontkowski, P.: Tips on technique: Hairspray as a pre-fixative for cytocentrifuge specimens. Cytotech. Bull., *13*:60–61, 1976.

Plott, A.E., Martin, F.J., Cheek, S.W., Yobs, A.R., and Wood, R.J.: Measuring screening skills in gynecologic cytology: Results of voluntary self-assessment. Acta Cytol., *31*:911–923, 1987.

Plowden, K.M., and Gill, G.W.: Pitfalls in cytopreparation with membrane filters. Cytotech. Bull., *12*:8–10, 1975.

Pollock, P.G., Valicenti, J.F., Jr., Meyers, D.S., Frable, W.J., and Durham, J.B.: The use of fluorescent and special staining techniques in the aspiration of nocardiosis and actinomycosis. Acta Cytol., *22*:575–579, 1978.

Preece, A.: Manual for Histologic Technicians. ed. 3. Boston, Little, Brown & Co., 1972.

Pundel, J.P., and Lichfus, C.: Modifications de la coloration cytologique des frottis vaginaux a l'hématoxyline-Shorr. Gynaecologia [Suppl.], *144*:58–60, 1957.

Qin, D.: Use of neostigmine to increase the rate of lung cancer detection by sputum cytology. Acta Cytol., *30*:547–548, 1986.

Quality control in the cytology laboratory. Symposium by mail. Cytotech. Bull., *12*:(2), 1–7, and (3), 1–8, 1975.

Rappaport, S.M., and Campbell, E.E.: The interpretation and application of OSHA carcinogen standards for laboratory operations. Am. Ind. Hyg., Assoc. J., *37*:690–696, 1976.

Rasmussen, K.: Tips on technique. (Letter to Editor.) Cytotech. Bull., *13*:30, 1976.

Reddish, G.F. (ed.): Antiseptics, Disinfectants, Fungicides and Chemical and Physical Sterilization. Philadelphia, Lea & Febiger, 1954.

Reynaud, A.J., and King, E.B.: A new filter for diagnostic cytology. Acta Cytol., *11*:289–294, 1967.

Richardson, H.L., Koss, L.G., and Simon, T.R.: Evaluation of concomitant use of cytological and histocytological techniques in recognition of cancer in exfoliated material from various sources. Cancer, *8*:948–950, 1955.

Richardson, H.L., Queen, F.B., and Bishop, F.H.: Cytohistologic diagnosis of material aspirated from stomach; accuracy of diagnosis of cancer, ulcer and gastritis from paraffin-embedded washings. Am. J. Clin. Pathol., *19*:328–340, 1949.

Riva, H.L., and Turner, T.R.: A ten-second acridine-orange staining technic for cytologic cancer screening. Obstet. Gynecol., *20*:451–458, 1962.

Rodney, M.B.: Data control and quality of the human cytoscreening function. Health Lab. Sci., *9*:215–224, 1972.

Rombach, J.J., Cranendonk, R., and Velthuis, F.J.J.M.: Monitoring laboratory performance by statistical analysis of rescreening cervical smears. Acta Cytol., *31*:887–894, 1987.

Rosebury, T.: Microorganisms Indigenous to Man. New York, McGraw-Hill, 1961.

Ross, K.F.A.: Cell shrinkage caused by fixatives and paraffin-wax embedding in ordinary cytological preparations. Q. J. Micro. Sci., *94*:125–139, 1953.

Rubio, C.A.: False negatives in cervical cytology: Can they be avoided? Acta Cytol., *25*:199–201, 1981.

Rubio, C.A., Knock, Y.R.A., and Berglund, K.: Studies of the distribution of abnormal cells in cytologic preparations: I. Making the smear with a wooden spatula. Acta Cytol., *24*:49–53, 1980.

Sachdeva, R., and Kline, T.S.: Aspiration biopsy cytology and special stains. Acta Cytol., *25*:678–683, 1981.

Saccomanno, G., Saunders, R.P., Ellis, H., Archer, V.E., and Wood, B.G.: Concentrations of carcinoma or atypical cells in sputum. Acta Cytol., *7*:305–310, 1963.

Saccomanno, G., Saunders, R.P., Archer, V.E., Auerbach, O., Kuschner, M., and Beckler, P.A.: Cancer of the lung: The cytology of sputum prior to the development of carcinoma. Acta Cytol., 9:413–423, 1965.

Safety in Academic Chemistry Laboratories. Prepared by the American Chemical Society Committee on Chemical Safety, March, 1974.

Sagi, E.S., and MacKenzie, L.L.: The use of acetone as a fixative in exfoliative cytological studies. Am. J. Obstet. Gynecol., 73:437–439, 1957.

Saulvester, E.L.: Retrieval of follow-up data in a diagnostic cytology laboratory. Cytotech. Bull., 13:17–18, 1976.

Schade, R.O.K.: Gastric Cytology, Principles, Methods, and Results. London, Edward Arnold, 1960.

Seal, S.H.: A method for concentrating cancer cells suspended in large quantities of fluid. Cancer, 9:866–868, 1956.

———: Silicone flotation: Simple quantitative method for isolation of free-floating cancer cells from blood. Cancer, 12:595–599, 1959.

———: A sieve for the isolation of cancer cells and other large cells from the blood. Cancer. 17:637–642, 1964.

Selbach, G.J., and Bondar, M.: Cytological filtration technics. Acta Cytol., 6:311–313, 1962.

Setterington, R.: The specification of a standard microscope coverglass. J. R. Micr. Soc., 73:69–76, 1953.

Shackelford, R.I., and Jones, J.L.: An embedding medium for permanent sections of exudative material and fragments of tissue removed for biopsy. Tech. Bull. Regist. Med. Techn., 29:155–156, 1959.

Sheffner, A.L.: The reduction in vitro in viscosity of mucoprotein solutions by a new mucolytic agent, N-acetyl-L-cysteine. Ann. N.Y. Acad. Sci., 106:298–310, 1963.

Sherman, A.B., Koss, L.G., Wyschogrod, D., Melder, K.H., Eppich, E.M., and Bales, C.E.: Bladder cancer diagnosis by computer image analysis of cells in the sediment of voided urine using a video scanning system. Anal. Quant. Cytol., 8:177–186, 1986.

Shorr, E.: New technic for staining vaginal smears. III. Simple differential stain. Science, 94:545–546, 1941.

———: Evaluation of clinical applications of vaginal smear method. J. Mt. Sinai Hosp., 12:667–688, 1945.

Smith, J.W., and Hughes, W.T.: A rapid staining technique for Pneumocystis carinii. J. Clin. Pathol., 25:269–271, 1972.

Smith, M.J., Kini, S.R., and Watson, E.: Fine needle aspiration and endoscopic brush cytology: Comparison of direct smears and rinsings. Acta Cytol., 24:456–459, 1980.

Smith, M.J., and Naylor, B.: A method for extracting ferruginous bodies from sputum and pulmonary tissue. Am. J. Clin. Pathol., 58:250–254, 1972.

Smith Fourshee, J.H., Kalnins, Z.A., Dixon, F.R., Girsh, S., Morehead, R.P., O'Brien, T.F., Pribor, H., and Tattory, C.: Gastric cytology: Evaluation of methods and results in 1,670 cases. Acta Cytol., 13:399–406, 1969.

Solomon, C., Amelar, R.D., Hyman, R.M., Chaiban, R., and Europa, D.L.: Exfoliated cytology of urinary tract; new approach with reference to isolation of cancer cells and preparation of slides for study. J. Urol., 80:374–382, 1958.

Spalsbury, C., Brodetsky, A.M., and Teplitz, R.L.: Discontinuous Ficoll gradient separation of normal and malignant cells: Cytologic applicability. I. Acta Cytol., 17:522–532, 1973.

Spriggs, A.I.: A simple density gradient method for removing red cells from haemorrhagic serous fluids. Acta Cytol., 19:470–472, 1975.

Spriggs, A.I.: Positive rate for sputum cytology. Acta Cytol., 27:703–704, 1983.

Spriggs, A.I., and Alexander, R.F.: An albumin gradient method for separating the different white cells of blood, applied to the concentration of circulating tumor cells. Nature, 188:863–864, 1960.

Spriggs, A.I., and Boddington, M.M.: The Cytology of Effusions. ed. 2. New York, Grune & Stratton, 1968.

Stark, E., and Wurster, U.: Preparation procedure for cerebrospinal fluid that yields cytologic samples suitable for all types of staining, including immunologic and enzymatic methods. Acta Cytol., 31:374–376, 1987.

Steere, N.V.: Handbook of Laboratory Safety. ed. 2. Cleveland, The Chemical Rubber Co., 1971.

Sun, T., and Chess, Q.: Fluorescence is not specific for Pneumocystis carinii. Acta Cytol., 30:549–552, 1986.

Sun, T., Chess, Q., and Tanenbaum, B.: Morphologic criteria for the identification of Pneumocystis carinii in Papanicolaou-stained preparations. Acta Cytol., 30:80–81, 1986.

Sykes, G. Disinfection and Sterilization. ed. 2. Philadelphia, J.B. Lippincott, 1967.

Sykes, J.A., Whitecarver, J., Briggs, L., and Anson, J.H.: Separation of tumor cells froom fibroblasts with use of discontinuous density gradients. J.N.C.I., 44:855–864, 1970.

Symmers, W. St. C.: Deep-seated fungal infecions currently seen in the histopathologic service of a medical school laboratory in Britain. Am. J. Clin. Pathol., 46:514–538, 1966.

Szczepanik, E., and Helpap, B.: Comparison of suspicious and positive colposcopic, cytologic and histologic findings in the uterine cervix. Acta Cytol., 27:241–244, 1983.

Taft, P.D., and Lojananond, P.: Evaluation of fluorescence microscopy in gynecologic exfoliative cytology. Am. J. Clin. Pathol., 37:334–337, 1962.

Thompson, A.B., Robbins, R.A., Ghafouri, M.A., Linder, J., and Rennard, S.I.: Bronchoalveolar lavage fluid processing: Effect of membrane filtration preparation on neutrophil recovery. Acta Cytol., 33:544–549, 1989.

Tutuarima, J.A., Hische, E.A.H., Sylva-Steenland, R.M.R., and van der Helm, H.J.: A cytopreparatory method for cerebrospinal fluid in which the cell yield is high and the fluid is saved for chemical analysis. Acta Cytol., 32:425–427, 1988.

United States Pharmacopeia. Rockland, Md., Pharmacopeial Convention, Inc., 1975.

van der Graaf, Y., Vooijs, G.P., Gaillard, H.L.J., and Go, D.M.D.S.: Screening errors in cervical cytologic screening. Acta Cytol., 31:434–438, 1987.

von Haam, E.: A comparative study of the accuracy of cancer cell detection by cytological methods. Acta Cytol., 6:508–518, 1962.

Vooijs, G.P., Elias, A., van der Graaf, Y., and Poelen-van der Berg, C.T.: The influence of sample takers on the cellular composition of cervical smears. Acta Cytol., 30:251–257, 1986.

Vooijs, G.P., van der Graaf, Y., and Elias, A.G.: Cellular composition of cervical smears in relation to the day of the menstrual cycle and the method of contraception. Acta Cytol., 31:417–426, 1987.

Wachtel, E., And Gordon, H.: An improved sampling device for cervical cytology. Lancet, July 6, 26–27, 1974.

Wade, A., and Reynolds, J.E.F. (eds.): Martindale, The Extra Pharmacopeia. ed. 27. London. The Pharmaceutical Press, 1977.

Watson, P.: A slide centrifuge—an apparatus for concentrating cells in suspension onto a microscope slide. J. Clin. Lab. Med., 68:494–501, 1966.

Wenger, J., and Raskin, H.F.: Diagnosis of cancer of pancreas, biliary tract, and duodenum by combined cytologic and secretory methods. II. Secretin test. Gastroenterology, 34:1009–1017, 1958.

West, W.F.: Cytopreparatory Method—Pneumocystis. In

Keebler, C.M., Reagan, J.W., and Wied, G.L. (eds.): Compendium on Cytopreparatory Techniques. ed. 4. pp. 95–96. Chicago, Tutorials of Cytology, 1976.

Whitaker, D.: Hyaluronic acid in serous effusion smears. Acta Cytol., *30*:90–91, 1986.

Wied, G.L.: Quality assurance measures in cytopathology. Acta Cytol., *32*:287, 1988.

Wied, G.L.: Replies to questions on quality assurance measures in cytopathology (multiple authors). Acta Cytol., *32*:913–939, 1988.

Wied, G.L., Bartels, P.H., Bibbo, M., and Keebler, C.M.: Frequency and reliability of diagnostic cytology of the female genital tract. Acta Cytol., *25*:543–549, 1981.

Wilander, E., Norhein, I., and Oberg, K.: Application of silver stains to cytologic specimens of neuroendocrine tumors metastatic to the liver. Acta Cytol., *29*:1053–1057, 1985.

Willcox, F., de Somer, M.L., and Roy, J.V.: Classification of cervical smears with discordance beween the cytologic and/or histologic rating. Acta Cytol., *31*:883–886, 1987.

Windholz, M., Budavari, S., Stromtsas, L.Y., and Fertig, M.N. (eds.): The Merck Index. ed. 9. Rahway, N.J., Merck & Co., Inc., 1976.

Wolman, M.: Problems of fixation in cytology, histology, and histochemistry. Int. Rev. Cytol., *4*:79–102, 1955.

Wood, R.J., and Hicklin, M.D.: Rescreening as a quality control procedure in cytopathology. Atlanta, Georgia, HEW, Center for Disease Control, March 17, 1976.

Woodruff, K.H.: Cerebrospinal fluid cytomorphology using cytocentrifugation. Am. J. Clin. Pathol., *60*:621–627, 1973.

Wottawa, Von A., Klein, G., and Atlmann, H.: A method for the isolation of human and animal lymphocytes with Ficoll-Urografin. Wien. Klin. Wochenschr., *86*:161–163, 1974.

Yobs, A.R., Plott, A.E., and Hicklin, M.D.: Retrospective evaluation of gynecologic cytodiagnosis: II. Interlaboratory reproducibility as shown in rescreening large consecutive samples of reported cases. Acta Cytol., *31*:900–910, 1987.

Zajicek, J.: Aspiration Biopsy Cytology. Part I. Cytology of Supradiaphragmatic Organs. Basel, S. Karger, 1974. (See also Chap. 29 in this book).

34

Immunochemistry in Cytology

Margaret B. Listrom, M.D., and
Cecilia M. Fenoglio-Preiser, M.D.

A reliable cytologic diagnosis represents an educated opinion based on a number of subjective criteria; hence, it is dependent on the experience of the interpreter. When the cytologist cannot reach a diagnosis with any degree of confidence, ancillary techniques may be applied. The most common of these ancillary techniques is immunocytochemistry, a method based on the selective binding of immunologic reagents to specific antigenic determinants on a cell in a precise lock and key mechanism. It is the unique recognition of an antigen by an antibody that led to the emergence of immunohistochemistry and immunocytochemistry as powerful diagnostic techniques in the routine practice of pathology. This has been facilitated by the availability of many reliable, commercially produced antibodies. Numerous modifications of the basic methods have allowed increasing applicability in a wide range of diagnostic settings. Immunocytochemical approaches offer the potential of making a specific diagnosis when the usual cytologic criteria do not allow one to form a definite opinion. However, immunocytochemical reactions should not be the sole basis of diagnosis because unanticipated false-positive or false-negative reactions may result in significant diagnostic errors. Further, the results of immunocytochemical staining should never be allowed to contradict an opinion based on the clinical presentation and experienced assessment of the cytologic features. Factors to be taken into account when rendering an immunocytochemical diagnosis are listed in Table 34-1.

In this chapter the structure and types of antibodies are reviewed. This is followed by a discussion of technical factors associated with the performance of the immunocytochemical reactions. In the second half of the chapter, the application of the methodology to the diagnosis of tumors and infectious diseases is presented. The section on tumors is further divided into a discussion of the most common markers used in the diagnostic setting, followed by their application to specific types of cytologic preparations.

Table 34–1
Pitfalls of Immunocytochemistry

False-Positive Reactions
Nonspecific ionic binding of antibodies and reagents
Cross-reacting natural antibodies
Existence of same or similar epitopes on different antigens
Drying of cells between steps
Inappropriate fixation
Ineffective blocking of endogenous enzymes
Endogenous biotin
Nonspecific binding of avidin
Nonspecific staining of crushed tissue, dead cells, and debris

False-Negative Reactions
Inappropriate fixative
Drying of cells between steps
Omission of one or more antibodies
Specimen contains crushed, degenerated, or necrotic elements
Incorrect preparation of substrate-chromogen mixture

ANTIBODIES

Structure

Antibodies are proteins (immunoglobulins) with two main functions: the binding of antigen via the antigen-combining site and the mobilization of defense mechanisms via the portion of the molecule, designated as Fc. When antibodies are used in diagnostic assays, one takes advantage of the first function. Immunoglobulin molecules are glycoproteins composed of four protein chains, a pair of heavy chains, and a pair of light chains (Fig. 34–1).

Most antibodies used diagnostically belong to the immunoglobulin G (IgG) class; the remainder are IgM antibodies. Digestion of the immunoglobulin molecule with the enzyme pepsin produces two identical Fab regions [F(Ab′)2] and degrades the Fc fragment. The two antigen combining sites, located in the Fab region, consist of a light chain (either kappa or lambda) and a portion of the heavy chain. Antigen binding is restricted to that region on the Fab fragment that contains the variable domains of both the heavy and light chains. Over 100 genes encode the amino acids of the variable region, including the hypervariable (HV) regions and

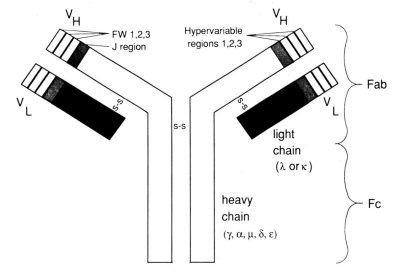

FIGURE 34–1. A simplified model for a human antibody molecule. V_L indicates the variable region of the light chains; V_H indicates the variable region of the heavy chains. Digestion of the molecule with pepsin produces one [(Fab)′]$_2$ molecule composed of two Fab units with intact interheavy chain disulfide bonds (S-S). Proteolytic digestion with papain yields two antigen-binding fragments (Fab′) and one crystalline fragment (Fc). The antigen-binding region includes the hypervariable regions and the surrounding framework residues (FW).

the surrounding framework (FW) residues (see Fig. 34–1). Diversity of antigen specificity results from recombinational arrangements of the light and heavy chain gene sequences (see Chapter 3). The Fc part of the antibody molecule contains only heavy chains and does not bind antigen, but it attaches to Fc receptors on the surfaces of many cells, triggering such functions as phagocytosis, complement fixation, and mediator secretion. The antibody may also bind to cellular Fc receptors, causing nonspecific reactions and generating false-positive results (Fig. 34–2).

Antigen Recognition

Most antibodies produced for immunocytochemical staining react with a limited, relatively unique cell region or site of a peptide antigen called an *epitope*, which usually consists of three to eight amino acids. However, because substantial homology exists among families of peptides, cross-reactivities between or among similar proteins can occur. This has become a problem, for example, in the widespread application of antibodies to intermediate filaments. Therefore, in interpreting immunoreactivity, it is well to keep in mind that tissues and cells contain known and unknown cross-reacting antigens that may account for unexpected positive reactions. A modification of cellular epitopes during specimen processing may also have a major impact on their reactivity. Changes in pH, buffers, temperature, or types of fixative may alter the recognition of an epitope by an antibody, resulting in a false-positive or false-negative reaction.

Polyclonal Antibodies

Polyclonal antibodies are produced by multiple injections of a foreign substance (an immunogen) into an animal. This process stimulates the proliferation of different B-lymphocyte clones, each responding to a unique epitope present in the immunizing mixture and each producing a single antibody with specificity for the epitope toward which it is directed. The serum from the animal is then tested against the immunizing antigen to determine the antibody titer. When an antibody with a sufficiently strong titer is present, the animal is bled. The antiserum produced in this way contains a mixture of antibodies recognizing multiple epitopes of multiple antigens; each of the antibodies has a different antigenic specificity and affinity (Fig. 34–3). Next, the antiserum is absorbed with antigens known to be present in the immunizing mixture but unwanted in the final reagent. Attempts to remove all unwanted or cross-reacting specificities from the antiserum are usually only partially successful. Residual cross-reactivities may cause false-positive reactions that may not be appreciated when the antibody is used for diagnostic purposes. Because each animal differs in its antibody responses, the unique serologic properties of these antisera cannot be reproduced in other animals. These animals also have pre-existing antibodies that were present before the animal was immunized and that will be present in the final antiserum. This results in batch-to-batch and animal-to-animal variability in the quality of the antibodies produced.

Monoclonal Antibodies

Hybridoma technology, first described by Köhler and Milstein in 1975, revolutionized the process of making customized monoclonal antibodies (MAbs) because it offered a means of producing a reliable antibody of reproducible qualities.

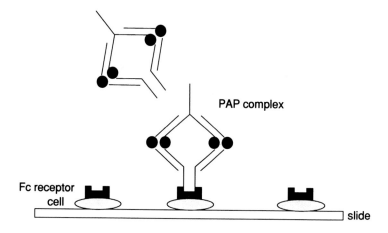

FIGURE 34–2. Diagram of interaction of the Fc portion of immunoglobulin with Fc receptors. In most applications, overt Fc-binding occurs in lightly fixed or unfixed smears and is a result of the peroxidase-antiperoxidase complex binding to the Fc receptors.

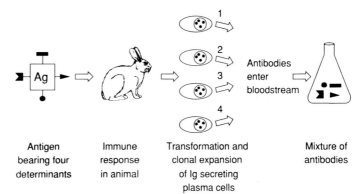

FIGURE 34–3. Conventional method of producing polyclonal antibodies (see text for details).

Antigen bearing four determinants — Immune response in animal — Transformation and clonal expansion of Ig secreting plasma cells — Antibodies enter bloodstream — Mixture of antibodies

Hybridomas are produced by fusing immuno-globulin-producing cultured myeloma cells with antigen-sensitized spleen cells, obtained by immunization of an animal. The immune spleen cells convey their antigen specificity to the myeloma cells and program them to secrete immunoglobulins directed against the immunizing antigen. Each hybridoma has its own antigenic specificity, and each recognizes only a single epitope present in the immunizing mixture; all subsequent progeny produce an identical antibody (Fig. 34–4). The hybridoma producing the antibody of interest is separated from the other antibody-producing clones and propagated to produce large quantities of the desired antibody. Hybridoma clones grow indefinitely in tissue culture or mouse ascitic fluid, or they can be frozen and stored for future use. In this way, pure antibodies are indefinitely produced without batch-to-batch variability.

Many MAbs are raised against whole cells or tissues so that often the precise nature of the antigen is unknown. The specificity of such MAbs is defined by their tissue-binding characteristics, which in turn are dependent on the thoroughness with which one maps the immunoreactivity patterns. Keeping this in mind, it is not surprising that unexpected patterns of immunoreactivity may emerge as these antibodies are applied to a wider range of normal and abnormal tissues with closely related molecules. However, as the purification and immunogenicity of the antigens are improved, the problems of unsuspected cross-reactivity and low affinity of MAbs may be resolved. Furthermore, antibodies increasingly are being generated against synthetically produced antigens whose structures are predicted by cloning and sequencing of the genes encoding the antigens in question.

The intensity of the immunoreaction is usually weaker with MAbs than with polyclonal antibodies, probably because the number of reactive determinants on MAbs is smaller. However, it is possible to intensify the reaction product in the detection systems (see below) to overcome this problem. In some instances, immunostaining with a MAb results in a stronger reaction than when a polyclonal antibody is used. This occurs most commonly when the antigen is localized to a specific region in the cell. The demonstration of the

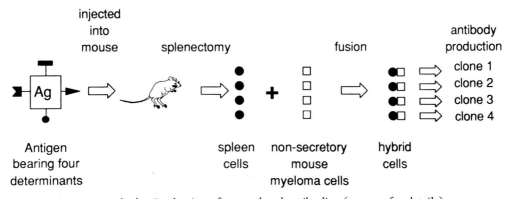

FIGURE 34–4. Production of monoclonal antibodies (see text for details).

immunoreactive sites produces less background or nonspecific staining when MAbs are used. This stems from the higher specificity of the MAbs and the fact that each MAb has an even binding pattern to its antigenic determinant. It is possible that when polyclonal antibodies bind to the cell, the different antibodies present in the antiserum compete with one another for binding to the different antigenic epitopes and may interfere with one another's attachment to the epitope, thereby resulting in unstable and less clearly defined binding reactions.

Since MAbs react with only a single antigenic determinant, any modification of that determinant in the tissue or cell sample may result in a negative stain. Such modifications may occur as the result of specimen processing, as noted earlier. However, they may also occur because of the presence of tissue proteases in the specimen or occur with phenotypic changes occurring during neoplastic transformation. To broaden the narrow band of reactivity characteristic for MAbs and to yield more information in diagnostic settings, mixtures of MAbs may be pooled; such reagents recognize several different epitopes on the same antigen,

thereby increasing the chances of a positive reaction if the antigen is present. This approach has been applied, for example, in some of the reagents used for the detection of cytokeratins.

Other Types of Antibodies

The newest antibodies include single domain antibodies (DAbs), biosynthetic antibodies (BAbs), chimeric antibodies, and molecular recognition units. DAbs differ from naturally occurring antibodies by being single domain antibodies that represent only one side of an antibody binding site (Fig. 34–5). Chimeric antibodies are typically composed of a human immunoglobulin, with another immunoglobulin from an animal source (i.e., mouse) providing a portion of the antigenic binding site. BAbs are single-stranded molecules that contain biosynthetic binding sites constructed through computer modeling. The DNA sequences for MAbs are generated, and the clones for only the binding site are isolated. As a result, the BAb is approximately one sixth the size of a MAb. Molecular recognition units are even smaller than BAbs and

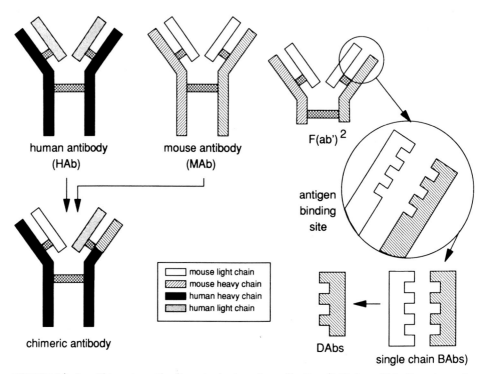

FIGURE 34–5. Chimeric antibodies, single domain antibodies (DAbs), and binding site antibodies (BAbs) are some of the newest developments in antibody production. The molecules are much smaller than routinely used immunoglobulins and typically are composed of highly selected antigen-binding sites.

consist of short peptide sequences that represent a fraction of the size of an antibody. All of these antibodies have been designed to target specific substances and, at the same time, to reduce their overall immunogenicity. Their role in histologic and cytologic diagnoses remains to be determined.

TECHNICAL FACTORS

Because each cytology practice is unique, individual laboratories must establish a number of basic parameters concerning their use of immunocytochemical methods. Among the points to be evaluated are (1) the optimal way to preserve cytologic morphology while still maintaining the antigenicity of the cell markers; (2) which antibodies, or battery of antibodies, are most cost-effective for the identification of specific cell lineages; (3) the most appropriate immunocytochemical approach to be used for evaluating different antigens in different cell- and specimen types; and (4) the changes in the expression of a given antigen when applied to normal, hyperplastic, or malignant cells of the same lineage. Specificity and sensitivity under different conditions must be assessed since artifacts and technical problems can give rise to misleading results.

The methods of performing immunostaining on the different types of cytologic specimens are not as standardized as they are for tissue specimens. Cytology specimens are collected by diverse medical personnel, ranging from nurses to clinicians, and including gynecologists, urologists, gastroenterologists, pulmonologists, surgeons, neurologists, radiologists, and pathologists. These people differ markedly in their understanding of the need for an adequate specimen preparation and fixation. The types of specimens received also vary widely. Finally, discrepancies among cytology laboratories may be due to differences in fixation techniques, staining procedures, or the choice of antibodies. These differences underline still further the need to establish and use consistent, well-defined, and well-controlled conditions in performing the immunocytochemical procedures. For example, smears prepared from effusions with a high protein content (as is often the case in malignant effusions) may have heavy background staining that interferes with the interpretation of the result if the cells are not washed in normal saline solution. Cell smears, imprints, cell blocks, and cytocentrifuge preparations are all used in our laboratory for immunostaining. However, it has been our experience that filter preparations tend to have unsolvable background problems that mask the cellular reaction and therefore are unsuitable for diagnostic interpretation.

Fixatives

As noted, adequate fixation is critical for preserving both the cytologic characteristics of the cells and their antigenicity. Specific factors detrimental to the preservation of surface antigens include fixation delays, an acid pH, prolonged fixation, and temperatures over 40°C. Air drying of cells before fixation may result in inconsistent results, either false-negative or false-positive. Inherent differences in the fixation and processing techniques used for cytology specimens as compared with their histologic counterparts can cause the results of the immunostaining reactions to differ in the cytologic preparation when compared with the histologic preparation from the same case. The most widely used fixative in cytology is alcohol. Alcohol preserves most cytoplasmic antigens, including intermediate filaments, peptides, and hormones, but many surface antigens are typically lost after alcohol fixation and diminished reactivity with antibodies against the protein S-100 has been reported. Air-dried smears or cytospins for surface markers may be fixed in acetone, methanol-acetone (1:1), or buffered 1:1 formol-acetone mixtures. Some authors have found that fixation with 0.05% glutaraldehyde offers optimal results.

Cells from needle aspirations may be collected in the cell culture medium RPMI 1640, Hanks' balanced salt solution, or phosphate-buffered saline (PBS), pH 7.4. After centrifugation the cell pellets are usually resuspended in buffer, and monolayer cytocentrifuge preparations are made (see Appendix).

Various fixatives have been tested on thin-needle aspirates to improve the accuracy and reliability of immunohistochemical techniques. We have found that the use of acetone or buffered formol-acetone provides excellent and consistent morphologic and immunocytochemical results on aspirates. Sections cut from cell blocks prepared from the aspirates are treated in the same manner as routine tissue sections. We do not routinely use enzyme digestion procedures, although some authors have found them to be useful.

For the best immunocytochemical results, air drying should be avoided since some authors have found that it significantly influences the quality of the immunoreactivity: complete loss of immunoreactivity and false-positive staining, particularly with antibodies directed against cytoskeletal components, have been recorded.

Optimally, if one could anticipate the need for immunocytochemical analyses before obtaining a cytology specimen, one could plan to fix the specimen in such a way as to preserve the antigens in question. This is possible in some situations and should be done routinely when a hematologic malignancy is suspected, when one deals with breast cancer that requires steroid receptor analysis, or when a possible metastasis from a known primary cancer is anticipated. This approach stresses the importance of a dialogue between the individual obtaining the specimen and the individual interpreting it. It also allows for advanced planning to maximize the use of the cell sample for additional ancillary studies, such as microbiologic or molecular biologic analyses.

Immunostaining of Previously Stained Slides

On many occasions the necessity for performing immunohistochemical reactions becomes apparent only after the Papanicolaou-stained preparation is examined. In these instances, the cover glass can be removed, the specimen destained in acid-alcohol, and then immunostained in a routine manner. However, this approach does not always work since sometimes the previous staining interferes with the immunoreactivity. Thus, the results are somewhat inconsistent, particularly for unstable antigens. Nonetheless, it is sometimes worth trying this approach, especially in those situations in which an additional sample would be difficult to obtain (see Color Plate 34–2 *E, F*).

Stains

Since the number of cytologic slides is usually limited, we typically use one slide, if available, as a negative control. However, unless several sequential sections of a cell block are available, one must remember that not all cytology preparations are identical, a problem that usually does not exist with histologic specimens. This makes it difficult to guarantee that the cell population of interest is present on all slides. An alternative is to use the same slide for both immunostaining and as a negative control. In this approach, the slide is divided in half by using a wax pencil or nail polish. The primary antibody is applied to one half of the slide but not to the other. Subsequently the two halves of the slide are processed in the same way. However, even with this approach the problems inherent in uneven cell distribution may still be present. A good source of known positive controls is a tissue section containing the antigen in question and fixed and processed in the same manner as the cytologic preparation.

DETECTION SYSTEMS OF IMMUNE STAINING

Immunohistochemical techniques have evolved from the simplest reaction, introduced in 1941 by Coons, who used a direct immunohistochemical assay, to one in which multiple bridging antibodies are used. The original techniques employed fluorescent labels that gave very poor resolution of the cytologic details. They also required specially processed tissue. These problems were partially addressed by the introduction of enzyme-labeled methods. Only those techniques most commonly applied to cytologic specimens are surveyed here.

Peroxidase-Antiperoxidase

The peroxidase-antiperoxidase (PAP) method involves the sequential use of a primary antibody, a second unlabeled antibody (referred to as the linking antibody), and an antibody to horseradish peroxidase generated in the same animal species as was the primary antibody (Fig. 34–6). The primary antibody is placed on the slide. After washing of the slide, the secondary antibody is added in great excess, compared with the amount of the primary antibody. This facilitates the binding of only one of the secondary antibody's antigen combining sites, leaving the second site free to bind the next reagent, a labeled immunoglobulin generated in the same species as the primary antibody. The labeled immunoglobulin is added in the form of a stable immune complex, that is, an antibody against horseradish peroxidase and horseradish peroxidase antigen (PAP). The immunoglobulins bound to the antigen are then localized by adding a substrate, usually hydrogen peroxide, and a chromogen, either diaminobenzidine (DAB) or aminoethyl carbazol. This results in a brown or red deposit localized over the antigenic sites.

Avidin-Biotin Peroxidase

In many laboratories, the avidin-biotin peroxidase (ABC) technique has replaced the PAP method.

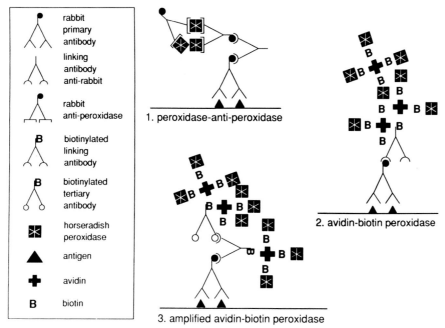

FIGURE 34-6. (1) The peroxidase-antiperoxidase (PAP) method relies on the interaction of a preformed enzyme immune complex reacting with the linking antibody. The primary antibody and the antibody of the enzyme immune complex must be produced in the same species. (2) The avidin-biotin (ABC) methods use preformed avidin-biotin enzyme complex (ABC) reacting with biotinylate secondary antibody. (3) The amplified ABC technique uses two linking antibodies.

The ABC reaction exploits the high affinity between the vitamin biotin and the egg white glycoprotein, avidin. The slide is first incubated with the primary antibody, followed sequentially by a biotinylated secondary antibody and a preformed avidin-biotin-horseradish peroxidase complex (see Fig. 34-6). We employ a modification of the ABC procedure that uses strepavidin, a protein produced by the bacterium *Streptomyces avidinii*. In our hands, with this approach, there is less nonspecific background staining; the use of streptavidin also allows us to dilute the primary antibody further than is possible with the original ABC technique. Strepavidin has a neutral isoelectric point that decreases the likelihood of nonspecific binding to highly charged molecules present on the slide. In contrast, egg white avidin has an isoelectric point that is close to 10, allowing nonspecific binding to many tissue constituents, particularly nucleic acids. Further, streptavidin does not contain those carbohydrate moieties, present in avidin, that are capable of binding to lectin-like substances ubiquitous in normal tissues.

The ABC method may be further improved by sequentially overlaying the sections with an avidin-rich, biotin-rich peroxidase complex. This enhances the sensitivity of the reaction, and conceivably, may allow to dilute the expensive primary antibodies still further. A third biotinylated antibody layer may be added to the already sensitive ABC system (see Fig. 34-6) to amplify the reaction product.

Alkaline Phosphatase

Alkaline Phosphatase (ALP) methods can be used as an alternative to the immunoperoxidase methods or in conjunction with immunoperoxidase double-immunostaining procedures. In this technique, the enzyme ALP replaces horseradish peroxidase. ALP acts on the naphthol AS:B1 phosphate substrate, coupled to the diazonium dye (fast red), which results in an insoluble precipitate at the antigenic site. The advantage of using ALP is that the use of DAB, which is believed to be weakly carcinogenic, is eliminated. Furthermore, it usually circumvents problems associated with endogenous peroxidases present in tissues. However, drawbacks also exist with ALP. The color fades over time, the slides cannot be dehydrated in organic solvents, and some tissues contain endogenous ALP.

Immunogold with Silver Enhancement

This method is based on the observation that gold particles are easily absorbed to proteins to form stable gold conjugates. Immunogold detection systems were originally used in electron microscopy, but they have been recently widely adopted for histology. The impetus for this popularity came from the observation that gold-labeled antibodies used in conjunction with silver-enhancing methods, increase the sensitivity of the reaction more than 200 times above that of standard immunoperoxidase techniques. The gold label is usually placed on the secondary antibody. Immunogold-silver techniques may represent the most sensitive and efficient light microscope immunocytochemical method currently available.

False-Positive and False-Negative Reactions

False-positive and false-negative results occur with immunocytochemical staining reactions and thereby hamper the cytologic interpretation (see Table 34–1). False-positive results occur as the result of antibody cross-reactivity with antigens other than the one being looked for, drying of the cells at any time during the collection, fixation or staining procedures, inappropriate fixation, ineffective blocking of the endogenous enzyme, binding to endogenous biotin, nonspecific binding of the antibody to Fc receptors, or binding of the biotinylated label to avidin in the tissues. False-negative reactions occur when outdated reagents are used or in situations in which the antigenicity of the specimen is not preserved. Antigens are destroyed by air drying of specimens, inappropriate or prolonged fixation, fixation delays, or overheating (in the case of sections cut from cell blocks).

Quantitative Immunocytochemistry

Immunohistochemical reactions performed on cytology specimens most often require only a qualitative evaluation, that is, whether an antigen is present or absent. However, situations are emerging in which the localization and quantification of a protein could be advantageous. By combining either image analysis or flow cytometric analysis with immunohistochemistry, one can derive an estimate of the amount of antigen present. Flow cytometry is discussed in Chapter 36 and image analysis in Chapter 35. Image analyses allow an assessment of the number of positive cells as well as the intensity of the reaction of those cells. This type of quantitative information is useful in those situations in which the amount of protein product present is of prognostic value. Such analyses include cell proliferation markers (Ki 67, cyclin), estrogen-receptor protein, progesterone-receptor protein, and proteins encoded for by the HER 2/neu oncogene in breast cancer, N-myc in neuroblastoma, and other oncoproteins (see p. 1595). These determinations can be made on aspirates of primary or metastatic tumors or on effusions. As with any immunologic assay, antibody specificity is a major concern and good quality-control practices must be adhered to. Furthermore, there is the need to standardize such factors as intensity of the light source and the computer programs used. Specimen thickness, important in tissue sections, plays no role in smears but must be determined in cell block preparations.

IMMUNOCYTOCHEMISTRY IN TUMOR DIAGNOSIS

During the past decades, a major change has occurred in the role of the pathologist vis-à-vis clinical oncology. In part, this is the result of wide application of aspiration biopsy, which has substantially improved early diagnosis of primary tumors and detection of local recurrences and metastases. Immunohistochemical analyses applied to these specimens can provide physicians with more precise diagnoses and with prognostic information such as DNA content, tumor cell proliferative activity, steroid-receptor analyses, tumor subtype, immunologic phenotypes, differentiation markers, drug resistance, and detection of occult metastases.

Choice of Markers

The cytologic diagnosis of malignancy is based primarily on nuclear changes, using known criteria for the diagnosis of cancer in conjunction with an adequate history and an adequate sample, as discussed elsewhere in this book. In most instances, the definitive diagnosis can be made. However,

Color Plates 34–1 to 34–3

Plate 34–1. (*A*) A gastric brushing of a small cell neoplasm present in the stomach of a 57-year-old man. (Papanicolaou stain, ×600) (*B*) Many of these uniform, round cells show peripheral rim staining with anticytokeratin stain, performed on an alcohol-fixed smear. The erythrocytes in the background stain brown because of endogenous peroxidase, but their presence does not hinder the interpretation of this smear. (Anticytokeratin–methylene blue–DAB, ×1,000) (*C*) Histologic section of the gastric carcinoid. (H&E, ×300) (*D*) Cell block preparation from a malignant pleural effusion in a 40-year-old woman with an unknown primary tumor. (H&E, ×400) (*E, F*) The cells are strongly positive with anti-carcinoembryonic antigen (*E*) and Leu M1 (*F*) antibodies (methylene blue–DAB, ×800), suggestive of an adenocarcinoma, perhaps of gastrointestinal tract of origin. (*G*) Cell block preparation from thin-needle aspiration of a liver mass revealed the classic histologic features of hepatoma. (H&E, ×200) (*H*) Carcinoembryonic antigen localizes to the luminal surfaces of the cells, a pattern that can be seen in adenocarcinoma. (CEA–methylene blue, ×650) (*I*) Alpha-fetoprotein stain in the same case. (×200) (*J*) Diff-Quik-stained cytospin of another malignant pleural effusion revealed numerous large atypical cells. (Diff-Quik, ×1,000) (*K*) These cells were determined to be malignant and of lymphoid origin because of positive lymphocyte common antigen (LCA) and kappa stains. (anti-kappa-hematoxylin–alkaline phosphatase–fast red, ×1,000) (*L*) The lambda stain was negative. (Hematoxylin, ×400. All photographs enlarged × 2)

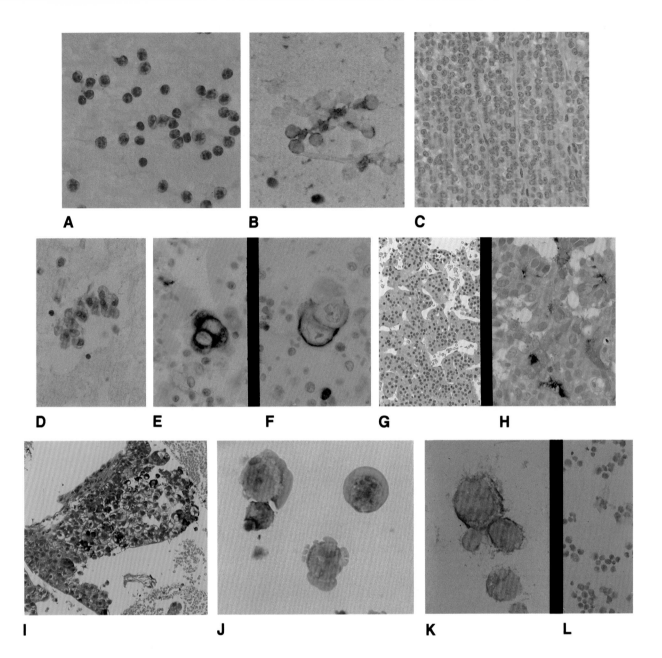

Plate 34–2. (*A, B*) A fine-needle aspiration from a large neck mass. The patient was a 50-year-old HIV-positive man. Leukocyte common antigen (LCA) stain, performed on the air-dried smears, identified the large neoplastic cells as of hematopoietic and not epithelial origin. A diagnosis of an immunoblastic sarcoma was made prior to treatment. (*A*, Diff-Quik stain, ×650; *B*, anti-LCA–hematoxylin–aminoethyl carbazol, ×1000) (*C*) Benign breast mass diagnosed by fine-needle aspiration. The muscle-specific actin antibody (HHF35) shows the myoepithelial cells in close proximity to the benign ductal cells. (alcohol fixation, methylene blue-DAB, ×800) (*D*) Histologic section of the same case showing fibrocystic disease. An actin stain on a paraffin section demonstrated an intact, myoepithelial layer surrounding the benign ducts. (Methylene blue–DAB, ×200) (*E*) Cells obtained from a thin-needle aspiration of a neck mass. Rare groups of cells were found in a background of pigmented macrophages and lymphocytes. The only history given was "cervical neck mass." (Papanicolaou stain, ×1,000) (*F*) The coverslip was removed from one of the smears, and an antithyroglobulin antibody was applied. The cells were intensely positive. (Methylene blue–DAB, ×1,000) (*G*) In histologic sections, cysts were lined by cuboidal epithelium, which was also positive with thyroglobulin antibody. A papillary carcinoma was found at thyroidectomy. (Methylene blue–DAB, ×400) (*H*) Medullary carcinoma of the thyroid. There are groups of spindle and oval cells. (Papanicolaou stain, ×800) (*I*) Calcitonin immunoreactivity is demonstrated after removing the coverslip and rehydrating the smear. The background stain is high but does not interfere with the interpretation. (Papanicolaou DAB, ×650). (*J*) Infiltrative nests of calcitonin positive cells are seen in the histologic sections. (Methylene blue-DAB, ×400. All photographs enlarged × 2)

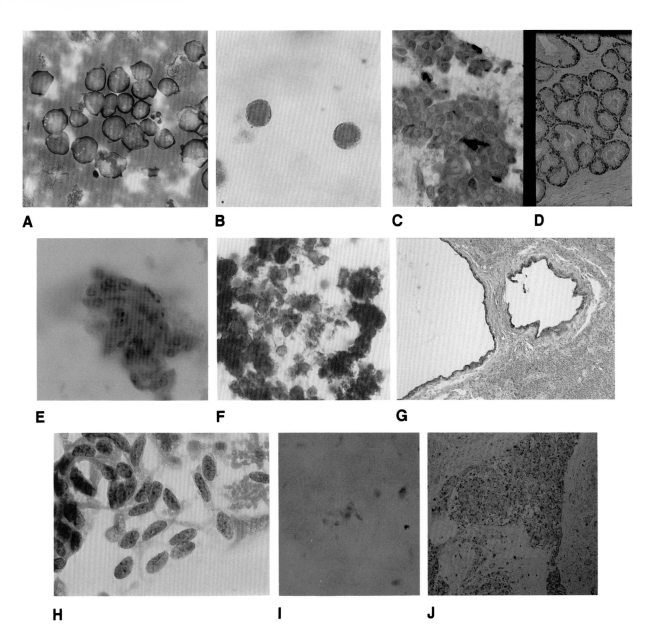

A

B

C

D

E

F

G

H

I

J

Plate 34–3. (*A*) Demonstration of HPV DNA in CIN cells by in situ hybridization (ISH) of an archival smear from 1979. (3–3′ diaminobenzidine with hematoxylin counterstain, original magnification ×400) (*B*) Demonstration of HPV DNA in a koilocytotic cell by ISH of an archival (1979) smear. (3–3′ diaminobenzidine with hematoxylin counterstain, original magnification ×400) (*C*) Demonstration of HPV-positive CIN cells in an archival cervical PAP smear. (3–3′ diaminobenzidine with hematoxylin counterstain, original magnification ×200) (*D*) Demonstration of HPV-positive CIN cells in a corresponding tissue biopsy of patient from (*C*). (3–3′ diaminobenzidine with hematoxylin counterstain, original magnification ×100) (*E*) Positive human genomic control using biotinylated human placental DNA. (3–3′ diaminobenzidine with hematoxylin in counterstain, original magnification ×400) (*F*) Negative control using biotinylated PBR 322. (3–3′ diaminobenzidine with hematoxylin counterstain, original magnification ×400. All photographs enlarged × 2. Reproduced with permission from Liang, X.-M., Wieczorek, R. L., and Koss, L. G.: In situ hybridization with human papillomavirus using biotinylated DNA probes on archival cervical smears. J. Histochem. Cytochem., *39*:771–775, 1991)

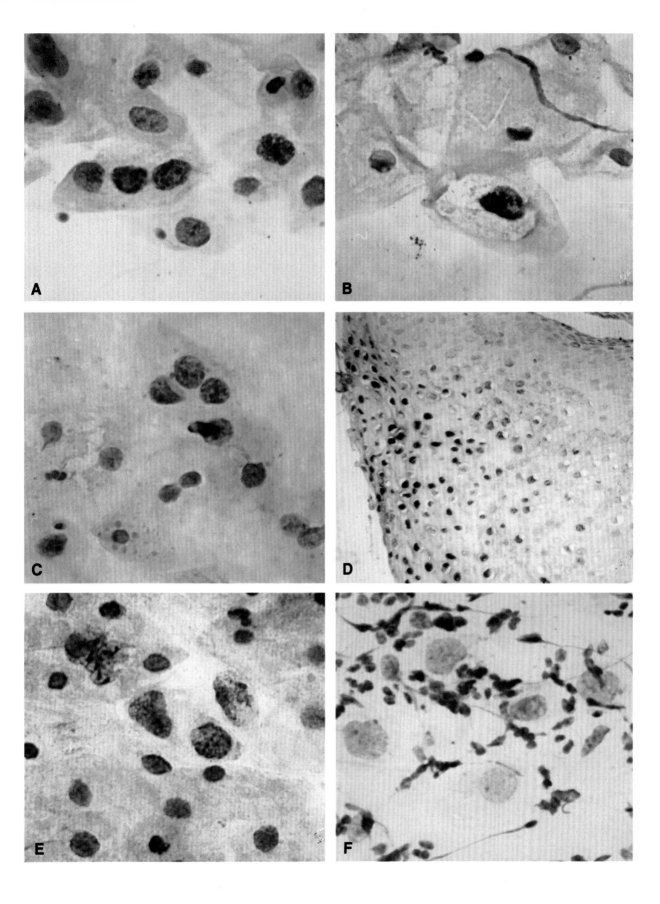

there are times when the use of immunocytochemical markers is useful or even necessary. The judicious choice of a panel of antibodies allows one to identify the cell of origin of many anaplastic round cell, small cell, and spindle cell tumors (Table 34–2). These antibody panels should be constructed in such a way that positive and negative staining results reinforce one another. These panels are usually designed to determine if the cell lineage is epithelial, neuroendocrine, mesenchymal, or lymphoid. Once this general distinction is made, the lineages can be further divided into (1) squamous, glandular, or melanoma; (2) muscular, fibrous, histiocytic, or neural; and (3) T cell, B cell, or null-cell. In some instances, a specific tissue of origin may be suggested by using antibodies to tissue-specific antigens such as thyroglobulin or prostate-specific protein. However, such antibodies cannot be used to determine whether the cells are benign or malignant. Some currently popular antibodies, such as those to S-100 protein, react with many cell lineages. When using such antibodies, it is imperative to know the underlying clinical picture before making a diagnostic interpretation with such broadly reactive reagents (Table 34–3). The combined use of multiple antibodies in a panel further narrows down the diagnostic possibilities.

Intermediate Filaments

Antibodies to intermediate filaments (IFs) are usually part of these panels since they allow one to distinguish several major tumor groups (Table 34–4).

As a rule, tumor cells retain their IF profiles in metastatic foci. Cytokeratins form a family of 19 related proteins that can be divided into subfamilies on the basis of sequence homologies, electrical charge, and immunoreactivities (Table 34–5). A characteristic feature of cytokeratins is their defined pattern of expression in different epithelial cell types and at different stages in their differentiation. Cytokeratins appear in combinations characteristic for certain types of tumors. High-molecular-weight cytokeratins are expressed in highly complex epithelia such as stratified squamous epithelium or squamous cell carcinomas. Low-molecular-weight cytokeratins are more characteristic of glandular epithelium and adenocarcinoma. As a result, antibodies to cytokeratins fall into two general groups: those that are broadly reactive, recognizing many classes of cytokeratins and therefore capable of recognizing epithelial cells in general, and those that are more selective (i.e., high molecular weight and low molecular weight), which might allow the discrimination of an adenocarcinoma from a squamous cell tumor (see also Chap. 1).

Antibodies recognizing low-molecular-weight keratin classes are the most useful diagnostically, since these keratins are expressed by many epithelial neoplasms (see Table 34–5, Color Plate 34–1 *B*). Because nonepithelial tumors such as leiomyosarcomas, rhabdomyosarcomas, and plasmacytomas can react with antibodies to cytokeratins, a panel of markers is required to verify the cell lineage.

Vimentin is found predominantly in mesenchymal cells and initially was used to differentiate

Table 34–2
Diagnostic Dilemmas Assisted by Immunocytochemistry

Differential Diagnosis	*Markers*
Carcinoma vs. lymphoma	LCA, T, B cell markers (lymphoma) keratin, CEA (carcinoma)
Melanoma vs. carcinoma	Keratin, CEA (carcinoma) S-100, HMB-45 (melanoma)
Carcinoma vs. mesothelioma	CEA, Leu M1 (carcinoma), EMA (mesothelioma)
Sarcoma vs. carcinoma	Keratin, CEA, EMA (carcinoma) vimentin, desmin, HHF-35, S-100 (sarcoma with exceptions, see text)
Neuroendocrine tumor	Chromogranin, synaptophysin, NSE, peptides, hormones
Metastatic carcinoma of unknown primary origin	PSA, PSAP (prostate)
	ER, PR (breast, endometrium)
	Thyroglobulin (thyroid)
	hCG (germ cell)
	GFAP (glial tumors)

LCA = leukocyte common antigen; CEA = carcinoembryonic antigen; HMB-45 = anti-melanoma; EMA = epithelial membrane antigen; HHF-35 = muscle-specific actin; NSE = neuron-specific enolase; PSA = prostate-specific antigen; PSAP = prostate-specific acid phosphatase; ER = estrogen-receptor protein; PR = progesterone-receptor protein; hCG = human chorionic gonadotropin; GFAP = glial fibrillary acidic protein.

Table 34–3
Distribution of Some Commonly Used Antibodies in Normal and Neoplastic Tissues

Antibody	Normal	Tumors
AA1T	Histiocytes (macrophages), mast cells, liver, lung, pancreatic islets, gastrointestinal tract, Paneth's cells, Brunner's glands	Histiocytic lesions; hepatocellular, gastric, germ cell, ovarian tumors
AACT	Histiocytes (macrophages), reticulum cells, gastric antrum, bronchial glands, Brunner's glands, exocrine pancreas, renal tubules, mesothelial cells	Carcinoma (various sites), hepatocellular, Wilms's, mesotheliomas, malignant fibrous histiocytoma, histiocytic lesions
ACTH	Normal pituitary gland	Pituitary adenomas, assorted tumors
Actin-muscle specific (HHF-35)	Skeletal, cardiac, smooth muscle, myofibroblasts	Rhabdomyosarcomas, leiomyosarcomas, Triton tumors*, mixed müllerian tumors*
AFP	Fetal liver, yolk sac, regenerating liver	Germ cell, hepatocellular, gastric carcinoma
Calcitonin	C cells, some dispersed endocrine cells	Medullary carcinoma, other endocrine tumors
CEA	Fetal and adult colon, small bowel, lung, regenerating liver and colon	Carcinoids, carcinomas of neuron sites, lung, endocervix, ovary, endometrium, pancreas, breast, prostate
Cytokeratins**	Epithelium	Epithelial cancers**
Chromogranin	Adrenal medulla, diffuse endocrine system, parathyroid, C cells, pituitary gland	Neuroendocrine tumors, pituitary tumors, medullary tumors of the thyroid
Desmin	Skeletal, cardiac, smooth muscle	Rhabdomyosarcomas, leiomyosarcomas
EMA	Fetal skin, adult renal tubules, pancreas, gastrointestinal tract, bile ducts, gynecologic tract, sweat glands, some mesenchymal cells	Neuroblastoma; renal cell, breast, gastrointestinal tract, bladder, germ cell tumors; carcinoids; mesothelioma; some mesenchymal tumors; numerous epithelial cancers; some B-cell lymphomas; some mesenchymal tumors
Factor VIII–related antigen	Endothelium	Angiosarcomas
Gastrin	Normal gut, epithelium, gastrointestinal tract nerves	Islet cell tumors, endocrine tumors
GFAF	Glial cells	Glial and astrocytic neoplasms, pleomorphic adenoma
Glucagon	Pancreas	Endocrine neoplasms
hCG	Normal placenta	Numerous tumors, mainly those containing elements of choriocarcinoma
HMB-45	Fetal and neonatal melanocytes	Junctional nevi, melanoma, dysplastic nevi, blue nevi
Immunoglobulins	Plasma cells, B cells	B-cell lymphomas
Insulin	Beta cells	Numerous tumors with endocrine features
LCA (PD7/26)	Histiocytes (macrophages), lymphocytes, granulocytes	Hematopoietic tumors
Leu M1	Monocytes, granulocytes	Reed-Sternberg cells, T-cells, adenocarcinomas
Leu-7 (HNK-1)	Natural killer, killer cells, diffuse endocrine system, prostate	T-cell lymphomas; neuroendocrine, neuroectodermal, prostate tumors
Myoglobin	Striated muscle	Rhabdomyomas, rhabdomyosarcomas
NSE	Neurons, diffuse endocrine system, adrenal medulla, nerves, smooth muscle	Neuroendocrine, neuroectodermal tumors; many carcinomas; lung, breast, gastrointestinal tract, ovarian, kidney tumors
PLAP	Trophoblasts	Trophoblastic elements, germ cell tumors
PSA	Prostate	Prostate tumors

continued

Table 34-3 *(continued)*

Antibody	Normal	Tumors
PSAP	Prostate, erythrocytes, lymphocytes, gastrointestinal tract	Prostate tumors, carcinoids, islet cell tumors
S-100	Melanocytes, Schwann's cells, glial cells, neurons, salivary glands, myoepithelial cells, chondrocytes, adipocytes	Breast, gastrointestinal tract, pancreas, lung tumors; melanoma; schwannoma; cartilaginous lesions; histiocytes (macrophages); renal cell cancer; liposarcoma; large cell lymphomas; salivary gland tumors
Somatostatin	Pancreas, gastrointestinal tract	Numerous endocrine tumors or carcinomas containing endocrine cells
Thyroglobulin	Thyroid	Thyroid tumors
Vimentin***	Mesenchymal cells	Mesenchymal tumors, some epithelial tumors

AA1T = alpha$_1$-antitrypsin; AACT = alpha$_1$-antichymotrypsin; ACTH = adrenocorticotropic hormone; AFP = alpha-fetoprotein; CEA = carcinoembryonic antigen; EMA = epithelial membrane antigen; GFAF = glial fibrillary acidic proteins; hCG = human chorionic gonadotropin; HMB-45 = antimelanoma; LCA = leukocyte common antigen; NSE = neuron-specific enolase; PLAP = placental alkaline phosphatase; PSA = prostate-specific antigen; PSAP = prostatic acid phosphatase; * = stains rhabdomyoblasts; ** = stains nonepithelial tumors such as melanoma, leiomyosarcomas, Ewing's sarcoma; *** = coexpressed with cytokeratin in some epithelial tumors.

nonepithelial from epithelial neoplasms. With increased testing of these antibodies, it became evident that rapidly growing epithelial cells may express vimentin. In fact, the widespread application of the use of panels of antibodies to IFs to various types of tumors has shown that many tumors coexpress more than one type of IF (Table 34-6). However, tumors coexpressing several IF types within a single cell must be distinguished from tumors expressing several IFs because they contain a mixture of two or more cell types, each expressing a different IF. Multiple types of IF may also be recognized if normal cells are admixed with neoplastic ones.

Desmin is a useful marker for rhabdomyosarcoma and is well preserved in alcohol-fixed samples. A complementary antibody useful in identifying all types of contractile cells, including muscle cells, myofibroblasts, and myoepithelium is muscle-specific actin (clone HHF-35).

Three polypeptides of differing molecular weights constitute the neurofilament class of IFs seen in neural tissues. Most neural neoplasms express this IF. Neuroendocrine cells may coexpress the lower-molecular-weight neurofilament protein with keratin. Antibodies to glial fibrillary acidic protein (GFAP) are useful in the study of central nervous system tumors. GFAP can be used on smears from brain tumors to distinguish astrocytic tumors from malignant lymphomas and from metastases of anaplastic carcinomas, even when fibril formation is absent.

Table 34-4
Intermediate Filaments

Name	Molecular Weight (kd)	Distribution
Acidic cytokeratins	40-60	Epithelial cells
Neutral/basic cytokeratins	40-68	Epithelial cells
Vimentin	57	Mesenchymal cells, some epithelial cells
Glial, fibrillary, and protein	55	Glial, Schwann's cells
Desmin	53	Muscle cells
Neurofilament	60, 68, 200	Neurons

Table 34–5
Distribution of Cytokeratin Polypeptides

Polypeptide Moll No.	(Molecular Weight × 10^{-3})	Tissue Specificity
1, 2, 10	(68, 65, 56.5)	Keratinizing epithelium
3, 12	(64, 55)	Corneal epithelium
4, 13	(59, 54)	Nonkeratinizing stratified squamous epithelium
5, 14, 15	(58, 50, 50')	Stratified epithelium
6, 16	(56, 48)	Proliferating keratinocytes
7, 17	(54, 46)	Simple and some stratified epithelia
8, 18	(52, 45)	Simple epithelium, hepatocellular carcinomas
19	(40)	Simple epithelium

Primary Panel of Antibodies

A primary panel of antibodies against vimentin, leukocyte common antigen (LCA), cytokeratin, S-100, and HMB-45 is recommended for initial evaluation in difficult cases (see Table 34–2 and Color Plates 34–1*K, L* and 34–2*A, B*). LCA is a cell surface glycoprotein, also known as CD45, that is expressed on lymphocytes and hematopoietic cells. The antigen cannot be used to distinguish be-

Table 34–6
Tumors Coexpressing Intermediate Filaments

	Keratin	Vimentin	NF	GFAP	Desmin
Carcimomas					
Ovary	+	+			
Breast	+	+			
Adenal	+	+			
Lung+	+	+			
Endometrium	+	+			
Thyroid	+	+			
Kidney	+	+			
Salivary gland*	+	+		+	
Prostate	+	+			
Neuroendocrine	+	+	+		
Sarcomas					
Synovial	+**	+			
Epithelioid	+**	+			
Leiomyosarcoma	+	+			+
Wilms's tumor	+**	+			+
Rhabdomyosarcomas	+				+
Germ cell tumors					
Seminoma	+***	+			
Embryonal	+	+			
Other					
Melanoma	+	+			
Mesothelioma	+	+			

+ = usually adenocrcinoma; * = usually pleomorphic adenoma, although rarely mucoepidermoid and adenoid cystic carcinoma; ** = glandular areas keratin-positive; *** = occasionally seen in multinucleated cells; NF = neurofilament; GFAP = glial fibrillary acidic protein.

nign from malignant proliferation, but it does differentiate lymphoid from nonlymphoid tumors. HMB-45 recognizes a 7-kd cytoplasmic peptide and is helpful in the diagnosis of melanoma (Fig. 34–7).

HMB-45 has a higher degree of specificity than S-100 for melanoma, a tumor often considered in the differential diagnosis of undifferentiated epithelial cancers. However, HMB-45 is less sensitive for spindle cell and desmoplastic melanomas. The recent demonstration of HMB-45 reactivity in occasional samples of normal and malignant breast tissue indicates the need to exercise caution in the interpretation of the immunoreactivity of this antibody.

Other antibodies often used in antibody panels include epithelial membrane antigen (EMA), neuron-specific enolase (NSE), chromogranin, and carcinoembryonic antigen (CEA). EMA, also known as human milk fat globulin (HMFG) antigen, was originally identified as a membrane antigen of human milk fat globules. It is also present on mammary epithelium. Antibodies to EMA recognize many adenocarcinomas. However, because EMA reactivity has been described in epithelioid sarcomas, leiomyosarcomas, and lymphomas, EMA positivity should not be used as the sole marker for epithelial derivation.

NSE is an isoenzyme of the glycolytic enzyme enolase that was originally considered to be a marker for nerve and for endocrine cells of the APUD family. However, numerous published papers suggest, and our own data confirm, that NSE stains so many tissue types that it cannot be used as the sole marker for neural or neuroendocrine differentiation.

In our experience, chromogranin is far more reliable than NSE as a neuroendocrine marker. Three chromogranin proteins have been identified. They represent major secretory proteins of neurosecretory granules in both normal and neoplastic cells. These proteins identify diverse types of endocrine and neuroendocrine cells. Chromogranin positivity occurs even in neuroendocrine tumor cells that are not producing their usual hormones, making this reaction very useful as a general marker of neuroendocrine differentiation (Fig. 34–8).

CEA is a useful marker in some situations. It was originally expected that it would be a specific marker of colon cancer, but this has not proved true. It is not even specific for malignancy, since it is found in many regenerating tissues. CEA is most often used to distinguish between metastatic adenocarcinoma and malignant mesothelioma (see below).

Differentiation Markers

Differentiation markers have been extensively applied to the evaluation of hematologic malignan-

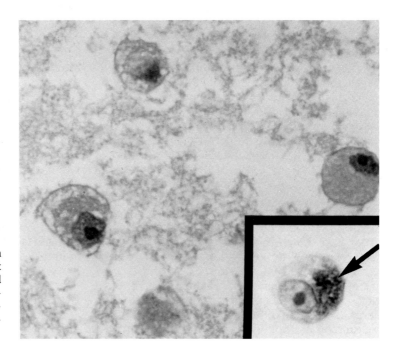

FIGURE 34–7. Pleural effusion with metastatic malignant melanoma of soft parts (H&E, ×800). The large, round tumor cells were strongly HMB-45 positive (*arrow in inset*). (Cell block preparation, methylene blue–diaminobenzidine [DAB], ×800).

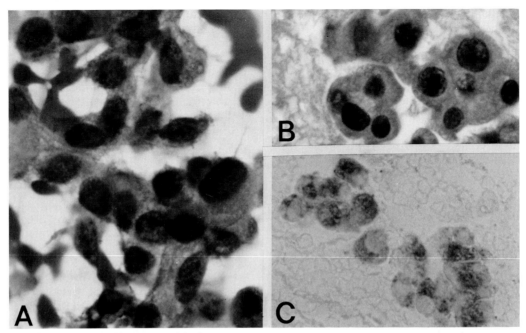

FIGURE 34–8. (*A*) Thin-needle aspiration of a peripancreatic mass revealed a neuroendocrine tumor. Note the uniform cells with eccentric nuclei in an acinar arrangement. (Papanicolaou stain, ×1,000) (*B*) Cell block from the same case. There is moderate anisonucleosis, but the rosette formation is still apparent. (H&E, ×800) (*C*) The cells are chromogranin positive, confirming their neuroendocrine histogenesis. A glucagon stain was also positive in this case. (Uncounterstained-DAB, ×650)

cies. They have allowed us to identify acute leukemias as well as the T- and B-cell lymphomas. This was made possible by the development of reagents that recognize stages of differentiation of B and T cells.

The antigens present on tumor cells variably reflect those present on the cell of origin. With the emergence of the neoplastic phenotype, antigens may be modified, lost, or gained.

Lectins are the prototypic markers that change in their reactivity with evolving neoplastic phenotypes. In part, this relates to the fact that neoplastic cells alter the glycosylation of surface determinants involved in the processes of invasion and metastasis. Lectins are carbohydrate-binding proteins, nonimmunologic in origin, that agglutinate cells and/or precipitate glycoconjugates (see p. 139). They have been used widely to study glycoconjugates on human tumor cell surfaces. Four general types of changes are recognized using these reagents: (1) loss of normal components; (2) increased amounts of normal components; (3) altered distribution of normal components; and (4) appearance of components that are not present on

the cells from which the tumor has arisen. The reagents most commonly used are Ulex-europeaus 1 (UEA1), which stains vascular tumors and reagents that recognize blood group antigens. The latter were particularly popular in the evaluation of bladder cancer since early studies suggested that the loss of blood group antigen expression relates to a poorer prognosis in these tumors (see p. 988).

Changes in antigens expressed on cancer cells are more dramatic with decreasing tumor differentiation. Tumors may also arise from stem cells that never acquired differentiation-related markers. It is also well known that tumors are capable of producing ectopic "inappropriate" products. Many carcinomas make various peptide hormones, and yet one would not classify them as arising from the normal site of production for that peptide. A classic example is production of adrenocorticotropic hormone (ACTH) by a lung carcinoma, which is never thought of as a pituitary tumor.

Similarly, the presence of antigens not usually found in normal tissue does not exclude the origin of a tumor from this tissue because such antigens may be expressed only in regenerative or neoplastic states. An example is the expression of EMA by inflamed or malignant stratified squamous epithelium. Because of these factors, there will always be a small percentage of tumors in which the cell of origin will remain in doubt.

In addition to determining the cell of origin, it is often useful to determine the proliferative activity of a given tumor since this is known to be an important prognostic variable.

Cell Proliferation Markers

Cell proliferation was traditionally measured by counting mitotic figures or by calculating a thymidine-labeling index. Newer techniques for making this assessment have emerged, including S-phase analysis using the flow cytometer (see Chapter 36) or the use of MAb directed against proliferation-associated antigens. The two most studied reagents are Ki-67 and a MAb against PCNA/cyclin. Both of these MAbs react with unknown nuclear antigens associated with cell proliferation, and they are expressed only in nuclei of proliferating cells. They allow one to determine (and quantitate) the growth fraction of tumors by immunostaining, even in minute tissue samples (Fig. 34–9).

Sources of Errors

One should always keep in mind that immunocytochemical studies do not distinguish between those antigens synthesized by the cell and those acquired elsewhere. Some antigens can be bound to cell surfaces via receptors (i.e., growth factors or hormones); others are nonspecifically adsorbed. In addition, some cells such as macrophages, histiocytes, or tumor cells are phagocytic, and endocytosis of numerous substances occurs. Finally, some cells that rapidly export their secreted products may be negative if such products are not stored in the cell.

Tumor-Specific Antibodies

In the preceding paragraphs we have outlined some general approaches that can be taken using immunologic reagents that can enhance cytologic diagnosis. However, one of the disappointing areas continues to be in the development of "tumor-specific" reagents. The saga of this disappointment began with CEA, which, as already indicated, was thought to be specific for colon cancer but is specific neither for colon cancer nor for cancer in general. Periodically, new reagents emerge that are actively promoted as being specific for a specific tumor type and eventually share the fate of CEA. Recently, B72.3, which recognizes a cellular glycoprotein, has received a great deal of attention. This reagent was actively promoted as being capable of distinguishing benign from malignant cells, particularly on cytologic specimens. Subsequent testing has shown that several benign tissues, such as on-

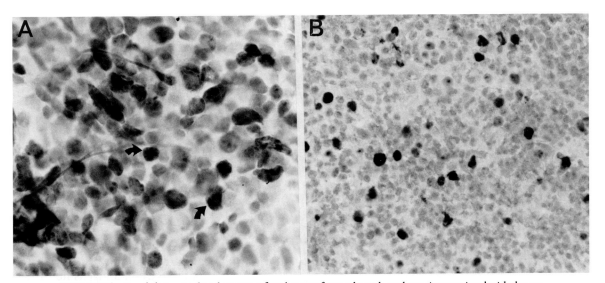

FIGURE 34–9. (*A*) An air-dried acetone-fixed smear from a lymph node aspirate stained with the proliferation marker Ki-67. The number of positive nuclei (*arrows*) on the smear correlates well with the percentage seen on the Ki-67 stain from a frozen section of the excised lymph node (*B*). (*A*, Ki-67–methylene blue–DAB, ×650; *B*, Ki-67–hematoxylin–DAB, ×400)

cocytes and endometrium, are also reactive with this reagent. In fact, numerous reagents were developed that recognize cellular glycoproteins, for example Ca1 (epitectin). The antigens recognized by these reagents either are unknown or constitute a part of a polysaccharide chain on a glycoprotein or a lipoprotein. These tumor-specific MAbs are usually classified by their predominant immunoreactivities with specific tumors. Two popular antibodies, among the many that exist, are CA 19-9, which reacts with determinants on gastrointestinal carcinoma, and OC-125, which is often used in patients with ovarian cancer.

In the following sections we describe the use of some of these reagents and others in specific types of cytology specimens.

EFFUSIONS

Cytologic examination of effusions (see also Chaps. 25 and 26) contributes to the identification of cancers involving the pleural, peritoneal, or pericardial cavities. However, the mesothelial cells, macrophages, and metastatic carcinoma cells may vary widely in their morphology, resulting in difficulty distinguishing among these three cells types in some cases. This problem is compounded by the fact that reactive mesothelial hyperplasia often occurs when a tumor is present and the atypical mesothelial cells intermingle with the neoplastic cells in the cytology specimen. In this setting, judicious use of antibodies may help resolve diagnostic uncertainties. To avoid misdiagnosis, one should always be sure that the interpretation of the immunohistochemical reaction in each cell takes into account whether the cell being analyzed is benign or malignant according to conventional cytologic criteria.

Adenocarcinoma is the most common cancer to be identified in malignant effusions, followed by large cell undifferentiated carcinoma and lymphoma or leukemia. In problem cases, the usual dilemmas facing the cytologist are (1) to determine whether malignant cells are present and (2) if cancer is present, to give the best estimate as to cancer type. To make both of these determinations — that is, to distinguish between metastatic adenocarcinoma and atypical mesothelial cells — and to determine the tumor type, immunocytochemical techniques may provide the most sensitive and specific approach.

Numerous studies substantiate that CEA positivity of cells in body fluids is virtually diagnostic of metastatic carcinoma since mesothelial cells, benign or malignant, do not express CEA (see Color Plate 34–1 *D–F*). One should note that if a cross-reacting antigen in polymorphonuclear leukocytes in effusions results in staining with polyclonal antibodies to CEA. We have eliminated this problem by using a MAb to CEA.

Another marker, Leu M1, a macrophage and Reed-Sternberg cell marker (CD 15), is expressed by numerous malignant tumors, particularly adenocarcinomas, but not by mesothelial cells. The presence of CEA and Leu M1 indicates the presence of metastatic carcinoma but does not suggest the site of origin of the primary tumor.

Additional support for distinction between mesothelial cells and metastatic carcinoma derives from the use of antibodies to EMA. EMA may be weakly and inconsistently visualized on mesothelial cells but is strongly expressed by most metastatic carcinomas. Still, published results with MAbs and EMA have generated conflicting results. Most of these reports used HMFG-2, a MAb to delipidated milk fat globules. A reliable MAb antibody against EMA (clone E29) is one that was raised against human milk fat globule membranes. EMA (E29) has a distinctive pattern of staining in malignant mesothelial cells when compared with metastatic carcinoma (Fig. 34–10). In mesothelial cells, thick cell membrane staining occurs along the periphery of cell clusters and *circumferentially around individual cells* in a pattern corresponding to the distribution of microvilli. When these thick membranes are present around the circumference, not only is the mesothelial origin of the cells confirmed but a malignant change may be suggested. Adenocarcinomas display strong, *diffuse cytoplasmic staining*, in contrast to the weak cytoplasmic staining present in mesothelial cells. It must be noted that negativity for CEA, Leu M1, or EMA does not exclude the diagnosis of adenocarcinoma, because, as already indicated, tumor cells may lose their antigens.

Identifying specific antigens may help define the origin of a metastatic cancer in selected cases. Chromogranin immunoreactivity indicates the presence of a neuroendocrine lesion (see Fig. 34–8). Metastatic prostate cancer is identified by positive immunostaining for prostate-specific antigen (PSA) and prostatic acid phosphatase (PSAP); thyroid cancer can be diagnosed using antibodies to thyroglobulin. PSA has been detected in most prostate cancers and their metastases (in excess of 95%). Specificity is high, and the antigen is not expressed in other adenocarcinomas, although

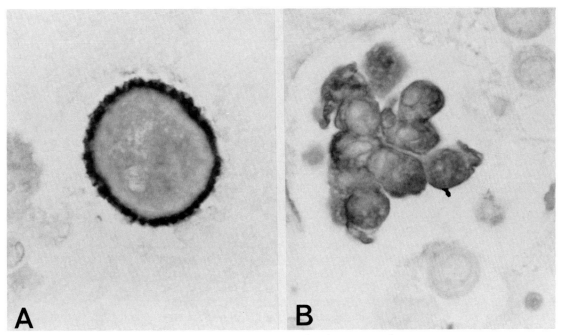

FIGURE 34–10. (*A*) Malignant mesothelioma stained with anti-EMA, demonstrating an intense circumferential staining pattern. (Methylene blue–DAB, ×1,000) (*B*) Metastatic adenocarcinoma cells have diffuse cytoplasmic immunoreactivity with the same anti-EMA antibody. (Methylene blue–DAB, ×1,000)

it may sometimes occur in urothelial tumors. These and other commonly used antibodies are listed in Table 34–3.

One marker that has been extensively studied in effusions in an effort to distinguish benign from malignant cells is B72.3, a MAb generated against a membrane-enriched extract of breast cancer. As noted above, B72.3 has been reported to be a marker for cancer cells, but most users have found that it also reacts with some benign cells. Therefore, it is not useful, in our opinion, for making this distinction.

Effusions containing numerous lymphoid cells often cause diagnostic dilemmas since it is difficult to distinguish reactive from malignant lymphocytes on purely cytologic grounds. The differential diagnosis usually includes an inflammatory process (i.e., tuberculosis), a nonspecific reaction to other diseases (i.e, carcinoma), or the presence of chronic lymphocytic leukemia or lymphoma. The application of a panel of antibodies to lymphocyte surface antigens often discloses the lymphocytic phenotype and indicates the reactive or neoplastic nature of the cells. Therefore, T- and B-cell enumeration and an evaluation of the monoclonality of staining for immunoglobulins are useful in establishing the diagnosis of malignant lymphoproliferative disease (see Color Plate 34–1*J–L*).

Pitfalls in Interpretation

When interpreting immunohistochemical reactions performed on effusion specimens, certain pitfalls should be kept in mind. These include weak false-positive staining limited to cell margins, nucleus, or extracellular background in degenerating cells. False-positive reactions can also occur when cells shed their antigens into the effusion fluid. These can become adsorbed to the surface of all cells present in the effusion, whether benign or malignant. These antigens, as well as dead tumor cells containing them, may also be phagocytosed by macrophages or mesothelial cells. The presence of brown intracellular pigment such as hemosiderin may also impart a false impression of a positive immunostain. Under these circumstances, stains for iron or melanin are useful in identifying the nature of pigment. Finally, if the cells contain large vacuoles, it may be difficult to interpret an immunoreaction because of the scanty extravacuolar cytoplasm present in such cells. This problem may occur when dealing with cytoplasmic antigens.

CEREBROSPINAL FLUID

Cytologic examination of cerebrospinal fluid (CSF) in patients with intracranial metastases provides a useful means of evaluating leptomeningeal involvement by tumors (see also Chapter 27). In some cases, however, morphologic examination alone may be insufficient to recognize the nature and origin of the cells, especially when they are large and mononuclear. In patients without prior documentation of cancer who present with malignant cells in the CSF, the distinction between metastatic carcinomas, lymphoma, or leukemia and a primary central nervous system (CNS) tumor may be difficult. A panel of MAbs capable of determining the general tumor classification (see above) may be of diagnostic help. The markers most useful for primary CNS tumors are GFAP, which stains all glial tumors, and S-100, which stains most such tumors. Glial tumors are also positive for vimentin and with antibodies to neuroendocrine markers. Neurofilaments and cytokeratins are usually negative. The presence of cytokeratin or desmin does not always imply the presence of a metastasis because primitive neuroectodermal tumors may express all IF types besides endocrine markers. In the CSF, however, the volume of fluid and the number of cells available for study are usually small, restricting the effectiveness of immunocytochemical techniques.

Immunostaining is best performed on cytospins prepared at 500 to 800 rpm for five to seven minutes. The optimal cellularity of the specimen is 50 to 100 cells per mm³. In specimens of sparse cellularity, the cells often become distorted or rupture. In contrast, when highly cellular preparations are spun, the smears may contain cell clumps and aggregates, making evaluation of the cytologic features difficult. Therefore, one should assess the cellularity of the sample by using an initial smear prior to spinning the specimen. The appropriate adjustments can then be made by either concentrating or diluting the specimen (see also comments in Chap. 33 on p. 1465).

Some observers suggest that the indirect alkaline phosphatase method is preferable for CSF specimens because the peroxidase (PAP) methods produce high background staining (see p. 1539).

URINE CYTOLOGY

Urine cytology (see also Chaps. 22, 23, and 33) is routinely used in the screening and follow-up of patients with bladder cancer. It has a high degree of accuracy in high-grade tumors. However, detection of low-grade urothelial (transitional cell) carcinomas is not reliable. Because of this, numerous MAbs have been evaluated immunochemically on urine specimens in an attempt to make this diagnosis more objective. One antibody, BL2-10D1, detects low-grade urothelial tumors and carcinoma in situ. Preliminary results suggest that the combination of routine cytology and immunostains with this antibody increases the probability of a correct diagnosis. Other MAbs with encouraging results include MAb 344 and MAb 486 P3/12. These MAbs have been applied to cytocentrifuge-prepared slides, fixed in 95% ethanol prior to staining. More extensive studies are necessary before any of these markers may be proposed as an adjunct to improve the diagnostic sensitivity of urine sediment in low-grade tumors. Another series of urothelial and renal monoclonal antibodies (Table 34–7) directed against glycoproteins or the cell surface membrane has been developed but not extensively tested in cytologic specimens.

As noted earlier, bladder cancers have been intensively investigated with respect to the distribution of blood group antigens in an attempt to develop prognostic indicators. There is a strong correlation between the presence of blood group antigens and the absence of invasion; however, the correlation between blood group substances and recurrence of low-grade bladder tumors is not secure. In general, blood group antigens do not seem to provide clinically useful information beyond that obtained by more readily available diagnostic techniques, including careful determination of tumor grade and stage, follow-up cytologic evaluation, and determination of DNA ploidy status.

PULMONARY CYTOLOGY

The high detection rates for pulmonary neoplasms obtained by cytologic examination (see also Chaps. 19 and 20) are offset by considerable observer variability regarding classification of the cells into precise cytomorphologic types. Accuracy in correlating cytologic and histologic typing of lung tumors ranges from 75% to 94% for squamous cell carcinoma, 68% to 92% for adenocarcinoma, 42% to

Table 34–7
Distribution of Urothelial Monoclonal Antibodies

Monoclonal Antibody	Molecular Weight	Immunizing Cell Line	Normal Tissue Reactivity	Neoplastic Tissue Reactivity
URO-1	140,000 120,000 30,000	Bladder cancer	Glomerulus, basal layer of transitional urothelium, skin	All bladder tumors; renal cell, colon, ovary, lung, and breast cancers
URO-2	160,000 Glycoprotein	Renal cancer	Proximal tubules, glomerulus	Renal cell carcinoma
URO-4	120,000 Adenosine-deaminase-binding protein	Renal cancer	Henle's loop, glomerulus, prostate epithelium	Renal cell carcinoma, lymphoma, rare prostate carcinoma
URO-5	48,000 42,000 Glycoprotein	Bladder cancer	Henle's loop; distal tubules; collecting ducts; transitional epithelium of prostate, breast ducts, skin, esophagus	Bladder, breast, and lung cancer
URO-9	Unknown	Fresh uncultured bladder cancer		Low-grade bladder cancers
URO-10	85,000	Bladder cancer	Proximal tubules, basal layer of skin, esophagus	Invasive bladder tumors; renal, colon, lung, and breast cancer

91% for large cell undifferentiated carcinoma (LCUC), and 83% to 96% for small cell carcinoma. The phenotypic heterogeneity of LCUC contributes to the diagnostic inaccuracy of this group of pulmonary tumors. MAbs against the various molecular-weight cytokeratins and some selected neuroendocrine markers may enhance the cytopathologist's ability to accurately classify pulmonary carcinomas. Two groups of LCUC can be identified by using antibodies of high- and low-molecular-weight keratins. The development of monoclonal antibodies against each cytokeratin type makes it possible to fingerprint these carcinomas. Our laboratory recently analyzed a series of LCUCs with MAbs to CK 8 (52.5 kd) and CK 1 (68 kd) against low- and high-molecular-weight cytokeratins, respectively (Fig. 34–11). Twenty-six percent (4 of 15) of LCUCs had evidence of squamous differentiation based on the presence of high-molecular-weight cytokeratin. On two of these patients tissue was available for histologic examination; both patients had squamous cell carcinomas (see Fig. 34–10).

Besides primary lung cancers, metastatic tumors may be the source of malignant cells. In some cases, the patient may have another known primary tumor, such as a prostatic carcinoma, and the question arises whether the lung lesion is a metastasis or a new primary tumor. In this setting, staining with several antibodies (to prostate-specific antigen and prostatic acid phosphatase) will usually provide the answer. If the patient is suspected of having an occult primary tumor, the specimen should be submitted to an "undifferentiated tumor workup" as outlined previously. In addition, the use of a panel of tumor-specific antibodies may provide a clue as to the site of the primary tumor. The panel could include reagents such as Br6.2 (for breast tumors), OC-125 (for ovarian tumors), URO-2 (for renal cell tumors), and CA19.9 (for gastrointestinal tumors).

NEEDLE-ASPIRATION BIOPSIES

The increasing use of aspiration biopsies to establish a diagnosis without surgical removal of tissue places on the pathologist the burden of establishing a precise diagnosis on a limited sample of cells (see also Chap. 29). When the diagnosis is in doubt, ancillary techniques such as immunocytochemistry may play a valuable role in reaching a conclusive verdict. The more secure a diagnosis is on conventional cytologic examination, the less likely it is that immunocytochemistry will play a significant diagnostic role. Indeed, immunostains of samples in which the diagnosis is not in doubt should be discouraged unless they provide additional in-

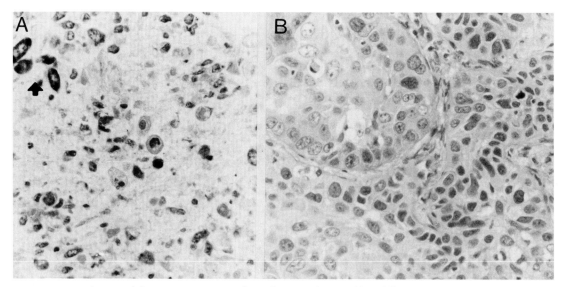

FIGURE 34–11. (*A*) Aspiration smear of a pulmonary large cell undifferentiated carcinoma. Rare cells are positive (*arrow*) with high-molecular-weight cytokeratin antibody 3BH12. (Methylene blue – DAB, ×800) (*B*) Histologic section illustrating a poorly differentiated squamous cell carcinoma. (H&E, ×400)

formation. On the other hand, immunocytochemistry may play a major role in establishing prognostic parameters such as steroid-receptor content or proliferative index. It is important to recognize, however, that the use of immunocytochemistry will usually not "rescue" the diagnosis on a sample that is basically inadequate or was handled in a suboptimal manner.

The small amount of material obtained in aspirated samples usually limits the range of ancillary studies. Nonetheless, the sample is usually adequate to perform a limited number of tests required to determine the antigenic phenotype of most tumors.

Additional unstained smears should be prepared when it is anticipated that additional studies will be required. When there is doubt and if sufficient material is available, additional unstained smears should be prepared, which, if unused, can be thrown away. At times, only stained slides are available. In this situation, either we use the destaining procedure or occasionally we immunostain a previously stained slide without destaining. However, as noted, results obtained by this approach should be interpreted with caution because of the possibility of false-negative or false-positive results.

To optimize the aspirated samples for possible subsequent special studies, we collect all samples in 50% alcohol and the tissue culture medium RPMI 1640 or Hanks' balanced salt solution.

All tissue fragments are embedded in agar and paraffin. The initial sections are stained with hematoxylin and eosin, and additional sections are available for immunoperoxidase studies. Cytospins are prepared from the residual material for Wright-Giemsa stains and for marker studies. Papanicolaou-stained smears are obtained from the alcohol-fixed material.

Lymph Nodes

Aspiration of lymph nodes is becoming increasingly common to evaluate lymphadenopathy, to identify disease processes such as metastatic or primary cancer, to stage a cancer, or to obtain material needed for immunophenotyping, flow cytometry, or genetic analysis. Aspiration of intra-abdominal or retroperitoneal lymph nodes is an attractive alternative to major surgery. The use of immunocytochemistry contributes to diagnostic accuracy by immunophenotyping undifferentiated tumors and by establishing immunocytochemical profiles in malignant lymphomas and related disorders (see Color Plate 34–2*A*, *B*).

Leukemias and Lymphomas

Immunophenotyping of leukemias and lymphomas has revealed a heterogeneity that was unsuspected on purely morphologic examination.

This heterogeneity became apparent with the development of MAbs that recognize precise stages in lymphocyte and granulocyte differentiation. Hundreds of MAbs are now available, directed against leukocytic determinants. Most are differentiation-related antigens appearing (and disappearing) during leukocyte ontogeny. The presence of well-defined sets of markers, correlating with specific stages of leukocyte maturation, forms the basis of immunophenotyping of lymphomas and leukemias. The antibodies to these immune determinants have been grouped according to the differentiation patterns into clusters of differentiation (CD) groups. The 45 CD groups can be assembled into three supergroups representing myeloid, B-cell, and T-cell lineages.

Cells exhibiting monocytoid differentiation are recognized by antibodies detecting the CD-14 group and by anti-Ia antibodies. Histiocytes (macrophages) are recognized by antibodies to lysozyme, alpha$_1$-antitrypsin, and chymotrypsin, but these markers are not reliable: many other cell types can be positive, including myeloid cells, lymphomas, and carcinomas. Antibodies recognizing CD-13 and CD-33 are useful in differentiating myeloid from lymphoid lineages, and the myeloid antigens CD-13 and CD-14 appear to have prognostic value.

Common acute lymphoblastic leukemia antigen (CALLA) is commonly used in the evaluation of B-cell malignancies. This antigen is identical to the enzyme neutral endopeptidase, which is also present in some nonlymphoid tissues.

B cells can be recognized by detecting surface or cytoplasmic immunoglobulins. Antibodies to CD-19 represent an excellent general B-cell marker, and antibodies to CD-10, CD-20, CD-22, and CD-5 antigens allow the recognition of B-cell subsets. Antibodies to CD-19, CD-20, and CD-22 detect antigens present on normal B cells and pre – B cells; their value resides in the recognition of B-cell lineages in cells that are negative for immunoglobulins.

T-cell lineage is often identified with antibodies to CD-2, CD-3, CD-4, CD-7, and CD-8. T-cell helper and suppressor cell subsets are distinguished by antibodies to CD-4 and CD-8, respectively. The ratio between CD-4 and CD-8 subsets is useful in evaluating non-neoplastic proliferations such as those occurring in patients with acquired immunodeficiency syndrome (AIDS).

Three to five separate lymph node preparations are usually required to obtain enough cells for immunophenotyping. The specimen is collected in 5 ml of RPMI 1640 tissue culture medium, with 1% fetal calf serum. The mononuclear cells are isolated by Ficole-Hypaque or by Lymphoprep density gradient separation. On this enriched specimen, surface marker and flow cytometry studies can be performed. Surface marker studies are performed on air-dried cytocentrifuged slides fixed in acetone or buffered formol-acetone. Cell morphology is evaluated on a Wright-Giemsa – stained preparation. The simple lymphoid screening panel we use in our laboratory includes antibodies that identify B-cell markers (CD-19, CD-20, lambda, kappa) and the T markers CD2, CD3, and CD5. A mixture of T cells and kappa and lambda light-chain-bearing cells in physiologic distribution (kappa : lambda <3 : 1 or lambda : kappa <2 : 1) is indicative of a polyclonal or a reactive process. Monoclonality is defined as kappa : lambda or lambda : kappa >6 : 1 (see Color Plate 34 – 1 *J–L*). The diagnosis of T-cell lymphoma is suggested if the atypical cells express a dominant T-cell phenotype (either helper CD4 or suppressor CD8) or if there is a loss of one or more of the pan — T markers (CD5, CD3). Hodgkin's disease is diagnosed when Reed-Sternberg cells are identified. A polyclonal B-cell population of lymphocytes with T-helper cells and Leu M1 positive cells is usually also present. Leu M1 and Ki-1 antibodies stain the membranes and cytoplasm of Reed-Sternberg cells and their variants. Peripheral T-cell lymphomas may be difficult to distinguish from Hodgkin's disease, and a conclusive diagnosis may not be possible in such cases. Interpretative problems arise (1) when the focal involvement of the lymph node is not sampled by the aspiration procedure or if the small component of monoclonal cells is overshadowed by the polyclonal population; (2) when there are numerous T cells in a T-cell-rich B-cell lymphoma; (3) when there are technical artifacts due to problems in specimen handling or background staining; or (4) when the large anaplastic cell lymphoma (Ki-1) mimicking melanoma or carcinoma is present. In difficult cases, excisional biopsy of the lymph node is recommended.

As noted, aspiration biopsy is an attractive way to accurately diagnose mediastinal, retroperitoneal, and intra-abdominal lymphomas (Fig. 34 – 12). An 86% correlation between biopsy diagnosis and FNA has been noted by one group of investigators. Cafferty et al. showed that the sensitivity of this procedure was approximately 66% and the predictive value of a positive test was 99%, whereas the predictive value of a negative test was 42%. These data were derived from a series of 238 aspirations of intra-abdominal masses suspected of being lymphoma. Seventy-nine percent of cases could be

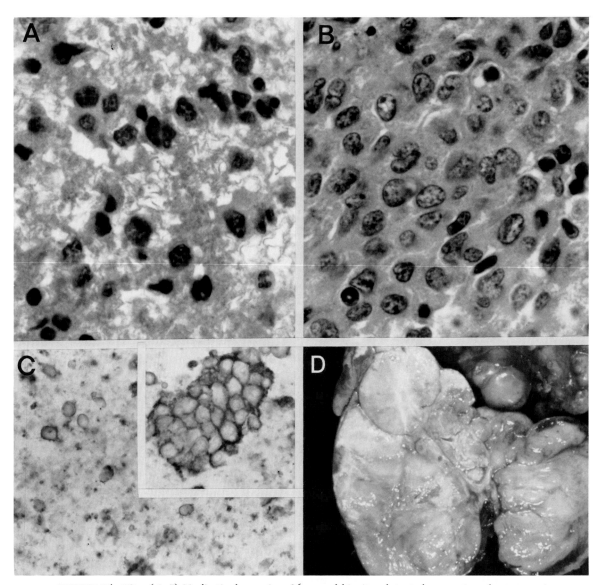

FIGURE 34–12. (*A, B*) Mediastinal mass in a 26-year-old janitor detected on routine chest x-ray. A thin-needle aspiration was performed. The specimen contained poorly differentiated neoplastic cells, forming cohesive sheets (*B*) or lying singly (*A*). The differential diagnosis was a thymoma versus lymphoma. (*A,* H&E cell block, ×650, *B* ×1,000) (*C*) The scattered tumor cells and the solid clusters (*inset*) were positive for leukocyte common antigen and L26 (B cell marker). (L26–methylene blue–DAB, ×400). The mass was surgically removed, and histology confirmed the needle aspiration diagnosis of B cell lymphoma. (*D*) The tumor was a 13-cm firm, fleshy, lobulated mass.

classified as T- or B-cell lymphoma on the basis of a small panel of immunomarkers.

Metastatic Tumors

Metastatic carcinomas and melanomas involving lymph nodes must often be considered in the differential diagnosis of lymphadenopathy. The work-up can be based on the antibody panels outlined previously. The detection of cytokeratin-positive cells is a very strong indicator that metastatic carcinoma is present. Cytokeratin-positive cells in a benign lymph node occur only in the presence of benign epithelial cell inclusions, an exceptional event. Some melanocytic markers may be positive in lymph nodes containing benign nevus cells under the capsule, another extremely rare event. In both situations, a positive staining reaction should not pose a diagnostic dilemma since the cells in the aspirate are benign. Some of the same interpretive problems that occur with lymphomas may also occur with lymph nodes containing metastatic disease. For example, a small metastasis may be missed in the aspirate. In the future the concept of detection of minimal malignant disease by cytologic techniques may be revolutionized by the polymerase chain reaction, followed by molecular hybridization (see Chap. 2). With this approach, the genetic sequence of interest, if it is known and/ or present, may be amplified to a level that can be detected by a hybridization reaction. Thus, for example, if a metastatic carcinoma is suspected, the DNA could be amplified and hybridized using a probe to the cytokeratin gene(s). The presence of a cytokeratin gene would strongly suggest that a carcinoma was present. This technology is still in experimental stages.

Infectious Processes

A certain number of lymphadenopathies are the result of infectious processes. If an organism is present in the nodal tissue (and the adenopathy is not merely a reaction to the infection), then immunocytochemistry may be of diagnostic value to identify the specific infectious agent by appropriate MAbs.

Liver

Aspiration biopsy is an accurate method of diagnosing space occupying lesions of the liver, especially when used in combination with radiologic imaging techniques. By this approach, one can diagnose primary and secondary tumors as well as some infections. The most common differential diagnosis is between a primary hepatoma and a metastatic tumor. The immunocytologic approach to the diagnosis of metastatic tumors was described previously, a process always made easier by knowledge of clinical data. When the metastasis is from an organ for which well-defined tissue markers exist (i.e., prostate or thyroid), the identification of the primary site is easy. In other cases the immunocytologic identification of the primary site is nearly impossible, except on morphologic and clinical grounds (see Chap. 29).

The distinction among varying degrees of hepa-

tocellular atypia (dysplasia), hepatocellular carcinoma (HCC), and regenerative liver cells is often difficult. These distinctions are better evaluated on the basis of cytologic features rather than immunocytochemistry (see Chapter 29). However, immunocytochemistry can be quite valuable in differentiating between HCC and a metastatic carcinoma. Several markers of hepatocellular differentiation are commonly used, none of which is unequivocally specific for liver cells.

Alpha-fetoprotein (AFP), if positive, is a reliable marker for HCC (see Color Plate 34–1*G–I*), provided a metastatic germ cell neoplasm has been excluded. This marker is positive in 25% to 75% of HCC, although the presence and degree of positivity of AFP do not always correlate with the serum levels. Regenerating and atypical (dysplastic) liver cells may also be positive. Alpha$_1$-antitrypsin is another marker useful in recognizing HCC, but it is not as reliable as AFP. Furthermore, a positive reaction to alpha$_1$-antitrypsin is seen in many other tumor types, including germ cell tumors (see Table 34–3).

Carcinoembryonic antigen CEA is variably positive in regenerating liver, primary, and metastatic tumors. In some situations, the pattern of CEA staining may be helpful in distinguishing tumor types, but we find these patterns to be unreliable (see Color Plate 34–1*G–I*, Fig. 34–3). In contrast, the use of different MAbs to cytokeratins may help in differentiating HCC, cholangiocarcinoma, and metastatic tumors. In general, HCCs are immunoreactive with the commercially available antikeratin MAb cocktails, 35BH11 and CAM 5.2, but not with AE1. Metastatic tumors and cholangiocarcinomas are positive with AE1 and CAM 5.2. Both 35BH11 and CAM 5.2 have antibodies against cytokeratin 8, a low-molecular-weight keratin, whereas cytokeratin 8 is not recognized by AE1.

Sarcomas

The immunocytochemical analysis of soft part and bone sarcomas is less rewarding than that of lymphomas or carcinomas. Sarcomas often demonstrate divergent patterns of differentiation, and many of these tumors contain poorly differentiated or undifferentiated cells that do not react with any specific antibody.

When the tumors are better differentiated, a mesenchymal phenotype can be detected. The usual markers of a mesenchymal phenotype are desmin, vimentin, myoglobin, actin, factor VIII–related antigen, UEA1, and neural or glial markers, as described previously. Many studies have shown that benign and malignant smooth and skeletal muscle tumors retain the desmin expression of their progenitor cells. We find that antibodies to desmin, in conjunction with those to myoglobin, are useful in diagnosing rhabdomyosarcoma (Table 34–8). However, we have also seen occasional cases in which we were certain that skeletal muscle differentiation was present on morphologic grounds, that were negative with both antibodies. Furthermore, one must keep in mind that some smooth muscle tumors are positive with antibodies to low-molecular-weight cytokeratins.

Actin is found in the cytoplasm of all cell types. Six different isoforms are expressed in various cell types. Gamma alpha actin isoforms are present in the cytoplasm of smooth muscle and nonmuscle cells, contrasting with alpha sarcomeric actin, which is expressed only in cardiac and skeletal muscle cells.

Vimentin is expressed in most connective tissue, stromal cells, and tumors arising from them. However, this intermediate filament may be coexpressed with other IFs, including cytokeratin (see Table 34–6). Both factor VIII–related antigen and UEA-I are used as markers of endothelial differentiation in angiosarcomas. UEA-I is a more sensitive marker, especially in less well differentiated tumors. However, UEA-I has the disadvantage of staining mucin-producing adenocarcinomas and therefore is less specific in establishing the diagnosis of angiosarcoma.

Breast Tumor Markers

Thin needle aspiration of breast masses has gained acceptance as an efficient, cost-effective diagnostic technique to evaluate breast disease. On adequate samples neoplastic disorders can be differentiated from benign diseases. In difficult cases, the use of immunocytochemistry can provide additional information. For example, the loss of myoepithelial cells, characteristic of most malignant processes, can be documented by the absence of cells positive for muscle-specific actin. Conversely, the identification of actin-positive myoepithelial cells closely associated with ductal cells provides supporting evidence for the presence of a benign lesion (see Color Plate 34–2C,D).

In lesions that are predominantly composed of lymphocytes, the immunocytochemical approach outlined on p. 1553 serves to separate neoplastic and non-neoplastic lesions. Tumors that can cause considerable diagnostic difficulties are those containing a prominent mesenchymal component, either alone or admixed with epithelial cells. The epithelial cells can be identified by their cytokeratin immunoreactivity, but it is important to remember that breast cancer cells are among those carcinomas known to express vimentin; consequently, vimentin positivity alone does not necessarily indicate the presence of a mesenchymal component in the tumor.

Prognosis in Mammary Carcinoma

Immunocytochemistry can also be used to assess prognosis in breast cancer. Estrogen receptors (ERs) and progesterone receptors (PRs) are both well recognized as prognostic indicators in breast cancer. Immunocytochemical localization studies on steroid receptors allow one to simultaneously evaluate the tissue for the presence of tumor cells as well as to localize the receptor protein to a specific cell population. It also allows ER content evaluation by image analysis on tissue fragments that are too small to be extracted for biochemical analysis. Furthermore, detection of steroid receptors on aspirated specimens may reduce the need for a sur-

Table 34–8
Immunocytochemical Markers in Small, Round Cell Tumors

	Keratin	*Vimentin*	*NF*	*Desmin*	*Actin*	*LCA*	*NSE*
Neuroblastoma	−	+	+**	−	−	−	+
Lymphoma	−	+	−	−	−	+	−
Rhabdomyosarcoma	−	+	−	+	+	−	+/−
Small cell carcinoma	+	−	+/−	−	−	−	+
Ewing's sarcoma	+*	+	−	−	−	−	+/−
Wilms's tumor	+***	+	−	−	−	−	−

* = rare; ** = may be seen on frozen sections only; +/− Variable immunoreactivity; *** = Positive in tubular component; NF = neurofilament; LCA = lymphocyte common antigen; NSE = neuron-specific enolase.

gical biopsy of the tumor. A direct correlation exists between positive ER staining and response to endocrine therapy in women with advanced disease. Therefore, ERs are generally accepted for selection of patients for endocrine therapy. Commercially available antibodies now exist that reliably detect ER and PR at the cellular level. Using these antibodies, many investigators have shown that the degree of immunocytochemical staining correlates with biochemical determination of ER content in the tissues (see also Chap. 35).

PR status in patients with primary breast cancer is also a significant independent prognostic factor for disease-free survival as well as for overall survival. Patients with detectable PR levels, whether high or low, have a generally better prognosis than those who are PR negative. Localization of PR on needle-aspirated specimens decreases the need for expensive biochemical assays (Fig. 34–13) and may reduce the need for a surgical procedure. Furthermore, tumors too small for biochemical assay can easily be aspirated and the ER status assessed by immunocytology performed on the smear. The results may vary in small samples because the ER distribution may be quite heterogeneous. There are also some drawbacks to the use of an immunocytochemical approach for ER or PR analysis of aspirates. One of the dilemmas is that the aspirated sample may not be representative of the tumor when compared with the results of a biochemical analysis performed on a larger portion of tissue.

Occasionally, ERs are detected only by immunostains when biochemical methods are negative. This occurs in patients on hormone therapy with tamoxifen, an antiestrogen drug known to block the active site of the receptor, thereby preventing biochemical analysis. To standardize the evaluation of ERs in tumor samples and cytologic material, the immunostains may be quantitated by image analysis techniques (see Chap. 35).

Technical difficulties also have been reported, such as the loss of cells from coated slides and loss of antigenicity in smears, after exposure to room temperature for variable periods of time before analysis. False-negative results may occur on needle aspirates in the presence of a large stromal component and low numbers of cancer cells.

Other prognostic markers include the nuclear protein recognized by the antibody Ki-67, which allows one to evaluate the growth fraction of the tumor, as indicated previously. Vimentin has been shown to correlate inversely with tumor ER content and directly correlates with tumor grade. The growth factor receptor encoded for by the onco-

gene HER2/*neu* may also prove to be a valuable prognostic indicator. Amplification of this gene appears to be particularly useful as a marker of prognosis in patients with positive lymph nodes. It is probable that staining of needle aspirates for the HER2/*neu* protein may prove to be clinically useful, particularly if combined with image analysis quantification techniques and as a component of a breast cancer prognostic panel (see Chap. 35).

The highly controversial antibody B72.3 has also been employed as a diagnostic adjunct in breast aspirates. The MAb, previously described, is reported to be 90% sensitive in detecting infiltrating breast cancer on aspirates with excellent specificity. However, benign apocrine cells also react positively with this antibody. Still, the reaction in benign apocrine cells is typically confined to the cell membrane, whereas in malignant cells the immunoreactivity is usually cytoplasmic.

Small Cell Tumors of Childhood

A number of highly malignant tumors composed of small, round cells, usually occurring in children but occasionally also in young adults, may be observed in a variety of cytologic specimens.

Neuroblastoma, rhabdomyosarcoma of embryonal type, Ewing's sarcoma, Wilms' tumor, and medulloblastoma may have a very similar cytologic presentation in a variety of fluids and aspirates. Because of very different treatment regimens, these tumors should be differentiated from one another and from malignant lymphomas. Additional points of differential diagnosis include small cell carcinomas and some endocrine carcinomas, including the Merkel cell tumor of the skin, usually seen in adults but occasionally also in children. The morphologic features of these tumors were discussed in the appropriate chapters. Table 34–8 lists the immune markers that may be useful in the differential diagnosis of these tumors.

Keratin staining is usually positive in carcinomas and in the epithelial components of Wilms' tumor (nephroblastoma). Neurofilaments are common in neuroblastomas (and in medulloblastomas). In neuroendocrine carcinomas (including Merkel cell tumors), keratin and chromogranin are usually positive (see Table 34–2).

INFECTIOUS DISEASE

Clinically useful immunocytochemical techniques have been described for rapid recognition of sev-

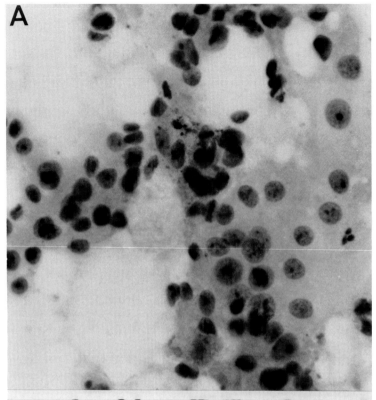

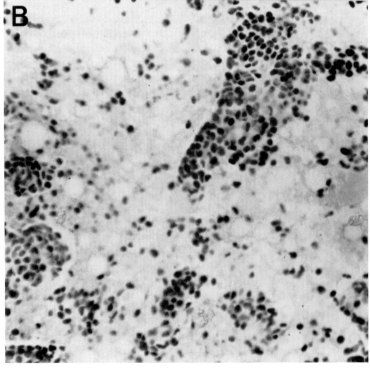

FIGURE 34–13. (*A*) A poorly differentiated invasive ductal carcinoma of the breast diagnosed by thin-needle aspiration. (Papanicolaou stain, ×800) (*B*) The tumor cells were strongly progesterone-receptor positive. (Progesterone - receptor - uncounterstained-DAB, ×400. Courtesy of Dr. Sue A. Bartow, University of New Mexico School of Medicine, Department of Pathology, Albuquerque, N.M.)

eral microorganisms that may otherwise be difficult to identify in cytologic preparations.

Infestation with *Trichomonas vaginalis* regardless of the location or state of preservation of the organism or previous staining of the preparation, can be diagnosed in genital and extragenital sites by using a specific antibody (see p. 345). Immunostaining of previously stained smears yields reproducible and permanent preparations.

The immunoperoxidase technique for the detection of herpes simplex virus (HSV) infections can be highly specific. However, a careful review of routinely stained smears may yield better results. The presence of the classic multinucleated giant cells in routine Papanicolaou smears is a finding with a high degree of sensitivity (90%) and specificity for HSV infection (95%) (see p. 351). Although alcohol fixation and 0.3% HC1 decolorizing steps have minimal effect on the sensitivity of immunoperoxidase techniques, the clinical stage of HSV lesions seems to be a factor. Numerous studies have indicated that the technique is more sensitive for early-stage lesions and less so for later-stage lesions. Cultures of later-stage lesions also tend to be negative. The immunoperoxidase technique is useful for the confirmation of the presence of HSV when routine smears are negative or equivocal. Monitoring of pregnant women known to harbor HSV is of particular concern because of the unpredictability of asymptomatic shedding of the virus. Infection in the birth canal can lead to herpetic encephalitis and other serious sequelae in the infant. Current methods for the diagnosis of HSV infection include viral cultures, immunofluores-

cence, and routine vaginocervical screening cytology. Immunoperoxidase methods can be applied to routine Papanicolaou smears, allowing a permanent documentation of HSV positivity. The presence of HSV may lead to delivery by a cesarean section. The techniques of identification of *human papillomavirus* are described in Chapter 11 and in Appendix II to this chapter. Identification techniques of human polyomavirus are described in Chapter 22.

Chlamydia trachomatis is an important infectious agent that may cause pelvic inflammatory disease in women. A positive culture is currently used as the gold standard to diagnose chlamydial infections because Papanicolaou smears are not a sensitive technique (see p. 342). Certain patient populations, including pregnant women and neonates suspected of having a chlamydial infection, may benefit from the immunocytochemical staining of destained Papanicolaou-stained smears to confirm the diagnosis of *Chlamydia* infection. The advantage of performing the immunostains on Papanicolaou smears is a correlation with the cytomorphologic findings.

Another area in which immunocytochemistry has played a role in infectious disease has been in the documentation of viral hepatitis. Specific antibodies exist against the various hepatitis viruses as well as against other viruses, and their use may be particularly beneficial in patients with mixed or atypical infections. The antibodies may also be used to confirm a diagnosis made on standard histologic criteria.

Appendix I:
Immunocytochemical
Methods

The following procedures are used in our laboratory as noted. Each laboratory, however, must experiment with immunostaining procedures.

AVIDIN-BIOTIN-PEROXIDASE STAINING PROCEDURE

Body Fluids

1. Body fluids: cytocentrifuge 200 ml of fresh fluid for 5 to 7 minutes between 500 and 800 rpm. (Less volume may be used if large amounts are unavailable.) Air-dry the preparations for at least 2 hours or overnight at room temperature. Some antigens may be retained up to 2 weeks if air-dried preparations are kept at 4°C. Some authors have reported that fixation of cell smears, imprints, and cytospins immediately after preparation reduces the loss of antigens.

2. Fix in cold, buffered formol-acetone at 4°C for 30 seconds or cold acetone at 4°C for 1 minute. Fixed slides may be stored at -20°C for up to 5 years. Fix stored slides in cold (-20°C) acetone immediately before use.

3. Rinse in phosphate-buffered saline (PBS) solution, pH 7.4 (1 minute).

4. Cover slides with 5% normal serum in PBS solution. Use the same animal species as that of the linking antibody. Incubate in humidity chamber for 10 minutes at room temperature.

5. Remove excess of normal serum (do not rinse).

6. Apply 50 to 100 μl of primary antibody in appropriate dilution. Incubate in humidity chamber for 60 minutes at room temperature.

7. Wash in PBS solution for 5 minutes.

8. Add biotinylated linking antibody (usually from kit). We use Biogenex strepavidin universal kits. Incubate for 30 minutes in humidity chamber at room temperature.

9. Wash in PBS solution for 5 minutes.

10. Add strepavidin-biotin-peroxidase complex. Incubate for 30 minutes at room temperature.

11. Wash in PBS solution for 5 minutes.

12. Incubate slides with 0.15 mg of diamino-benzidine dissolved in 20 ml of PBS solution with 40 μl of 30% H_2O_2 for 2 to 10 minutes at room temperature.

13. Wash with distilled water for 5 minutes.

14. Counterstain with Mayer's hematoxylin.

15. Wash in tap water, dehydrate slides and coverslip with Permount. Endogenous peroxidase activity may decrease the specificity of the staining by increased background. A 3% H_2O_2 PBS solution may be applied to smears for 10 minutes at room temperature before the normal serum block. This step, however, may result in loss of cells from slides.

INDIRECT IMMUNOALKALINE PHOSPHATASE PROCEDURE

1. Prepare smears as indicated in avidin-biotin procedure.
2. We use the Dakopatts APAPP kit.
3. Incubate smears for 30 minutes with primary antibody diluted in TRIS buffer, pH 7.5. All incubations are carried out in a humidity chamber.
4. Rinse in TRIS buffer for 1 minute.
5. Apply linking antibody (Dakopatts), and incubate for 30 minutes at room temperature.
6. Rinse in TRIS buffer for 1 minute.
7. Apply the APAPP complex (Dakopatts), and incubate slides for 30 minutes.
8. Rinse in TRIS buffer for 1 minute.
9. Incubate the slides in the following filtered medium for 20 minutes at room temperature: Fast Red chromogen, naphthol AS phosphate substrate, and levamisole (inhibits endogenous alkaline phosphatase).
10. Rinse in distilled water for 5 minutes.
11. Counterstain in Mayer's hematoxylin.
12. Rinse in water and coverslip with a prewarmed aqueous mounting medium (glycerol jelly).

PREPARATION OF THIN-NEEDLE ASPIRATES

Any excess material from FNA can be flushed into 3 to 5 ml of RPMI 1640 (Flow Laboratories) tissue culture media, Hanks' balanced salt solution, or phosphate buffered saline. Cytospin preparations are made using a Shandon cytospin between 500 and 800 rpm for 5 to 7 minutes, using approximately 200 μl of the cell suspension depending on the cellularity. These smears are air-dried over-night at room temperature or stored at -20°C until stained. The staining procedure is as previously described. Cells obtained from suspected lymphomas may be concentrated by Ficoll-Hypaque or Lymphoprep density gradient. This concentrated mixture may be divided for cytospins, flow cytometry, or other studies.

FIXATIVE

A buffered mixture of acetone and formalin: (pH 6.6) 15 mg of N_2HPO_4, 120 mg of KH_2PO_4, 30 ml of H_2O, 45 ml of acetone, and 25 ml of 40% formaldehyde. This is kept at 2° to 6°C and is stable up to 1 month.

Acknowledgments

We gratefully acknowledge the technical assistance of Joanne Hart, the photographic expertise of the Medical Media Service at the VA Medical Center, and the editorial assistance of Agnes Truske.

BIBLIOGRAPHY

Antibodies

Huber R.: Structural basis for Ag-Ab recognition. Science, *233*:702–703, 1986.

Köhler, G., and Milstein, C.: Continuous cultures of fused cells secreting antibody of predefined specificity. Nature, *256*:495–497, 1975.

Larsson, L.-I.: *Immunocytochemistry: Theory and Practice.* pp. 1–36. Boca Raton, Fla., CRC Press, 1988.

Technical Factors

Chess, Q., and Hajdu, S.I.: The role of immunoperoxidase staining in diagnostic cytology. Acta Cytol. *30*:1–7, 1986.

Dinges, H.P., Wirnsberger, G., and Hofler, H.: Immunocytochemistry in cytology, comparative evaluation of different techniques. Anal. Quant. Cytol. Histol., *11*:22–32, 1989.

Domagala, W.M., Markiewski, M., Tuziak, T., Kram, A., Weber, K., and Osborn, M.: Immunocytochemistry on fine needle aspirates in paraffin mini-blocks. Acta Cytol., *34*:291–296, 1990.

Elias, J.M., Margiotta, M., and Gaborc, D.: Sensitivity and detection efficiency of the peroxidase antiperoxidase (PAP), avidin-biotin peroxidase complex (ABC) and peroxidase-labeled avidin-biotin (LAB) procedures. Am. J. Clin. Pathol., *92*:62–67, 1989.

Gustafsson, B., and Manson J.-C.: Methodological aspects and application of the immunoperoxidase staining technique in diagnostic fine-needle aspiration cytology. Diagn. Cytol., *3*:68–73, 1987.

Li, C.-Y., Ziesmer, S.C., Yam, L.T., English, M.C., and Janckila, A.J.: Practical immunocytochemical identification of human blood cells. Am. J. Clin. Pathol., *81*:204–212, 1984.

Nadji, M.: The potential value of immunoperoxidase techniques in diagnostic cytology. Acta Cytol. *24*:442–447, 1980.

Pettigrew, N.M.: Techniques in immunocytochemistry application to diagnostic pathology. Arch. Pathol. Lab. Med., *113*:641–644, 1989.

Pollard, K., Lunny, D., Holgate, C.S., et al.: Fixation, processing and immunochemical reagent effects on preservation of T lymphocyte surface membrane antigen in paraffin embedded tissue. J. Histochem. Cytochem., *35*:1329–1338, 1987.

Puchtler, H., and Meloan, S.N.: On the chemistry of formaldehyde fixation and its effects on immunohistochemical reactions. Histochemistry, *82*:201–204, 1985.

Riederer, B.M.: Antigen preservation tests for immunocytochemical detection of cytoskeletal proteins: Influence of aldehyde fixatives. J. Histochem. Cytochem., *37*:675–681, 1989.

To, A., Coleman, D.V., Dearnaly, D.P., Omerod, M.G., Steele, K., and Neville, A.M.: Use of antisera to epithelial membrane antigen for the cytodiagnosis of malignancy in serous effusion. J. Clin. Pathol., *34*:1326–1332, 1981.

Detection Systems of Immune Reactions

Cattoretti, G., Berti, E., Schiro, R., et al.: Improved avidin-biotin-peroxidase complex (ABC) staining. Histochem. J., *20*:75–80, 1989.

Colley, M., Kommoss, F., Bibbo, M., Dytch, H.E., Franklin, W.A., Holt, J.A., and Wied, G.L.: Assessment of hormone receptors in breast carcinoma by immunocytochemistry and image analysis. II. Estrogen receptors. Anal. Quant. Cytol. Histol., *11*:307–314, 1989.

DeWaele, M., Demay, J., Reynaert, P., et al.: Detection of cell surface antigens in cryostat sections with immunogold-silver staining. Am. J. Clin. Pathol., *85*:573–578, 1986.

Duffy, A.M., Stevens, M.W., and McLennan, G.: The immunogold staining technique for the measurement of lymphocyte subpopulations in bronchoalveolar lavage fluid. Acta Cytol. *30*:152–156, 1986.

Faulk, W., and Taylor, G.: An immunocolloid method for the electron microscopy. Immunochemistry, *8*:1081–1083, 1971.

Fishman, W.H.: Perspectives on alkaline phosphatase isoenzymes. Am. J. Med., *56*:617–650, 1974.

Gupta, P.K., Myers, J.D., Baylin, S.B., Mulshire, J.L., Guttitta, F., and Gazdar, A.F.: Improved antigen detection in ethanol-fixed cytologic specimens. A modified avidin-biotin-peroxidase complex (ABC) method. Diagn. Cytopathol., *1*:133–136, 1985.

Hsu, S.M., Raine, L., and Fanger, H.: Use of avidin-biotin-peroxidase complex (ABC) in immunoperoxidase techniques: A comparison between ABC and unlabeled antibody (PAP) procedures. J. Histochem. Cytochem., *29*:577–580, 1981.

Konmoss, F., Bibbo, M., Colley, M., Dytch, H.E., Franklin, W.A., Holt, J.A., and Wied, G.L.: Assessment of hormone receptors in breast carcinoma by immunocytochemistry and image analysis. I. Progesterone receptors. Anal. Quant. Cytol. Histol., *11*:298–305, 1989.

Ormanns, W., and Schaffer, R.: An alkaline-phosphatase staining method in avidin-biotin immunohistochemistry. Histochemistry, *82*:421–424, 1985.

Springall, D.R., Lackie, P., Levene, M.M., et al.: The potential of the immunosilver staining method for paraffin sections. Histochemistry, *81*:603–608, 1984.

Sternberger, L.A., Hardy, P.H., Jr., Cuculis, J.J., and Meyer, H.G.: The unlabeled antibody enzyme method of immunohistochemistry. Preparation and properties of soluble antigen-antibody complex (horseradish peroxidase-antihorseradish peroxidase) and its use in identification of spirochetes. J. Histochem. Cytochem., *18*:315–333, 1970.

Yam, L.T., Janckila, A.J., Epremian, B.E., and Li, C.-Y.: Diagnostic significance of levamisole-resistant alkaline phosphatase in cytochemistry and immunocytochemistry. Am. J. Clin. Pathol., *91*:31–36, 1989.

Tumor Diagnosis

Battifora, H., and Kopinska, M.I.: Distinction of mesothelioma from adenocarcinoma. An immunohistochemical approach. Cancer, *55*:1679–1685, 1985.

Borowitz, M.J., and Stein, R.B.: Diagnostic applications of monoclonal antibodies to human cancer. Arch. Pathol. Lab. Med., *108*:101–105, 1984.

Damjanov, I., and Knowles, B.B.: Biology of disease. Monoclonal antibodies and tumor associated antigens. Lab. Invest., *48*:510–525, 1983.

Gould, V.E., Rorken, L.B., Jansson, D.S., Molenay, W.M., Trojanowski, J.Q., Lee, V.M., Heyderman, E., Warren, P.J., and Haines, A.M.R.: Immunocytochemistry today—problems and practice. Histopathology, *15*:655–658, 1989.

Johnston, W.W.: Applications of monoclonal antibodies in clinical cytology as exemplified by studies with monoclonal antibody B72.3. Acta Cytol. *31*:537–556, 1987.

Klug, T.L., Bast, R.C., Jr., Niloff, J.M., et al.: Monoclonal antibody immunoradiometric assay for an antigenic determinant (CA125) associated with human epithelial ovarian carcinomas. Cancer Res., *44*:1048–1053, 1984.

Koprowski, H., Herlyn, M., Steplewski, Z., et al.: Specific antigen in serum from patients with colon carcinoma. Science, *212*:53, 1981.

Leong, A.S.-Y., and Milios, J.: An assessment of a melanoma-specific antibody (HMB-45) and other immunohistochemical markers of malignant melanoma in paraffin-embedded tissues. Surg. Pathol., 2:132–145, 1989.

Listrom, M.B., Little, J.V., McKinley, M., and Fenoglio-Preiser, C.M.: Immunoreactivity of tumor associated antigen (TAG-72) in normal, hyperplastic and neoplastic colon. Hum. Pathol., 20:994–1000, 1989.

Martin, S.E., Moshiri, S., Thor, A., Vilasi, V., Chir, E.W., and Schlom, J.: Identification of adenocarcinoma in cytospin preparations of effusions using monoclonal antibody B72.3. Am. J. Clin. Pathol., 86:10–18, 1986.

Nuti, M., Teramoto, Y.A., Mariani-Constantine, R., et al.: A monoclonal antibody (B72.3) defines patterns of distribution of a novel tumor-associated antigen in human mammary carcinoma cell populations. Int. J. Cancer, 29:539–545, 1982.

Osamura, R.Y., Watanabe, K., and Akatsuka, Y.: Peroxidase-labeled antibody staining for carcinoembryonic antigen of cytologic specimens for light and electron microscopy. Acta Cytol. 29:254–256, 1985.

Parker, R.J., and Franke, W.W.: Primitive neuroectodermal tumors of the central nervous system express neuroendocrine markers and all classes of intermediate filaments. Hum. Pathol., 21:245–252, 1990.

Thomas, P., and Battifora, H.: Keratins versus epithelial membrane antigen in tumor diagnosis: An immunohistochemical comparison of five monoclonal antibodies. Hum. Pathol., 18:728–734, 1987.

Tron, V., Wright, J.L., and Schurg, A.: Carcinoembryonic antigen and milk-fat globulin protein staining of malignant mesothelioma and adenocarcinoma of the lung. Arch. Pathol. Lab. Med., 111:291–293, 1987.

Walts, A.E., Said, J.W., Shintaku, I.P., and Lloyd, R.V.: Chromogranin as a marker of neuroendocrine cells in cytologic material—an immunocytochemical study. Am. J. Clin. Pathol., 84:273–277, 1985.

Effusions

Bauman, M.D., Borowitz, M.F., and Johnston, W.W.: Immunoglobulin evaluation of lymphoid aspirates and effusions. Acta. Cytol. 28:628–629, 1985.

Ghosh, A.K., Spriggs, A.I., and Mason, D.Y.: Immunocytochemical staining of T and B lymphocytes in serous effusions. J. Clin. Pathol., 38:608–612, 1988.

Heyderman, E., Strudley, I., Powell, G., Richardson, T.C., Cordell, J.L., and Mason, D.Y.: A new monoclonal antibody to epithelial membrane antigen (EMA)-E29. A comparison of its immunocytochemical reactivity with polyclonal EMA antibodies and with another monoclonal antibody HMFG-2. Br. J. Cancer, 52:355–361, 1985.

Lauritzen, A.F.: Diagnostic value of monoclonal antibody B72.3 in detecting adenocarcinoma cells in serous effusions. APMIS, 97:761–766, 1989.

Lauritzen, A.F.: Distinction between cells in serous effusions using a panel of antibodies. Virchows Arch. [A.], 411:299–304, 1987.

Leong, A.S.-Y., Parkinson, R., and Millios, J.: Thick cell membranes revealed by immunocytochemical staining: A clue to the diagnosis of mesothelioma. Diagn. Cytopathol., 6:9–13, 1990.

Li, C.-Y., Lazcano-Villarreal, O., Pierre, R.V., and Yam, L.T.: Immunocytochemical identification of cells in serous effusions. Technical considerations. Am. J. Clin. Pathol., 88:696–706, 1987.

Li, C.-Y., Ziesmer, S.C., Wong, Y.-C., and Yam, L.T.: Diag-

nostic accuracy of the immunocytochemical study of body fluids. Acta Cytol., 33:667–673, 1988.

Mason, M.R., Bedrossian, C.W.M., and Fahey, C.A.: Value of immunocytochemistry in the study of malignant effusions. Diagn. Cytopathol., 3:251–221, 1987.

Sheibani, K., Battifora, H., Burke, J.S., and Rappaport, H.: Leu-M1 antigen in human neoplasms. Am. J. Surg. Pathol., 10:227–236, 1986.

Spriggs, A.I., and Vanhegan, R.I.: Cytological diagnosis of lymphoma in serous effusions. J. Clin. Pathol., 34:1311–1325, 1981.

Szpak, C.A., Johnston, W.W., Lottich, S.C., Kufe, D., Thor, A., and Schlom, J.: Pattern of reactivity of four novel monoclonal antibodies (B72.3, FS, B1-1, B6.2) with cells in human malignant and benign effusions. Acta Cytol., 28:356–367, 1984.

Walts, A.E., and Said, J.W.: Specific tumor markers in diagnostic cytology, immunoperoxidase studies of carcinoembryonic antigen, lysozyme, and other tissue antigens in effusions, washes, and aspirates. Acta Cytol., 27:408–416, 1983.

Walts, A.E., Said, J.W., and Shintakir, I.P.: Epithelial membrane antigen in the cytodiagnosis of effusions and aspirates: Immunocytochemical and ultrastructural localization in benign and malignant cells. Diagn. Cytopathol., 3:41–49, 1987.

Cerebrospinal Fluid

Bigner, S.H., and Johnston, W.W.: The cytopathology of cerebrospinal fluid. II. Metastatic cancer, meningeal carcinomatosis and primary central nervous system neoplasia. Acta Cytol. 25:461–678, 1981.

Kobayashi, T.K., Yamaki, T., Yoshiro, E., Higuchi, T., and Kamachi, M.: Immunocytochemical demonstration of carcinoembryonic antigen in cerebrospinal fluids with carcinomatous meningitis from rectal cancer. Acta Cytol. 28:430–434, 1984.

Vick, W.W., Wikstrand, C.J., Kemshead, J., Coakham, H.B., et al.: The use of a panel of monoclonal antibodies in the evaluation of cytologic specimens from the central nervous system. Acta Cytol. 31:815–824, 1987.

Yam, L.T., English, M.C., Janckila, A.J., Ziesmer, S., and Li, C.Y.: Immunocytochemistry of cerebrospinal fluid. Acta Cytol. 31:825–833, 1987.

Urine Cytology

Chopin, D.K., deKerndon, J.B., Rosenthal, D.L., and Fahey, J.L.: Monoclonal antibodies against transitional cell carcinoma for detection of malignant urothelial cells in bladder washings. J. Urol., 134:260–265, 1985.

Cordon-Cardo, C., Bander, N.H., and Fradet, Y.: Immunoanatomic dissection of the human urinary tract by monoclonal antibodies. J. Histochem. Cytochem., 32:1035–1043, 1984.

Fradet, Y., Islam, N., Boucher, L., et al.: Polymorphic expression of a human superficial bladder tumor antigen defined by mouse monoclonal antibodies. Proc. Natl. Acad. Sci. U.S.A., 84:7227–7231, 1987.

Huland, H., Arndt, R., Huland, E., et al.: Monoclonal antibody 486 P3/12: A valuable bladder carcinoma marker for immunocytology. J. Urol., 137:654–659, 1987.

Longin, A., Fontaniere, B., Berger-Dutrieer, X.N., Devone,

C.M., and Laurent, J.-C.: A useful monoclonal antibody (BL2-10D1) to identify tumor cells in urine cytology. Cancer, 65:1412–1417, 1990.

Stein, B.S., and Kendall, A.R.: Blood group antigens and bladder carcinoma: A perspective. Urology, 20:229–233, 1982.

Summers, J.L., Coon, J.S., Falor, W.H., Ward, R.A., Miller, A.W., and Weinstein, R.S.: Prognosis in carcinoma of the urinary bladder based upon tissue ABH and T antigen status and karyotype of the initial tumor. Cancer Res., 43:934–939, 1983.

Tomaszewski, J.E., and Kornstein, M.J.: Sensitivity and specificity of URO antibodies in diagnostic surgical pathology. (Abstract.) Lab. Invest., 52:68A, 1985.

Pulmonary Cytology

Banner, B.F., Gould, V.E., Radosevich, J.A., Ma, Y., et al.: Application of monoclonal antibody 44-3A6 in the cytodiagnosis and classification of pulmonary carcinomas. Diagn. Cytopath., 1:300–306, 1985.

Kyrkou, K.A., Iatriclis, S.G., Athanassiadou, P.P., Lambropoulou, S., and Liossi, A.: Immunodetection of neuron-specific enolase and keratin in cytological preparations as an aid in the differential diagnosis of lung cancer. Diagn. Cytopathol., 2:217–220, 1986.

Mottolese, M., Venturo, I., Rinaldi, M., Camptoni, N., Aluffi, A., Curcio, C.C., Donnarso, R.P., and Natali, P.G.: Combinations of monoclonal antibodies can distinguish primary lung tumors from metastatic lung tumors sampled by fine needle aspiration biopsy. Cancer, 64:2493–2500, 1989.

Tao, L.C., Sanders, D.E., Weisbrod, G.L., Ho, C.S., and Wilson, S.: Value and limitations of transthoracic and transabdominal fine-needle aspiration cytology in clinical practice. Diagn. Cytopathol., 2;271–276, 1986.

Needle Aspirates

Battifora, H.: Clinical applications of the immunohistochemistry of filamentous proteins. Am. J. Surg. Pathol., 12:24–42, 1988.

Battifora, H., and Trowbridge, I.S.: A monoclonal antibody useful for the differential diagnosis between malignant lymphoma and nonhematopoietic neoplasma. Cancer, 51:816–821, 1983.

Collins, V.P.: Monoclonal antibodies to glial fibrillary acidic protein in the cytologic diagnosis of brain tumors. Acta Cytol., 28:401–406, 1984.

Domagala, W., Lasota, J., Chosia, M., Szadowska, A., Weber, K., and Osborn, M.: Diagnosis of major tumor categories in fine-needle aspirates is more accurate when light microscopy is combined with intermediate filament typing. Cancer, 63:504–507, 1989.

Domagala, W., and Osborn, M.: Immunocytochemistry. In: Koss, L.G., Woyke, S., and Olszewski, W.: Aspiration Biopsy: Cytologic Interpretation and Histologic Bases, 2nd ed. New York, Igaku-Shoin, 1992.

Domagala, W., Weber, K., and Osborn, M.: Diagnostic significance of coexpression of intermediate filaments in fine needle aspirates of human tumors. Acta Cytol., 32:49–59, 1987.

Droese, M., Altmannsberger, M., Kehl, A., Lankisch, P.G., Weiss, R., Weber, K., and Osborn, M.: Ultrasound guided percutaneous fine needle aspiration biopsy of abdominal and retroperitoneal masses. Accuracy of cytology in the diagnosis of malignancy, cytologic tumor typing and use of antibodies to intermediate filaments in selected cases. Acta Cytol., 28:368–384, 1984.

Gould, V.E., Rorke, L.B., Jansson, D.S., Molenaar, W.M., Trojanowski, J.Q., et al.: Primitive neuroectodermal tumors of the central nervous system express neuroendocrine markers and may express all classes of intermediate filaments. Hum. Pathol., 21:245–252, 1990.

Katz, R.L., Raval, P., Brook, T.E., and Ordonez, N.G.: Role of immunocytochemistry in diagnosis of prostatic neoplasia by fine needle aspiration biopsy. Diagn. Cytopathol., 1:28–31, 1985.

Keshgegian, A.A., and Kline, T.S.: Immunoperoxidase demonstration of prostatic acid phosphatase in aspiration-biopsy cytology (ABC). Am. J. Clin. Pathol., 82:586–589, 1984.

Koss, L.G., Woyke, S., and Olszewski, W.: Aspiration biopsy: Cytologic Interpretation and Histologic Bases. pp. 191–222. New York, Igaku-Shoin, 1984.

Leong, A.S.-Y., Kan, A.E., and Milios, J.: Small round cell tumors in childhood: Immunohistochemical studies in rhabdomyosarcomas, neuroblastoma, Ewing's sarcoma, and lymphoblastic lymphoma. Surg. Pathol., 2:5–17, 1989.

Michie, S.A., Spagnolo, D.V., Dunn, K.A., Warnke, R.A., and Rouse, R.V.: A panel approach to the evaluation of the sensitivity and specificity of antibodies for the diagnosis of routinely processed histologically undifferentiated human neoplasms. Am. J. Clin. Pathol., 88:457–462, 1987.

Miettinen, M., Lehto, V.P., and Virtanen, I.: Antibodies to intermediate filament proteins in the diagnosis and classification of human tumors. Ultrastruct. Pathol., 7:83–107, 1984.

Miettinen, M., Lehto, V.-P., and Virtanen, I.: Immunofluorescence microscopic evaluation of the intermediate filament expression of the adrenal cortex and medulla and their tumors. Am. J. Pathol., 118:360–366, 1985.

Mukai, M., Torikata, C., and Iri, H.: Expression of neurofilament triplet proteins in human renal tumors. Am. J. Pathol., 122:28–35, 1986.

Osborn, M., Altmannsberg, M., Debus, E., and Weber, K.: Differentiation of the major human tumor groups using conventional and monoclonal antibodies specific for individual intermediate filament proteins. Ann. N.Y. Acad. Sci., 455:649–668, 1985.

Ostrzega, N., Cheng, L., and Layfield, L.: Glial fibrillary and protein immunoreactivity in fine-needle aspiration of salivary gland lesions. A useful adjunct for the differential diagnosis of salivary gland neoplasms. Diagn. Cytopathol., 5:145–149, 1989.

Ramaekers, F., Haag, D., Jap, P., and Vooijs, P.G.: Immunochemical demonstration of keratin and vimentin in cytologic aspirates. Acta Cytol., 28:385–392, 1984.

Tani, E.M., Christensen, B., Porwit, A., and Skog, L.: Immunocytochemical analysis and cytomorphologic diagnosis on fine needle aspirates of lymphoproliferative diseases. Acta Cytol., 32:209–215, 1988.

Travis, W.D., and Wold, L.E.: Immunoperoxidase staining of fine needle aspiration specimens previously stained by the Papanicolaou technique. Acta Cytol., 31:517–520, 1987.

Lymph Nodes

Caffert, L.L., Katz, R.L., Ordonez, N.F., Canasco, C.H., and Cabanillas, F.R.: Fine needle aspiration diagnosis of intra-abdominal and retroperitoneal lymphomas by a morphologic and immunocytochemical approach. Cancer, *65*:72–77, 1990.

Dang, D.D., Kamat, D., Zaleski, S., Goeken, J., and Dick, F.R.: Analysis of immunoglobulin and T-cell receptor gene rearrangement in cytologic specimens. Acta Cytol., *33*:483–446, 1989.

Hu, E., Horning, S., Flynn, S., Brown, R., and Sklar, J.: Diagnosis of B-cell lymphoma by analysis of immunoglobulin gene rearrangements in biopsy specimens obtained by fine needle aspiration. J. Clin. Oncol., *4*:278–283, 1986.

Katz, B.L., Cabanillas, F., Sneige, N., Fanning, T., Goodance, A., Patrak, S., and Lee, M.: The value of fine needle aspiration in lymphoma for cytogenetic and molecular studies. (Abstract) Acta Cytol., *30*:574, 1986.

Katz, R.L., Fritsman, A., Fanning, C.V., Dekmezian, R.H., and Butler, J.J.: Fine needle aspiration cytology of peripheral T cell lymphoma: A cytologic, immunologic and cytometric study. Am. J. Clin. Pathol., *91*:120–131, 1989.

Lubiński, J., Chosia, M., Kotońska, K., and Huebner, K.: Genotypic analysis of DNA isolated from fine-needle aspiration biopsies. Anal. Quant. Cytol. Histol., *10*:383–390, 1988.

Robey, S.S., Cafferty, L.L., Beschorneg, W.E., and Gupta, P.K.: Value of lymphocyte marker studies in diagnostic cytopathology. Acta Cytol., *31*:454–459, 1987.

Sneige, N.: Diagnosis of lymphoma and reactive lymphoid hyperplasia by immunocytochemical analysis of fine needle aspiration biopsy. Diagn. Cytopathol., *6*:39–43, 1990.

Sneige, N., Dekmezian, R.H., Katz, R.L., Fanning, T.V., Lukeman, J.L., Ordonez, N.F., and Cabanillas, F.F.: Morphologic and immunocytochemical evaluation of 220 fine needle aspirates of malignant lymphoma and lymphoid hyperplasia. Acta Cytol., *34*:311–322, 1990.

Tani, E.M., Christensson, B., Porwit, A., and Skoog, L.: Immunocytochemical analysis and cytomorphologic diagnosis on fine needle aspirates of lymphoproliferative disease. Acta Cytol., *32*:209–215, 1988.

Liver

Bedrossian, C.W.M., Davila, R.M., and Merenda, G.: Immunocytochemical evaluation of liver fine needle aspirations. Arch. Pathol. Lab. Med., *113*:1225–1230, 1989.

Frable, W.J.: Needle aspiration biopsy: Past, present and future. Hum. Pathol., *20*:504–517, 1989.

Johnson, D.E., Herndier, B.G., Medeiros, L.J., et al.: The diagnostic utility of keratin profiles of hepatocellular carcinoma and cholangiocarcinoma. Am. J. Surg. Pathol., *12*:187–197, 1988.

Kojior, M., Kawano, Y., Isomura, T., and Nakashima, T.: Distribution of albumin and/or alpha-fetoprotein-positive cells in hepatocellular carcinoma. Lab. Invest., *44*:221–226, 1981.

Van Eyken, P., Sciot, R., Paterson, A., et al.: Cytokeratin expression in hepatocellular carcinoma: An immunohistochemical study. Hum. Pathol., *19*:562–568, 1988.

Sarcomas

Gown, A.M., Vogel, A.M., Gordon, D., and Lu, P.L.: A smooth muscle-specific monoclonal antibody recognizes smooth muscle actin isozymes. J. Cell Biol., *100*:807–813, 1985.

Norton, A.J., Thomas, J.A., and Isaacson, P.G.: Cytokeratin-specific monoclonal antibodies are reactive with tumors of smooth muscle derivation. An immunocytochemical and biochemical study using antibodies to intermediate filament cytoskeletal proteins. Histopathology, *11*:487–499, 1987.

Schurch, W., Skalli, O., Seemayer, T.A., and Gabbrani, G.: Intermediate filament proteins and actin isoforms as soft markers for soft tissue tumor differentiation and origin. I. Smooth muscle tumors. Am. J. Pathol., *130*:515–531, 1987.

Wick, M.R., Manivel, J.C., and Swanson, P.E.: Contributions of immunohistochemistry to the diagnosis of soft tissue tumors. *In* Fenoglio-Preiser, C.M., Wolff, M., and Rilke, F. (eds.): Progress in Surgical Pathology. volume 8. pp. 197–250. Philadelphia, Field and Wood, Inc., 1988.

Breast Tumors (see also Chapter 35, breast cancer profile)

Brown, D.C., Gatter, K.C., Dunnill, M.S., and Mason, D.Y.: Immunocytochemical analysis of cytocentrifuged fine needle aspirates. A study based on lung tumors in vitro. Acta Cytol., *11*:140–145, 1989.

Domagala, W., Lasota, J., Bartkowiak, J., Weber, K., and Osborn, M.: Vimentin is preferentially expressed in human breast carcinomas with low estrogen receptor and high Ki-67 growth fraction. Am. J. Pathol., *136*:219–227, 1990.

Gerdes, J., Lelle, R.J., Pichartz, H., et al.: Growth factors in breast cancers determined in situ with monoclonal antibody Ki-67. J. Clin. Pathol., *39*:977–980, 1986.

Gusterson, B., Warburton, M.J., Mitchel, D., Ellison, M., Neville, A.M., and Rudland, P.S.: Distribution of myoepithelial cells and basement membrane proteins in the normal breast and in benign and malignant breast diseases. Cancer Res., *42*:4763–4770, 1982.

Heyderman, E., Ebbs, S.R., Larkin, S.E., Brown, B.M.E., Haines, A.M.R., and Bates, T.: Response of breast carcinoma to endocrine therapy predicted using immunostained pelleted fine needle aspirates. Br. J. Cancer, *60*:630–633, 1989.

Hijazi, Y.M., Lessard, J.L., and Weiss, M.A.: Use of anti-actin and S-100 protein antibodies in differentiating benign and malignant sclerosing breast lesions. Surg. Pathol., *2*:125–135, 1989.

Lozowski, M., Greene, G.L., Sadie, D., Starick, D., Pai, P. Harris, M.A., and Lundy, J.: The use of fine needle aspirates in the evaluation of progesterone receptor content in breast cancer. Acta Cytol., *34*:27–30, 1990.

Lundy, J., Kline, T.S., Lozowski, M., and Chao, S.: Immunoperoxidase studies by monoclonal antibody B72.3 applied to breast aspirates. Diagnostic consideration. Diagn. Cytopathol., *4*:95–98, 1988.

McGurrin, J.F., Doria, M.I., Dawson, P.J., Karrison, T., Stein, H.O., and Franklin, W.A.: Assessment of tumor-cell kinetics by immunohistochemistry in carcinoma of the breast. Cancer, *59*:1744–1750, 1987.

Raymond, W.A., and Leong, A.S.-Y.: Vimentin—A new prognostic parameter in breast carcinoma. J. Pathol., *158*:107–114, 1989.

Reiner, A., Reiner, G., Spona, J., Teleky, B., Kolb, R., and Holzner, J.H.: Estrogen receptor immunocytochemistry for preoperative determination of estrogen receptor status or fine needle aspirates of breast cancer. Am. J. Clin. Pathol., *88*:399–404, 1987.

Silverman, J.F., Dabbs, D.J., and Falbert, C.F.: Fine needle aspiration cytology of adenosis tumor of the breast: With immunocytochemical and ultrastructural observations. Acta Cytol., *33*:181–187, 1989.

Slamon, D.J., Gololphon, W., Jones, L.A., Holt, J.A., Wong, S.G., Kietz, D.E., Levin, W.J., Stuart, S.G., Udove, J., Ullrich, A., and Press, M.J.: Studies of the HER-2/neu proto-oncogene in human breast and ovarian cancer. Science, *24*:707–713, 1989.

Tavassoli, F.A., Jones, M.W., Majeste, R.M., and O'Leary, T.J.: Immunohistochemical staining with monoclonal Ab B72.3 in benign and malignant breast disease. Am. J. Surg. Pathol., *14*:128–133, 1990.

Tsuchiya, S., Maruyama, Y., Koike, Y., Yamada, K., et al.: Cytologic characteristics and origin of naked nuclei in breast aspirate smears. Acta Cytol., *31*:285–290, 1987.

Weintraub, J., Weintraub, D., Redard, M., and Vassilakos, P.: Evaluation of estrogen receptors by immunocytochemistry on fine needle aspiration biopsy specimens from breast tumors. Cancer, *60*:1163–1172, 1987.

Van Netten, J.P., Algard, F.T., Coy, P., et al.: Heterogeneous estrogen receptor levels detected via multiple microsamples from individual breast cancer. Cancer, *56*:2019–2024, 1985.

Infectious Disease

Anderson, G.H., Matistic, J.P., and Thomas, B.A.: Confirmation of genital herpes simplex infection by an immunoperoxidase technique. Acta Cytol., *29*:695–700, 1985.

Giampaolo, C., Murphy, J., Benes, S., and McCormack, W.N.: How sensitive is the Papanicolaou smear in the diagnosis of infection with *Chlamydia trachomatis*? Am. J. Clin. Pathol., *80*:844–849, 1983.

O'Hara, C.M., Gardner, W.A., and Bennett, B.D.: Immunoperoxidase staining of *Trichomonas vaginalis* in cytologic material. Acta Cytol., *24*:448–451, 1980.

Silverman, J.F., Smitz, N., Unverfertz, M., and Carney, M.: The value of immunoperoxidase staining for *Chlamydia* on Papanicolaou stained smears. Acta Cytol., *29*:903–905, 1985.

Wingorson, L.: Two new tests for *Chlamydia* get quick results without culture. J.A.M.A., *250*:2257–2259, 1983.

Wong, J.Y., Zaharopoulos, P., and Dinh, T.V.: Diagnosis of herpes simplex virus in routine smears by an immunoperoxidase technique. Acta Cytol., *29*:701–705, 1985.

Appendix II: In Situ DNA Hybridization of Smears and Tissues

*Rosemary L. Wieczorek, M.D.,
Xiao-Man Liang, M.D., and
Leopold G. Koss, M.D.*

DEMONSTRATION OF VIRAL DNA IN CYTOLOGIC SAMPLES

In recent years, particularly in reference to human papillomavirus infection, several techniques have been developed to document the presence of viral DNA and RNA in tissue and cell samples. The principles of several of these techniques, such as Southern and Northern blotting, dot blotting, and in situ hybridization, were discussed in Chapter 2. The demonstration of viral DNA by in situ hybridization documents that viral genome is present in a cell but sheds no light on the activity of the virus. The documentation is easier when the cells contain a large number of viral copies (ten or more per cell) than when the number of viral copies is smaller. Demonstration of viral RNA suggests that the messages for viral protein were or are being transcribed. The use of RNA antisense probes docu-

ments that the protein transcription is active (see Chapter 2). More recently, the very sensitive polymerase chain reaction (PCR) has been used to amplify viral DNA and document its presence in tissues and cell samples. The principles of this technique were also discussed in Chapter 2.

In this summary, a technique of in situ hybridization of archival or recent, alcohol-fixed cell samples for demonstration of DNA of human papillomavirus is described.

PRINCIPLES

The presence of viral genome in an unknown sample of tissues or cells is documented by molecular hybridization, in which a match between the nucleotide sequences of a viral probe with the target strand of DNA is achieved (see p. 76 and Fig. 2–

1567

24). The hybridization process follows the same principles of nucleotide pairing that govern the replication and reannealing of normal DNA (i.e., G-C and A-T), and the molecules are aligned in the 5' to 3' direction.

The annealing of the known probes with the target molecule of DNA may occur under *stringent* and *nonstringent* conditions. Under stringent conditions, only the presence of the specific type of DNA is revealed. Under nonstringent conditions, nonspecific signals can be recorded, indicating the presence of viral DNA of a variety of related types. These conditions are created in the laboratory and depend on the melting temperature of DNA (Tm), defined by McConaughy et al.* as the point at which 50% of any given double-stranded DNA will "melt," that is, the two strands will be separated. The melting temperature depends on the size of the probe (in kilobases), the salinity of the probe, and formamide concentration, according to the formula

$$Tm \text{ (degrees C)} = 81.5 + 16.6(\log Na^+) + 0.41 \text{ (\%G + C)} - 0.72 \text{ (\% formamide)} - \frac{650}{\text{length of DNA probe}} \text{ (bp)}$$

in which C stands for cytosine, G for guanosine, bp for base pairs, and Na^+ for concentration of sodium ions.

In general, in situ hybridization occurs below Tm. At Tm $- 35°C$, low stringency conditions are achieved. At Tm $- 18°C$, stringent conditions are achieved.

Preparation of Target DNA

To separate the two strands of DNA, the target tissue or cells must be either treated with hydrochloric acid or heated to 95°C during the hybridization process. The separation of strands is usually preceded by stripping DNA of histones and other DNA-associated proteins by proteinase K (Sigma, St. Louis, Mo.).

Preparation of Probes

DNA probes for in situ hybridization may be provided in plasmids (see Chapter 2), containing in-

serts of viral DNA. The probes must be separated from the plasmid by lysis and purified. Subsequently, the probes must be nick-translated; that is, one of the two strands of the viral DNA must be broken and a label must be inserted. Either single virus types or a mixture of types can be used. The label can be either a radioactive substance, such as radioactive sulfur, tritiated thymidine, or a biotin-labeled probe. The use of radioactive probes requires that the specimen after hybridization be covered with a sensitive photographic emulsion for several days in the dark, and the results are seen as radioautographs (see Fig. 11 – 6A). The use of biotin-labeled probes allows for biotin-avidin-enzyme-chromogen reaction to take place, with the advantage of speed and avoidance of exposure to radioactive substances (see Fig. 11 – 6B).

Hybridization Cocktails

The hybridization cocktails contain formamide (50% for stringent conditions of hybridization or 10% for nonstringent condition of hybridization), in the presence of saline sodium citrate (SSC) buffer (1 X SSC is 0.15M sodium chloride, 0.015M sodium citrate) or SSPE buffer (0.75M sodium chloride, 0.05M sodium phosphate, 0.005M ethylenediaminetetra-acetic acid [EDTA]), 10% dextran sulfate, $400\mu g/ml$ of salmon DNA. The buffers facilitate and stabilize the reaction.

METHOD OF HYBRIDIZATION OF RECENT OR ARCHIVAL SMEARS WITH HUMAN PAPILLOMAVIRUS (HPV) DNA WITHOUT DESTAINING†

The method is applicable to alcohol-fixed, stained or unstained, recent or archival cervical smears. It does not require destaining, and therefore, the cell loss is minimal with the use of an adhesive agent 3 APTES. It can also be applied to paraffin sections.

Materials

Xylene
Rehydration system of archival smears (absolute ethanol, 50% ethanol, water)
Paraformaldehyde 4% in phosphate-buffered sa-

McConaughty, B.L., Laird, C.D., McCarthy, B.J.: Nucleic acid reassociation in formamide. Biochemistry, 8:3289–3295, 1969.

†*Liang, X.-M., Wieczorek, R.L., and Koss, L.G.: In situ hybridization with human papillomavirus using biotinylated DNA probes on archival cervical smears. J. Histochem. Cytochem., 39:771–775, 1991.*

line (PBS) solution, pH 7.5 (Sigma, St. Louis, MO)

Phosphate buffered saline (PBS), pH 7.2 (Sigma)

Proteinase K buffer (10-mM Tris, pH 7.5, 2mM CaCl$_2$) (Sigma)

Proteinase K, 5 mg/ml, in proteinase K buffer (Sigma)

Distilled water

Acetone (Fisher, Fair Lawn, N.J.)

3-Aminopropyltriethoxysilane (3 APTES) (2% in acetone) (Sigma)

Glutaraldehyde 1% in PBS (Matheson, Norwood, Ohio)

Triton X-100 (0.1% in PBS) (Sigma)

0.1M triethanolamine buffer, pH 8.0 (Sigma)

Acetic anhydride (Sigma)

HPV probes in PBR 322 plasmid (in HB 101 cells). Single types or a mixture of types can be used.

Polyethylene glycol (8000, Fisher, Raritan, N.J.)

Biotin nick-translation kit (Enzo, New York, N.Y.)

HPV hybridization cocktail (final concentration 2.0-μg biotinylated viral DNA/ml)

Saline sodium citrate buffer (SSC), pH 7.0 (Sigma)

Glycine (0.2% in PBS) (Sigma)

Procedure

1. Soak archival or recent smears in xylene for 2 to 3 days.
2. Remove coverslip.
3. Rehydrate in absolute alcohol, 50% alcohol, water (5 minutes each)
4. Air-dry smears.
5. Place in 4% paraformaldehyde/PBS, pH 7.5, at 25°C for 10 minutes.
6. Wash in PBS × 3, 5 minutes each wash.
7. Proteinase K buffer (10-mM Tris, pH 7.5, 2mM CaCl$_2$), 10 minutes, 25°C.
8. Proteinase K (5 mg/ml) in proteinase K buffer, 60 minutes, 25°C.
9. Wash in distilled water (3 to 5×).
10. Air dry smears.
11. Acetone × 2, 10 minutes each, 25°C.
12. 2% 3-APTES in acetone, 10 minutes, 25°C.
13. Air-dry.
14. 1% Glutaraldehyde in PBS, pH 7.2, 10 minutes, 25°C.
15. 0.1% Triton X-100 in PBS, 10 minutes, 25°C.
16. Wash in distilled water × 3.
17. To 50-ml bath of 0.1-M triethanolamine buffer, pH 8.0, add 126 μl of acetic anhydride immediately before use. Incubate slides for 10 minutes at room temperature.

19. Dehydrate in 50% alcohol, 100% alcohol, and air-dry.
20. Prepare HPV probes by alkaline lysis method with purification by polyethylene glycol.
21. Nick-translate PBR 322 plasmids containing HPV type or types of interest, according to manufacturer with Biotin 11 dUTP.
22. Prepare hybridization cocktail (2.0 μg of biotinylated DNA/ml of cocktail), according to the method of Beckmann et al. (J. Med. Virol., *16*:265, 1983).
23. Place 20 μl of hybridization cocktail on 1 cm^2 of slide.
24. Cover with siliconized glass coverslip.
25. Seal coverslip with rubber cement, let dry.
26. Denature cell DNA at 100°C for 15 minutes.
27. Incubate for 3 days (66 hours at 42°C).
28. Use controls: biotinylated human placental DNA (human genomic positive control) and biotinylated in PBR 322 plasmid (negative control). Use Caski and HeLa cell lines as HPV positive controls. Spin down culture and prepare a cell block.
29. Remove coverslip after incubation and wash with nonstringent method (2X SSC pH 7.0, 4 times 10 minutes each, 25°C).
30. Probe detection by avidin-biotin technique:

   a. 0.2% glycine in PBS, pH 7.2, 10 minutes, room temperature.
   b. Avidin DN 1:100, 15 minutes (Vector Laboratories Burlingame, Calif.), 42°C.
   c. Wash in PBS, pH 7.2, 5 minutes, X 3 (all PBS washes are at 25°C).
   d. Biotin, undiluted 15 minutes (from avidin-biotin blocking kit, Vector Laboratories), 42°C.
   e. Wash in PBS, pH 7.2, 5 minutes, X 3.
   f. Mouse antibiotin (1:25 or 1:50), 15 minutes (Dako, Carpinterica, Calif.), 42°C.
   g. Wash in PBS, pH 7.2, 5 minutes, X 3.
   h. Biotinylated horse-antimouse IgG (1:200) (Vector Laboratories), 15 minutes, 42°C.
   i. Wash in PBS, pH 7.2, 5 minutes, X 3.
   j. Use ABC Elite complex (1:100) (Vector Laboratories), 15 minutes at 42°C.
   k. Wash in PBS, pH 7.2, 5 minutes X 3.
   l. Use 3-3′ diaminobenzidine (Dako) as a chromogen, according to manufacturer's instructions.

31. Counterstain in hematoxylin, clear, and mount.

Results: HPV DNA containing nuclei stain brown.

Application to Tissue Sections and Cell Blocks of Control Cells

1. Place 3- to 6-μm-thick tissue sections on slides pretreated with 3-APTES and air-dried (58°C overnight).
2. Dewax in xylene. Rehydrate in alcohol and water.
3. Digest with 1% pepsin in 0.4 N HCl for 20 minutes (room temperature).
4. Wash in distilled water 5 X, 3 minutes each.

Continue with step 15 described for smears.

Results

The results of hybridization of archival smears and tissues are shown in Color Plate 34–3. The brown precipitate in the nuclei indicates a positive reaction with viral DNA (*A–D*). Control studies are shown in *E* and *F*. See legends to the plate.

COMMENT

The value and efficacy of in situ hybridization with human papillomavirus (HPV) were discussed in Chapter 11. The method described above is but one example of this technique; several other methods were mentioned in Chapters 2 and 11. There are also commercial kits that may be applied to smears and to biopsies. As stated in Chapter 11, the clinical value of these procedures is questionable because the infection per se can not be cured and most lesions of the genital tract associated with HPV require treatment, or at least close follow-up, regardless of viral type, as discussed in Chapter 12.

In situ hybridization techniques are not limited to HPV and may be used to document the presence of other DNA viruses such as herpesvirus (see Chap. 10, p. 351) and human polyomavirus (see Chap. 22, p. 909). Other applications of this technique include chromosome identification, as described in Chapter 5, p. 132. At the time of this writing (1991), some genetic probes to normal and defective genes are available, and others are being developed. The presence of such genes may now be documented by the various methods described in Chapter 2 and may soon enter the mainstream of diagnostic cytology.

A selected short bibliography, covering some of the methods and contributions to the techniques of in situ hybridization, is appended. Additional references pertaining to HPV may be found in Chapters 2 and 12. Other applications of in situ hybridization techniques are discussed in the appropriate chapters.

BIBLIOGRAPHY

Burk, R.D., Kadish, A.S., Calderin, S., and Romney, S.L.: Human papillomavirus infection of the cervix detected by cervicovaginal lavage and molecular hybridization: Correlation with biopsy results and Papanicolaou smear. Am. J. Obstet. Gynecol., *154*:982–989, 1986.

Cohen, P.S., Seeger, R.C., Triche, T.J., and Israel, M.A.: Detection of N-myc gene expression in neuroblastoma tumors by in situ hybridization. Am. J. Pathol., *131*:391–397, 1988.

Del Mistro, A., Braunstein, J.D., Halwer, M., and Koss, L.G.: Identification of human papillomavirus types in male urethral condylomata acuminata by in situ hybridization. Hum. Pathol., *18*:936–940, 1987.

Griffin, N.R., Dockey, D., Lewis, F.A., and Wells, M.: Demonstration of low frequency of human papillomavirus DNA in cervical adenocarcinoma and adenocarcinoma in situ by the polymerase chain reaction and in situ hybridization. Int. J. Gynecol. Pathol., *10*:36–43, 1991.

Gupta, J.W., Gupta, P.K., Rosenshein, N., and Shah, K.V.: Detection of human papillomavirus in cervical smears. A comparison of *in situ* hybridization, immunocytochemistry and cytopathology. Acta Cytol., *31*:387–396, 1987.

Liang, X.-M., Wieczorek, R.L., and Koss, L.G.: In situ hybridization with human papillomavirus using biotinylated DNA probes on archival cervical smears. J. Histochem. Cytochem., *39*:771–775, 1991.

Lorincz, A.T., Lancaster, W.D., Kurman, R.J., Jenson, A.B., and Temple, G.F.: Characterization of human papillomaviruses in cervical neoplasias and their detection in routine clinical screening. *In* Peto, R., zur Hausen, H. (eds.): Viral Etiology of Cervical Cancer: Banbury Report 21. Cold Spring Harbor, N.Y.: Cold Spring Harbor Laboratory, pp. 225–237, 1986.

Nagai N., Nuovo G., Friedman, D., and Crum, C.P.: Detection of papillomavirus nucleic acids in genital precancers with in situ hybridization technique. Int. J. Gynecol. Pathol., *6*:366–379, 1987.

Rentrop, M., Knapp, B., Winter, H., and Schweizer, J: Aminoalklsilane treated glass slides as support for in situ hybridization of keratin cDNAs to frozen tissue sections under varying fixation and pretreatment conditions. Histochem J., *18*:271–276, 1986.

Rule, A.H., Naber, S.P., Perry, C., Waters, G., Coburn, E.W., Moblaker, H., DeLellis, R., and Wolfe, H.: Cells and tissues covalently bound to silanized glass slides. Lab. Invest., *60*:81A, 1989.

Sambrook, J., Fritsch, E., and Maniatis, T.: Molecular Cloning. A Laboratory Manual. 2nd ed. Cold Spring Harbor, New York: Cold Spring Harbor Laboratory Press, 1989.

Schneider, A.: Methods of identification of human papillomaviruses. *In* Syrjanen, K., Gissmann, L., and Koss, L.G. (eds): Papillomaviruses and Human Disease. Springer-Verlag, 1987.

Schneider, A., Meinhardt, G., Kirchmayr, R., and Schneider, V.: Prevalence of human papillomavirus genomes in tissues from the lower genital tract as detected by molecular in situ hybridization. Int. J. Gynecol. Pathol., *10*:1–14, 1991.

Shibata, D.K., Arnheim, N., and Martin, W.J.: Detection of human papillomavirus in paraffin-embedded tissue using the polymerase chain reaction. J. Exper. Med., *167*:225–230, 1988.

Stoler, M.H., and Broker, T.R.: In situ hybridization detection of human papillomavirus DNAs and messenger RNAs in genital carcinomas and a cervical carcinoma. Hum. Pathol., *17*:1250–1258, 1986.

Syrjänen, S., Partanen, P., Mäntyjärvi, R., and Syrjänen, K.: Sensitivity of in situ hybridization technique using biotin and S-35 labeled human papillomavirus (HPV) DNA probes. J. of Virol. Meth., *19*:225–238, 1988.

Syrjänen, K., Gissmann, L., and Koss, L.G. (eds): Papillomaviruses and Human Disease. New York, Springer-Verlag, 1987.

Unger, E.R., Budgeon, L.R., Myerson, D., and Brigate, D.J.: Viral diagnosis by in situ hybridization. Description of a rapid simplified colorimetric method. Am. J. Surg. Pathol., *10*:1–8, 1986.

Vallejos, H., Del Mistro, A., Kleinhaus, S., Braunstein, J.D., Halwer, M., and Koss, L.G.: Characterization of human papilloma virus types in condylomata acuminata in children by in situ hybridization. Lab. Invest., *56*:611–615, 1987.

Van Prooijen-Knegt, A.C., Raap, A.K., Van Der Burg, M.J., Vrolijk, J., and Van der Ploeg, M.: Spreading and staining of human metaphase chromosomes on aminoalklsilane treated glass slides. Histochem J., *14*:333–344, 1982.

35

Image Analysis and Its Applications to Cytology

*Gunter F. Bahr, M.D., Peter H. Bartels, Ph.D.,
Harvey E. Dytch, S.B., Leopold G. Koss, M.D.,
and George L. Wied, M.D.*

Objective analysis of microscopic images of cells and tissues for purposes of classification and of measurements of cell components has been a goal of human pathology and cytology since the middle of the 19th century. Early work in this area consisted of simple linear measurements of cell- and nuclear sizes, followed by calculations of cell- and nuclear volumes. A major step in quantitative cytology was the observations by Caspersson (1936), who correlated measurements of specific fluorescence of nucleic acids with cell function (see also Chaps. 1 and 5). The historical developments of this research were summarized by Koss (1982, 1985, 1987) and need not be repeated here.

The recent spectacular developments in objective analysis of cells, cell components, and, to some extent, histologic tissue sections relate to the developments in computer sciences that allowed for automation of many functions previously requiring manual calculations. There are today three specific approaches to automated, computer-based systems of cell and tissue analysis: morphometry, image analysis, and flow cytometry.

1. Morphometry has been applied mainly to microscopic analysis of histologic sections for purposes of tumor grading and prognosis. The method requires human input in the selection of the target area. The measurements of nuclear sizes, configuration, and DNA content are computerized. The method has been successfully applied to tissue sections of ovarian, mammary, and bladder tumors (summaries in Baak and Oort, 1983; Baak, 1984, 1987; Collan et al., 1987; Baak et al., 1989; van Diest et al., 1989). Except for brief comments the method is not further discussed in this book.

2. Image analysis is discussed in this chapter.

3. Flow cytometry is discussed in Chapter 36.

PURPOSES OF IMAGE ANALYSIS

The initial target of image analysis of human cells had to do with objective classification of human leukocytes (Prewitt and Mendelsohn, 1966). This work led to the developments of several automated instruments for purposes of differential blood counts.

Wied et al. (1968) introduced a concept of automated classification of cells in cervical smears by a system known as the taxonomic intracellular analysis system (TICAS) to be discussed in some detail below. TICAS and derivative systems have been subsequently applied to other cytologic targets, discussed later in this chapter.

The initial purpose of TICAS was to classify cells in cervical smears, with the ultimate goal of automation of the screening process. Subsequent developments, however, led to the application of image analysis to *quantitation of cell components* such as DNA. At the time of this writing (1991) virtually any cell component that can be visualized by means of an immunochemical reaction can be quantitated. The methods have found numerous applications in human cancer, for example, breast and bladder, and in experimental work (see p. 1595).

As an incidental recent development in new computer and software technology, the initial purpose of TICAS, that is, the automated screening of the cervical smear, has been recently revived. Contemporary machines based on principles of image analysis and artificial intelligence software (described below) may prove helpful in quality control or prescreening of cervical smears but will not be likely to replace cytotechnologists or cytopathologists.

TARGETS OF IMAGE ANALYSIS

Theoretically, any microscopic object ranging from bacteria, chromosomes, and intracellular components to whole cells and tissue sections can be studied by image analysis.

Practical targets of application of this technology in the context of this book are cells in the form of smears. A number of cell features and components are particularly suitable for this approach.

Table 35–1 lists a number of cell properties that may be measured by automated means, regardless of methodology. The italicized entries mark subject areas that, in the authors' opinion, hold promise for further development of useful descriptors or markers.

Table 35–1
Measurable Parameters for Whole Cells, the Cytoplasm, the Nucleus, and Resolvable Organelles

Volume
Shape, appendages (cilia, pseudopodia)
Mass, *distribution of mass in volume* } (Morphology)
Viability
Susceptibility:
   To hypo- or hypertonic media
   To toxic substances and drugs, radiation
   To enzymes
Electrophoretic mobility
Deformability
Light scattering
Effects on polarized light
Indices of refraction
Cytochemically accessible properties:
   DNA, RNA, protein, lipid
   Chromatin configuration
   Glycogen, mucopolysaccharides
   Pigments, inorganic molecules
   *-SH,-S-S-*groups
   Cyclic amino acids
   Enzymes
Stainability-reactivity with light-absorbing and with fluorescent dyes, intravitally or after fixation
   Immunologic properties:
   Reaction with highly specific antibodies at cell surface and/or cell interior
   Gene expression with use of specific monoclonal antibodies and fluorescent or light-absorbing staining reactions.

BASIC PRINCIPLES OF IMAGE ANALYSIS

Computers cannot see but can manipulate and analyze numbers with speed and efficiency vastly surpassing that of humans. Therefore, the basic task of computerized automated image analysis is to transform microscopic images into a form suitable for computer analysis, that is, into numbers. The summary of this sequence of events is shown in Fig. 35–1.

All high-resolution systems for the objective measurement and analysis of cells are based on a common approach to the problem. The process may be divided into several well-defined stages:

- 1. Image acquisition and digitization
- 2. Scene segmentation
- 3. Feature extraction
- 4. Feature analysis
- 5. Object classification

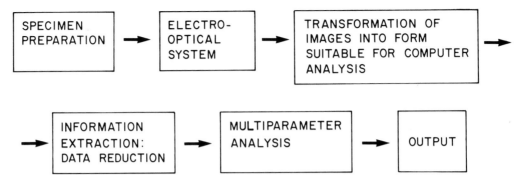

FIGURE 35-1. Sequence of events in image analysis (high-resolution automated cytology).

In short, after conversion of the microscope cell image into numbers suitable for use by a computer, the boundaries of objects of interest, such as the nuclear and cytoplasmic envelopes, must be found. The raw numbers derived from the image must be converted into more generalized and meaningful data such as measures of size and mass and then compared to previously measured cells of known type. This sequence of events in image analysis is summarized in Fig. 35-2.

This process, on one hand, parallels the traditional cytomorphologic method and, on the other, is radically different in certain respects and is based on principles of pattern recognition. Many of the cell features that are measured, such as size, shape, and texture, closely parallel the structures normally examined by the eye. The radically different aspects of this approach are

- 1. Instead of the microscopic image, the digital image is examined.
- 2. The examination is performed and analyzed by computer.
- 3. Features or strictly quantitative descriptors are extracted from the digital image.
- 4. Some features based on mathematical and statistical calculations have little, if any, analogy to those normally assessed by the human eye.

A signal advantage of image analysis is the preservation of the objects of the study, that is, stained smears or histologic sections. This allows for visual selections or correlations of the results of computer analysis with morphology of the target. In fact, the analysis and the correlation may be performed many times on the same target, allowing for selections of the optimal computer parameters for the specific purpose.

Image Acquisitions

The images of microscopic objects are acquired for analysis by measuring light transmission or absorption, using a comparatively simple set-up described on p. 1602. Depending on the type of measurement to be performed, the light source may be visible light, useful in analysis of stained images, or ultraviolet light, required in analysis of fluorescent signals. The very slow, older image analysis systems that required the recording of the measurements point-by-point have now been largely replaced by television cameras and computers. A further advantage of television technology is the option of recording the data in the three basic colors, i.e., red, green, and blue, enhancing still further the analytical potential. The new systems also display the objects to be measured on a television screen, allowing for visual control and selection of targets.

Principles of Quantitation of Light-Absorbing Substances: Beer's Law

Quantitation of cell components by image analysis is based on measurements of light absorption. These measurements are subject to Beer's law.

When the amount of light-absorbent stain doubles, the amount of light absorbed (lost) is more than double. For example, if the concentration of a stain increases fivefold, the transmitted light is reduced more than sevenfold. These relationships are described by *Beer's Law* (1852) and by Bunsen and Roscoe (1862). As a consequence, it is important to recognize that a single measurement of a microscopic object with areas of variable density is

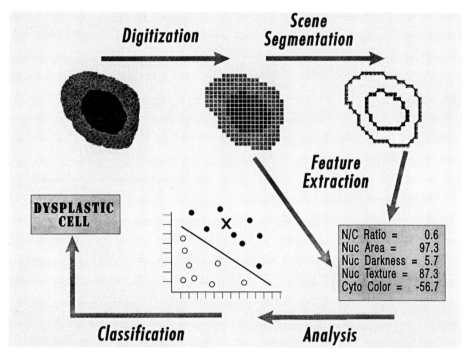

FIGURE 35-2. A schematic depiction of the important stages in high-resolution image analysis. The microscopic optical image of a cell is digitized (converted into numbers associated with discrete points), the boundaries of nucleus and cytoplasm are established, and these data are used to compute cell features associated with morphologic properties of the cell of diagnostic value. The data are then analyzed graphically and statistically to categorize groups of cells according to these features. On the basis of this analysis, a diagnostic classification may be attempted.

inaccurate. For example, in a cell nucleus, each area of density must be measured separately because the amount of light transmitted for each area is not proportional to the overall density of the stain.

In the past the results of multiple measurements had to be tediously calculated according to Beer's law. Contemporary computer-based image analysis systems contain appropriate software adjustments that perform the calculations automatically.

Image Digitization

The complex relationship between the absorbing substances and the transmitted light is discussed above. It may be recalled that a single global measurement of light absorption of a whole cell or a whole nucleus is an inaccurate reflection of the chemical makeup of the target because of Beer's law. The problem may be solved by measuring

consecutive small portions of the cellular area and then putting them together (summation or integration) to achieve an estimated total cellular absorption of the incident illumination. A sequence of such measurements taken at equispaced points along a straight line is called a *scan line of pixel* (picture element) values. A collection of such lines, spaced as far apart as are the individual pixels along the line, reflects closely the image of the cell (Fig. 35-3). Because every scan line contains the same number of pixels, the image can be considered a *rectangular array* of equispaced pixel values.

There are two common techniques for making these measurements: scanning photometry and video photometry. The first method uses a computer-controlled microscope stage, moving the target cell through the light path in small, reproducible steps (see Fig. 35-3). At the end of each step a measurement of transmitted light intensity (or incident light diminution) is taken. Each such measurement applies only to the portion of the cell in-

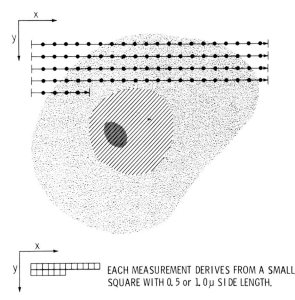

FIGURE 35–3. Schematic diagram of scanning measurement of a cell. In the depicted instance the object slide with a cell on it moves rapidly from right to left. At each interval, marked by a black dot, a measurement is taken. One file of measurements is called a scan line, which in the result appears to have moved from left to right. The cell is covered by measured points (pixels), which are actually square in the shown application.

tersecting the light path. This cellular portion is tightly confined by admitting to the photosensor only a narrow pencil of well-collimated light by means of an aperture placed in the light path. The second means of acquiring these individual pixel values is video technology. This technique projects the optically magnified microscopic image of the cell of interest on the tube(s) of a standard television camera. In a charge-coupled device (CCD) camera, a two-dimensional matrix of individual photoelectronic elements provides a conversion of light intensity to electronic signal, whereas in a tube camera the same result is achieved by electronically scanning the face of the tube.

Whichever means is used to acquire this two-dimensional array of a microscopic image the values can be expressed in a variety of physical units, such as optical density or light transmission, or as "gray values" that are purely measures of relative brightness. Beer's law can be used to calculate from the values the total amount of substance contained within the two-dimensional projection of the cell or nucleus (or any other region of the cell). This can be performed by summation of the pixel mass for all positions lying within the cellular con-

tour. These calculations are now performed by a computing device or a computer, to be discussed below.

Under consideration for the moment is not so much the quantitative aspects of the scanning but the fact that, by the procedure described, the image can be reconstituted from these pixel elements, as has been done with a photograph transmitted by a teleprinter (Fig. 35–4) or with extraterrestrial images received by space probes and transmitted as a string of signals in the form of a radio message.

In Fig. 35–4*B* one can actually discern small white and black squares. The effect of grayness in Figure 35–4*A* is created by having the black square shrink to a small dot, thereby making that image area appear lighter. Conversely, by making the black square larger, spilling its black successively into the adjoining white areas until these are eventually filled, a fully black area is created. This mode of handling gray is prevalent in printed black-and-white pictures. Although the preceding example illustrates how a photograph image can be composed of small elements, the sensing of image points from a cell (see Fig. 35–3) involves gray values, obtained by subdividing the scale of intensity from white to black. Modern systems can generally measure at least 256 shades of gray.

In the next operational step, numbers or numerical values are assigned to each gray value and in this fashion the cellular image has been converted into one consisting of numbers only (Fig. 35–5). The process is called digital conversion or digitization, and the distribution on the points of density reflecting the image of the cell has been transformed into a digital matrix. Although the partial cellular image in Fig. 35–5*B* (*bottom*) is represented by numbers, with relatively little knowledge of the geometry of the actual object scanned, one can roughly distinguish the clear background of the slide (values ranging from 0 to 2), the cytoplasm (values ranging from 5 to 18), and the nucleus (values greater than 20). Other arbitrary number systems may be used as well.

Most modern cytometry systems also allow the measurement of color information through the use of multiple photomultipliers or color television cameras. The principles are the same, but now three two-dimensional arrays of numbers representing cell image data must be stored: one each for pixel values as measured in the red, green, and blue regions of the optical spectrum.

A wide variety of image processing algorithms now exist for the manipulation of the raw image before scene segmentation or feature extraction.

(text continues on page 1579)

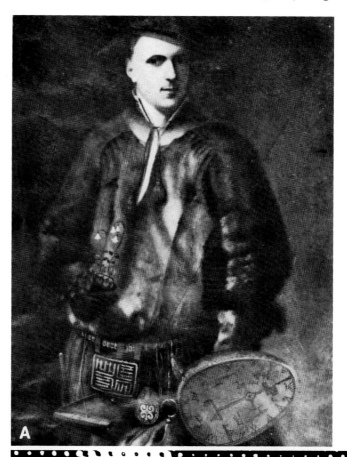

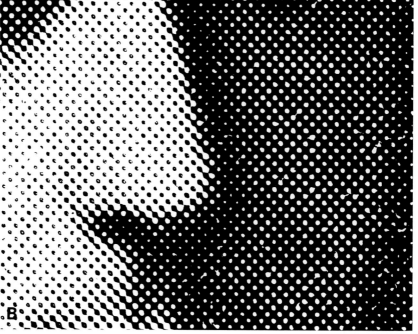

FIGURE 35–4. Two magnifications of the same picture. (*A*) The image consists of printed squares that appear to fuse to continuous tones in human vision. (*B*) An enlargement demonstrates the nature of the picture elements, apparently varying in intensity from white to black with shades of gray in between. (Illustration Carl v. Linne, Linnaeus, Bettman Archive, Courtesy of Scientific American. S. von Reis Altschul: Sci. Am., *236*:96–105, 1977)

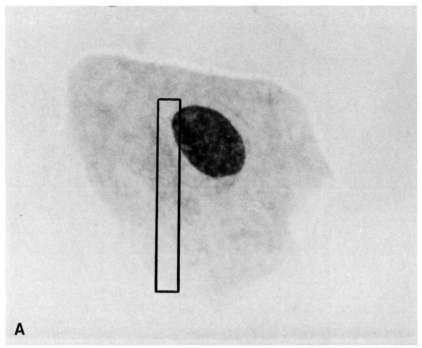

A

```
10  10  10  11  12  14  13
10  10  10  11  12  13  15
10  10  12  11  12  14  17
11  11  11  13  15  22  33
10  11  12  13  16  26  36
10  11  13  17  25  34  35
11  12  14  18  28  34  37
12  15  19  28  33  39  47
13  15  17  24  29  32  35
13  16  23  30  31  34  39
12  15  20  31  33  35  36
14  16  25  34  38  38  39
11  13  18  30  33  35  42
11  14  20  31  32  37  40
10  12  14  22  29  35  38
11  12  13  21  30  33  36
11  11  11  12  17  26  31
10  10  10  11  13  16  18
11  10  10  10  11  13  15
10  10  10   9  10  12  15
10   9  10  10  10  10  11
10  10  11  10  10  10  10
10  10  10  10  10  10  10
10  10  10  10  10  10  10
10  11  10  10   9   9  10
 9  10  11  10   9   9  11
10  10  11  11  10  10   9
11  11  11  10   9   9  10
11  11  11  11  10  11  10
11  11  11  11  11  11  11
11  11  11  11  11  11  11
11  12  12  11  11  11  11
11  12  12  13  12  11  11
13  14  14  13  12  13  12
12  12  12  13  12  13  13
11  10  10  10  11  12  12
11  11  11  11  10  11  11
10  11  11  11  12  11  11
10  10  11  11  12  11  11
10  10  11  11  11  11  11
 9  10  11  11  10  11  11
 9  10  10  10  10  11  10
 9   9   9  10  10  11  11
 9   9   9   9  10  10  11
 8   9   9   9   9  10  11
 6   8   8   8   9   9  10
 5   6   7   7   8   9   9
 5   5   5   6   7   7   7
 4   4   5   6   6   6   7
 3   3   3   5   6   6   6
 6   4   3   3   3   3   4
 0   0   0   4   3   4   3
 0   0   0   3   3   4
```

FIGURE 35–5. An intermediate squamous cell is shown (*A*) at high magnification (×2,700). The entire cell was scanned, but the mass of digital values cannot be reproduced. Therefore, a black rectangle serves to indicate the area from which the density values of (*B*) were derived. The geometry of the digital image is distorted because the printer compresses in the vertical and expands in the horizontal direction. One can identify the nuclear border in the digital image by the relative abrupt increase in density. In the area surrounding the cellular body values drop to zero. **B**

These allow the selective enhancement of various elements of the image, such as particular darkness levels or contrast regions. As an example, in Fig. 35–6, the cell image on a slide is digitized, magnified, and enhanced to bring out nuclear detail and enhanced to determine edge regions of high contrast.

Scene Segmentation

For the digital image to be analyzed by computer, the areas of interest within the field must be distinguished. Among other parameters, the cell and nuclear border may be identified (see Fig. 35–6). Such boundaries may be determined interactively, with operator assistance aided by visual observation of a graphic display of cellular image. However, computer programs that search through the pixels of the digitized image and automatically find important areas or demarcation lines are usually employed when large numbers of cells must be examined.

A variety of methods have been developed for automating this process. The computer may search for regions that are locally homogeneous in terms of such properties as optical density, color, or texture. Alternatively, it may look for regions of rapid *change* in terms of such properties. Generally, such abrupt swings in gray value or another property indicate structural edges, such as cytoplasmic or nuclear borders (Prewitt and Mendelsohn, 1966; Mendelsohn et al., 1968; Prewitt, 1972). Procedures that can be implemented on computers,

called *edge-finding algorithms,* have been devised for the express purpose of finding those pixel positions that constitute boundaries of cytologic interest (Taylor et al., 1975). If the pixels within a particular region of interest are relatively uniform in terms of optical density and quite different from other areas, as in the case of a darkly stained nucleus within much lighter cytoplasm, a histogram of optical density will show these regions as distinct peaks. The valleys between these peaks then represent those pixels with optical density values appropriate to the bordering edges of the larger contiguous areas and can be used as a beginning in determining the appropriate boundaries (Pratt, 1981). More complicated but more robust methods may employ techniques known as hierarchic thresholding using color information, two-dimensional histogram threshold, and the incorporation of a priori knowledge about the expected scene (Liedtke et al., 1987). The interested reader is referred to the original source for further technical information.

Feature Extraction

Once scene segmentation has taken place and appropriate boundaries are identified, it becomes a relatively easy matter to compute such quantities as cellular area, nuclear area, total nuclear optical mass, and so on. Cellular characteristics that can be quantitatively evaluated in the digital image of any cell are referred to as *features,* and the process by which a computer program examines a given digi-

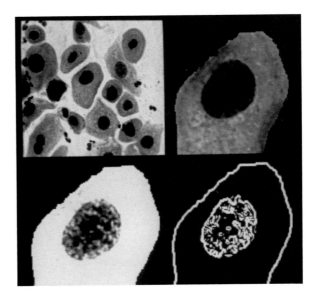

FIGURE 35–6. Image processing in high-resolution cytometry. *Clockwise, from top left*: Raw cell image embedded in the context of the slide; cell isolated and digitally magnified (note individual pixels); cell with histogram equalization to bring out nuclear features; cell after Laplacian transform to identify edge regions of rapid change in optical density.

tal image and computes such features is called *feature extraction.* These features, which are expressed numerically, may include a wide variety of diagnostic parameters, some of which are summarized in Table 35–2.

The cell and nuclear areas are computed inside their respective boundaries. The cytoplasmic area is the difference between the area of the cell and the area of the nucleus. Any desired ratio, including nucleocytoplasmic (N:C) ratio, can be determined using two of the previously extracted features. From the cell and nuclear boundaries, the cellular and nuclear edge lengths are computable. Since these borders embody the relative position and shape of the cellular and nuclear edges, such features as geometric centers of the cell or of the nucleus, centers of optical mass for the cell and the nucleus, and the relationship (e.g., distance) between cell and nuclear centers—whether geometric or optical—are within practical computational reach.

If the combination of stain and illumination wavelength is chosen propitiously, then the relative or absolute mass of nuclear DNA may be determined. There are difficulties, however, with highly atypical cells (Taylor et al., 1974; Tanaka et al., 1977) because portions of the cytoplasm often stain as deeply as the nucleus, whereas a nucleus containing areas of chromatin "clearing" or rare-

Table 35–2
Types of Descriptive Features Used in
High-Resolution Cytometry

Global Features
Global thresholded area
Scan-line optical density data
Total nuclear optical density
Optical density frequency distributions
Optical density differences

Size and Shape Descriptors
Nuclear, cytoplasm areas
Nucleocytoplasmic ratio
Roundness measures
Elongation measures
Fourier-shape descriptors

Texture Features
Optical density (OD) transition probability matrix features
Radial chromatin distribution measures
Run-length measures
Chromatin clumping measures
Homogeneity, heterogeneity measures

Color Features
Simple color features: keratinization measures
Nonlinear color measures: marker features
Measures in hue/saturation/intensity space

faction may be difficult to separate from the cytoplasm. Some of these problems can be successfully handled when image acquisition is performed simultaneously in three colors (i.e., three wavelengths) (Taylor et al., 1978).

More complex features concerned with cell shape and texture can also be evaluated. Some of these methods require considerable mathematical experience for their understanding. Roughly, a textural feature describes some aspect of gray value distribution in some region of the image. The space in which the distribution takes place depends on the feature being evaluated. There exist, for example, textural features quantitating various aspects of chromatin granularity. Ingenuity in devising features has allowed quantitation of most aspects of what was formerly purely qualitative morphologic analysis. A true quantitative morphologic analysis for cells is at hand.

It is possible to sort the gray values from a particular region in an image, for example, from the nucleus. Each gray value is placed in a "bin" or an interval, placed on a line representing the total range of gray values. The resulting graph or histogram represents the distribution of the gray values observed within a given nucleus. The height of each bar of the histogram shows the frequency of gray values found in that range, whereas the number of bars on the horizontal line represents the range of gray values within the nucleus (Fig. 35–7). As is apparent is this graph, an entirely new aspect of nuclear morphology has been gained, generated by computer. Obviously, the human eye cannot transform the visual impression of a nucleus into anything resembling a histogram, thus genuinely new information has been gained for the diagnostic process. The relationship between individually measured image points within the nucleus is also of interest. For example, in a finely granular nucleus the density values adjacent to each other are at the same or only slightly different levels. If one considers the value 38 in Fig. 35–5B, it is likely that the preceding and the following values will be 38 or close to 38, for example, 36 or 40. A precipitous drop to 10 is not to be expected within this nucleus. Another nucleus that shows steep rises and falls of density values will be of a different configuration, and a coarse chromatin pattern may be anticipated. Histograms and probabilities of change in density can be captured numerically, and the extracted features can be used as descriptors (Pressman, 1976).

The use of color video technology and multispectral photomultiplier scanning allows the computation of color features, usually derived from

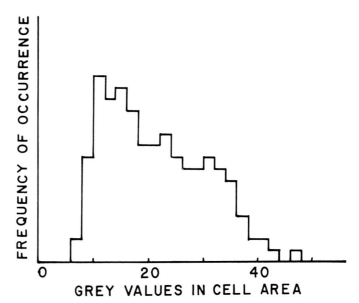

FIGURE 35–7. Histogram of optical densities. Numerical density or gray values derived from a cell are ranked, and the frequency of their respective occurrence is noted. The result is a histogram. Histograms are used as cell descriptors or for the derivation of more complex descriptors.

optical density measurements in each of the red, green, and blue bands (Brugal and Adelh, 1982; Bibbo, 1983). These may then be analyzed by examining normalized differences between the various spectral optical densities in a particular region of the image or by converting these images to hue, intensity, and saturation measures.

The features discussed so far parallel those perceived by the human observer at the microscope. Clearly, the human eye cannot make the precise quantitative evaluations, but a rough approximation of the quantitative results can be achieved. In a cell's picture, an observer can roughly guess at the approximate geometric center, notice where the density tends to concentrate, and estimate the length or size of the cell or of the nucleus. Qualitative and quantitative estimations of nucleocytoplasmic ratio have been recorded in clinical cytology for many years. The principal differences between machine and human determination of these parameters are that the machine is more accurate, is more consistent, does not become fatigued, and provides rapid calculations of the cell features of interest.

With the use of mathematics and statistics, many descriptors can be extracted from a digitized cell image. More than 300 descriptors are now available in the laboratory at the University of Chicago and affiliated laboratories. Parenthetically, it is of interest to note that rarely more than ten descriptors are used at any one time. It may be concluded that a cell can be objectively analyzed in mathematical terms and the accuracy of this analysis can be assessed by a statistical evaluation.

Contextual Features

The features discussed so far have been associated with a single entity: cell, nucleus, cytoplasm, and so on. Another kind of mathematical descriptor of diagnostic importance is the contextual feature. These features relate cells or nuclei to each other and to the larger context within which they appear, be it a cell cluster in an aspirate or a position of the nucleus within a stratified epithelium or gland.

For example, in the meso-TICAS software system for stratified epithelia (Dytch et al., 1987; Dytch and Wied, 1990) not only are basic karyometric features computed, but the orientation and relative position of each nucleus are recorded, along with information on the positions of the layer of basal cells and tissue surface. Thus, features can be studied as a function of epithelial depth, and measures of polarity, nuclear crowding, and regularity of nuclear spacing can be computed. Weighted measures of mitotic density are also calculated. Bibbo et al. (1987) used this system to study renal cell carcinomas. Detweiler et al. (1988) found that contextual analysis of nuclei in cell clusters from aspiration biopsy smears of mammary cancer made an important contribution to correct diagnosis and found a combined classifier using both contextual and high-resolution information to yield the best results. Garcia et al. (1987) found contextual analysis to be useful in classifying cervical smears. Hutchinson et al. (1989) employed contextual analysis for the examination of prostate aspirates, as described below.

Subvisual Diagnostic Clues

One of the promises of high-resolution computer evaluation of cell images, which is just beginning to be fulfilled, is the ability to discriminate specimens and cell types on the basis of diagnostic information that is difficult or impossible for a human observer to perceive. Statistical analyses may be able to appreciate very slight but consistent differences in nuclear size, for example, that are too subtle for a cytologist to notice. If these differences are expressed throughout an entire sample, they may allow accurate discrimination from other specimens. Such features can be understood conceptually and even used to great advantage in classifying cells. Yet the services of a high-speed computational device are required to bring them to the attention of the human observer in the first place.

One of the most intriguing examples of such a subvisual clue is the marker features for neoplastic events in the uterine cervix that appear to be expressed in otherwise normal-appearing intermediate cells from patients with intraepithelial neoplasia. These changes have been noted by Burger et al. (1981), Wied et al. (1980, 1982), and others (Bibbo et al., 1981; Vooijs et al., 1982; Bartels et al., 1983; Rosenthal et al., 1983; Boon et al., 1986; Katzko et al., 1987; Hall et al., 1988). If validated on a large clinical sample of patients, these findings may have an important effect on cervical cancer prescreening. The relatively rare tumor cells on a sample would not need to be identified, but rather an alarm could be given if ancillary changes were detected in a statistically valid sample of intermediate cells. Rosenthal et al. (1987) found that marker features were of predictive value in assessing cases of moderate dysplasia in routinely prepared cervical smears. Such marker features have also been detected in other organ sites, as discussed below.

Sample Analysis and Cell Classification

The primary goal of machine detection of a cancer cell among normal cells is still based on identification of a property or marker that reliably signals when a cell is a cancer cell, without resorting to assistance from the human eye. Unfortunately, no single chemical or physical marker for the detection of cancer is currently available. Similarly, no single descriptor will unequivocally signal the presence of the malignant state. However, mathematical analysis of cellular morphology may yield statistical differentiation of cell classes, including classes of malignant cells, with a high degree of confidence.

The task of investigators in automation is to discover features that can be used to statistically discriminate one class of cells from all others (Prewitt and Mendelsohn, 1966; Lipkin et al., 1966; Sandritter et al., 1967). The historical development of cell image analysis has been reviewed by Preston (1977). Many approaches are available to identify relevant features. These include standard statistical techniques such as parametric and nonparametric significance tests, and linear discriminant analysis. The use of appropriate computer graphics displays may also aid in the selection of suitable feature sets (Dytch, 1982).

Since even diversely classified cells have many features in common, the first step is to discriminate a given class of cells from all others. For example, in a cervical sample the superficial squamous cells may be identified and separated from all other cells. Once a class is recognized, its members can be removed from the population under consideration. The procedure of cell classification continues as before but on a reduced cell population, disregarding the cell class previously culled from the original population. After a sufficient number of these cycles, all the possible cell classes having been considered, no more images remain to be classified, and every image has been placed in a class.

For any one of these discrimination rules, the optimum set of features is selected. In some cases simple features, such as area measurements, may suffice; in others, composite discriminators involving complex textural descriptors of chromatin granularity have to be employed. For example, normal superficial squamous cells can be recognized by size and nucleocytoplasmic ratio alone. We see a decision sequence develop in which one decision may or may not lead to further decisions (Taylor et al., 1974). In Fig. 35–8, such a hierarchical decision sequence and the results of computer classification of cell classes from the uterine cervix are shown.

Artificial Intelligence Techniques

Among the more recent additions to the arsenal of techniques available to the researcher in analytic cytometry are tools associated with the branch of computer science known as artificial intelligence (AI). AI technologies such as *expert systems* and *artificial neural networks* may be conveniently contrasted with traditional algorithmic computational methods, in which step-by-step "hard-

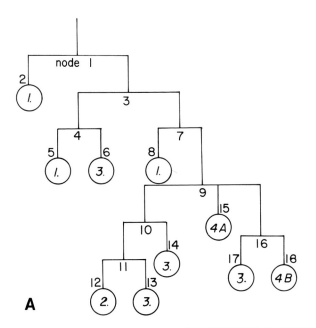

A

CONFUSION MATRIX (%)
0.5 μm. steps

	1	2	3	4A	4B	UNKN
SUP	100.0	0.0	0.0	0.0	0.0	0.0
SUB	100.0	0.0	0.0	0.0	0.0	0.0
INT	100.0	0.0	0.0	0.0	0.0	0.0
MTM	95.1	1.6	3.3	0.0	0.0	0.0
PAR	1.1	78.2	11.5	4.6	0.0	4.6
MTI	1.2	63.5	25.9	3.5	3.5	2.4
DSK	0.0	7.5	92.5	0.0	0.0	0.0
DSN	0.0	4.6	81.5	0.0	1.5	12.3
DSM	0.0	7.2	20.6	40.2	17.5	14.4
CIS	0.0	1.2	3.6	67.5	14.5	13.3
INV	1.2	0.0	9.9	11.1	61.7	16.0

B

FIGURE 35–8. (*A*) A typical decision tree, which, in this example, contains eight decision points, called *nodes* (1, 3, 4, 7, 9, 10, 11, 16), utilizes ten separate decision nodes, and results in five possible classifications (1–4, plus an unknown category). The first two categories include mature squamous cells (superficial and intermediate cells) as well as immature cells (i.e., parabasal cells and immature metaplastic cells). The third category comprises the dysplastic cells, and the fourth category is used to represent tumor cells, with a subdivision into a class of in situ and invasive tumor cells. (*B*) Percentage of correct and incorrect classifications tabulated in a confusion matrix. At the lefthand margin abbreviations are listed for cell categories: SUP = superficial cell red cytoplasm; SUB = superficial cell blue cytoplasm; INT = intermediate cell; MTM = mature metaplastic cell; PAR = parabasal cell; MTI = immature metaplastic cell; DSK = dysplastic keratinized cell; DSN = dysplastic nonkeratinized cell; DSM = dysplastic cell in metaplasia, usually markedly dysplastic; CIS = carcinoma in situ; IVN = invasive cancer. The numbers in the top line mean: 1 = absolutely normal; 2 = immature cells but benign; 3 = immature or dysplastic cells; 4AB = tumor cells (with the attempt to have invasive carcinoma identified as 4B). One can see that all superficial cells were correctly identified; so were intermediate cells. Mature metaplastic cells were considered 95.1% mature, 1.6% immature, and 3.3% dysplastic. Malignant cells in category 4 were identified correctly in 70% to 80%. Although this percentage of identifying a single carcinoma cell appears low, the probability of making a correct diagnosis on a case containing ten cells becomes extremely high.

wired" procedures are followed in arriving at results. Although both AI techniques are nonalgorithmic, each employs quite different means to achieve its goals, which are briefly discussed.

Expert Systems

In general terms an expert system (Forsyth, 1984; Buchanan et al., 1984; Waterman, 1986; Jackson, 1986; Graham and Jones, 1988; Parsaye and Chaynell, 1988) is defined as a computer program that can provide advice or solve problems relating to a specific field. Such devices use inference procedures (a system of logical assumptions) based on in-depth knowledge of that field. An expert system may perform at a level of sophistication that ordinarily would require a very experienced and qualified human authority. The field within which the expert system is competent is said to be its *domain*.

The symbolic inference procedures that it employs are software programs known as the expert system's *inference engine*. The body of knowledge that the expert system possesses, embodied in rules, facts, and relationships, is called its *knowledge base*.

The inference engine is the central element of the expert system, governing the flow of information between the knowledge base and the user and providing logical conclusions to the queries.

A sketch of a prototypic expert system functioning in the role of an expert cytometric diagnostic adviser is shown in Fig. 35–9. Data provided in the form of numerical cytometric data and past history data from a patient data base are converted into symbolic facts that can be used by the expert system. The expert system interacts with the cytopathologist-user through the use of an interface

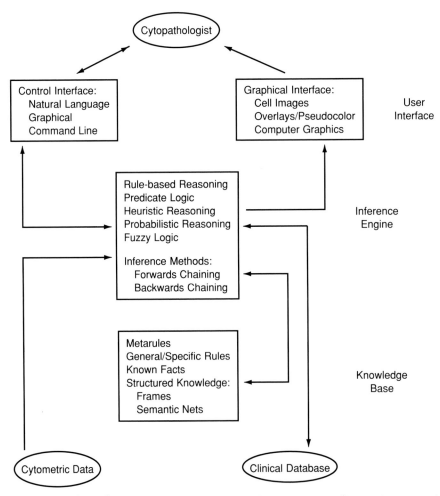

FIGURE 35–9. Outline of a prototypic expert system acting as an expert diagnostic cytometric adviser, showing major components. See text for further explanation.

and may use computer-generated color graphics for cell image display and interpretative aid.

Depending on requirements, the expert systems can be constructed with various types of inferencing mechanisms and knowledge bases. Basic expert systems are often simply "rule-based" systems in which the body of knowledge is formulated as an assumption of rules and facts, which allow the system to arrive at conclusions. These conclusions are then incorporated into the system as new facts, and the system continues until this process has exhausted the logical deductions possible with the given knowledge. An example of a simple rule in the expert diagnostic cytometry system might be:

If
The nuclear-cytoplasmic ratio of the cell is very high
and
the total optical density suggests that the nucleus is markedly aneuploid,
then
the cell is probably a neoplastic cell (0.85 certainty).

This rule raises several points about such systems. First, the meaning of such symbolic terms as "very high" and "markedly aneuploid" must be defined either in terms of the numerical cytometric variables themselves or by the user. Additional rules may provide this capability. Second, the system may be able to estimate the probable accuracy of a particular conclusion based on the accuracy of the facts that led to that deduction. There is still a great deal of controversy regarding the appropriate methods by which to deal with this quantified inexactness. Approaches include the use of a number of mathematical techniques such as classic probability combination, fuzzy logic, certainty theory, confidence factors, possibility theory, and Bayesian belief networks. The reader is referred to other sources, listed in bibliography, for further explanation of these techniques.

Once rules and facts have been established, a methodical approach to matching them by some inference method is still needed. There are two basic types of inference logic methods known as *forward chaining* and *backward chaining*. In a forward chaining approach to a given problem, the basic facts and rules currently available are examined, analyzed, and used to produce conclusions in the form of new facts, as described above. This process continues until a conclusion (in this example a diagnosis) has been achieved or until all data are exhausted. Thus, in a sense, the flow of logic anticipates (is forward to) the goal. In a backward chaining approach, the initial goal is a hypothesis, and the system is asked what facts need to be established for that hypothesis to be true. These facts (or subhypotheses) are in turn examined to see if the necessary conditions for their existence are met. Thus, in a sense, the flow of the logic corresponds to a movement backward from the hypothetical diagnostic conclusion to data. Depending on the type of problem and facts available, each of these methods may be appropriate.

A very important AI technique is that of appropriately *structuring* and representing knowledge. In a general sense, facts and rules, as illustrated above, may be viewed as rudimentary knowledge structuring techniques. Another very important technique for representing knowledge in expert systems is the use of *frames,* or software structures that contain the known sequence of events (hierarchies) in the domain under study. Frames are a logical way of representing objects and their relationships and the attributes that each object possesses. These attributes are known as *slots,* which can be filled with values appropriate for the specific attribute. The various frames of a system are linked in a parent-child lattice, in which properties of a "child node" may be *inherited* from a parent node. Thus the slots and the values of those slots in a child node representing, for example, a dysplastic cell, might be inherited from a parent node representing the notion of a cell in general. As the actual expert system begins working on data, *instances* of these frames are formed and are used in the logical deduction process. The use of such techniques can greatly simplify the knowledge representation process.

The development of expert systems in the recent past often required the use of specialized programming languages such as LISP and PROLOG to initiate the building of the appropriate knowledge representation schemes and inference mechanisms. The services of a "knowledge-engineer", a person familiar with AI techniques and able to develop the often elusive heuristic rules that the domain expert uses in problem solving was also a necessary requirement. Today, the availability of microcomputer-based expert system "shells," which incorporate the basic building blocks of expert systems and which often provide simple data-entry and knowledge elicitation mechanisms, has made the development of expert systems much more accessible to persons not versed in AI techniques.

Artificial Neural Networks

Neurocomputers or *neural nets* represent a different nonalgorithmic approach to artificial intelligence (Rumelhart, 1986; Grossberg, 1987; Anderson and Rosenfeld, 1988). These techniques attempt to mimic the function of the human brain. Although the computational abilities of the brain are much inferior to that of a computer, the brain is capable of many functions that escape the ordinary computer; in the context of this narrative, chief among them is the ability to identify and classify images, solve problems, and learn from experience. It is generally thought that these functions of the brain are vested in neurons interconnected with one another by axons and dendrites.

Neural nets are composed of a large number of relatively simple computing elements known as *processing elements* (PEs), which are arranged in *layers* or slabs and are extensively interconnected. Hence the neural nets are an offshoot of the *connectionist* approach to complex computational problems. The neural nets are composed of an input layer that receives data to be analyzed and an output layer providing the results of the analysis. Between the input and the output, the PEs are arranged in "hidden layers" that may vary in number from a few to several hundred (Fig. 35 – 10). Each PE receives signals from adjacent PEs; its function is to compute these signals and convey them to other PEs. Therefore each PE is in a state of *activation.* According to the strength of the signals received and the strength of the connections, the PEs have *weights* that are adjustable by "experience," as in the learning process. As in the brain, these weights may be positive or negative, hence excitatory or inhibitory. The strength of neurocomputing is vested in the weights. For example, cytometric data may be fed into the input layer of an artificial neural network trained as a diagnostic adviser. The PEs in this input layer, which are activated proportionally to the strength of these data, feed the second layer of processing elements. Each one of the second layer elements will variously weigh these inputs before combining them and achieving a new state of activation. The process is repeated for the next hidden layer and so on. This process of weighting, combining, and signal output cascades forward throughout the network until the output layer is reached. The pattern of PE activity in this output layer will then correspond to the symbolic correct diagnosis based on the cytometric input data if the net is functioning correctly. Assuming that some combination of weights exists that will "solve" a particular problem (and there is good mathematical evidence that this will be true for most well-defined problems), the obvious question is how to determine those weights. The neurocomputer solution is to *teach* the network the correct weights through example.

Artificial neural networks learn by example: they are adaptive processing tools, adjusting their knowledge in response to training prototypes. For example, the supervised learning situation that often occurs in diagnostic cytology, a network would be shown sets of cytometric data together with the desired response of the output layer. Ordinarily, many presentations of many examples are required for a net to adjust its weights. It changes these weights slowly in accordance with a *learning rule* that describes how to make these adjustments. One of the most popular learning rules is variously known as the delta rule, Widrow-Hoff rule, or LMS rule, and it simply states that the input weights to a PE are adjusted proportionally to the difference between the current activity of that PE and the desired activity. A generalization of this rule results in one of the most popular current networks, the *back-propagation* network, in which errors and weight modifications are computed during training, moving backward from the output layer toward the input. Often several hundred cycles of adjustments may be required (Fig. 35 – 11). The cumulative error of the network gradually decreases during training, until weights are adjusted to their final values, and the net is ready to actually produce useful results with unknown input data (see Fig. 35 – 11).

The promise of neural networks is that, because of their novel architecture, they will be able to deal with classes of problems that have proved difficult to solve by traditional algorithmic computation and symbolic AI methods. These include many of the tasks that humans do superbly, in spite of their very slow (relative to computers) computational abilities. Examples of this kind of problem include visual understanding, language, and memory recall. These kinds of problems abound in cytology research.

The preceding examples represent a characteristic *pattern recognition* problem. A typical neural net solution may use a vector of preprocessed cytometric features as input to a feed-forward network, producing an output vector of PE activity representing a particular diagnosis. In Fig. 35 – 12 there is a *Hinton diagram* of such a network, trained to make a diagnostic assessment of cervical tissue specimens on the basis of their DNA ploidy spectra. The network consists of a 16-element input layer representing the DNA histogram, a hidden layer of eight PEs, and a three-element output layer representing the diagnostic categories with which the network was trained. The strengths of the weights of the various elements are represented by the size of the various boxes in the diagram, with

(text continues on page 1589)

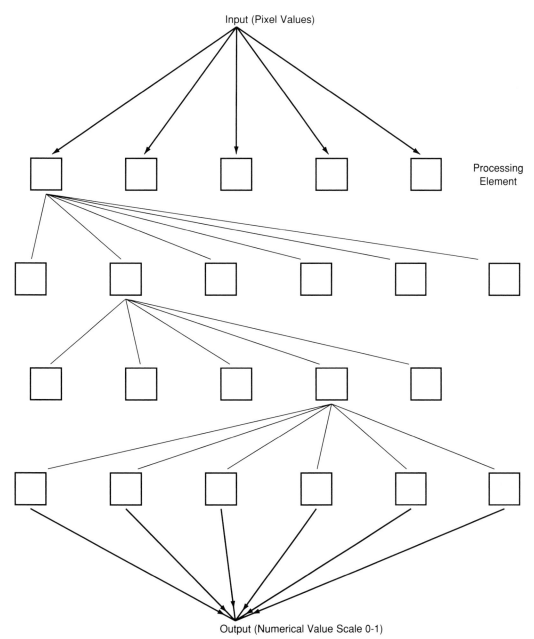

FIGURE 35-10. A schematic, much-simplified representation of an artificial neural network. In this example, the input is the value of pixels in an image-processing system. The output is in arbitrary units that can be programmed and adjusted to suit the user's needs. The core of the system is composed of several "hidden" layers or slabs of adjustable processing elements (PEs) that are connected with one another. For the sake of simplicity only four layers of processing elements are shown; in an actual working system fewer or more such layers may be used. In this drawing, only one processing element in each layer shows connections to the next layer of processing elements: in an actual system, all of the processing elements in all the layers are connected to one another.

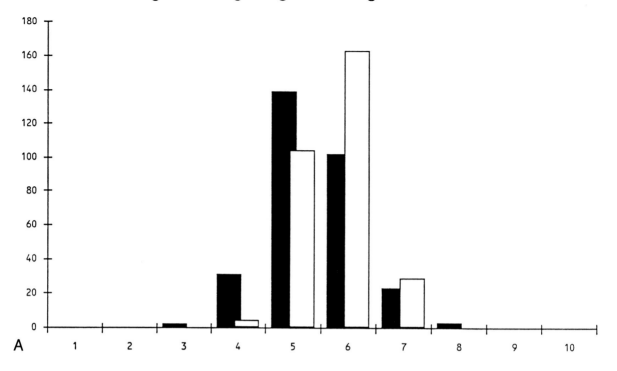

Training Set - Beginning of Training of A.I. Circuits

A

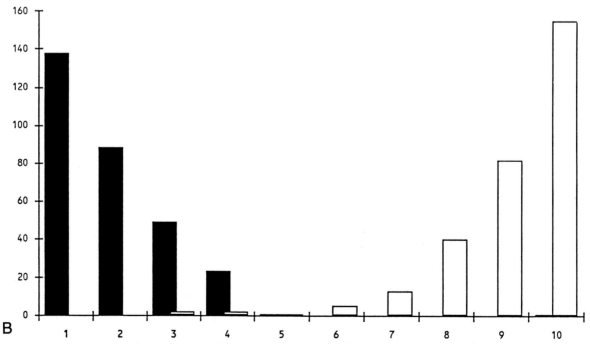

Training Set - End of Training of A.I. Circuits

B

FIGURE 35-11. Results of training of an artificial neural network. In (*A*), images of malignant cervical cells (*black bars*) and benign cervical cells (*clear bars*) were fed into the network. The network was unable to separate the two sets of images. (*B*) shows the results of training of the network after about 200 cycles. The images of the malignant and benign cells are well separated with only a minimal overlap.

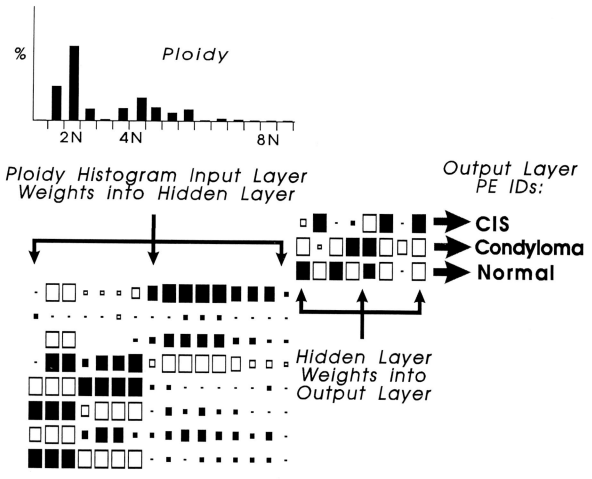

FIGURE 35–12. Artificial neural network trained to classify cervical DNA ploidy spectra, shown as a Hinton diagram. See text for further explanation.

positive connections indicated by solid boxes and negative ones by open boxes. For example, one can see in the network the association of the concept of aneuploidy in the strong positive connections between the region of the DNA spectrum above 5N and the second, sixth, and eighth hidden-layer PEs, which in turn are strongly connected to the carcinoma in situ (CIS) diagnostic output element. Artificial neural networks such as this may use as input diverse cytologic, cytometric and clinical data ranging from nuclear texture to patient age and may be able to deal appropriately with complex diagnostic decisions that are difficult to solve with traditional statistical methods.

Artificial neural networks may also be used to analyze the complex relationships between two very large sets of data, for example, clinical data and cytometric data derived from cells in cervical smears. The results may reveal hidden relation-ships of disparate clusters of information that will be embedded in the synaptic strength of the net. Such systems are known as *distributed databases* and are based on software known as *content addressable memory* (CAM). Such neural nets have a different architecture, inasmuch as the PEs are connected not only with other PEs but also with selves. Once established, such neural nets may be able to generalize, i.e., deal with incomplete or erroneous sets of data by filling in the gaps and pointing out possible errors. Such systems are therefore capable of intelligent guesses.

Machine vision is one of the most exciting possibilities of neurocomputing. In its most extreme forms, machine vision should be able to "see" and identify objects without the need for intermediate steps such as image segmentation and feature extraction. Early work includes the construction of the Perceptron by Frank Rosenblatt (Rosenblatt,

1958, 1962; Minsky and Papert, 1969), the Neocognitron (Fukushima et al., 1983) and the work of David Marr (1982).

These investigators constructed artificial retinae composed of a grid of photoreceptors and output units and documented some of the properties of neural nets, such as the ability to generalize or process faulty signals. The machines failed, however, in processing many simple problems of logic, and the assessment of their future by Minsky and Papert was pessimistic. Many of the difficulties encountered by the early investigators have since been overcome, resulting in the construction of the contemporary machines described above. Using sophisticated new software (preattentional network, short-term memory), machine vision has become a reality. Classified military target recognition and handwriting recognition are some of the current applications of this technology.

Neural networks possess properties that make them highly appropriate for this type of application because of their ability to generalize and handle novel input and their capacity to handle degraded data, perhaps in the form of images with extraneous noise. A simple low-resolution network operating on binary cell images was used by Dytch and Wied (1990) to illustrate this kind of approach to cytologic image data.

Neither of these AI approaches is a panacea, however. Each has strengths and weaknesses. Expert systems require explicit formulation of heuristic rules that may be difficult to obtain, whereas neural networks can generalize and learn how to solve problems directly from a training set of examples. On the other hand, because of the way knowledge is embodied in each, expert systems can provide access to the reasoning behind a diagnostic recommendation, while examination of the "reasoning" behind a neural network's decision may be hidden in the complex pattern of weighted interconnections that contain its knowledge. It is likely that a combination of these techniques, along with traditional statistics and algorithmic computational methods, will provide the best approach to the development of complex expert advisory systems in cytology.

Applications of these tools in high-resolution image analysis have included their use in scene segmentation and pattern recognition and classification. Wied et al. (1986, 1987) and Bartels et al. (1986) used expert systems technology in the role of a diagnostic adviser applied to diagnostic histopathology and cytopathology. Weber et al. (1988) applied these techniques to the diagnosis of colonic lesions. Bartels et al. (1987, 1989) have employed an expert system–based approach to scene segmentation in tissue, especially colonic sections. The use of expert system technology for the construction of a computer-assisted tutoring tool in cervical cytology was discussed by Tang et al. (1988). Dytch et al. (1988, 1990) applied artificial neural network pattern recognition paradigms to the classification of cervical histopathologic specimens. Dytch and Wied (1990) discussed the integration of these approaches in hybrid systems for expert diagnostic assistance. In some contemporary commercial instruments (PAPNET), artificial intelligence computers were combined with algorithmic machines for analysis of cells in cervical smears (see p. 1593).

HIGH-RESOLUTION SYSTEMS OF CELL CLASSIFICATION BY IMAGE ANALYSIS

In 1966 Prewitt and Mendelsohn suggested that the recording of high-resolution digitized images and subsequent analysis by a digital computer could lead to the automated recognition and classification of five principal types of leukocytes. This classic paper applied new concepts to microscopic image analysis in that the photometric information collected from each image point was used to compute descriptors, which in turn were subjected to statistical classifications in a three-dimensional space (Mendelsohn et al., 1968).

In 1968 several authors of this chapter initiated in Wied's laboratory the TICAS project (*T*axonomic *I*ntra*C*ellular *A*nalysis *S*ystem) with the aim of bringing machine objectivity to clinical cytology (Wied et al., 1968). The objectives of the project were (1) reproducibility and greater objectivity in diagnostic decision making; (2) better definition of cytomorphologic characteristics in disease, with concomitant improvement in prognostication; (3) improved international classification of disease entities, particularly with respect to premalignant states and cancer; (4) detection of subpopulations of cells with differing function within a parent population of cells having indistinguishable morphologic characteristics when observed by the eye; (5) detection of new or variant disease entities; and (6) assistance in difficult differential diagnosis for cases in which visual cytomorphologic evidence is marginal.

Although TICAS was originally designed for cytologic samples from the female genital tract, it has found many applications to cells derived from other organs. It has undergone many changes in terms of hardware and software during the past 20-plus years, evolving from the early giant, relatively simple computers to the sophisticated personal computers now in use. The principles of the system, however, have remained much the same. Cell images are digitized and stored on magnetic or optical storage media and analyzed on a dedicated computer. More than 300 features based either on basic features of cells (e.g., cell size, nuclear size, chromatin texture) or on mathematical derivatives based on optical density histograms are available for analysis. The concept of "computable image (cell) information," first suggested by Prewitt and Mendelsohn, was greatly extended and systematically explored under the TICAS project (Bartels et al., 1969, 1970, 1971, 1973, 1974, 1979–1983, 1980, 1981; Bibbo et al., 1984, 1985; Wied et al., 1981, 1982, 1983, 1985, 1989).

The program complex of TICAS contains decisions on data recording, image editing and preprocessing, extensive programs for feature extraction, feature selection and evaluation, statistical analysis, and three major program subsystems: the supervised learning programs, the unsupervised learning programs, and the automated cell classification programs.

The supervised learning programs rely on external "truth" (i.e., cells are first identified by visual observation as belonging to a certain class). Self-learning by computer in the context of a cell-identifying program system implies the assembly of programs and subprograms into a master program with the purpose of completely replacing human choice in the selection of suitably discriminating image properties in a given cell population (Bartels et al., 1970). These objective methods result in a final numerical value, such as a probability ratio, for the correctness of a decision as it is applied to an individual cell or group of cells. The program has been successfully applied to the identification of many classes of squamous cells from the uterine cervix, glandular cells of endocervical and endometrial origin, urothelial cells, mesothelial cells, and various classes of leukocytes. *The unsupervised learning programs* accept for classification by computer data sets on which no prior information is supplied as to the existence of natural groups of cells.

This program complex of TICAS also contains mathematical routines to test for the homogenicity of a set of examined cells by means of grouping algorithms or the so-called clustering procedures. The aim of the latter is the detection of persistent groups of outliers within the hierarchic order in a set of cells represented by multidimensional vectors (Bartels et al., 1970).

APPLICATIONS OF HIGH-RESOLUTION IMAGE ANALYSIS SYSTEMS TO CELL IDENTIFICATION

Differential White Blood Count

The pioneering work of Prewitt and Mendelsohn (1966) with the CYDAC system estimated the proportions of five or more groups of leukocytes and erythrocytes in specially prepared films of peripheral blood. Two hundred to 500 cell images, from 7 to 25 μm in diameter, were typically examined. Reproducibility, objectivity, and, to some extent, speed were realized in automatic white cell counters using pattern recognition (Preston, 1962; Ingram and Preston, 1970; Bacus, 1971; Dew et al. 1974; Megla, 1973).

More complex diagnostic and identification problems in hematology and immunology have also been studied (Kiehn, 1972; Prewitt, 1972; Bahr et al., 1974; Brenner, 1974; Olson et al., 1974; Bartels et al., 1974, 1975; Andersen et al., 1975; Bacus et al., 1976).

Automated differential blood counters represented the first successful clinical application of automated cytology. Automated cytology of epithelial cells represents a much more difficult task.

Classification of Cells in Cervical Smears

It was initially erroneously inferred from the early success with blood films, with their relatively simple cell components, that cervical (Pap) smears could be analyzed with the same or similar machines. Although the principles are comparable for both targets, the difficulties of the respective tasks differ by many orders of magnitude (Wied, Bahr, and Bartels, 1970). The automated device is faced with a search situation for a possibly rare event—the occurrence of abnormal cells. This means that sample sizes of from 40,000 to 100,000 cells may have to be examined. The cell images are typically 40 to 70 μm in diameter, and they may represent up to 16 different cell categories or classes. Biologically, the changes in cells undergoing malignant transformation probably represent a continuous spectrum. The traditional classification of cells by structural features constitutes, at best, an approximation of their biologic significance. It is not surprising, therefore, that the use of high-resolution imagery in a prescreening device for the detection of cervical cancer was deemed impractical. Only a few years ago competent engineers concluded from their assessment of technology that neither the required data rates nor the massive computational power could be provided in a cost-effective manner.

Nonetheless, the TICAS devised by Wied et al. and described previously has been successfully used in automated classifications of cells derived from the uterine cervix.

Although much effort was initially invested in discriminating between two populations (i.e., benign and malignant cells), it is clear that the cervical sample contains many possible cell classes. By 1973 it has clearly been established that computer algorithms could recognize all major cervical cell types of epidermoid derivation with good reliability (Bibbo et al., 1973).

Squamous cells from eight categories recognized in cervical cytology (i.e., superficial, intermediate, parabasal, metaplastic, metaplastic-dysplastic, and nonkeratinizing dysplastic cells; cells from carcinoma in situ; and cells from invasive carcinoma) were analyzed by Bartels et al. (1973). A continuous transition from category to category of cells was confirmed in an objective manner by cell image analysis (see Fig. 35–8). Still, visually recognized classes of cells can be clearly correlated with computer-generated classes (Bibbo et al., 1973). Subsequently, other methods of cell classification by computer were devised and successfully applied to sort the cervical squamous cells into 11 classes (Taylor et al., 1974).

Although the early TICAS system laid the scientific bases for automated analysis of the sample from the uterine cervix, it was too slow and complex for clinical application. Therefore, as a forerunner, a fully integrated unit of microscope and special-purpose multiple-processor computer was designed (Wied et al., 1975) for the demonstration of automatic real-time identification of any of 16 types of squamous epithelial cells, whether normal or abnormal, at the push of a button. This unit, the TICAS-RTCIP (real-time cell identification processor), further served to present the advantages and feasibility of designing analytical systems with a network of microprocessors operating in parallel.

This system was followed by development of a two-stage screening system. The system employed a monolayer device, the TICAS-MLD (Wied et al., 1981), to prepare a dispersed monolayer specimen, and a cell detection module, the CDM (Read et al., 1979), to provide a dry enrichment of the sample by prescreening the slide at lower resolution to detect suspicious objects before high-resolution scanning.

The more recent evolution of the TICAS has seen the development of several microcomputer workstation versions—micro-TICAS for basic analyses and meso-TICAS for contextual measurements and analyses of stratified epithelia (Puls et al., 1986; Dytch et al., 1986, 1987; Bibbo et al., 1986; Dytch and Wied, 1990). These video-based systems provide rapid cytometric analyses with redundant capabilities that far exceed those of the minicomputer-based TICASs of only a decade or so ago. Current work is aimed at integrating the large clinical data base collected at the University of Chicago with these objective cytometric measurements through the use of AI techniques (Wied, et al. 1987; Wied et al., 1990).

Nuclear DNA ploidy measurements in cervical specimens have proved useful for diagnosis and prognosis (Bibbo et al., 1985, 1989). The use of high-resolution cytometric data for comparison and quality control of cytologic and histologic diagnoses of cervical lesions was described by Bibbo et al. (1983). Dytch et al. (1983) found that high-resolution features, including color features, could be used to reject the noncellular artifacts that often are a problem in screening machines. Rosenthal et al. (1984) found that visually similar moderate dysplasia cells from cervical specimens could be separated by high-resolution image analysis into clusters dependent on the parent lesion. Hall et al. (1988) found canonical analysis to be a useful technique for the classification of high-resolution images of Papanicolaou-stained cervical cells. Linear discriminant analysis based on features derived from high-resolution cervical cell images was found useful in the prediction of regression or progression by Rosenthal et al. (1987).

In 1969 a national program for automation of cervical cytology was launched in the United States (Melamed, 1969). Similar programs were developed in other countries. In Japan a single-purpose system, CYBEST, with a very high speed of data acquisition was described by Tanaka et al. (1973–1977, 1987) as the first industrial prescreening device. CYBEST, which has been discontinued, used a flying spot device for prescreening of smears and the search for abnormal cell images, which were then evaluated by high-resolution scanning. The recognition of abnormal cells by the flying spot device was based on nuclear size and density. The high-resolution scanning was based on nuclear chromatin pattern and nuclear boundary outline. The features of abnormal cells, the edge-finding routine for nuclear and cytoplasmic boundary, caused some difficulties (Tanaka et al., 1977), resulting in up to 20 percent of cells falsely labeled as abnormal.

In Germany four major laboratories made a concerted effort to develop a system of automatic tumor diagnosis (TUDAB) through image processing (*Tumor Diagnose durch Automatische Bild*

*V*erarbeitung). Essentially, the approach combined coherent optical and high-resolution absorption analysis with the use of an optoelectronic hybrid system in the cell-finding step and image preprocessing by coherent optical computing (i.e., by means of matched spatial filtering in the Fourier domain) (Reuter et al., 1976; Burger, 1976). The diffraction pattern of single cells on photographs or on slides was obtained and analyzed with the use of software masks by special hardware detectors, such as a segmented, circular solid-state detector, or by a TV camera of special design.

Other automatic or semiautomatic systems for prescreening or screening of the cervical sample have been developed in various countries. Some examples of these systems are the BIOPEPR (Zahniser, 1979), CERVIFIP (1983), FAZYTAN (Reinhardt, 1982), and LEYTAS (Ploem, 1987) systems. Their principles remain much the same, and the technical details are beyond the scope of this summary. At the time of this writing (1991), several new systems for the automation of cervical screening have appeared in the United States. Some of these systems use monolayer preparations. The PAPNET system incorporates image processing and artificial neural network techniques to analyze ordinary Papanicolaou-stained cervical smears (see Color Plates 12–3, 12–4, and 12–5). The performance of this and other machines is still being tested.

Classification of Urothelial Cells in Urine

Koss et al. have used high-resolution image analysis to study urothelial cells in urinary sediment in an ongoing program (1975, 1977, 1978, 1980, 1983, 1984, 1987, 1989). It has clearly been demonstrated that benign and malignant cells of human urothelium can be discriminated with small error rates by computer. Differences in nuclear texture were one of the most useful descriptors. Supervised learning algorithms have disclosed that atypical urothelial cells form a distinct, although ill-defined, family of cells that differs from normal and malignant cells (see Chap. 23). Studies of patients' profiles by scanning of sequential, well-preserved urothelial cells in the urinary sediment yielded promising diagnostic data (Koss et al., 1978, 1989). It is possible to classify high-resolution images obtained from sediments of voided urine by using such techniques as hierarchical analysis (Koss et al., 1980) and a selective mapping algorithm (Wong et al., 1989). Subvisual marker features have also been detected in urothelial cells

by Sherman and Koss (1983). A semiquantitative technique of preserving and processing urothelial cells used in these studies was developed by Bales (see Chap. 33).

Cell Classification in Immunology and Hematology

It had long been known that the granularity, arrangement, state of condensation, and specific pattern of distribution of nuclear chromatin carry significant diagnostic information, which is evident to the readers of this volume. Early measurement for the objective description of such information were performed by Sandritter et al. (1974, 1967) and Kiefer et al. (1973). What had not been known was the high discriminatory power derived from assessing stochastic (i.e., statistical assessment of random distribution) image properties. It could be demonstrated convincingly that granularity, state of condensation, and specific patterns of distribution of nuclear chromatin granules that do not appear different to the human eye can be mapped through computation into well-separated regions of a pattern space formed by the parameters derived from the texture of chromatin. These properties of image analysis have been successfully applied to discrimination of groups of cells that cannot be separated from one another by visual analysis. An excellent example is the identification of T and B lymphocytes. Image analysis of chromatin patterns in Feulgen-stained preparations of chicken lymphocytes allowed the differentiation of the subgroups T and B with a high degree of precision (Olson et al., 1973, 1974). When thoracic duct lymphocytes from CBA mice and from athymic nude mice were compared, the likelihood of distinguishing B cells from T cells was found by Bartels et al. (1975) to be 135 to 1, whereas the likelihood of distinguishing T cells from B cells was as high as 730 to 1. More interesting still is the discovery that a number of subsets could be distinguished in the pure T population but not among pure B cells. This agrees well with the present biologic and immunologic concepts.

Clearly, in the realm of mathematics and beyond the reach of human vision are algorithms using the "higher order" statistical properties of gray values of pixels. Such properties may be used for cell discrimination. For example, Bartels et al. (1974) used the mutual dependencies of gray values in the nucleus for the study of Papanicolaou-stained benign lymphocytes and cells of malignant lymphoma. Here, the dependencies in strings of values no longer than ten pixels were sufficient to achieve cell recognition with acceptable error rates.

A high-resolution scanning system for leukocyte recognition has been described by Vastola et al. (1974) and Brenner et al. (1974, 1976) in which the instrumentation and software systems designed by Neurath were applied to Wright-stained blood films. Three maturity levels of the myeloid series and three grades of maturity in the lymphomonocytic series could be identified with satisfactory probabilities. The principal algorithm searched for changes in density from one pixel to the next, following one scan line. In this respect a methodologic analogy exists to the line scan transition probability profiles of Bartels et al. (1969).

In a methodologic study by Jarkowski et al. (1971) proof was provided that supervised and nonsupervised learning programs are capable of recognizing the cells of asymptomatic chronic lymphocytic leukemia over normal lymphocytes and of showing variances, possibly subgroups of cells, within the population of leukemic cells. The supervised learning section, aimed at secure identification of individual cells, resulted in a very high likelihood for recognition of a cell as either normal or leukemic. The nonsupervised section of the program identified subsets of cells with different properties, with an acceptably low error rate. Zajicek et al. (1972) analyzed lymphocytes aspirated from lymph nodes in well-differentiated lymphocytic lymphoma, lymphadenitis, and peripheral blood. Although preliminary, the results showed that discrimination of these look-alike conditions by computer programs is possible and invites future studies.

These results are cited for historical interest only. The high-resolution image analysis techniques of hematopoietic cells have been replaced by immunologic, cytochemical, and molecular biologic techniques (see Chaps. 2 and 34).

Cell Classification in Other Cytologic Targets

A variety of cytologic targets have proved amenable to study by means of high-resolution image analysis. Jahoda et al. (1973) correctly classified a very high percentage of normal and reactive mesothelial cells, histiocytes, and cells of metastatic adenocarcinoma of lung and breast origin in effusions as well as a high percentage of mesothelial cells and ovarian cancer cells in peritoneal fluids. Zajicek et al. (1973) studied fine-needle aspirates from patients with breast cancer by TICAS rou-

tines and found significant predictors of response to radiotherapy. Bibbo et al. (1987) found differences in histologic grade of renal cell carcinomas to be significantly associated with several variables such as nuclear area, shape, crowding, elongation, and frequency of mitosis. Poor survival was associated with high mitotic rate and elongated and crowded nuclei. Boon et al. (1982) used image analysis to classify follicular adenoma and carcinoma of the thyroid on aspiration smears. Studies of fine-needle aspirates of invasive follicular carcinoma of the thyroid and microinvasive follicular carcinoma of the thyroid have indicated the presence of subvisual marker features associated with these lesions (Bibbo et al., 1986, 1990; Galera-Davidson et al., 1990). Several studies have established the value of high-resolution cytometry combined with DNA analysis (see below) in making an objective and reproducible assessment of prostatic carcinoma (Sprenger et al., 1974; Auer et al., 1984; Bibbo et al., 1989; Schultz et al., 1990). Hutchinson et al. (1989) achieved correct classification of 22 of 26 prostate aspirates by using contextual analysis. Many researchers have used objective cytometric techniques to study carcinoma of the breast (Sprenger et al., 1979). Hutchinson et al. (1989) used contextual analysis to achieve a correct classification in 15 of 18 breast aspirates. Subvisual marker features in foam cells from breast exudate were reported by King et al. (1982). Mansi et al. (1988) used the LEYTAS system to automate screening for micrometastases of breast cancer in bone marrow smears. Baak et al. (1985, 1987) showed the value of morphometric features in providing prognostic information on ovarian cancer patients. Fleming et al. (1990) have used image analysis to assess nuclear atypia in dysplastic nevi and melanomas. Many more examples could be cited, but it is clear that image cytometry is capable of providing diagnostically and prognostically relevant information regarding disease from a wide variety of body sites. It is equally clear, however, that many years may be required to fully realize the potential of these techniques (Koss, 1982, 1985, 1987, 1990).

Image Analysis of Histologic Sections

High-resolution analysis of histologic section represents a very complex undertaking in image analysis, as first pointed out in Lipkin et al. (1966) and Kirsch (1971). Several approaches are possible. One is based on the identification within a complex "scene" (i.e., tissue pattern) of individual, simple components or cells that may be related to each other by contextual histometry, as discussed above. Nuclear features may be related to nuclear position relative to the tissue architecture, gland placement pattern, and other nuclei. The gland placement pattern as a whole may be characterized. Another approach is the analysis of the global features of the tissue. The latter approach may quantitate a tissue component or components that can be identified by special stains. For example, it may prove possible to calculate the amount of amyloid or other similar deposit by computing precisely the area occupied by the foreign substance.

The goal of such analyses is to interpret tissue patterns in terms of a diagnostic decision similar to that rendered by a pathologist. This may be accomplished by a low-power pattern recognition procedure or, for more precise diagnostic decisions, by analysis of cell components of a tissue. In the latter case, cells must be visually or automatically recognized as an entity. Some cells are naturally isolated in the section from others and from interfering debris, but this is not true for most cells. Methods of cell isolation are needed, and for this purpose manual-visual procedures (Wied et al., 1970) and procedures based on AI have been described (Taylor et al., 1975). The isolation of single cells from digitized sections of tissue is an extension of such methods. Prewitt and Wu (1978) have studied the structure of sections of bladder tumor tissue. Preston (1980) has reviewed several examples of the analysis of images of tissue sections, including the counting of nuclei, boundary detection of corneal epithelial cells, and classification of normal and abnormal cells in the human liver. Baak et al. (1981) analyzed the histology of ovarian tumors and endometrial hyperplasia and carcinoma using imaging techniques. Bartels et al. (1987, 1989) have employed expert system techniques to analyze such sections, as previously described. Contextual techniques were employed by Dytch et al. (1987) and by Dytch and Wied (1990) to analyze stratified epithelia, as discussed earlier, and Bibbo et al. (1989) found contextual analysis to be of value in analyzing prostatic carcinoma. Bibbo et al. (1990) found subvisual markers in normal-appearing glands adjacent to adenocarcinoma in the human colon and in tissue adjacent to invasive (1989) and in situ cervical carcinomas (Montag et al., 1989). Measurements of both architectural and high-resolution features were found to enable accurate grading of prostatic cancer sections by Bibbo et al. (1990). At the time of this writing (1991) image analysis of tissue sections is still in developmental stages.

APPLICATION OF HIGH-RESOLUTION IMAGE ANALYSIS SYSTEMS TO QUANTITATIVE ANALYSIS OF CELLS AND CELL COMPONENTS

A major development in the use of image analysis systems has been their application to measurements of cell components, listed in Table 35–1.

The oldest of these applications is the quantitation of nucleic acids. Caspersson (1936) was the first to observe that when subjected to ultraviolet light of a specific wavelength the cellular DNA, RNA, and proteins could be measured by densitometry. For this purpose Caspersson used microscopes with quartz optics to photograph cells under ultraviolet light. In photographs thus obtained the nucleus was sharply contrasted with the cytoplasm because of high differential ultraviolet light absorption by DNA. When the cytoplasm contained large quantities of RNA, it too would absorb strongly. A laborious procedure made it possible to translate absorptive properties of DNA and RNA into the respective quantities of these substances per nucleus or cytoplasm (Caspersson, 1950, Caspersson and Lomakka, 1962).

Caspersson and Santesson (1942) also documented major cytochemical differences between benign and malignant cells (see Chap. 5).

The very tedious, and time-consuming techniques developed by Caspersson have now been replaced and have found wide application in human pathology and cytology. At the time of this writing, (1991), image analysis instruments can be applied efficiently and rapidly to quantitation of a broad range of cell components—from DNA to cell genes and their products.

General Principles

Image analysis systems require that the target to be measured be isolated (segmented) from its background. The easiest way to accomplish this task is to use a stain specific for its target and not to use a counterstain for the background. A perfect example is the use of Feulgen stain for DNA without a counterstain (see Fig. 1–28). Only the nuclei will be visible because mitochondrial DNA occurs in such small quantities that it can be disregarded for all practical purposes. The nuclei can be digitized by the procedure described above and their light absorption (adjusted for Beer's law) and area determined. The summary of the measurements of several nuclei can be expressed as a histogram. By complex calculations and use of appropriate controls, the amount of DNA per nucleus can be calculated.

If the target of the measurements cannot or should not be selectively stained, the choice of the counterstain becomes very important: it should be visible only at a wavelength that is significantly different from the wavelength that renders the target visible. Under these circumstances, after the identification of the target, the background stain can be eliminated by the use of appropriate optical filters.

A third method is the use of contrasting ordinary laboratory stains, such as Papanicolaou stain, in which the target (the nucleus) can be identified by scene segmentation techniques, identical to those described for cell classification analysis (see p. 1591).

Finally, with the use of specific fluorescent stains and appropriately equipped microscopes the amount of fluorescence can be measured. This last technique has found wide application in flow cytometry (see Chapter 36). Selected specific applications of quantitative image analysis are described below.

Measurements of Cellular DNA

Measurements of DNA may be performed using specific stains such as the Feulgen stain (see p. 1502) or gallocyanin-chromalum stain. Approximate measurements can be obtained by the use of customary laboratory nuclear stains such as hematoxylin in various combinations. The latter approach does not offer quantitative analysis and is appropriate only for comparison of two targets, such as a cervical smear and cervical biopsy to determine the concordance of DNA patterns (Wied et al., 1983; Bibbo et al., 1985).

Generally, however, the basic purpose of DNA measurements is to determine the ploidy of the target cells. Of particular value is the measurement of DNA in some human cancers wherein the DNA content may prove to be of prognostic value, for example, in bladder tumors or in mammary carcinoma.

Studies of Fresh Material

Fresh material, be it an aspirate, a fluid sample, or a tissue culture, can nearly always be processed to form a smear, which is an ideal way to measure DNA. Touch preparation smears or smears of aspirates obtained by means of a very thin needle can be prepared from tissues. For DNA analysis it does not matter whether the smear is air-dried or fixed in alcohol or acetone because the DNA molecule remains preserved for many years (Auer and Zetterberg, 1984). However, in air-dried preparations, the cells become flattened on slides, and the nuclei are significantly larger when compared with those of fixed cells, an important point if the DNA content is to be calculated per unit of nuclear surface. The best stain for DNA analysis is Feulgen stain. The stain does not fade perceptibly after some months of storage (Auer and Zetterberg, 1984).

Archival Material

DNA can also be measured in stained archival smears, after destaining, rehydration, and restaining with Feulgen. Thus retrospective studies of DNA distribution are possible and have been reported by Auer and Zetterberg (1984) and by others in reference to breast and prostate cancers.

It is also possible to process paraffin-embedded tissue by image analysis. A modification of Hedley's method, described in Chapter 36, may be used (Amberson et al., 1987). The result of the procedure is a suspension of nuclei that can be processed as a cytocentrifuge preparation, stained with Feulgen.

Measuring DNA in archival histologic sections is a much more difficult target. The principal reason for it is the presence of cross sections of nuclei. Thus, dealing with nuclei of various sizes in a tissue section, one is never certain whether the cross section is representative of a small nucleus or of a tangential cross section of a large nucleus. Several approaches to this dilemma have been proposed. For example, Fu et al. (1979, 1981, 1985) used 10- to 14-μ-thick sections and focused on whole nuclei. This method may be difficult to implement if the microscope lens has a shallow focusing distance. In thin (3- to 5-μm) sections it is necessary to perform a large number of measurements on cross sections of nuclei with the hope that the mean values achieved in this fashion will represent the DNA content of whole nuclei. Mikel et al. (1985) calculated the number of measurements required, depending on the thickness of the section.

Selection of Targets

As described, image analysis offers the advantage of visual control of the cells or nuclei selected for measurements. In virtually all instruments available today the cells may be visualized either under a microscope or on a television screen. For DNA measurements in smears of tumors a selection of large nuclei must be made because these are most likely to represent tumor cells. Broken or fractured nuclei and nuclear debris must be avoided. In tumors with very fragile cells this may sometimes be difficult. Unfortunately, in Feulgen stain that is not counterstained with a cytoplasmic dye, the entire cell may be difficult to visualize and therefore the selection of nuclei may be fraught with error. A light counterstain with cresyl blue or a similar stain has limited impact on DNA measurements and may help in cell identification.

It is quite helpful if nuclei of polymorphonuclear leukocytes can be identified in the same smear since these may give guidance as to the nuclear size and also serve as measurement control (see below). Unfortunately, lymphocytes may be difficult to identify as such, particularly in small-cell neoplasms.

Controls of DNA Measurements

Establishing appropriate controls of DNA measurements by image analysis is a difficult and often underestimated task. Unfortunately, inactive lymphocytes that represent an excellent diploid control in flow cytometry are too compact to be of value in image analysis. In virtually all image analysis systems available today the mean DNA content of inactive lymphocytes is nearly always much lower than the value of diploid cells. Therefore, lymphocytes constitute a very poor control. Polymorphonuclear leukocytes, which are easier to recognize and spread better on glass than lympho-

cytes, can be used as controls, but the complex shape of their nuclei may not always be captured by the cell analysis systems. Other controls are benign epithelial cells or fibroblasts of the same origin, but here again the recognition of these cells may be difficult in Feulgen-stained preparations. Some manufacturers, notably Cell Analysis System, Inc. (909 S. Rt. 83, Elmhurst, Ill. 60126-4944), provide slides with built-in controls consisting of animal liver or kidney cells with a known DNA content. Again, caution must be exercised in assessing the value of animal cells as controls in human cell samples, but perhaps this is, at present, the best approach to a vexing problem.

Histogram Interpretation

The purpose of DNA measurements is to determine whether a given population of cells has a DNA distribution similar to normal or whether it is abnormal. As shown in the uninterrupted curve in Fig. 35–13, any normal cycling cell population may have a broad range of normal values, with most cells residing in the G_0/G_1 compartment, some in the G_2/M compartment, and some in the intermediate S compartment (see Chap. 36). Thus the DNA values of an abnormal population must either form abnormal peaks, outside of the customary compartments, or have a skewed distribution of cell in the various compartments. Histograms with clearly abnormal peaks or obvious maldistribution of DNA values are easily classified as aneuploid. Histograms with normal distribution of cells are classified as diploid or euploid. There

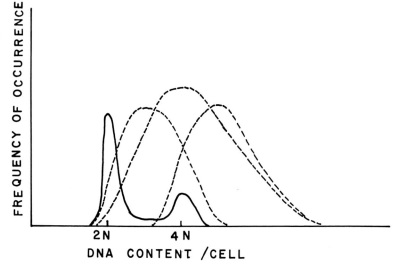

FIGURE 35–13. Distribution of DNA values in populations of cells. *Solid line* represents a growing and dividing normal population of cells. Most cells are at the resting state 2N (diploid), others have doubled their DNA and are ready to divide: 4N or tetraploid. In between 2N and 4N S-phase cells are located. *Broken lines* represent the DNA distribution in three carcinomas. Although, as a population, each one of the tumors differs clearly from normal, a single cell found at 4N could be either a tumor cell or a proliferating normal cell. Another designation of N is C, used in Figs. 35–14 and 35–15.

are, however, many histograms with only slight deviation from normal, and these may constitute a major problem in classification.

Histograms of DNA content in a given smear or a cytocentrifuge preparation are usually constructed on the basis of 100 to 200 primary measurements and 20 to 50 controls. The DNA absorption values are placed in computer-generated slots or "bins," which are arbitrarily defined and may contain values within 10% or more of the target. Because of the limited number of entries, the histograms are often "rough," with ragged edges, and resemble building blocks (Fig. 35–14). The histograms can be smoothed, that is, replaced by computer-generated curves that help little in the interpretation. As can be seen in Fig. 35–13, there is, in smoothed histograms, a major overlap in DNA values between a benign cell population and cancer cells. Auer et al. (1980), cognizant of this problem, preferred to classify DNA histograms according to type, rather than labeling them as diploid, polyploid, tetraploid, or aneuploid (Fig. 35–15).

Another means of histogram classification is the estimation of hyperdiploid cell fraction, or excess of 2N (or 2C) (diploid) cells or excess of hypertetraploid cells (excess of 4N or 4C). For all intents and purposes it may be safely stated that any cell population with cells with DNA values above 4C is malignant (see Fig. 35–15, *bottom*). The exceptions to this rule are few and pertain to megakaryocytes and other rare multinucleated cells, usually readily recognized under the microscope or on the television screen.

Regarding the diagnostic or prognostic value of DNA histograms, the reader is referred to the discussion in Chapter 36. However, the following must be noted: under some circumstances, studies of DNA distribution by image analysis disclose the presence of abnormal clones of cells that may not be apparent in flow cytometry. This has been shown to be true in reference to effusions (Schneller et al., 1987), to bladder washings (Koss et al., 1989), and to aspirates of mammary cancer (Cornelisse and Van Driel-Kulker, 1985) (Fig. 35–16). The differences are particularly obvious if the population of cells with a high DNA content is very small and is therefore not seen in flow cytometric histograms. For further discussion of these problems, see Chapter 36.

Quantitation of Cell Receptors and Genes

With the developments in immunocytochemistry and specific monoclonal antibodies (Mabs) directed against an array of cell components it became possible to visualize a number of reactions using either the peroxidase-antiperoxidase system or one of its variants described in Chapter 34. At the time of this writing (1991), an array of Mabs combine with a variety of cell receptors, such as estrogen and progesterone receptors, and a variety of gene products, including oncoproteins. Among others, antibodies to Her2/neu, Ha *ras*, c-*myc*, and c-*fos* oncoproteins are commercially available. Most recently, an antibody to the retinoblastoma (Rb gene, see Chapter 2) gene product was tested (Cance et al., 1990). Antibodies to Ki 67 and cyclin cell proliferation factors are also available.

As mentioned at the beginning of this chapter, any cell product that can be visualized can also be measured. Labeling of the cell product with a fluorescent compound allows it to be measured in a quantitative microscope system under ultraviolet light or by flow cytometry. It is also possible to measure the precipitate by image analysis with equivalent results (Czerniak et al., 1990). A number of essential precautions must be taken. Primarily, the specificity of the antibody must be tested by precipitating it with the protein to which it is di-

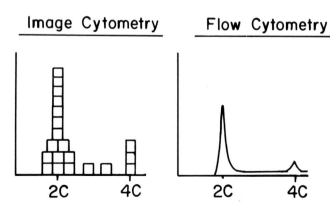

Image Cytometry   Flow Cytometry

FIGURE 35–14. Histograms of DNA content, obtained by image analysis (*left*) and by flow cytometry (*right*). The histograms obtained by image analysis are "rough" because of relatively few measurements, placed in "boxes" or bins. The very large number of measurements obtained by flow cytometry (usually in excess of 10,000) account for the "smooth" contours of the histogram.

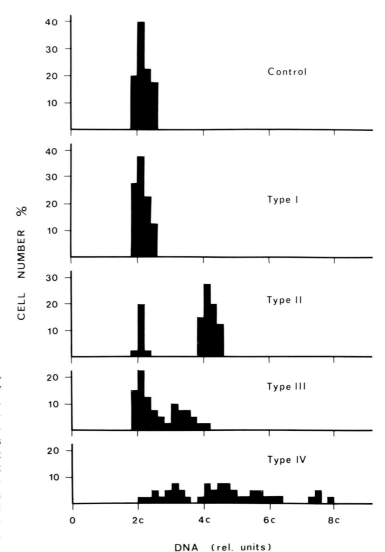

FIGURE 35–15. Classification of DNA histograms of breast carcinoma cells by image analysis suggested by Auer et al. (1980). Instead of classifying the histograms as diploid and aneuploid, these authors classified them as types I to IV. It was subsequently documented (Fallenious et al., 1988) that the prognosis of breast cancer was better with type I and II histograms than with type III and IV. (From Auer, G., Caspersson, T., and Wallgren, A.: DNA content and survival in mammary carcinoma. Anal. Quant. Cytol. *3*:161–165, 1980; with permission)

rected (Western blot). Negative controls must also be provided, either by using an irrelevant antibody or by blocking the antibody with the specific protein (see Figs. 2–27, 35–18 and 35–19).

Of the two measuring systems, image analysis is easier to implement because it can be performed on smears. However, great care must be exercised in preparing, staining, and counterstaining of the preparations. In reference to the oncoproteins, some are located in the nucleus (for example, c-*fos* protein p55 and c-*myc* protein p62) and others in the cell membrane or cytoplasm (for example, *ras* protein p21 and c-*erb* protein p185) (Fig. 35–17). We found that methyl green counterstain was ex-

cellent for the demonstration of the precipitates located in the nucleus, whereas fast green was used for the demonstration of membrane and cytoplasmic proteins (Czerniak et al., 1990).

The actual measurements of the density of the precipitate (corresponding to the amount of the product) must be performed with a masking system that eliminates the counterstain and measures only the density of the precipitate. Needless to say, the principles of Beer's law must be observed, and the correction is built into commercially available machines. An example of the staining is shown in Fig. 35–17 and of the results of the measurements in Figs. 35–18 and 35–19.

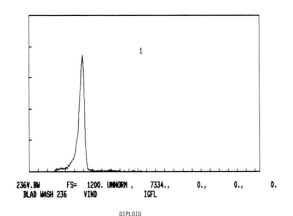

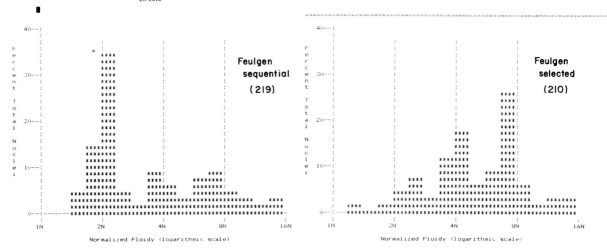

FIGURE 35–16. Comparison of DNA distribution by flow cytometry and image analysis in the same specimen of bladder washings from a patient with a history of urothelial carinoma grade III. The flow cytometric histogram (>5,000 cells, propidium iodide stain, *top*) had a single peak in the diploid range. Feulgen-stained cytocentrifuge preparations of nuclei were examined by MICROTICAS image analysis system (acquired from Dr. George Wied, University of Chicago) in two modes: sequential mode (219 nuclei, *bottom left*) and selection mode (selection of 210 larger nuclei, *bottom right*). Image analysis disclosed the presence of nuclei with hyperdiploid values, not seen in the flow histogram. The diploid values were reduced, and the aneuploid values of the histogram were enhanced by the selection process (*bottom right*). (From Koss, L. G., Predictive value of DNA measurements in bladder washings. Comparison of flow cytometry image cytophotometry and cytology of voided urine in urothelial tumors. Cancer, *64*:916–924, 1989; reproduced with permission from Cancer)

Clinical Applications

At the time of this writing (1991) the most common application of image analysis to cell products is to carcinoma of the breast. There is evidence that *breast cancer panel* may be of clinical and prognostic value. The makeup of the breast cancer panel at the time of this writing is as follows:

1. DNA ploidy
2. Estrogen-receptor binding
3. Progesterone-receptor binding
4. Expression of HER/neu oncoprotein
5. Proliferation index measured by reaction with the antibody to Ki 67

Undoubtedly, with time, other parameters will be measured. The techniques used in these measurements are the same as those described above for oncoproteins (see Figs. 35–17 to 35–19).

The rationale behind the breast cancer panel is as follows. There is evidence that carcinomas of the

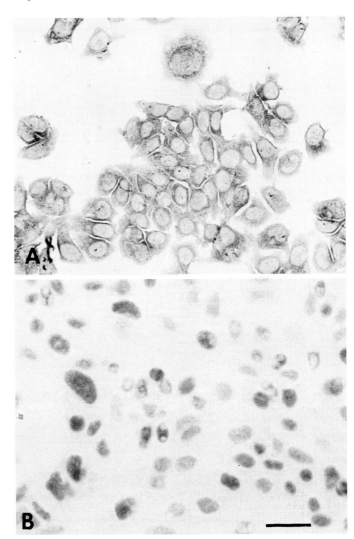

FIGURE 35–17. Immunocytologic documentation of the c-*ras* oncogene product (p21), demonstrated by avidin-biotin-immunoperoxidase assay, in the cell membrane (*A*), and of the c-*fos* oncogene product (p55) in the nuclei of cultured human carcinoma cell line MCF7-KO (*B*). The results of the measurements of these two oncogene products are shown in Figs. 35–18 and 35–19. (Czerniak, B., et al.: Quantitation of oncogene products by computer-assisted image analysis and flow cytometry. J. Histochem. Cytochem., *38*:463–466, 1990; with permission)

breast with a diploid DNA content and a small proliferation fraction (measured as S phase in a flow cytometry or as Ki 67 index in image analysis) have a better prognosis than aneuploid breast cancers with a high level of proliferating cells. Such tumors are also provided with estrogen receptors and thus respond to hormonal manipulation. There is also evidence that tetraploid tumors, of intermediate degree of aggressive behavior, express high levels of HER/neu oncogene. On the other hand, highly aggressive tumors that are aneuploid, have no estrogen or progesterone receptors, and have a low level of HER/neu protein expression respond to chemotherapy, even though the response may be only temporary (Bur et al., 1987; Franklin et al., 1987; Doria et al., 1987; Colley et al., 1989; Follenius et

al., 1988; Kommoss et al., 1989; Bacus et al., 1988, 1989, 1990).

There are other examples of human cancer in which measurement of cell components appears to be of prognostic value. Bladder tumors with a diploid DNA content and low expression of *Ha ras* oncogene produce have a better prognosis than aneuploid tumors with a high level of oncogene product (Czerniak et al., 1990). Carcinomas of the prostate with a diploid DNA content appear to be less aggressive than aneuploid carcinomas (Amberson et al., 1987). The expression of high levels of *myc* protein carries with it an unfavorable prognosis in neuroblastoma (Cohen et al., 1988). These are but a few examples of early applications of quantitative image analysis to human cancer. With progress in

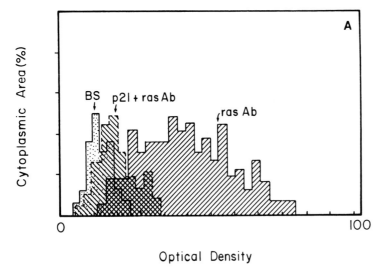

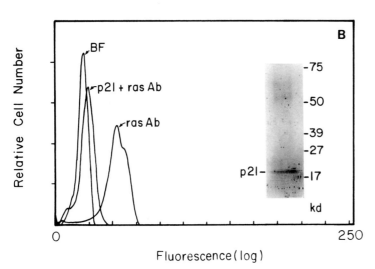

FIGURE 35-18. Quantitation of the c-*ras* oncogene product p21 located in the cell membrane (see Fig. 35-16*A*) by image analysis (*A*) and by flow cytometry (*B*). The specificity of the antibody used (Y13-259, from Oncogene Science, Inc. Manhasset, N.Y.) was tested by a Western blot (*B*, *right*). (*A*) BS = background staining; p21 + *ras* Ab = optical density of cells incubated with anti-*ras* antibody absorbed with p21 protein (control experiment); *ras* Ab = excess optical density of measured c-*ras* oncogene product p21. The dark hatched area at the bottom of the diagram indicates the overlapping areas of the three measurements. (*B*) BF = background fluorescence; p21 + *ras* Ab = antibody absorbed with *ras* p21 protein (control measurement); *ras* Ab = increased fluorescence level with unopposed anti-*ras* antibody. Both measurements (expressed as arbitrary units) show an increase of c-*ras* expression over control measurements, (*A*) in arithmetic scale, (*B*) in log scale. (Czerniak, B., et al.: Quantitation of oncogene products by computer-assisted image analysis and flow cytometry. J. Histochem. Cytochem., *38*:463-466, 1990; with permission)

cell biology and recognition and sequencing of additional genes, this repertoire of reactions undoubtedly will increase. Still, the principles described in this chapter will probably remain the same.

IMPLEMENTATION OF HIGH-RESOLUTION CYTOMETRY

Hardware and Software

High-resolution image analysis systems based on microcomputer technology have become quite affordable. Although several commercial systems are available, it is quite possible for a researcher to assemble the required components from readily available "off-the-shelf" items. The basic modules of such a system and the state of the image signal at each are summarized in Fig. 35-20. An ordinary laboratory microscope serves as a platform for mounting an ordinary video camera, usually a color camera with independent sensors, and possibly a small charge coupled device (CCD) camera. Depending on the application, different objectives may be used; oil-immersion objectives reduce the effects of spherical abberation. The optical image from the microscope optics is converted in the camera into an analog signal (usually red-green-blue [RGB] for reasons of quality) and transferred

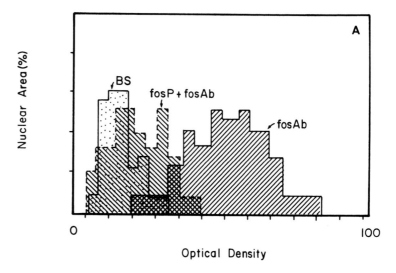

FIGURE 35–19. Quantitation of the c-*fos* oncogene product p55, located in the nucleus (see Fig. 35–16*B*) by image analysis (*A*) and by flow cytometry (*B*). The specificity of the antibody used (DCX 821 from Cambridge Research Biochemical) was tested by Western blot (*A, right*). The explanation of abbreviations is the same as in Fig. 35–17, except that *fos* is used instead of *ras*. An increase in the expression of this oncoprotein over controls is documented by both types of measurements. (Czerniak, B., et al.: Quantitation of oncogene products by computer-assisted image analysis and flow cytometry. J. Histochem. Cytochem., *38*:463–466, 1990; with permission)

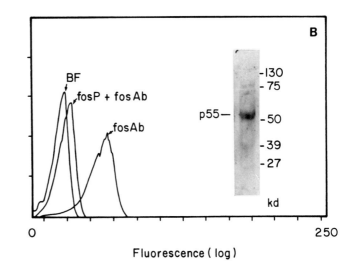

FIGURE 35–20. A typical microcomputer-based video image cytometry system, showing the main components and the state of the image signal during processing. The raw microscopic optical signal is converted by a video camera to an analog electronic signal, which is in turn digitized by an imaging board located within a microcomputer. The digital signal is then available in the local memory of the microcomputer for analysis, and may be converted, with overlaid graphic information, for display on a color monitor.

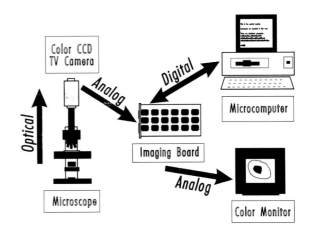

to an imaging board located in the chassis of a microcomputer. One of the roles of the imaging board is to act as a display buffer and to convert the analog electronic television signal into a digital image, which is then stored locally. Pixel values from this digital image may then be transferred to the main memory of the host microcomputer for scene segmentation, feature extraction, and analysis. The digitized cell image, possibly enhanced and manipulated, is displayed on a color RGB monitor, and control of the image processing software is directed through an ordinary computer display.

It is important to choose components that are matched to one another in terms of capabilities and resolution. A very-high-resolution imaging board is wasted if used with low-grade microscope optics or a low-resolution video camera. In choice of camera and image board it is as important to have sufficient control over the electronics as to establish suitable response for microphotometry, which is often *not* the setup of the camera used for broadcast work. For example, if geometric accuracy is to be achieved, the normal 4:3 aspect ratio of the standard camera must be changed, and the response of the camera to light must linear. Likewise, if the camera compensates for low light levels, the photometric accuracy of measurements of dark nuclei will not be of the desired quality.

The most expensive and high-quality hardware in the world is of no value without the driving software that enables its use as a tool to make the desired measurements. With a turnkey system, software is provided as part of the package — indeed, perhaps the most essential part. If the system has been built from off-the-shelf hardware components, the choice is between programming the system oneself or buying an existing software package. Depending on the image board chosen, general to specific software packages are available for accomplishing various image processing tasks. The trade-off is between the generality of most such programs and the specific needs for the project at hand.

BIBLIOGRAPHY

Amberson, J.B., Schreiber, K., Wersto, R., Koizumi, J.H., Detich, D., Freed, S., Vaughan, E.D., and Koss, L.G.: Image cytometry in prostatic carcinoma. Acta Cytol. *31*:682, 1987.

Andersen, R.E., Olson, G.B., Shank, C., Howarth, J.L., Wied, G.L., and Bartels, P.H.: Computer anaysis of defined populations of lymphocytes irradiated in vitro. Evaluation of murine thoracic duct lymphocytes. Acta Cytol., *19*:126–133, 1975.

Anderson, J.A., and Rosenfeld, E.: Neurocomputing. Cambridge, Mass. 1988, MIT Press.

Ansley, H.R., and Ornstein, L.: Enzyme histochemistry and differentiated white cell counts on the Technicon Hemalog-D. *In* Advances in Automated Analysis, Vol. 1. Miami, Thurman Associates, 1971, pp 437–452.

Atkin, N.B.: Modal DNA value and chromosome number in ovarian neoplasia. Cancer, *27*:1064–1073, 1971.

Atkin, N.B., Mattinson, G., and Baker, M.C.: A comparison of the DNA content and chromosome number of fifty human tumors. Br. J. Cancer, *30*:87–101, 1966.

Atkin, N.B., and Richards, B.M.: Deoxyribonucleic acid in human tumors as measured by microspectrophotometry of Feulgen stain: A comparison of tumors arising at different sites. Br. J. Cancer, *10*:769–786, 1956.

Atkin, N.B., Richards, B.M., and Ross, A.J.: The deoxyribonucleic acid content of carcinoma of the uterus: An assessment of its possible significance in relation to histopathology and clinical course, based on data from 165 cases. Br. J. Cancer, *13*:773–787, 1959.

Auer, G., Caspersson, T., and Wallgren, A.: DNA content and survival in mammary carcinoma. Anal. Quant. Cytol., *3*:161–165, 1980.

Auer, G.U., and Zetterberg, A.: The prognostic significance of nuclear DNA content in malignant tumors of breast, prostate and cartilage. *In* Koss, L.G., and Coleman, D.V. (eds.): Advances in Clinical Cytology. 2nd ed. pp. 123–134. New York, Masson Publishing USA, 1984.

Baak, J.P.A.: Basic points in and practical aspects of application of diagnostic morphometry. Pathol. Res. Pract., *179*:193–199, 1984.

Baak, J.P.A.: The principles and advances of quantitative pathology. Anal. Quant. Cytol. Histol., *9*:89–95, 1987.

Baak, J.P.A., Blanco, A.A., Kurver, P.H.J., Langley, F.A., Boon, M.E., Lindeman, J., Overdiep, S.H., Niwuwlaat, A., and Brekelmans, E.: Quantitation of borderline and malignant ovarian tumours. Histopathology, *5*:353–360, 1981.

Baak, J.P.A., Kurver, P.H.J., Overdiep, S.H., Delemarre, F.J.M., Boon, M.E., Lindeman, J., and Diegenbach, P.C.: Quantitative microscopical, computer-aided diagnosis of endometrial hyperplasia or carcinoma in individual patients. Histopathology, *5*:689–695, 1981.

Baak, J.P.A., Noteboom, E., and Koevoets, J.J.M.: The influence of fixatives and other variations in tissue processing on nuclear morphometric features. Anal. Quant. Cytol. Histol., *11*:219–224, 1989.

Baak, J.P.A., and Oort, J.: Morphometry in Diagnostic Pathology. Berlin, Springer Verlag, 1983.

Baak, J.P.A., Wisse-Brekelmans, E.C.M., Uyterlinde, A.M., and Schipper, N.W.: Evaluation of the prognostic value of morphometric features and cellular DNA content in FIGO I ovarian cancer patients. Anal. Quant. Cytol. Histol., *9*:287–290, 1987.

Baak, J.P.A., Fox, H., Lanagley, F.A., and Buckley, C.H.: The prognostic value of morphometry in ovarian epithelial tumors of borderline malignancy. Int. J. Gynecol. Pathol., *4*:186–191, 1985.

Bacus, J.W.: An automated classification of the peripheral blood leukocytes by means of digital image processing. Ph.D. thesis. Chicago, University of Illinois, 1971.

Bacus, J.W., Belanger, M.C., Aggarwal, R.K., and Trobaugh, F.E.: Image processing for automated erythrocyte classification. J. Histochem. Cytochem., *24*:195–201, 1976.

Bacus, S.S., Bacus, J.W., Slamon, D.J., and Press, M.F.: HER-2/Neu oncogene expression and DNA ploidy analysis in breast cancer. Arch. Pathol. Lab. Med., *114*:164–169, 1990.

Bacus, S.S., Flowers, J.L., Press, M.F., Bacus, J.W., and McCarty, J.S., Jr.: The evaluation of estrogen receptor in primary breast carcinoma by computer assisted image analysis. Am. J. Clin. Pathol., *90*:233, 1988.

Bacus, S.S., Goldschmidt, R., Chin, D., Moran, G., Wienberg, D., and Bacus, J.W.: Biologic grading of breast cancer using antibodies to proliferating cells and other markers. Am. J. Pathol., *135*:783–792, 1989.

Bahr, G.F, Bartels, P.H., Bibbo, M., de Nicolas, M., and Wied, G.L.: Evaluation of the Papanicolaou stain for computer assisted cellular pattern recognition. Acta. Cytol., *17*:106–112, 1973.

Bahr, G.F., Taylor, J., Bartels, P.H., and Wied, G.L.: Distinguishing normal human blood lymphocytes from lymphocytes in dengue and typhoid fever. Virchows Arch. [Cell Pathol.,] *16*:205–210, 1974.

Bartels, P.H.: Numerical evaluation of cytologic data. A series of tutorial articles in vols. *1* through *5* of Anal. Quant. Cytol., 1979–1983.

Bartels, P.H., Bahr, G.F., Bellamy, T.C., Bibbo, M., Richards, D.L., and Wied, G.L.: A self-learning computer program for cell recognition. Acta. Cytol., *14*:486–494, 1970.

Bartels, P.H., and Bahr, G.F., Griep, J., Rappaport, H., and Wied, G.L.: Computer analysis of lymphocytes in transformation. A methodological study. Acta. Cytol., *13*:557–568, 1969.

Bartels, P.H., Bahr, G.F., Bibbo, M., and Wied, G.L.: Objective cell image analysis. J. Histochem. Cytochem., *20*:239–254, 1972.

Bartels, P.H., Bhattacharya, P.K., Bellamy, T.C., Bahr, G.F, Bibbo, M., and Wied, G.L.: Computer generated, synthetic cell images. Acta. Cytol., *18*:155–164, 1974.

Bartels, P.H., Bahr, G.F., and Wied, G.L.: Cell recognition from line scan transition probability profiles. Acta Cytol., *13*:210–217, 1969.

Bartels, P.H., Bibbo, M., Bahr, G.F., Taylor, J., and Wied, G.L.: Cervical cytology: Descriptive statistics for nuclei of normal and atypical cell types. Acta Cytol., *17*:449–453, 1973.

Bartels, P.H., Bibbo, M., Dytch, H.E., Pishotta, F.T., and Wied, G.L.: Marker features for malignancy in ectocervical cells —statistical evaluation. Cell Biophys., *5*:71–78, 1983.

Bartels, P.H., Bibbo, M., Taylor, J., and Wied, G.L.: Cell recognition from statistical dependence of gray values in digitized images. Acta Cytol., *18*:165–169, 1974.

Bartels, P.H., Graham, A., Kuhn, W., Paplanus, S., and Wied, G.L.: Knowledge engineering in quantitative histopathology. Appl. Optics, *26*:3330–3337, 1987.

Bartels, P.H., Graham, A., Paplanus, S., Dytch, H.E., and Wied, G.L.: Computer assessment of cells and tissues: Classification procedures and expert systems. Morphometry, stereology, and image analysis. *In* Mary, F.V., and Rigaut, F.P. (eds.): Cancer Cytology and Histopathology International Conference Proceedings. pp. 113–123. Villejuif, France, Elsevier, 1986.

Bartels, P.H., Koss, L., and Wied, G.L.: Automated cell diagnosis in clinical cytology. pp. 314–342. *In* Koss, L.G., and Coleman, D.V. (eds.): Advances in Clinical Cytology. London, Butterworths and Co., 1980.

Bartels, P.H., Kuhn, W.P., Saffer, J., Paplanus, S.H., and Graham, A.R.: Training and learning in an expert system for scene segmentation. IEEE Proceedings, EMBS-EMSA, pp. 1548–1550. Boston, November 1987.

Bartels, P.H., Layton, J.M., Jarkowski, T.L., Bellamy, J.C., Bahr, G.F., and Wied, G.L.: Cell recognition by multivariate gray value analysis in digitized images. Acta Cytol., *15*:284–288, 1971.

Bartels, P.H., Olson, G.B., Jeter, U.S., and Wied, G.L.: Evaluation of unsupervised learning algorithms in the computer analysis of lymphocytes. Acta Cytol. *18*:376–388, 1974.

Bartels, P.H., Oldon, G.B., Layton, J.M., Anderson, T.E., and Wied, G.: Computer discrimination of T and B lymphocytes. Acta Cytol., *19*:53–57, 1975.

Bartels, P.H., and Thompson, D.: Expert systems in histopathology. III. Representation of knowledge as "structured objects." Anal. Quant. Cytol. Histol., *11*:367–374, 1989.

Bartels, P.H., and Wied, G.L.: Computer analysis and biomedical interpretation of microscopic images: Current problems and future directions. Proc. IEEE, *65*:252–262, 1977.

Bartels, P.H., and Wied, G.L.: Automated image analysis in clinical pathology. Am. J. Clin. Pathol., *75*:489, 1981.

Bastos, A.L., Vigario, J.D., Moura Numes, J.F., Margus, D., Terrinha, A.M., and da Silva, J.A.F.: Inducible fluorescent reaction as an approach for cell identification. *In* Evans, D.M.D. (ed.): Cytology Automation. London, E.G.S. Livingstone, 1970.

Beer, A.: Bestimmung der Absorption des roten Lichtes in farbigen Fluessigkeiten. Ann. Phys., *86*:78, 1852.

Bhattacharya, P.K., Bartels, P.H., Bahr, G.F., and Wied, G.L.: A test statistic for detecting the presence of abnormal cells in a sample. Acta Cytol., *15*:533–544, 1971.

Bhattacharya, P.K., Bartels, P.H., Bibbo, M., Taylor, J., and Wied, G.L.: Estimation procedure for the cellular composition of cervical smears. Acta Cytol., *19*:366–373, 1975.

Bhattacharya, P.K., Bartels, P.H., Taylor, J., and Wied, G.L.: A decision procedure for automated cytology: Test statistic for detecting sample abnormality and inadequacy. Acta Cytol., *17*:538–548, 1973.

Bibbo, M., Bartels, P.H., Bahr, G.F., Taylor, J., Wied, G.L.: Computer recognition of cell nuclei from the uterine cervix. Acta Cytol., *17*:340–350, 1973.

Bibbo, M., Bartels, P.H., Chen, M., Harris, M.J., Truttmann, B.J., and Wied, G.L.: The numerical composition of cellular samples from the female reproductive tract. I. Carcinoma in situ. Acta Cytol., *19*:438–447, 1975.

Bibbo, M., Bartels, P.H., Chen, M., Harris, M.J., Truttmann, B.J., and Wied, G.L.: The numerical composition of cellular samples from the female reproductive tract. II. Cases with invasive squamous carcinoma of uterine cervix. Acta Cytol., *20*:239–242, 1976.

Bibbo, M., Bartels, P.H., Chen, M., Harris, M.J., Truttmann, B.J., and Wied, G.L.: The numerical composition of cell samples from the female reproductive tract. III. Cases with mild and moderate dysplasia of uterine cervix. Acta Cytol., *20*:565–572, 1976.

Bibbo, M., Bartels, P.H., Chen, M., Harris, M.J., Truttmann, B.J., and Wied, G.L.: The numerical composition of cellular samples from the female reproductive tract. IV. Carcinoma in situ cases exhibiting other than normal vaginal flora. Acta Cytol., *21*:705–709, 1977.

Bibbo, M., Bartels, P.H., Sychra, J.J., and Wied, G.L.: Chromatin appearance in intermediate cells from patients with uterine cancer. Acta Cytol., *25*:23–28, 1981.

Bibbo, M., Bartels, P.H., Dytch, H.E., Pishotta, F.T., and Wied, G.L.: High-resolution color video cytophotometry. Cell Biophys., *5*:61–70, 1983.

Bibbo, M., Bartels, P.H., Dytch, H.E., and Wied, G.L.: Computed cell image information. *In* Greenberg, S.D. (ed.): Survey and Synthesis of Pathology Research. pp. 62–100. Basel, Karger, 1984.

Bibbo, M., Bartels, P.H., Dytch, H.E., and Wied, G.L.: Ploidy measurements by high-resolution cytometry. Anal. Quant. Cytol. Histol., *7*:81–88, 1985.

Bibbo, M., Bartels, P.H., Dytch, H.E., and Wied, G.L.: Ploidy patterns in cervical dysplasia. Anal. Quant. Cytol. Histol., *7*:213–217, 1985.

Bibbo, M. Bartels, P.H., Galera-Davidson, H., Dytch, H.E., and

Wied, G.L.: Markers for malignancy in the nuclear texture of histologically normal tissue from patients with thyroid tumors. Anal. Quant. Cytol. Histol., 8:168–176, 1986.

Bibbo, M., Dytch, H.E., Puls, J.H., Bartels, P.H., and Wied, G.L.: Clinical applications for an inexpensive microcomputer-based DNA-cytometry system. Acta Cytol., 30:372–378, 1986.

Bibbo, M., Dytch, H.E., Alenghat, E., Bartels, P.H., and Wied, G.L.: DNA ploidy profiles as prognostic indicators in CIN lesions. Am. J. Clin. Pathol., 92:261–265, 1989.

Bibbo, M., Galera-Davidson, H., Dytch, H.E., Gonzalez de Chaves, J., Lopez-Garrido, J., Bartels, P.H., and Wied, G.L.: Karyometry and histometry of renal-cell carcinoma. Anal. Quant. Cytol. Histol., 9:182–187, 1987.

Bibbo, M., Galera-Davidson, H., Dytch, H.E., Lerma-Puertas, E., Bartels, P.H., and Wied, G.L.: Quantitative contextual karyometry in prostate carcinoma. *In* Karr, J.P., Coffey, D.S., Gardner, W., Jr. (eds.): Prognostic Cytometry and Cytopathology of Prostate Cancer. pp. 200–217. New York, Elsevier, 1989.

Bibbo, M., Bartels, P.H., Salguero, M., Dytch, H.E., Lerma-Puertas, E., and Galera-Davidson, H.: Karyometric marker features in fine needle aspirates of microinvasive follicular carcinoma of the thyroid. Anal. Quant. Cytol. Histol., 12:42–47, 1990.

Bibbo, M., Kim, D.H., Galera-Davidson, H., di-Loreto, C., and Dytch, H.E.: Architectural, morphometric and photometric features and their relationship to the main subjective diagnostic clues in the grading of prostatic cancer. Anal. Quant. Cytol. Histol., 12:85–90, 1990.

Bibbo, M., Michelassi, F., Bartels, P.H., Dytch, H., Bania, C., Lerma, E., and Montag, A.G.: Karyometric marker features in normal-appearing glands adjacent to human colonic adenocarcinoma. Cancer Res., 50:147–151, 1990.

Bibbo, M., Montag, A.G., Lerma-Puertas, E., Dytch, H.E., Leelakusolvong, S., and Bartels, P.H.: Karyometric marker features in tissue adjacent to invasive cervical carcinomas. Anal. Quant. Cytol. Histol., 11:281–285, 1989.

Boddington, M.M.: Scanning area required for screening cervical smears. *In* Evans, D.M.D. (ed.): Cytology Automation. London, E.G.S. Livingstone, 1970.

Bohm, N., and Sandritter, W.: DNA in human tumors: A cytophotometric study. *In* Current Topics in Pathology. vol. 6. pp. 152–219. New York, Springer-Verlag, 1975.

Boon, M.E., Juetting, U., Rodenacker, K., Gais, P., and Kok, L.P.: Differences in chromatin pattern of benign cells in smears with condylomatous CIN I and III. *In* Proceedings, Fifth International Conference on Automation of Diagnostic Cytology and Histology, p. 23, Brussels, Belgium, 1986.

Boon, M.E., Trott, P.A., Kaam, H.V., Kurver, P.H.J., and Baak, J.P.A.: Computation of preoperative diagnosis probability for follicular adenoma and carcinoma of the thyroid on aspiration smears. Anal. Quant. Cytol. Histol., 4:1–5, 1982.

Boveri, T.H.: Zur Frage der Entstehung Maligner Tumoren. Jena, Germany, Fischer, 1914.

Brandao, H.J.S.: DNA content in epithelial cells of dysplasia of the uterine cervix. Acta Cytol., 13:232–237, 1969.

Brugal, G., and Adelh, D.: SAMBA 200: An industrial prototype for high resolution analysis of colored cell images. International Conference on High Resolution Cell Image Analysis, pp. 24–26, Los Angeles, 1982.

Buchanan, B.G., and Shortliffe, E.H.: Rule-Based Expert Systems. Reading, Massachusetts, Addison-Wesley, 1984.

Bunsen, R.W., and Roscoe, H.E.: Photochemische Untersuchungen. Poggendorfs Ann., 117:529, 1862.

Bur, M., Bibbo, M., Dytch, H.E., Holt., J.A., Greene, G.L., Lorincz, M., Wied, G.L., and Press, M.: Computerized image analysis of estrogen receptor quantitation in FNA of breast cancer: A preliminary report. Lab. Invest., 56:9A, 1987.

Burger, G.: Combination of coherent optical and high resolution absorption analysis. *In*: Goerttler, K., and Herman, Ch.J. (eds.): Technologies for Automation in Cervical Cancer Screening. pp. 126–131. Heidelberg, German Cancer Center Publication, 1976.

Burger, G., Juetting, U., and Rodenacker, K.: Changes in benign cell populations in cases of cervical cancer and its precursors. Anal. Quant. Cytol., 3:261–271, 1981.

Cance, W.G., Brennan, M.F., Dudas, M.E., Huang, C.M., and Cordon-Cardo, C.: Altered expression of the retinoblastoma gene product in human sarcomas. N. Engl. J. Med., 323:1457–1462, 1990.

Caspersson, T.: Ueber den chemischen Aufban der Strukturen des Zellkernes. Scand. Arch. Phys. [Suppl.], 8:73, 1936.

Caspersson, T.: Cell Growth and Function. New York, Norton, 1950.

Caspersson, T., and Lomakka, G.M.: Scanning microscopy techniques for high resolution quantitative cytochemistry. Ann. N.Y. Acad. Sci., 97:449–463, 1962.

Caspersson, T., and Santesson, L.: Studies on protein metabolism in the cells of epithelial tumors. Acta Radiol. [Suppl.], 46:1–105, 1942.

Cassidy, M., Yee, C., and Costa, J.: Automated analysis of antigen-stimulated lymphocytes. J. Histochem. Cytochem., 24:373–377, 1976.

Castleman, K.R., Melnyk, J., Frieden, H.L., Persinger, G.W., and Wall, R.J.: Computer assisted karyotyping. J. Reprod. Med., 17:53–58, 1976.

Chacho, M.S., Eppich, E., Wersto, R., and Koss, L. G.: Influence of human papillomavirus on DNA ploidy determination in genital condylomas. Cancer, 65:2291–2294, 1990.

Clark, G.M., Dressler, L.G., and Owends, M.A.: Predictions of relapse or survival in patients with node-negative breast cancer by flow cytometry. N. Engl. J. Med., 320:627–633, 1989.

Cohen, P.S., Seeger, R.C., Triche, T.J., and Israel, M.A.: Detection of N-myc gene expression in neuroblastoma tumors by in situ hybridization. Am. J. Pathol., 131:391–397, 1988.

Collan, Y., Torkkeli, T., Kosma, V.M., Pesonen, E., Kosunen, O., Jantunen, E., Mariuzzi, G.M., Montironi, R., Marinelli, F., and Collina, G.: Sampling in diagnostic morphometry. Pathol. Res. Pract., 182:401–406, 1987.

Colley, M., Kommoss, F., Bibbo, M., Dytch, H.E., Holt, J. Wied, G.L., and Franklin, W.A.: Estrogen and progesterone receptors and KI-67 growth fraction in breast carcinoma: Quantitation of hormone receptors by image analysis and comparison with cytosolic methods. Lab. Invest., 60:19A, 1989.

Colley, M., Kommoss, F., Bibbo., M., Dytch, H.E., Franklin, W.A., Holt, J., and Wied, G.L.: Assessment of hormone receptors in breast carcinoma by immunocytochemistry and image analysis: II. Estrogen receptors. Anal. Quant. Cytol. Histol., 11:307–314, 1989.

Cornelisse, C.J., and Ploem, J.S.: A new type of two-color fluorescence staining for cytology specimens. J. Histochem. Cytochem., 24:72–81, 1976.

Cornelisse, C.J. and Van Driel-Kulker, A.M.: DNA image cytometry on machine-selected breast cancer cells and a comparison between flow cytometry and scanning cytophotometry. Cytometry, 6:471–477, 1985.

Czerniak, B., Herz, F., and Koss, L.G.: DNA distribution patterns in early gastric carcinomas. A Feulgen cytometric study of gastric brush smears. Cancer, *59*:113–117, 1987.

Czerniak, B., Herz, F., Wersto, R.P., Alster, P., Puszkin, E., Schwarz, E., and Koss, L. G.: Quantitation of oncogene products by computer-assisted image analysis and flow cytometry. J. Histochem. Cytochem., *38*:463–466, 1990.

Czerniak, B., Deitch, D., Simmons, H., Etkind, P., Herz, F., and Koss, L.G.Ha-*ras* gene codon 12 mutation and DNA ploidy in urinary bladder carcinoma. Br. J. Cancer, *62*:762–763, 1990.

Detweiler, R., Zahnizer, D.J., Garcia, G.L., and Hutchinson, M.L.: Contextual analysis complements single cell analysis in the diagnosis of breast cancer in fine needle aspirates. Anal. Quant. Cytol. Histol., *10*:10–15, 1988.

Doria, M.I., Dytch, H.E., Puls, J.H., Franklin, W.A., Bibbo, M., and Wied, G.L.: Computer analysis of cell proliferation rates in sections stained with the monoclonal antibody Ki-67. Lab. Invest., *56*:90, 1987.

Dytch, H.E., Bartels, P.H., Bibbo, M., Pishotta, F.T., and Wied, G.L.: Computer graphics in cytodiagnosis. Anal. Quant. Cytol., *4*:263–268, 1982.

Dytch, H.E., Bartels, P.H., Bibbo, M., Pishotta, F.T., and Wied, G.L.: The rejection of noncellular artifacts in Papanicolaou-stained slide specimens by an automated high-resolution system: Identification of important cytometric features. Anal. Quant. Cytol., *5*:241–250, 1983.

Dytch, H.E., Bibbo, M., Puls, J.H., Bartels, P.H., and Wied, G.L.: Software design for an inexpensive, practical, microcomputer-based DNA cytometry system. Anal. Quant. Cytol. Histol., *8*:8–18, 1986.

Dytch, H.E., Bibbo, M., Bartels, P.H., Puls, J.H., and Wied, G.L.: An interactive microcomputer-based system for the quantitative analysis of stratified tissue sections. Anal. Quant. Cytol. Histol., *9*:69–78, 1987.

Dytch, H.E., Bibbo, M., Puls, J.H., and Wied, G.L.: A PC-based system for the objective analysis of histologic specimens through quantitative contextual karyometry. App. Optics, *26*:3270–3279, 1987.

Dytch, H.E., Wied, G.L., and Bibbo, M.: Artificial neural nets as tools for expert systems in objective histopathology. Proceedings of the IEEE Engineering in Medicine and Biology Society 10th International Conference, 1375CH2566-8/88/0000-1375, 1988.

Dytch, H.E., and Wied, G.L.: Integrating expert systems and neural nets (Abstract). Anal. Quant. Cytol. Histol., *12*:190, 1990.

Dytch, H.E., and Wied, G.L.: Contextual histometry (Abstract). Anal. Quant. Cytol. Histol., *12*:190, 1990.

Dytch, H.E., and Wied, G.L.: Neurocomputing: Artificial neural nets as AI tools for quantiative pathology. *In* Baak, J.P.A. (ed.): Expert Systems in Cytopathology. pp. 485–502. New York, Springer Verlag, 1990.

Dytch, H.E., and Wied, G.L.: Artificial neural networks and their use in quantitative pathology. Anal. Quant. Cytol. Histol., *12*:379–393, 1990.

Emson, H.E., and Kirk, H.: Value of deoxyribonucleic acid (DNA) in evolution of carcinomas of the human breast. Cancer, *20*:1248–1252, 1967.

Fallenious, A.G., Auer, G.U., and Carstensen, J.M.: Prognostic significance of DNA measurements in 409 consecutive breast cancer patients. Cancer, *62*:331–341, 1988.

Fallenius, A.G., Franzén, S.A., and Auer, G.U. Predictive value of nuclear DNA content in breast cancer in relation to clinical and morphologic factors. Cancer, *62*:521–530, 1988.

Fleming, M.G., Wied, G.L., and Dytch, H.E.: Nuclear image analysis of dysplastic nevi. Anal. Quant. Cytol. Histol., *12*:191, 1990.

Fleming, M.G., Wied, G.L., and Dytch, H.E.: Image analysis cytometry of dysplastic nevi. J. Invest. Dermatol., *95*:287–291, 1990.

Forsyth, R.: Expert Systems. London, Chapman and Hall, 1984.

Franklin, W.A., Bibbo, M., Doria, M.I., Dytch, H.E., Toth, J., DeSombre, E., and Wied, G.L.: Quantitation of estrogen receptor and Ki-67 in breast carcinoma by the microTICAS image analysis system. Anal. Quant. Cytol. Histol., *9*:279–286, 1987.

Fu, Y.S., and Hall, T.L.: DNA ploidy measurements in tissue sections. Anal. Quant. Cytol., *7*:90–95, 1985.

Fu, Y.S., Reagan, J.W., and Richart, R.M.: Definition of precursors. Gynecol. Oncol., *12*:s220–s231, 1981.

Fu, Y.S., Reagan, J.W., Richart, R.M., and Townsend, D.E.: Nuclear DNA and histologic studies of genital lesions in diethylstilbestrol-exposed progeny. I. Intraepithelial squamous abnormalities. Am. J. Clin. Pathol., *72*:503–514, 1979.

Fu, Y.S., Hall, T.L., Berek, J.S., Hacker, N.F., and Reagan, J.W.: Prognostic significance of DNA ploidy and morphometric analyses of adenocarcinoma of the uterine cervix. Anal. Quant. Cytol. Histol., *9*:16–24, 1987.

Fukushima, K., Miyake, S., and Takayuki, I.: Neocognitron: A neural network model for a mechanism of visual pattern recognition. IEEE Transactions on Systems, Man, and Cybernetics, SMC-13:826–834, 1983.

Galera-Davidson, H., Bartels, P.H., Fernandez-Rodriguez, A., Dytch, H.E., Lerma-Puertas, E., and Bibbo, M.: Karyometric marker features in fine needle aspirates of invasive follicular carcinoma of the thyroid. Anal. Quant. Cytol. Histol., *12*:35–41, 1990.

Garcia, G.L., Kuklinski, W.S., Zahniser, D.J., Oud, P.S., Vooys, P.G., and Brenner, J.F.: Evaluation of contextual analysis for computer classification of cervical smears. Cytometry, *8*:210–216, 1987.

Garcia, A.M.: The one-wavelength, two area method in ultraviolet cytophotometry. Acta Cytol, *17*:224–232, 1973.

Gill, J.E., and Jotz, M.M.: Deoxyribonucleic acid cytochemistry for automated cytology. J. Histochem. Cytochem., *22*:470–477, 1974.

Graham, I., and Jones, P.L.: Expert Systems: Knowledge, Uncertainty and Decision. London, Chapman and Hall, 1988.

Gray, J.W.: Cell cycle analysis from computer synthesis of deoxyribonucleic acid histograms. J. Histochem. Cytochem., *22*:642–650, 1974.

Grossberg, S.: The Adaptive Brain, I-II. New York, Elsevier/North-Holland, 1987.

Gustavson, B., and Enerback, L.: Cytofluorometric quantitation of 5-hydroxytryptamine and heparin in individual mast cell granules. J. Histochem. Cytochem., *26*:47–54, 1978.

Hall, T.L., Castleman, K.R., and Rosenthal, D.L.: Canonical analysis of cells in normal and abnormal cervical smears. Anal. Quant. Cytol. Histol., *10*:161–165, 1988.

Hanselaar, A.G.J.M., Vooijs, G.P., Oud, P.S., Pahlplatz, M.M.M., and Beck, J.L.: DNA ploidy patterns in cervical intraepithelial neoplasia grade III, with and without synchronous invasive squamous cell carcinoma: Measurements in nuclei isolated from paraffin-embedded tissue. Cancer, *62*:2537–2545, 1988.

Helin, H.J., Helle, M.J., Helin, M.L., and Isola, J.J.: Immunocytochemical detection of estrogen and progesterone receptors in 124 human breast cancers. Am. J. Clin. Pathol., *89*:137–142, 1988.

Hrushovetz, S.B., and Lauchlan, S.C.: Comparative DNA content of cells in the intermediate and parabasal layers of cervical intraepithelial neoplasia studied by two-wavelength Feulgen cytophotometry. Acta Cytol., *14*: 68–77, 1970.

Hutchinson, M.L., Schultz, D.S., Stephenson, R.A., Wong, K.L., Harry, T., and Zahnizer, D.J.: Computerized microscopic analysis of prostate fine needle aspirates: Comparison with breast aspirates. Anal. Quant. Cytol. Histol., *11*:105–110, 1989.

Ingram, M., and Preston, K., Jr.: Automatic analysis of blood cells. Sci. Am., *223*:72, 1970.

Jackson, P.: Introduction to Expert Systems. Wokingham, United Kingdom, Addison-Wesley, 1986.

Jahoda, E., Bartels, P.H., Bibbo, M., Bahr, G.F., Holzner, J.H., and Wied, G.L.: Computer discrimination of cells in serous effusions. I. Pleural fluids. Acta Cytol., *17*:94–105, 1973.

Jahoda, E., Bartels, P.H., Bibbo, M., Bahr, G.F., and Holzner, J.H.: Computer discriminations of cells in serous effusions. II. Peritoneal fluid. Acta Cytol., *17*:533–537, 1973.

Jarkowski, T.L., Layton, J.M., Bahr, G.F., Wied, G.L., Bellamy, J.C., and Bartels, P.H.: Computer recognition of cells from asymptomatic lymphocytic leukemia. I. Methodological study. Acta Cytol., *14*:147–153, 1971.

Kallioniemi, O.P., Blanco, G., and Alavaikko, M.: Improving the prognostic value of DNA cytometry in breast cancer by combining DNA index and S-phase fraction. Cancer, *62*:183–190, 1988.

Kamentsky, L.A., Melamed, M.R., and Derman, H.: Spectrophotometer: New instrument for ultrarapid cell analysis. Science, *150*:630–631, 1965.

Kasten, F.H.: Cytochemical studies with acridine orange and the influence of dye contaminants in the staining of nucleic acids. Intern. Rev. Cytol., *21*:141–202, 1967.

Katzko, M.W., Pahplatz, M.M., Oud, P.S., and Vooijs, P.G.: Carcinoma in situ specimen classification based on intermediate cell measurements. Cytometry, *8*:9–13, 1987.

Kiefer, R., Kiefer, G., Salm, R., Rossner, R., and Sandritter, W.: A method for the quantitative evaluation of eu- and heterochromatin in interphase nuclei using cytophotometry and pattern analysis. Br. J. Pathol., *150*:163–173, 1973.

Kiehn, T.E.: Computer analysis of transforming lymphocytes. Ph.D. dissertation. Department of Microbiology, University of Arizona, 1972.

King E. B., Chu, K.L., Mayall, B., and Petrakis, N.: Foam cell measurements may be useful in diagnosis of breast cancer. Sixth International Symposium on Flow Cytometry. Schloss Elmau, Bavaria, October 1982.

Kirsch, R.A.: Computer determination of the constituent structure of biological images. Comput. Biomed. Res., *4*:315–328, 1971.

Klintenberg, C., Stal, O., Nordenskjold, B., Wallgren, A., Arvidsson, S., and Skoog, L.: Proliferative index, cytosol estrogen receptor and axillary node status as prognostic predictors in human mammary carcinoma. Breast Cancer Res. Treat., *7*:S99–S106, 1986.

Kohen, E., Thorell, B., Kohen, C., and Michaelis, M.: Rapid microfluorometry for biochemistry of the living cell in correlation with cytomorphology and transport phenomena. *In* Thaer, A.A., and Sernetz, M. (eds.): Fluorescence Techniques in Cell Biology. pp. 219–234. New York, Springer-Verlag, 1972.

Kohen, E., Kohen, C., Thorell, B., and Wagener, G.: Quantitative aspects of rapid microfluorometry for the study of enzyme reactions and transport mechanisms in single living cells. *In* Thaer, A.A., and Sernetz, M. (eds.): Fluorescence Techniques in Cell Biology. pp. 207–218. New York, Springer-Verlag, 1972.

Kommoss, F, Bibbo, M., Colley, M., Dytch, H.E., Franklin, W.A., Holt, J., and Wied, G.L.: Assessment of hormone receptors in breast carcinoma by immunocytochemistry and image analysis. I. Progesterone receptors. Anal. Quant. Cytol. Histol., *11*:298–306, 1989.

Koss, L.G.: Analytical and quantitative cytology. A historical perspective. Anal. Quant. Cytol., *4*:251–256, 1982.

Koss, L.G.: High resolution automated microscopy. Anal. Quant. Cytol., *7*:2–3, 1985.

Koss, L.G.: Automated cytology and histology: A historical perspective. Anal. Quant. Cytol. Histol., *9*:369–374, 1987.

Koss, L.G.: The future of cytology. The Wachtel lecture for 1988. Acta Cytol., *34*:1–9, 1990.

Koss, L.G., Bartels, P.H., Bibbo, M., Freed, S.Z., Sychra, J.J., Taylor, J., and Wied, G.L.: Computer analysis of atypical urothelial cells. I. Classification by supervised learning algorithms. Acta Cytol., *21*:247–260, 1977.

Koss, L.G., Bartels, P.H., Bibbo, M., Freed, S.Z., Taylor, J., and Wied, G.L.: Computer discrimination between benign and malignant urothelial cells. Acta Cytol., *19*:378–391, 1975.

Koss, L.G., Bartels, P.H., Sherman, A., Sychra, J.J., Schreiber, K., Moussouris, H., and Wied, G.L.: Computer identification of degenerated urothelial cells. Anal. Quant. Cytol., *2*:107–111, 1980.

Koss, L.G., Bartels, P.H., Sherman, A., Sychra, J.J., Schreiber, K., Moussouris, H., and Wied, G.L.: Computer identification of multinucleated urothelial cells. Anal. Quant. Cytol., *2*:112–116, 1980.

Koss, L.G., Bartels, P.H., Sychra, J.J., and Wied, G.L.: Computer analysis of atypical urothelial cells. II. Classification by unsupervised learning algorithms. Acta Cytol., *21*:261–265, 1977.

Koss, L.G., Bartels, P.H., Sychra, J.J., and Wied, G.L.; Computer discriminant analysis of atypical urothelial cells. Acta Cytol., *22*:382–386, 1978.

Koss, L.G., Bartels, P.H., Sychra, J.J., and Wied, G.L.: Diagnostic cytologic sample profiles in patients with bladder cancer using TICAS system. Acta Cytol., *22*:392–397, 1978.

Koss, L.G., Bartels, P.H., and Wied, G.L.: Computer-based diagnostic analysis cells in the urinary sediment. J. Urol., *123*:846–849, 1980.

Koss, L.G., Dembitzer, H.M., Herz, F., Herzig, N., Schreiber, K., and Wolley, R.C.: The monodisperse cell sample: Problems and possible solutions. *In* Wied, G.L., Bahr, G.F., and Bartels, P.H. (eds.): The Automation of Uterine Cancer Cytology. pp. 54–60. Chicago, Tutorials of Cytology, 1976.

Koss, L.G., Eppich, E.M., Melder, K.H., and Wersto, R.: DNA cytophotometry of voided urine sediment. Comparison with results of cytologic diagnosis and image analysis. Anal. Quant. Cytol. Histol., *9*:398–404, 1987.

Koss, L.G., Sherman, A., Bartels, P.H., Sychra, J.J., and Wied, G.L.: Hierarchical analysis of multiple types of urothelial cells by computer. Anal. Quant. Cytol., *2*:166–174, 1980.

Koss, L.G., Sherman, A.B., and Adams, S.E.: The use of hierarchic classification in the image analysis of a complex cell population. Experience with the sediment of voided urine. Anal. Quant. Cytol., *5*:159–166, 1983.

Koss, L.G., Sherman, A.B., and Eppich, E.: Image analysis and DNA content of urothelial cells infected with human polyomavirus. Anal. Quant. Cytol., *6*:89–95, 1984.

Koss, L.G., Wersto, R.P., Simmons, D.A., Deitch, D., Herz, F., and Freed, S.Z.: Predicative value of DNA measurements in bladder washings. Comparison of flow cytometry, image cytophotometry, and cytology in patients with a past history of urothelial tumors. Cancer, *64*:916–924, 1989.

Koss, L.G., Wolley, R.C., Schreiber, K., and Mendecki, J.: Flow-microfluorometric analysis of nuclei isolated from various normal and malignant human epithelial tissues. J. Histochem. Cytochem., *25*:565–572, 1977.

Kraayenhof, R.: Atebrin and related fluorochromes as quantitative probes of membrane energization. *In* Thaer, A.A., and Sernetz, M. (eds.): Fluorescence Techniques in Cell Biology. pp. 381–394. New York, Springer-Verlag, 1972.

Kramer, P.M., Deaven, L.L., Crissman, H.A., Steinkamp, H.A., and Pedersen, D.F.: On the nature of heteroploidy. Cold Spring Harbor Symposia on Quantitative Biology, *38*:133–144, 1974.

Ladinsky, J.L., Sarto, G.E., and Peckham, B.M.: Cell size distribution patterns as a means of uterine cancer detection. J. Lab. Clin. Med., *64*:970–976, 1964.

Liedtke, C.E., Gahm, T., Kappei, F., and Aeikens, B.: Segmentation of microscopic cell scenes. Anal. Quant. Cytol., *9*:197–211, 1987.

Lief, R.C., Clay, S.P., Gratzner, H.G., Haines, H.G., and Vallarino, L.M.: Markers for instrumental evaluation of cells of the female reproductive tract: Existing and new markers. *In* Wied, G.L., Bahr, G.F., and Bartels, P.H. (eds.): The Automation of Uterine Cancer Cytology. pp. 313–344. Chicago, Tutorials of Cytology, 1976.

Lipkin, L.E., Watt, W.C., and Kirsch, R.A.: The analysis, synthesis and description of biological images. Ann. N.Y. Acad. Sci., *128*:984–1012, 1966.

Mansi, J.L., Mesker, W.E., McDonnell, T., Van Driel-Kulker, A.M.J., Ploem, J.S., and Coombes, R.C.: Automated screening for micrometastases in bone marrow smears. J. Immunol. Methods, *112*:105–111, 1988.

Marr, D: Vision. San Francisco, W.H. Freeman, 1982.

Mayall, B.H.: Monodisperse cell samples: The problem and possible solutions. *In* Wied, G.L., Bahr, G.F., and Bartels, P.H. (eds): The Automation of Uterine Cancer Cytology. pp. 61–68. Chicago, Tutorials of Cytology, 1976.

Mayall, B.H., and Mendelsohn, M.L.: Deoxyribonucleic acid cytophotometry of stained human leukocytes. The mechanical scanner of CYDAC, the theory of scanning photometry and the magnitude of residual errors. J. Histochem. Cytochem., *18*:383–407, 1970.

Mayer, J.S., and Coplin, M.D.: Thymidine labelling index, flow cytometric S-phase measurements, and DNA index in human tumors. Am. J. Clin. Pathol., *89*:586–599, 1988.

Melamed, M.R.: State-of-the-art workshop on automated Papanicolaou smear analysis. *In* Ramsey-Klee, (ed.): Washington, D.C.: United States Government Printing Office, United States Public Health Service, 1969.

Melamed, M.R.: The automation of uterine cancer cytology. *In* Wied, G.L., Bahr, G.F., and Bartels, P.H. (eds.): The Automation of Uterine Cancer Cytology. pp. 399–401. Chicago, Tutorials of Cytology, 1976.

Melamed, M.R., and Kamentsky, L.A.: Automated cytology. Int. Rev. Exp. Pathol., *14*:205–295, 1975.

Melnyk, J., Persinger, G.W., Mount, B., and Castleman, K.R.: A semiautomated specimen preparation system for cytogenetics. J. Reprod. Med., *17*:59–68, 1976.

Mendelsohn, M. L.: The two-wavelength method of microspectrophotometry. I. A microspectro-photometer and tests on model systems. J. Biophys. Biochem. Cytol., *4*:407–414, 1958.

Mendelsohn, M.L.: The two-wavelength method of microspectrophotometry. II. A set of tables to facilitate the calculations. J. Biophys. Biochem. Cytol., *4*:415–424, 1958.

Mendelsohn, M.L.: The two-wavelength method of microspectrophotometry. III. An extension based on photographic color transparencies. J. Biophys. Biochem. Cytol., *4*:407–414, 1958.

Mendelsohn, M.L., Mayall, B.H., Prewitt, J.M.S., Bostrom, R.S., and Holcomb, W.G.: Digital transformation and computer analysis of microscopic images. *In* Barer, R., and Cosslett, V.E. (eds.): Advances in Optical and Electron Microscopy. New York, Academic Press, 1968.

Meyer, J.S., Friedman, E., McCrate, M.M., and Bauer, W.C.: Prediction of early course of breast carcinoma by thymidine labeling. Cancer, *51*:1879–1886, 1983.

Miescher, F.: Die Histochemischen und Physiologischen Arbeiten. Leipzig, Vogl., 1897.

Mikel, U.V., Fishbein, W.N., and Bahr, G.F.: Some practical considerations in quantitative absorbance microspectrophotometry: Preparation techniques in DNA cytophotometry. Anal. Quant. Cytol. Histol., 7:107–118, 1985.

Minsky, M., and Papert, S.: Perceptrons. Cambridge, Mass., MIT Press, 1969.

Montag, A.G., Bartels, P.H., Lerma-Puertas, E., Dytch, H.E., Leelakusolvong, S., and Bibbo, M.: Karyometric marker features in tissue adjacent to in situ cervical carcinomas. Anal. Quant. Cytol. Histol., *11*:275–280, 1989.

O'Brien, R., Pino, I., Sambuccetti, L., and Weeramantry, A.: Spectral characteristics of human leukocytes and their relevance to automated cell identification. II. Monocytes. Acta Cytol. *20*:557–564, 1976.

Olson, G.B., Anderson, R.E., and Bartels, P.H.: Differentiation of murine thoracic duct lymphocytes into T and B subpopulations by computer cell-scanning techniques. Cell. Immunol., *13*:347–355, 1974.

Olson, G.B., Wied, G.L., and Bartels, P.H.: Differentiation of chicken thymic and bursal lymphocytes by cell image analysis. Acta Cytol., *17*:454–461, 1973.

Olson, G.B., Wied, G.L., and Bartels, P.H.: Differentiation of lymphoid tissue by analysis of digitized images. Acta Cytol., *17*:89–93, 1973.

Ornstein, L.: The distributional error in microspectrophotometry. Lab. Invest., *1*:250–265, 1952.

Ornstein, L., and Ansley, H.R.: Spectral matching of classical cytochemistry to automated cytology. J. Histochem. Cytochem., *22*:453–469, 1974.

Papadimitriou, J.M., Van Duijn, P., Brederoo, P., and Streefkerk, J.G.: A new method for the cytochemical demonstration of peroxidase for light, fluorescence and electron microscopy. J. Histochem. Cytochem., *22*:452–469, 1974.

Parry, J.S., Cleary, B.K., Williams, A.R., and Evans, D.M.: Ultrasonic dispersal of cervical cell aggregates. Acta Cytol., *15*:163–166, 1971.

Parsaye, K., and Chagnell, M.: Expert Systems for Experts. New York, John Wiley & Sons, 1988.

Patau, K.: Absorption microphotometry of irregular shaped objects. Chromosoma, *5*:341–362, 1952.

Patten, S.F.: Sensitivity and specificity of routine diagnostic cytology. *In* Wied, G.L., Bahr, G.F., and Bartels, P.H. (eds.): The Automation of Uterine Cancer Cytology. pp. 406–419. Chicago, Tutorials of Cytology, 1976.

Peckham, B., and Ladinsky, J.: Cellular metabolic activity—a new basis for screening of vaginal cytology? Am. J. Obstet. Gynecol., *87*:418–424, 1964.

Perrot-Applanant, M.G.T., Lorenze, F., Jolivet, A., Hai, V., Pallud, C., Spyratos, F., and Milgrom, F.: Immunocytochemical study with monoclonal antibodies to progesterone receptor in human breast tumors. Cancer Res., *47*:2652–2661, 1987.

Ploem, J.S., van Driel-Kulker, A.M.J., and Verwoerd, N.P.: LEYTAS: A cytology screening system using the new modular image analysis computer (MIAC) from Leitz. *In* Burger, G., et al. (eds.): Clinical Cytometry and Histometry. pp. 24–35. London, United Kingdom, Academic Press, 1987.

Pollister, A.W., and Ornstein, L.: The photometric chemical

analysis of cells. *In* Mellors, R.C. (ed.): Analytical Cytology. pp. 431–518. New York, McGraw-Hill, 1959.

Pratt, W.K.: Digital Image Processing. New York, John Wiley & Sons, 1981.

Pressman, N.K.: Markovian analysis of cervical cell images. J. Histochem. Cytochem., 24:138–144, 1976.

Preston, K.: Machine techniques for automatic leukocyte pattern analysis. Ann. N.Y. Acad. Sci., 97:482–490, 1962.

Preston, K.: Digital image analysis in cytology. *In* Rosenfeld, A.(ed.): Digital Image Analysis. New York, Springer-Verlag, 1977.

Preston, K.: Tissue section analysis: Feature selection and image processing. Pattern Recog., 13:17–36, 1980.

Prewitt, J.M.S.: Parametric and non-parametric recognition by computers: An application to leukocyte image processing. Adv. Computers, 12:285–414, 1972.

Prewitt, J.M.S., and Mendelsohn, M.L.: The analysis of cell images. Ann. N.Y. Acad. Sci., 128:1035–1043, 1966.

Prewitt, J.M.S., and Wu, S.C.: An application of pattern recognition to epithelial tissues. pp. 15–25. Proceedings of the 2nd Annual Symposium on Computer Applications in Medical Care, IEEE Computer Society, 1978.

Puls, J.H., Bibbo, M., Dytch, H.E., Bartels, P.H., and Wied, G. L.: MicroTICAS: The design of an inexpensive video-microphotometer computer system for DNA ploidy studies. Anal. Quant. Cytol. Histol., 8:1–7, 1986.

Read, J.S., Boravec, R.T., Bartels, P.H., Bibbo, M., Puls, J.H., Reale, F.R., Taylor, J., and Wied, G.L.: A fast image processor for locating cell nuclei in uterine specimens. *In* Pressman, N.J., and Wied, G.L. (eds.): The Automation of Cancer Cytology and Cell Image Analysis. pp. 143–156. Proceedings of the 2nd International Conference on the Automation of Cancer Cytology. Tokyo, International Academy of Cytology, 1979.

Reinhardt, E.R., Blanz, W.E., Erhardt, R., Greiner, W., Hornstein, B., Kringler, W., Lenz, R., Schmipf, I., Schipf, W., Schwarzmann, P., Stressl, G., and Bloss, W.H.: Automated classification of cytologic specimens based on multistage pattern recognition. Proceedings of the 6th International Conference on Pattern Recognition, Munchen, FRG:153–159, 1982.

Reuter, B., Hutzler, P., and Kinder, J.: Real time optical processing and a microscope. *In* Goerttler, K., and Herman, Ch.J. (eds.): Technologies for Automation in Cervical Cancer Screening. pp. 94–97. Heidelberg, German Cancer Research Center, 1976.

Rosenblatt, F.: The Perceptron: A probablistic model for information storage and organization in the brain. Psychol. Rev., 65:386–408, 1958.

Rosenblatt, F.: Principles of Neurodynamics. Washington, D.C., Spartan, 1962.

Rosenthal, D.L., Leibel, J., Meyer, D.J., Woods, S.D., McLatchie, C., Suffin, S.C., and Castleman, K.R.: The effect of filtration on the loss of abnormal cervical cells in specimen preparation for automated cytology. Anal. Quant. Cytol., 5:236–240, 1983.

Rosenthal, D.L., and Suffin, S.C.: Predictive value of digitized cell images for the prognosis of cervical neoplasia. Monogr. Clin. Cytol., 9:163–180, 1984.

Rosenthal, D.L. Suffin, S.C., Missirlian, N., McLatchie, C., and Castleman, K.R.: Cytomorphometric differences among individual "moderate dysplasia" cells derived from cervical intraepithelial neoplasia. Anal. Quant. Cytol., 6:189–195, 1984.

Rosenthal, D.L., and Manjikian, V.: Techniques in the preparation of a monolayer of gynecologic cells for automated cytology. An overview. Anal. Quant. Cytol. Histol., 9:55–59, 1987.

Rosenthal, D.L., Philippe, A., Hall, T.L., Harami, S., Missirlian, N., and Suffin, S.C.: Prognosis of moderate dysplasia. Predictive value of selected markers in routinely prepared cervical smears. Anal. Quant. Cytol. Histol., 9:165–168, 1987.

Rosenthal, D.L., Missirlian, N., McLatchie, C., Suffin, S., and Castleman, K.R.: Predicting cervical epithelial disease states using subcategories on intermediate cells. Anal. Quant. Cytol., 5:217, 1983.

Ruch, F., and Bosshard, U.: Photometrische Bestimmung von Stoffmengen im Fluoreszenzmikroskop. Z. Wiss. Mikr., 65:335–341, 1963.

Rumelhart, D.E., Hinton, G.E., and Williams, R.J.: Parallel Distributed Processing: Explorations in the Microstructures of Cognition (Vol I-II). Cambridge, Mass., 1986. MIT Press.

Salzman, G.C.: Analysis of gynecological specimen by multiangle light scattering. *In* Goerttler, K., and Herman, Ch.J. (eds.): Technologies for Automation in Cervical Cancer Screening. pp. 91–93. Heidelberg, German Cancer Research Center, 1976.

Sandritter, W., and Bohm, N.: Ploidy of normal and malignant cells. *In* Wied, G.L., Bahr, G.F., and Bartels, P.H. (eds.): The Automation of Uterine Cancer Cytology. pp. 289–304. Chicago, Tutorials of Cytology, 1976.

Sandritter, W, Carl, M., and Ritter, W.: Cytophotometric measurements of the DNA content of human malignant tumors by means of the Feulgen reaction. Acta Cytol., 10:26–30, 1966.

Sandritter, W., Kiefer, G., Kiefer, R., Salm, R., Moore, G.W., and Grimm, H.: DNA in heterochromatin. Cytophotometric pattern recognition image analysis among cell nuclei in duct epithelium and in carcinoma of the human breast. Beitr. Pathol., 151:87–96, 1974.

Sandritter, W., Kiefer, G., Schluter, G., and Moore, W.: Eine cytophotometrische Methode zur Objektivierung der Morphologie von Zellkernen. Histochemistry, 10:341–352, 1967.

Schneller, J., Eppich, E., Greenebaum, E., Elequin, F., Sherman, A., Wersto, R., and Koss, L.G.: Flow cytometry and Feulgen cytophotometry in evaluation of effusions. Cancer, 59:1307–1313, 1987.

Schultz, D.S., Harry, T., Wong, K.L., Stilmant, M.M., Zahnizer, D.J., and Hutchinson, M.L.: Computer-assisted grading of adenocarcinoma in prostatic aspirates. Anal. Quant. Cytol. Histol., 12:91–97, 1990.

Seger, G.: Feature extraction by diffraction pattern sampling. *In*: Goerttler, K., and Herman, Ch.J. (eds): Technologies for Automation in Cervical Cancer Screening. pp. 76–87. Heidelberg, German Cancer Research Center, 1976.

Sherman, A.B., and Koss, L. G.: Morphometry of benign urothelial cells in the presence of cancer. Anal. Quant. Cytol. Histol., 5:332, 1983.

Silverman, A.D., Rubio, C.A., and Thorell, B.: Rapid-flow cytofluorometry of exfoliated cervicovaginal cell suspensions from mice. Acta Cytol., 21:63–67, 1977.

Sprenger, E., Moore, G.W., Naujoks, H., Schluter, G., and Sandritter, W.: DNA content and chromatin pattern analysis on cervical carcinoma in situ. Acta Cytol., 17:27–31, 1973.

Sprenger, E., Ulrich, H., and Schoendorf, H.: The diagnostic value of cell-nuclear DNA determination in aspiration cytology of benign and malignant lesions of the breast. Anal. Quant. Cytol., 1:29–36, 1979.

Sprenger, E., Volk, L., and Michaelis, W.E.: The significance of nuclear DNA measurements in the diagnosis of prostatic carcinomas. Beitr. Pathol., 53:370–378, 1974.

Spriggs, A.I., Diamond, R.A., and Meyer, E.W.: Automated screening for cervical smears. Lancet, 1:359, 1968.

Steinkamp, J.A., and Crissman, H.A.: Automated analysis of

deoxyribonucleic acid, protein and nuclear to cytoplasmic relationships in tumor cells and gynecologic specimens. J. Histochem. Cytochem., *22*:616–621, 1974.

Stohr, M.: On the correlation of chromosome number and DNA content in Hela cell clones. Acta Cytol., *19*:299–305, 1975.

Swift, H.: The desoxyribose nucleic acid content of animal nuclei. Physiol. Zool., *23*:169–198, 1950.

Swift, H., and Rasch, E.: Microphotometry with visible light. Phys. Tech. Biol. Res., *3*:353–400, 1956.

Sychra, J.J., Bartels, P.H., Taylor, J., Bibbo, M., and Wied, G.L.: Computerized recognition of cells by cytoplasmic and nuclear shape analysis. Acta Cytol., *20*:68–78, 1976.

Tanaka, N., Ikeda, H., Ueno, T., Takahashi, M., Imosato, Y., Watanabe, S., and Kashida, R.: Fundamental study of automatic cytoscreening for uterine cancer. I. Feature evaluation for the pattern recognition system. Acta Cytol., *21*:72–78, 1977.

Tanaka, N., Ikeda, H., Ueno, T., Takahashi, M., Urabe, M., Imasato, V., Watanabe, S., Youeyama, T., Genchi, H., Matozaki, T., and Kashida, R.: Fundamental study for approaching the continuation of cytological diagnosis in cancer and new automatic cytoscreening apparatus. Jpn. J. Clin. Pathol., *22*:757–768, 1973.

Tanaka, N., Ikeda, H., Ueno, T., Watanabe, S., and Imasato, Y.: Fundamental study of automatic cytoscreening for uterine cancer. II. Segmentation of cells and computer simulation. Acta Cytol., *21*:79–84, 1977.

Tanaka, N., Ikeda, H., Ueno, T., Watanabe, S., Imasato, Y., and Kashida, R.: Fundamental study on automatic cytoscreening for uterine cancer. III. New system of automated apparatus (CYBEST) utilizing pattern recognition method. Acta Cytol., *21*:85–89, 1977.

Tanaka, N., Ikeda, H., Ueno, T., Watanabe, S., Imasato, Y., and Tsuneckawa, S.: Fundamental study of automatic cytoscreening for uterine cancer. IV. Sample requirements for CYBEST and simulation test of cell dispersion. Acta Cytol., *21*:531–535, 1977.

Tanaka, N, Ikeda, H., Ueno, T., Watanabe, S., Imasato, Y., and Kashida, R.: Fundamental study of automatic cytoscreening for uterine cancer. V. Data analysis for improvement of CYBEST. Acta Cytol., *21*:536–538, 1977.

Tanaka, N., Ikeda, H., Ueno, T., Mukawa, A., Watanabe, S., Okomoto, K., Hosoi, S., and Tsunekawa, S.: Automated cytologic screening system (CYBEST model 4) and integrated image cytometry system. Appl. Optics, *26*:3301–3307, 1987.

Tang, Z.Y., Savino, A., Wong, E.K., Koss, L.G., and Shaw, L.G.: An expert system designed as a tutoring tool in cervical cytology: TTCC-1 system. Anal. Quant. Cytol. Histol., *10*:417–422, 1988.

Taylor, J., Bahr, G.F., Bartels, P.H., Bibbo, M., Richards, D.L., and Wied, G.L.; Development and evaluation of automatic nucleus finding routines; threshold of cervical cytology images. Acta Cytol., *19*:289–298, 1975.

Taylor, J., Bartels, P.H., Bibbo, M., Bahr, G.F., and Wied, G.L.: Implementation of a hierarchical cell classification procedure. Acta Cytol., *18*:515–521, 1974.

Taylor, J., Puls, J.H., Sychra, J.J., Bartels, P.H., Bibbo, M., and Wied, G.L.: A system for scanning biological cells in three colors. Acta Cytol., *22*:29–35, 1978.

Tolles, W.E.: A multidimensional analysis of some quantitative characteristics of exfoliated cells in Papanicolaou smears. Boston, Second Annual Meeting of the Inter-Society Cytology Council, 1954.

Tolles, W.E.: Quantitation of the rate-zonal sedimentation spectrum. J. Histochem. Cytochem., *24*:6–10, 1976.

den Tonkelaar, E.M., and Van Duijn, P.: Photographic color-

imetry as a quantitative cytochemical method. Histochemie, *4*:1–9, 1964.

Tucker, J.H., and Shippey, G.: Basic performance tests on the CERVIFIP linear array prescreener. Anal. Quant. Cytol., *5*:129–137, 1983.

Tycko, D.H., Anbalagan, S., Liu, H.C., and Ornstein, L.: Automatic leukocyte classification using cytochemically stained smears. J. Histochem. Cytochem., *24*:178–194, 1976.

van de Vijver, M.J., Peterse, J.L., Mooi, W.J., Wisman, P., Lomans, J., Dalesio, O., and Nusse, R.: Neu-Protein overexpression in breast cancer. N. Engl. J. Med., *319*:1239–1245, 1988.

van Diest, P.J., Smeulders, A.W.M., Thunnissen, F.B.J. M., and Baak, J. P.A: Cytomorphometry. A methodologic study of preparation techniques, selection methods and sample sizes. Anal. Quant. Cytol. Histol., *11*:225–231, 1989.

Vastola, E.F., Hertzberg, R., Neurath, P., and Brenner, J.: Description by computer of texture in Wright-stained leukocytes. Acta Cytol., *18*:231–247, 1974.

Vielh, P., Chevillard, S., Mosseri, V., Donatini, B., and Magdelenat, H.: Ki67 index and S-phase fraction in human breast carcinomas. Comparison and correlations with prognostic factors. Am. J. Clin. Pathol., *94*:681–686, 1990.

Vooijs, G.P., Oud, P.S., Zahniser, D.J., Pahlplatz, M.M., Hermkens, H.G., van der PlasCats, M., and Herman, C.J.: Chromatin measurements in Feulgen stained intermediate cells from normal and abnormal cervical smears. Anal. Quant. Cytol., *4*:154, 1982.

Wagner, D., Sprenger, E., and Merkle, D.: Cytophotometric studies in suspicious cervical smears. Acta Cytol., *20*:366–371, 1976.

Waterman, D.A.: A Guide to Expert Systems. Reading, Mass., Addison-Wesley, 1986.

Watson, J.D., and Crick, F.H.C.: Genetical implications of the structure of deoxyribonucleic acid. Nature, *171*:964–967, 1953.

Weber, J.E., Bartels, P.H., Griswold, W., Kuhn, W., Paplanus, S.H., and Graham, A.R.: Colonic lesion expert system: Performance evaluation. Anal. Quant. Cytol. Histol., *10*:150–159, 1988.

West, S.S.: Potential of fluorescent molecular probes for instrumental evaluation of cells in the female reproductive tract. *In* Wied, G.L., Bahr, G.F., and Bartels, P.H. (eds.): The Automation of Uterine Cancer cytology. pp. 345–362. Chicago, Tutorials of Cytology, 1976. (See also the immediately following discussion by H.M. Shapiro, Z. Darzynkiewicz, and B.D.Halpern.)

Wheeless, L.L., Jr., Pattern, S.F., and Cambier, M.A.: Slit-scan cytofluorometry: Data base for auomated cytopathology. Acta Cytol. *19*:460–464, 1975.

Wheeless, L.L., Jr., and Onderdonk, M.A.: Preparation of clinical gynecologic specimens for automated analysis: An overview. J. Histochem. Cytochem., *22*:522–525, 1974.

Wied, G.L., Bahr, G.F., and Bartels, P.H.: Automatic analysis of cell images by TICAS. *In* Wied, G.L., and Bahr, G.F.(eds.): Automated Cell Identification and Cell Sorting. pp. 195–360. New York, Academic Press, 1970.

Wied, G.L., Bahr, G.F., Bibbo, M., Puls, J.H., Taylor, J.H., and Bartels, P.H.: The TICAS-RTCIP real time cell identification processor. Acta Cytol., *19*:286–288, 1975.

Wied, G.L., Bahr, G.F., Griep, J., Rappaport, H., and Bartels, P.H.: Computer discrimination of blood cells from two cases of "leukemic" lymphosarcoma. Acta Cytol., *13*:688–695, 1969.

Wied, G.L., Bahr, G.F., Oldfield, D.G., and Bartels, P.H.: Computer-assisted identification of cells from uterine adenocarcinoma. A clinical feasibility study with TICAS. Acta Cytol., *12*:357–370, 1968.

Wied, G.L., Bahr, G.F., Oldfield, D.G., and Bartels, P.H.: Computer-assisted identification of cells from uterine adenocarcinoma. II. Measurements at 590 nm. Acta Cytol., 13:21–26, 1969.

Wied, G.L., and Bartels, P.H.: International standardization of cell images: Automation of cytodiagnostic assessment. *In* Wied, G.L., Bahr, G.F., and Bartels, P.H. (eds.): The Automation of Uterine Cancer Cytology. pp. 429–441. Chicago, Tutorials of Cytology, 1976.

Wied, G.L., Bartels, P.H., Bahr, G.F., and Oldfield, D.G.: Taxonomic intracellular analytic system (TICAS) for cell identification. Acta Cytol., 12:180–204, 1968.

Wied, G.L., Bartels, P.H., Bahr, G.F., and Reagan, J.W.: TICAS assessment of cells from atypical hyperplasia of endometrium. Acta Cytol., 13:552–556, 1969.

Wied, G.L., Bartels, P.H., Bibbo, M., and Dytch, H.E.: Rapid DNA evaluation in clinical diagnosis. Acta Cytol., 27:33–37, 1983.

Wied, G.L., Bartels, P.H., Bibbo, M., Dytch, H.E., and Pishotta, F.T.: Rapid high-resolution cytometry. Anal. Quant. Cytol., 4:257–262, 1982.

Wied, G.L., Bartels, P.H., Bibbo, M., and Sychra., J.: Cytomorphometric markers for uterine cancer in intermediate cells. Anal. Quant. Cytol., 2:257–263, 1980.

Wied, G.L., Bartels, P.H., Dytch, H.E., Pishotta, F.T., Yamauchi, K., and Bibbo, M.: Diagnostic marker features in dysplastic cells from the uterine cervix. Acta Cytol., 26:475–483, 1982.

Wied, G.L., Bartels, P.H., Weber, J., and Dytch, H.E.: Expert systems design under uncertainty of human diagnosticians. IEEE Proceedings (8th Annual Conference on Engineering in Medicine and Biology 1986), CH 2368-9. vol. 25. pp. 757–760.

Wied, G.L., Bartels, P.H., Bibbo, M., and Dytch, H.E.: Image analysis in quantitative cytopathology and histopathology. Hum. Pathol., 20:549–571, 1989.

Wied, G.L., Bibbo, M., and Bartels, P.H.: Computer analysis of microscopic images: Application in cytopathology. *In* Rosen, P.P. (ed.): Pathology Annals. vol. 16. pp. 367–409. New York, Appleton-Century-Crofts, 1981.

Wied, G.L., Bibbo, M., Bahr, G.F., and Bartels, P.H.: Computerized microdissection of cellular images. Acta Cytol., 14:418, 1970.

Wied, G.L., Bibbo, M., Bahr, G.F., and Bartels, P.H.: Computerized recognition of uterine glandular cells. I. Assessment of a self-optimizing recognition program. Acta Cytol., 13:611–619, 1969.

Wied, G.L., Bibbo, M., Bahr, G.F., and Bartels, P.H.: Computerized recognition of uterine glandular cells. II. The application of a self-learning program. Acta Cytol., 13:662–671, 1969.

Wied, G.L., Bibbo, M., Bahr, G.F., and Bartels, P.H.: Computerized recognition of uterine glandular cells. III. Assessment of the efficiency of 1 μ vs. 0.5 μ spot sizes. Acta Cytol., 14:136–141, 1970.

Wied, G.L., Bibbo, M., and Bartels, P.G.: Computer analysis of microscopic images: Application in cytopathology. Pathol. Annu., 16:387, 1981.

Wied, G.L., Bibbo, M., Dytch, H.E., and Bartels, P.H.: Computer grading of cervical intraepithelial neoplastic lesions: I. Cytologic indices. Anal. Quant. Cytol. Histol., 7:52–60, 1985.

Wied, G.L., Legorreta, G., Mohr, D., and Rauzy, A.: Cytology of invasive cervical carcinoma and carcinoma in situ. Ann. N.Y. Acad. Sci., 97:759–766, 1962.

Wied, G.L., Messina, A.M., and Rosenthal, E.: Comparative quantitative DNA measurements on Feulgen stained cervical epithelial cells. Acta Cytol., 10:31–37, 1966.

Wied, G.L., Weber, J.E., Dytch, H. E., Bibbo, M., and Bartels, P.H.: TICAS-STRATEX, an expert diagnostic system for stratified cervical epithelium. IEEE Proceedings, EMBS-EMSA, Boston, November 1987.

Wied, G.L., Weber, J.E., and Bartels, P.H.: Expert systems as classifiers in diagnostic cytopathology. IEEE Proceedings, EMBS-EMSA, Boston, November 1987.

Wilbanks, G.D., Richart, R.M., and Terner, J.Y.: DNA content of cervical intraepithelial neoplasia studied by two-wavelength Feulgen cytophotometry. Am. J. Obstet. Gynecol., 98:792–799, 1967.

Wilson, E.B.: The Cell in Development and Heredity. New York, Macmillan, 1896.

Wooley, R.C., Dembitzer, H.M., Herz, F., Schreiber, K., and Koss, L.G.: The use of a slide spinner in the analysis of cell dispersion. J. Histochem. Cytochem., 25:11–15, 1976.

Wong, E.K., Liang, E.H., Lin, E.K., Simmons, D.A., and Koss, L. G.: A selective mapping algorithm for computer analysis of voided urine cell images. Anal. Quant. Cytol. Histol., 11:203–210, 1989.

Wyatt, P.J.: Differential light scattering: A physical method for identifying living bacterial cells. Appl. Optics, 7:1879–1896, 1968.

Zahniser, D.J.: The development of a fully automatic system for the prescreening of cervical smears. Ph.D. thesis. Netherlands, Nijmegen, 1979.

Zajicek, J., Bartels, P.H., Bahr, G.F., Bibbo, M., Jakobson, P.A., and Wied, G.L.: Computer analysis of needle aspirates from breast carcinomas during radiotherapy. Acta Cytol., 17:179–187, 1973.

Zajicek, J., Bartels, P.H., Bahr, G.F., Bibbo, M., and Wied, G.L.: Computer analysis of lymphocytes from cases with lymphadenitis and lymphocytic lymphoma. Acta Cytol., 16:284–296, 1972.

36

Flow Cytometry*

Flow cytometry is an analytic technique based on the principle of measurements of fluorescence in single particles, such as cells or nuclei, suspended in a mantle of fluid, passing one by one (flowing) across a narrow beam of fluorescent light (Fig. 36–1). The intensity of the fluorescence of each particle is recorded and entered into a computer. Because the flow of particles is very rapid, a large number of measurements can be performed in a few minutes. The results of the measurements are presented as a histogram, a scattergram, or a three-dimensional display of fluorescence (see Figs. 36–5 to 36–7).

For this goal to be accomplished, the target of study, if not composed of single particles, has to be disaggregated. The single particles must then be combined with a suitable fluorescent substance (fluorochrome or fluorescent probe) that tags the cell component to be measured, for example, DNA. With two sources of fluorescence or the splitting of one beam of fluorescent light into two wavelengths, two synchronous measurements of different features of the cells can be performed. Such measurements require the use of two fluorochromes, each tagging a different component of the cell, provided that they fluoresce at different wavelengths (Fig. 36–2). In experimental instruments three or more cell components can be measured, but this technique is generally not available on commercial instruments. A summary of the sequence of events in flow cytometry is shown in Figure 36–3.

Most contemporary instruments also include an option of sorting the particles or cells, based on their fluorescent properties. Other applications of flow cytometry include measurements of certain optical features and sizes of the particles by using the technique of light scatter or by recording the time necessary for a particle to cross the fluorescent beam, the time being in proportion to the size of the particle. The technical principles and the appli-

*This chapter is based in part on "Flow cytometric measurements of DNA and other cell components in human tumors. A critical appraisal," by L.G. Koss, B. Czerniak, F. Herz, and R.P. Wersto, Hum. Pathol., 20:528–548, 1989; with permission of W. B. Saunders Co.

SCHEMATIC REPRESENTATION
OF A FLOW CYTOMETER

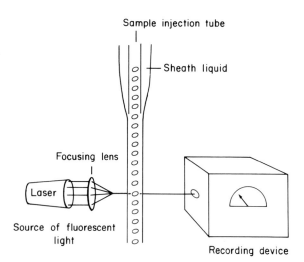

FIGURE 36-1. A highly simplified schematic diagram of a flow cytometer and its fundamental components: a capillary flow chamber, a source of fluorescent light, that may be a laser or a mercury lamp, and a recording device. The particles stained with a fluorescent dye are suspended in a jet of fluid and flow (pass) one by one across the focused beam of fluorescent light. The emitted fluorescence is recorded. The level of fluorescence is measured individually for each particle. The sum of measurements is presented as a histogram of fluorescence (see Fig. 36-5), as a scattergram of fluorescence (see Fig. 36-6), or as a tridimensional display (see Fig. 36-7).

cation of these techniques to research and clinical practice are described below.

HISTORICAL DEVELOPMENTS

Many fields of science, such as microscopy, optics, chemistry, physics, mathematics, computer technology, engineering, biology, and medicine, contributed to developments in quantitative cytology, including flow cytometry (for an analysis of the historical developments see Koss, 1982, 1987). The conceptual ideas of flow cytometry were based on observations of Caspersson, who used ultraviolet light to measure components fluorescing at different wavelengths in unstained cells (Caspersson, 1936; Caspersson and Santesson, 1942; Caspersson, 1950). Nucleic acids and proteins were measured by densitometry on photographs of cells in ultraviolet light (see p. 47). This tedious and time-consuming work made major contributions to the understanding of the relationship of cell components in benign and malignant cells.

The development of the first commercially available flow cytometer, the Cytofluorograf, was based on the idea conceived in 1960 by Herbert Derman, a pathologist, and John Hoffer, an engineer working at IBM. The primary purpose of the system was the automation of the cervical smear (Papanicolaou smear) for the detection of carcinomas and precancerous states of the uterine cervix. The construction of the system was entrusted to a physicist, Louis Kamentsky, then working at

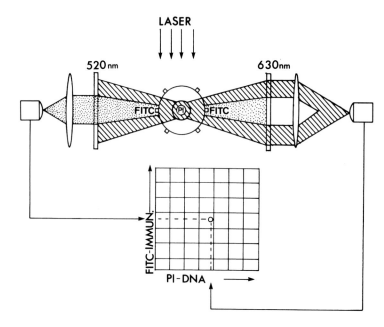

FIGURE 36-2. Principles of simultaneous measurement of immunofluorescence and DNA content for quantitating expression of various cellular components in relation to the cell cycle. The component of interest is stained via a direct or an indirect immunostaining procedure using fluoresceinated antibodies (*FITC*, green fluorescence). Then the cells are counterstained for DNA using propidium iodide (*PI*, red fluorescence). During the measurements, the two color components of each cell are separated with the use of appropriate filters and captured by two photomultipliers. Coordinates for the two parameters of each cell are stored in list mode array for subsequent analysis.

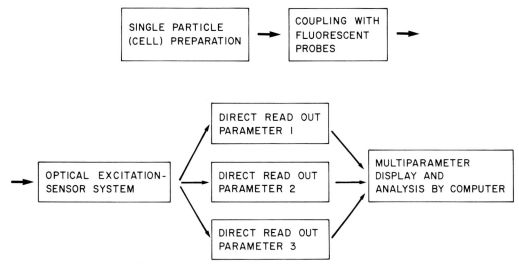

FIGURE 36-3. Sequence of events in flow cytometry.

the IBM Watson Research Center in New York City. The initial measurements of fluorescence on cells in cervical smears were performed in a static system that documented different distribution of nucleic acids in benign and abnormal cells (Fig. 36–4). In a series of papers published in *Science*, the fundamental principles of flow cytometry and cell sorting were described (Kamentsky et al., 1963, 1965, 1967). Kamentsky's essential contribution was the construction of an apparatus that combined fluorescence, as observed in the static system, with Coulter's idea of electronic assessment of cell properties in cell suspensions (Coulter, 1956). The result was a flow cytometry system, whereby the fluorescent properties of nucleic acids and proteins could be measured in a suspension of cells, after enhancement of the cell components by staining with appropriate fluorescent dyes.

FIGURE 36-4. Absorption patterns of three cells from a cervical smear at different wavelengths. Scanning at 2,652 Å corresponds to absorption by nucleic acids; scanning at 2,976 Å corresponds to absorption by certain other proteins; scanning at 5,460 Å corresponds to visible light. The cell on the left is a normal squamous cell, whereas the cells designated as A and B represent varying degrees of abnormality. Cell A is dyskaryotic, closely resembling the benign cell on the left, except for an enlarged and hyperchromatic nucleus. Yet its absorption pattern in ultraviolet light (2,652 Å) reveals a marked increase in the cytoplasmic content of nucleic acids. In Cell B, which is a frank squamous cancer cell, there is a further increase of the cytoplasmic nucleic acids to the point of partial obliteration of the nuclear peak. (Modified from Kamentsky, L. A., et al.: Ultraviolet absorption of epidermoid cancer cells. Science, *142*:1580–1583, 1963)

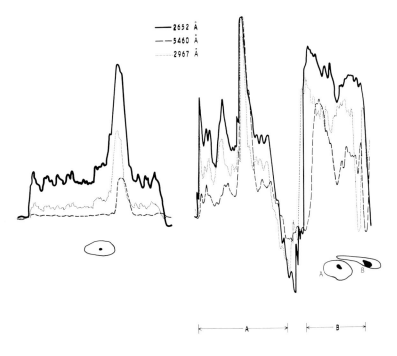

The initial application of the machine, namely the automation of the analysis of the cell sample from the uterine cervix, was a failure (Koenig et al., 1968). Still, the machine proved a valuable clinical and research tool in other areas of cell biology and pathology.

PRINCIPLES OF FLOW CYTOMETRY

In contrast to cytophotometry or image cytometry, which are inherently slow techniques based on the analysis of optical parameters of cells spread on a glass slide, flow cytometry allows rapid measurements of one or more parameters of individual particles such as cells and therefore is applicable to studies of large cell populations. The principal features of the two systems are compared in Table 36–1. As mentioned, flow cytometers are machines constructed to measure and record fluorescence. The measurements are usually performed on particles (cells) stained with an appropriate fluorochrome, flowing past an excitation source (see Fig. 36–1). The fluorescence level of the stained cells is captured by a photomultiplier tube and digitally converted to an electronic pulse. Precise measurements of fluorescence are achieved because the cells or particles pass through the excitation source one by one, in single file, within a laminar flow jet of a liquid suspension medium to control positional accuracy. The excitation source can be either a xenon-mercury arc lamp or a laser, usually an argon-ion or krypton-ion laser producing monochromatic light between wavelengths of 450 to 600 nm, sufficient to excite the absorption maxima of most fluorescent dyes used for the analysis of cellular components. In the case of cells stained with two or more fluorochromes (multiparameter flow cytometry), either two sources of fluorescent or, using a single source, optical dichroic mirrors are used to separate the color components of light into two or more wavelengths, which are recorded by two or more photomultipliers (see Fig. 36–2).

Usually, cells are analyzed at rates of 100 to 200 cells per second (although the machines are capable of more rapid analysis), and the resulting fluorescence measurements are stored in a computer for subsequent analysis of correlated parameters. Besides fluorescence, cell size can be measured, a feature useful in the analysis of complex cell populations. There are several methods to accomplish this goal in flow systems. Electronic Coulter volume measurements, based on differences in the electrical conductibility of cells and the saline solution in which they are suspended, are proportional to some extent to the size of cells (Coulter, 1956). In some instances, mainly in very homogeneous cell populations, similar information can be obtained by the measurement of light scattering at small angles (see Melamed et al., 1979, 1990; Shapiro, 1985). Cell sizes can also be measured by the determination of pulse width or time in flow by objects passing through the beam of light.

Table 36–1
Comparison of High-Resolution (Image Analysis) Systems with Flow Cytometry

Features	Image Analysis	Flow Cytometry
Applicability to routine cytologic material on smears	Yes	No
Correlation with cell morphology	Yes	Possible with cell sorters
Cell orientation	Important	Important
Measurement of multiple parameters	Yes	Limited
Speed	Slow	Very fast
Measurements of cell components such as DNA	Yes	Yes
Use of fluorescent probes	Limited	Yes
Use of absorbent probes	Yes	No
Autoradiography	Yes	No
Bioassays quantitation	Yes*	Yes†
Tissue analysis	Yes	No

*With monoclonal antibodies and peroxidase-antiperoxidase reaction
†With fluorescent tagging.

A major limitation of flow cytometry is the inability of morphologic corroboration of the identity of the measured objects; this is particularly vexing in mixed cell populations obtained from human samples. This drawback can be overcome to some extent by cell sorting, which makes possible the isolation of cell populations with precisely defined fluorescent characteristics.

Cell Sorting

The sorting method commonly used is based on the principle of jet printing. The stream of fluid exiting from the capillary tube is broken into droplets, and electrostatic charges are applied to droplets containing cells with previously defined characteristics, such as the level of fluorescence (Kamentsky et al., 1965; Fulwyler, 1965, 1969). The charged droplets are deflected into a collecting vessel by an electrostatic field. The sorted cells can be studied directly under the microscope or in cell culture systems. However, cell sorting, although valuable in research, is a time-consuming and difficult technique that cannot be applied routinely to clinical specimens.

PREPARATION OF BIOLOGIC MATERIAL FOR FLOW CYTOMETRY

Flow cytometric analysis can be performed on any cell suspension, such as leukocytes or bone marrow cells, and on cell samples obtained directly from the patient by thin-needle aspiration techniques or, indirectly, by aspiration of surgically removed tissue samples. In malignant tumors there is evidence that needle aspiration techniques may selectively sample nondiploid cell populations; hence, these cells may be more representative of tumor abnormalities than single tissue samples (Greenebaum et al., 1984). Fresh or archival tissue samples may also be processed. Regardless of the source of cells, the preparation of cell suspensions for flow cytometry requires strict attention to technical details and, for solid tissues, may be time-consuming, requiring the services of a skilled technologist. (See also Appendix.)

Cell Suspensions

One of the major limitations of flow cytometry is the requirement that the specimen to be measured be in the form of a single cell suspension. Cells that normally lack intercellular junctions (peripheral blood cells, bone marrow cells, lymphoid tissue) are ideal for flow cytometric measurements and require little special effort; cell suspensions are relatively easy to prepare by differential centrifugation techniques. It is also relatively easy to obtain single cell suspensions from cultured cells. However, preparation of a suspension of intact whole cells from benign or malignant solid human and animal tissues is much more difficult. The results may vary, depending on the organ. Whole cells can be relatively easily obtained from parenchymal organs such as the liver by using a perfusion method (Blobel and Potter, 1966). By contrast, epithelial cells bound by desmosomes are extremely difficult to isolate by mechanical means, such as syringing across a small-caliber needle, because the tough cell junctions cannot be dissociated without significant damage to cell cytoplasm and membrane (Koss et al., 1976; Wolley et al., 1976; Thornthwaite et al., 1980; Bijman et al., 1985; Ensley et al., 1987).

Several enzymatic and/or detergent treatment protocols are available for the preparation of cell suspensions (see Appendix). Thus, treatment of tissues with ethylenediaminetetra-acetic acid (EDTA), pepsin, trypsin, collagenase, and so on, have been proposed, but no single method is universally applicable (Wolley et al., 1979; McDivitt, 1984; Slocum et al., 1981; Smeets et al., 1987). Even with these disaggregation methods the cytoplasm may be severely damaged. In general, tissues composed of cells with a substantial cell skeleton rich in keratin filaments, such as squamous or urothelial cells, will withstand the disaggregation procedure better than fragile cells, such as mucus-producing glandular cells. Consequently, the results obtained with cell dissociation procedures are poorly reproducible and must be extensively tested according to target tissue. The reliability of the results should always be confirmed by a microscopic and, preferably, electron microscopic examination of the dissociated cells to ascertain the degree of damage.

Nuclear Isolation Techniques

To circumvent the problems of cell isolation from solid animal tissues, methods have been developed for the isolation of intact nuclei that permit flow cytometric analysis of nuclear components, such as DNA.

Fresh Material

The first nuclear isolation technique described for flow cytometry was the use of citric acid–sodium citrate buffer (CASC), a low pH solution that effectively disrupts desmosomes, destroys the cytoplasm in squamous and other epithelial human cells, and effectively permeabilizes the nuclei to allow penetration of fluorochromes (Koss et al., 1977). Several other techniques were also introduced, often combining the use of low pH solutions (Krishnan, 1975) and detergents (Vindelöv et al., 1983) with fluorochromes. Although the nuclear isolation techniques are more reproducible than whole cell isolation techniques, their applicability to various targets must be individually tested. For example, the CASC method was found to be adequate for nuclear isolation from the squamous epithelium and the epithelium of the colon (Wersto et al., 1988). In targets of lesser cellularity, however, such as bladder washings, the cell loss with CASC was too great and Vindelöv's technique proved superior. If possible, cell loss should be assessed for each sample because not all cells in the suspension may react in the same way and the sample may favor one cell type over another.

Archival Material

A method for the preparation of isolated nuclei from paraffin-embedded tumor tissues, described by Hedley, has been widely used for flow cytometric analysis of the DNA content in archival material (Hedley et al., 1983, 1984, 1985, 1989). This approach allows retrospective studies of patients with known clinical course of disease and helps to overcome limitations imposed by a small patient number and insufficient period of follow-up in prospective studies. The method is based on the deparaffinization of thick (30 to 50 μm) sections of tissue, rehydration in descending series of alcohols to water, and dissociation of the sample by enzymatic action (trypsin or pepsin) before staining with a fluorochrome. The rehydration procedure can be automated in a tissue processor (Amberson et al., 1991). With some modifications, the method can be used to isolate nuclei from microscopically selected areas of a tissue sample (Oud et al., 1986).

The reproducibility of the method was tested in a multilaboratory study by processing several aliquots of the same tissue blocks of bladder tumors by somewhat different technical approaches and using different flow cytometers (Coon et al., 1988). A surprisingly high degree of reproducibility of results was achieved, even though minor differences in histogram construction and interpretation were noted.

A great deal has been written about the clinical value of retrospective DNA measurements in human tumors (see below), but at the time of this writing (1991), it is still not known how accurate these determinations are. The success of the measurements on archival material depends to a large extent on the size and fixation of the original tissue sample (only formalin-fixed material can be used because formalin stabilizes DNA-associated proteins) and the conditions and length of storage. In many instances the nuclei disintegrate completely, resulting in debris that precludes the interpretation of the results. It is also possible that storage and paraffin embedding affect the DNA content of the tissue. In a large study of colonic cancer, the DNA content of freshly processed tissues and of paraffin-embedded tissues was compared; losses in the aneuploid component were observed in paraffin-embedded material in 19% of the tumors with resulting shift of the DNA values toward the diploid range. On the other hand, in 3% of the tumors, aneuploid patterns of DNA not seen in fresh material were observed in paraffin blocks (Koss and Wersto, unpublished data, 1991). It is evident, therefore, that similar comparisons should be established for all archival tissues studied, before the results of these studies can be evaluated and considered to be of clinical value.

Staining

The most common clinical applications of flow cytometry pertain to the identification of subgroups of lymphohematopoietic cells, such as lymphocytes, and to the measurements of nucleic acids, chiefly DNA. Depending on the goal of the study, the cell or nuclear suspension requires staining with a fluorochrome that will selectively bind to the cell component of interest.

For immunologic studies there is now a large selection of commercially produced monoclonal and polyclonal antibodies that selectively bind to specific cell types (such as subgroups of T lymphocytes) and to a broad variety of membrane or cytoplasmic proteins. The specificity of these antibodies should be tested before use with Western immunoblots by combining the antibody with the target protein under appropriately controlled circumstances (see Figs. 35–18 and 35–19). A fluorescent molecule, such as fluorescein isothiocyanate (FITC), can be covalently attached to virtually any antibody for direct measurements of fluorescence. Another approach is to visualize the bound primary antibody with a secondary antibody labeled with an appropriate fluorochrome. Using two fluorochromes, fluorescing at two wavelengths sufficiently divergent to be simultaneously and distinctly measured may be used for dual-parameter analysis (see above and Thornthwaite et al., 1984; Horan et al., 1986; Czerniak et al., 1987; Cohen et al., 1988). The knowledge of the distinct characteristics of the fluorochromes is essential in these endeavors because any cross-fluorescence will obscure the results.

Single-parameter measurements based on direct staining of cellular components such as the DNA, RNA, or protein can be accomplished with several known fluorochromes. Propidium iodide (PI), ethidium bromide, and diamidinophenylindole (DAPI) are commonly used for DNA analysis (Table 36–2). The use of these dyes requires pretreatment of the samples with ribonuclease (RNAse) to prevent fluorochrome binding to RNA. Acridine orange (AO), which binds differently to DNA and RNA, can be used for the simultaneous analysis of both components under strict experimental conditions (Darzynkiewicz et al., 1984; Darzynkiewicz, 1986).

The reader is referred to standard textbooks for a complete list of available fluorochromes and for an analysis of the staining techniques (Melamed et al., 1979, 1990; Shapiro, 1985). The most common techniques used in this laboratory are listed in the Appendix.

As with the preparation of the cell sample, meticulous attention to detail is necessary in the use of fluorochromes. There is comparatively little information on the suitability of various fluorochromes for specific tissue targets, and individual laboratories tend to retain one staining method with which their technical staff are best acquainted. The results obtained with a given fluorochrome may also be modified by a different method of cell processing and may not necessarily be reproducible in other laboratories or on other instruments.

Inter- and intralaboratory differences have been evaluated by a Network of laboratories, sponsored by the National Cancer Institute (U.S.A.), using bladder tumor tissues and bladder washings as a primary target. The DNA measurements performed by five laboratories on paraffin-embedded tissues were discussed previously (Coon et al., 1988). The results of DNA measurements on "cocktails" of cells disclosed significant intra- and interlaboratory differences (Wheeless et al., 1989). The clinical significance of these differences must still be explored.

Table 36–2
Principal Fluorescent Probes*

	Excitation Wavelength (nm)	Maximum Emission Wavelength (nm)
Acridine orange	500	530 (green)
		640 (red)
Ethidium bromide	520	610
Propidium iodide	520	590
Hoechst 32258†	356	460
Chromomycin A_3‡	430	570
7 Amino-actinomycin D_3‡	550	655
Quinacrine§	455	500
Duanomycin§	510	600
4′,6′Diamidinophenylindole (DAPI)	350	475

* Based in part on data provided by the late Dr. Samuel Latt, The Children's Hospital Medical Center, Harvard Medical School, Boston.
† Binds predominantly or exclusively to A-T pairs in DNA.
‡ Binds predominantly or exclusively to G-C pairs in DNA.
§ Quantum yield A-T-specific.

ANALYSIS OF DATA

Display of Data

The data generated by flow cytometers are either displayed instantaneously on a video screen or stored in the computer for further analysis. The results of single-parameter measurements are usually displayed as a frequency histogram in which the number of stained cells is plotted as a function of fluorescence energy expressed in channel numbers (Fig. 36–5). The channel designation is pro-

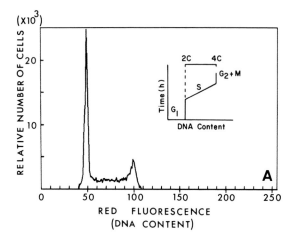

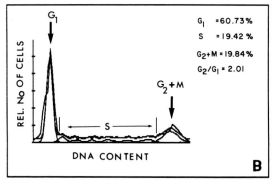

FIGURE 36–5. DNA distribution pattern during the cell cycle. (*A*) Histogram showing the DNA distribution of exponentially proliferating HeLa S3 cells in culture. The histogram was generated by flow cytometric measurement of cells stained with propidium iodide, which intercalates stoichiometrically into the DNA backbone. The major peak represents cells in G_1 and the smaller second peak cells in $G_2 + M$ phase of the cycle. Cells between the two peaks are in S phase. The insert depicts the theoretical chronologic changes in DNA content of a single cell traversing the cell cycle. (*B*) Data from (*A*) showing computer-derived cell cycle distribution. The percentage of cells in the various cell cycle phases and the ratio of G_2/G_1 cells are indicated in the upper right.

vided by the manufacturer of the instruments and is usually adjustable. For example, one can select channel 50, corresponding to the position of the first (diploid) peak, and channel 100, corresponding to the position of the second (tetraploid) peak (see Fig. 36–5). For an explanation of the significance of the peaks, see below.

In the case of simultaneous measurements of several parameters (usually two), the results are presented as scattergraphs or as three-dimensional contour maps showing the relationship between the measured features (Figs. 36–6 and 36–7).

In immunologic studies, the proportion of cells binding to a given fluorescent antibody is easily ascertained as a percentage of the cell population screened. For example, the proportion of T-suppressor or helper cells in a population of lymphocytes may be directly determined. Similar principles apply to a broad variety of specific antibodies used in studies of bromodeoxyuridine (BrdU) incorporation (cell cycle studies), Ki-67 (proliferation antigen), proteins reflecting the presence of oncogene products, tissue-specific markers, and tumor-associated antigens (examples in Gratzner, 1982; Valet et al., 1984; Czerniak and Koss, 1985; Feitz et al., 1985; Darzynkiewicz, 1986; Jacobberger et al., 1986; Wersto et al., 1988; Rabinovitch et al., 1988; Czerniak et al., 1990).

Among the most common measurements is the DNA content of a given cell population. The interpretation of the DNA patterns in a given human cell population follows the assumption (not always correct—see below) that the quantitation of DNA is related to the number of chromosomes (46 in humans; see Chapter 6). The term *stem line* is also used to define the dominant (or most important) lineage in a complex population of cells. Fig. 36–8 indicates the principal designations of ploidy patterns that may be observed in human benign or malignant tissues. The results of the measurements are usually displayed as histograms, interpreted in accordance with ploidy standards, that is, 2C (or 2N) = diploid (euploid), 4C (or 4N) = tetraploid, and so on (see Fig. 36–5), in which C or N indicates a haploid number of chromosomes found in a gamete (ovum or spermatozoon), which is 23 in humans. With normal cells, certain assumptions are being made in such displays, namely that the diploid peak corresponds to the diploid number of normal chromosomes (46 in human samples) and the tetraploid peak to twice that number (92 in human samples). In reality, the measurements of normal cells, such as inactive lymphocytes, always follow gaussian distribution within at least 1% or 2% off the center of the peak. The results are usu-

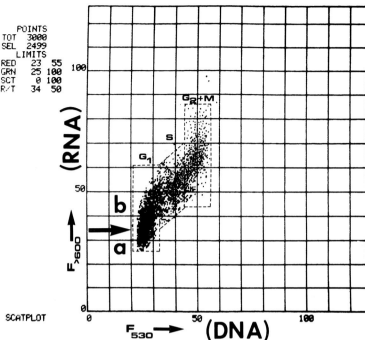

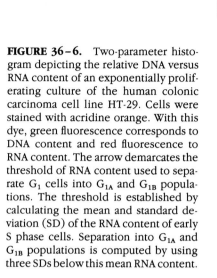

FIGURE 36–6. Two-parameter histogram depicting the relative DNA versus RNA content of an exponentially proliferating culture of the human colonic carcinoma cell line HT-29. Cells were stained with acridine orange. With this dye, green fluorescence corresponds to DNA content and red fluorescence to RNA content. The arrow demarcates the threshold of RNA content used to separate G_1 cells into G_{1A} and G_{1B} populations. The threshold is established by calculating the mean and standard deviation (SD) of the RNA content of early S phase cells. Separation into G_{1A} and G_{1B} populations is computed by using three SDs below this mean RNA content.

ally analyzed by using the coefficient of variation (CV; see below, Quality of Histograms). It is not known whether the gaussian distribution is a function of a variable DNA content in normal human cells or is an instrumental or measurement error. Further, as discussed below, the position of the diploid peak in apparently normal human epithelial samples may vary by ± 10% from the mean.

DNA Index

Another way of presenting DNA data is the DNA index (DI). This formula is used to compare the position of a histogram peak (in fluorescence intensity scale, expressed as channel number) in reference to the position of the diploid peak, also in channel number (see Fig. 36–5). For example, if the position of the diploid peak is in channel 50 on the fluorescence intensity scale and the position of the tetraploid peak in channel 100, the DI of the tetraploid peak is $100:50 = 2$. The position of abnormal peaks is determined in the same fashion. For example, if an abnormal peak is located in channel 75 and the diploid peak in channel 50, the DI of the abnormal peak is $75:50 = 1.5$. The DI serves to identify abnormal peaks and is mainly useful in the interpretation of histograms with a nearly normal distribution of cycling cells (see Fig. 36–9B). Still, in practice the position of the diploid

peak is not always secure, and it is customary to consider deviations of ±10% as normal. These are highly arbitrary decisions, not based on controlled studies (see below), that often cast doubt on the interpretation of histograms of DNA fluorescence in tumors.

Controls

One of the fundamental issues in flow cytometry is the use of appropriate controls. In immunologic studies the control is provided by the level of fluorescence of cells not binding the antibody, which must be subtracted from the fluorescence level of cells binding the antibody. Alternately, the antibody may be blocked by the addition of a specific protein before staining to determine the level of nonspecific background fluorescence. Background fluorescence may also be determined by staining the cells with an irrelevant (i.e., unrelated) antibody of the same isotype, such as mouse-mouse or rat-rat (see examples in Czerniak et al., 1987; Wersto et al., 1988).

In DNA measurements the controls may be external or internal. External controls of the diploid peak position may be provided by obtaining a population of normal inactive lymphocytes, preferably from the same patient. Internal controls are cells

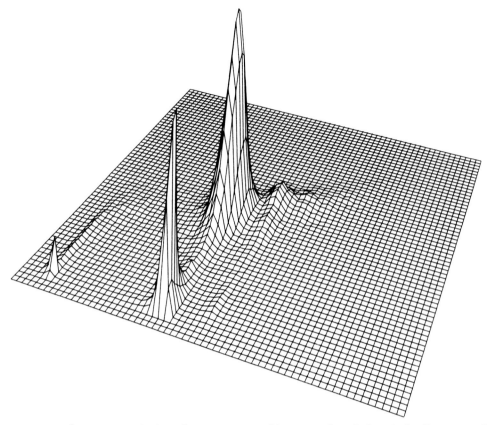

FIGURE 36–7.   Isometric view of a two-parameter histogram of cervical-vaginal cells measured by flow cytometry. The histogram is generated by determining chromomycin A_3 fluorescence intensity as a measure of cellular DNA content (abscissa in the plane) and 90° light scatter intensity as a measure of cell size (ordinate in the plane) simultaneously on each cell. The number of cells is plotted vertically. Thus the location on the plane shows DNA content and cell size while the height above the plane shows the relative frequency of occurrence. To best define the features in the histogram, intensities of the fluorescence and scatter signals are measured and presented logarithmically. With the use of an electronic cell sorter it is possible to identify the cell types that give rise to these features. The small peak and shoulder at the far left corner of the histogram (i.e., lowest values of fluorescence and scatter) are due to cell debris and bacteria. The sharp peak in the foreground with a higher fluorescence intensity, characteristic of a diploid amount of DNA, and low scatter results from white blood cells; signals at equal fluorescence intensity but higher values of scatter generated by the larger epithelial cells produce the large peak in the middle of the histogram. Small shoulders to the right of the white cell and epithelial cell peaks are due to cell aggregates. Cells of carcinoma in situ and invasive carcinoma contain elevated amounts of DNA and tend to be intermediate in size between white cells and epithelial cells. Thus a large fraction of the abnormal cells display fluorescence and scatter intensities well separated from signals produced by the majority of the normal cells. These signals are localized to a region of the histogram to the right of the main peaks in fluorescence intensity and between them in scatter intensity. By sorting from this area a 10- to 20-fold enrichment of abnormal cells can be obtained for microscopic analysis. However, since some signals from normal cells and aggregates also appear in this region, this technique of automated diagnosis of cervical carcinoma is not completely reliable. To increase the potential accuracy of automated cytologic diagnosis, a new independent marker correlated with cellular abnormality must be included as a third parameter in the analysis. (Courtesy of Dr. Ronald J. Hensen, Lawrence Livermore Laboratory, University of California, Livermore, California)

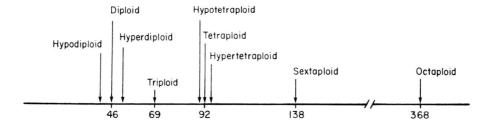

Number of Chromosomes

FIGURE 36-8. Designation of ploidy patterns in human tissues as a function of the number of chromosomes (see also Chapter 35). The diploid peak is often designated as 2C or 2N, the tetraploid peak as 4C or 4N (cfr. Fig. 36-5A). The term *stem line* is used to designate the dominant (or most important) pattern in a complex cell population that, in tumors, may comprise several coexisting DNA ploidy designations.

with known DNA content, and hence position in the channel number of fluorescence intensity, that are added to the unknown sample. Nucleated chicken or trout erythrocytes are commonly used (see Fig. 36-9) (Shackney et al., 1979; Jakobsen, 1983; Vindelöv et al., 1983).

It is not certain whether normal human lymphocytes are a suitable control for DNA analysis of solid human tumors. They do not fulfill this role when compared with cultured human cells (Wolley et al., 1982). It is therefore preferable to obtain suitable controls from the benign component of the same tissue harboring the tumor. Such control tissues are sometimes difficult to obtain, and the results of DNA analysis may be surprising. A large study of 188 samples of benign colonic epithelium from the periphery of colons, surgically resected for carcinoma, disclosed unexpected variations in the position of the diploid peak (Wersto et al., 1988). In about 25% of the cases, the DI was below or above (by more than 10% in channel numbers) the calculated normal mean channel position. The findings were not related to the distance from the tumor or to the grade or stage of the tumor. It is likely that such observations represent individual variations in DNA content or in accessibility of DNA to fluorescent dyes. Similar variability of DI was observed in lymphocytes from different donors by Mayall et al. (1984). It is evident, therefore, that variations in the position of the diploid peak must not necessarily be construed as representing DNA abnormalities, unless a series of reliable control measurements has been conducted. Otherwise, claims of abnormality may be invalid. It is recommended that the control sample be obtained from the same patient and, preferably, from the same tissue, from which the unknown sample is derived.

The difficulty of obtaining adequate controls is enhanced in measuring the DNA content in archival, formalin-fixed, and paraffin-embedded tissues. Probably the best way of securing control samples is by attempting to identify within the same tissue block an area of clearly benign component and measure its DNA content on the assumption that it is diploid. The assumption may or may not be correct.

Quality of Histograms

Several mathematical calculations are commonly used to evaluate the quality of flow cytometric measurements. These are the coefficient of variation (CV), skewness, and kurtosis.

The Coefficient of Variation

CV is a measure of tightness of the curve in the first left peak of the histogram of fluorescence intensity. CV is determined by dividing the mean channel position (channel number) by its standard deviation, obtained by multiple measurements. The result is expressed as a percentage. CV can be determined on the full width of the peak or on half-width by dividing the peak in two by means of a vertical line. The smaller the CV, the tighter the curve. For example, theoretically, the measurements of DNA content of inactive lymphocytes should all fall into one channel, such as channel 50 (see Fig. 36-5), and the standard deviation of this measurement should be zero. In this purely theoretical situation, the value of CV = 0%. In practice CVs of less than 1% are exceptional. More commonly, a CV of 2% to 3% will be observed for inactive lymphocytes or internal controls. For less homogeneous cell populations, such as human tumors, the CVs are often much larger, from 4% to 6%. If the CV is very large, that is, greater than 7% or 8%, the peak may be composed of two or more populations of cells that cannot be resolved in the machine. Very large CVs, of 10% or more, are not considered acceptable and are likely to represent tumor heterogeneity or deterioration of the DNA measurement system, owing to either sample failure or machine failure.

Skewness

In histograms with a CV of 3% or more, the shape of the curve (skewness) becomes important. If the peak is symmetrical, that is, if both arms are equidistant from the center, it is nearly certain that the peak represents a single population. If the position of the two arms of the peak is asymetrical, that is, one arm is more distant from the center than the other, the skewness of the peak is high and the possibility of the presence of two overlapping cell populations must be considered. Skewness of the histogram is also important in cell cycle analysis (see below).

Kurtosis

Kurtosis is a statistical function providing information on the shape of the peak, that is, whether it is sharp or flattened. Deviations from an integer value of 3 or more indicate a flat peak (decrease in peakedness). The value of kurtosis can be determined only by an appropriate analytical computer program.

As mentioned, in virtually any measurement of human tissues or cells, there are deviations from the hypothetical normal that cannot be explained at this time. The clinical significance of these variations is unknown at this time (1991).

Cell Cycle by DNA Analysis

One of the common applications of flow cytometry is the analysis of cell cycle in an unknown cell population. Much of the information available today is based on measurements of exponentially growing tissue cultures and stimulated lymphocytes. The information thus obtained has been applied to other human tissues, but the value of this comparison remains uncertain and should undergo further scrutiny (see below).

As discussed in Chapter 6, actively growing cells, particularly cells in culture, undergo a number of changes during the events of the cell cycle, during which the DNA of the mother cell doubles. These changes can be roughly identified by measuring DNA in a cell population, and the histogram of flow cytometric measurement can be divided into the three basic cell cycle compartments: G_1, S, and G_2 + M (see Fig. 6-1). The DNA content of normal dividing (G_1), or nondividing, quiescent (G_0) cells is representative of the diploid or 2C (or 2N) modal chromosome number of somatic cells (see Fig. 36-5). During the S (synthesis) phase of the cell cycle, there occurs a duplication of DNA to ensure that each daughter cell will receive a full complement of the genetic material of the mother cell. Thus, during the ensuing G_2 and M phases of the cycle, the DNA content of the cells will be double that in G_0/G_1 phases of the cycle (4C or 4N). Fig. 36-5A shows a typical DNA distribution of exponentially growing cultured cells. The first peak on the left represents the G_0/G_1 population, the smaller peak to the right the G_2 + M populations. The S-phase cells are residing in between these two peaks. An analysis of the histogram into each of the cell cycle compartments, using a computer model, is shown in Fig. 36-5B. The cell cycle distribution in a human diploid mammary carcinoma is shown in Fig. 36-9A. The similarities of the cell distribution between Figs. 36-6A and 36-9A are evident, except for a much lower S-phase compartment in the human epithelial sample, suggesting a lower replication rate. The significance of S-phase cells in the human tissue samples is discussed below.

Additional information about the cell cycle distribution can be obtained with the use of the metachromatic dye, acridine orange (AO), which binds to DNA and RNA in a different fashion. Under stoichiometric conditions, binding of AO to DNA results in green fluorescence and binding to RNA results in red fluorescence, allowing for synchronous measurements of the two cell components (Darzynkiewicz et al., 1980, 1982; Darzynkiewicz, 1983). Fig. 36-6 illustrates the typical distribution of DNA versus RNA content of an exponentially growing cell population in culture. The distribution shows that cells in the G_1 phase contain variable amounts of RNA. Arbitrarily, such cells can be divided into two groups: a group with low levels of RNA (group A) and a group with high levels of RNA (group B). It has been postulated that cells must accumulate high levels of RNA before they can enter the S phase of the cycle, and hence begin the synthesis of DNA (Darzynkiewicz, 1983). Similar observations have been made in reference to total protein content. This technique also disclosed that in some situations the noncycling cells with low RNA content may have a DNA content typical

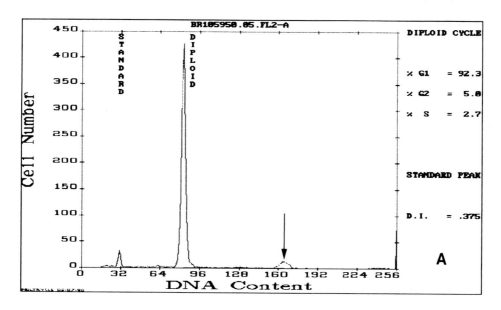

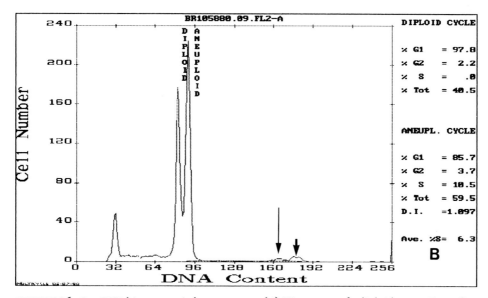

FIGURE 36–9. DNA histograms in breast cancer. (*A*) Histograms of a diploid tumor. Formalin-fixed calf thymocytes were used as internal control (left small peak in channel 32 identified as standard). The G_0G_1 peak, located at channel 90 of this instrument, contained 92.3% of all cells, and the coefficient of variation (CV) of the measurement was 2.1%, very low for human tumor samples. The small G_2 peak (*arrow*) is located in channel position 170, hence somewhat below the anticipated position in channel 180. A small proportion of cells (2.7%) were contained between the two peaks. Computer analysis of the cell cycle compartments is displayed to the right of the histogram. (*B*) Histogram of an aneuploid tumor in which the *DNA* index (DI) of the aneuploid hyperdiploid cell population was only a few channels distant from the diploid peak (DI = 1.097). The CV of the diploid peak was a very low 1.7%. With a larger CV the second peak would have been difficult to identify. Both the diploid and hyperdiploid (aneuploid) cell populations were cycling, and therefore the histograms show two G_2M peaks, one corresponding to the diploid cell population (*long arrow*) and one corresponding to the hyperdiploid cell population (*short arrow*). Internal controls standard (calf thymocytes) is shown in channel 32. A computer analysis of the cell cycle in the diploid and aneuploid cell population is shown to the right of the histogram. (Histograms courtesy of Dr. Robert Wersto, Bethesda, Md.)

of S or G_2 cells. It is assumed that these cells are noncycling cells with abnormally high DNA content, perhaps cells not progressing normally through the cell cycle. It is thus possible that cells are not equally endowed at birth: some, with high levels of RNA, are destined to re-enter the cell cycle without a pause, and others, with low levels of RNA, linger as G_0 cells, perhaps as a reserve population. It is of interest, as shown by us, that the distribution of several oncogene products and tumor-associated antigens in some human cancer cell lines follows the pattern of RNA and protein distribution across the cell cycle (Czerniak et al., 1984, 1987).

Another method of analysis of the S phase of the cell cycle is based on incorporation of bromodeoxyuridine (BrdU) into cycling cells. BrdU replaces the thymidine molecule during the replication of DNA, and thus its presence indicates cells replicating their DNA. With the use of a monoclonal antibody to BrdU, the proportion of S-phase cells can be determined (Gratzner, 1982). Several modalities of this technique have been described (summary in Gray and Mayall, 1985; Schutte et al., 1987; Rabinovitch et al., 1988). Unfortunately, the addition of BrdU to cycling cells is possible only in a tissue culture system because its incorporation into other types of cell suspension or tissue fragments yields insecure results. Attempts have been made, mainly in Japan, to inject BrdU into patients before harvesting cells for purposes of cell cycle analysis. This practice is not recommended until the toxicity and appropriate dosage of the drug are better defined.

Cell Cycle in Normal Human Cells

Direct cell cycle analysis of human cells is relatively simple in suspensions of lymphocytes and other hematopoietic cells. The DNA analysis usually results in "clean" DNA histograms in which there is a clear-cut distribution of cell cycle compartments. Computer programs are available that calculate the percentage of cells in each cell cycle compartment (Figs. 36–5 and 36–9) (Dean and Jett, 1974; Bagwell et al., 1979; Kosugi et al., 1988).

Cell cycle analysis of benign solid human tissues is often performed as a baseline study before the DNA analysis of a malignant tumor of the same origin (see previous section on Controls). A suspension of disaggregated single cells or nuclei is required and may be very difficult to obtain if the normal tissue is fibrotic, cartilaginous, or bony. In most published studies, the "normal" was composed of a limited number of samples, usually de-

fined as "diploid." A study of 188 samples of benign colonic epithelium, mentioned previously, revealed that the histograms of cell cycle distribution were similar to those of exponentially growing cells, and hence normal. The first (G_0/G_1) peak contained approximately 90% of all cells. However, in about 25% of cases, the position of the diploid peak varied from the mean by more than 10% in channel numbers (Wersto et al., 1988). Cell cycle analysis of human tumors is discussed below.

DNA PLOIDY IN HUMAN TUMORS

With the introduction of quantitative analytic techniques in the 1940s, DNA measurements in populations of cells of solid malignant human tumors disclosed that in most, but not nearly all of them, the DNA content is abnormal, corresponding to chromosomal abnormalities (see Chapters 5 and 7).

The terminology describing such tumors is based on the interpretation of histograms of DNA distribution (see Fig. 36–8). Human tumors can be divided into two major groups: diploid and aneuploid. If the main peak of the DNA histogram centers on the 2C region and the overall DNA distribution is similar to that of normal somatic cells, the tumor is classified as a diploid or, better, *diploid-range* tumor (see Fig. 36–9A). By contrast, DNA histograms with an anomalous position of the first major peak or the presence of one or more anomalous peaks not corresponding in channel position or number of cells to the cell cycle distribution of normal diploid cells are considered to be nondiploid or *aneuploid* (see Fig. 36–9B). Nondiploid distribution patterns can be either *unimodal*, with one major cell population having an abnormal DNA content, or *multimodal* or *mosaic*, with several distinct abnormal cell populations differing in their DNA contents (Figs. 36–9B and 36–10). Quite often, a cell population with an abnormal DNA content accompanies another population in the diploid range (see Fig. 36–10). If the abnormal cell populations are cycling, several G_2+M peaks in abnormal positions may also be observed (see Fig. 36–9B). The validity of the observations depends to a large extent on the adequacy of the sample and the excellence of the preparatory technique. It is generally accepted that a flow cytometric histogram composed of less than 5,000 cells is not adequate and not necessarily representative of the abnormality.

Another important issue in reference to solid

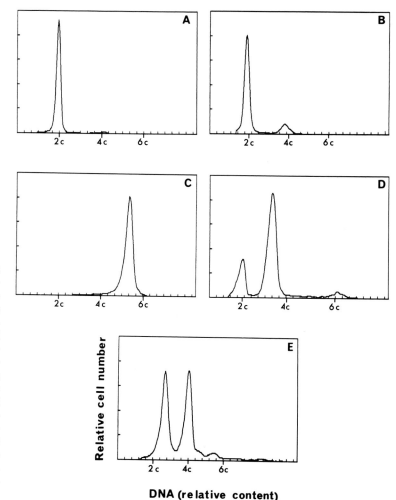

FIGURE 36-10. DNA distribution patterns in benign and malignant prostate lesions. (*A*) DNA histogram of benign prostatic hyperplasia with the major peak in the 2c region corresponding to G_0/G_1 cells. The small second peak in the 4c region represents $G_2 + M$ cells. (*B*) Diploid carcinoma with a DNA distribution pattern similar to that of benign tissue. (*C*) Aneuploid carcinoma with unimodal DNA distribution pattern. (*D*) Aneuplid carcinoma with one diploid (normal) and one heteroploid (abnormal) cell population. (*E*) Aneuploid carcinoma with a mosaic pattern of two heteroploid (abnormal) cell populations.

human tumors is the number of samples. Many solid tumors are complex and may show a different DNA distribution in different samples. In a study of colon cancer, performed in this laboratory, a single diploid-range sample carried with it an error of about 20%. In other words, in almost one quarter of the tumors judged to be in the diploid range on a single sample, additional sampling would have disclosed nondiploid DNA patterns (Wersto et al., 1991).

A further comment pertains to a comparison of fresh samples and samples embedded in paraffin. As discussed on p. 1618, in a large study of colonic cancer based on 335 samples, there was a loss of aneuploidy in 19% of the paraffin-embedded samples, presumably because of poor preservation or destruction of larger nuclei. On the other hand, in 3% of the samples, the paraffin-embedded material showed aneuploidy patterns not seen in fresh tissue, presumably because of sampling of a somewhat different region of the tumor. An incomplete survival analysis of these patients suggested that, using paraffin-embedded samples, a significant survival bias in favor of the diploid-range samples would prevail. This example shows how difficult it is to correlate DNA ploidy patterns with clinical data. Similar large studies have not been performed on cancers of other organs. It is therefore possible that many reported studies based on archival paraffin blocks may not necessarily represent the true ploidy of the tumors studied, although the differences in DNA content and distribution between diploid-range and aneuploid tumors are generally considered to be of biologic and clinical significance. This matter is discussed further below.

Interpretation of DNA Histograms

The principles of histogram interpretation based on cell cycle compartments and the DNA index have been generally applied to the interpretation of DNA histograms in human tumors as well. These principles are applicable to some tumors with a clean, well-defined histogram and low coefficient of variation (see Fig. 36–9). Still, this type of analysis has major limitations.

Currently available flow cytometers can resolve two cell populations in the G_1 peak, provided there is at least a 4% difference in DNA content between them (see Fig. 36–9B). Thus, karyotype abnormalities pertaining to one or two chromosomes usually cannot be detected by this method in commercially available machines. In fact, chromosomal hybridization studies by in situ hybridization documented that in bladder tumors with diploid DNA content, extra chromosomes 1 and 18 may be found (Hopman et al., 1988). Although it may be argued that the chromosomal probes used in this work were not fully reliable, further work along these lines is likely to confirm the presence of chromosomal abnormalities in many diploid-range malignant tumors and in some benign tumors as well (see also Chapters 5 and 7 and Fig. 5–8). Further, DNA studies of diploid tumors do not account for molecular abnormalities such as translocations that are not reflected in DNA quantitation. For example, a Burkitt's lymphoma may have a diploid DNA content that will not shed light on the translocation between chromosomes 8 and 14 (see Chaps. 2 and 7). Similar comments are applicable to many forms of leukemia. Thus, the classification of tumors as diploid is, at best, a biologic approximation.

These difficulties are compounded in tumors with abnormal DNA content. In such tumors the correlation between numerical abnormalities of chromosomes and flow cytometric DNA content disclosed a rough correspondence between the two sets of data (Barlogie et al., 1987; Coon et al., 1986). Similar correlations were observed by Atkin and others with regard to chromosomal number and Feulgen cytophotometry in tumors of the female genital tract (summary in Atkin, 1984). Unfortunately, the technical difficulties in cytogenetic analysis of solid human tumors, described in detail in Chapter 7, account for the fact that such studies are few in number and limited. Further, the mere correlation between chromosomal numbers and DNA values sheds little light on the molecular mechanisms in primary or secondary chromosomal abnormalities.

Position of the Diploid Peak

In practice, the interpretation of the histograms of human tumors may be very difficult. Truly diploid histograms in which the DNA distribution and CV are precisely the same as those of control lymphocytes or control benign cells of the same origin (DI = 1.0, CV = 2% to 3%) are rare (see Fig. 36–9A). As described, even with normal tissues shifts in position of the G_0/G_1 peak by 10% (in channel numbers) and sometimes slightly more may occur. For example, if the G_0/G_1 of channel position of control cells is 50, positions from 45 to 55 are often considered to be within normal limits. These assumptions are not well documented because the reasons for these shifts are not clear. They may reside in packaging of chromatin, individual variations in the binding of the fluorochromes to DNA, techniques of cell or nuclear preparation, or perhaps other, not yet understood factors (Wersto et al., 1988).

Distribution of Cells in Cell Cycle Compartments

A truly diploid G_0/G_1 peak of cycling cells should contain about 90% of the cells, and the remaining cells should be approximately evenly distributed between the S and G_2+M compartments (see Fig. 36–9A). The question of interpretation of samples that contain less than 90% of the cells in the G_0/G_1 peak has not been satisfactorily resolved, and the lower limit of acceptability has not been objectively established. Melamed et al. proposed that the limit of normal for samples of bladder washings is 85% of cells in the G_0/G_1 compartment of the histogram. Samples with fewer than 85% of cells in the first peak of the histogram were considered "abnormal" (Devonec et al., 1982; Klein et al., 1982). Others who followed the same arbitrary definition observed a large proportion of samples with "abnormal" DNA patterns in the absence of tumors. The reported rate of such false-positive measurements was 38% (deVere White et al., 1986) and 28% (Murphy et al., 1986). We have shown in a comparative study that about 20% of DNA histograms considered to be in the diploid range by flow cytometry contained aneuploid cell populations as documented by image cytometry and that this observation was of clinical value (Koss et al., 1989) (see Fig. 35–16). Similar results were previously obtained in our laboratories with DNA measurements in cancerous effusions (Schneller et al., 1987). Clearly, for each organ or organ system a large series of control measurements may be required, before the precise level of normal range can be defined.

If the second (G_2+M) peak of a diploid histogram exceeds 5% of the cell population, a new dilemma must be faced: does this peak represent an aneuploid cell population, doublets (i.e., two nuclei stuck together), or merely a polyploid pattern that is either permanent or transient? After all, polyploidy is known to occur in normal tissues, such as liver, which has a large proportion of tetraploid and even octaploid cells (Mendecki et al., 1978).

Depending on the organ studied, cell sample, preparatory techniques, instrument, or skill of the operator, the frequency of histograms difficult to interpret may be high or low. The clinical significance of borderline DNA patterns must yet be established and may be organ or tissue dependent. In samples containing a large proportion of benign cells, small populations of aneuploid cells may not be detected by routine flow cytometric measurements. Such populations can be identified by cytophotometric measurement of Feulgen-stained selected cells under visual control (Cornelisse and van Driel-Kulker, 1985; Strang et al., 1985; Stal et al., 1986; Schneller et al., 1987; Koss et al., 1989). Therefore, in laboratories equipped with flow and static cytophotometric systems, the measurements of DNA should be performed by both techniques to enhance the accuracy of tumor classification based on DNA distribution patterns.

S-Phase Analysis

In many studies attempts have been made to use flow cytometric cell cycle analysis, mainly the calculation of the proportion of S-phase cells, to predict the clinical behavior of human tumors. The assumption of these studies is that the percentage of cells synthesizing DNA (S-phase cells) is a direct reflection of tumor proliferation, and hence aggressive behavior (Terz et al., 1971; Bauer et al., 1986; Christensson et al., 1986). The calculation of S-phase cells by computer programs is again relatively simple with "clean" histograms with low CV and low skewness of the first peak. The assessment is much more complicated in histograms with high CV and high skewness of the peak(s).

In such histograms the separation of S-phase cells from a slanting G_0/G_1 and the G_2+M peaks is often quite arbitrary and based on visual assessment of the histogram by the placement of

markers. Two methods of analysis are illustrated in Fig. 36–11. It is evident that different S values will be obtained depending on the judgment of the analyst and the analytic method employed. Furthermore, computation of the proportion of S-phase cells, especially in highly aneuploid tumors in which several cycling populations may overlap each other, is still more difficult and far from accurate.

The other dilemma is the possibility that cells with a DNA content in the S-phase area are not cycling, whether dead or alive. The discovery, in experimental cell systems, of noncycling cells with the DNA content corresponding to the S-phase cells (S_q cells) strongly supports this possibility (Darzynkiewicz et al., 1983, 1986). As discussed, in experimental cell systems, proliferating cells can be identified by the use of techniques based on BrdU incorporation. Proliferation antigens such as the one recognized by the antigen Ki-67 may also be used for this purpose (Wersto et al., 1988). The efficacy of these approaches to solid human tissues must still be determined, although the use of Ki-67 in breast cancer and other tumors is widespread (see Chapter 35). Unfortunately, incorporation of tritiated thymidine (3H), which in experienced hands defines the S-phase component in solid human tumors (Meyer et al., 1978; Meyer, 1986), is not applicable to flow cytometry. Preliminary data suggest, however, that the thymidine labeling index is roughly comparable to the S-phase cell fraction measured by flow cytometry in suitable targets (Meyer and Coplin, 1988).

Regardless of these difficulties, several studies on record document that an increase in the proportion of S-phase cells in some human tumors may be related to malignant behavior, mainly in leukemias and lymphomas (Holdrinet et al., 1983; Ffrench et al., 1987; Riccardi et al., 1986). In solid human tumors, similar correlations were suggested for mammary carcinoma (McGuire, 1989; Sigurdsson, 1990), particularly for low-stage, diploid tumors (Clark et al., 1989). However, there are also reports of highly malignant tumors with relatively low proliferation rates and poor prognosis, thus casting doubt on the universal value of S-phase analysis as the predictor of the clinical behavior of all human tumors (Frankfurt et al., 1984; Volm et al., 1988; Hedley et al., 1987). Therefore, although flow cytometric cell cycle analysis is a powerful tool for studying cell proliferation characteristics in experimental systems, its application for clinical purposes (i.e., assessment of tumor behavior) cannot be considered conclusive at the time of this writing (1991).

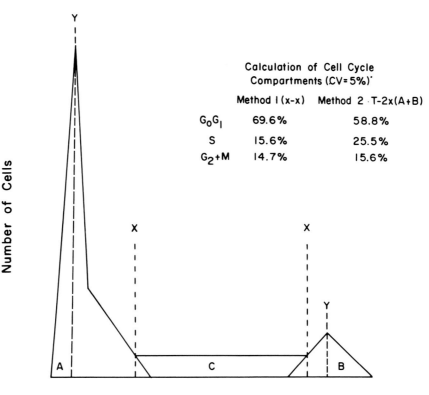

FIGURE 36–11. A theoretical geometric DNA histogram showing the distribution of cells in the phases of the cell cycle with a right "shoulder" in the G_0/G_1 peak. The CV of the $G_0 G_1$ peak was defined at 5%. The proportion of cells in S phase, expressed as a percentage of the area of the histogram, depends on the location and/or overlap of this fraction into the G_0/G_1 or $G_2 + M$ fractions and can be estimated in two ways. One approach assumes no overlap between the cell cycle boundaries (at the cut-off points indicated as X) and calculates the overlap of G_0/G_1 and $G_2 + M$ as a part of the S fraction. The second method is based on the assumption that the true G_0/G_1 component is hidden in the slanted peak and is best estimated by drawing a vertical divider (Y) and multiplying area A by 2. The same procedure is used for the $G_2 + M$ peak (area B). The formula used for the second calculation is total area of histogram (T) $- 2 \times$ (A + B). The difference in the calculated proportion of cells in the S cell cycle compartment may be quite substantial depending on the method used: using the first method the S fraction is 15.6%; with the second method it is 25.5%.

DNA PLOIDY AS A PROGNOSTIC FACTOR IN HUMAN CANCER

A great many studies on the application of flow cytometric DNA measurements to human tumors have been published. Even though few of these studies address the issues of histogram interpretation, the general trend has been to classify human cancers as diploid or aneuploid. Generally, tumors

with modal patterns close to diploid appear to have a more favorable prognosis than tumors with tetraploid, aneuploid, or mosaic DNA distribution. Normal or near-normal DNA modes often correlate with a high degree of histologic differentiation. However, the diagnostic and prognostic significance of DNA distribution patterns depends on the primary site of origin of a given tumor and its histologic type. Further, most of the studies published were retrospective and based either on studies of archival aspiration smears by image cytometry or on processing of paraffin blocks by image or flow cytometry. As discussed, the precise value of these measurements, when compared with those of fresh tissues, has not been adequately established, and for many organs and tumor types, prospective studies are still needed to confirm the predictive value of DNA analysis. The possible clinical value of these measurements is summarized in Table 36–3. The value judgments expressed are the author's and should not be considered binding. A brief summary of the principal observations follows, according to the listing in Table 36–3.

Tumors with Strong Correlation of Prognosis with DNA Patterns

Carcinoma of the Bladder and Related Tumors

The DNA content of epithelial tumors and neoplastic conditions of the urinary bladder has been extensively studied by flow cytometry, notably by

Tribukait et al. (Tribukait et al., 1982; Gustafson et al., 1982; Tribukait, 1984; Tribukait, 1987). In retrospective and prospective studies, it was shown that there is an excellent correlation between DNA ploidy patterns, histologic classification, and behavior, and hence prognosis, of most tumors. Grade I papillary tumors unlikely to progress to invasive cancer are, for the most part, diploid. Grade III tumors, nonpapillary carcinoma in situ and deeply invasive carcinomas are for the most part aneuploid. The grade II tumors are about equally divided into diploid and aneuploid tumors, suggesting that this group of tumors is heterogeneous. Distribution of DNA ploidy pattern by tumor stage documented that diploid-range tumors, though capable of recurrences, are not likely to progress to invasive and metastatic cancer, although exceptions to this rule have been noted. Highly aneuploid tumors of the bladder have a strong propensity to progress to invasive and metastatic growth. A small proportion of grade II and III tumors had a predominantly tetraploid DNA distribution, and this pattern appears to express an intermediate grade of clinical malignancy, with a high recurrence rate and moderate invasive tendencies.

Table 36–3
Value of DNA Ploidy as Prognostic Factor In Selected Groups of Human Tumors

Primary Site and Type of Tumor	Relationship to Prognosis	Favorable DNA Pattern
Bladder carcinoma	Strong	Diploid
Prostatic carcinoma	Strong	Diploid
Ovarian carcinoma	Strong	Diploid
Endometrial carcinoma	Strong	Diploid
Cutaneous melanoma	Probable	Diploid
Breast carcinoma	Probable	Diploid
Colorectal carcinoma	Probable	Diploid
Sarcoma	Probable	Diploid
Nephroblastoma	Probable	Diploid
Germ cell tumor	Probable	Diploid
Oncocytoma	Probable	Diploid
Brain tumor	Probable	Diploid
Lung carcinoma	Weak	Diploid
Renal carcinoma	Weak	Diploid
Cervical carcinoma	Weak	Diploid?
Squamous carcinoma of head and neck	Weak	Aneuploid
Thyroid carcinoma	None	—
Gastric carcinoma	None	—
Lymphoma and leukemia	Varies with type of tumor and patient's age	Varies with type of tumor and patient's age

Thus, DNA ploidy in urothelial tumors is rather well correlated with potential for invasion and metastases, previously established by histologic and clinical studies, and clarifies the unpredictable behavior of grade II tumors (see also Chap. 23).

It must be noted, however, that the term "diploid" in reference to bladder tumors does not necessarily reflect a normal chromosomal content. As has been shown by Hopman et al. (1988) by in situ hybridization technique, multiple copies of chromosomes 1 and 18 may be observed in the nuclei of such tumors (see Fig. 5–8). As probes to other chromosomes become available, it may be anticipated that other chromosomal abnormalities will be observed. For further discussion of this issue, see p. 132.

Within recent years it has been proposed that measuring DNA in bladder washings or barbotage by flow cytometry is a superior method of monitoring patients with bladder tumors (Devonec et al., 1982; Klein et al., 1982). A series of papers documented that DNA pattern analysis provides information similar to that from the cytologic examination of the sediment of voided urine and provides reliable guidance in patients treated by immunotherapy for flat carcinoma in situ of the bladder (Melamed, 1984; Melamed and Klein, 1984; Badalament et al., 1986, 1987). Histogram interpretation in this material and the avoidance of false-positive results were discussed previously. It is also difficult to obtain adequate bladder washing specimens with a sufficient number of cells for a reliable analysis from patients who are not under anesthesia and who may have significant discomfort during the procedure. The value of bladder washings as a replacement for the customary monitoring methods (i.e., cytology and cystoscopy) has not been settled, and the procedure must be considered experimental at this time (Koss et al., 1989).

It is of interest that DNA distribution patterns in bladder tumors were correlated with the results of cytology of voided urine samples: diploid-range tumors are extremely unlikely to shed cells that could be recognized as abnormal, whereas cells derived from tetraploid and aneuploid tumors are readily recognized as cancer cells (see Chapter 23). Some ultrastructural features and tumor antigen expression could also be correlated with DNA ploidy. Aneuploid bladder carcinomas have higher density and higher total number of nuclear pores, suggesting an increased rate of nuclear and cytoplasmic exchange in this group of tumors (Czerniak et al., 1984). With the use of flow cytometric measurements it was also shown that aneuploid bladder carcinoma cells have an increased proportion of Ca antigen (epitectin) binding cells, when compared with diploid tumors (Czerniak et al., 1985). It is not clear at present, however, whether these ancillary findings represent information of prognostic value, above and beyond DNA ploidy. In most recent work from this laboratory, molecular techniques have been applied in an attempt to further subclassify the diploid and nondiploid tumors of the bladder according to the codon substitution in the Ha-*ras* oncogene (Czerniak et al. 1990).

Prostatic Carcinoma

In prospective and retrospective studies the overall prognosis for prostatic carcinomas with DNA ploidy pattern in the diploid range appears to be significantly better than that for aneuploid tumors (Koss, 1988). For technical reasons, flow cytometry and image cytometry of cells in prostatic aspirates have been used in such studies. DNA ploidy in prostatic carcinoma has an interesting, and possibly important, relationship to clinical stage: most tumors in stage A appear to be diploid, whereas most tumors in stages C and D are aneuploid or tetraploid. Tumors in stage B appear to be intermediate between these two groups. It is of interest that even in stages C and D the relatively uncommon diploid tumors appear to be less aggressive than aneuploid tumors (Stephenson et al., 1987; Winkler et al., 1988). It has been postulated that few diploid tumors of low stage will progress to metastatic cancer, accounting for the large proportion of occult prostatic cancers observed in autopsy material of elderly men. The correlation of ploidy with Gleason's histologic grading is, at best, adequate for low- and high-grade tumors; it fails for the common, intermediate-grade carcinomas.

Additional evidence for the prognostic value of DNA ploidy is provided by studies of patients with prostatic carcinoma in whom the combination of ploidy values with histologic grading was used to predict which patients would die from their tumors and which patients would die from other causes (Lundberg et al., 1987). In another retrospective study it was documented that only 15% of diploid tumors progressed locally or metastasized, whereas 75% of the tumors with abnormal DNA distribution patterns progressed during the follow-up period, ranging from 5 to 19 years; none of the patients with diploid tumors died of prostatic carcinoma during the period of observation (Fordham et al., 1986).

The clinical implications of these observations are significant, particularly for patients with incidentally discovered prostatic cancers. The selection of such patients for treatment may be facilitated by establishing DNA patterns of their tumors.

Carcinoma of the Ovary

In retrospective studies of ovarian carcinoma, DNA ploidy was repeatedly shown to be a major determinant of survival. The survival rates of patients with diploid or near-diploid carcinomas were significantly better than those of women with aneuploid tumors (Friedlander et al., 1983, 1984, 1988; Blumenfeld et al., 1987). In a retrospective study of paraffin-embedded tissues, the relative risk of death was shown to be twofold higher for tumors with a single aneuploid DNA mode and sixfold higher for tumors with mosaic aneuploidy when compared with near-diploid tumors. Tetraploid tumors exhibited low-risk ratio, whereas hypertetraploid tumors were clinically aggressive with a high risk of death from disease (Iverson, 1988). DNA ploidy correlated to some extent with stage of disease. In one study, all advanced carcinomas were aneuploid, whereas only 40% of early-stage tumors had aneuploid cell populations (Friedlander et al., 1983). It was also shown that diploid DNA pattern is associated with good prognosis only in reference to tumors in stage III and below, whereas stage IV tumors had a poor prognosis irrespective of DNA ploidy (Friedlander et al., 1988). In reference to histologic grading, diploid DNA modes correlated well with low or borderline tumor types (Friedlander, 1984). This information correlates well with that from cytophotometric studies conducted by Atkin (1984) and with information derived from histologic classification and grading of ovarian carcinomas (see Chapter 16). Although there is still a need for a large prospective flow cytometric study with extensive sampling of tumors, the accumulated evidence is not controversial since it correlates well with other known prognostic parameters.

Endometrial Carcinoma

The information about endometrial carcinoma is based mainly on retrospective studies, most conducted by cytophotometry (summary in Atkin, 1984) and a very few by flow cytometry (Geisinger et al., 1986; Iversen, 1986; Lindahl et al., 1987). In general, the survival rates of patients with diploid or near-diploid endometrial carcinomas were significantly better than those of women with aneuploid tumors. Aneuploidy was observed predominantly in poorly differentiated tumors, whereas well-differentiated tumors were predominantly diploid. Tumors of intermediate degrees of differentiation were for the most part diploid. DNA ploidy could also be correlated with disease stage: high-stage tumors were for the most part aneuploid, particularly in advanced disease (stage IV tumors), suggesting that aneuploid tumors have a greater tendency to progress. Approximately 60% to 70% of all endometrial carcinomas responding to progesterone therapy were shown to be diploid. As with ovarian cancer, data on DNA ploidy show good correlation with other known prognostic parameters, such as tumor grade, stage, and response to progestational agents. Still, a large, long-term prospective study should be performed to confirm the retrospective data.

Human Cancers with Probable but Not Definite Correlation with DNA Ploidy Patterns

Carcinoma of the Breast

The first fundamental retrospective study of the value of DNA ploidy in the prognosis of mammary carcinoma was presented by Auer et al. (1980). Breast tumors were classified into four major groups according to cytophotometric DNA distribution patterns in aspiration biopsy smears (see Chap. 35). The groups ranged from diploid tumors (group I) with good ten-year survival to tumors with pronounced aneuploidy and survival of less than two years (group IV). Groups II and III represented tumors with tetraploid or a combination of tetraploid and diploid DNA modes exhibiting an intermediate degree of clinical malignancy (see Fig. 35–15). The initial observations were confirmed by Fallenius et al. (1988). In another cytophotometric study by the same group, Fallenius et al. (1984) documented that clinically occult small mammary carcinomas discovered by stereotactic mammography are for the most part diploid. Diploid tumors were also reported to have a high level of estrogen receptors. Hence, it is concluded that diploid mammary cancers have a better prognosis than aneuploid tumors.

Breast cancer is, however, a complex chronic disease, and the evidence presented by the Swedish group clearly required confirmation by further retrospective and prospective studies. Several such studies using flow cytometry have been published (Olszewski et al., 1981; Coulson et al., 1984; Thorud et al., 1986; McGuire, 1989; Clark et al., 1989; Sigurdsson et al., 1990). In general, these studies suggested that tumors in the diploid range were better differentiated (inasmuch as this histologic parameter can be applied to mammary carcinoma), have a high level of estrogen receptors, and appear to be somewhat less aggressive over the short term (5 years) than aneuploid tumors. On the other hand, the studies are contradictory in reference to the correlation of the DNA ploidy patterns with stage of disease, lymph node status, relapse rate, long-term significance, and other clinical factors such as age at diagnosis. Bacus et al. (1990) pointed out that the expression of HER-2/*neu* oncogene is associated mainly with tetraploid tumors and not with either diploid or aneuploid cancers. Clark et al. (1989) observed a good correlation of elevated S-phase fraction with aggressive disease patterns in diploid, low-stage cancers. This observation was in keeping with prior data by Meyer (1978, 1986). See also the comments on "breast profile" in Chapter 35.

A major, well-controlled prospective study with multiparameter analysis of the many known prognostic factors is obviously still needed before DNA ploidy in breast cancer can be accepted as an independent prognostic variable. Until such time, the value of DNA measurements in mammary carcinoma must be considered experimental, although it is likely that this parameter may enhance the value of other prognostic parameters of documented clinical value such as tumor size, presence or absence of metastases, and family history of breast cancer.

Cutaneous Melanomas

In several retrospective studies of cutaneous melanomas, DNA ploidy apparently correlated with survival and recurrence rate and, to some extent, with the stage of disease (Sondergaard et al., 1983; von Roenn et al., 1986; Coon et al., 1987). In one report, aneuploidy was seen only in Clark's level IV and V lesions (von Roenn et al., 1986). In another study, aneuploidy was shown to be a bad prognostic sign in stage I melanoma, suggesting a high tendency for recurrence (Coon et al., 1987). Aneuploidy in skin melanoma appeared to correlate strongly with recurrence and shorter disease-free intervals. For tumors stratified by thickness, DNA ploidy was the most significant independent prognostic factor among all commonly recognized parameters (Coon et al., 1987). In more recent studies, this evidence was questioned, and the results must be considered tentative. A prospective study is still needed to confirm the DNA data reported so far. It remains to be seen whether the DNA ploidy information is an acceptable guide to treatment, above and beyond the established histologic and clinical criteria.

Colorectal Carcinoma

The first prospective study on the value of DNA ploidy measurements in colonic carcinoma was published from this laboratory on a group of 33 patients observed for up to five years (Wolley et al., 1982). There was a remarkable difference in behavior between tumors in the diploid range of DNA and aneuploid tumors, regardless of stage of disease. The patients with diploid-range tumors had few recurrences and, even in the presence of metastases, occasional long-term survival. All but one patient with aneuploid tumors died of disease within three years. Subsequent unpublished follow-up data on the survivors confirmed that patients with diploid-range tumors continued to live longer, and after six years, half of them were free of disease. Unfortunately, the group of patients was too small to warrant statistical analysis. There is but one other prospective study (Melamed et al., 1986) in which another group of 33 patients with rectal carcinoma was observed for three years; the study failed to disclose significant differences in pattern of metastases or survival according to DNA ploidy patterns. More recently, several major retrospective studies found a statistically significant relationship between near-diploid DNA modes and better prognosis of patients with carcinoma of the large bowel and rectum (Armitage et al., 1985; Kokal et al., 1986). The differing results make it difficult to assess at this time the prospective value of DNA measurements as prognostic factors in colorectal carcinomas. A resolution of these questions requires prospective studies with a large number of patients. One such study is in progress in our laboratories.

Additional studies from this laboratory pointed out some problems with flow cytometric measurements of ploidy as a prognostic factor in colonic cancer. The issue of variation in the position of the

G_0/G_1 peak in control measurements and the loss of aneuploidy in paraffin-embedded tumor tissue when compared with fresh tissue were discussed on pp. 1626 and 1627. In my opinion, the value of ploidy determination in colon cancer remains open.

Sarcomas

In limited retrospective flow cytometric studies of primary bone and soft part sarcomas, aneuploidy was found in most malignant tumors (Kreicbergs et al., 1984; Xiang et al., 1987). It was shown that patients with diploid chondrosarcoma had a significantly longer survival than those with aneuploid tumors (Alho et al., 1983). In a recent prospective study of 26 patients with osteosarcoma, Look et al. (1988) reported that the presence of near-diploid tumor stem lines, whether or not associated with hyperdiploid (aneuploid) stem lines, was of favorable prognostic value in terms of response to chemotherapeutic agents, occurrence of metastases, and survival.

In retrospective studies, leiomyosarcomas appear to have generally better prognosis if they are near-diploid (Tsushima et al., 1987). On the other hand, studies from this laboratory (Agarval et al., 1991), disclosed aneuploid DNA patterns in several benign neoplastic and reactive soft part lesions, such as schwannoma, pseudosarcomatous fasciitis, and reparative granulomas. These observations suggest that use of DNA ploidy patterns in the assessment of the benign or malignant nature of a difficult soft part lesion is unlikely to be successful. At this time it is premature to assess the true significance of DNA ploidy as a prognostic factor in bone and soft tissue lesions.

Other Tumors

In some other human tumors DNA ploidy patterns may prove to be of prognostic value. These are listed in Table 36–3. In the rare nephroblastomas and related neoplasms of childhood and in germ cell tumors, aneuploid DNA patterns appear to be an unfavorable prognostic sign (Rainwater et al., 1987; Schmidt et al., 1986).

DNA ploidy pattern may prove to be of value in attempting to assess the behavior of some human tumors in which histologic patterns fail in this regard. Oncocytic tumors of the salivary glands, thyroid, and kidneys may belong here. In retrospective studies it was shown that salivary gland oncocytomas with benign behavior had a DNA ploidy pattern in the diploid range; none of the patients with diploid-range oncocytomas of the thyroid (Hürthle cell tumors) or the kidney died of disease. On the other hand, 58% of patients with aneuploid Hürthle cell tumors of the thyroid died of disease, and several patients with aneuploid renal oncocytomas had metastases (Rainwater et al., 1986). Although such predictions are still of limited scope, they should be pursued further.

High-grade gliomas, tumors with an extremely poor prognosis, have been shown to be aneuploid (Wolley et al., 1979; Zaprianov and Christov, 1988). Clearly, the low-grade gliomas, although diploid, are rarely curable but may be consistent with longer survival. In medulloblastoma, on the other hand, aneuploid DNA pattern was shown to be consistent with a better response of tumor to therapy (Tomita et al., 1988).

Tumors with Weak Association of DNA Ploidy with Prognosis

Carcinoma of the Lung

Lung cancer, regardless of type, is a group of diseases with highly unfavorable prognosis, except for the rare cases of small, surgically excised cancers without metastases (see Chapter 20). Hence, measuring DNA in these tumors is, at best, a matter of scientific curiosity. Still, it appears that treated squamous cell carcinomas and adenocarcinomas appear to show a somewhat better survival pattern when they are near-diploid (Bunn et al., 1983; Volm et al., 1985, 1988). However, at least 80% of these types of tumors are nondiploid. Small cell carcinomas can also be classified as near-diploid and nondiploid, and here again there appears to be some correlation of DNA ploidy to clinical behavior (Abe, 1985).

Renal Carcinomas

In retrospective studies, only about 20% of patients with diploid renal cell carcinomas had metastases compared with about 90% of those with aneuploid tumors within a follow-up period of one to four years (Otto et al., 1984). It was also shown that surgical excision of metastases in patients with diploid tumor could be of significant benefit since these patients may stay alive and free of disease for a relatively long period (Ljungberg et al., 1986). In a study of a large number of cases, it became evident that aneuploidy in renal carcinoma has significant correlation with subsequent development of metastatic disease independent of tumor grade and stage. However, in the same study, long-term (up to ten years) survival differences for the two groups of patients were not fully persuasive: 62% and 37% for diploid and aneuploid tumors, respectively (Rainwater et al., 1987). In other studies, however, the overall survival rates of patients with diploid and aneuploid tumors were not significantly different (Ekfors et al., 1987). Again, a long-term prospective study is needed to ascertain the clinical value of DNA measurements.

Carcinoma of the Uterine Cervix

Original information concerning survival rates and DNA distribution patterns in invasive epidermoid cervical carcinomas treated by radiotherapy was provided by Atkin and Richards (1962) using cytophotometry. These studies showed that in cervical carcinoma diploid DNA mode did not correlate with response to radiotherapy, and hence prognosis. On the contrary, it was shown that aneuploid-triploid tumors have a better response to radiotherapy than diploid-range tumors. These observations were confirmed by Dyson et al. (1987). Different results were obtained with flow cytometric measurements applying different criteria of tumor classification according to their DNA distribution pattern (Jakobsen, 1984). In all stages of squamous carcinoma of the cervix, aneuploid tumors had higher recurrence rates and lower survival rates when a DI above 1.5 was arbitrarily used to identify a high-risk group. In low-stage cervical carcinomas, aneuploidy correlated with a high frequency of lymph node metastases and recurrence after treatment (Jakobson, 1984). On the other hand, Rutgers et al. (1986) reported that squamous cancers of the cervix with diploid or tetraploid DNA patterns had a less favorable prognosis than nondiploid and nontetraploid tumors.

Hanselaar et al. (1988) observed that early invasive cervical carcinomas could be either diploid or aneuploid and that the same DNA pattern was observed in adjacent carcinomas in situ, presumably the source of origin of the invasive cancer. The observation was correlated with age of patients, inasmuch as aneuploid carcinomas were more prevalent in older women.

It is evident from this brief review that the prognostic value of DNA patterns in cervical carcinoma has not been fully established. Because of the current rarity of invasive cervical cancer in institutions performing flow cytometry, a prospective study on a large group of patients is unlikely, unless material could be obtained from countries with a persisting high rate of this disease. Such a study would probably suffer from inadequate follow-up information. Thus the prognostic significance of DNA ploidy in cervical cancer may remain a mystery for some time yet.

Squamous Carcinomas of the Head and Neck Area

In squamous cell carcinoma of the upper aerodigestive tract, including laryngeal carcinoma, DNA aneuploidy correlates with favorable response to treatment (Goldsmith et al., 1986, 1987; Lampe et al., 1987) as compared with diploid tumors. Another study showed that there is a high-risk correlation between abnormal DNA ploidy values and histologic abnormalities in precancerous lesions of the larynx (Bjelkenkrantz et al., 1983).

Tumors with No Evidence of Association of DNA Ploidy Value and Prognosis

Thyroid Carcinomas

In thyroid carcinomas, DNA ploidy is not a prognostic factor of value. In well-differentiated thyroid carcinomas (i.e., papillary, follicular, and medullary) diploid DNA pattern is more common than aneuploid (Johanessen et al., 1981; Tangen et al., 1983; Joensuu et al., 1986). In fact, even metastatic tumors may be diploid. On the other hand, many encapsulated follicular lesions, and hence adenomas, are aneuploid (Greenebaum et al., 1985). DNA ploidy in this group of tumors has virtually no predictive value when compared with conventional factors such as capsular invasion or lymph node status. Because of the extremely slow evolution of thyroid cancer, it is unlikely that a significant prospective study could be organized to ascertain the prognostic value of DNA ploidy measurements in this group of diseases.

Gastric Carcinomas

Advanced, invasive gastric carcinomas, regardless of histologic type and grade, represent a group of tumors with highly unfavorable prognosis. In these tumors the DNA ploidy does not correlate with response to therapy or with survival rates (Deinlein et al., 1983; Macartney et al., 1986; Odegaard et al., 1987). Early (intramucosal) gastric cancers are an exception to this rule because of a generally excellent prognosis that is not ploidy dependent. Measuring DNA in early tumors is purely a matter of scientific curiosity.

Lymphomas and Leukemias

Generally, in these types of tumor, DNA ploidy per se is not a particularly strong and independent prognostic factor. However, in several types of lymphohematopoietic disorders, DNA ploidy may be used as an ancillary method to predict clinical behavior or response to therapy (Barlogie et al., 1987). In acute lymphoblastic leukemia (ALL) of childhood, hyperdiploid (aneuploid) DNA modes correlate with favorable prognosis (Smets et al., 1985). In adult type of ALL, abnormal (hyperdiploid) DNA content correlates with compound karyologic abnormalities and is associated with shorter survival time. In contrast, patients with myelogenous leukemia with an abnormal DNA content may have a more favorable prognosis (Barlogie et al., 1987).

Several reports pointed out that in the most common types of non-Hodgkin's lymphoma aneuploidy did not correlate with age of the patients, site or stage of disease, or survival rates (Roos et al., 1985; Young et al., 1987). In some less common types of non-Hodgkin's lymphoma, such as mycosis fungoides or gastrointestinal lymphoma, DNA aneuploidy correlated with rapid progression of disease and shorter survival times (Bunn et al., 1980; Joensuu et al., 1987). It was also shown that diploid-range myelomas respond better to chemotherapy. Hypodiploid or multimodal myelomas respond poorly to chemotherapy and have significantly shorter survival rates when compared with diploid tumors (Barlogie et al., 1983). Preliminary data also suggest that the same relationship between DNA distribution patterns, survival rates, and response to therapy may exist in Burkitt's lymphoma (Lehtinen et al., 1987).

DNA Ploidy in Benign and Premalignant Lesions

DNA aneuploidy is not a feature found only in malignant tumors. Aneuploid cell populations have been found in several benign tumors of various origins and in reactive or inflammatory lesions (Agarwal et al., 1991; Deinlein et al., 1983; see also Chap. 7). Also of interest is the frequent presence of cell populations with abnormal DNA content in intraepithelial or intramucosal neoplastic lesions. Such populations have been found in some cervical intraepithelial neoplasias of the uterine cervix, regardless of grade (Jakobsen et al., 1983), skin (Newton et al., 1986), larynx (Bjelkenkrantz et al., 1983), esophagus (Reid et al., 1987), stomach (Macartney et al., 1986), and colon (Hammarberg et al., 1984; Petrova et al., 1986; Quirke et al., 1986). The prognostic clinical significance of these changes is unknown, particularly since Hanselar et al. (1988) observed invasive cervical cancer derived from diploid preinvasive lesions.

FLOW CYTOMETRIC MEASUREMENTS OF CELLULAR CONSTITUENTS OTHER THAN DNA

With the introduction of highly specific probes, such as monoclonal antibodies (MAbs), that can be labeled with fluorescent dyes and the ever-increasing sensitivity of flow cytometers, accurate quantitation of cellular components other than nucleic acids and total protein became feasible (Watson, 1987). Of particular importance in this regard is the analysis of cell surface markers that define the various subsets of lymphohematopoietic cells (Thornthwaite et al., 1984; Horan et al., 1986; Cohen et al., 1988). Thus, the flow cytometric procedures, now widely used, permit the evaluation of the patient's immunologic status and may contribute to the classification of the malignant lymphomas and leukemias. An example of an analysis is shown in Fig. 36–12, representing selected fluorescent profiles obtained with cells of a malignant lymphoma exposed to various antibodies of the Leu series. Another application of flow cytometry is the analysis of subgroups of T lymphocytes. The ratio of the helper-suppressor cells (see Chap. 34) is of value in establishing the diagnosis and in monitoring patients with acquired immunodeficiency syndrome (AIDS). The procedure is performed by means of specific fluorescent antibodies identifying the epitopes of these cells. The helper T lymphocytes are characterized by the presence of CD4 protein, which, along with other proteins, may facilitate the entry of the human immunodeficiency virus (HIV, types I and II), leading to the destruction of these cells that play a key role in the cellular immunologic response. This results in a relative increase of suppressor T cells, characterized by the presence of a CD8 protein (summary in Levy,

1989). The results of the analysis are displayed in a manner similar to that shown in Fig. 36–13.

Because of a possible contamination of the flow cytometer with HIV, a dedicated instrument should be used for these analyses under appropriate conditions in ensuring the safety of laboratory personnel.

Recently, progress has been made in extending flow cytometric measurements of surface and cytoplasmic markers in solid tumors (Valet et al., 1984; Czerniak and Koss, 1985; Czerniak et al., 1985; Fietz et al., 1985). Preliminary attempts have been made to use this approach for the identification of malignant cells by having several antibodies react with tumor-associated antigens (Fig. 36–15). The same approach could also be used for tissue typing and differentiation. The limitation of this procedure is mainly due to the difficulty in obtaining suspensions of single, intact cells from solid tumor for surface-marker typing. Another limitation is imposed by the lack of fully specific tumor cell markers that are expressed only on malignant cells. Usually, as shown in Fig. 36–14, benign cells react to some extent with an antibody raised to tumor-associated antigens. Quantitation of cytoplasmic or nuclear components with antibodies is more difficult and requires cell membrane permeabilization (Clevenger et al., 1985; Hayden et al., 1988). Standard procedures to permeabilize

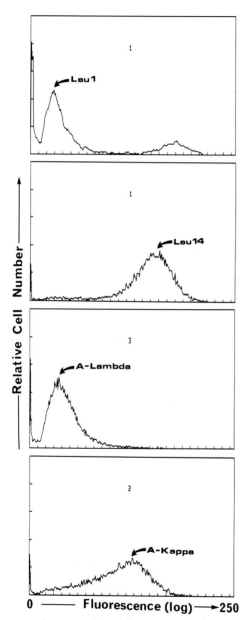

FIGURE 36–12. Selected fluorescent profiles of lymphoma cells obtained with monoclonal antibodies of the Leu series. Strong reactivity (shift to the right) is seen with Leu-14 (*second panel*) and A-kappa (*bottom panel*) antibodies. This indicates that the tumor is of B cell origin and confirms the production by the lymphoma cells of a kappa immunoglobulin chain.

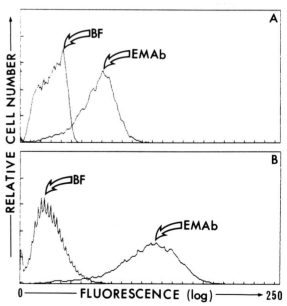

FIGURE 36–13. Indirect immunofluorescence profiles of short-term cultures of benign (*A*) and malignant (*B*) prostate cells exposed to an antibody against epithelial membrane antigen (EMAb). BF indicates nonspecific background fluorescence of cells treated with the second antibody only. The strong positive reaction with EMAb in both panels confirms the epithelial origin of the cells.

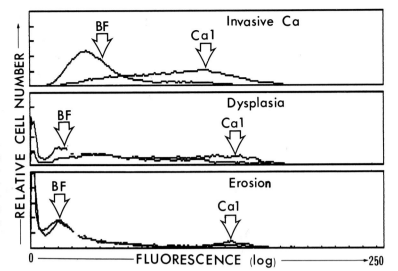

FIGURE 36–14. Reactivity of Ca1 monoclonal antibody, specific for Ca antigen (epitectin) with malignant, dysplastic, and benign cells in cervical samples. Strongly positive immunofluorescence is seen with invasive squamous carcinoma cells and with dysplastic cells. However, there is also some reactivity with benign cells in a case of cervical erosion.

cells with alcohol or acetone, however, induce unacceptably high background levels of nonspecific fluorescence. For several intracellular antigens, satisfactory results have been reported with fixation in cold methanol (−10°C). Some antigens destroyed by alcohol fixation could be measured with the use of paraformaldehyde and detergent fixation or permeabilization protocols. As described and shown in Chapter 35, MAbs specific for oncoproteins are now commercially available and can be applied to quantitative studies by flow cytometry in experimental cell systems (Czerniak et al., 1990). Flow cytometric analysis of human cancer cells depends on the location of the oncoprotein and preservation of cells during processing. Oncoproteins located in the nucleus, such as *c-myc*, can be quantitated (Watson, 1987), but membrane and cytoplasmic oncoproteins require a degree of cell preservation achievable only in lymphomas and leukemias but not in solid tumors.

The simultaneous analysis of cellular antigens versus DNA content using multiparameter flow cytometry offers the possibility of correlating the expression of cell components with the cell cycle (Czerniak et al., 1987; Lehman et al., 1988). The principle of cell staining and measurement in this approach is schematically shown in Fig. 36–2. The antigen is stained with FITC-labeled antibody using direct or indirect immunofluorescence procedure. The cells are then counterstained for DNA with propidium iodide. Cells so prepared emit two color signals (green and red) corresponding respectively to the antigen and the DNA contents. Of po-

tentially great biologic importance is the application of this technique to study cell cycle–related expression of the proteins involved in growth control, proliferation, differentiation, and malignant transformation. An example in Fig. 36–15 shows the relationship between the expression of the Ha-*ras* oncogene product (protein p21) and cell cycle progression in a cultured human tumor cell line. The application of this type of analysis to solid human tumors is in its beginnings and will require ingenious technical developments before it can be applied in a clinical laboratory.

COMMENTS

Flow cytometry is a quantitative and analytic cytologic technique that has received increasing attention within the recent years. Other areas of current interest are image analysis and image cytometry (see Chap. 35). The historical events leading to these developments were briefly summarized in the opening pages of this chapter and Chapter 35. The reasons for the current interest in these methods are multiple. One is the preoccupation with the application of technologic innovations to a better, more precise, and more reproducible diagnosis of human diseases. Another is the recognition of limits of microscopy as a prognostic method in human cancer. Perhaps the most important reason is the natural human desire to probe the secrets of life, using whatever technology is

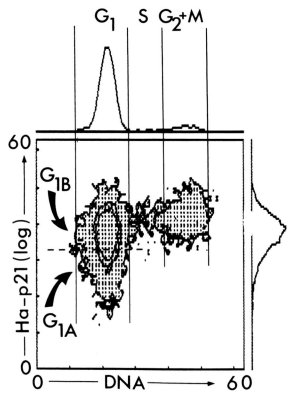

FIGURE 36–15. An example of the approach described in Fig. 36–2. The product of Ha-*ras* oncogene, a 21,000-dalton protein (p21) of the human bladder carcinoma cell line T24, is stained with an appropriate primary antibody and with a second antibody labeled with FITC. The cell cycle distribution is obtained by a simultaneously generated DNA histogram of the same cells stained with propidium iodide. Cell cycle compartments are graphically separated according to their DNA content (*vertical continuous lines*). The *dashed horizontal line* indicates p21 threshold level and separates two subcompartments of the $G_0 G_1$ cells, one with a low level (G_{1A}) and the other with a high level of the oncoprotein (G_{1B}). The p21 content remains essentially constant during the remaining phases of the cell cycle.

available. With the unraveling of the structure of the DNA molecule by Watson and Crick in 1953 and the advent of molecular biology, it was expected that the fundamentals of normal cell function would be rapidly unraveled, leading to an equally rapid understanding of disease processes, such as cancer. Viewed from the perspective of 1991, these hopes are very far from being realized. As stated in an editorial (Koss and Greenebaum, 1986), the prognosis of human cancer depends on the disease and on the patient. Since the means of

assessing the individual's response to cancer are extremely limited, we study the disease and, in this instance, the cancer cells.

With the developments in flow cytometry, it became fashionable to apply these high-technology instruments to measurements of various cell components — notably DNA and to a lesser extent RNA, proteins, and an ever-increasing number of other cell constituents. The technique offers some significant advantages: the measurements are rapid, and the results are displayed in the form of scattergrams and histograms that appear easy to interpret. The users of flow cytometry have rarely stressed the difficulties with the use, tuning, and maintenance of these instruments that usually require highly trained technical supervision. Difficulties with sample preparation, the choice of optimal processing method that may vary from tissue to tissue, sample preservation and fixation, and the selection of optimal fluorochromes have been rarely stressed.

In reference to DNA measurements, histograms of fluorescence are fairly easy to obtain. In "clean" histograms, the cell cycle components may be identified. Perhaps the most difficult questions pertain to interpretation of DNA histograms that deviate from normal by proportion of cells in the first peak, by the DI, or by a large CV. Several questions must be asked. What constitutes a diploid histogram, and when does aneuploidy begin? What degree of variation from normal is acceptable and offers important clinical guidance? Is it true that the presence of 90% of cells in the G_0/G_1 peak is prognostically different from 85% of cells? Is the position of the diploid peak that varies 10% from the presumed normal still normal? What about variations by 11% or 12%. Is the histogram truly representative of the tumor? How many tumor samples must be studied to arrive at the correct conclusions? Hopman et al. (1988) have recently pointed out that even in bladder tumors with a clean diploid type of histogram, multiple copies of chromosomes 1 and 18 may be observed by in situ hybridization with chromosome-specific probes. Thus, even in diploid-range tumors there are major disturbances in karyotypic structure.

Our own work in comparing the results of DNA measurements of the same samples by flow cytometry and image cytophotometry repeatedly revealed that small populations of aneuploid cells may be missed in DNA histograms generated by flow cytometry and discovered under visual control (see Fig. 35–16).

Despite these fundamental reservations, there is clinical evidence that DNA distribution approaching the pattern of normal diploid cell population is, in many but not all malignant tumors, a favorable prognostic sign.

What makes the diploid-range tumors behave differently from aneuploid tumors? Only speculation can be offered. For example, it is possible that there is a better preservation of tumor-suppressing genes (such as the retinoblastoma or Rb gene; see Chap. 2) in diploid-range tumors than in aneuploid tumors. It is also possible that these beneficial genes are selectively destroyed, mutated, or blocked during the development of aneuploid cell clones. Tumor cells in the diploid range may be better recognized and controlled by the host.

The same questions in reverse could be asked in reference to aneuploid tumors. What makes them proliferate, invade, and metastasize more readily? Chromosomal abnormalities and aneuploidy may also be observed in some benign tumors and in some non-neoplastic lesions (see Chapter 7). Further, aneuploid DNA patterns may also be observed in preinvasive intraepithelial lesions — for example, in the uterine cervix — that may or may not progress to invasive cancer. Thus, aneuploidy

may be reversible in some instances and is, per se, not a sufficient condition to declare a cell population to be malignant in the clinical sense (see also Chap. 7).

Yet another mystery is raised in reference to those rare malignant human conditions that respond better to therapeutic measures when aneuploid or offer a better prognosis when diploid-range cell populations accompany hyperdiploid populations, as noted for osteosarcoma (Look et al., 1988).

It is evident from this summary that measuring DNA and other cell components in human cancer, although potentially useful for the prognosis of malignant tumors in some organs and of prognostic benefit in other organs, raises a number of fundamental biologic questions that cannot be answered at this time. Obviously, a great deal of additional fundamental work is necessary to understand why measuring DNA sometimes gives answers of clinical value. The same reservation applies to other cell components and genes. Despite some progress at the molecular level, the mysteries of human cancer have not yet been penetrated.

Appendix: Essential Technical Methods in Flow Cytometry*

EQUIPMENT OF LABORATORY

Large Items
Flow cytometer
Refrigerated centrifuge with swinging bucket rotor
Coulter cell counter or equivalent instrument (may be replaced by a manual hemocytometer)
Micropipettor
Microcentrifuge

Small Items
Pasteur pipettes, various lengths. The most useful are 5¾-inch-long (about 15 cm) pipettes.
Disposable serologic pipettes, various sizes
Disposable syringes, 1 ml, with fitting 21-caliber needles
Nylon mesh, 47 to 53 μm, cut into 1 × 1-inch (2.5 × 2.5 cm) squares
Disposable centrifuge tubes, conical, 15 ml
Microcentrifuge tubes, various sizes

Note: The nylon mesh removes larger fragments of tissue from the nuclear suspension. The optimal

Protocols established by Robert P. Wersto, Ph.D., during his tenure at the Montefiore Medical Center, Albert Einstein College of Medicine, Bronx, N.Y.

way of processing, proposed by Wersto, is to aspirate the suspension into an *unarmed* syringe, place the nylon mesh on the tip of the syringe, and then fit the needle hub onto the syringe. The liquid expressed from the syringe is filtered across the nylon mesh, before entering the needle.

DNA ANALYSIS

Specimen Collection

The following options are available:

1. *Fresh material:* Fresh material, not otherwise preserved, must be processed within 30 to 60 minutes after removal.
2. *Fresh material, methods of preservation:*
   a. phosphate-buffered saline (PBS)
   b. bone marrow transport medium (RPMI 1640 with 10% calf serum and 14.3 U of sodium heparin/ml) (Gibco, Grand Island, N.Y. 14072)
   c. 70% ethanol or methanol

Processing should occur within 24 hours of collection.

3. *Fresh material,* snap frozen in liquid nitrogen, or at least frozen to $-20°C$, can be kept indefinitely before processing.

4. *Archival material:* Only tissue or fluids fixed in 10% buffered formalin for at least 24 hours are suitable for processing. If paraffin-embedded material is processed, the same principles of fixation apply. Smaller paraffin-embedded samples give better and cleaner histograms than large tissue blocks.

General Principles

With few exceptions, the measurements of DNA in human material are performed on nuclei stripped of cytoplasm. The cytoplasm is destroyed either by acid (citric acid–sodium citrate [CASC] procedure, Krishnan's procedure) or by proteolytic enzymes (Vindelöv's procedures, see below). If an enzyme is used, the reaction must be timed and stopped. *All samples must be treated by RNAse, to avoid binding of the fluorochrome to RNA.*

If RNA measurements are desirable, DNAse must be used.

Control Cells

All flow cytometric measurements must be carefully controlled.

Peripheral blood lymphocytes, preferably from the same donor, must be prepared by the Ficoll-Hypaque method from heparinized blood. Samples can be stored at $-70°C$ in a buffer composed of dimethyl sulfoxide (Sigma) with 10% calf serum. Aliquots of the stored lymphocytes can be diluted for use with the buffer used for the DNA procedure (i.e., CASC, Vindelöv's buffer, Krishnan's buffer —see below). The deep-frozen samples can be used for 6 to 12 months after preparation. There is a slightly lower DNA content in males than in females (a Y chromosome is somewhat smaller than an X chromosome), and matching the sex of the donor with the sex of the lymphocyte sample may be advisable.

Nucleated erythrocytes (chicken erythrocytes, Environmental Diagnostics, Burlington, N.C. 27215) or trout erythrocytes (no constant source of supply) may also be used and should be mixed with the unknown sample before use (see p. 1645).

RNAse Solution and Use

Reagents.   RNAse (ribonuclease A), type 1-A, bovine pancreas (Sigma). Phosphate buffered saline (PBS).

Preparation of Solution.   Dissolve 100 mg of RNAse in 10 ml of PBS. Store at $4°C$ (lasts 1 week).

Method of Procedure.   To the fluorochrome-stained sample in PBS, add $10\,\mu l$. of the RNAse solution and incubate for 30 minutes at $37°C$ in the dark. Store incubated samples at $4°C$ for at least 2 hours before DNA analysis (samples remain stable for 72 hours if stored in the dark).

METHODS OF SAMPLE PROCESSING

Citric Acid–Sodium Citrate Method (CASC)

The CASC method was initially developed to isolate nuclei from squamous epithelial cells, which often resist other methods of processing (Koss et al., 1977). The method is applicable to a number of cell-rich tissues, and it offers the advantage of simplicity.

Reagents

Preparation of 0.01M solution of citric acid: Dissolve 2.10 gm of citric acid monohydrate (formula weight 210.14) in 1 L of distilled water. Store at $4°C$.

Preparation of 0.09M solution of sodium citrate: Dissolve 26.47 gm of sodium citrate (formula weight 294.10) in 1 L of distilled water. Store at $4°C$.

Procedure

For use, mix in equal parts. Mince tissues in about 5 ml of the solution. Centrifuge for 10 minutes at $220 \times g$; discard supernatant. Add 50 ml of CASC and incubate for 30 minutes, using a magnetic stirrer. Filter through gauze or nylon mesh and syringe, as described above. Incubate with RNAse. The sample can be processed with any fluorochrome for DNA analysis.

For general comments on flow cytometric procedure, see below, p. 1645.

Vindelöv's Procedure

Principle

DNA analysis is performed on nuclei, stripped free of cytoplasm, using trypsin. Trypsin inhibitor is used to stop the reaction, and the nuclei are treated with RNAse before staining with propidium iodide. The following reagents are needed:

Reagent/Grade	Source	Catalog No.
Citric acid, trisodium salt	Sigma*	C-7254
Propidium iodide	Calbiochem†	537059
Dimethyl sulfoxide, ACS reagent	Sigma	D-8779
Nonidet P-40 (NP-40)	Sigma	N-3516
RNAse (ribonuclease A), type 1-A, bovine pancreas	Sigma	R-4875
Spermine tetrahydrochloride	Sigma	S-2876
Sucrose, enzyme grade	Sigma	
Tris buffer, free base, reagent grade	Sigma	T-1503
Trypsin, type IX, from porcine pancreas	Sigma	T-0134
Trypsin inhibitor, type II-O, from chicken egg white	Sigma	T-9253

*Sigma Chemical Company, P.O. Box 14508, St. Louis, Mo. 63178-9916.
†Calbiochem Brand Biochemicals, Behring Diagnostics, P.O. Box 12087, San Diego, Calif. 92112-4180.

Reagent Preparation

1. Sample storage buffer:
     85.50 gm sucrose (250 mM)
     11.76 gm citric acid, trisodium salt (40 mM)
     50 ml dimethyl sulfoxide (DMSO)
   Dissolve the first two reagents in approximately 800 to 900 ml of distilled water and add the DMSO. Add additional distilled water to bring the volume to 1,000 ml. Adjust the pH to 7.60, and date and store at 4°C. (Normally, 250 ml of this solution is made up.)
   Label as Vindelöv Storage Buffer, with the date of preparation and an expiration date (90 days).

2. Staining buffer:
     2.0 gm citric acid, trisodium salt (3.4 mM)
     1.044 gm spermine tetrahydrochloride (1.5 mM)
     0.121 gm Tris buffer, free base (0.5 mM)
     2.0 ml Nonidet P40 (NP 40) (0.1%)
   Dissolve all reagents in 2,000 ml of distilled water and adjust the pH to 7.60. This solution becomes the buffer solution for the preparation of Vindelöv solutions A, B, and C and is used immediately. Excess is discarded.

3. Solution A:
     15 mg trypsin
   Dissolve in 500 ml of staining buffer (step 2), adjust pH to 7.60, and store aliquots in 15-ml centrifuge tubes. Usually aliquots of 3, 5, and 10 ml are useful. Label tubes on sides and on caps with A, date batch, and immediately store in a −70°C freezer. Make about 500 ml.

4. Solution B:
     250 mg trypsin inhibitor
     50 mg RNAse A
   Dissolve in 500 ml of staining buffer, adjust pH to 7.60. Usually aliquots of 3, 5, and 10 ml are useful. Label tubes on sides and on caps with B, date batch, and immediately store in a −70°C freezer. Make about 500 ml, and aliquot and freeze as described for Solution A.

5. Solution C:
     208 mg propidium iodide (PI)
     580 mg spermine tetrahydrochloride
   Dissolve in 500 ml of staining buffer, and adjust pH to 7.60. If the PI is purchased from Sigma Chemical Co., the purity is 95% to 97%, and some insoluble matter will be noted. Before freezing aliquots, filter Solution C through a 0.2 μl sterile filter unit. PI purchased from Calbiochem requires no filtering. Usually aliquots of 3, 5, and 10 ml are useful. Label tubes on sides and on caps with C, date batch, and immediately store in a −70°C freezer. Make about 500 ml, and aliquot and freeze as described for Solution A. Make about 500 ml. Protect the PI solution at all times from light.

6. *General reagent notes.* The pH should be adjusted to 7.60 ± 0.5 units, although it appears to work better on the low side (7.53 to 7.58) than over pH 7.60. All solutions are stored frozen. If the freezer thaws, make new solutions. Usually when the enzyme solutions start to deteriorate, the G_1 coefficient of variation (CV) of control lymphocytes increases. Each batch *must* be tested with lymphocyte controls before use on clinical samples. Staining solutions that yield CVs above 4% on lymphocytes that had CVs of 2% to 3% with prior batches of stain indicate that an error was made and the solutions should be remade. Reagents with specific catalog numbers should not be substituted.

Procedure

1. Transport frozen aliquots of solutions A, B, and C on ice (and covered with aluminum foil) after removal from the −70°C freezer. Using warm water (≤37°C), rapidly thaw these frozen solutions by constantly inverting the tubes under a stream of warm water. Solutions A and B can be placed in a rack at room temperature for up to 10 to 15 minutes before use. The thawed Solution C is stored *on ice* and covered.

2. To 200 μl (0.2 ml) of thawed sample, containing 5×10^5 cells, add the following:

   a. 1.8 ml of Solution A. Set a timer for 10 minutes and start it immediately after the addition of Solution A to the first tube. *Incubate 10 minutes at room temperature, inverting several times during this period.*

   b. 1.5 ml of Solution B. Start timer as above, and *incubate for 10 minutes at room temperature, inverting several times during this period.*

   c. 1.5 ml of Solution C. Start timer as above, and *incubate for 15 minutes on ice in the dark (or covered), inverting several times during this period.*

3. Centrifuge samples at $500 \times g$ (1,500) rpm at 4° to 10°C for 5 minutes to concentrate samples and transfer the centrifuged tubes with pellets, *undisturbed*, to an ice bucket, which is covered at all times or left uncovered in a totally darkened flow laboratory (or one with a background yellow or red darkroom light). Samples should be analyzed within 3 hours of preparation. For large numbers of samples, it is a good idea to prepare them in batches.

4. To analyze the sample, gently remove most of the clear supernatant using a clean Pasteur pipette so that approximately 0.5 ml of supernatant remains. This volume is dependent on the sample concentration and can be altered upward or downward to achieve an adequate concentration. This prevents an increase in sample pressure on the instrument. Resuspend the pellet in the remaining supernatant using the same Pasteur pipette, and transfer the solution to a 1.5-ml microcentrifuge tube. Using a 1-ml plastic syringe (with the needle removed), fill the syringe with the cell suspension and place a piece of 47 to 53 μm nylon mesh (approximately 1 to 2 cm square) between the barrel of the syringe and the hub of a 27-gauge needle. Tighten the needle and slowly filter the cell suspension through the mesh into a 0.5-ml microcentrifuge tube that has the cap removed (in order to fit in the flow cytometer's sample holder). Keep the filtered sample in the dark and on ice at all times before analysis.

General Notes and Comments

I. Long-Term Storage of Cells. Besides yielding DNA histograms with good resolution in terms of CVs, the other benefit of Vindelöv's procedure is the long term-storage of clinical specimens, which permits batch-type analysis. Generally, solid tissues are finely minced in a small Petri dish, flooded with some sample storage buffer (DMSO/sucrose/citrate), and filtered through a 350-μm mesh. The filtrate is then counted and adjusted so that the cell number is 2.5×10^6 cells per ml. Counting minced tumor samples is often difficult, and the sample density can be estimated by eye or by comparison with that of the lymphocytes used as external DNA standards. The specimens at all times are kept on ice and immediately transferred to a −70°C freezer, where they may be kept for up to 6 months to 1 year before analysis. For thin-needle aspirates of the breast, colon, or prostate, generally no counting or mincing is necessary and the sample can be directly resuspended in 200 μl of the sample storage buffer and frozen. The same applies to touch or scrape preparations as well as bladder washings. The samples may be "snap" or quick frozen in liquid N_2 and then transferred to the −70°C freezer.

II. Internal Standards. For accurate DNA analysis, all clinical samples must have an internal standard admixed with the test specimen to control for stain and instrument variability. Nucleated chicken erythrocytes (CRBC) are useful (see above). Usually, 50 ml of CRBCs shipped in citrate will last for several years. On receipt, wash 10 to 15 ml of the solution two to three times with a large volume of the Vindelöv's sample storage buffer (DMSO/sucrose/citrate) or until the supernatant is clear. Decant the supernatant and resuspend the pellet in 10 ml of the sample storage buffer and count an aliquot of the CRBCs. Freeze 50 to 100 μl aliquots of the cells in 0.5-ml microcentrifuge tubes at −70°C. For use, thaw a frozen tube in your hand (about 15 seconds) and add an appropriate amount to the clinical specimen. Based on our experience, the CRBC concentration should be 5% to 10% of the total cell number. Therefore, 5 μl of the concentrated cells is placed in 4.5 ml of the sample storage buffer. Mix well and add 5 to 10 μl of the diluted CRBC to 200 μl of the clinical sample. It is best to check the dilutions by analyzing control lymphocytes with various dilutions of the CRBCs.

III. External Standards. Peripheral blood lymphocytes from a "normal" donor are used as external standards for defining the channel position of the G_0/G_1 peak of the clinical sample. These are prepared by centrifugation of 10 ml of whole heparinized blood (or diluted 1:1 with RPMI 1640 tissue culture medium) onto a pad of 10 ml of Ficoll-Hypaque for 30 minutes at $300 \times g$ at 22°C. The interface containing the cells is removed using a Pasteur pipette or a spinal tap needle and washed three times (10 minutes, 1,100 rpm at 4° to 8°C; $200 \times g$) with a large volume of cold RPMI 1640 (at least 40 to 50 ml each time). After the final wash, the pellet is resuspended in 2 to 5 ml of the medium, counted, and recentrifuged. At this point, slowly pour off the supernatant, place the inverted tube on a clean paper towel for about a minute, invert to upright, and tap the pellet to dislodge it. Add the appropriate amount of sample storage buffer (DMSO/sucrose/citrate) so that the lymphocyte concentration is 2.5×10^6 cells per ml or 5×10^5 cells per 400 μl. Pour aliquots of 500-μl samples into 0.5-ml microcentrifuge tubes on ice and immediately freeze in a −70°C freezer. It is a good idea to test each batch against a previous batch with known good CV. If possible, lymphocytes from the same patient from whom the clinical sample was obtained should be used.

IV. Flow Cytometry: General Comments

1. Try to use as few optical filters as possible to analyze the sample. The Coulter EPICS instruments require a 510-nm interference filter, 515-nm-long pass filter, and 590-nm-long pass filter (in this order toward the photomultiplier tube). If the 515-nm-long pass filter has no defects, the 590-nm one can be omitted. For other instruments, follow the manufacturer's directions.
2. For optimal resolution, sample flow rates should be 30 to 50 events per second (75 to 100 per second is acceptable).
3. The sample sheath fluid is distilled water. Since the sample is kept on ice before analysis, it is advantageous to configure the flow cytometer with temperature control of both the sheath and sample and run samples at 4°C.
4. Instrument optical alignment is accomplished with DNA check microspheres (10 μm, Fine Particle Division, Coulter Electronics, Hialeah, Fla.), which on linear fluorescence and forward-angle light scatter have a CV of less than 2%.
5. For practical purposes, the high voltage of the fluorescent signal required for the selected probe should be adjusted for the mean channel position of the G_0/G_1 peak of control lymphocytes to be near channel 70 (± 5 channels). In this case, the diploid (2N) peak is in channel 70, a tetraploid peak in channel 140, and an aneuploid (6N) peak in channel 210. This setup gives both good positioning of aneuploid peaks in the $>2N$ and $<5N$ range, which account for nearly all possible aneuploid combinations. If the 2N peak is in channel 70, the peak position of admixed CRBC should be in channel 25. Thus, the ratio of the diploid 2N peak position to that of the CRBCs is always 2.8 ± 0.05, and variation outside of this range indicates either poor staining or a nonlinear fluorescent signal. Notwithstanding, the position of the diploid (2N) peak is a trade-off. If one were to analyze cancer cells that may be in the 8N range, these would be off-scale with lymphocytes in channel 70 ($4 \times 70 =$ channel 280). However, positioning of the CRBCs in channels below 25 would prevent setting the discriminator high enough to gate out debris.

Krishnan's Technique for Fresh/Frozen Tissue

Principle

DNA analysis is performed on nuclei, stripped free of cytoplasm, using hypotonic lysis in dilute citric acid. The technique works best on nonfixed fresh or frozen tissue. The nuclei are treated with RNAse before staining with propidium iodide. The following reagents are needed:

Reagent/Grade	Source	Catalog No.
Citric acid, trisodium salt, Molecular Biology grade	Sigma*	C-8532
Propidium iodide (PI)	Calbiochem†	537059
Nonidet P-40 (NP-40)	Sigma	N-3516
RNAse (ribonuclease A), type 1-A, bovine pancreas	Sigma	R-4875

*Sigma Chemical Company, P.O. Box 14508, St. Louis, Mo. 63178-9916.
†Calbiochem Brand Biochemicals, Behring Diagnostics, P.O. Box 12087, San Diego, Calif. 92112-4180.

Reagent Preparation — Modified Krishnan Buffer

To 250 ml of distilled water, add the following:
0.25 gm sodium citrate
   (0.1% final concentration)
0.005 gm RNAse
   (0.02 mg/ml final concentration)
0.75 ml NP-40   (0.3% final concentration)
0.0125 gm PI
   (0.05 mg/ml final concentration)
Although pH is not critical, the pH of the buffer should be 7.4 before the addition of the PI. Cover the buffer with aluminum foil and store in the dark at 4°C. Label as Modified Krishnan Buffer with the preparer's initials, the date of preparation, and an expiration date (3 weeks).

Procedure

1. With a pipette place 1-ml aliquots of the dissociated tumor tissue containing $1-2 \times 10^6$ cells into a 12 mm $\times$ 75 mm conical centrifuge tube and centrifuge at $250 \times g$ (1,000 rpm) for 5 minutes at 4°C.
2. Remove the supernatant from the tubes, and add 1 ml of the Modified Krishnan Buffer per 1×10^6 cells. Vortex each sample for 10 seconds.
3. Incubate samples for a minimum of 30 minutes to 1 hour at 4°C in an ice bucket, which is covered with aluminum foil to protect the samples from photobleaching.
4. Remove samples from ice bath and centrifuge at $250 \times g$ (1,000 rpm) for 5 minutes at 4°C.

5. Remove the supernatant from the tubes, and add 1 ml of fresh Modified Krishnan Buffer per 1×10^6 cells. Vortex each sample for 10 seconds and syringe each sample through a 47 to 53-μm nylon mesh, which is placed between the barrel of a 1-ml syringe and the hub of a 27-gauge needle, before analysis on the flow cytometer.

General Notes

1. Samples are stable for at least 3 hours on ice in the dark.
2. Distilled water is used as the instrument sample sheath.
3. See general comments on Vindelöv's procedure, above.

DNA Analysis of Paraffin-Embedded Samples (Hedley's Procedure Modified by Amberson and Wersto, Semiautomated)

Principle

DNA analysis is performed on nuclei, stripped free of cytoplasm using pronase, from deparaffinized tissue sections that have been fixed in formalin. The technique was originally designed by Hedley et al., specifically for single-parameter DNA analysis from archival material. The nuclei are treated with RNAse before staining with propidium iodide.

The following reagents are needed:

Reagent/Grade	Source	Catalog No.
MgCl$_2$, hexahydrate	Sigma* (or Mallinchrod)	
Pronase	Sigma	P-8038
Propidium iodide (PI)	Calbiochem†	537059
RNAse (ribonuclease A), type 1-A, bovine pancreas	Sigma	R-4875
Sodium azide	Sigma (or Fisher)	
Tris hydrochloride		

* Sigma Chemical Company, P.O. Box 14508, St. Louis, Mo. 63178-9916.
†Calbiochem Brand Biochemicals, Behring Diagnostics, P.O. Box 12087, San Diego, Calif. 92112-4180.

Reagent Preparation

1. Pronase Solution: To 50 ml of PBS, add 50 mg of Pronase (Protese type XXI, Sigma). Make an aliquot of the solution and freeze at −70°C. Label as Pronase Solution with the date of preparation and an expiration date (6 months). Once thawed, the solution should be used immediately, and the remainder discarded.

2. PI stain, archival:
   To 100 ml of distilled water, add the following:

MgCl$_2$	0.102 gm
PI	0.5 mg
Sodium azide	0.100 gm
Tris	0.121 gm

   Dissolve well, and adjust the pH to 7.4. Store in an aluminum foil–wrapped bottle in the dark at 4°C. Label the date of preparation and an expiration date (1 week).

3. RNAse solution, archival:
   To 10 ml of PBS, add 100 mg of RNAse (final concentration is 10 mg/ml). Store at 4°C for no more than 1 week, or make an aliquot and freeze for long-term storage of up to 3 months. Label with the date of preparation and an expiration date (1 week).

Procedure

1. Select tissue blocks showing the least amount of necrosis and the highest cellularity.

2. Cut two to three 50- to 100-μm sections, and place the sections from each patient sample into an embedding paper bag and then into a plastic tissue cassette

3. Deparaffinize and hydrate the cut sections by running the samples through a tissue processor following this schedule, *usually overnight:*

a.	Xylene	3 hours
b.	Xylene	4 hours
c.	100% ethanol	3 hours
d.	100% ethanol	2 hours
e.	95% ethanol	2 hours
f.	70% ethanol	1 hour
g.	50% ethanol	1 hour
h.	Distilled H$_2$O	1 hour
i.	Distilled H$_2$O	1 hour
j.	Distilled H$_2$O	Until removed

4. Remove the cassettes from the processor, and immediately place them in PBS. Change this solution after approximately 10 minutes.

5. Carefully transfer the dewaxed tissue sections to a 15-ml centrifuge tube, either manually or with forceps or by removing the specimen from the embedding bag with 3 to 5 ml of PBS. If the latter technique is used, centrifuge the specimen at 250 × g (1,100 rpm) for 5 minutes, before proceeding to the next step.

6. Add 1 to 2 ml of Pronase Solution to the deparaffinized sections in the centrifuge tube and incubate at 37°C for 30 minutes, vortexing every 5 to 10 minutes. A cloudy solution is indicative of a successful cellular digestion.

7. Filter each specimen through a piece of 47- to 53-μm nylon mesh into a clean 4.5-ml conical centrifuge tube.

8. Centrifuge the sample at 300 × g (1,300 to 1,500 rpm) for 5 minutes at 4°C.

9. Remove the supernatant and add 2 ml of PBS, vortexing gently. Repeat steps 8 and 9, with a final resuspension of the samples in PBS.

10. Samples can now either be stored in PBS at 4°C for up to 2 days or centrifuged as described in step 8 and, after decanting the supernatant, resuspended in 1 ml of the PI stain for immediate analysis.

11. Stain the sample for 30 minutes at 4°C in the dark.

12. Add 10 μl of the RNAse solution to each of the stained samples and incubate for 30 minutes at 37°C. Store the samples wrapped in aluminum foil in the dark at 4°C for at least 2 hours before analysis. Stained samples are stable for 72 hours at 4°C when stored in the dark. RNAse and PI can be added to the sample at the same time.

General Notes

1. Distilled water is used as the instrument sample sheath.

2. See general comments for Vindelöv's procedure.

3. *Diploid lymphocytes or chick red blood cells cannot be used as standards. In all instances, benign tissue from the same block or a fixed specimen of benign tissue from the same organ site and patient must be used for calculation of the tumor DNA index.*

IMMUNOFLUORESCENCE STAINING FOR THE SIMULTANEOUS MEASUREMENT OF INDIVIDUAL PROTEINS AND DNA CONTENT BY FLOW CYTOMETRY*

Stock Solutions

1. 0.01M phosphate-buffered saline solution (PBS, pH 7.4)
2. 0.5% paraformaldehyde in PBS
3. 100% methanol (−20°C)

Method developed by B. Czerniak, M.D., and F. Herz, Ph.D.

4. 5% albumin in PBS
5. Primary antibody (specificity must be tested by Western blotting)
6. Fluorescein isothiocyanate (FITC)-conjugated secondary antibody
7. Propidium iodide (PI) solution (100 µg/ml in PBS).

Procedure

1. Dilute the primary and secondary antibodies in PBS containing 5% albumin. Working dilution varies depending on the type of antibody and its source.
2. Fix the cells (in suspension) for 5 minutes at 4°C with 0.5% paraformaldehyde in PBS.
3. Wash the cells three times with PBS at 4°C and centrifuge.
4. Permeabilize the cells by resuspension in 100% methanol (5 minutes at −20°C).
5. Count the cells and transfer an aliquot containing 1×10^6 cells into a 5-ml conical test tube.
6. Centrifuge the cells and resuspend in 200 µl of the primary antibody solution.
7. Incubate at room temperature for 1 hour or at 4°C overnight.
8. Wash the cells three times with PBS and centrifugate.
9. Resuspend the cells in 200 µl of the secondary antibody solution.
10. Incubate the cells with the secondary antibody for 30 minutes at room temperature.
11. Wash the cell three times in PBS followed by centrifugation.
12. Resuspend the cells in 0.9 ml of PBS.
13. Immediately before the measurements, add 0.1 ml of stock (PI) solution (final concentration: 10 µl/ml) and keep at 4°C for 5 minutes.
14. Perform flow cytometric measurements of green (FITC) and red (PI) fluorescence.

Control samples are prepared following the same protocol, except that instead of being incubated with primary antibody (step 7), the cells are incubated with 5% albumin solution in PBS. For inhibition assays in step 7, the cells are exposed to the primary antibody, which was preincubated overnight at the working dilution with its corresponding immunogen at a molar antibody:immunogen ratio >2.

BIBLIOGRAPHY

Abe, S., Makimura, S., Itabashi, K., Nagai, T., Tsuneta, Y., and Kawakami, Y.: Prognostic significance of nuclear DNA content in small cell carcinoma of the lung. Cancer, 56:2025–2030, 1985.

Agarwal, V., Greenebaum, E., Wersto, R.P., and Koss, L.G.: DNA ploidy of spindle cell soft tissue tumors and its relationship to histology, Arch. Path. Lab. Med., 115:558–562, 1991.

Alho, A., Connor, J.F., Mankin, H.J., Schiller, A.L., and Campbell, C.J.: Assessment of malignancy of cartilage tumors using flow cytometry. A preliminary report. J. Bone Joint Surg., 65:779–785, 1983.

Allison, D.C., Yuhas, J.M., Ridolpho, P.F., Anderson, S.L., and Johnson, T.C.: Cytophotometric measurement of the cellular DNA content of [3H]thymidine-labelled spheroids. Demonstration that some non-labelled cells have S and G2 DNA content. Cell Tissue Kinet., 16:237–246, 1983.

Amberson, J.B., Wersto, R.P., Agarwal, V., Suhrland, M., and Koss, L.G.: Preparation of paraffin-embedded tissue for flow cytometric analysis: An improved and more efficient procedure. (Submitted for publication.)

Andreeff, M., Beck, J.D., Darzynkiewicz, Z., Traganos, F., Gupta, S., Malamed, M.R., and Good, R.A.: RNA content in human lymphocyte subpopulations. Proc. Natl. Acad. Sci., 75:1338–1942, 1978.

Armitage, N.C., Robins, R.A., Evans, D.F., Turner, D.R., Baldwin, R.W., and Hardcastle, J.D.: The influence of tumour cell DNA abnormalities on survival in colorectal cancer. Br. J. Surg., 72:828–830, 1985.

Atkin, N.B.: Prognosic value of cytogenetic studies of tumors of the female genital tract. *In* Koss, L.G., and Coleman, D.V. (eds.): Advances in Clinical Cytology vol. 2. pp. 103–122, New York, Mason Publishing, 1984.

Atkin, N.B., and Richards, B.M.: Clinical significance of ploidy in carcinoma of cervix: Its relation to prognosis. Br. Med. J., 2:1445–1446, 1962.

Auer, G.U., Caspersson, T.O., and Wallgren, A.S.: DNA content and survival in mammary carcinoma. Anal. Quant. Cytol., 2:161–165, 1980.

Augenlicht, L.H., and Baserga, R.: Changes in the Go state of WI-38 fibroblasts at different times after confluence. Exp. Cell Res., 89:255–262, 1974.

Baak, J.P., Wisse-Brekelmans, E.C., Uyterlinde, A.M., and Schipper, N.W.: Evaluation of the prognostic value of morphometric features and cellular DNA content in FIGO I ovarian cancer patients. Anal. Quant. Cytol. Histol., 9:287–290, 1987.

Bacus, S.S., Bacus, J.W., Slamon, D.J., and Press, M.F.: HER-2/neu oncogene expression and DNA ploidy analysis in breast cancer. Arch. Pathol. Lab. Med., 114:164–169, 1990.

Badalament, R.A., Gay, H., Whitmore, W.R., Jr., Herr, H.W., Fair, W.R., Oettgen, H.F., and Melamed, M.R.: Monitoring intravesical bacillus Calmette-Guérin treatment of superficial bladder carcinoma by serial flow cytometry. Cancer, 58:2751–2757, 1986.

Badalament, R.A., Hermansen, D.K., Kimmel, M., Gay, H., Herr, H.W., Fair, W.R., Whitmore, W.F., and Melamed, M.R.: The sensitivity of bladder wash flow cytometry, bladder wash cytology, and voided cytology in the detection of bladder cacinoma. Cancer, 60:1423–1427, 1987.

Badalament, R.A., Kimmel, M., Gay, H., Cibas, E.S., Whitmore, W.F., Jr., Herr, H.W., Fair, W.R., and Melamed, M.R.: The sensitivity of flow cytometry compared with conventional cytology in the detection of superficial bladder carcinoma. Cancer, 59:2078–2085, 1987.

Bagwell, C.B., Hudson, J.L., and Irvin, G.L.: Nonparametric flow cytometry analysis. J. Histochem. Cytochem, 27:293–296, 1979.

Baisch, H., Göhde, W., and Linden, W.A.: Analysis of PCP-data to determine the fraction of cells in the various phases of the cell cycle. Radiat. Environ. Biophys. *12*:31–39, 1975.

Barlogie, B., Alexanian, R., Gehan, E.A., Smallwood, L., Smith, T., and Drewinko B.: Marrow cytometry and prognosis in myeloma. J. Clin. Invest., *72*:853–861, 1983.

Barlogie, B., McLaughlin, P., and Alexanian, R.: Characterization of hematologic malignancies by flow cytometry. Anal. Quant. Cytol. Histol., *9*:147–155, 1987.

Barlogie, B., Stass, S., Dixon, D., Keating, M., Cork, A., Trujillo, J.M., McCredie, K.B., and Freireich, E.J.: DNA aneuploidy in adult acute leukemia. Cancer Genet. Cytogenet., *28*:213–228, 1987.

Bauer, H.C.F., Kreicbergs, A., and Tribukait, B.: DNA microspectrophotometry of bone sarcomas in tissue sections as compared to imprint and flow DNA analysis. Cytometry, *7*:544–550, 1986.

Bijman, J.T., Wagener, D.J.T., van Rennes, H., Wessels, J.M.C., and van den Broek, P.: Flow cytometric evaluation of cell dispersion from human head and neck tumors. Cytometry, *6*:334–341, 1985.

Bjelkenkrantz, K., Lundgren, J., and Olofsson, J.: Single-cell DNA measurement in hyperplastic, dysplastic and carcinomatous laryngeal epithelia, with special reference to the occurrence of hypertetraploid cell nuclei. Anal. Quant. Cytol., *5*:184–188, 1983.

Blobel G., and Potter, V.R.: Nuclei from rat liver; isolation method that combines purity with high yield. Science, *154*:1662–1665, 1966.

Blomjous, C.E., Schipper, N.W., Baak, J.P., van Galen, E.M., de Voogt, H.J., and Meyer, C.J.: Retrospective study of prognostic importance of DNA flow cytometry of urinary bladder carcinoma. J. Clin. Pathol., *41*:21–25, 1988.

Blomjous, E.C., Schipper, N.W., Baak, J.P., Vos, W., De Voogt, H.J., and Meijer, C.J.: The value of morphometry and DNA flow cytometry in addition to classic prognosticators in superficial urinary bladder cacinoma. Am. J. Clin. Pathol., *91*:243–248, 1989.

Blumenfeld, D., Braly, P.S., Ben-Ezra, J., and Klevecz, R.R.: Tumor DNA content as a prognostic feature in advanced epithelial ovarian carcinoma. Gynecol. Oncol., *27*:389–402, 1987.

Braunstein, J.D., Good, R.A., Hansen, J.A., Sharpless, T.K., and Melamed, M.R.: Quantitation of lymphocyte response to antigen by flow cytofluorometry. J. Histochem. Cytochem., *24*:378–382, 1976.

Brunsting, A., and Mullaney, P.F.: Differential light scattering: A possible method of mammalian cell identification. J. Colloid Interface Sci., *39*:492, 1972.

Buchner, T., Hiddemann, W., Wormann, B., Kleinemeier, B., Schumann, J., Göhde, W., Ritter, J., Muller, K.M., von Bassewitz, D.B., Roessner, A., and Grundmann, A.: Differential patterns of DNA-aneuploidy in human malignancies. Pathol. Res. Pract., *179*:310–317, 1985.

Brunn, P.A., Jr., Carney, D.N., Gazdar, A.F., Whang-Peng, J., and Matthews, M.J.: Diagnostic and biologic implications of flow cytometric DNA content analysis in lung cancer. Cancer Res., *43*:5026–5032, 1983.

Bunn, P.A., Jr., Whang-Peng, J., Carney, D.N., Schlam, M.L., Knutsen, T., and Gazdar, A.F.: DNA content analysis by flow cytometry and cytogenetic analysis in mycosis fungoides and Sézary's syndrome. J. Clin. Invest., *65*:1440–1448, 1980.

Caspersson, T., and Santesson, L.: Studies of protein metabolism in the cells of epithelial tumors. Acta Radiol. (Suppl.), *46*:1–105, 1942.

Caspersson, T.: Cell Growth and Function. New York, Norton, 1950.

Caspersson, T.: Uber den chemischen Aufbau der Strukturen des Zellkernes. Scand. Arch. Phys. Suppl., *8*:73, 1936.

Christensson, B., Tribukait, B., Linder, I.L., Ullman, B., and Biberfeld, P.: Cell proliferation and DNA content in non-Hodgkin's lymphoma. Flow cytometry in relation to lymphoma classification. Cancer, *58*:1295–1304, 1986.

Christov, K., and Zapryanov, Z.: Flow cytometry in brain tumors. I. Ploidy abnormalities. Neoplasma, *88*:49–55, 1986.

Cibas, E.S., Malkin, M.G., Posner, J.B., and Melamed, M.R.: Detection of DNA abnormalities by flow cytometry in cells from cerebrospinal fluid. Am. J. Clin. Pathol., *88*:570–577, 1987.

Clark, G.M.,., Dressler, L.G., Owens, M.A., Pounds, G., Oldaker, T., and McGuire, W.L.: Predictions of relapse or survival in patients with node-negative breast cancer by DNA flow cytometry. N. Engl. J. Med., *320*:627–633, 1989.

Clevenger, C.V., Bauer, K.D., and Epstein, A.L.: A method of simultaneous nuclear immunofluorescence and DNA content quantitation using monoclonal antibodies and flow cytometry. Cytometry, *6*:208–214, 1985.

Clevenger, C.V., Epstein, A.L., and Bauer, K.D.: Quantitative analysis of a nuclear antigen in interphase and mitotic cells. Cytometry, *8*:280–286, 1987.

Cohen, J.H.M., Aubrey, J.P., Bancherau, J., and Revillard, J.P.: Identification of cell subpopulations by dual-color surface immunofluorescence using biotinylated and unlabeled monoclonal antibodies. Cytometry, *9*:303–308, 1988.

Collste, L.G., Devonec, M., Darzynkiewicz, Z., Traganos, F., Sharpless, T.K., Whitmore, W.F., Jr., and Melamed, M.R.: Bladder cancer diagnosis by flow cytometry. Correlation between cell samples from biopsy and bladder irrigation fluid. Cancer, *45*:2389–2394, 1980.

Coon, J.S., Bines, S., Kheir, S., and Soong, S.-J.: DNA flow cytometry in stage I cutaneous melanoma. Cytometry, *1*(Suppl):55, 1987.

Coon, J.S., Deitch, A.D., DeVere White, R.W., Koss, L.G., Melamed, M.R., Reeder, J.E., Weinstein, R.S., Wersto, R.P., and Wheeless, L.L.: Interinstitutional variability in DNA flow cytometric analysis of tumors. The National Cancer Institutes flow cytometry network experience. Cancer, *61*:126–130, 1988.

Coon, J.S., Landay, A.L., and Weinstein, R.S.: Advances in flow cytometry for diagnostic pathology. Lab. Invest., *57*:453–479, 1987.

Coon, J.S., Lanay, A.L., and Weinstein, R.S.: Flow cytometric analysis of paraffin-embedded tumors. Implications for diagnostic pathology. Hum. Pathol., *117*:435–437, 1986.

Coon, J.S., Schwartz, D., Summers, J.L., Miller, A.W., and Weinstein, R.S.: Flow cytometric analysis of deparaffinized nuclei in urinary bladder carcinomas. Comparison with cytogenetic analysis. Cancer, *57*:1594–1601, 1986.

Cornelisse, C.J., and van Driel-Kulker, A.M.: DNA image cytometry on machine-selected breast cancer cells and a comparison between flow cytometry and scanning cytophotometry. Cytometry, *6*:471–477, 1985.

Cornelisse, C.J., van de Velde, C.J.H., Caspers, R.J.C., Moolenaar, A.J., and Hermans, J.: DNA ploidy and survival in breast cancer patients. Cytometry, *8*:225–234, 1987.

Coulson, P.B., Thornthwaite, J.T., Woolley, T.W., Sugarbaker, E.V., and Seckinger, D.: Prognostic indicators including DNA histogram type, receptor content, and staging related to human breast cancer patient survival. Cancer Res., *44*:4187–4196, 1986.

Coulter, W.H.: Proceed. Natl. Electr. Conf., *12*:1034, 1956.

Cram, L.S., and Lehman, L.M.: Flow microfluorometric DNA

content measurements of tissue culture cells and peripheral lymphocytes. Hum. Genet., *37*:201–206, 1977.

Crissman, H.A., and Tobey, R.A.: Cell-cycle analysis in 20 minutes. Science, *184*:1297–1298, 1974.

Croonen, A.M., van der Valk, H.C.J., and Lindeman, J.: Cytology, immunology and flow cytometry in the diagnosis of pleural and peritoneal effusions. Lab. Invest., *58*:725–731, 1988.

Czerniak, B., Darzynkiewicz, Z., Stoiano-Coico, L., Herz, F., and Koss, L.G.: Expression of Ca antigen in relation to cycle in cultured human tumor cells. Cancer Res., *44*:4342–4346, 1984.

Czerniak, B., Deitch, D., Simmons, H., Efkin, P., Herz, F., and Koss, L.G.: Ha-*ras* gene codon 12 mutation and DNA ploidy in urinary bladder. Brit. J. Cancer, *62*:762–763, 1990.

Czerniak, B., Herz, F., Wersto, R.P., and Koss, L.G.: Expression of Ha-ras oncogene p21 protein in relation to the cell cycle of cultured human tumor cells. Am. J. Pathol., *126*:411–416, 1987.

Czerniak, B., Herz, F., Wersto, R.P., and Koss, L.G.: Modification of Ha-ras oncogene p21 expression and cell progression in the human colonic cancer cell line HT-29. Cancer Res., *47*:2826–2830, 1987.

Czerniak, B., Herz, F., Wersto, R.P., Alster, P., Puszkin, E., Schwartz, E., and Koss, L.G.: Quantitation of oncogene products by computer-assisted image analysis and flow cytometry. J. Histochem. Cytochem., *38*:463–466, 1990.

Czerniak, B., and Koss, L.G.: Expression of Ca antigen on human urinary bladder tumors. Cancer, *55*:2380–2383, 1985.

Czerniak, B., Koss, L.G., and Sherman, A.: Nuclear pores and DNA ploidy in human bladder carcinomas. Cancer Res., *44*:3752–3756, 1984.

Czerniak, B., Papenhausen, P.R., Herz, F., and Koss, L.G.: Flow cytometric identification of cancer cells in effusions with Ca1 monoclonal antibody. Cancer, *55*:2783–2788, 1985.

Darona, M., Riccardi, A., Mazzini, G., Ucci, G., Gaetani, P., Silvani, V., Knerich, R., Butti, G., and Ascari, E.: Ploidy and proliferative activity of human brain tumors. A flow cytofluorometric study. Oncology, *44*:102–107, 1987.

Darzynkiewicz, Z.: Metabolic and kinetic compartments of the cell cycle distinguished by multiparameter flow cytometry. *In* Skehan, P., and Friedman, S.J., (eds.): Growth, Cancer, and the Cell Cycle. pp. 291–336 Clifton, N.J., Humana Press, 1986.

Darzynkiewicz, Z.: Molecular interactions and cellular changes during the cell cycle. Pharmacol. Ther., *21*:143–188, 1983.

Darzynkiewicz, Z., Andreeff, M., Traganos, R., Sharpless, T., and Melamed, M.R.: Discrimination of cycling and noncycling lymphocytes by BudR-suppressed acridine orange fluorescence in a flow cytometric system. Exp. Cell Res., *115*:1938–1942, 1978.

Darzynkiewicz, Z., Crissman, H., Traganos, F., and Steinkamp, J.: Cell heterogeneity during the cell cycle. J. Cell Physiol., *113*:465–474, 1982.

Darzynkiewicz, Z., Traganos, F., Kapuscinski, J., Stoiano-Coico, L., and Melamed, M.R.: Accessibility of DNA in situ to various fluorochromes: Relationship to chromatin changes during erythroid differentiation of Friend leukemia cell. Cytometry, *5*:355–363, 1984.

Darzynkiewicz, Z., Traganos, F., and Melamed, M.R.: New cell cycle compartments identified by multiparameter flow cytometry. Cytometry, *1*:95–108, 1980.

Dean, P.H., and Jett, J.H.: Mathematical analysis of DNA dis-

tributions derived from flow microfluorometry. J. Cell Biol., *60*:523–527, 1974.

Dean, P.J., and Murphy, W.M.: Importance of urinary cytology and future role of flow cytometry. Urology, *26*(Suppl.):11–15, 1985.

Deinlein, E., Schmidt, H., Riemann, J.F., Grassel-Pietrusky, R., and Hornstein, O.P.: DNA flow cytometric measurements in inflammatory and malignant human gastric lesions. Virchows Arch. [A], *402*:185–193, 1983.

deVere White, R.W., Deitch, A.D., Baker, W.C., Jr., and Strand, M.A.: Urine: A suitable sample for deoxyribonucleic acid flow cytometry studies in patients with bladder cancer. J. Urol., *139*:926–928, 1988.

deVere White, R.W., Olsson, C.A., and Deitch, A.D.: Flow cytometry: Role in monitoring transitional cell carcinoma of bladder. Urology, *28*:15–20, 1986.

Devonec, M., Darzynkiewicz, Z., Whitmore, W.F., and Melamed, M.R.: Flow cytometry for followup examinations of conservatively treated low stage bladder tumors. J. Urol., *126*:166–170, 1981.

Devonec, M., Darzynkiewicz, Z., Kostyrka-Claps, M.L., Collste, L., Whitmore, W.F., Jr., and Melamed, M.R.: Flow cytometry of low stage bladder tumors: Correlation with cytologic and cytoscopic diagnosis. Cancer, *49*:109–118, 1982.

Dyson, J.F., Joslin, C.A., Rothwell, R.I., Quirke, P., Khoury, G.G., and Bird, C.C.: Flow cytofluorometric evidence for the differential radioresponsiveness of aneuploid and diploid cervix tumours. Radiother. Oncol., *8*:263–272, 1987.

Ekfors, T.O., Lipasti, J., Nurmi, M.J., and Eerola, B.: Flow cytometric analysis of the DNA profile of renal cell carcinoma. Pathol. Res. Pract., *182*:58–62, 1987.

Ensley, J.F., Maciorowski, Z., Pietraszkiewicz, H., Hasan, M., Kish, J., Al-Sarraf, M., Jacobs, J., Weaver, A., Atkinson, D., and Crissman, J.: Solid tumor preparation for clinical application of flow cytometry. Cytometry, *8*:488–493, 1987.

Ewers, S.B., Langstrom, E., Baldetorp, B., and Killander, D.: Flow-cytometric DNA analysis in primary breast carcinomas and clinicopathological correlations. Cytometry, *5*:408–419, 1984.

Fallenius, A.G., Askensten, U.G., Skoog, L.K., and Auer, G.U.: The reliability of microspectrophotometric and flow cytometric nuclear DNA measurements in adenocarcinomas of the breast. Cytometry, *8*:260–266, 1987.

Fallenius, A.G., Auer, G.U., and Carstensen, J.M.: Prognostic significance of DNA measurements in 409 consecutive breast cancer patients. Cancer, *62*:331–341, 1988.

Fallenius, A.E., Skoog, L.K., Svane, G.E., and Auer, G.U.: Cytophotometrical and biochemical characterization of nonpalpable, mammographically detected mammary adenocarcinomas. Cytometry, *5*:426–429, 1984.

Feichter, G.E., Kuhn, W., Czernobilsky, B., Muller, A., Heep, J., Abel, U., Haag, D., Kaufmann, M., Rummel, H.H., Kubli, F., et al.: DNA flow cytometry of ovarian tumors with correlation to histopathology. Int. J. Gynecol., Pathol., *4*:336–345, 1985.

Feichter, G.E., Mueller, A., Kaufman, M., Haag, D., Born, I.A., Abel, U., Klinga, K., Kubli, F., and Goerttler, K.: Correlation of DNA flow cytometric results and other prognostic factors in primary breast cancer. Int. J. Cancer, *41*:823–828, 1988.

Ffrench, M., Manel, A.M., Magaud, J.P., Fiere, D., Adeleine, P., Guyotat, D., and Bryon, P.A.: Adult acute lymphoblastic leukemia: Is cell proliferation related to other clinical and biological features. Br. J. Haematol., *36*:11–17, 1987.

Fietz, W.F.J., Beck, H.L.M., Smeets, A.W.G.B., Debruyne, F.M.J., Vooijs, G.P., Herman, C.J., and Ramaekers, F.C.S.:

Tissue-specific markers in flow cytometry of urological cancers: cytokeratins in bladder carcinoma. Int. J. Cancer, 36:349–356, 1985.

Finch, P.D.: Substantive difference and the analysis of histograms from very large samples. J. Histochem. Cytochem., 27:800, 1979.

Fordham, M.V., Burdge, A.H., Matthews, J., Williams, G., and Cooke, T.: Prostatic carcinoma cell DNA content measured by flow cytometry and its relation to clinical outcome. Br. J. Surg., 73:400–403, 1986.

Fosså, S.D., Thorud, E., Vaage, S., and Shoaib, M.C.: DNA cytometry of primary breast cancer. Comparison of microspectrophotometry and flow cytometry and different preparation methods for flow cytometric measurements. Acta Pathol. Microbiol. Immunol. Scand. [A], 91:235–243, 1983.

Frankfurt, O.S., Arbuck, S.G., Chin, J.L., Greco, W.R., Pavelic, Z.P., Slocum, H.K., Mittelman, A., Piver, S.M., Pontes, E.J., and Rustum, Y.M.: Prognostic application of DNA flow cytometry for human solid tumors. Ann. N.Y. Acad. Sci., 468:276–290, 1986.

Frankfurt, O.S., Greco, W.R., Solcum, H.K., Arbuck, S.G., Gamarra, M., Pavelic, Z.P., and Rustum, Y.M.: Proliferative characteristics of primary and metastatic human solid tumors by DNA flow cytometry. Cytometry, 5:629–635, 1984.

Friedlander, M.L., Hedley, D.W., and Taylor, I.W.: Clinical and biological significance of aneuploidy in human tumours. J. Clin. Pathol., 37:961–974, 1984.

Friedlander, M.L., Hedley, D.W., Taylor, I.W., Russell, P., Coates, A.S., and Tattersall, M.H.N.: Influence of cellular DNA content on survival in advanced ovarian cancer. Cancer Res., 44:397–400, 1984.

Friedlander, M.L., Hedley, D.W., Swanson, C., and Russell, P.: Prediction of long-term survival by flow cytometric analysis of cellular DNA content on patients with advanced ovarian cancer, J. Clin. Oncol., 6:282–290, 1988.

Friedlander, M.L., Russell, P., Taylor, I.W., Hedley, D.W., and Tattersal, M.H.N.: Flow cytometric analysis of cellular DNA content as an adjunct to the diagnosis of ovarian tumours of borderline malignancy. Pathology, 16:301–306, 1984.

Friedlander, M.L., Taylor, I.W., Russell, P., et al.: Ploidy as a prognostic factor in ovarian cancer. Int. J. Gynecol. Pathol., 2:55–63, 1983.

Fulwyler, M.J.: Electronic separation of biological cells by volume. Science, 150:910–911, 1965.

Fulwyler, M.J., Glascock, R.B., Hiebert, R.D., and Johnson, N.M.: Device which separates minute particles according to electronically sensed volume. Rev. Sci. Instrum., 40:42–48, 1969.

Geisinger, K.R., Homesley, H.D., Morgan, T.M., Kute, T.E., and Marshall, R.B.: Endometrial adenocarcinoma. A multiparameter clinicopathologic analysis including the DNA profile and the sex steroid hormone receptors. Cancer, 58:1518–1528, 1986.

Goldsmith, M.M., Cresson, D.H., Arnold, L.A., Postma, D.S., Askin, F.B., and Pillbury, H.C.: DNA flow cytometry as a prognostic indicator in head and neck cancer. Otolaryngol. Head Neck Surg., 96:307–316, 1987.

Goldsmith, M.M., Cresson, D.H., Postma, D.S., Askin, F.B., and Pillsbury, H.G.: Significance of ploidy in laryngeal cancer. Am. J. Surg., 152:396–402, 1986.

Gratzner, H.G.: Monoclonal antibody to 5-bromo- and 5-iododeoxyunidine: A new reagent for detection of DNA replication. Science, 218:474–475, 1982.

Gray, J.W., and Mayall, B.H. (eds.): Monoclonal Antibodies against Bromodeoxyuridine. New York, A.R. Liss, 1985.

Greenebaum, E., Koss, L.G., Sherman, A.B., and Elequin, F.: Comparison of needle aspiration and solid biopsy technics in the flow cytometric study of DNA distributions of surgically resected tumors. Am. J. Clin. Pathol., 82:559–564, 1984.

Greenebaum, E., Koss, L.G., Elequin, F., and Silver, C.E.: The diagnostic value of flow cytometric DNA measurements in follicular tumors of the thyroid gland. Cancer, 56:2011–2018, 1985.

Gustafson, H., Tribukait, B., and Esposti, P-L: DNA pattern, histological grade, and multiplicity related to recurrence rate in superficial bladder tumours. Scand. J. Urol. Nephrol., 16:135–139, 1982.

Haag, D., Feichter, G., Goerttler, K., and Kaufmann, M.: Influence of systematic errors on the evaluation of the S phase portions from DNA distributions of solid tumors as shown for 328 breast carcinomas. Cytometry, 8:377–385, 1987.

Haggitt, R.C., Reid, B.J., Rabinovitch, P.S., and Rubin, C.E.: Barrett's esophagus—correlation between mucin histochemistry, flow cytometry, and histologic diagnosis for predicting increased cancer risk. Am. J. Pathol., 131:53–61, 1988.

Hammarberg, C., Rubio, C., Slezak, P., Tribukait B., and Ohman, U.: Flow-cytometric DNA analysis as a means for early detection of malignancy in patients with chronic ulcerative colitis. Gut, 25:905–908, 1984.

Hammarberg, C., Slezak, P., and Tribukait, B.: Early detection of malignancy in ulcerative colitis. A flow-cytometric DNA study. Gut, 53:291–295, 1984.

Hanselaar, A.G.J.M., Vooijs, G.P., Oud, P.S., Pahlplatz, M.M.M., and Beck, J.L.M., DNA ploidy patterns in cervical intraepithelial neoplasia grade III, with and without synchronous invasive squamous cell carcinoma: Measurements in nuclei isolated from paraffin-embedded tissue. Cancer, 62:2537–2545, 1988.

Hayden, G.E., Walker, K.Z., Miller, J.F.A.P., Wotherspoon, J.S., and Raison, R.L.: Simultaneous cytometric analysis for the expression of cytoplasmic and surface antigens in activated T cells. Cytometry, 9:44–51, 1988.

Hedley, D.W.: Flow cytometry using paraffin-embedded tissue: Five years on. Cytometry, 10:229–241, 1989.

Hedley, D.W., Friedlander, M.L., and Taylor, I.W.: Application of DNA flow cytometry to paraffin-embedded archival material for the study of aneuploidy and its clinical significance. Cytometry, 6:327–333, 1985.

Hedley, D.W., Friedlander, M.L., Taylor, I.W., Rugg, C.A., and Musgrove, E.A.: DNA flow cytometry of paraffin-embedded tissue. Cytometry, 5:1660, 1984.

Hedley, D.W., Friedlander, M.L., Taylor, I.W., Rugg, C.A., and Musgrove, E.A.: Method for analysis of cellular DNA content of paraffin-embedded pathological material using flow cytometry. J. Histochem. Cytochem., 31:1333–1335, 1983.

Hedley, D.W., Rugg, C.A., and Gelber, R.D.: Association of DNA index and S-phase fraction with prognosis of nodes positive early breast cancer. Cancer Res., 47:4729–4735, 1987.

Helio, H., Karaharju, E., and Nordling, S.: Flow cytometric determination of DNA content in malignant and benign bone tumours. Cytometry, 6:165–171, 1985.

Hiddemann, W., Schumann, J., Andreeff, M., Barlogie, B., Herman, C.J., Leif, R.C., Mayall, B.M., Murphy, R.F., and Sandberg, A.: Convention on nomenclature for DNA cytometry. Cancer Genet, Cytogenet., 13:181–183, 1984.

Holdrinet, R.S.G., Pennings, A., Drenthe-Schonk, A.M., van Egmond, J., Wessels, J.M.C., and Haanen, C.: Flow cytometric determination of the S-phase compartment in adult acute leukemia. Acta Haematol. (Basel), 70:369–378, 1983.

Hopman, A.H.N., Ramaekers, F.C.S., Raap, A.K., Beck, J.L.M., Devilbe, P., van der Ploeg, M., and Vooijs, G.P.: In situ hybridization as a tool to study numerical chromosome aberrations in solid bladder tumors. Histochemistry, 89:307–316, 1988.

Horan, P.K., Slezak, S.E., and Poste, G.: Improved flow cytometric analysis of leukocyte subsets: Simultaneous identification of five cell subsets using two-color immunofluorescence. Proc. Natl. Acad. Sci. U.S.A., 83:8361–8365, 1986.

Horan, P.K., and Wheeless, L.L.: Quantitative single cell analysis and sorting. Science, 198:149–157, 1977.

Horsfall, D.J., Tilley, W.D., Orell, S.R., Marshall, V.R., and Cant, E.L.: Relationship between ploidy and steroid hormone receptors in primary invasive breast cancer. Br. J. Cancer, 53:23–28, 1986.

Iverson, O.E.: Flow cytometric deoxyribonucleic acid index: A prognostic factor in endometrial carcinoma. Am. J. Obstet. Gynecol., 155:770–776, 1986.

Iverson, O.E.: Prognostic value of the flow cytometric DNA index in human ovarian carcinoma. Cancer, 61:971–975, 1988.

Jacobberger, J.W., Fogelman, D., and Lehman, J.M.: Analysis of intracellular antigens by flow cytometry. Cytometry, 7:356–364, 1986.

Jakobsen, A.: Ploidy level and short-time prognosis of early cervix cancer. Radiother. Oncol., 1:271–275, 1984.

Jakobsen, A.: Prognostic impact of ploidy level in carcinoma of the cervix. Am. J. Clin. Oncol., 7:475–480, 1984.

Jakobsen, A.: The use of trout erythrocytes and human lymphocytes for standardization in flow cytometry. Cytometry, 4:161–165, 1983.

Jakobsen, A., Kristensen, P.B., and Poulsen, H.K.: Flow cytometric classification of biopsy specimens from cervical intraepithelial neoplasia. Cytometry, 4:166–169, 1983.

Joensuu, H., Klemi, P., Eerola, E., and Touminen, J.: Influence of cellular DNA content on survival in differentiated thyroid cancer. Cancer, 58:2462–2467, 1986.

Joensuu, H., Soderstrom, K.K., P.J., and Eerola, B.: Nuclear DNA content and its prognostic value in lymphoma of the stomach. Cancer, 60:3042–3048, 1987.

Johannessen, J.V., Sobrinho-Simoes, M., Tangen, K.O., and Lindmo, T.: A flow cytometric deoxyribonucleic acid analysis of papillary thyroid carcinoma. Lab. Invest., 45:336–341, 1981.

Johnson, D.A., White, R.A., and Barlogie, B.: Automatic processing and interpretation of DNA distributions. Comparison of several techniques. Comput. Biomed. Res., 11:393–404, 1978.

Jovin, T.M., Morris, S.J., Striker, G., Schultens, H.A., Digweed, M., and Arndt-Jovin, D.J.: Automatic sizing and separation of particles by ratios of light scattering intensities. J. Histochem. Cytochem., 24:269–283, 1976.

Kallioniemi, O.P., Blanco, G., Alavaikko, M., et al.: Improving the prognostic value of DNA cytometry in breast cancer by combining DNA index and S-phase fraction. Cancer, 62:183–190, 1988.

Kallioniemi, O.P., Punnonen, R., Mattila, J., Lehtien, M., and Koivula, T.: Prognostic significance of DNA index, multiploidy, and S-phase fraction in ovarian cancer. Cancer, 61:334–339, 1988.

Kamel, O.W., Franklin, W.A., Ringus, J.C., and Meyer, J.S.: Thymidine labeling index and Ki-67 growth fraction in lesions of the breast. Am. J. Pathol., 1134:107–113, 1989.

Kamentsky, L.A., Derman, H., and Melamed, M.R.: Ultraviolet absorption of epidemoid cancer cells. Science, 142:1580–1583, 1963.

Kamentsky, L.A., Melamed, M.R., and Derman, H.: Spectro-photometer: New instrument for ultrarapid cell analysis. Science, 150:630–631, 1965.

Kamentsky, L.A., Melamed, M.R., and Derman, H.: Spectrophotometric cell sorter. Science, 156:1364–1365, 1967.

Kaplow, L.S., Dauber, H., and Lerner, E.: Assessment of monocyte esterase activity by flow cytophotometry. J. Histochem. Cytochem., 24:363–372, 1976.

Klein, F.A., Herr, H.W., Sogani, P.C., Whitmore, W.F., Jr., and Melamed, M.R.: Detection and follow-up of carcinomas of the urinary bladder by flow cytometry. Cancer, 50:389–395, 1982.

Klein, F.A., Herr, H.W., Whitmore, W.F., Sogani, P.C., and Melamed, M.R.: An evaluation of automated flow cytometry (FCM) in detection of carcinoma in situ of the urinary bladder. Cancer, 50:1003–1008, 1982.

Klintenberg, C., Stal, O., Nordenskjold, B., Wallgren, A., Arvidsson, S., and Skoog, L.: Proliferative index, cytosol estrogen receptor and axillary node status as prognostic predictors in human mammary carcinoma. Breast Cancer Res., Treat., 7:S99–S106, 1986.

Koenig, S.H., Brown, R.D., Kamentsky, L.A., Sedlis, A., and Melamed, M.R.: Efficacy of a rapid cell spectrophotometer in screening for cervical cancer. Cancer, 21:1019–1026, 1968.

Kokal, W., Sheibani, K., Terz, J., and Harada, J.R.: Tumor DNA content in the prognosis of colorectal carcinoma. J.A.M.A., 255:3123–3127, 1986.

Koss, L.G.: Analytical and quantitative cytology: A historical perspective. Anal. Quant. Cytol. Histol., 4:251–256, 1982.

Koss, L.G.: Automated cytology and histology: A historical perspective. Anal. Quant. Cytol. Histol., 9:369–374, 1987.

Koss, L.G.: The puzzle of prostatic carcinoma. Mayo Clin. Proc., 63:193–197, 1988.

Koss, L.G., Czerniak, B.H.F., and Wersto, R.P.: Flow cytometric measurements of DNA and other cell components in human tumors: A critical appraisal. Hum. Pathol., 20:528–548, 1989.

Koss, L.G., Dembitzer, H.M., Herz, F., Herzig, N., Schreiber, K., and Wolley, R.C.: The monodisperse cell sample. I. Problems and possible solutions. In Wied, G.L., and Bahr, G. (eds.): Proceedings of the International Conference on Automation of Uterine Cervix Cytology. Chicago, University of Chicago Press, 1976.

Koss, L.G., and Greenbaum, E.: Measuring DNA in human cancer. J.A.M.A., 255:3158–3159, 1986.

Koss, L.G., Wersto, R.P., Simmons, D.H., Deitch, D., and Freed, S.Z.: Predictive value of DNA measurements in bladder washings. Comparison of flow cytometry image cytophotometry and cytology of voided urine in urothelial tumors. Cancer, 64:916–924, 1989.

Koss, L.G., Wolley, R.C., Schreiber, K., and Mendecki, J.: Flow microfluorometric analysis of nuclei isolated from various normal and malignant human epithelial cells. J. Histochem. Cytochem., 25:565–572, 1977.

Kosugi, Y., Sato, R., Genka, S., Shitara, N., and Takakura, K.: An interactive multivariate analysis of FCM data. Cytometry, 9:405–408, 1988.

Kreicbergs, A., Silfersward, C., and Tribukait, B.: Flow DNA analysis of primary bone tumors. Relationship between cellular DNA content and histopathologic classification. Cancer, 53:129–136, 1984.

Krishnan, A.: Rapid flow cytofluorometric analysis of mammalian cell cycle by propidium iodide staining. J. Cell Biol., 66:188–193, 1975.

Lacombe, F., Belloc, F., Bernard, P., and Boisseau, M.R.: Evaluation of four methods of DNA distribution data analysis based on bromodeoxyuridine/DNA bivariate data. Cytometry, 9:245–253, 1988.

Lampe, H.B., Flint, A., Wolf, G.T., and McClatchey, K.D.: Flow cytometry: DNA analysis of squamous cell carcinoma of the upper aerodigestive tract. J. Otolaryngol., *16*:371–376, 1987.

Latt, S.A.: Fluorescent probes of chromosome structure and replication. Can. J. Genet. Cytol., *19*:603–623, 1977.

Lehman, J.M., Laffin, J., Jacobberger, J.W., and Fogelman, D.: Analysis of simian virus 40 infection of permissive CV-1 cells by quantitative two-color fluorescence with flow cytometry. Cytometry, *9*:52–59, 1988.

Lehtinen, T., Lehtinen, M., Aine, R., Kallioniemi, O.P., Leino, T., Hakala, T., Leinikki, P., and Alavaikko, M.: Nuclear DNA content of non-endemic Burkitt's lymphoma. J. Clin. Pathol., *40*:1201–1205, 1987.

Lennert, P., Roos, G., Johansson, H., Lindh, J., and Dige, V.: Non-Hodgkin lymphoma. Multivariate analysis of prognostic factors including fraction of S-phase cells. Acta Oncol., *26*:179–183, 1987.

Lindahl, B., Alm, P.K., D., Langstrom, B., and Thorpe, C.: Flow cytometric DNA analysis of normal and cancerous human endometrium and cytological-histopathological correlations. Anticancer Res., *7*:781–789, 1987.

Lindahl, B., Alm, P., Ferno, M., Killander, D., Langstrom, B., Norgren, A., and Trope, C.: Prognostic value of flow cytometrical DNA measurements in stage I–II endometrial carcinoma: Correlations with steroid receptor concentration, tumor myometrial invasion, and degree of differentiation. Anticancer Res., *7*:791–797, 1987.

Ljungberg, B., Stenling, R., and Roos, G.: Prognostic value of deoxyribonucleic acid content in metastatic renal cell carcinoma. J. Urol., *136*:801–804, 1986.

Look, A.T., Douglass, E.C., and Meyer, W.H.: Clinical importance of near-diploid tumor stem lines in patients with osteosarcoma of an extremity. N. Engl. J. Med., *318*:1567–1572, 1988.

Lundberg, S., Carstensen, J., and Rundquist, I.: DNA flow cytometry and histopathological grading of paraffin-embedded prostate biopsy specimens in survival study. Cancer Res., *47*:1973–1977, 1987.

Macartney, J.C., Camplejohn, R.S., and Powell, G.: DNA flow cytometry of histological material from human gastric cancer. J. Pathol., *148*:273–277, 1986.

Macartney, J.C., and Camplejohn, R.S.: DNA flow cytometry of histological material from dysplastic lesions of human gastric mucosa. J. Pathol., *150*:113–118, 1986.

Mayall, B.H., Carrano, A.V., Moore, D.H., II, Ashworth, L.K., Bennett, D.E., and Mendelsohn, M.L.: The DNA-based karyotype. Cytometry, *5*:376, 1984.

McDivitt, R.W., Stone, K.R., and Meyer J.S.: A method for dissociation of viable human breast cancer cells that produce flow cytometric kinetic information similar to that obtained by thymidine labeling. Cancer Res., *44*:2628–2633, 1984.

McGuire, W.L.: Adjuvant therapy of node-negative breast cancer. N. Engl. J. Med., *320*:525–527, 1989.

Melamed, M.R.: Flow cytometry of the urinary bladder. Urol. Clin. North Am., *11*:599–608, 1984.

Melamed, M.R., Enker, W.E., Banner, P., Janov, A.J., Kessler, G., and Darzynkiewicz, Z.: Flow cytometry of colorectal carcinoma with three-year follow-up. Dis. Colon Rectum, *29*:184–186, 1986.

Melamed, M.R., and Kamentsky, L.A.: Automated cytology. Int. Rev. Exp. Pathol., *14*:205–295, 1975.

Melamed, M.R., and Klein, F.A.: Flow cytometry of urinary bladder irrigation specimens. Hum. Pathol., *15*:302–305, 1984.

Melamed, M.R., Mullaney, P.R., and Mendelsohn, M.L.: Flow Cytometry and Sorting. New York, John Wiley & Sons, 1979.

Melamed, M.R., Lindmo, T., and Mendelsohn, M.L.: Flow Cytometry and Sorting, 2d ed. New York, Wiley-Liss, 1990.

Mendecki, J., Dillman, W., Wolley, R.C., Oppenheimer, J.H., and Koss, L.G.: Effect of thyroid hormone on the ploidy of rat liver nuclei as determined by flow-cytometry. Poc. Soc. Exp. Biol. Med., *158*:63–67, 1978.

Merkel, D.E., Dressler, L.G., and McGuire, W.L.: Flow cytometry, cellular DNA content, and prognosis in human malignancy. J. Clin. Oncol., *5*:1690–1703, 1987.

Meyer, J.S.: Cell kinetics of histologic variants of in situ breast cancer. Breast Cancer Res. Treat., *7*:171–180, 1986.

Meyer, J.S., Bauer, W.C., and Rao, B.R.: Subpopulation of breast carcinoma defined by S-phase fraction, morphology, and estrogen receptor content. Lab. Invest., *39*:225–235, 1978.

Meyer, J.S., and Coplin, M.D.: Thymidine labeling index, flow cytometric S-phase measurement, and DNA index in human tumors. Comparisons and correlations. Am. J. Clin. Pathol., *89*:586–595, 1988.

Meyer, J.S., Friedman, E., McCrate, M.M., and Bauer, W.C.: Prediction of early course of breast carcinoma by thymidine labeling. Cancer, *51*:1879–1886, 1983.

Mullany, P.F., VanDilla, M.A., Coulter, J.R., and Dean, P.N.: Cell sizing: A light scattering photometer for rapid volume determination. Rev. Sci. Instrum., *40*:1029, 1969.

Murphy, W.M., Emerson, L.D., Chandler, R.W., Moinuddin, S.M., and Soloway, M.S.: Flow cytometry versus urinary cytology in the evaluation of patients with bladder cancer. J. Urol., *136*:815–819, 1986.

Nervi, C., Badaracco, G., Morrelli, M., and Starace, G.: Cytokinetic evaluation in human head and neck cancer by autoradiography and DNA cytofluorometry. Cancer, *45*:452–459, 1980.

Newton, J.A., Camplejohn, R.S., and McGibbon, D.H.: Aneuploidy in Bowen's disease. Br. J. Dermatol., *114*:691–694, 1986.

Odegaard, S., Hostmark, J., Skagen, D.W., Schrumpf, E., and Laerum, O.D.: Flow cytometric DNA studies in human gastric cancer and polyps. Scand. J. Gastroenterol., *22*:1270–1276, 1987.

Olszewski, W., Darzynkiewicz, Z., Rosen, P.P., Schwartz, M.K., and Melamed, M.R.: Flow cytometry of breast carcinoma: I. Relationship of DNA ploidy level to histology and estrogen receptor. Cancer, *48*:980–984, 1981.

Olszewski, W., Darzynkiewicz, Z., Rosen, P.P., Schwartz, M.K., and Melamed, M.R.: Flow cytometry of breast carcinoma: II. Relation of tumor cell cycle distribution to histology and estrogen receptor. Cancer, *48*:985–988, 1981.

Otto, U., Baisch, H., Huland, H., and Kloppel, G.: Tumor cell deoxyribonucleic acid content and prognosis in human renal cell carcinoma. J. Urol., *132*:237–239, 1984.

Oud, P.S., Hanselaar, T.G.J.M., Reubsaet-Veldhuizen, J.A.M., Meijer, J.W.R., Gemmink, A.H., Pahlplatz, M.M.M., Beck, H.L.M., and Vooijs, G.P.: Extraction of nuclei from selected regions in paraffin-embedded tissue. Cytometry, *7*:595–600, 1986.

Petrova, A.S., Subrichina, G.N., Tschistjakova, O.V., Rottenberg, V.I., Weiss, H., Jacobasch, K.H., Streller, B., and Wildner, G.P.: DNA ploidy and proliferation characteristics of bowel polyps analysed by flow cytometry compared with cytology and histology. Arch. Geschwulstforsch, *56*:179–191, 1986.

Pontes, J.E., Wajsman, Z., Huben, R.P., Wolf, R.M., and Englander, L.S.: Prognostic factors in localized prostatic carcinoma. J. Urol., *134*:1137–1139, 1985.

Quirke, P., Fozard, J.B.J., Dixon, M.F., Dyson, J.E.D., Giles, G.R., and Byrd, C.C.: DNA aneuploidy in colorectal adenomas. Br. J. Cancer, *53*:477–481, 1986.

Rabinovitch, P.S., Kubbies, M., Chen, Y.C., Schindler, D., and Hoehn, H.: BrdU-Hoechst flow cytometry: A unique tool for quantitative cell cycle analysis. Exp. Cell Res., *174*:309–318, 1988.

Rainwater, L.M., Farrow, G.M., Hay, I.D., and Lieber, M.M.: Oncocytic tumours of the salivary gland, kidney, and thyroid: Nuclear DNA patterns studied by flow cytometry. Br. J. Cancer, *53*:799–804, 1986.

Rainwater, L.M., Hosaka, Y., Farrow, G.M., and Lieber, M.M.: Well differentiated clear cell renal carcinoma: Significance of nuclear deoxyribonucleic acid patterns studied by flow cytometry. J. Urol., *137*:15–20, 1987.

Rainwater, L.M., Hosaka, Y., Farrow, G.M., Kramer, S.A., Kelalis, P.P., and Lieber, M.M.: Wilms tumors: Relationship of nuclear deoxyribonucleic acid ploidy to patient survival. J. Urol., *138*:974–977, 1987.

Reid, B.J., Haggitt, R.C., Rubin, C.E., and Rabinovitch, P.S.: Barrett's esophagus. Correlation between flow cytometry and histology in detection of patients at risk for adenocarcinoma. Gastroenterology, *93*:1–11, 1987.

Riccardi, A., Danova, M., Montecucco, C., Ucci, G., Cassano, E., Giordano, M., Mazzini, G., and Giordano, P.: Adult acute nonlymphoblastic leukaemia: Reliability and prognostic significance of pretreatment bone marrow, S-phase size determined by flow cytofluorometry. Scand. J. Haematol., *36*:11–17, 1986.

Rodenburg, C.J., Cornelisse, C.J., Heintz, P.A., Hermans, J., and Fleuren, G.J.: Tumor ploidy as a major prognostic factor in advanced ovarian cancer. Cancer, *59*:317–323, 1987.

Roos, G., Dige, V., Lenner, P., Lindh, J., and Johansson, H.: Prognostic significance of DNA-analysis by flow cytometry in non-Hodgkin's lymphoma. Hematol., Oncol., *3*:233–242, 1985.

Rutgers, D.H., van der Linden, P.M., and van Peperzeel, H.A.: DNA-flow cytometry of squamous cell carcinoma from the human uterine cervix: The identification of prognostically different subgroups. Radiother. Oncol., *7*:249–258, 1986.

Ryan, D.H., Fallon, M.A., and Horan, P.K.: Flow cytometry in the clinical laboratory. Clin. Chim. Acta, *171*:125–197, 1988.

Sahni, K., Tribukait, B., and Einhorn, N.: Comparative study of proportion of S-phase cells in ascites and pleural effusions in ovarian carcinoma using antibromodeoxyuridine monoclonal antibody and DNA flow-cytometry. Acta Oncol., *28*:705–708, 1989.

Sahni, K., Tribukait, B., and Einhorn, N.: Flow cytometric measurement of ploidy and proliferation in effusions of ovarian carcinoma and their possible prognostic significance. Gynecol., Oncol., *35*:240–245, 1989.

Schmidt, D., Wiedemann, B., Keil, W., Sprenger, E., and Harms, D.: Flow cytometric analysis of nephroblastomas and related neoplasms. Cancer, *58*:2494–2500, 1986.

Schneller, J., Eppich, E., Greenebaum, E., Elequin, F., Sherman, A., Wersto, R., and Koss, L.G.: Flow cytometry and Feulgen cytophotometry in evaluation of effusions. Cancer, *59*:1307–1313, 1987.

Schutte, B., Reynders, M.M.J., van Assche, C.L.M.V.J., Hupperets P.S.G.J., Bosman, F.T., and Blijham, G.H.: An improved method for the immunocytochemical detection of bromodeoxyuridine labeled nuclei using flow cytometry. Cytometry, *8*:372–376, 1987.

Shackney, S.E., Erickson, B.W., and Skramstad, K.S.: The T-lymphocyte as a diploid reference standard for flow cytometry. Cancer Res., *39*:4418–4427, 1979.

Shapiro, H.M.: Laser noise and news. Cytometry, *8*:248–250, 1987.

Shapiro, H.M.: Multistation multiparameter flow cytometry: A critical review and rationale. Cytometry, *3*:227–243, 1983.

Shapiro, H.M.: Practical Flow Cytometry. 2nd Ed. New York, Alan R. Liss, 1988.

Shapiro, H.M.: Technical developments in flow cytometry. Hum. Pathol., *17*:649–651, 1986.

Sharpless, T.K., and Melamed, M.R.: Estimation of cell size from pulse shape in flow cytofluorometry. J. Histochem. Cytochem., *24*:257–264, 1976.

Sigurdsson, H., Baldetorp, B., Borg, A., Dalberg, M., Ferno, M., Killander, D., and Olsson, H.: Indicators of prognosis in node-negative breast cancer. N. Engl. J. Med., *323*:1045–1053, 1990.

Sledge, G.W., Jr., Eble, J.N., Roth, B.J., Wuhrman, B.P., and Einhorn, L.H.: Flow cytometry derived DNA content of the primary lesions of advanced germ cell tumours. Int. J. Androl., *10*:115–120, 1987.

Slocum, H.K., Pavelic, Z.P., Rustrum, Y.M., Creaven, P.J., Karakousis, C., Takita, H., and Greco, W.R.: Characterization of cells obtained by mechanical and enzymatic means from human melanoma, sarcoma, and lung tumors. Cancer Res., *41*:1428–1434, 1981.

Smeets, A.W.G.B., Pauwels, R.P.E., Beck, H.L.M., Feitz, W.F.J., Geraedts, J.P.M., Debruyne, F.M.J., Laarakkers, L., Vooijs, G.P., and Ramaekers, F.C.S.: Comparison of tissue disaggregation techniques of transitional cell bladder carcinomas for flow cytometry and chromosomal analysis. Cytometry, *8*:14–19, 1987.

Smets, L.A., Slater, R.M., Behrerdt, H., Van't-Veer, M.B., and Homan-Blok, J.: Phenotypic and karyotypic properties of hyperdiploid acute lymphoblastic leukaemia of childhood. Br. J. Haematol., *61*:113–123, 1985.

Sondergaard, K., Larsen, J.K., Moller, U., Christiansen, I.J., and Hou-Jensen, K.: DNA ploidy-characteristics of human malignant melanoma analysed by flow cytometry and compared with histology and clinical course. Virchows Arch. [Cell Pathol.], *42*:43–52, 1983.

Spaar, F.W., Blech, M., and Ahyai, A.: DNA-flow fluorescence-cytometry of ependymomas. Report on ten surgically removed tumours. Acta Neuropathol. (Berl.), *69*:153–160, 1986.

Stal, O., Klintenberg, C., Franzen, G., Risberg, B., Arvidsson, S.B.K., Skoog, L., and Nordenskjold, B.: A comparison of static cytofluorometry and flow cytometry for estimation of ploidy and DNA replication in human breast cancer. Breast Cancer Res. Treat., *7*:15–22, 1986.

Steinkamp, J.A., Hansen, K.M., and Crissman, H.A.: Flow microfluorometric and light-scatter measurement of nuclear and cytoplasmic size in mammalian cells. J. Histochem. Cytochem., *24*:292–297, 1976.

Steinkamp, J.A., Romero, A., and Van Dilla, M.A.: Multiparameter cell sorting: Identification of human leukocytes by acridine orange fluorescence. Acta Cytol. (Baltimore), *17*:113–117, 1973.

Stephenson, R.A., James, B.C., Gay, H., Fair, W.R., Whitmore, W.F., Jr., and Melamed, M.R.: Flow cytometry of prostate cancer: Relationship of DNA content to survival. Cancer Res., *47*:2504–2507, 1987.

Strang, P., Eklund, G., Stendahl, U., and Frankendal, R.: S-phase rate as a predictor of early recurrences in carcinoma of the uterine cervix. Anticancer Res., *7*:807–810, 1987.

Strang, P., Lindgren, A., and Stendhahl, U.: Comparison between flow cytometry and single cell cytophotometry for DNA content analysis of the uterine cervix. Acta. Radiol. [Oncol.], *24*:337–341, 1985.

Stuart-Harris, R., Hedley, D.W., Taylor, I.W., Leven, A.L., and Smith, I.E.: Tumour ploidy, response and survival in patients receiving endocrine therapy for advanced breast cancer. Br. J. Cancer, *51*:573–576, 1985.

Tangen, K.O., Lindmo, T., Sobrinho-Simoes, M., and Johannessen, J.V.: A flow cytometric DNA analysis of medullary thyroid carcinoma. Am. J. Clin. Pathol., 79:172–177, 1983.

Tannenbaum, E., Cassidy, M., Alabaster, O., and Herman, C.: Measurement of cellular DNA mass by flow microfluorometry with use of a biological internal standard. J. Histochem., Cytochem., 26:145–148, 1978.

Terz, J.J., Curutchet, H.P., and Lawrence, W.J., Jr.: Analysis of the cell kinetics of human solid tumors. Cancer, 28:1100–1110, 1971.

Thornthwaite, J.F., Seckinger, D., Sugarbaker, E.V., Rosenthal, P.K., and Vazquez, D.A.: Dual immunofluorescent analysis of human peripheral blood lymphocytes. Am. J. Clin. Pathol., 82:48–56, 1984.

Thornthwaite, J.T., Sugarbaker, E.V., and Temple, W.J.: Preparation of tissues for DNA flow cytometric analysis. Cytometry, 1:229–237, 1980.

Thorud, E., Fossa, S.D., Vaage, S., Kaalhus, O., Knudsen, O.S., Bormer, O., and Shoaib, M.C.: Primary breast cancer. Flow cytometric DNA pattern in relation to clinical and histopathological characteristics. Cancer, 57:808–811, 1986.

Tomita, T., Yasue, M., Engelhard, H.H., McLone, D.G., Gonzalez-Crussi, F., and Bauer, K.D.: Flow cytometric DNA analysis of medulloblastoma. Prognostic implication of aneuploidy. Cancer, 61:744–749, 1988.

Traganos, F.: Flow cytometry. Principles and applications. II. Cancer Invest., 2:239–258, 1984.

Traganos, F., Darzynkiewicz, Z., Sharpless, T., and Melamed, M.R.: Erythroid differentiation of Friend leukemia cells as studied by acridine orange staining and flow cytometry. J. Histochem. Cytochem., 27:382–389, 1979.

Tribukait, B.: Flow cytometry in surgical pathology and cytology of tumors of the genito-urinary tract. *In* Koss, L.G., and Coleman, D.V. (eds.): Advances in Clinical Cytology. vol. 2. pp. 163–189. New York, Masson Publishing, 1984.

Tribukait, B.: Flow cytometry in assessing the clinical aggressiveness of genito-urinary neoplasms. World J. Urol., 5:108–122, 1987.

Tribukait, B., Gustafson, H., and Esposti, P-L. The significance of ploidy and proliferation in the clinical and biological evaluation of bladder tumours: a study of 100 untreated cases. Br. J. Urol., 54:130–135, 1982.

Tsushima, K., Rainwater, L.M., Goellner, J.R., van Heerden, J.A., and Lieber, M.M.: Leiomyosarcomas and benign smooth muscle tumors of the stomach. Nuclear DNA patterns studied by flow cytometry. Mayo Clin. Proc., 62:275–280, 1987.

Tsushima, K., Stanhope, C.R., Gaffey, T.A., and Lieber, M.M.: Uterine leiomyosarcomas and benign smooth muscle tumors: Usefulness of nuclear DNA patterns studied by flow cytometry. Mayo Clin. Proc., 63:248–255, 1988.

Unger, K.M., Rabes, M., Bedrossian, C.W.M., Stein, D.A., and Barlogie, B.: Analysis of pleural effusions using automated flow cytometry. Cancer, 52:873–877, 1983.

Valet, G., Russmann, N.L., and Wirsching, R.: Automated flow-cytometric identification of colorectal tumour cells by simultaneous DNA, CEA-antibody and cell volume measurements. J. Clin. Chem. Clin. Biochem., 22:935–942, 1984.

Van Dilla, M.A., Trujillo, T.T., Mullaney, P.F., and Coulter, J.R.: Cell microfluorometry: A method for rapid fluorescence measurement. Science, 163:1213–1214, 1969.

Vindelöv, L.L., Christensen, I.J., and Nissen, N.I.: A detergent-trypsin method for the preparation of nuclei for flow cytometric DNA analysis. Cytometry, 3:323–327, 1983.

Vindelöv, L.L., Christensen, I.J., and Nissen, N.J.: Standardization of high-resolution flow cytometric DNA analysis by the simultaneous use of chicken and trout red blood cells as internal reference standards. Cytometry, 3:328–331, 1983.

Volm, M., Bak, M., Hahn, E.W., Mattern, J., and Weber, E.: DNA and S-phase distribution and incidence of metastasis in human primary lung carcinoma. Cytometry, 9:183–188, 1988.

Volm, M., Drings, P., Mattern, J., Sonka, J., Vogt-Moykopf, I., and Wayss, K.: Prognostic significance of DNA patterns and resistance-predictive tests in non-small cell lung carcinoma. Cancer, 56:1396–1403, 1985.

Volm, M., Mattern, J., Sonka, J., Vogt-Schaden, M., and Wayss, K.: DNA distribution in non-small-cell lung carcinomas and its relationship to clinical behavior. Cytometry, 6:348–356, 1985.

Volm, M., Matten, J., Muller, T., and Drings, P.: Flow cytometry of epidermoid lung carcinomas: Relationship of ploidy and cell cycle phases to survival. A five year follow-up study. Anticancer Res., 8:105–112, 1988.

von Roenn, J.M., Kheir, S.M., Walter, J.M., and Coon J.S.: Significance of DNA abnormalities in primary malignant melanomas and nevi; a retrospective flow cytometric study. Cancer Res., 46:3192–3195, 1986.

Watson, J.V.: Quantitation of molecular and cellular probes in populations of single cells using fluorescence. Mol. Cell. Probes, 1:121–136, 1987.

Watson, J.V.: Practical Flow Cytometry. Oxford, Blackwell, 1991

Watson, J.V., Stewart, J., Cox, H., Sikora, K., and Even, G.I.: Flow cytometric quantitation of the c-*myc* oncoprotein in archival neoplastic biopsies of the colon. Mol. Cell. Probes, 1:151–157, 1987.

Wersto, R.P., Greenebaum, E., Deitch, D., Kerstenberger, K., and Koss, L.G.: Deoxyribonucleic acid ploidy and cell cycle events in benign colonic epithelium peripheral to carcinoma. Lab. Invest., 58:218–225, 1988.

Wersto, R.P., Herz, F., Gallagher, R.E., and Koss, L.G.: Cell cycle-dependent reactivity with the monoclonal antibody Ki-67 during myeloid cell differentiation. Exp. Cell Res., 179:79–88, 1988.

Wersto, R.P., Liblit, R.,L., Deitch, D., and Koss, K.G.: Variability of DNA. Measurements in multiple tumor samples of human colonic carcinoma. Cancer, 67:106–115, 1991.

Wheeless, L.l., Coon, J.S., Deitch, A.D., et al.: Comparison of automated and manual techniques for analysis of DNA frequency distributions in bladder washings. Cytometry, 9:600–604, 1988.

Wheeless, L.L., Coon, J.S., Cox, C., Deitch, A.D., White, R.W.D., Koss, L.G., Melamed, M.R., O'Connell, M.J., Reeder, J.E., Weinstein, R.S., and Wersto, R.P.: Measurement variability in DNA flow cytometry of replicate samples. Cytometry, 10:731–738, 1989.

Wheeless, L.L., Pattern, S.F., and Cambier, M.A.: Slit-scan cytofluorometry: Data base for automated cytopathology. Acta Cytol., 19:460–464, 1975.

Winkler, H.Z., Rainwater, L.M., Myers, R.P., Farrow, G.M., Therneau, J.M., Zincke, H., and Leiber, M.M.: Stage D1 prostatic adenocarcinoma: Significance of nuclear DNA ploidy patterns studied by flow cytometry. Mayo Clin. Proc., 63:103–112, 1988.

Wolley, R.C., Dembitzer, H.M., Herz, F., Schreiber, K., and Koss, L.G.: The use of a slide spinner in the analysis of cell dispersion. J. Histochem. Cytochem., 24:11–15, 1976.

Wolley, R.C., Herz, F., and Koss, L.G.: Caution on the use of lymphocytes as standards in the flow cytometric analysis of cultured cells. Cytometry, 2:370–372, 1982.

Wolley, R.C., Herz, F., Dembitzer, H.M., Schreiber, K., and Koss L.G.: The monodisperse cervical smear. Quantitative analysis of cell dispersion and loss with enzymatic and chemical gents. Anal. Quant. Cytol., *1*:43–49, 1979.

Wolley, R.C., Kawamoto, K.,,. Herz, F., Hirano, A., and Koss, L.G.: Flow cytometry of human brain tumors. *In* Zimmerman, H.M. (ed.): Progress in Neuropathology vol. 4. pp. 267–276, New York, Raven Press, 1979.

Wolley, R.C., Schreiber, K., Koss, L.G., Karas, M., and Sherman, A.: DNA distribution in human colon carcinomas and its relationship to clinical behavior. J.N.C.I., *69*:15–22, 1982.

Xiang, J.H., Spanir, S.S., Benson, N.A., and Braylan, R.C.: Flow cytometric analysis of DNA in bone and soft-tissue tumors using nuclear suspensions. Cancer, *59*:1951–1958, 1987.

Young, G.A., Hedley, D.W., Rugg, C.A., and Iland, H.J.: The prognostic significance of proliferative activity in poor histology non-Hodgkin's lymphoma: A flow cytometry study using archival material. Eur. J. Cancer Clin. Oncol., *23*:1497–1504, 1987.

Zaprianov, Z., and Christov, K.: Histological grading, DNA content, cell proliferation, and survival of patients with astroglial tumors. Cytometry, *9*:380–386, 1988.

Index

Vol. 1: pp. 1–889; Vol. 2: pp. 890–1657

Page numbers followed by f *indicate figures; those followed by* t *indicate tabular material.*

1

ISBN 0-397-51222-8

90000